Male Reproductive Dysfunction

Male Reproductive Dysfunction

Pathophysiology and Treatment

Edited by
FOUAD R. KANDEEL
City of Hope National Medical Center, Duarte, California, USA
David Geffen School of Medicine at the University of California, Los Angeles, USA

Associate Editors
RONALD S. SWERDLOFF
Harbor-UCLA Medical Center, Torrance, California, USA
David Geffen School of Medicine at the University of California, Los Angeles, USA

JON L. PRYOR
University of Minnesota Medical School, Minneapolis, USA

informa
healthcare

New York   London

Informa Healthcare USA, Inc.
52 Vanderbilt Avenue
New York, NY 10017

© 2007 by Informa Healthcare USA, Inc.
Informa Healthcare is an Informa business

No claim to original U.S. Government works
Printed in the United States of America on acid-free paper
10 9 8 7 6 5 4 3 2 1

International Standard Book Number-10: 1-57444-848-X (Hardcover)
International Standard Book Number-13: 978-1-57444-848-1 (Hardcover)

Library of Congress Cataloging-in-Publication Data

Male reproductive dysfunction : pathophysiology and treatment / [edited by]
   Fouad R. Kandeel.
     p. ; cm.
   Includes bibliographical references.
   ISBN-13: 978-1-57444-848-1 (hardcover : alk. paper)
   ISBN-10: 1-57444-848-X (hardcover : alk. paper)
   1. Infertility, Male. 2. Impotence. I. Kandeel, Fouad R.
   [DNM: 1. Infertility, Male. 2. Genital Diseases, Male--Complications.
  3. Infertility, Male--therapy. WJ 709 M24555 2007]

   RC889.M3558 2007
   616.6'92--dc22   2007005802

Visit the Informa Web site at
www.informa.com

and the Informa Healthcare Web site at
www.informahealthcare.com

This volume is dedicated to those who have helped shape the path of my academic and professional career in the hope that the information contained herein will enrich the knowledge of others.

Preface

Given the finite nature of the human lifespan, it is possible to argue that an individual man's most precious and lasting gift to the world is the legacy created by his offspring. It is no wonder, then, that the purely reproductive function of fertility has become inextricably tied to the human male's impression of his own masculinity. The fact of being childless is often an extremely emotional issue for patients and their families, and ameliorating such a cause is certainly worthy of our efforts. Each day, great strides are made in the ever-evolving body of knowledge that comprises the whole science and practice of medicine, allowing men to live longer, healthier lives; thus, retaining sexual and reproductive health even well into their later years has taken on increased importance for many men, and, consequently, for the physicians who treat them.

Yet, with the benefit of increased longevity, there must simultaneously exist an increased likelihood that the male reproductive tract will be subjected to greater levels of stress resulting from longer exposure to harmful environmental agents, poor lifestyle choices, and new diseases and infections. Additionally, the therapeutic drugs and regimens prescribed for these conditions frequently diminish sexual and reproductive capacities to an even greater degree. For example, a male patient who survives cancer and its treatment often falls victim to sexual, reproductive, and interpersonal difficulties that may further compromise his quality of life.

Due to the wide range of impairments that may impact a man's reproductive health throughout his lifespan, by necessity, the field of reproductive medicine is a multidisciplinary specialty comprised of andrology, endocrinology, urology, gynecology, radiology, psychology, and sociology. The vast array of data and the complexity of new technologies constantly being produced in so many different areas are often bewildering. Therefore, the chief goal in creating this first edition of *Male Reproductive Dysfunction: Pathophysiology and Treatment* has been to assimilate the most pertinent and important scientific knowledge gained from the complementary expertise of more than 70 individual leaders in all related disciplines into a single, comprehensive source, and to present this information from a clinical viewpoint, not only for the benefit of those actively involved in managing male patients with reproductive disorders, but also for the considerable numbers of physicians and healthcare providers who are likely to encounter and care for such men, regardless of etiology or precipitating factors. We hope to educate our readers with both the science behind these complex disorders and to equip them with practical tools for the effective and rational management of these conditions.

Based on the most recent data available, *Male Reproductive Dysfunction: Pathophysiology and Treatment* presents historical, psychosocial, behavioral, medical, and surgical perspectives in an unparalleled 43-chapter guide to the assessment and treatment of the male patient with reproductive dysfunction. Logically divided into five parts, the book begins with an extensive review of the normal anatomy and physiology of the male reproductive system, including a chapter on the effect of aging on testosterone production. Building on this foundation, the second part details the many etiologies, mechanisms, and clinical manifestations of male reproductive disorders. Both common and rare conditions of male reproductive dysfunction are covered, from genetic defects and childhood developmental abnormalities to other causes of hypogonadism, including the adverse effects of substance abuse, malnutrition, environmental toxins, and the iatrogenic effects of cancer treatments and other pharmacotherapies on the hypothalamic-pituitary-testicular axis. Also highlighted are problems that occur later in life, such as the complications of systemic diseases, obstructive and mass lesions of the reproductive tract, and sperm allergy.

With this information well in hand, the third part invaluably outlines strategies for the complete assessment of the hypogonadal and/or infertile male patient, from obtaining the initial history and physical exam, to ordering blood-work and semen analyses, to interpreting advanced imaging studies and performing testicular biopsies. The multitude of illustrations, images, algorithms, and tables elucidate these complex topics even more clearly. Of special note are the chapters dedicated to the evaluation of immunological factors that may be contributing to infertility and the effective use of imaging technology in the diagnosis of male reproductive tract pathology.

The fourth part then provides extensive guidelines for the treatment of male reproductive dysfunction depending on the individual pathology, including specialized situations such as patients who are cancer survivors or have spinal cord or other neurological injury. The details of various surgical sperm retrieval methods as well as assisted reproduction techniques (ART) are described step-by-step. Several chapters feature additional information that is unique to this book, such as the latest progress in male contraception, micromanipulation procedures for the treatment of the subfertile male, the psychological effects of infertility and its treatment, and the management of immunological factors in male infertility.

The final, fifth part is devoted to a full discussion of the mass lesions of the male reproductive tract, including testicular, penile, prostate, and male breast cancers. The problems of prostate hyperplasia, prostatitis, and gynecomastia are also addressed.

Most importantly, each chapter in this volume considers the future aims of its particular topic, opening the doorway for continued thought and discussion as new research is added to the current armamentarium. It is hoped that this book will become an essential, self-contained desk reference for both new and seasoned clinicians involved in the care of male patients with all forms of reproductive dysfunction, and that by enriching the current body of knowledge, our work will provide the starting point for future generations of medical professionals to learn, study, develop, and discover.

Fouad R. Kandeel

Acknowledgments

The editors are very grateful to the following individuals and would like to acknowledge their assistance in the preparation of this volume: Chakriya Anunta, Jeannette Hacker, Bernard de la Cruz, Karen Ramos, and Angela Hacker.

Contents

Part V.   Mass Lesions of the Male Reproductive System

Contributors

Paul David Abel   Division of Surgery, Oncology, Reproduction and Anesthesia, Imperial College School of Medicine, London, U.K.

Chakriya D. Anunta   Department of Diabetes, Endocrinology and Metabolism, City of Hope National Medical Center, Duarte, California, U.S.A.

Stephen J. Assinder   Discipline of Physiology, School of Medical Sciences, University of Sydney, New South Wales, Australia

Anthony Atala   Department of Urology, Wake Forest University School of Medicine, Wake Forest Institute for Regenerative Medicine, Winston-Salem, North Carolina, U.S.A.

H. W. Gordon Baker   Department of Obstetrics and Gynaecology, University of Melbourne and The Royal Women's Hospital, Carlton, Victoria, Australia

Carol Bennett   Department of Urology, Greater Los Angeles VA Medical System and David Geffen School of Medicine, University of California, Los Angeles, California, U.S.A.

Benjamin K. Canales   Department of Urologic Surgery, University of Minnesota Medical School, Minneapolis, Minnesota, U.S.A.

Peter T. K. Chan   Department of Urology, McGill University Health Centre, Montreal, Quebec, Canada

Monique M. Cherrier   Department of Psychiatry and Behavioral Sciences, University of Washington School of Medicine and Veterans Administration Puget Sound Health Care System, Seattle, Washington, U.S.A.

Bartley G. Cilento, Jr.   Department of Urology, Children's Hospital and Department of Surgery, Harvard Medical School, Boston, Massachusetts, U.S.A.

Gary N. Clarke   Andrology Laboratory Division of Laboratory Services, The Royal Women's Hospital, Carlton, Victoria, Australia

Jean-Louis Dacheux   Equipe "Spermatozoides," UMR INRA-CNRS 6073, Institut National de la Recherche Agronomique, Nouzilly, France

John W. Davis   Department of Urology, The University of Texas M.D. Anderson Cancer Center, Houston, Texas, U.S.A.

Helen M. Fenlon   Department of Radiology, Mater Misericordiae Hospital, Dublin, Ireland

Harry Fisch   College of Physicians and Surgeons, Columbia University and Male Reproductive Center, Columbia-Presbyterian Medical Center, New York, New York, U.S.A.

Kenneth Gannon   School of Psychology, University of East London, Stratford, London, U.K.

Claire Garrett   Department of Obstetrics and Gynaecology, University of Melbourne, and The Royal Women's Hospital, Carlton, Victoria, Australia

Chhanda Ghosh   Department of Oncology, University of Edinburgh, Edinburgh, Scotland, U.K.

Sarah K. Girardi   Department of Urology, Weill Medical College of Cornell University, North Shore University Hospital, Manhasset, New York, U.S.A.

Lesly Glover   Department of Clinical Psychology, The University of Hull, Hull, U.K.

Marc Goldstein   Cornell Institute for Reproductive Medicine, Department of Urology, New York-Presbyterian Hospital and Weill Medical College of Cornell University, New York, New York, U.S.A.

Erik T. Goluboff   College of Physicians and Surgeons, Columbia University and New York-Presbyterian Hospital, New York, New York, U.S.A.

Jeannette Hacker   Department of Diabetes, Endocrinology and Metabolism, City of Hope National Medical Center, Duarte, California, U.S.A.

Timothy B. Hargreave   Department of Oncology, University of Edinburgh, Western General Hospital, Fertility Problems Clinic, Edinburgh, Scotland, U.K.

Khashayar Hematpour   St. Luke's-Roosevelt Hospital Center, Columbia University College of Physicians and Surgeons, New York, New York, U.S.A.

Avner Hershlag   Department of Obstetrics and Gynecology, North Shore University Hospital, New York University School of Medicine, Manhasset, New York, U.S.A.

Ramon Hinojosa   Department of Sociology, University of Florida, Gainesville, Florida, U.S.A.

Simon J. Howell   Department of Endocrinology, Christie Hospital NHS Trust, Withington, Manchester, U.K.

Russell C. Jones   Discipline of Biological Sciences, The University of Newcastle, New South Wales, Australia

Fouad R. Kandeel   Department of Diabetes, Endocrinology and Metabolism, City of Hope National Medical Center, Duarte, California and David Geffen School of Medicine, University of California, Los Angeles, California, U.S.A.

Jeremy Kaufman   Department of Urology, The New York-Presbyterian Hospital, New York Center for Biomedical Research and The Rockefeller University Hospital, New York, New York, U.S.A.

Daniel M. Keenan   Department of Statistics, University of Virginia, Charlottesville, Virginia, U.S.A.

Jeffrey B. Kerr   Department of Anatomy and Cell Biology, Monash University, Victoria, Australia

Edward D. Kim   Department of Surgery, Division of Urology, University of Tennessee Medical Center, Knoxville, Tennessee, U.S.A.

Vivien Koussa   H.C. Healthcare Management and Development, Inc., Long Beach, California, U.S.A.

Ewa Kuligowska   Department of Radiology, Boston Medical Center, Boston, Massachusetts, U.S.A.

Ann Lavers   Department of Urologic Surgery, University of Minnesota Medical School, Minneapolis, Minnesota, U.S.A.

Lucille Leong   Division of Medical Oncology, City of Hope National Medical Center, Duarte, California, U.S.A.

Swee-Lian Liow   Embryonics International, Gleneagles Hospital, Singapore

De Yi Liu Department of Obstetrics and Gynaecology, University of Melbourne, and The Royal Women's Hospital, Carlton, Victoria, Australia

Peter Y. Liu Division of Endocrinology, Harbor-UCLA Medical Center, Torrance, California, U.S.A. and Department of Andrology, ANZAC Research Institute, University of Sydney, New South Wales, Australia

Donald F. Lynch Department of Urology, East Virginia Medical School, Norfolk, Virginia, U.S.A.

William Marsiglio Department of Sociology, University of Florida, Gainesville, Florida, U.S.A.

Brett C. Mellinger Department of Clinical Urology, SUNY Stony Brook, Stony Brook, New York, U.S.A.

John E. Morley Department of Medicine, Adelaide University, Australia and Division of Geriatric Medicine, St. Louis University School of Medicine and GRECC, St. Louis VA Medical Center, St. Louis, Missouri, U.S.A.

Nissrine Nakib Department of Urologic Surgery, University of Minnesota Medical School, Minneapolis, Minnesota, U.S.A.

Durwood E. Neal, Jr. Department of Urology, University of Missouri Medical School, Columbia, Missouri, U.S.A.

Erik N. Nelson Department of Radiology, Massachusetts General Hospital, Boston, Massachusetts, U.S.A.

Jason Ng Division of Endocrinology, Department of Medicine, Queen Elizabeth Hospital, Hong Kong, Special Administration Region, P.R. China

Soon-Chye Ng O & G Partners Fertility, Gleneagles Hospital, Singapore

Helen D. Nicholson Department of Anatomy and Structural Biology, Otago School of Medical Sciences, University of Otago, Dunedin, New Zealand

Christopher C. Oakes Departments of Pharmacology and Therapeutics, and Obstetrics and Gynecology, McGill University, Montreal, Quebec, Canada

Nan B. Oldereid Department of Obstetrics and Gynecology, Rikshospitalet–Radiumhospitalet Medical Center, Oslo, Norway

Horace M. Perry III Department of Internal Medicine–Geriatrics, St. Louis University School of Medicine, St. Louis, Missouri, U.S.A.

Jon L. Pryor Department of Urologic Surgery, University of Minnesota Medical School, Minneapolis, Minnesota, U.S.A.

Sandeep K. Reddy Los Alamitos Hematology/Oncology Medical Group, Inc., Los Alamitos, California, U.S.A.

Erick J. Richmond Pediatric Oncology, National Children's Hospital, San Jose, Costa Rica

Bernard Robaire Departments of Pharmacology and Therapeutics, and Obstetrics and Gynecology, McGill University, Montreal, Quebec, Canada

Alan D. Rogol Clinical Pediatrics, University of Virginia, Charlottesville, Virginia, U.S.A.

Paul F. Schellhammer Department of Urology, Eastern Virginia Medical School, Norfolk, Virginia and Prostate Cancer Center, Sentara Cancer Institute, Hampton, Virginia, U.S.A.

Peter N. Schlegel Departments of Urology and Reproductive Medicine, Weill Medical College of Cornell University, New York, New York, U.S.A.

Steve M. Shalet Department of Endocrinology, Christie Hospital NHS Trust, Withington, Manchester, U.K.

Rebecca Z. Sokol Keck School of Medicine, University of Southern California, Los Angeles, California, U.S.A.

Tanya M. Stewart Department of Obstetrics and Gynaecology, University of Melbourne, and The Royal Women's Hospital, Carlton, Victoria, Australia

Ronald S. Swerdloff Division of Endocrinology and Metabolism, Harbor-UCLA Medical Center, Torrance, California and Department of Medicine, David Geffen School of Medicine, University of California, Los Angeles, California, U.S.A.

Paul J. Turek Departments of Urology, Obstetrics, Gynecologic and Reproductive Sciences, Male Reproductive Laboratory, University of California, San Francisco, California, U.S.A.

Johannes D. Veldhuis Endocrine Research Unit, Mayo Clinic College of Medicine, Rochester, Minnesota, U.S.A.

Christina Wang General Clinical Research Center, Harbor-UCLA Medical Center, Torrance, California and Department of Medicine, David Geffen School of Medicine, University of California, Los Angeles, California, U.S.A.

Stephen H. Weinstein Director of Clinical Skills, University of Missouri Medical School, Columbia, Missouri, U.S.A.

Stephen J. Winters Division of Endocrinology and Metabolism, University of Louisville, Louisville, Kentucky, U.S.A.

Gary A. Wittert School of Medicine, Discipline of Medicine, University of Adelaide; Hanson Research Institute; and Discipline of Medicine, Royal Adelaide Hospital, Adelaide, Australia

Ekaterina V. Zubkova Departments of Pharmacology and Therapeutics, and Obstetrics and Gynecology, McGill University, Montreal, Quebec, Canada

Part I

Physiology of Male Reproductive Function

Reproduction is perhaps the most evolutionarily significant activity a man can perform in his lifetime. It is no wonder, then, that the successful achievement of new life from the combined events of spermatogenesis, sexual arousal, sexual intercourse, and the penetration and fertilization of the female ovum is so tightly regulated at every step in the process—a feat nothing short of biologically extraordinary. Yet, because intact reproductive function requires the synchronous coordination of myriad anatomical, vascular, neurologic, psychologic, endocrine, immunological, systemic, and even environmental and nutritional factors, defects may easily occur in any one or more of these individual components, resulting in some type of solely male-factor reproductive dysfunction, as detailed in Part II of this volume. Due to breakthroughs in bench research studies and the development of state-of-the-art anatomical and functional imaging techniques, however, much progress has been made in the understanding of the physiology of male reproductive function, resulting in a greater appreciation of the intricate neurohormonal mechanisms that govern sexual maturation and spermatogenesis. Similar innovations in surgical and microsurgical techniques have enabled previously infertile men to have children, via, e.g., the operative relief of ejaculatory duct obstruction (including vasectomy reversal), and the ability to harvest healthy sperm for in vitro fertilization or intracytoplasmic sperm injection. Therefore, it is imperative that the reproductive health professional remains abreast of the ever-evolving data in this exciting field. The chapters in Part I of this volume carefully describe the most up-to-date knowledge regarding the physiology of male reproductive health at all stages of the life cycle in the hopes of providing a thorough scientific and psychosocial understanding for any clinician involved in the care of the infertile male patient.

1

Male Reproduction: Evolving Concepts of Procreation and Infertility Through the Ages

Jeannette Hacker

Department of Diabetes, Endocrinology and Metabolism, City of Hope National Medical Center, Duarte, California, U.S.A.

Fouad R. Kandeel

Department of Diabetes, Endocrinology and Metabolism, City of Hope National Medical Center, Duarte, California and
David Geffen School of Medicine, University of California, Los Angeles, California, U.S.A.

□ INTRODUCTION

Human perspectives on reproductive function seem to have evolved along with an increased capacity for learning and the ability to reason. As brain function and thought processes began to advance, so too did our ancestors' understanding of their roles in reproduction, albeit with some interesting misnomers along the way. A detailed review of evolving concepts of human reproduction through the ages would require the dedication of an entire text and is beyond the scope of the current volume. Therefore, this chapter seeks to provide a synopsis of milestones that have shaped mankind's understanding of procreation and infertility and inevitably influenced the practice of modern reproductive medicine (Table 1).

□ EVOLVING CONCEPTS OF HUMAN REPRODUCTION

Early humans likely perceived childbirth as a spontaneous process. From the beginning, the female role in reproductive events was highly regarded, probably due to the obvious physical growth witnessed during gestation and the nature of the birth process itself. Therefore, the worship of "Mother Earth" and other personified female objects was predominant in ancient cultures. Originally, many cultures believed that the earth was born from the female sea. Some cultures thought that the sun itself fathered human children, because it was observed that the warm rays of the sun could make things grow. Others surmised that the moon, or a male personification of it, impregnated a woman (1).

Sexual interaction with a man was eventually recognized as being essential for the "magical" feat of procreation, and the male role in reproduction was given precedence over the female one. For more than 1000 years, common belief held that the male seed carried the power of new life, and women were thought to serve only as a nesting ground within which this new life could be nurtured; this may be due to the fact that the man's contribution to the reproductive process (the emission of semen) could be tangibly perceived, whereas the woman's contribution of the egg could not. The only visible physical sign of the woman's contribution was the monthly flow of menstrual blood, which came to be interpreted as another indicator of her purely nutritive function in pregnancy. Metaphors such as the "seed" and "soil" were symbols commonly used to represent male semen and the female womb. Intercourse was sometimes poetically described as "cultivating the soil."

Greco-Roman Philosophy

Western concepts of human reproduction were largely shaped by theories presented by the prominent Greek philosophers/physicians Aristotle, Hippocrates, and Galen from the fifth century B.C. through the first century A.D. In addition to their many other contributions to philosophy and medicine, these men individually strove to answer more complex questions about how human life began.

The first of the three philosophers, Aristotle (384–322 B.C.), promoted what has been referred to as the "one-seed theory" of conception. As in previous male-dominated preconceptions of procreation, Aristotle thought male seed (semen) was responsible for the generation of new life, while women provided merely the matter (menstrual blood) that nourished the seed once it was implanted in the womb through sexual intercourse. Because women only donate nutrient matter, Aristotle held that women were able to conceive in the absence of orgasm, and thus concluded that their role was less significant. He likened the reproductive process to that of curdling cheese, comparing the menstrual blood to inert milk and active semen to the rennin that activates it (2).

The Greek physician Hippocrates (460–377 B.C.), the "Father of Medicine," was one of the first Western philosophers to recognize the contributions of both

Table 1 Historical Milestones Toward Understanding Human Reproduction

Pre-history	Concept of spontaneous birth prevails. Ancient humans likely believed that women were impregnated by forces of nature, such as the sun or moon.
500 B.C.	Aristotle theorizes that the male seed is the source of new life, while females provide only nutrient matter.
400 B.C.	Hippocrates, "Father of Medicine," argues that similar reproductive fluids are secreted by both sexes and that new life is created through mixture of these fluids during the intensity of sexual pleasure. He uses this to explain the common observation that a child could resemble both his/her father and mother.
200 A.D.	Based on his anatomical studies, Galen combines the concepts of Aristotle and Hippocrates to promote "two-seed" theory, which dominates Western thought for the next 1500 years.
1672	Marcello Malpighi concludes that the female egg is the source of life based on his studies of embryologic development in chicken eggs.
1672	Renier de Graaf discovers what he believes are eggs in the rabbit ovary, structures that are later identified as Graafian follicles, or the fluid-filled vesicles in the mammalian ovary that contain a maturing egg.
1677	Antoni van Leeuwenhoek, the "Father of 'Microbiology," discovers spermatozoa using a rudimentary microscope of his own creation.
~1780	Dr. John Hunter reports first successful human artificial insemination.
1827	Karl Ernst von Baer first identifies mammalian ovum in dissected female dog.
1861	Karl Gegenbaur discovers that the vertebrate ovum is unicellular.
1875	Oscar Hertwig discovers fertilization involves the combination of the nuclei from male and female gametes.
1877	Hermann Fol observes entry of sperm into the egg of a sea urchin, finally demonstrating how pregnancy occurs.
1891	H. Henking describes accessory chromosomes and their role in sex determination.
1900	Three European scientists re-examine observations on plant hybridization published by Gregor Mendel between 1856–1866 to develop the Mendelian theory of inheritance, which later evolved into what is now known as classical genetics.
1960	Landrum Shettles publishes photographic atlas of the human egg, which included the first images of human fertilization in process.

sexes in conception (2,3). He argued that the intensity of pleasure involved in the sexual act resulted in the distillation of seminal fluids derived from all parts of the partners' bodies. Unlike Aristotle, Hippocrates thought that the two reproductive fluids were similar in nature and that the production of new life was achieved by mixing them. As a result, traits in the child could be inherited from each parent, a fact that troubled Aristotelian theory. For conception to occur, Hippocrates believed that both sexes must experience orgasm for the male and female fluids to mix properly.

Another famous Greek physician, Galen (129–200 A.D.), who practiced extensively in Rome, introduced the concept of experimentation to medicine and used vivisection of animals to develop his ideas on functional anatomy (4). Galen integrated and built upon the ideas of Aristotle and Hippocrates to formulate his "two-seed theory" of human reproduction (2,5). In tune with Hippocrates, Galen believed that both sexes were equally responsible for conception and that orgasm was necessary in both partners for conception to occur. He argued that the female seed moved much like the male's, and adduced that a woman who had her ovaries removed could not bear children as proof that a woman served as more than a mere nest in procreation. Through his studies of dissected apes, Galen also noted similarities in male and female reproductive structures and labeled the penis as homologous to the clitoris and the testicles as homologous to the horns of the uterus (ovaries). (See Chapter 2, Fig. 1.) Although Galen acknowledged the contributions of both sexes in the reproductive process, he continued to believe that the male seed was superior, possessing unique spiritual qualities that the female seed lacked. Galen's two-seed theory dominated Western thought for the next 1500 years.

Preformation

Although Galen's theory on human reproduction was generally accepted, the details regarding how human conception occurred remained elusive and a source of intense debate. In line with Galen, some believed that new life was created de novo upon combination of the male and female secretions (epigenesists). Others believed that new life was preformed and then incubated into being (preformists).

The doctrine of preformation took root in the late 17th and early 18th centuries as methods of scientific study advanced. Marcello Malpighi, who investigated embryological development in chicken eggs, came to the conclusion that the female egg was the source of life but required the energy of male semen to grow (2). The idea that women possessed miniature, preformed offspring was further promoted in England in 1672 by Renier de Graaf, who discovered what were later named Graafian follicles, which hold the mammalian egg. At this time, the function of semen in reproduction was thought to be limited to nourishing the egg, shaking the egg free, or exciting the egg into life (2).

The idea that preformed life existed solely in the female egg was not long lived. The concept was countered in 1677 when Antoni van Leeuwenhoek invented the microscope and became the first person to see spermatozoa, which he described as containing completely formed miniature beings. These tiny beings were aptly named "homunculi" and were later sketched as a miniature man curled up within the spermatozoan head (Fig. 1) (6). This furthered the idea that a woman's role

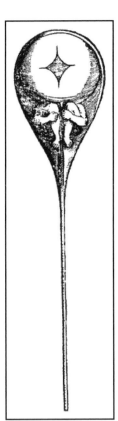

Figure 1 Homunculus (little man). Spermatozoa were first seen by Leeuwenhoek in 1677 and were later sketched as tiny preformed men by Hartsoeker in 1694. *Source*: From Ref. 6.

in conception was purely a nutritive one since this "proved" that men donated fully developed miniature humans.

Cell Biology and Genetics

The mammalian egg was first identified by Karl Ernst von Baer in 1827 during the dissection of a female dog (7). His discovery lent credence to the possibility that men and women contributed equally to the development of life. Although largely dismissed at the time, von Baer's discovery of the mammalian ovum set the stage for a series of pivotal cellular and genetic discoveries made during the century and a half that followed (3). This included confirmation that the egg and later the sperm were unicellular; identification of human chromosomes and the role of genes in gender assignment and trait inheritance in the late 19th and early 20th centuries; and the first photomicrographs of fusion between the male sperm and female egg during early in vitro fertilization experiments (Table 1) (8).

Religious Doctrines on Human Reproduction

Conception is commonly revered as a blessing from God. Religious texts provide detailed guidelines regarding how the faithful should go about properly conceiving a child. Due to the prevailing influence religion has on cultural practices, it is worthwhile to consider the religious teachings and how they have contributed to mankind's understanding of the reproductive process.

A shared belief among the Judaic, Christian, and Islamic faiths is that human life on Earth arrived from God's creation of Adam from dust of the earth, and later Eve, from one of Adam's ribs: "And the rib, which the LORD God had taken from man, made he a woman, and brought her unto the man. And Adam said, 'This [is] now bone of my bones, and flesh of my flesh: she shall be called Woman, because she was taken out of Man'" (Bible, King James Version, Gen. 2:22–23). Given this perspective, it is easy to understand how humankind held to the concept of man as the source of new life for so long.

Communicated in the sixth century, well before the development of modern technological advances (i.e., the microscope), the Qur'an offers striking insights into the human reproductive process. In *The Bible, The Qur'an and Science* (9), Dr. Maurice Bucaille summarizes some notable descriptions of conception in the Qur'an from fertilization through childbirth. First, life is said to begin as a mixed *nutfah* (or drop) of fluid (Qur'an 76:2). The mixed drop of fluid can be interpreted as the mixture of the sperm and egg or perhaps as a reference to the various components of semen (spermazoa plus secretions of the seminal vesicles, prostate gland, and bulbourethral glands). The drop is described as developing into *alaqah* (a leech-like structure) (Qur'an 22:5), an apt metaphor to describe how the embryo attaches to the endometrium of the uterus for blood supply, similar to how a leech derives blood from its host by clinging to the skin. The *alaqah* develops into a *mudghah* (chewed lump) (Qur'an 23:14), which seems to serve as a possible description of the human embryo during the fourth week of gestation, when somites (early fetal structures that eventually become the vertebrae) appear. These somites have been described as resembling teeth marks. "We made out of the chewed lump, bones and clothed the bones in flesh" (Qur'an 23:14); "And He gave you hearing and sight and feeling and understanding" (Qur'an 32:9). These Qur'anic excerpts are thought to describe the developing fetus, and accurately cite the order in which the fetal parts develop, starting with bone, muscle, and then the sensing organs of the ear, then eyes, and lastly the brain. The fetus is said to be made "in the wombs of your mothers in stages, one after another, in three veils of darkness," interpreted by some as representing the amniotic membrane, uterine wall, and abdominal wall. The fetus is said to rest in the womb "for an appointed term" (Qur'an 22:5). Thus, religions have also utilized the description of the reproductive process as evidence for the vulnerability and weakness of human beings during fetal development, and God's power over the regulation and permission of such developments to take place.

☐ FERTILITY AS A SYMBOL OF MASCULINITY

Across most cultures, a man's success in fathering children has often been perceived as a benchmark of male potency, strength, virility, and sexual prowess. As the "active" sex responsible for planting the life-giving seed, the completion of this task (birth of a healthy child) serves as a tribute to his success in performing his manly duties. Typically, the more children a man has sired, the more potent he is perceived to be. Having a healthy brood of children also serves to validate the traditional male role as breadwinner for the family by showing how effective he is in both creating and supporting a large number of offspring. Across most cultures throughout history, and still today, sons have been valued more highly than daughters for their ability to continue the family name and legacy. It was commonly believed that stronger sperm led to the development of male heirs, while less virile sperm resulted in the development of weaker female progeny (10). This furthered the preconception that strong, powerful men produced sons. Alternatively, the inability to sire children brought into question a man's very nature. Links between fertility and a man's sense of self persist in present-day cultures around the world (11,12).

Given that semen was thought to be totally responsible for the regeneration of life, it is no wonder that it became a substance of prized worth and value. Some ancient rites required a daily offering of semen to the gods and the vital fluid was provided by masturbation, which sometimes took place in groups accompanied by music (1). In other societies, boys ingested semen during fellatio rituals to induce male puberty (13). In ancient Greece and Rome, semen was considered the source of strength and masculinity (14). It was thought that excessive sexual activity and emission of semen would drain a man of his manliness, power, and worth. Excessive ejaculation was also thought to cool a man's hot/dry nature, making him more cool/wet and, thus, more feminine. Therefore, precautions were taken not to waste the precious substance for fear of losing one's physical, mental, and spiritual stamina.

Semen was also viewed negatively at times. Although semen was recognized and valued for its reproductive function, many authors in the medieval period thought that abstinent behavior resulted in a buildup of excess semen that could diminish health and regarded sexual release as a necessary excretory function. Sexual abstinence was thought to be unhealthy for men and women alike, and as a result, masturbation was commonly practiced by both sexes during this time period (15). The religious texts contain other examples of negative perceptions of semen (1). For example, the Bible lays down strict rules regarding ejaculation outside of intercourse as being "unclean" and requiring those who emitted semen anywhere other than the vagina to be isolated and purified (Bible, King James Version, Leviticus) (15).

Likely due to fascination by its ability to grow erect and revered as the instrument that delivers the male seed, the penis is a frequent symbol of masculinity found across cultures (16). Around the world, we find examples of phallic idolization and worship in the form of artwork and reverence for natural wonders resembling the penis, such as trees and rocks. Gods of fertility were often depicted with exaggerated, erect phalluses, such as the Greek god, Priapus, and the Egyptian god, Min.

□ INFERTILITY

Throughout much of history, infertility was commonly blamed on the woman and her barren womb. This may be due to the fact that whether it contained viable sperm or not, semen was seen to be emitted; therefore, the inability to conceive a child was blamed on the woman's inability to support and nurture the male seed. Impotence constituted the only situation under which the man could take responsibility for infertility. Otherwise, if he was able to penetrate and ejaculate, his job was considered done. We have since learned that up to 50% of infertility cases are at least partially related to a male factor (17).

As mentioned above, bearing children is considered by many to be a blessing from God; therefore, failure to procreate could be viewed as a sign of God's disfavor or as punishment for sin. Impotence, infertility, and miscarriage were often blamed on witchcraft (2,10). Some present-day cultures continue to believe that infertility is caused by evil spirits (18). Male and female infertility were also sometimes attributed to age or imbalances in heat, cold, moisture, and dryness (2). Theories such as Galen's that contended a woman must experience orgasm to conceive led to the belief that a woman could be rendered barren by lack of enjoyment or disgust with the sexual act (2). In the 1960s, the work of William Masters and Virginia Johnson (19,20) served to clarify the distinction between the sexual and reproductive functions, thereby opening the door to the development of a clearer understanding of human reproductive dysfunction.

□ FERTILITY TREATMENTS

In ancient times, when pregnancy was still considered a mystical act of the deities, treatment for infertility appears to have focused on worshiping aspects of nature thought to be connected to reproduction (i.e., sun, moon, and rain) or worshiping animals known to be fecund, such as the virile bull and the cat (21). The polytheistic faiths produced a host of gods thought to enhance fertility. Exploration of literary references to "fertility gods" yields documentation of dozens of individual deities across cultures that were heralded for the ability to promote conception. Fertility gods and goddesses were depicted in many forms: as all-powerful and life-giving forces, such as the gods that ruled over the sun, rain, and the moon; as symbols of male virility, such as the Egyptian gods Sobek and

Khnum (featured on the cover of this volume); or as ultrafeminine, sensual, and often pregnant goddesses that ruled over love and pregnancy, such as the Greek goddess Aphrodite.

As mankind realized that they were involved in the reproductive process, various strategies were employed to try to improve one's odds of conceiving (2). Diet and herbal remedies were used to balance excessively hot, cold, dry, or moist natures or as aphrodisiacs to entice a sterile man or woman into amorous behavior. Eating grapes and other seed-bearing fruits and grains were thought to, in turn, increase production of the male seed and improve virility (21).

The first case of artificial insemination reportedly occurred in the late 1700s, when Dr. John Hunter instructed a male patient with hypospadias to inject his semen into his wife's vagina with a syringe, which succeeded in inducing pregnancy (10). More than 100 years would pass before the procedure could be reliably reproduced in livestock and humans. Several decades later, in vitro fertilization and other assisted-reproduction technologies (ART) were established. It is estimated that more than 200,000 children have been born using ART (22). While providing happy endings to many would-be parents, these new infertility treatments raise a host of new questions related to their psychological, legal, and social impact (23). Thus, the field of reproductive medicine continues to evolve and remains a topic of philosophic debate.

□ CONCLUSION

Throughout the ages, the miracle of human reproduction has engaged man's curiosity and imagination. Although procreation was initially attributed to supernatural forces, mankind's growing understanding that they were actively involved in the procreation event led to increasingly more complex questions about conception and eventually inspired the scientific studies of human anatomy, physiology, cellular biology, embryology, and reproductive medicine. Despite scientific and medical advances in our understanding of human reproduction, deep-seated beliefs and misconceptions continue to color the thoughts and feelings of men regarding their role in procreation.

□ ACKNOWLEDGMENTS

The authors would like to acknowledge the comprehensive summaries of human reproduction provided by Angus McLaren in his volume entitled *Reproductive Rituals: The Perception of Fertility in England from the Sixteenth to the Nineteenth Century* and by P. Loizos and P. Heady in *Conceiving Persons: Ethnographies of Procreation, Fertility and Growth*, which served as invaluable resources in the preparation of the synopsis of reproduction theories presented in this chapter.

□ REFERENCES

1. Brasch R. How Did Sex Begin? The Sense and Nonsense of the Customs and Traditions That Have Shaped Men and Women Since Adam and Eve. New York: David McKay Company, Inc., 1973.
2. McLaren A. Reproductive Rituals: The Perception of Fertility in England from the Sixteenth Century to the Nineteenth Century. New York: Methuen & Co., 1984.
3. Stonehouse J. Procreation, patriarchy and medical science: resistance to recognizing maternal contributions in European embryological thought. In: Loizos P, Heady P, eds. Conceiving Persons: Ethnographies of Procreation, Fertility and Growth. London: The Athlone Press, 1999:219–242.
4. Galen (Translated by May MT). Galen on the Usefulness of the Parts of the Body. Ithaca: Cornell University Press, 1968.
5. http://www.iep.utm.edu/g/galen.htm (accessed October 2006).
6. Hartsoeker N. Essai de deoptrique, Paris, 1694.
7. von Baer KE. De ovi mammalium et hominis genesi. Lipsiae: Epistola ad Academiam Imperialem Sciantiarum Petropolitanam, 1827.
8. Shettles LB. Ovum Humanum. New York: Hafner Publishing Company, Inc., 1960.
9. Bucaille M. The Bible, the Qur'an and Science: The Holy Scriptures Examined in the Light of Modern Knowledge. 7th ed. New York: Tahrike Tarsile Qur'an, 2003.
10. Bullough VL, Bullough B. Sexual Attitudes: Myths and Realities. New York: Prometheus Books, 1995.
11. Gannon K, Glover L, Abel P. Masculinity, infertility, stigma and media reports. Soc Sci Med 2004; 59(6): 1169–1175.
12. Inhorn MC. Middle Eastern masculinities in the age of new reproductive technologies: male infertility and stigma in Egypt and Lebanon. Med Anthropol Q 2004; 18(2):162–182.
13. Gilmore DD. Manhood in the Making: Cultural Concepts of Masculinity. New Haven: Yale University Press, 1990.
14. Martin DB. Contradictions of masculinity: ascetic inseminators and menstruating men in Greco-Roman culture. In: Finucci V, Brownlee K, eds. Generation and Degeneration: Tropes of Reproduction in Literature and History from Antiquity through Early Modern Europe. Durham: Dale University Press, 2001:81–108.
15. Bullough VL, Brundage JA. Handbook of Medieval Sexuality. New York: Garland Publishing, Inc., 1996.

16. Daniélou A: The Phallus: Sacred Symbol of Male Creative Power. Rochester: Inner Traditions International, 1995.

17. Thonneau P, Marchand S, Tallec A, et al. Incidence and main causes of infertility in a resident population (1,850,000) of three French regions (1988–1989). Hum Reprod 1991; 6(6):811–816.

18. Papreen N, Sharma A, Sabin K, et al. Living with infertility: experiences among urban slum populations in Bangladesh. Reprod Health Matters 2000; 8(15):33–44.

19. Masters W, Johnson V. Human Sexual Response. Boston: Little Brown, 1966.

20. Masters WH, Johnson VE. Human Sexual Inadequacy. Boston: Little, Brown and Company, 1970.

21. Franklin R. Baby Lore: Superstitions and Old Wives Tales from the World Over Related to Pregnancy, Birth and Motherhood, 2nd ed. West Sussex: Diggory Press, 2006.

22. Zegers-Hochschild F, Nygren KG, Adamson GD, et al. The International Committee Monitoring Assisted Reproductive Technologies (ICMART) glossary on ART terminology. Fertil Steril 2006; 86(1):16–19.

23. Austin CR. Legal, ethical and historical aspects of assisted human reproduction. Int J Dev Biol 1997; 41(2):263–265.

2

Anatomy of the Male Reproductive Tract

Fouad R. Kandeel

Department of Diabetes, Endocrinology and Metabolism, City of Hope National Medical Center, Duarte, California and David Geffen School of Medicine, University of California, Los Angeles, California, U.S.A.

Vivien Koussa

H.C. Healthcare Management and Development, Inc., Long Beach, California, U.S.A.

Ewa Kuligowska

Department of Radiology, Boston University School of Medicine, Boston, Massachusetts, U.S.A.

□ INTRODUCTION

The complex individual organs that comprise the male reproductive system have but a single evolutionary goal: to deliver spermatozoa to the female reproductive tract (1). Haploid germ cells originate in the testis and travel through the epididymis and into the vas deferens, eventually reaching the ampulla, where the mixing of seminal vesicle secretions occurs. The vas deferens then becomes the ejaculatory duct as it winds through the prostate to empty into the prostatic urethra. The germ cells, now additionally mixed with ejaculatory secretions from the accessory sex glands (seminal vesicles, prostate, and bulbourethral gland), then exit the body through the penile urethra. The entire system is dependent on neuroendocrine regulation from the pituitary and hypothalamus. Knowledge of the anatomy and embryologic origins of each of the components of the male reproductive tract is important in developing a basic and thorough understanding of the system as a whole. This chapter provides a brief overview of the male external and internal genital organs, with the intention of providing the foundation for the better diagnosis and treatment of male reproductive dysfunction. For more information on spermatogenesis, the neuroendocrine control of the male reproductive system, and the physiology of the prostate and epididymis, please refer to other chapters contained in Part I of this volume.

□ MALE EXTERNAL GENITAL ORGANS
The Penis
Structure

The penis arises from the genital tubercle (Fig. 1) (2), a region just cranial to the cloacal folds in the embryo. Under the influence of androgens produced by the fetal testis (see below), the cells of the genital tubercle proliferate, causing elongation of the tubercle into the primitive phallus. The penile urethra is formed from the urethral folds as the phallus elongates. In the adult penis, the urethra is divided into the membranous portion, which extends through the urogenital diaphragm, and the pendulous portion, which courses through the penis (Fig. 2). Lateral to the urethra are the paired corpora cavernosa, which, when engorged with blood, become the main functional components of penile erection (4–7). The corpora cavernosa comprise the bulk of the penis and consist of two cylinders of sponge-like tissue fused distally for approximately three-quarters of their length, with a common septum in between, separating at the proximal portion of each corpus cavernosum (the crus), which is attached to the inferior surface of the ischial ramus on the corresponding side (Figs. 2 and 3) (3). The septum is perforated by vessels that allow free passage of blood from one cylinder to the other, permitting the two cavernosal bodies to function as a single unit.

The erectile tissues of the corpora cavernosa are surrounded by a dense, nondistensible fascial sheath known as the tunica albuginea (Fig. 2). Emissary veins that carry the returned blood from the corporeal bodies traverse the tunica albuginea. Tensing of the tunica albuginea during erection by the expanded corporeal tissue compresses the subtunical plexus and emissary veins, reducing blood outflow.

Inferior to the corpora cavernosa lies the corpus spongiosum (Figs. 2 and 3), which contains the urethra and extends distally to form the majority of the glans penis. The penile corporeal tissue is surrounded by another dense fascial sheath (Buck's fascia), which anchors the penis to the symphysis pubis, and compresses the circumflex veins during the erectile responses, thereby further limiting the venous drainage. Histologically, the tissue of the corpora cavernosa consists of bundles of smooth muscle fibers intertwined in a collagenous extracellular matrix. Interspersed within this parenchyma is a complex network of endothelial cell-lined sinuses (lacunae), helicine arteries, and nerve terminals (Fig. 2) (9).

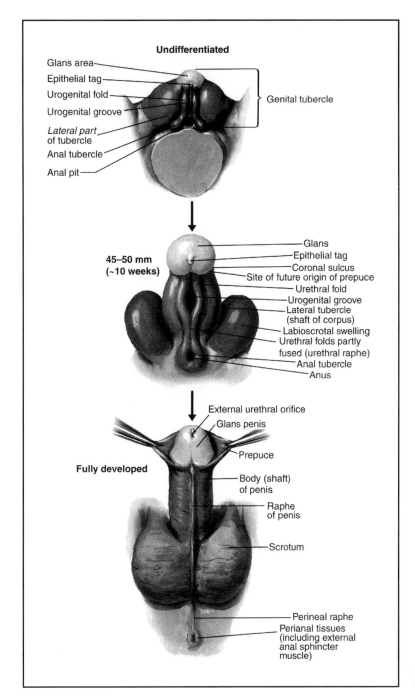

Undifferentiated

Glans area
Epithelial tag
Urogenital fold
Urogenital groove
Lateral part of tubercle
Anal tubercle
Anal pit

Genital tubercle

45–50 mm (~10 weeks)

Glans
Epithelial tag
Coronal sulcus
Site of future origin of prepuce
Urethral fold
Urogenital groove
Lateral tubercle (shaft of corpus)
Labioscrotal swelling
Urethral folds partly fused (urethral raphe)
Anal tubercle
Anus

Fully developed

External urethral orifice
Glans penis
Prepuce
Body (shaft) of penis
Raphe of penis
Scrotum
Perineal raphe
Perianal tissues (including external anal sphincter muscle)

Figure 1 (*See color insert*.) Differentiation of fetal penis and male gonads. *Source*: From Ref. 2.

The skin overlying the penis is exceptionally mobile and expandable, enabling it to accommodate the considerable increase in girth and length that occurs during erection (3). This lack of adherence makes the penis relatively susceptible to edema. In its distal portion, the penile skin extends forward to form the prepuce before folding backwards and attaching to the corona of the glans penis.

The pendulous portion of the penis is supported and stabilized by the suspensory ligament. Division of this structure makes the penis appear longer in its flaccid state, but it will not enhance the proportions of the organ when erect.

Vasculature

The terminal branches of the paired internal pudendal arteries (Figs. 4A, 4B) supply the penis with blood. Each internal pudendal artery arises from the anterior division of the respective internal iliac (hypogastric) artery, and arborizes into four branches (10–12): the bulbar artery, which supplies the urethral bulb, the posterior portion of the corpus cavernosum, and the bulbo-urethral gland; the urethral (spongiosal) artery, which supplies the urethral and the corpus spongiosal tissue; the deep penile (corpus cavernosal or profunda) artery, which supplies the corpus cavernosum; and finally, the deep dorsal artery, which supplies the skin and the

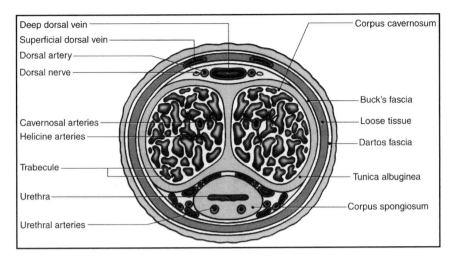

Deep dorsal vein
Superficial dorsal vein
Dorsal artery
Dorsal nerve

Cavernosal arteries
Helicine arteries

Trabecule

Urethra

Urethral arteries

Corpus cavernosum

Buck's fascia
Loose tissue

Dartos fascia

Tunica albuginea

Corpus spongiosum

Figure 2 (*See color insert.*) Cross section of the male penis showing the various structures. Note that the erectile tissue consists of two corpora cavernosa. Each corpus cavernosum is surrounded by a thick, fibrous sheath, the tunica albuginea. Each corpus has a centrally running cavernosal artery that supplies blood to the multiple lacunar spaces, which are interconnected and lined by vascular endothelium. *Source*: From Ref. 3.

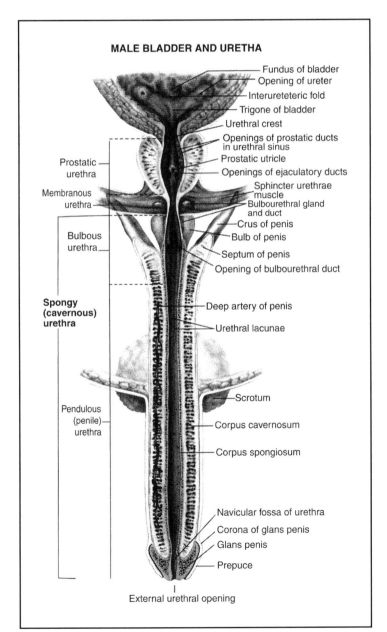

MALE BLADDER AND URETHA

Fundus of bladder
Opening of ureter
Interureteteric fold
Trigone of bladder
Urethral crest
Openings of prostatic ducts in urethral sinus
Prostatic utricle
Openings of ejaculatory ducts
Sphincter urethrae muscle
Bulbourethral gland and duct
Crus of penis
Bulb of penis
Septum of penis
Opening of bulbourethral duct

Prostatic urethra

Membranous urethra

Bulbous urethra

Spongy (cavernous) urethra

Deep artery of penis
Urethral lacunae

Pendulous (penile) urethra

Scrotum

Corpus cavernosum

Corpus spongiosum

Navicular fossa of urethra
Corona of glans penis
Glans penis
Prepuce

External urethral opening

Figure 3 (*See color insert.*) Male bladder and urethra: longitudinal section of the male penis, prostate, and bladder. The cross section through the penis also shows the urethra. *Source*: From Ref. 8.

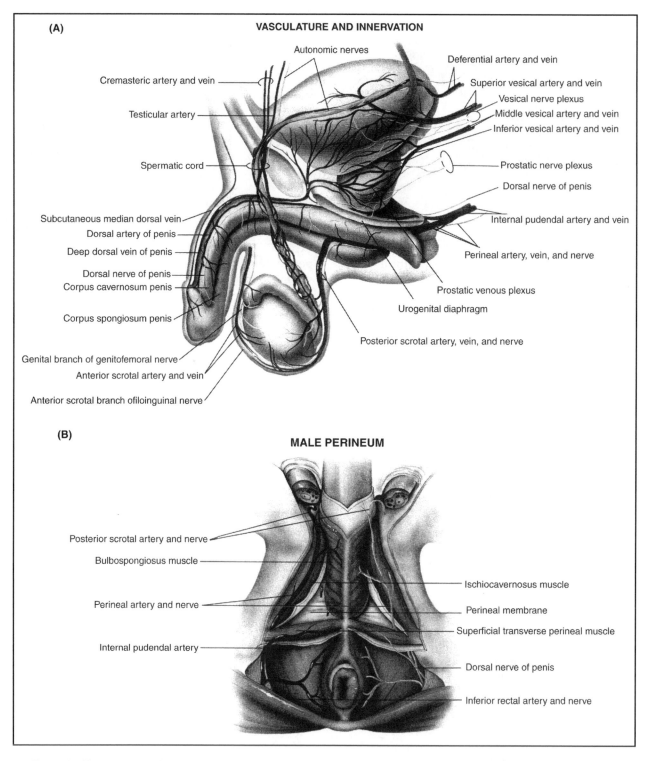

(A) VASCULATURE AND INNERVATION

Autonomic nerves
Cremasteric artery and vein
Testicular artery
Spermatic cord
Subcutaneous median dorsal vein
Dorsal artery of penis
Deep dorsal vein of penis
Dorsal nerve of penis
Corpus cavernosum penis
Corpus spongiosum penis
Genital branch of genitofemoral nerve
Anterior scrotal artery and vein
Anterior scrotal branch ofiloinguinal nerve

Deferential artery and vein
Superior vesical artery and vein
Vesical nerve plexus
Middle vesical artery and vein
Inferior vesical artery and vein
Prostatic nerve plexus
Dorsal nerve of penis
Internal pudendal artery and vein
Perineal artery, vein, and nerve
Prostatic venous plexus
Urogenital diaphragm
Posterior scrotal artery, vein, and nerve

(B) MALE PERINEUM

Posterior scrotal artery and nerve
Bulbospongiosus muscle
Perineal artery and nerve
Internal pudendal artery

Ischiocavernosus muscle
Perineal membrane
Superficial transverse perineal muscle
Dorsal nerve of penis
Inferior rectal artery and nerve

Figure 4 (*See color insert.*) Vasculature and innervation of the male genitalia (**A**) and male perineum (**B**). *Source*: From Ref. 8.

glans penis. The deep penile artery lies centrally within the corpus cavernosum and measures 600 to 1000 μm in diameter during the flaccid state. The deep penile artery gives rise to many perpendicular branches called helicine arterioles (150 μm in diameter) that supply the cavernous sinusoidal space (13). During erection, the deep penile artery dilates to twice its diameter. Several normal anatomic variations in the arterial supply of

the penis have been described (14–18), including the presence of an accessory internal pudendal artery and the presence of bridging, cross-flowing, and collateral routing. The penile arteries are interconnected by anastomoses along their entire course.

The venous drainage of the penis occurs through two major systems, the superficial and the deep (Figs. 2 and 4A) (4–7,10,19–21). The skin is serviced mainly by the superficial system, which gives rise to a single superficial dorsal penile vein. This eventually empties into the external iliac vein via the external pudendal, saphenous, and femoral veins. The deep venous drainage system drains the corpora cavernosa, the corpus spongiosum, and the urethra. The distal and middle portions of the corpora cavernosa are drained by the subtunical plexus and emissary veins. The emissary veins enter the circumflex veins at the lateral borders of the penis. The circumflex veins empty into a single deep dorsal vein that drains into the pudendal plexus or periprostatic plexus (Santorini's plexus), and finally into the internal iliac vein. The proximal corpora cavernosa are drained via the cavernous and crural veins into the periprostatic plexus and the internal pudendal veins. The superficial dorsal vein has many collaterals to the deep dorsal penile vein. Urethral veins that empty into the internal pudendal vein drain the corpus spongiosum and urethra. Direct arteriovenous anastomoses also exist. Similarly, the presence of communication between the spongiosal and cavernosal vascular compartments of the penis has been suggested (3).

Lymphatic Drainage

Lymph is drained from the penis by lymphatics that pass into the superficial and deep inguinal lymph nodes of the femoral triangle (3). In turn, these nodes, which may become secondarily involved in patients who have carcinoma of the penis, drain into the external and internal iliac lymphatic chains. Conditions that obstruct these lymphatic channels, such as metastatic prostate cancer, may result in gross penile and scrotal edema.

Innervation

The penis is innervated by somatic and autonomic nerve fibers (Figs. 2, 4A, and 4B) (4,5,7,22–30). The somatic innervation supplies the penis with sensory fibers and the perineal skeletal muscles with motor fibers. The paired dorsal nerve of the penis carries the somatosensory afferent inputs for transmission to the intermediolateral cell column in the lumbosacral spinal cord and subsequently to the brain cortex. The right and left dorsal nerves travel in close apposition to one another, within 1 cm, directly on the surface of the tunica albuginea of the corpus cavernosum, beneath the Buck's fascia. The axons of each nerve are arranged in two populations, one traveling to the glans and one arborizing over the surface of the penile shaft, with some fibers terminating in the urethra (28). The nerve terminals in the glans penis are numerous and are present as free nerve endings (FNEs) in almost every dermal papilla, as well as being scattered throughout the deep dermis. The ratio of FNEs to corpuscular receptors in the glans is approximately 10:1. Genital end bulbs are also present throughout, but are most abundant in the corona and near the frenulum. The unique corpuscular receptor of the glans consists

of axon terminals that resemble a tangled skein of FNEs. The glans is relatively insensitive to tactile and mechanical stimuli, but its FNEs can sense deep pressure and pain (22). In contrast, penile skin is rich in fine-touch neuroceptors that carry sensory input from the penile shaft. A band of ridged mucosa, located at the junction of true penile skin with the smooth inner surface of the prepuce, contains more Meissner's corpuscles than does the rest of the smooth preputial mucosa, and thus exhibits features of specialized sensory mucosa. This band constitutes an important component of the overall sensory mechanism of the penis (23). Fibers from the urethral innervation appear to carry afferent information necessary for sustaining reflex bulbocavernosus muscle contractions until expulsion of seminal fluid is complete (28). The dorsal penile nerves have an undulating course, to accommodate the significant change in penile length during erection. Proximally, the dorsal nerves pass through the suspensory ligaments, along the inferior pubic ramus on the inferior surface of the urogenital diaphragm, joining other sensory fibers from the perineal and inferior rectal nerves at the pudendal canal, to form the pudendal nerve. Fibers from the somesthetic receptors of the glans penis and frenulum (specialized genital corpuscles and Pacinian corpuscles) as well as those from the penile skin (noncapsulated spray-like FNEs) pass through numerous networks on the dorsum of the penile shaft to form the right and left dorsal nerves (27). Proximally, the dorsal nerves pass through the suspensory ligaments to follow their respective internal pudendal arteries along the inferior pubic ramus on the inferior surface of the urogenital diaphragm. Additional sensory fibers from other genital nerves, including the perineal and inferior rectal nerves, join in at the pudendal canal to form the pudendal nerve. The pudendal nerve fibers enter the dorsal roots of the sacral spinal cord segments S2–S4. Fibers then ascend into the spinal cord to synapse in the corticomedullary junction and the thalamus, and then terminate in the contralateral primary sensory area deep in the interhemispheric tissue. The somatic motor innervation supplies the perineal skeletal muscles (the bulbocavernosus and ischiocavernosus muscles that surround the corporeal bodies), the external sphincter, and the levator ani muscles. The motor fibers originate from the sacral segments S2–S4 and exit the spinal cord together with the pudendal nerve in the posterior portion of the pudendal canal to form the deep perineal nerve, which passes alongside the perineal artery (26). Contraction of the perineal skeletal muscles during erection leads to a temporary increase in corporeal body pressure to a level above the mean systolic pressure, and thus helps to increase penile firmness.

The autonomic innervation of the penis is both parasympathetic and sympathetic. The major efferent parasympathetic pathway originates in the intermediolateral aspect of the sacral cord (S2–S4), traveling in the pelvic nerve (Nervi Erigentes) to supply a vasodilating innervation to the corporeal bodies. The higher centers for the parasympathetic pathway include the cingulate gyrus, the gyrus rectus, the medial forebrain bundle, the anterior medial portion of the thalamus, the hippocampus, the septum pellucidum, the paraventricular nucleus, and the mamillothalamic tracts. Outflow neural messages travel through the substantia nigra to the ventrolateral portion of the pons and descend to the sacral parasympathetic nuclei. After the parasympathetic nerve fibers exit the spinal cord, they run in the retroperitoneal space in the lateral aspect of the rectum and bladder, then pass inferiorly and laterally toward the prostate and urogenital diaphragm. The cavernous nerve enters the corporeal body alongside the cavernous artery at the crura of the corpora as preganglionic nerve fibers. The most likely neurotransmitter at the synaptic end of these fibers is acetylcholine. The postganglionic nerve fiber segments terminate either on the vascular smooth muscle of the corporeal arterioles or on the nonvascular smooth muscle of trabecular tissue surrounding the corporeal lacunae (26). The sacral parasympathetic neurons are chiefly responsible for the erectile function and are influenced by a cortical–sacral efferent pathway. Penile erection can be initiated with a single episode of electrical stimulation of the pelvic nerve. Maintenance of erection for an extended period of time without significant changes in corporeal body blood gases can be achieved with repetitive stimulation for 40 to 50 seconds, with a minimum latency period between stimuli of 50 seconds (26). The sympathetic outflow originates in the thoracolumbar region of the spinal cord (T11–L2) and passes through the inferior mesenteric, hypogastric, and pelvic plexuses. The sympathetic innervation of the penis mediates the detumescence following orgasmic relief, and in the absence of sexual arousal, it maintains the penis in the flaccid state. Evidence suggests that activation of the postsynaptic alpha-1 and alpha-2 adrenergic receptors by norepinephrine and epinephrine is involved in the local control of corpus cavernosum smooth muscle tone (21,22). Sympathetic innervation of the prostate, the seminal vesicles, and related structures is the chief neural system involved in regulation of ejaculation. Stimulation of the postganglionic fibers leads to contraction of the ejaculatory duct, with a concomitant contraction of the bladder neck musculature, resulting in expulsion of the seminal fluid and prevention of the seminal fluid from retrograde deposition into the bladder.

The Testes

The testes are central to the male reproductive system (1). These organs generate the haploid germ cell by the process of spermatogenesis (see Chapter 5), and are also the site of androgen production.

The testes (Fig. 5) are paired ovoid structures that are suspended in the scrotum by the spermatic cord. Usually, the left testis hangs more inferiorly than the right testis. Each testis is contained within a thick fibrous capsule called the tunica albuginea and the thin tunica vaginalis visceralis, which also covers the epididymis. The parietal layer of the tunica vaginalis, adjacent to the internal spermatic fascia, is more extensive than the visceral layer and extends superiorly for a short distance into the distal part of the spermatic cord. A posterior invagination of the tunica albuginea, called the mediastinum testis, contains entering testicular vessels and exiting efferent ductules. Each testis is attached from its inferior pole to the scrotal sac by the gubernaculum testis. The testis itself is divided into hundreds of lobules of seminiferous tubules (Figs. 5 and 6) that converge into the tubuli recti, rete testes, and then efferent ductules at the mediastinum. The efferent ductules drain into the epididymis, posterior to the testis.

By the fourth week of embryonic life, the Wolffian (mesonephric) duct arcs anteriorly to join the ventral portion of the cloaca, which subsequently differentiates into the urogenital sinus. The ureter develops concurrently as an outgrowth from the posteromedial aspect of the Wolffian duct, 4 to 6 cm cephalad to its insertion at the urogenital sinus. The segment of the Wolffian duct lying between the urogenital sinus and the ureteral bud is called the combined nephric duct in the embryonic stage. Along with the downward migration of the combined nephric duct to the urogenital sinus, both the ureteral bud and the Wolffian ducts migrate inferiorly and finally achieve independent openings into the urogenital sinus. The combined nephric duct is then progressively absorbed into the urogenital sinus until, by the seventh week, it forms the bladder trigone (31–33).

From this point onward, the orifices of the Wolffian duct and the ureteral bud migrate apart, with the ureteral orifice moving upward and laterally and the Wolffian duct orifice moving downward and medially. As a result, the Wolffian duct—the embryonic equivalent of the vas deferens (see subsequently)—will cross over the ureter. This process of separation and rotation is complete by the eighth week of development. By the twelfth week, the ureteral orifice and the Wolffian duct will have reached their final locations (31–33).

Induced by the Wolffian ducts during the fifth fetal week, the Mullerian ducts migrate caudally and fuse in the midline with an outgrowth of the urogenital sinus to form the prostatic utricle—which, being the male homologue of the female uterus, has no further biologic function. The Sertoli cells of the developing testes further promote Mullerian duct involution by secreting Mullerian regression factor. The only remnants of the Mullerian duct present in the developing male fetus are the prostatic utricle and the appendix of the testis (31–33).

Under the influence of the Y chromosome and testis-determining factor, the embryo's previously indifferent gonad will develop proliferating testis cords deep within the gland's medulla at approximately six weeks of age. The cords elongate and lose contact with the gland surface, progressively getting separated from the superficial epithelium by tubular

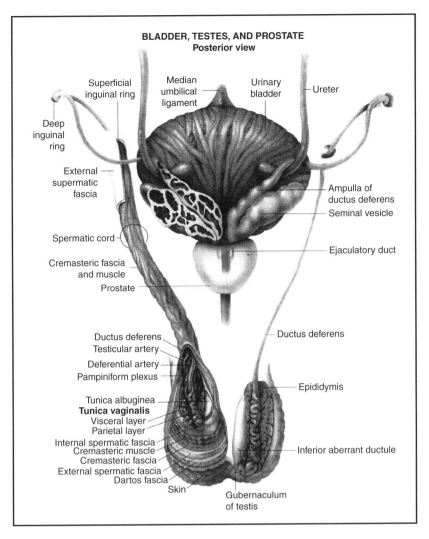

Figure 5 (*See color insert*.) Bladder, testes, and prostate gland. *Source*: From Ref. 8.

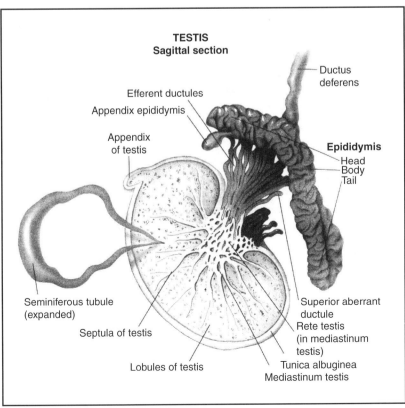

Figure 6 (*See color insert*.) Testis and the epididymis, sagittal section. *Source*: From Ref. 8.

rete testis cords at the hilum and by the fibrous tunica albuginea elsewhere. During the second trimester, the testis cords invaginate and proliferate into large groups of germ cells and Sertoli cells, the latter of which manufacture the Mullerian-inhibiting substance that suppresses further development of the paramesonephric duct. Meanwhile, the development of the mesonephric ducts (the future epididymis and vas deferens) is induced by testosterone, which is produced by the interstitial cells of Leydig that line the spaces between the testis cords. Dihydrotestosterone similarly stimulates growth of the penis, scrotum, and prostate. In puberty, the testis cords become canalized to from the seminiferous tubules (34).

The fetal testis is attached to the posterior abdominal wall by the urogenital mesentery, which is comprised of the caudal genital ligament and the gubernaculum. An inferior, extra-abdominal portion of the gubernaculum grows toward the developing scrotum during the second and third months of gestation, and the testes progressively migrate from the level of the kidneys toward the inguinal ring. The coelomic cavity peritoneum evaginates along the course of the gubernaculum testis into the scrotum, forming the processus vaginalis and the inguinal canal. Around the time of birth, the testes will descend through their respective inguinal rings, each testis becoming covered, in turn, by the tunica vaginalis, internal spermatic fascia, cremasteric fascia and muscle, and external spermatic fascia as it migrates into the scrotum (Figs. 1 and 5). The constituents of the spermatic cord are the ductus deferens, the testicular artery (supplies testis and epididymis), the artery of the ductus deferens (arises from inferior vesical artery), the cremasteric artery (arises from inferior epigastric artery), the pampiniform plexus (a venous network formed by up to 12 veins), sympathetic nerve fibers (on arteries, plus both sympathetic and parasympathetic fibers on the ductus deferens), the genital branch of the genitofemoral nerve (supplying cremaster muscle), and lymphatic vessels (draining the testis and closely associated structures into lumbar lymph nodes).

Because the testis develops abdominally, successful descent into the scrotum is essential for fertility (1). The scrotum is a cutaneous sac consisting of two layers: heavily pigmented skin and the closely related dartos fascia, a layer of smooth muscle responsible for the rugose (wrinkled) appearance of the adult scrotum. The scrotum is formed as coelomic epithelium that penetrates the abdominal wall and protrudes into the genital swelling as the processus vaginalis. An outgrowth of each layer of the abdominal wall is carried with this epithelium, giving rise to the fascial layers of the scrotum. The testis then descends behind the processus vaginalis, and the layers of fascia covering the testis on each side fuse to form the scrotum with the overlying skin of the genital swelling.

The scrotum is supplied primarily by the testicular, deferential, and cremasteric arteries, all of which are contained within the spermatic cord. The pampiniform plexus serves as the major venous drainage of the scrotum, continuing as the testicular veins; the left testicular vein joins the left renal vein, while the right testicular vein drains directly into the inferior vena cava (35).

Normal Penile and Testicular Size in Adult Males

Wessells et al. (36) have reviewed the normative data on penile size in the adult human male. The studies ranged in sample size from 50 to 2770 subjects, with an age range between 17 and 91 years. The average unstretched flaccid length ranges from 8.85 to 10.70 cm, stretched flaccid length ranges from 12.45 to 16.74 cm, and erection length ranges from 12.89 to 15.50 cm.

Reports on penile volume are limited, and have relied either upon the measurement of penile circumference manually (37–39) or upon penile cross-section by ultrasound techniques (36,40,41). In the latter studies, the average penile volume ranged from 17.15 to 43.62 mL in the flaccid state, and from 69.41 to 80.16 mL in the erect state (induced by intracorporeal injection of vasoactive agents). The average volume increase between these two phases of the erectile cycle ranged from 27.87 to 56.35 mL. The average mid-shaft circumference for the flaccid and erect penises was 9.71 and 12.30 cm, respectively. Average pubic fat-pad depth was 2.85 cm, which when added to the average erect penis length, rendered the average functional penile length 15.74 cm. Stretched flaccid penile length correlated strongly with the erect length in this series. Further, pubic fat-pad was greater in depth in men older than 40 years of age. The increase in central obesity may contribute to the occasionally reported decrease in penile length with age. Differences in methods of data gathering (subject self-reporting, single versus multiple examiners, single versus repeated stretching of the penis prior to measurement) and/or differences in populations studied (men with normal sexual function versus men with sexual dysfunction, different ethnic or age groups) could have contributed to some of the differences seen in the average values reported in the above studies. There is a loss of tensile strength of the tunica as men grow older, but no loss of the tunica albuginea itself.

Based on the available data, Wessells et al. (36) considered adult men with penile length of greater than 4 cm in the unstretched flaccid state or greater than 7.5 cm in the stretched flaccid state or the erect state to have a normal penile length. No parallel suggestions were made for penile girth or volume.

Normally, the testis increases in size from 1 to 3 mL during the neonatal period of life to 15 to 30 mL in adulthood. The germ cells and seminiferous tubules represent 90% of the testicular volume while Leydig cells contribute to less than 1%. A normal-size adult testis has dimensions of 4.1 to 5.2 cm in length and 2.5 to 3.3 cm in width (42).

A national probability sample of 1410 American men aged 18 to 59 years (National Health and Social

Life Survey) conducted in 1992 found that 77% of 1284 U.S.-born men were circumcised, compared with 42% of 115 non–U.S.-born men. Caucasians had a higher rate of circumcision than African Americans or Hispanics (81% vs. 65% or 54%; respectively), and these differences remained significant after controlling for confounding variables. Further, circumcision rates varied significantly with the level of education attained by the person's mother (62% of men whose mothers did not finish high school were circumcised vs. 84–87% for others), suggesting that the practice of circumcision is directly related to socioeconomic class (43).

☐ MALE INTERNAL GENITAL ORGANS
Epididymis

The epididymis, vas deferens, and seminal vesicles all have their origin in the mesonephric duct (Wolffian duct) (1). Initially serving as the early embryonic excretory system, the mesonephric duct is comprised of the longitudinal duct as well as a series of tubules that branch from the duct toward the developing gonad. Although most will degenerate, several of these tubules persist and anastomose with the seminiferous tubules (rete testis), forming the efferent ducts (or ductuli efferentes) through which spermatozoa exit the testis (Figs. 5 and 6). The portion of the mesonephric duct closest to the ductuli efferentes elongates, becomes extensively convoluted, and forms the epididymis. Because it arises from a single duct, the epididymis, unlike the testis, consists of a single tubule through which all spermatozoa must pass. The epididymis remains in close contact with the testis and descends with the testis into the scrotum.

Each epididymis has a thick triangular head, a thin elongated body, and a narrow tail. The appendix epididymis is a pedunculated structure arising from the epididymal head (44,45).

Testicular spermatozoa are nonmotile and incapable of fertilization. The function of the epididymis is to bring testicular spermatozoa to maturity. (For more information on this topic, see Chapter 6.)

Vas Deferens and Ejaculatory Ducts

The portion of the mesonephric duct extending from the caudal end of the epididymis to the seminal vesicles (see below) becomes thickened and muscular, forming the vas deferens (or ductus deferens) (Fig. 5) (1). The portion of the mesonephric duct that continues distal to the seminal vesicle is known as the ejaculatory duct, and this section is contained entirely within the prostate gland (see below). In its course, the vas deferens ascends from the scrotum with the vessels that vascularize the testis and epididymis, through the inguinal canal, over the pubic ramus, over the superior lateral aspect of the bladder medial to the ureter, and enters the superior aspect of the prostate, just distal to the seminal vesicle on that side. The primary function of the vas deferens and ejaculatory duct is to transport mature spermatozoa and seminal vesicle secretions to the prostatic urethra. The arterial supply of the vas deferens and ejaculatory ducts is provided by the tiny deferential artery (which usually arises from the inferior vesical artery). The veins accompany the arteries and have corresponding names. Lymphatic vessels from the vas deferens and ejaculatory ducts drain into the external iliac lymph nodes. The nerves of the ejaculatory ducts derive from the inferior hypogastric plexus.

Seminal Vesicles

The mature seminal vesicles reside immediately above the prostate gland (Fig. 5). Their arterial supply is derived from the inferior vesical and middle rectal arteries. The veins accompany the arteries and corresponding similar names. Lymph is drained into the internal iliac lymph nodes. The walls of the seminal vesicles also contain a plexus of nerve fibers and some sympathetic ganglia.

The seminal vesicles develop between the fifth and sixth weeks of embryonic life as lateral outgrowths at the caudal end of each Wolffian duct, migrating to lie posterior to the developing bladder and inferolateral to the vas deferens and ureter. Consequently, these glands share a common embryologic origin with the epididymis and vas deferens. Though initially a simple, saccular structure, each seminal vesicle will eventually develop complex internal convolutions corresponding to the folds of the very active secretory epithelium. In fact, the seminal vesicle contributes to the majority of the fluid volume of the ejaculate (1). Seminal vesicle secretions are rich in fructose and prostaglandins. While fructose may be an important energy source for spermatozoa, the role of the prostaglandins remains unknown. The seminal vesicle also produces several androgen-dependent secretory proteins that are involved in the rapid clotting of the ejaculate.

Prostate

The prostate (Figs. 5 and 7) is a walnut-sized exocrine gland located in the space below the bladder and above the urogenital diaphragm. It is separated posteriorly from the rectum by the rectovesical (Denonvillier's) fascia. Because it is located immediately anterior to the rectum, the prostate can be palpated and biopsied from the rectal canal. The prostate is homologous to the female Skene's glands. The prostatic arteries are mainly branches of the internal iliac artery, especially the inferior vesical artery, but also the internal pudendal and middle rectal arteries. The prostatic venous plexus, located on the sides and base of the prostate between the fibrous capsule of the prostate and the prostatic sheath, drains into the internal iliac veins. The prostatic plexus is continuous superiorly with the vesical venous plexus and communicates posteriorly with the internal vertebral venous plexus. The lymphatic vessels of the prostate terminate chiefly in the internal iliac and sacral lymph nodes.

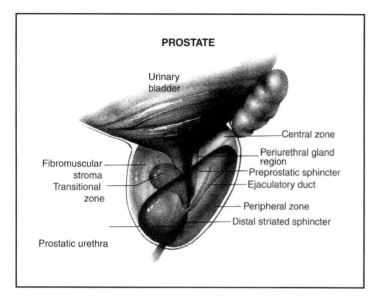

PROSTATE

Urinary
bladder

Central zone

Periurethral gland
region

Fibromuscular
stroma

Preprostatic sphincter

Transitional
zone

Ejaculatory duct

Peripheral zone

Distal striated sphincter

Prostatic urethra

Figure 7   (*See color insert*.) The prostate gland. *Source*: From Ref. 8.

The prostate arises from several distinct sets of tubules that evaginate from the primitive posterior urethra (1). Each set of tubules develops into a separate lobe: the right and left lateral lobes (the largest), the middle lobe, and the anterior and posterior lobes (very small). The lobes are further comprised of alveoli that are lined with a secretory epithelium. These drain through a series of converging tubules into the prostatic urethra. Although the lobes arise independently, they are continuous in the adult male, with no apparent gross or morphologic distinctions. Consequently, a more useful subdivision of the prostate has been developed that distinguishes prostatic zones based on morphologic and functional properties (Fig. 7). The peripheral zone is the subcapsular portion of the posterior aspect of the prostate gland that surrounds the distal urethra and comprises up to 70% of the normal prostate gland in young men. It is from this portion of the gland that more than 70% of prostatic cancers originate. The central zone (CZ) constitutes approximately 25% of the normal prostate gland and surrounds the ejaculatory ducts; CZ tumors account for more than 25% of all prostate cancers. The transition zone (TZ) is responsible for 5% of the prostate volume and is very rarely associated with carcinoma. The TZ surrounds the proximal urethra and is the region of the prostate gland that grows throughout life and is generally responsible for the occurrence of benign prostatic enlargement. (For further information on prostate cancer, see Chapter 41.)

Prostatic secretions contribute up to one-third of the fluid volume of the ejaculate (1). These secretions are high in zinc, citric acid, and choline. While the actual function of these substances has not yet been determined, it is postulated that zinc has some antimicrobial activity. The prostate also secretes several proteins, including acid phosphatase, seminin, plasminogen activator, and prostate-specific antigen. It is presumed that these substances are important for the function and survival of spermatozoa during and after ejaculation, but the details remain unknown. (For further information on the physiology of the prostate, see Chapter 7.)

Bulbourethral Glands

Homologous to the female Bartholin's glands, the paired pea-sized bulbourethral (Cowper's) glands are compound tubuloalveolar exocrine glands that lie posterolateral to the intermediate (membranous) part of the urethra (Fig. 3). The ducts of the bulbourethral glands pass through the inferior fascia of the urethral sphincter (perineal membrane) with the urethra and open through minute apertures into the proximal part of the spongy urethra in the bulb of the penis. Their clear, viscous secretion (pre-ejaculate) enters the urethra during sexual arousal, and may contain a small number of sperm. This fluid aids in lubricating the urethra to facilitate the passage of sperm, and may also help to flush out any residual urine or other foreign matter. The glands appear to diminish in size with advancing age.

□ CONCLUSION

This brief introduction to the male reproductive tract demonstrates the integrated nature of the system. The entire unit is maintained by androgens, secreted by the testis under hypothalamic and pituitary control. It is important to note that many of these structures are embryologically distinct; thus, developmental abnormalities will manifest in these organs in different ways. Knowledge of the embryology and anatomy of the male reproductive tract will enable a better understanding of both the common and not-so-common disorders encountered in the clinic.

□ REFERENCES

1. The American Society of Andrology. Handbook of Andrology. San Francisco: American Society of Andrology, 1995.
2. Netter FH. The CIBA Collection of Medical Illustrations: A Compilation of Paintings on the Normal and Pathologic Anatomy of the Reproductive System. Vol 2. Summit, NJ: CIBA Pharmaceutical Products, Inc., 1954.
3. Kirby RS. An Atlas of Erectile Dysfunction: An Illustrated Textbook and Reference for Clinicians. New York: The Parthenon Publishing Group, 1999.
4. Myer JK. Disorders of sexual function. In: Wilson JD, Foster DW, eds. Williams Textbook of Endocrinology. 7th ed. Philadelphia: WB Saunders Company, 1985: 476–491.
5. Newman HF. Physiology of erection: autonomic consideration. In: Krane RJ, Goldstein I, eds. Male Sexual Dysfunction. Boston: Little, Brown and Company, 1983:1–7.
6. Krane RJ. Sexual function and dysfunction. In: Walsh PC, Perfmutter AD, Staney TA, eds. Campbell's Urology. 5th ed. Philadelphia: WB Saunders Company, 1986: 700–735.
7. Rivard DJ. Anatomy, physiology, and neurophysiology of male sexual function. In: Bennett AH, ed. Management of Male Impotence. Int Perspect Urol, vol 5. Baltimore: Williams & Wilkins, 1982:1–25.
8. Springhouse. Atlas of Human Anatomy. 1st ed. Springhouse, PA: Lipincott, Williams, and Wilkins, 2001.
9. Lerner SE, Melman A, Christ GJ. A review of erectile dysfunction: new insights and more questions. J Urol 1993; 149:1246–1255.
10. Wagner G. Erection: physiology and endocrinology. In: Wagner G GR, ed. Impotence: Physiological, Psychological, Surgical Diagnosis and Treatment. New York: Plenum Press, 1981:25–36.
11. Krysiewicz MB. The role of imaging in the diagnostic evaluation of impotence. AJR 1989; 153(6):1133–1139.
12. Lue TF, Tanagho EA. Hemodynamics of erection. In: Tanagho EA, McClure RD, eds. Contemporary Management of Impotence and Infertility. Baltimore: Williams & Wilkins, 1988:28–38.
13. Krane RJ, Goldstein I, Saenz de Tejada I. Impotence. N Engl J Med 1989; 321(24):1648–1659.
14. Aboseif SL, Lue TF. Hemodynamics of penile erection. Urol Clin North Am 1988; 15(1):1–7.
15. Rosen MP, Schwartz AN, Levine FJ, et al. Radiologic assessment of impotence: angiography, sonography, cavernosography, and scintigraphy. Am J Roentgenol 1991; 157(5):923–931.
16. Bookstein JL. Penile magnification pharmacoarteriography: details of intrapenile anatomy. Am J Roentgenol 1987; 148(5):883–888.

17. Gray RR, Keresteci AG, Louis ELS, et al. Investigation of impotence by internal pudendal angiography: experience with 73 cases. Radiology 1982; 144(4):773–780.
18. Rosen MP, Greenfield AJ, Walker TG, et al. Arteriogenic impotence: findings in 195 impotent men examined with selective internal pudendal angiography. Radiology 1990; 174(3):1043–1048.
19. Bodner D. Impotence: evaluation and treatment. Prim Care 1985; 12(4):719–733.
20. Althof SS. The evaluation and management of erectile dysfunction. Psychiatr Clin North Am 1995; 18(1):171–192.
21. Klein E. The anatomy and physiology of the normal male sexual function. In: Montague D, ed. Disorders of Male Sexual Function. Chicago: Year Book Medical Publishers Inc., 1988:2–19.
22. Federman DD. Impotence: etiology and management. Hosp Prac 1982; 17(3):155–159.
23. Siroky MB, Krane RJ. Neurophysiology of erection. In: Krane RJ, Siroky MB, Goldstein I, eds. Male Sexual Dysfunction. Boston: Little, Brown and Company, 1983:9–20.
24. Siroky MB, Krane RJ. Physiology of male sexual function. In: Krane RJ, Siroky MB, eds. Clinical Neuro-Urology. Boston: Little, Brown and Company, 1979:45–62.
25. Steers WD. Current perspectives in the neural control of penile erection. In: Lue TF, ed. World Book of Impotence. London/Niigata-Shi: Smith-Gordon/ Nishimura, 1992:23–32.
26. Goldstein I. Evaluation of penile nerves. In: Tanagho EA, Lue TF, McClure RD, eds. Contemporary Management of Impotence and Infertility. Baltimore: Williams & Wilkins, 1988:70–83.
27. Traish AM, Moreland RB, Huang YH, et al. Expression of functional alpha2-adrenergic receptor subtypes in human corpus cavernousm and in cultured travecular smooth muscle cells. Recept Signal Transduct 1997; 7:55–67.
28. Gupta S, Moreland RB, Yang S, et al. The expression of functional postsynaptic alpha2-adrenoceptors in the corpus cavernosum smooth muscle. Br J Pharmacol 1998; 123(6):1237–1245.
29. Giuliano FA, Benoit G, Rampin O, et al. Neural control of penile erection. Urol Clin North Am 1995; 22(4): 747–766.
30. Saenz de Tejada I, Goldstein I, Krane RJ. Local control of penile erection. Nerves, smooth muscle, and endothelium. Urol Clin North Am 1988; 15(1):9–15.
31. Parsons RB, Fisher AM, Bar-Chama N, et al. MR imaging in male infertility. Radiographics 1997; 17(3): 627–637.
32. Tanagho EA. Embryologic basis for lower ureteral anomalies: a hypothesis. Urology 1976; 7(5):451–464.
33. Moore KL. The Developing Human: Clinically Oriented Embryology. 3rd ed. Philadelphia: W. B. Saunders, 1982: 365–382.

34. Sadler TW. Langman's Medical Embryology. 7th ed. Baltimore: Williams & Wilkins, 1995:286–309.

35. Hattery RR, King BF Jr, Lewis RW, et al. Vasculogenic impotence. Duplex and color doppler sonography. Radiol Clin North Am 1991; 29(3):629–645.

36. Wessells H, Lue TF, McAninch JW. Penile length in the flaccid and erect states: guidelines for penile augmentation. J Urol 1996; 156(3):995–997.

37. Virag R, Bouilly P, Virag H. Dimensions, volume and rigidity of the penis. Fundamental elements in the study of the erection and its dysfunctions. [Article in French]. Ann Urol (Paris) 1986; 20(4):244–248.

38. Gobec CJ, Cass AS. Quantifcation of erection. J Urol 1981; 126:345–357.

39. Bancroft J, Bell C. Simultaneous recording of penile diameter and penile arterial pulse during laboratory-based erotic stimulation in normal subjects. J Psychosom Res 1985; 29(3):303–313.

40. Chen KK, Chou YH, Chang LS, et al. Sonographic measurement of penile erectile volume. J Clin Ultrasound 1992; 20(4):247–253.

41. Nelson RP, Lue TF. Determination of erectile penile volume by ultrasonography. J Urol 1989; 141(5):1123–1126.

42. Bondil P, Costa P, Daures JP, et al. Clinical study of the longitudinal deformation of the flaccid penis and of its variations with aging. Eur Urol 1992; 21(4):284–286.

43. Laumann EO, Paik A, Rosen RC. Sexual dysfunction in the United States. JAMA 1999; 281(6):537–544.

44. Brant WE. Genital tract and bladder ultrasound. In: Brant WE, Helms CA, eds. Fundamentals of Diagnostic Radiology. 2nd ed. Baltimore: Lippincott, Williams & Wilkins, 1999:859–880.

45. Gooding GA. Scrotal ultrasonography. Radiologist 1994; 1:297–307.

3

Neuroendocrine Control of Testicular Function

Stephen J. Winters

Division of Endocrinology and Metabolism, University of Louisville, Louisville, Kentucky, U.S.A.

☐ GONADOTROPIN-RELEASING HORMONE SYNTHESIS AND SECRETION

Gonadotropin-releasing hormone (GnRH) is the central regulator of reproduction. GnRH, a C-terminal amidated decapeptide (pGlu-His-Trp-Ser-Tyr-Gly-Leu-Arg-Pro-Gly-NH2), is found in a small number of neurons that are located diffusely throughout the anterior hypothalamus in primates (1). GnRH neurons send axons through subventricular and periventricular pathways to terminate in the capillary space within the median eminence. GnRH from these axons enters the capillaries and is transported in the hypothalamic portal blood to the cells of the anterior pituitary.

The amount of GnRH secreted is influenced by many factors. GnRH mRNA levels are determined by the rate of transcription of the pro-*GnRH* gene and by the stability (half-life) of GnRH mRNA in the cytoplasm. Transcription of the *GnRH* gene is controlled by the POU-homeodomain protein, Oct-1, adhesion-related kinase, and by retinoid-X receptors, among other factors (2). Studies in GT1-7 cells, a GnRH-producing murine neuronal cell line, suggest that mRNA stability plays an important role in maintaining *GnRH* gene expression. The increased level of GnRH mRNA in the hypothalamus of adult male monkeys following orchidectomy (3) indicates that the testis secretes endocrine hormones that suppress *GnRH* gene expression. Transcription of GnRH mRNA produces a pro-GnRH precursor peptide that is processed to the mature GnRH decapeptide. Posttranslational processing may take place either within a cell, at the cell surface, or after secretion, and may be physiologically regulated as well.

The mean concentration of GnRH in hypothalamic portal blood (in rams) is approximately 20 pg/mL (0.02 nM). GnRH, like most hypophysiotropic factors, is released into portal blood in bursts. GnRH levels in the hypothalamic portal blood in conscious sheep ranged from minimum values of lesser than 5 pg/mL to pulse peak values of about 30 pg/mL (4). In these studies, GnRH pulse amplitudes in intact, castrated, and testosterone-treated castrated rams were roughly equivalent, whereas GnRH pulse frequency varied. The implication of these findings is that GnRH secretion rises with testosterone deficiency primarily because GnRH pulse frequency is accelerated.

The GnRH pulse generator is a poorly understood but highly synchronized firing of neurons in the mediobasal hypothalamus. The idea that changes in membrane potentials predispose to bursts of GnRH release follows from the finding that bursts of electrical activity in this region of the brain in the nonhuman primate coincide with pulses of luteinizing hormone (LH) secretion (5). The coincident firing of multiple GnRH-expressing neurons may reflect communication by gap junctions, interneurons, or second messengers. The findings that GnRH neurons express GnRH receptors and that adding GnRH to these cultures depresses GnRH pulsatile release provides a possible framework for intraneuronal communication by GnRH itself (6).

The release of GnRH is influenced by many neurotransmitters (Fig. 1), including glutamate, gamma-aminobutyric acid (GABA), neuropeptide Y, opiates, dopamine, norepinephrine, cyclic adenosine monophosphate (cAMP), and nitric oxide (7). Receptors on GnRH neurons for most of these substances imply that they influence GnRH neurons directly. *N*-methyl D-aspartic acid receptors that mediate glutamate activation of GnRH may involve the nitric oxide signaling pathway. Neurotransmitters with receptors not expressed on gonadotrophs may regulate GnRH via synaptic connections between GnRH neurons and other interneurons. Regulation of GnRH secretion may also occur directly on neuronal axon terminals in the median eminence.

Structural variants of GnRH (e.g., GnRH-II) that were initially identified in nonvertebrates have also been found in the primate brain and in peripheral tissues, including the placenta, gonads, breasts, and prostate, where they may have a neuromodulatory function. These peptides appear to activate a unique GnRH-II receptor (8).

☐ GONADOTROPHS AND GnRH RECEPTORS

Gonadotrophs constitute 6% to 10% of the cells of the anterior pituitary (9). Gonadotrophs may be small and round or larger and ovoid and are diffcult to identify by morphological criteria. Instead, gonadotrophs are identified by immunostaining using specific antibodies for LH and follicle-stimulating hormone (FSH). From studies in rats, nearly all gonadotrophs are bihormonal

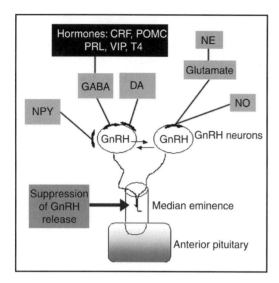

Figure 1 Diagram showing activation of GnRH neurons by neurotransmitters and their relation to the anterior pituitary. *Abbreviations*: CRF, corticotropin-releasing factor; DA, dopamine; GABA, gamma-aminobutyric acid; GnRH, gonadotropin-releasing hormone; NE, norepinephrine; NO, nitric oxide; NPY, neuropeptide Y; POMC, pro-opiomelanocortin; PRL, prolactin; T4, thyroxine; VIP, vasoactive intestinal polypeptide.

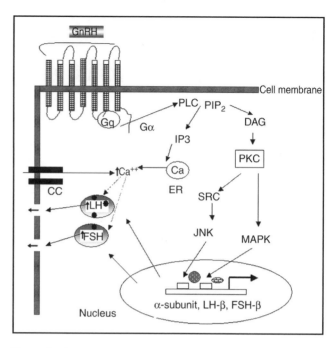

Figure 2 Signaling mechanisms initiated by activation of the GnRH receptor that result in gonadotropin synthesis and secretion. *Abbreviations*: Ca, calcium ion; CC, calcium channel; DAG, membrane diacylglycerol protein; ER, endoplasmic reticulum; FSH-β, follicle-stimulating hormone, β subunit; Gα, alpha subunit product of G protein; GnRH, gonadotropin-releasing hormone; G, G protein subtype that is associated with GnRH receptor; IP3, inositol triphosphate; JNK, member of the mitogen-activated protein kinases subfamilies; LH-β, luteinizing hormone, β subunit; MAPK, member of the mitogen-activated protein kinases subfamilies; PIP$_2$, phosphatidylinositol bisphosphate; PKC, protein kinase C; PLC, phospholipase C; SRC, family of protein tyrosine kinases.

(they express both LH-β and FSH-β subunit genes). A small fraction of cells appear to express LH or FSH selectively, but the biological significance of this finding is not known. Interestingly, some gonadotrophs produce growth hormone (GH) as well as the gonadotropic hormones.

GnRH activates gonadotrophs and thereby stimulates testosterone production and spermatogenesis through both short-term and long-term mechanisms. Upon reaching the pituitary, GnRH binds to and activates a cell-surface G protein coupled receptor (GnRH-R) that is specific for gonadotrophs (10). The receptor is a structurally unique member of the seven-transmembrane G protein–linked receptor family that lacks a long C-terminal intracellular tail typical of most GnRH-Rs (Fig. 2). This structure is important in the rapid desensitization of other GnRH-Rs, whereas downregulation of the GnRH receptor is a delayed event. Binding of GnRH to its receptor facilitates binding of a G protein to the receptor's third intracellular loop. The bound G protein exchanges GDP for GTP and dissociates into its constituent α and $\beta\gamma$ subunits. The α-subunits are unique to each G protein, whereas the β- and γ-subunits of the different G proteins are similar. The dissociated G protein α-subunit activates downstream signaling pathways (11). Gqα, the major G protein that associates with the GnRH-R, activates membrane-associated phospholipase C to hydrolyze membrane phosphoinositides and increase intracellular inositol phosphates including inositol triphosphate $(I_{1,4,5})$P3. IP3 rapidly mobilizes calcium from intracellular stores, and voltage-gated calcium channels open so that extracellular calcium enters the cell (10). The increase in intracellular free calcium is primarily responsible for the immediate release of LH and FSH

from the cell (12). GnRH receptors may interact with other G proteins as well.

The long-term stimulatory effects of GnRH are to increase transcription of the genes for the gonadotropin subunits and for the GnRH-R. These effects occur primarily because GnRH signaling also liberates membrane diacylglycerol, which in turn activates protein kinase C (PKC). The subsequent phosphorylation of subfamilies of mitogen-activated protein (MAP) kinases, including members of the ERK and JNK families, initiates nuclear translocation of proteins that bind directly to the 5′ regulatory regions of gonadotropin subunit and the *GnRH-R* genes, or serve as cofactors for promoter activation (13). Increased intracellular calcium may also contribute to the transcriptional effects of GnRH (14).

GnRH receptors are upregulated by pulsatile GnRH (15). Thus, when pulsatile GnRH secretion increases, as in castration or primary testicular failure, GnRH receptors increase, gonadotrophs become more responsive to GnRH, and the LH response to GnRH stimulation is amplified (16). With continuous GnRH treatment, GnRH receptors decline, followed by suppression of LH-β and FSH-β mRNAs. This "homologous desensitization" of the GnRH-R is regulated by several serine–threonine protein kinases [including protein kinase A (PKA) and PKC] as well as by G protein coupled receptor kinases. GnRH receptors also decline with GnRH deficiency.

□ THE GONADOTROPIC HORMONES

LH and FSH are members of the glycoprotein hormone family that also includes thyrotroph-stimulating hormone (TSH) and human chorionic gonadotropin (hCG). These heterodimeric hormones are composed of a common α-subunit and unique β-subunits. The subunits have oligosaccharide chains that are asparagine associated. Each of the subunits is encoded by a unique gene that is found on a separate chromosome. The human α-subunit gene has been localized to 6p21.1-23, LH-β to 19q13.3, and FSH-β to 11p13.

The production of LH and FSH is directly influenced by the levels of the gonadotropin subunit mRNAs. This relationship seems especially strong for FSH-β mRNA and FSH secretion. Each of the gonadotropin subunit mRNAs is increased by GnRH, and stimulation by GnRH of the β-subunit genes is primarily transcriptional. Complexes of transcription factors, including *SF-1*, *EGR-1*, and *SP1*, are activators of the *LHβ*-subunit gene (17), whereas the AP1 proteins fos/jun are important for the upregulation of FSH-β transcription by GnRH (18). In order to increase LH-β and FSH-β mRNA levels, GnRH stimulation must be pulsatile. Transcriptional regulatory proteins that control α-subunit expression include cAMP response element binding protein (CREB), MAP kinase/ERK1, and GATA-binding proteins (19). Alpha-subunit gene expression is increased robustly both by pulsatile and by continuous GnRH, and GnRH not only stimulates α-subunit transcription, but also prolongs α-subunit mRNA half-life (20). Thus, the requirements for α-subunit mRNA upregulation by GnRH are less stringent than are those for the β-subunit genes. These factors partly explain why α-subunits are synthesized in excess of β-subunits, and why β-subunits are rate limiting for gonadotropin synthesis.

Proteins destined for secretion, such as the gonadotropins, are synthesized on ribosomes bound to the endoplasmic reticulum (ER). During the translational process, preformed oligosaccharide chains are linked to the side chain amino group of asparagines on the gonadotropin subunits. As translation continues, sugar moieties are trimmed, and the subunits change configuration allowing for their combination. A region of the β-subunit, termed the "seatbelt," is wrapped around the α-subunit loop 2 (21). Dimeric LH and FSH are segregated in the ER and transferred to the Golgi where they are concentrated in secretory granules. These protein-rich vesicles subsequently fuse with the plasma membrane following stimulation by GnRH. This process is termed "exocytosis." There is evidence that granules containing FSH are also exported directly to the plasma membrane independent of GnRH pulsatile stimulation. This mode of secretion allows for FSH secretion between pulses. Gonadotrophs also secrete an uncombined α-subunit both in pulsatile and continuous modes, but whether the uncombined α-subunit has a biological function is not known.

□ PULSATILE GONADOTROPIN SECRETION

Experiments in ovariectomized rhesus monkeys rendered gonadotropin deficient with hypothalamic lesions first revealed that an intermittent pattern of GnRH administration was necessary for normal LH secretion (22). In those animals, GnRH administered as pulses stimulated LH secretion, but GnRH administered continuously was much less effective. The pulsatile nature of LH secretion was subsequently established in all species studied, including humans (23). Moreover, LH secretion is stimulated when GnRH is administered in pulses to gonadotropin-deficient patients, but not when GnRH is administered continuously (24). An understanding of these physiological mechanisms led to the use of pulsatile GnRH to stimulate fertility and to the development of long-acting GnRH analogs that produce a biochemical orchiectomy as a treatment for patients with prostate cancer and other androgen-dependent disorders. GnRH analogs with a long circulating plasma half-life initially stimulate gonadotropin secretion, but with continued treatment, gonadotropin secretion declines, and testosterone production falls to low levels (25).

With current assays, GnRH is undetectable in the peripheral circulation. Therefore, GnRH secretion cannot be studied directly in humans. Instead, changes in circulating LH levels are used to evaluate the activity of the human GnRH pulse generator. LH secretion is determined by the frequency, amplitude, and duration of the secretory pulses. Presumably because of its longer circulating half-life, pulses of FSH are less clearly defined in the peripheral blood than are LH pulses; FSH pulses are clearly evident in jugular blood in ewes where clearance effects are minimized (26).

As a model, cultured pituitary cells that are perifused with pulses of GnRH yield important information on the actions of GnRH and other factors that regulate gonadotropin secretion under controlled conditions (27). Using this experimental approach (Fig. 3), episodes of LH as well as FSH secretion are distinct and short lived, with a rapid upstroke and abrupt termination. LH pulse amplitude is directly proportional to the dose of GnRH administered and the median duration of an LH pulse of about 25 minutes.

In contrast to the regularity of LH pulses produced by an invariant dose of GnRH in vitro, LH pulses in the peripheral circulation in humans are irregular in amplitude (Fig. 4), and interpulse intervals vary. LH pulses in vivo also have a less rapid upstroke and a slower decline from the peak, presumably reflecting the dilution of secreted hormone by plasma in the general circulation and the influence of clearance of LH by the liver and kidney. Whether LH is released in the

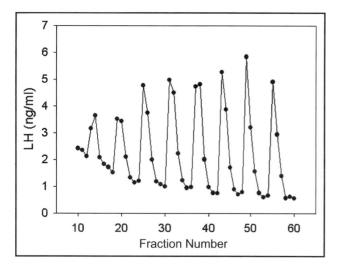

Figure 3 Secretion of LH by pituitary cells from adult male primates perifused with pulses of GnRH. Pulses of GnRH (2.5 nM) were applied to the cells every one hour for two minutes. Fractions of the column effluent were collected every 10 minutes, and LH was measured in the media by immunoassay. *Abbreviations*: GnRH, gonadotropin-releasing hormone; LH, luteinizing hormone. *Source*: From Ref. 27.

basal interval between GnRH-initiated secretory episodes has been debated, but this mode of secretion is minimal and is probably not biologically important.

Hormone pulse detection has been standardized by the development of computer algorithms (28). With this approach, objective assessment of the frequency and amplitude characteristics of hormone pulses has been possible. Pulses of LH secretion occur throughout the day and night in normal adult men. Estimates of the frequency of LH (GnRH) pulses in men have varied based on the intensity and duration of the blood sampling protocol, the assay used to measure LH, and the algorithm used to identify pulses. Most investigators have proposed an average frequency of one LH pulse every one to two hours for normal men, but there is a

large amount of variation between individuals (29). Because of the variation in pulse amplitude and frequency, the distinction between true and artifactual pulses can be diffcult. One approach is to coanalyze LH and uncombined α-subunit pulses, since the α-subunit is released into the circulation by GnRH together with LH and FSH (30). According to this logic, concordant LH and α-subunit fluctuations presumably reflect true GnRH pulsatile signals. There is generally a positive relationship between LH pulse amplitude and the preceding interpulse interval in part because a longer interval allows for the circulating level to decline to a lower baseline value. (For further details, see Chapter 4.)

In addition to the pulsatile pattern of LH secretion, there is a pronounced diurnal variation in circulating LH and testosterone levels in pubertal boys with increased LH levels during sleep, and increased testosterone levels in the early morning hours (31). While there is also a diurnal variation in plasma testosterone in adults, there is no clear diurnal rhythm for LH in most adult men (32), implying that the diurnal variation in testosterone levels in men is only partly LH controlled. The diurnal testosterone variation in men is disrupted by fragmented sleep (33), but the mechanism for this alteration has not been established. The diurnal variation in testosterone is blunted in older men (34) and in young men with testicular failure (35).

□ LUTEINIZING HORMONE CONTROL OF TESTOSTERONE SYNTHESIS

Testosterone, a C19 3-keto, 17β-hydroxy Δ4 steroid, is synthesized from cholesterol through a series of cytochrome P450- and dehydrogenase-dependent enzymatic reactions (Fig. 5) (36). The conversion of cholesterol to pregnenolone occurs within mitochondria and is catalyzed by P450scc, the cytochrome P450 side chain cleavage enzyme. P450scc catalyzes sequential hydroxylations of the cholesterol side chain at C22 and at C20 and subsequently cleaves the C20–22 bond to produce pregnenolone.

Pregnenolone exits the mitochondria and can be converted to testosterone by two alternative routes referred to as the Δ4-pathway or the Δ5-pathway, based on whether the steroid intermediates are 3-keto, Δ4 steroids (Δ4) or 3-hydroxy, Δ5 steroids (Δ5).

Classical experiments in which human testicular microsomes were incubated with radiolabeled steroids revealed that the Δ5-pathway predominates in the human testis. In that pathway, C17 hydroxylation of pregnenolone to form 17α-hydroxypregnenolone is followed by cleavage of the C17 to C20 bond of 17α-hydroxypregnenolone to produce dehydroepiandrosterone (DHEA). Both reactions are catalyzed by one enzyme, cytochrome P450 17α-hydroxylase/C17,20 lyase (P450c17). Oxidation of the 3β-hydroxy group and isomerization of the C5 to C6 double bond of DHEA by 3β-hydroxysteroid dehydrogenase/Δ5-Δ4

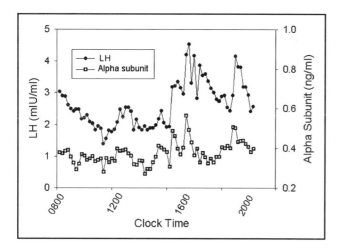

Figure 4 Circulating LH and alpha subunit levels in a normal adult man. Blood samples were drawn every 10 minutes for 12 hours beginning at 0800 hours and measured for LH using the Nichols Allegro LH 2-site assay and a specific double antibody immunoassay for the α-subunit. *Abbreviation*: LH, luteinizing hormone.

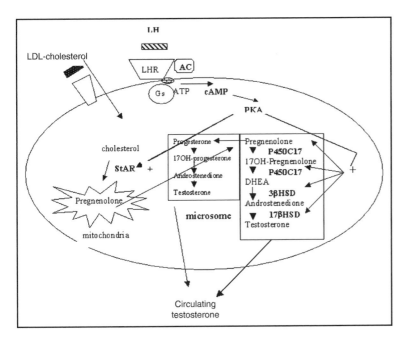

Figure 5 Regulation of testosterone biosynthesis in Leydig cells by LH. *Abbreviations*: 17βHSD, 17βhydroxy steroiddehydrogenase; 3βHSD, 3βhydroxysteroid dehydrogenase/Δ⁴-Δ⁵ isomerase; AC, adenylate cyclase; CAMP, cyclic adenosine monophosphate; DHEA, dehydroepiandrosterone; LHR, luteinizing hormone receptor; P450c17, 17αhydroxylase/c17,20 lyase; PKA, protein kinase A; StAR, steroidogenic acute regulatory protein.

isomerase (3βHSD) forms androstenedione. The C17 keto group of androstenedione is oxidized to a hydroxyl group by 17β HSD–producing testosterone.

In the Δ4-pathway that predominates in rodents, pregnenolone is metabolized to progesterone by 3βHSD. Progesterone is hydroxylated at C17 to produce 17α-hydroxyprogesterone, followed by cleavage of the C17 to C20 bond of 17α-hydroxyprogesterone to produce androstenedione. Cytochrome P450c17 catalyzes both reactions. Finally, the C17 keto group of androstenedione is oxidized to a hydroxyl group by 17β HSD to produce testosterone.

LH stimulates testosterone biosynthesis in Leydig cells through a G protein–associated seven-transmembrane receptor (37). LH binding initiates a signaling cascade by activating G proteins that stimulate adenylate cyclase activity in order to increase intracellular cAMP levels and activate cAMP-dependent PKA. cAMP-dependent PKA regulates testosterone synthesis in two ways. The acute response, which occurs within minutes of hormonal stimulation, is an increase in cholesterol transport into the mitochondria and is regulated by the steroidogenic acute regulatory (StAR) protein (38). StAR appears to function at the mitochondrial outer membrane, but the mechanism of action for its cholesterol transport is not yet known. The chronic response to LH, which requires several hours, involves transcriptional activation of the genes encoding the steroidogenic enzymes of the testosterone biosynthetic pathway, P450scc, P450c17, 3βHSD, and 17βHSD.

Other factors that stimulate testosterone synthesis directly include prolactin (PRL), GH, triiodothyronine (T3), pituitary adenylate cyclase-activating polypeptide (PACAP), vasoactive intestinal polypeptide, and inhibin. Factors that have been reported to reduce testosterone production by Leydig cells include glucocorticoids, estradiol, activin, arginine vasopressin, corticotropin-releasing factor (CRF) and interleukin (IL)-1. Although

early studies with purified FSH preparations suggested that FSH enhanced Leydig cell responsiveness to LH, more recent experiments using recombinant FSH have not supported that idea (39,40). The role of FSH in testosterone biosynthesis continues to be investigated.

The blood production rate of testosterone in normal adult men is estimated to range from 5000 to 7500 µg/24 hr (41), and levels of total testosterone among normal men range from 250 to 1000 ng/dL (10–40 nmol/L) in most assays. The level of testosterone in adult men declines by more than 95% if the testes are removed. The remainder of the testosterone is derived from the production of androstenedione and DHEA by the adrenal cortex.

☐ ESTROGENS IN MALES

In addition to testosterone, normal men produce about 40 µg of estradiol and 60 µg of estrone daily. Estradiol is produced from testosterone, and estrone is derived from androstenedione, by aromatase P450, the product of the *CYP19* gene (42). This microsomal enzyme oxidizes the C19 angular methyl group to produce a phenolic A-ring. Aromatase is expressed in adult Leydig cells, where it is upregulated by LH and hCG (43); however, most of the estrogen in men is derived from aromatase in adipose and skin stromal cells, aortic smooth-muscle cells, kidney, skeletal cells, and the brain. Regulation of extratesticular aromatase is less well understood. The promoter sequences of the testicular and extragonadal P450 aromatase genes are tissue specific due to differential splicing, but the translated protein appears to be the same in all tissues.

Exogenous estrogens are well known to suppress testosterone production and to disrupt spermatogenesis, but endogenous estrogens play a physiological role in men (44). The actions of estradiol are, for the most part, mediated by intracellular receptor proteins that bind to and activate the promoters of estrogen-responsive genes. It is now known that there are two forms of the estrogen receptor (ER) that play a role in reproduction and are encoded by separate genes (45). These genes have been designated *ER-α* and *ER-β*. *ER-α* is the dominant form in the pituitary and hypothalamus, whereas both *ER-α* and *ER-β* are found in the testis, prostate, and epididymis (46). Clinical findings in an adult man with an inactivating mutation of the *ER-α* and in two men with mutations of the *CYP19* aromatase gene (47), together with results from the development of mice that are lacking ERs or are deficient in aromatase (48), have expanded the understanding of the importance of estradiol in the neuroendocrine control of testicular function. Studies of the *ER-α* knock-out mouse have revealed dilatation and atrophy of the seminiferous tubules, implying an estrogen effect in the regulation of the efferent ductules of the testis. Although fertile in early life, aromatase-deficient mice subsequently develop infertility. Thus, estradiol appears to be essential for male fertility.

□ TESTICULAR CONTROL OF GONADOTROPIN SECRETION

Gonadotropin secretion, while upregulated by GnRH, is maintained at physiological levels through testicular negative feedback mechanisms (Fig. 6). Accordingly, plasma LH and FSH levels rise when negative feedback is disrupted by castration, and decrease following the administration of testosterone or estradiol.

The mechanisms for the negative feedback control of LH and FSH by gonadal steroids in males are partly species specific. There is considerable evidence

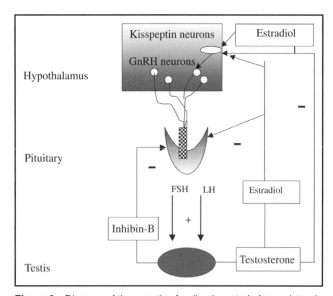

Figure 6 Diagram of the negative feedback control of gonadotropin secretion by testicular hormones. *Abbreviations*: FSH, follicle-stimulating hormone; GnRH, gonadotropin-releasing hormone; LH, luteinizing hormone.

that in primates, androgens suppress LH synthesis and secretion primarily through an action on the GnRH pulse generator. Peripheral blood pulse profiles reveal that LH pulse frequency and amplitude are elevated in castrates and are suppressed by testosterone replacement (49,50). In addition, expression of the mRNAs for GnRH (3), pituitary GnRH-receptors, and the gonadotropin subunit genes are increased in castrates (51). These effects contribute to the testosterone-induced reduction in LH pulse amplitude.

GnRH-deficient men have been used as a human model to examine the pituitary and hypothalamic effects of testicular negative feedback. In men with GnRH deficiency treated with fixed doses of GnRH (52), LH secretion was less effectively suppressed by testosterone than in normal men, indicating a role for testosterone in the control of GnRH secretion. Experiments in the nonhuman adult male primate (rendered gonadotropin deficient by a hypothalamic lesion and reactivated with pulses of GnRH) also demonstrated the importance of the GnRH pulse generator in the negative feedback control of LH secretion by testosterone. In that model, removal of both testes produced little change in LH secretion until the frequency of the applied GnRH pulses was increased (53). Moreover, when pituitary cells from adult male monkeys were stimulated with pulses of GnRH, no inhibition of GnRH-induced LH secretion by testosterone or dihydrotestosterone (DHT) was found. In pituitary cells from rats, on the other hand, the gonadotroph is a direct site of testosterone-negative feedback control, since GnRH-stimulated LH pulses were suppressed in amplitude by testosterone, and α-subunit gene expression was reduced (27). Thus, the primate pituitary is insensitive to negative feedback from androgens.

Whether or not testosterone—by itself and/or with the estradiol derived from testosterone by aromatase in the central nervous system or in peripheral tissues—controls LH secretion has been a subject of considerable interest. The finding that the nonaromatizable androgen, DHT, decreases LH pulse frequency strongly supports a role for androgens in the regulation of the GnRH pulse generator. Further, LH pulse frequency is increased in patients with nonfunctional androgen receptors (AR) in the complete androgen insensitivity (testicular feminization) syndrome, indicating that nuclear AR signaling somehow regulates GnRH pulse frequency (54).

It is now well established that estradiol also plays an important physiological role in the negative feedback control of gonadotropin secretion in men. This control mechanism was suggested by pharmacological studies using the estrogen antagonist, clomiphene (55), or the aromatase inhibitor, testolactone (56). When these drugs were administered to normal men, circulating LH and FSH levels rose together with plasma testosterone concentrations. More recently, gonadotropin and testosterone levels were reportedly increased in a man with an inactivating mutation of the *ER-α* (57), and in two men with mutations in the aromatase gene (Table 1) (58,59). Thus, even though androgen levels are increased, estrogen blockade or deficiency leads to increased gonadotropin secretion. Moreover, in one man with aromatase deficiency, serum gonadotropin levels were suppressed by estrogen treatment. The finding that clomiphene increased LH pulse frequency (55) indicated that a portion of the negative feedback action of estradiol was at the level of the GnRH pulse generator. This finding was recently confirmed and extended using the aromatase inhibitor, anastrozole (60). Estradiol treatment also decreases the LH response to GnRH stimulation in men (61) and in primate pituitary cells perifused with pulses of GnRH (27), indicating a direct negative effect on the pituitary, as well.

GnRH neurons appear by autoradiography and immunocytochemistry to lack both androgen and ERs. Steroid feedback is now believed to involve neurons that express kisspeptin.

□ FSH AND INHIBIN

There are both similarities and differences in the neuroendocrine control of FSH when compared to LH secretion. As for LH, the synthesis and secretion of FSH is upregulated by GnRH and is suppressed by gonadal steroid hormones; however, two paracrine factors, pituitary activin and follistatin, and testicular inhibin-B selectively regulate FSH secretion by regulating *FSH-β* gene expression (62). Because of these unique control mechanisms for FSH, LH and FSH secretion are sometimes dissociated.

Activin, a member of the transforming growth factor (TGF)-β family of growth factors, stimulates FSH-β mRNA transcription and prolongs FSH-β mRNA half-life. Activin is a dimeric peptide consisting of two similar subunits that were designated as β-subunits because the identification of activin followed the cloning of inhibin, an α-β heterodimer. There are at least four forms of the β subunit: βA, βB, βC, and βD. Activin is expressed in all tissues in the body and plays a role in neural and mesodermal morphogenesis, wound healing, vascular remodeling, and inflammation, as well as in reproductive function. The pituitary expresses βB, and activin-B (βBβB) is the form found in the pituitary, whereas most other tissues produce activin-A. Activin binds to a serine/threonine kinase receptor (activin receptor type II) that complexes with, and phosphorylates a type 1 activin receptor to initiate intracellular signaling (63). A group of intracellular proteins known as Smads mediate the actions of activin as well as TGF-β. Ultimately, the activin-stimulated Smad complex enters the nucleus and activates target genes including FSH-β.

The actions of activin are antagonized by follistatin, which binds to, and thereby neutralizes, the bioactivity of activin. Additionally, inhibin competes with activin for binding to the activin receptor (64). Inhibin is an antagonist of activin because it fails to initiate intracellular Smad signaling. Betaglycan, a membrane proteoglycan, appears to function as an accessory receptor-binding protein for inhibin as well as for TGF-β and plays a role in inhibin suppression of activin signaling (65). Follistatin is structurally unrelated to activin and inhibin, but like activin, is found in all tissues examined. In the rat pituitary, follistatin is upregulated by activin, GnRH, and PACAP, and is suppressed by testosterone and by follistatin itself—no doubt through binding to activin. One effect of pituitary follistatin is to influence the FSH and LH response to castration. Follistatin expression increases following orchiectomy in male rats (66), and there is a reciprocal relationship between follistatin and *FSH-β* gene expression that rises only two- to threefold in orchiectomized rats. This relation implies that follistatin attenuates the FSH castration response in that species. On the other hand, in male primates, including humans, FSH-β mRNA increases about 50-fold following bilateral orchiectomy, but follistatin mRNA levels are unchanged (50). Thus, follistatin appears to function as a brake on FSH production in male rodents but not in primates.

Inhibin is produced by Sertoli cells and by fetal Leydig cells and plays a fundamental role in the selective regulation of FSH (67). Inhibin may also be an intragonadal regulator, but that function of inhibin is less well understood. The term "inhibin" was first applied in 1932 to the aqueous extract of bull testis that prevented the development of castration cells within the anterior pituitary and was distinguished from "androitin" (what is now known as testosterone) that was present in the ether extract and stimulated prostate growth.

Inhibin is a heterodimer of an α-subunit and one of two β-subunits, βA and βB. Of these, only the βB subunit seems to be expressed by the testis, and therefore testicular inhibin is inhibin-B. The inhibin α-subunit gene is upregulated by FSH, whereas the factors regulating the βB subunit gene are not well understood. The level of inhibin/activin βB mRNA in the rat testis is unaffected by hypophysectomy or by FSH treatment (68). Transcription factors of the GATA-binding protein family were found to regulate both the

TABLE 1   Hormone Levels in a Man with a Mutation of the *ER*-α and Two Men Deficient in Aromatase

Age (yr)	Testosterone (ng/dL)	Estradiol (pg/mL)	LH (mIU/mL)	FSH (mIU/mL)	Ref.
28	445	119	37 (2.0–20)	33 (2.0–15)	(57)
24	2015	<7	26.1 (2.0–9.9)	28.3 (5.0–9.9)	(58)
31	523	<10	5.6 (1.4–8.9)	17.1 (1.7–6.9)	(59)

Note: LH and FSH levels in parentheses are the normal ranges reported in those references.
Abbreviations: LH, luteinizing hormone; FSH, follicle-stimulating hormone, ER, estrogen receptor.

inhibin β- and α-subunit promoters (69). Control of inhibin βB by a germ-cell factor is suggested by the abrupt decline in plasma inhibin-B levels but not inhibin-α subunit levels that follows destruction of germ cells by cancer chemotherapy (70).

Inhibin suppresses FSH secretion by decreasing the level of the mRNA for the FSH-β subunit (71). Based on this effect, plasma inhibin-B and FSH concentrations are inversely related among normal men and are more strikingly correlated when values from men with primary testicular failure are included in the analysis. The relationship between circulating inhibin-B and FSH is different, however, from that between serum LH and testosterone levels. Specifically, there is no correlation between circulating LH and testosterone among normal men. The different relationship between plasma LH with testosterone and FSH with inhibin-B levels was clearly demonstrated in experiments conducted by Ramaswamy et al. (72). These investigators removed one testis from adult male rhesus monkeys and observed that the plasma levels of both testosterone and inhibin-B decreased, but the decline in testosterone was brief and was restored to normal by a rise in LH, whereas inhibin-B levels remained at about 50% of the baseline value for up to six weeks even though FSH levels rose. Similarly, Anawalt et al. (73) found that very large doses were required for FSH to increase circulating inhibin-B levels in normal men. Thus, LH and testosterone form a classical feed-forward/feedback loop, whereas inhibin-B controls FSH but is less dependent on FSH stimulation.

Inhibin-B levels increase during the neonatal phase of development and again at puberty. Although plasma LH and FSH levels rise at these developmental stages, the number of Sertoli cells also increases. Studies in adult monkeys showed a strong positive correlation between circulating inhibin-B levels and Sertoli cell number (74). Thus, circulating inhibin-B appears to reflect the number and function of Sertoli cells and is less dependent on FSH stimulation.

FSH activates a G protein–associated seven-transmembrane Sertoli-cell receptor (75). The activated receptor stimulates adenylate cyclase and increases intracellular levels of cAMP. Numerous Sertoli-cell genes are activated by cAMP, most often through cAMP-dependent PKA, with subsequent phosphorylation of the cAMP response element CREB transcription factor. The role of FSH in spermatogenesis is, however, a matter of controversy. The classical view was that FSH stimulated spermatogenesis and that LH stimulated testosterone production by Leydig cells; however, spermatogenesis is qualitatively maintained by testosterone alone in hypophysectomized rats or in rats immunized against GnRH. More recently, men with an inactivating mutation of the FSH-R gene were identified in Finland. The testes of the five homozygotes were reduced in size, and the sperm count and/or motility was reduced, but two men were fertile (76). Moreover, an FSH-β–deficient mouse that was developed was likewise fertile (77), implying that FSH is not essential for male fertility. On the other hand, spermatogenesis is not quantitatively normal in these models, and FSH acts synergistically with testosterone in rodents or with hCG in men, implying a role for FSH in spermatogenesis as well. Species differences in the progression of undifferentiated spermatogonia and in the production of FSH independent of GnRH may explain why FSH seems to be less important in rodents than in primates.

☐ NEUROENDOCRINE MECHANISMS FOR THE DIFFERENTIAL CONTROL OF FSH AND LH

In addition to selective regulation of FSH-β mRNA levels by pituitary activin and follistatin and by testicular inhibin-B, other mechanisms may contribute to the differential secretion of FSH and LH. Results from studies in rats (78) and rat pituitary cell cultures (79) revealed that the frequency of GnRH pulses regulates LH and FSH syntheses differently, with very rapid GnRH pulse frequencies (every 15–30 minutes) favoring LH-β over FSH-β gene expression. This difference may be partly due to upregulation of follistatin mRNA levels by rapid GnRH pulse frequencies (79) with subsequent suppression by follistatin of activin-stimulated FSH-β gene expression. Although this mechanism seems to be applicable in rats, its importance in men is less well established. In men with congenital hypogonadotropic hypogonadism (CHH) (e.g., Kallmann's syndrome) who were treated long term with pulsatile GnRH, increasing the frequency of GnRH stimulation from every two hours to every 30 minutes for seven days increased serum LH levels threefold, but FSH levels rose by 50% (80). It is well established that the rise in LH exceeds the rise in FSH when normal men are administered a GnRH bolus. A second study in a similar population of men revealed that increasing the GnRH pulse frequency from every 1.5 hours to every 0.5 hours suppressed plasma FSH, but plasma LH levels were unchanged (81). In both studies, changes in testosterone, estradiol, and inhibin-B levels may have influenced the results. PACAP is a neuropeptide that stimulates α-subunit transcription and lengthens LH-β mRNA transcripts and presumably prolongs half-life but suppresses FSH-β mRNA levels by stimulating follistatin transcription (82). These observations in vitro suggest PACAP could also play a role in the differential production of FSH and LH. A third idea is that increasing the frequency of GnRH pulses modifies GnRH-receptor signaling pathways and thereby regulates FSH-β and LH-β gene expression differently (83).

☐ THE INTERNAL AND EXTERNAL ENVIRONMENT AND THE NEUROENDOCRINE CONTROL OF TESTICULAR FUNCTION

Changes in the internal or external environment may predispose to neuroendocrine testicular dysfunction through either an acceleration or a slowing in GnRH pulse frequency, or an increase or decline in GnRH pulse amplitude. So far, no abnormalities have been ascribed to GnRH pulses of abnormal duration. Because each LH pulse is initiated by a burst of GnRH secretion, a disturbance in LH pulse frequency is considered to indicate a change in function of the hypothalamic GnRH pulse generator. On the other hand, variations in LH pulse amplitude are consistent with either a change in GnRH secretion, a change in GnRH responsiveness due to changes in GnRH-receptor number or signaling mechanisms, or a change in gonadotropin subunit gene expression. Because LH interpulse intervals and LH secretory pulse amplitudes are variable both within and between subjects, distinguishing between hypothalamic and pituitary mechanisms of disease by evaluating pulse patterns in humans can be difficult. The LH response to pharmacological stimulation with GnRH is often unhelpful in distinguishing hypothalamic from pituitary disease, as well, since responsiveness to GnRH can be inversely proportional to GnRH frequency, can overlap with normal in some patients with pituitary disease, and is attenuated by prolonged GnRH deficiency.

In men with CHH, plasma LH levels are frequently undetectable, and LH pulses are absent (84). Other men have partial defects with evidence for testicular development, and circulating testosterone levels that are similar to those of boys during puberty (85). Some cases of CHH in men with Kallmann's syndrome are now understood to be due to hypothalamic GnRH deficiency, and other cases of CHH have been associated with mutations in the GnRH-receptor gene (86). Chromosomal mapping of the GnRH receptor to autosome 4q22.1 explains how CHH affects a small number of females. Gonadotropin deficiency also occurs in men with adrenal hypoplasia congenita, a disorder causing primary adrenal failure in neonates, which is now known to result from mutations in the gene for *DAX1*, a member of the orphan nuclear hormone superfamily (87). Studies in rodents support a role for *DAX1* and the related gene, steroidogenic factor-1 in the regulation of the LH-β and α-subunit as well as the GnRH receptor and adrenocorticotropic hormone (ACTH) receptor genes. Yet, most cases of CHH remain idiopathic.

Gonadotropin deficiency in adult men is acquired, rather than inherited, and results from tumors of the pituitary or suprasellar region, or from granulomatous or infiltrative disorders including sarcoidosis, histiocytosis, and hemochromatosis. Some cases of acquired hypogonadotropic hypogonadism have no evident explanation (88).

Nutritional factors play an important role in the neuroendocrine control of testicular function. In acute starvation, LH pulse frequency and amplitude decrease (89). Prolonged starvation, as in patients with anorexia nervosa, may be accompanied by a complete loss of LH pulsatile secretion (90). In fact, since adrenal androgen production also declines with starvation, serum testosterone levels in males with anorexia nervosa may

fall to levels usually observed in prepubertal boys. The nutritional signals that influence the neuroendocrine regulation of gonadal and adrenal androgens are a subject of active investigation.

There is evidence that leptin from fat tissue, which suppresses feeding behaviors, regulates neuroendocrine function (91). In many species, plasma leptin levels decline rapidly during caloric restriction and herald a decrease in gonadotropin production (92). Moreover, genetically obese ob/ob mice (lacking endogenous leptin) are infertile, and treatment of these animals with leptin stimulates the activity of the reproductive endocrine system and induces fertility (93). Similarly, treatment with leptin prevented the fasting-induced decline in LH pulse frequency in sheep (94). Leptin effects on both the pituitary and on GnRH neurons have now been reported, but the mechanism by which leptin may regulate gonadotropin secretion remains controversial. With decreased caloric intake, reduced leptin signaling activates neuropeptide Y (NPY) gene expression in the hypothalamic arcuate nucleus. Thus, leptin deficiency may suppress GnRH through an NPY-mediated mechanism. Orexins, recently discovered hypothalamic neuropeptides that stimulate feeding behavior, also suppress LH pulsatile secretion in rats. Hypoglycemic stress also suppresses pulsatile LH secretion in rodents.

Nutritional stress also increases CRF-ACTH mediated cortisol production. CRF, ACTH, and cortisol have each been implicated in stress-associated gonadotropin deficiency. Men with Cushing's syndrome are often hypogonadal (95), and prolonged glucocorticoid treatment of men with otherwise normal testicular function produces gonadotropin deficiency (96). Moreover, glucocorticoids suppress transcription of the mouse GnRH gene (97). Corticotropin-releasing hormone (CRH) also directly decreases GnRH mRNA. Testicular CRF negatively regulates LH action by inhibiting gonadotropin-induced cAMP generation and thereby decreases androgen production (98). CRH also increases IL-1 in Sertoli cells, and IL-1 inhibits Leydig cell steroidogenesis in vitro. In this way, testicular CRH may play a role in the decline in testosterone production that occurs with stress and inflammation.

β-endorphin is another product of the pro-opiomelanocortin gene, in addition to ACTH, that is increased with stress and is a likely regulator of the neuroendocrine reproductive system. This peptide has opiate-like bioactivity and inhibits GnRH secretion in experimental animals. In humans, endorphin antagonists increase pulsatile LH secretion (99). β-endorphin may also mediate CRF-induced gonadotropin deficiency.

PRL secretion also increases with stress. Studies using in situ hybridization techniques in rats with experimental hyperprolactinemia have demonstrated a reduction in GnRH mRNA levels per cell and a resulting decline in GnRH receptor concentration. In patients with PRL-producing pituitary tumors, pulsatile LH secretion is reduced (100) and is restored with pulsatile GnRH therapy (101).

The neuroendocrine regulation of testicular function is also altered by obesity. Low testosterone levels are common among obese men, partly because sex hormone binding globulin (SHBG) concentrations are reduced (102). Low levels of SHBG may result from hyperinsulinemia because insulin is known to suppress SHBG production in vitro (103), lowering circulating insulin levels with diazoxide increased plasma levels of SHBG (104); however, the inverse correlation between circulating insulin and SHBG is imperfect, implying that other factors related to insulin resistance in obesity could be important regulators of SHBG as well. Free and non-SHBG bound testosterone levels also decline with massive obesity. Because mean serum estrone and estradiol levels may be increased, one idea is that increased estrogen production from expression of aromatase in adipose tissue lowers testosterone production. A pituitary site of estradiol action is suggested because gonadotropin pulse amplitude is suppressed in obese men (105).

□ CONCLUSION

The proximate regulator of testicular function is GnRH produced in neurons scattered throughout the anterior hypothalamus. GnRH stimulates the synthesis and secretion of the pituitary gonadotropic hormones, LH and FSH. LH and FSH are released into the circulation in bursts and activate receptors on Leydig and Sertoli cells, respectively, in order to stimulate testosterone production and spermatogenesis. The system is tightly regulated and maintained at a proper set point by the negative feedback effects of testicular steroids and inhibin-B. Testicular function is also influenced by multiple internal and external environmental factors.

□ REFERENCES

1. Goldsmith PC, Thind KK, Song T, et al. Location of the neuroendocrine gonadotropin-releasing hormone neurons in the monkey hypothalamus by retrograde tracing and immunostaining. J Neuroendocrinol 1990; 2:157–168.

2. Kepa JK, Spaulding AJ, Jacobsen BM, et al. Structure of the distal human gonadotropin releasing hormone (hGnRH) gene promoter and functional analysis in Gt1-7 neuronal cells. Nucleic Acids Res 1996; 24(18): 3614–3620.

3. El Majdoubi M, Sahu A, Plant TM. Changes in hypothalamic gene expression associated with the arrest of pulsatile gonadotropin-releasing hormone release during infancy in the agonadal male rhesus monkey (Macaca mulatta). Endocrinology 2000; 141(9): 3273–3277.

4. Caraty A, Locatelli A. Effect of time after castration on secretion of LHRH and LH in the ram. J Reprod Fertil 1988; 82(1):263–269.

5. Knobil E. The electrophysiology of the GnRH pulse generator in the rhesus monkey. J Steroid Biochem 1989; 33(4B):669–671.

6. Krsmanovic LZ, Martinez-Fuentes AJ, Arora KK, et al. Local regulation of gonadotroph function by pituitary gonadotropin-releasing hormone. Endocrinology 2000; 141(3):1187–1195.

7. Urbanski HF, Kohama SG, Garyfallou VT. Mechanisms mediating the response of GnRH neurones to excitatory amino acids. Rev Reprod 1996; 1(3):173–181.

8. Neill JD, Duck LW, Sellers JC, et al. A gonadotropin-releasing hormone (GnRH) receptor specific for GnRH II in primates. Biochem Biophys Res Commun 2001; 282(4):1012–1018.

9. Childs GV. Division of labor among gonadotropes. Vitam Horm 1995; 50:215–286.

10. Stojilkovic SS, Reinhart J, Catt KJ. Gonadotropin-releasing hormone receptors: structure and signal transduction pathways. Endocr Rev 1994; 15(4): 462–499.

11. Shacham S, Harris D, Ben-Shlomo H, et al. Mechanism of GnRH receptor signaling on gonadotropin release and gene expression in pituitary gonadotrophs. Vitam Horm 2001; 63:63–90.

12. Conn PM, Janovick JA, Stanislaus D, et al. Molecular and cellular bases of gonadotropin-releasing hormone action in the pituitary and central nervous system. Vitam Horm 1995; 50:151–214.

13. Weck J, Anderson AC, Jenkins S, et al. Divergent and composite gonadotropin-releasing hormone-responsive elements in the rat luteinizing hormone subunit genes. Mol Endocrinol 2000; 14(4):472–485.

14. Haisenleder DJ, Yasin M, Marshall JC. Gonadotropin subunit and gonadotropin-releasing hormone receptor gene expression are regulated by alterations in the frequency of calcium pulsatile signals. Endocrinology 1997; 138(12):5227–5230.

15. Kaiser UB, Jakubowiak A, Steinberger A, et al. Regulation of rat pituitary gonadotropin-releasing hormone receptor mRNA levels in vivo and in vitro. Endocrinology 1993; 133(2):931–934.

16. Clayton RN, Catt KJ. Gonadotropin-releasing hormone receptors: characterization, physiological regulation, and relationship to reproductive function. Endocr Rev 1981; 2(2):186–209.

17. Kaiser UB, Halvorson LM, Chen MT. Sp1, steroidogenic factor 1 (SF-1), and early growth response protein 1 (egr-1) binding sites form a tripartite gonadotropin-releasing hormone response element in the rat luteinizing

hormone-beta gene promoter: an integral role for SF-1. Mol Endocrinol 2000; 14(8):1235–1245.

18. Strahl BD, Huang HJ, Sebastian J, et al. Transcriptional activation of the ovine follicle-stimulating hormone beta-subunit gene by gonadotropin-releasing hormone: involvement of two activating protein-1-binding sites and protein kinase C. Endocrinology 1998; 139(11): 4455–4465.

19. Maurer RA, Kim KE, Schoderbek WE, et al. Regulation of glycoprotein hormone alpha-subunit gene expression. Recent Prog Horm Res 1999; 54:455–484.

20. Chedrese PJ, Kay TW, Jameson JL. Gonadotropin-releasing hormone stimulates glycoprotein hormone alpha-subunit messenger ribonucleic acid (mRNA) levels in alpha T3 cells by increasing transcription and mRNA stability. Endocrinology 1994; 134(6):2475–2481.

21. Xing Y, Williams C, Campbell RK, et al. Threading of a glycosylated protein loop through a protein hole: implications for combination of human chorionic gonadotropin subunits. Protein Sci 2001; 10(2): 226–235.

22. Belchetz PE, Plant TM, Nakai Y, et al. Hypophysial responses to continuous and intermittent delivery of hypopthalamic gonadotropin-releasing hormone. Science 1978; 202(4368):631–633.

23. Nankin HR, Troen P. Repetitive luteinizing hormone elevations in serum of normal men. J Clin Endocrinol Metab 1971; 33(3):558–560.

24. Crowley WF Jr, McArthur JW. Simulation of the normal menstrual cycle in Kallman's syndrome by pulsatile administration of luteinizing hormone-releasing hormone (LHRH). J Clin Endocrinol Metab 1980; 51(1):173–175.

25. Labrie F. Endocrine therapy for prostate cancer. Endocrinol Metab Clin North Am 1991; 20(4): 845–872.

26. Padmanabhan V, McFadden K, Mauger DT, et al. Neuroendocrine control of follicle-stimulating hormone (FSH) secretion. I. Direct evidence for separate episodic and basal components of FSH secretion. Endocrinology 1997; 138(1):424–432.

27. Kawakami S, Winters SJ. Regulation of lutenizing hormone secretion and subunit messenger ribonucleic acid expression by gonadal steroids in perifused pituitary cells from male monkeys and rats. Endocrinology 1999; 140(8):3587–3593.

28. Veldhuis JD, Johnson M. Testing pulse detection algorithms with simulations of episodically pulsatile substrate, metabolite, or hormone release. Methods Enzymo 1994; 240:377–415.

29. Spratt DI, Carr DB, Merriam GR, et al. The spectrum of abnormal patterns of gonadotropin-releasing hormone secretion in men with idiopathic hypogonadotropic hypogonadism: clinical and laboratory correlations. J Clin Endocrinol Metab 1987; 64(2):283–291.

30. Winters SJ, Troen P. Pulsatile secretion of immunore-active alpha-subunit in man. J Clin Endocrinol Metab 1985; 60(2):344–348.

31. Boyar RM, Rosenfeld RS, Kapen S, et al. Human puberty. Simultaneous augmented secretion of lutein-izing hormone and testosterone during sleep. J Clin Invest 1974; 54(3):609–618.

32. Tenover JS, Matsumoto AM, Clifton DK, et al. Age-related alterations in the circadian rhythms of pulsatile luteinizing hormone and testosterone secretion in healthy men. J Gerontol 1988; 43(6): M163–M169.

33. Luboshitzky R, Zabari Z, Shen-Orr Z, et al. Disruption of the nocturnal testosterone rhythm by sleep fragmentation in normal men. J Clin Endocrinol Metab 2001; 86(3):1134–1139.

34. Bremner WJ, Vitiello MV, Prinz PN. Loss of circadian rhythmicity in blood testosterone levels with aging in normal men. J Clin Endocrinol Metab 1983; 56(6): 1278–1281.

35. Winters SJ. Diurnal rhythm of testosterone and luteinizing hormone in hypogonadal men. J Androl 1991; 12(3):185–190.

36. Payne AH, Youngblood GL. Regulation of expression of steroidogenic enzymes in Leydig cells. Biol Reprod 1995; 52(2):217–225.

37. Dufau ML. The luteinizing hormone receptor. Annu Rev Physiol 1998; 60(1):461–496.

38. Stocco DM. StAR protein and the regulation of steroid hormone biosynthesis. Annu Rev Physiol 2001; 63(1): 193–213.

39. Mannaerts B, de Leeuw R, Geelen J, et al. Comparative in vitro and in vivo studies on the biological characteristics of recombinant human follicle-stimulating hormone. Endocrinology 1991; 129(5):2623–2630.

40. Majumdar SS, Winters SJ, Plant TM. A study of the relative roles of follicle-stimulating hormone and luteinizing hormone in the regulation of testicular inhibin secretion in the rhesus monkey (Macaca mulatta). Endocrinology 1997; 138(4):1363–1373.

41. Vierhapper H, Nowotny P, Waldhausl W. Production rates of testosterone in patients with Cushing's syndrome. Metab: Clin Exp 2000; 49(2):229–231.

42. Jones ME, Simpson ER. Oestrogens in male reproduction. Baillieres Best Pract Res Clin Endocrinol Metab 2000; 14(3):505–516.

43. Brodie A, Inkster S, Yue W. Aromatase expression in the human male. Mol Cell Endocrinol 2001; 178(1–2):23–28.

44. O'Donnell L, Robertson KM, Jones ME, et al. Estrogen and spermatogenesis. Endocri Rev 2001; 22(3):289–318.

45. Couse JF, Curtis Hewitt S, Korach KS. Receptor null mice reveal contrasting roles for estrogen receptor alpha and beta in reproductive tissues. J Steroid Biochem Mol Biol 2000; 74(5):287–296.

46. Couse JF, Lindzey J, Grandien K, et al. Tissue distribution and quantitative analysis of estrogen receptor—alpha (ERalpha) and estrogen receptor-beta (ERbeta) messenger ribonucleic acid in the wild-type and ERalpha-knockout mouse. Endocrinology 1997; 138(11):4613–4621.

47. Grumbach MM, Auchus RJ. Estrogen: consequences and implications of human mutations in synthesis and action. J Clin Endocrinol Metab 1999; 84(12):4677–4694.

48. Robertson KM, O'Donnell L, Jones ME, et al. Impairment of spermatogenesis in mice lacking a functional aromatase (cyp 19) gene. Proc Natl Acad Sci USA 1999; 96(14):7986–7991.

49. Plant TM. Effects of orchidectomy and testosterone replacement treatment on pulsatile luteinizing hormone secretion in the adult rhesus monkey (Macaca mulatta). Endocrinology 1982; 110(6):1905–1913.

50. Winters SJ, Troen P. A reexamination of pulsatile luteinizing hormone secretion in primary testicular failure. J Clin Endocrinol Metab 1983; 57(2):432–435.

51. Winters SJ, Kawakami S, Sahu A, et al. Pituitary follistatin and activin gene expression, and the testicular regulation of FSH in the adult Rhesus monkey (Macaca mulatta). Endocrinology 2001; 142(7):2874–2878.

52. Finkelstein JS, Whitcomb RW, O'Dea LS, et al. Sex steroid control of gonadotropin secretion in the human male. I. Effects of testosterone administration in normal and gonadotropin-releasing hormone-deficient men. J Clin Endocrinol Metab 1991; 73(3):609–620.

53. Plant TM, Dubey AK. Evidence from the rhesus monkey (Macaca mulatta) for the view that negative feedback control of luteinizing hormone secretion by the testis is mediated by a deceleration of hypothalamic gonadotropin- releasing hormone pulse frequency. Endocrinology 1984; 115(6):2145–2153.

54. Naftolin F, Pujol-Amat P, Corker CS, et al. Gonadotropins and gonadal steroids in androgen insensitivity (testicular feminization) syndrome: effects of castration and sex steroid administration. Am J Obstet Gynecol 1983; 147(5):491–496.

55. Winters SJ, Troen P. Evidence for a role of endogenous estrogen in the hypothalamic control of gonadotropin secretion in men. J Clin Endocrinol Metab 1985; 61(5):842–845.

56. Marynick SP, Loriaux DL, Sherins RJ, et al. Evidence that testosterone can suppress pituitary gonadotropin secretion independently of peripheral aromatization. J Clin Endocrinol Metab 1979; 49(3):396–398.

57. Smith EP, Boyd J, Frank GR, et al. Estrogen resistance caused by a mutation in the estrogen-receptor gene in a man. N Engl J Med 1994; 331(16):1056–1061.

58. Morishima A, Grumbach MM, Simpson ER, et al. Aromatase deficiency in male and female siblings caused by a novel mutation and the physiological role of estrogens. J Clin Endocrinol Metab 1995; 80(12):3689–3698.

59. Carani C, Qin K, Simoni M, et al. Effect of testosterone and estradiol in a man with aromatase deficiency. N Engl J Med 1997; 337(2):91–95.

60. Hayes FJ, Seminara SB, Decruz S, et al. Aromatase inhibition in the human male reveals a hypothalamic site of estrogen feedback. J Clin Endocrinol Metab 2000; 85(9):3027–3035.

61. Santen RJ, Bardin CW. Episodic luteinizing hormone secretion in man. Pulse analysis, clinical interpretation, physiologic mechanisms. J Clin Invest 1973; 52(10):2617–2628.

62. Mather JP, Moore A, Li RH. Activins, inhibins, and follistatins: further thoughts on a growing family of regulators. Proc Soc Exp Biol Med 1997; 215(3): 209–222.

63. Pangas SA, Woodruff TK. Activin signal transduction pathways. Trends Endocrinol Metab 2000; 11(8): 309–314.

64. DePaolo LV. Inhibins, activins, and follistatins: the saga continues. Proc Soc Exp Biol Med 1997; 214(4): 328–339.

65. Lewis KA, Gray PC, Blount AL, et al. Betaglycan binds inhibin and can mediate functional antagonism of activin signalling. Nature 2000; 404(6776):411–414.

66. Kaiser UB, Chin WW. Regulation of follistatin messenger ribonucleic acid levels in the rat pituitary. J Clin Invest 1993; 91(6):2523–2531.

67. Burger HG, Robertson DM. Editorial: inhibin in the male—progress at last. Endocrinology 1997; 138(4):1361–1362.

68. Krummen LA, Toppari J, Kim WH, et al. Regulation of testicular inhibin subunit messenger ribonucleic acid levels in vivo: effects of hypophysectomy and selective follicle-stimulating hormone replacement. Endocrinology 1989; 125(3):1630–1637.

69. Feng ZM, Wu AZ, Zhang Z, et al. GATA-1 and GATA-4 transactivate inhibin/activin beta-B-subunit gene transcription in testicular cells. Mol Endocrinol 2000; 14(11):1820–1835.

70. Wallace EM, Groome NP, Riley SC, et al. Effects of chemotherapy-induced testicular damage on inhibin, gonadotropin, and testosterone secretion: a prospective longitudinal study. J Clin Endocrinol Metab 1997; 82(9):3111–3115.

71. Carroll RS, Corrigan AZ, Gharib SD, et al. Inhibin, activin, and follistatin: regulation of follicle-stimulating hormone messenger ribonucleic acid levels. Mol Endocrinol 1989; 3(12):1969–1976.

72. Ramaswamy S, Marshall GR, McNeilly AS, et al. Dynamics of the follicle-stimulating hormone (FSH)-inhibin B feedback loop and its role in regulating spermatogenesis in the adult male rhesus monkey (Macaca mulatta) as revealed by unilateral orchidectomy. Endocrinology 2000; 141(1):18–27.

73. Anawalt BD, Bebb RA, Matsumoto AM, et al. Serum inhibin B levels reflect Sertoli cell function in normal men and men with testicular dysfunction. J Clin Endocrinol Metab 1996; 81(9):3341–3345.

74. Ramaswamy S, Marshall GR, McNeilly AS, et al. Evidence that in a physiological setting Sertoli cell number is the major determinant of circulating concentrations of inhibin B in the adult male rhesus monkey (Macaca mulatta). J Androl 1999; 20(3):430–434.

75. Simoni M, Gromoll J, Nieschlag E. The follicle-stimulating hormone receptor: biochemistry, molecular biology, physiology, and pathophysiology. Endocr Rev 1997; 18(6):739–773.

76. Tapanainen JS, Vaskivuo T, Aittomaki K, et al. Inactivating FSH receptor mutations and gonadal dysfunction. Mol Cell Endocrinol 1998; 145(1–2):129–135.

77. Kumar TR, Wang Y, Lu N, et al. Follicle stimulating hormone is required for ovarian follicle maturation but not male fertility. Nat Genet 1997; 15(2):201–204.

78. Kirk SE, Dalkin AC, Yasin M, et al. Gonadotropin-releasing hormone pulse frequency regulates expression

of pituitary follistatin messenger ribonucleic acid: a mechanism for differential gonadotrope function. Endocrinology 1994; 135(3):876–880.

79. Besecke LM, Guendner MJ, Schneyer AL, et al. Gonadotropin-releasing hormone regulates follicle-stimulating hormone- beta gene expression through an activin/follistatin autocrine or paracrine loop. Endocrinology 1996; 137(9):3667–3673.

80. Spratt DI, Finkelstein JS, Butler JP, et al. Effects of increasing the frequency of low doses of gonadotropin- releasing hormone (GnRH) on gonadotropin secretion in GnRH-deficient men. J Clin Endocrinol Metab 1987; 64(6):1179–1186.

81. Gross KM, Matsumoto AM, Berger RE, et al. Increased frequency of pulsatile luteinizing hormone-releasing hormone administration selectively decreases follicle-stimulating hormone levels in men with idiopathic azoospermia. Fertil Steril 1986; 45(3):392–396.

82. Tsujii T, Ishizaka K, Winters SJ. Effects of pituitary adenylate cyclase-activating polypeptide on gonadotropin secretion and subunit messenger ribonucleic acids in perifused rat pituitary cells. Endocrinology 1994; 135(3):826–833.

83. Kaiser UB, Sabbagh E, Katzenellenbogen RA, et al. A mechanism for the differential regulation of gonadotropin subunit gene expression by gonadotropin-releasing hormone. Proc Natl Acad Sci USA 1995; 92(26):12280–12284.

84. Waldstreicher J, Seminara SB, Jameson JL, et al. The genetic and clinical heterogeneity of gonadotropin-releasing hormone deficiency in the human. J Clin Endocrinol Metab 1996; 81(12):4388–4395.

85. Boyar RM, Wu RH, Kapen S, et al. Clinical and laboratory heterogeneity in idiopathic hypogonadotropic hypogonadism. J Clin Endocrinol Metab 1976; 43(6):1268–1275.

86. Seminara SB, Hayes FJ, Crowley WF Jr. Gonadotropin-releasing hormone deficiency in the human (idiopathic hypogonadotropic hypogonadism and Kallmann's syndrome): pathophysiological and genetic considerations. Endocr Rev 1998; 19(5):521–539.

87. Habiby RL, Boepple P, Nachtigall L, et al. Adrenal hypoplasia congenita with hypogonadotropic hypogonadism: evidence that DAX-1 mutations lead to combined hypothalmic and pituitary defects in gonadotropin production. J Clin Invest 1996; 98(4):1055–1062.

88. Nachtigall LB, Boepple PA, Pralong FP, et al. Adult-onset idiopathic hypogonadotropic hypogonadism—a treatable form of male infertility. N Engl J Med 1997; 336(6):410–415.

89. Cameron JL, Weltzin TE, McConaha C, et al. Slowing of pulsatile luteinizing hormone secretion in men after forty-eight hours of fasting. J Clin Endocrinol Metab 1991; 73(1):35–41.

90. Tomova A, Kumanov P. Sex differences and similarities of hormonal alterations in patients with anorexia nervosa. Andrologia 1999; 31(3):143–147.

91. Ahima RS, Saper CB, Flier JS, et al. Leptin regulation of neuroendocrine systems. Front Neuroendocrinol 2000; 21(3):263–307.

92. Kopp W, Blum WF, von Prittwitz S, et al. Low leptin levels predict amenorrhea in underweight and eating disordered females. Mol Psychiatry 1997; 2(4):335–340.

93. Barash IA, Cheung CC, Weigle DS, et al. Leptin is a metabolic signal to the reproductive system. Endocrinology 1996; 137(7):3144–3147.

94. Nagatani S, Zeng Y, Keisler DH, et al. Leptin regulates pulsatile luteinizing hormone and growth hormone secretion in the sheep. Endocrinology 2000; 141(11):3965–3975.

95. Luton JP, Thieblot P, Valcke JC, et al. Reversible gonadotropin deficiency in male Cushing's disease. J Clin Endocrinol Metab 1977; 45(3):488–495.

96. MacAdams MR, White RH, Chipps BE. Reduction of serum testosterone levels during chronic glucocorticoid therapy. Ann Intern Med 1986; 104(5):648–651.

97. Chandran UR, Attardi B, Friedman R, et al. Glucocorticoid repression of the mouse gonadotropin-releasing hormone gene is mediated by promoter elements that are recognized by heteromeric complexes containing glucocorticoid receptor. J Biol Chem 1996; 271(34):20412–20420.

98. Dufau ML, Tinajero JC, Fabbri A. Corticotropin-releasing factor: an antireproductive hormone of the testis. Faseb J 1993; 7(2):299–307.

99. Veldhuis JD, Rogol AD, Johnson ML. Endogenous opiates modulate the pulsatile secretion of biologically active luteinizing hormone in man. J Clin Invest 1983; 72(6):2031–2040.

100. Winters SJ, Troen P. Altered pulsatile secretion of luteinizing hormone in hypogonadal men with hyperprolactinaemia. Clin Endocrinol (Oxf) 1984; 21(3):257–263.

101. Bouchard P, Lagoguey M, Brailly S, et al. Gonadotropin-releasing hormone pulsatile administration restores luteinizing hormone pulsatility and normal testosterone levels in males with hyperprolactinemia. J Clin Endocrinol Metab 1985; 60(2):258–262.

102. Glass AR, Burman KD, Dahms WT, et al. Endocrine function in human obesity. Metabolism 1981; 30(1): 89–104.

103. Plymate SR, Matej LA, Jones RE, et al. Inhibition of sex hormone-binding globulin production in the human hepatoma (Hep G2) cell line by insulin and prolactin. J Clin Endocrinol Metab 1988; 67(3):460–464.

104. Nestler JE, Barlascini CO, Matt DW, et al. Suppression of serum insulin by diazoxide reduces serum testosterone levels in obese women with polycystic ovary syndrome. J Clin Endocrinol Metab 1989; 68(6):1027–1032.

105. Vermeulen A, Kaufman JM, Deslypere JP, et al. Attenuated luteinizing hormone (LH) pulse amplitude but normal LH pulse frequency, and its relation to plasma androgens in hypogonadism of obese men. J Clin Endocrinol Metab 1993; 76(5):1140–1146.

4

Analysis of the Neuroendocrine Control of the Human Hypothalamo–Pituitary–Testicular Axis

Johannes D. Veldhuis
Endocrine Research Unit, Mayo Clinic College of Medicine, Rochester, Minnesota, U.S.A.

Daniel M. Keenan
Department of Statistics, University of Virginia, Charlottesville, Virginia, U.S.A.

□ INTRODUCTION

The appraisal of hypothalamo–pituitary–gonadal dynamics in men requires the assessment of the stimulation of luteinizing hormone (LH) secretion by gonadotropin-releasing hormone (GnRH), negative feedback on GnRH and LH output by testosterone (Te), and feedforward by LH on androgen biosynthesis. Quantitations of LH and Te time series, both separately and jointly, provide a window to these interactions. For example, analyses in aging men have disclosed a loss of normal orderliness of the LH-release process, erosion of LH pulse amplitude, accelerated LH peak frequency, and disruption of LH–Te coupling in the face of normal mean serum LH and total Te concentrations. Continuing developments should allow estimates of in vivo dose–response interfaces that link GnRH, LH, and Te and eventual prediction of the unobserved behavior of hypothalamic GnRH secretion.

□ OVERVIEW

Beyond the gametogenic component of the male reproductive axis, androgen secretion in the adult is driven by an ensemble of approximately 800 to 1200 hypothalamic GnRH neurons (and their multiple regulatory inputs), the LH-secreting gonadotrope-cell population in the anterior pituitary gland, and lutropin-responsive gonadal Leydig cells (1–4). The multisite nature of the GnRH–LH–Te feedforward and feedback axes has motivated more formalized biomathematical constructs of this dynamic system (5–9). The clinical application of such an integrative perspective will be illustrated here by analyses of LH and androgen secretion in the aging male, in whom a progressive reduction in Te bioavailability is mediated by an array of nonexclusive factors.

□ CLINICAL RESEARCH TOOLS
Monohormonal Secretory Disruption in the Aging Male

Multiple clinical research tools have become available in the last two decades to evaluate monohormonal secretion both objectively and reproducibly in health and disease; viz., high-frequency and extended blood-sampling paradigms to capture the full spectrum of LH and Te secretory activity (1,10–15); precise, sensitive, specific, and reliable automated assays of LH and Te (15–19); objective "discrete peak-detection" methods and deconvolution-based techniques to quantitate pulsatile hormone secretion (20–28); the approximate entropy (ApEn) (regularity) statistic to monitor the orderliness of feedback-dependent secretory patterns (29–32); validation of a selective steroidogenic inhibitor to induce reversible hypoandrogenemia and unleash endogenous GnRH/LH drive (33,34); pulsatile i.v. infusions of GnRH to impose a "hypothalamic GnRH clamp" (35–38); and measurements of selected other pituitary glycoproteins, such as free alpha–subunit (39,40), biologically active LH (41–45), and chromato-focused LH isoforms (46–48). The foregoing approaches have unveiled the subtle pathophysiology of the male gonadal axis in the absence of overt hypothalamic, pituitary, or gonadal failure.

Frequent and Extended Blood-Sampling Protocols

The GnRH–LH functional unit operates physiologically under intermittent, rather than continuous, hypothalamic drive (2,4,49,50). Thus, to the extent that endogenous GnRH–LH coupling is preserved, appraisal of pulsatile LH release provides a window to monitor episodic hypothalamic GnRH secretion indirectly (15,51). Clinical studies affirm that sampling blood at 5- or 10-minute intervals for 12 to 24 hours will capture the majority of detectable LH-secretory peaks in healthy

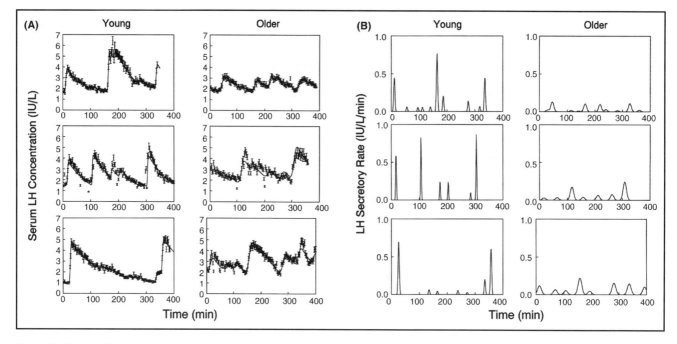

Figure 1 Serum LH concentration profiles in three young and three older men sampled at 2.5-minute intervals during the hours of sleep. The continuous lines are predicted by deconvolution analysis. Older individuals manifest more irregular, frequent, and low-amplitude LH-secretory pulses. *Abbreviation*: LH, luteinizing hormone. *Source*: From Ref. 57.

men (1,10–15,21). Intensive sampling methods have documented consistent blunting of high-amplitude pulsatile LH-secretion in healthy older men (3,17, 37,38,52–56). The erosion of large LH pulses in aging has been corroborated by sampling blood every 2.5 minutes overnight and by high-precision immunoradiometric assay and ultrasensitive chemiluminescence-based LH assays (Fig 1A, 1B) (31,52,53). The aged male Brown Norway rat also exhibits consistent loss of LH pulse height (58,59).

Impoverishment of high-amplitude LH-secretory pulses in the (aging) male could denote: (*i*) diminished hypothalamic GnRH drive; (*ii*) heightened negative-feedback restraint by androgens of GnRH and/or LH secretion; and/or (*iii*) reduced gonadotrope-cell responsiveness to physiological amounts of GnRH. To address the last consideration, recent clinical studies have implemented randomly ordered, prospective and separate-day acute i.v. GnRH dose–response analyses of LH secretion in young and older volunteers (40,60). Deconvolution analyses of GnRH-stimulated LH release have revealed equivalent (or amplified) maximal LH-secretory rates in older individuals, thus defining normal or augmented GnRH efficacy (40). Minimally stimulatory doses of GnRH were more effective in aging men, thus pointing to increased GnRH *potency* (heightened pituitary sensitivity to GnRH) (60). Preserved pituitary responsiveness to GnRH would exclude primary gonadotrope-cell failure in older men (61) and favor hypotheses of reduced hypothalamic GnRH feedforward of gonadotropes and/or heightened androgen–negative-feedback restraint of LH pulse amplitude (3). Extending the foregoing GnRH stimulation experiment to a two-week

paradigm of 90-minute i.v. pulsatile GnRH infusions established full pituitary responsiveness to short-term GnRH drive in older men (52).

Although not evident using a 20-minute sampling schedule (62), analyses based on 2.5- or 10-minute blood-sampling paradigms have disclosed an accelerated frequency of low-amplitude LH pulses in older men (3,18,37,38,53). Blunting of LH peak amplitudes also prevails in the aged male rat (58,63). A higher mean LH pulse frequency in the aging male could reflect a secondary rise in hypothalamic GnRH pulse-generator activity in the face of reduced feedback by lower bioavailable Te concentrations (2,18,53). The notion of normal androgenic repression of GnRH pulse frequency is supported by two experimental paradigms in young men: (*i*) administration of androgenic steroids suppresses LH pulse frequency (and reciprocally elevates LH pulse amplitude) (2,16,61,64–68); (*ii*) conversely, short-term androgen-receptor blockade with a nonsteroidal antiandrogen (flutamide) accelerates LH pulse frequency (69,70). Accordingly, a higher frequency of low-amplitude LH pulses in the aging male may result from (*i*) a primary reduction in the amount of GnRH secreted per pulse, or (*ii*) a secondary rise in GnRH pulse frequency due to reduced bioavailable-androgen feedback. This bipartite thesis does not exclude age-related simultaneous failure of GnRH secretion and Leydig-cell steroidogenesis (see below) (2,3,18,37,38,53,55,61,71–74).

Luteinizing Hormone Assays

Quantitation of serum LH concentrations requires a valid, reliable, specific, sensitive, and precise assay

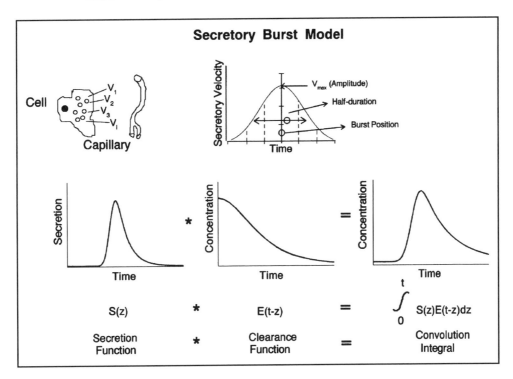

Figure 2 Schema illustrating the technique of deconvolution analysis applied to serum LH concentration profiles. Deconvolution analysis reconstructs underlying rates of basal and pulsatile neurohormone release. A secretory burst is defined by its position in time, maximum value (amplitude), and half-duration (duration at half-maximal amplitude) or skewness. The half-life is estimated simultaneously, since secretion rates and kinetics jointly specify the observed hormone concentration profile. Data represent immunoradiometric assay of serial (10 minutes) serum LH concentrations in young and older men. *Abbreviation*: LH, luteinizing hormone. *Source*: From Refs. 13, 23, 25–27.

with statistics-based data reduction. Recent immuno-radiometric (16,17,75) and immunofluorometric (15,18) methods achieve these requirements, and often correlate well with in vitro LH bioassays (39,41,45,46,76). For example, fluorescence- and chemiluminescence-based LH assays achieve 30- to 100-fold greater sensitivity than earlier radioimmuno assays (77), and thereby document a 30-fold rise in LH pulse height (or mass) in pubertal boys (17,78). For high assay precision, one should use a fully automated (robotics) procedure, and for statistical analysis, on-line model-free data reduction (79–81). To verify LH assay validity, one might apply a heterologous (e.g., rodent) in vitro Leydig cell bioassay of LH action (39,41,46), or a homologous recombinant human (rh) LH recep-tor–transfected human fetal kidney (cell line 293) cell bioassay (82).

Enumerating Serum LH Concentration Peaks and Quantitating Underlying LH-Secretory Bursts

Various computer-assisted discrete peak–detection technologies are available to identify peaks objectively in appropriately sampled and assayed serum LH concentration time series (1,14,20,67,83,84). Such meth-odologies are important for estimating putative GnRH pulsatility indirectly, assuming the presence of res-ponsive pituitary gonadotropes. One such (model-free) peak-detection technique is cluster analysis (20). This procedure identifies diminished LH peak amplitude

and increased LH peak frequency in the healthy aging male (52).

Observed serum LH concentration profiles are generated jointly by underlying LH secretion and hormone-specific kinetics, namely: (*i*) the amount (mass) of LH secreted within each pulse; (*ii*) the distri-bution volume and half-life of LH; (*iii*) any concurrent basal (or nonpulsatile) LH secretion; and (*iv*) earlier hormone secretion that still continues to decay (22–27). "Deconvolution analysis" provides a means to quan-titate the foregoing combined secretory and kinetic contributions to a hormone pulse profile (1,23,25,27), as illustrated in Figure 2.

Two complementary classes of deconvolution techniques exist: model-specific and waveform-inde-pendent methods (1,3,13,14,22–27,85–93). Like cluster analysis, both types of deconvolution procedures doc-ument a lower amplitude of pulsatile LH secretion in older men (3,18,53). Indeed, a third-generation decon-volution approach—using a random-effects model of basal LH secretion admixed with variable pulsatile LH-release episodes—also predicts suppressed LH-secretory pulse amplitude and increased LH-secretory burst frequency in older men (5,6,8,9).

Entropy or Orderliness of LH-Release Patterns

In addition to pulsatile secretion, the degree of regular-ity of subpatterns in the data characterizes moment-to-moment LH secretion (29,31,32,94). Orderliness of the

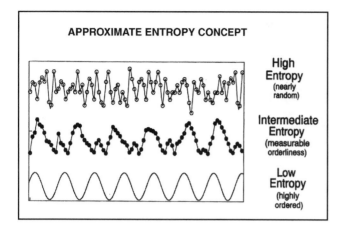

APPROXIMATE ENTROPY CONCEPT

High Entropy (nearly random)

Intermediate Entropy (measurable orderliness)

Low Entropy (highly ordered)

Figure 3 Concept of the ApEn statistic to quantify the relative orderliness of neurohormone time series. The three curves represent a simple cosine waveform (*bottom*), which denotes low ApEn or well-ordered patterns; less-regular serial data (*middle*); and an irregular (higher ApEn) profile (*top*). Aging is accompanied by consistently more disorderly LH and testosterone secretion as quantitated by higher ApEn (Fig. 4). *Abbreviation*: ApEn, approximate entropy.

hypothalamo–pituitary basis underlying putatively hypogonadotropic states; for example, aging, hyperprolactinemia, anorexia nervosa, Kallmann's syndrome, fasting-induced hypogonadism in men, etc. (37,40, 52,73,108–110). For example, pulsatile i.v. infusion of GnRH versus saline every 90 minutes for two weeks was imposed in a prospective, randomly ordered,

sample-by-sample hormone release process can be quantitated via the ApEn statistic (Fig. 3). ApEn represents a single number calculated for any given time series, which provides a sensitive barometer of irregularity due to feedback alterations within the interactive network (see below) (29–32,94–96). For example, the ApEn metric quantitates highly irregular tumoral production of adrenocorticotropic hormone (ACTH), growth hormone (GH), aldosterone, and prolactin (29,30,97–100); discriminates more disorderly GH release in the female than in the male (101); and quantitates more subtly variable ACTH, GH, and insulin secretion in aging men and women (102–105). ApEn calculations likewise disclose greater disorderliness of LH and Te release in the older male (Fig. 4A, upper) (3,31,52,96).

As an extension of the concept of ApEn for a single time series, cross-ApEn is used to assess the degree of coordinate or synchronous secretion of two hormones (Fig. 4A, lower). Cross-ApEn of paired LH- and Te-release profiles is elevated in aging men, denoting the disruption of within-axis bihormonal synchrony (31,52,106). The establishment of the precise locus (or loci) that drive(s) this disruption requires additional pertinent "localizing" experiments. For example, older men also manifest higher cross-ApEn of LH–prolactin, LH–follicle-stimulating hormone (FSH), LH–NPH, LH–sleep, and nocturnal penile tumescence (NPT)–sleep linkages (Fig. 4B) (107). This collection of two-variable asynchrony suggests a central nervous system (CNS) contribution to altered neurohormone outflow in the aging male.

GnRH "Clamp" Studies

The availability of GnRH as a synthetic decapeptide for clinical use has allowed clinical testing of the

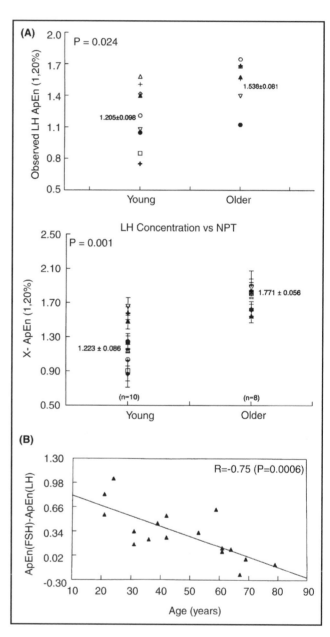

Figure 4 (**A**) Increased ApEn (1.20%) of overnight (2.5-minute sampled) serum LH concentration profiles in older men compared with young men. Higher ApEn denotes more disorderly gonadotropin outflow (*upper panel*). Elevated cross-ApEn of LH release and nocturnal penile tumescence oscillations in older men define loss of synchrony in aging (*lower panel*). (**B**) Erosion of the young-adult difference between FSH and LH ApEn with increasing age in men. The decline in bihormonal ApEn differences signifies uncoupling of the coordinate release of LH and FSH in older individuals. *Abbreviations*: ApEn, approximate entropy; FSH, follicle-stimulating hormone; LH, luteinizing hormone.

cross-over study to test putative gonadotrope failure in aging men (52). On day 14 of the saline (control) infusion, older men exhibited low-amplitude and high-frequency LH pulsatility with high ApEn, denoting more irregular LH release. Controlled pulsatile GnRH drive normalized pulsatile and entropic features of LH release in older men to values indistinguishable from those attained in identically infused younger individuals (52). GnRH-stimulated LH secretion, however, failed to increase Te output in older men, thus pointing to defective Leydig cell steroidogenesis and/or reduced biological activity of LH in aging. The latter hypothesis was not affirmed, since mean plasma LH concentrations assessed by in vitro Leydig cell bioassay were comparable in the two age cohorts (52). Thus, an exogenous GnRH "rescue" paradigm may be useful to unmask (i) reduced hypothalamic GnRH output, if sustained pulsatile i.v. GnRH infusions normalize low-amplitude pulsatile LH secretion; and (ii) impaired Leydig cell steroidogenic responsiveness to endogenous LH stimulation, if Te production fails to rise normally in the face of induced LH secretion (52).

Free Alpha-Subunit Measures

At high LH pulse frequencies (e.g., secretory bursts occurring every 45 to 60 minutes), conventional discrete-peak detection becomes more difficult analytically (1,14,22). In this situation, one might also measure free alpha-subunit levels, since this glycoprotein has a shorter half-life than that of intact LH (39,40,111–113). More rapid kinetics favor peak identification (13,22,25–27). Alpha-subunit measurements are not always necessary, since detection of LH-secretory bursts by deconvolution analysis is validated at higher event frequencies (15,23).

Ketoconazole-Induced Steroidogenic Blockade to Achieve Short-Term Androgen Deprivation

Reversible inhibition of adrenal and gonadal steroidogenesis with ketoconazole (KTCZ) provides a clinical test of hypothalamo–pituitary responsiveness to acute withdrawal of androgenic negative feedback (33,34, 106,114,115). Earlier studies in healthy young men showed that this antifungal drug can inhibit Te production by approximately 80% for periods of several days with attendant doubling or tripling of LH secretion (33,34,106,114,116,117). KTCZ blocks cytochrome P450–containing enzymes (116,118). At higher doses, this steroidogenic inhibitor lowers mean 24-hour serum Te concentrations below 100 ng/dL and effectively stimulates LH secretion (33,34). The latter patterns become more irregular (as monitored by higher ApEn values) and exhibit a higher mean pulse frequency, as ascertained by technically independent means (33,34). The specificity of Te as the steroidal feedback signal blocked by KTCZ has been affirmed by showing that i.v. infusion of androgen promptly normalizes the foregoing features of hypergonadotropism (34).

Pulsatile I.V. Infusions of rh LH During Inhibition of GnRH Action

Pulsatile i.v. infusions of rh LH will stimulate Te secretion within 20 to 40 minutes in leuprolide-suppressed young and older men (119). Older men show a 30% to 50% impairment in this response. In this paradigm, however, injected LH pulses do not normalize total serum Te concentrations even in young men. Incomplete responsiveness of the GnRH agonist–downregulated testis probably reflects withdrawal of the trophic actions of LH on sterol-transport protein, low-density lipoprotein receptor, and steroidogenic-enzyme gene expression, since GnRH agonists exert little, if any, direct inhibitory effects on the human (unlike the rodent) testis (1,2,120). In contrast, full gonadal responsiveness to LH pulses is maintained following acute injection of a pure GnRH antagonist, which suppresses LH and Te secretion within two to six hours (Fig. 5) (39,121–124).

GnRH–LH–Te Network Feedback Principles

Neuroendocrine systems comprise specialized arrays of discrete neural structures and corresponding glands, which communicate via intermittent blood-borne chemical signals (1,3,5,9,36,126). A hallmark of such dynamic autoregulatory systems is the operation of relevant neuroglandular interfaces; for example, hypothalamic (brain) signals impact pituitary (somatic) cells. Secreted pituitary hormones in turn activate downstream glandular loci, which release peripherally acting effector molecules. The latter typically feedback to the brain and/or pituitary gland to repress secretion. This concept of a classical "closed-loop" model is highlighted in Figure 6 for the male reproductive axis (2). The three pivotal regulatory nodes in this case include an ensemble of upper-brainstem electrically coupled GnRH-secreting neurons, specialized anterior-pituitary gonadotrope cells that synthesize and release LH, and testicular Leydig cells that secrete Te (4,9,49,127–129).

The GnRH–LH–Te network is driven by joint feedforward and feedback interfaces (1–3). In vitro data indicate that interface behavior can be approximated algebraically by nonlinear monotonic (logistic-like) functions (3,5,8,9,45,130,131). The foregoing multiply-coupled interactions and their time delays give rise to the dynamic output of GnRH, LH, and Te. Thus, analyzing any one component of the axis in isolation would fail to explain complete system behavior (5,9). Moreover, whereas GnRH release is not quantifiable in the human, a correct formulation of the foregoing dynamics should allow the reconstruction of unobserved GnRH signals based on simultaneously observed LH and Te secretion. In addition, an appropriately defined interactive model should ultimately permit estimation of in vivo neuroglandular interface (dose–response) functions (Table 1).

Viewed broadly from a neuroendocrine perspective, analytically tractable network models (above)

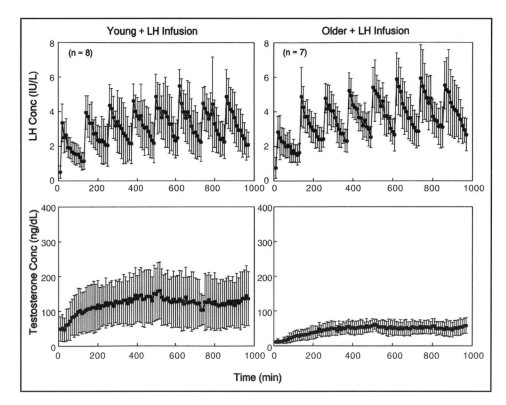

Figure 5 Recurrent intravenous infusions of recombinant human LH every two hours as six-minute square-wave pulses in eight young men (*left*) and seven older men (*right*) following leuprolide-induced downregulation of endogenous LH secretion. Data are serum LH and testosterone concentrations (mean ± SEM) obtained by sampling blood every 10 minutes for 16 hours. LH injections began after the first blood sample was withdrawn. *Abbreviation*: LH, luteinizing hormone. *Source*: From Ref. 125.

have several important biomedical implications in aging research. Firstly, establishing the essential interactive elements and the corresponding time delays of the relevant GnRH–LH–Te becomes an evolving process, which is subject to revision as knowledge grows. Secondly, a formalized construct of an intuitively complex system has utility in testing the

Table 1 Primary Goals of Neuroendocrine Modeling of Male Reproductive Axis

Infer behavior of unobserved signals (e.g., GnRH)
Estimate in vivo dose–response (interface) behavior (e.g., luteinizing hormone's feedforward on testosterone)
Assess system reaction to a particular parameter change (e.g., muted or enhanced feedback of testosterone on GnRH)
Revise concept of network based on emergent experimental data
Explicate clinical pathophysiology, species differences, or drug effects
Design parsimonious interventional experiments

Abbreviation: GnRH, gonadotropin-releasing hormone.

feasibility of clinical inferences. Thirdly, such formalism allows a priori predictions of interventional effects on the biological network. Lastly, a robust model formulation should guide more parsimonious planning of higher-yield experiments from a larger repertoire of intuitive choices, thereby potentially limiting cost, animal resources, and time expenditures (5,8,9,130).

Core Model Structure: Deterministic Interfaces, Time Delays, Stochastic Elements, Hormone Secretion, and Elimination
Deterministic Interfaces

Deterministic features of biological processes are critical in maintaining long-term system homeostasis. Here, deterministic denotes stable and generally reproducible input/output or cause-and-effect relationships. For example, extensive in vitro and in vivo

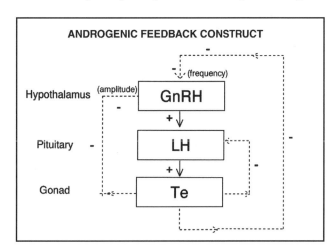

Figure 6 Schematized construct of the normal male hypothalamo–pituitary–gonadal axis. *Arrows* mark feedforward (+) or feedback (−) connections driven by corresponding interface (dose–response) functions. Leydig-cell Te feeds back to repress pituitary LH production and to inhibit both the amplitude and the frequency of hypothalamic GnRH pulsatility. *Abbreviations*: GnRH, gonadotropin-releasing hormone; LH, luteinizing hormone; Te, testosterone. *Source*: From Ref. 96.

animal experiments establish that sequential signaling by the hypothalamic peptide, GnRH, and the pituitary glycoprotein hormone, LH, drives secretion of Te. The latter occurs via monotonic receptor–dependent and target-cell specific responses to the lutropic stimulus (1–3,45,132–140). The implicit relationship between the (time-integrated) input signal and the secretory response can be approximated algebraically via a simple four-parameter logistic-like function; for example, as used in assay data–reduction software (3,5,8,9). For example, the latter algebraic form encapsulates the feedforward action of LH on Te secretion and the feedback of Te on GnRH release at the hypothalamic level (Fig. 7). This concept is extended for the trivariate GnRH/LH–Te interaction at the pituitary level to incorporate concurrent GnRH feedforward and Te feedback on LH, yielding a GnRH/LH–Te response surface (Fig. 7).

Time Delays

Interface functions within the interconnected GnRH–LH–Te axis operate after a relevant time delay, reflecting latencies inherent in the circulatory and cellular delivery of the effector hormone and unfolding of the

target-tissue response. The exact magnitude of such input–output latencies depends upon physical factors; for example, the circulatory delay is brief (seconds) for brain GnRH to reach pituitary LH–secreting cells due to a short portal capillary system (2). The whole-body circulatory delay is somewhat larger for LH to reach the testis and penetrate the interstitium to stimulate Leydig cells. Target-tissue response delays are more complex and variable, since they reflect the emergence of multiple sequential and parallel intracellular messenger pathways that supervise cellular changes (1–3,9).

Stochastic Elements

Measurements of GnRH, LH, and Te are confounded by *experimental uncertainty* (Fig. 8). In addition, there is preassay variability introduced by sample withdrawal and processing (nonuniform blood centrifugation, defibrination, serum separation, freeze–thaw artifacts, etc.). Estimates of the latter approach, in the range of 3% to 12%, are based on the coefficient of variation (CV) of 50 to 300 replicate assays of a continuously infused hormone or long-lived stable serum components, such as calcium or albumin, sampled frequently (1,3,14). The analytical assay usually introduces an additional CV of 3% to 7% (79,80).

Stochastic (random) variability also arises biologically. Hypothalamic pulses are generated episodically; that is, sequential GnRH/LH pulse waiting times (interpulse intervals) are uncorrelated (141–143). Indeed, ApEn values of successive interpulse-interval lengths approach mean empirically random (as estimated by 1000 random shuffles of each sequence) (144,145). Accordingly, the GnRH pulse-generator system exhibits no evident memory for preceding pulse times. In this setting, one might utilize a classical

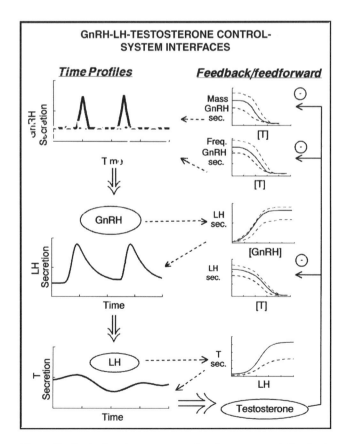

Figure 7   Illustrative dose–response functions encapsulating feedforward (LH's stimulation of Te secretion) and feedback (Te's inhibition of GnRH-stimulated LH secretion) connections within the GnRH–LH–Te axis. *Abbreviations*: GnRH, gonadotropin-releasing hormone; LH, luteinizing hormone; Te, testosterone. *Source*: From Ref. 35.

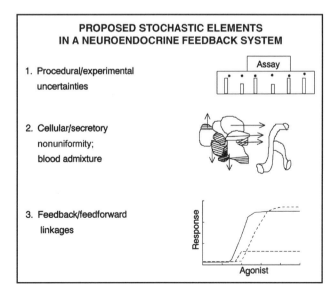

Figure 8   Schema highlighting various sources of random biological and experimental variations in an interlinked neurohormone system.

Poisson renewal ("counting") process to encapsulate the GnRH pulsing mechanism (5). Sex-steroid negative feedback and/or 24-hour rhythmic variation of GnRH pulse frequency also occurs, however, thereby requiring a nonstationary Poisson model (1,3,5,14,133,137, 138,140,146–148).

The Poisson probability density is also constrained by the equality of its mean and variance; i.e., a mean GnRH pulse frequency of 16 events per day has a Poisson-forced (definitional) CV of 25%. To address this limitation, the notion of a Poisson pulse generator can be extended to loosely coupled (rather than strictly independent) GnRH neuronal oscillators (149). This construction is modeled by the Weibull probability density, a member of the generalized Gamma function, which uncouples the mean pulsing intensity from its variance (8,9,144,145). Under simplifying conditions (gamma equals one), the Weibull distribution is equivalent to the classical Poisson density (5). The Weibull function thus accommodates a spectrum of interpulse variability (CV) at any given (probabilistic) mean frequency. This concept is important in explicating the anomalous pulsing behavior of GnRH/LH in the aging male (see below for further information).

Stochastic contributions also probably arise at feedforward/feedback interfaces—that is, any given theoretical (idealized) dose–response function occupies a parameter probability space. This concept incorporates expected variability in the micro- and macroenvironments of the secretory gland, circulation, and target organ; e.g., nonhomogeneous access of effector molecules to cells in the responding gland, unequal degrees of cellular reactivity to the effector signal, and variable stores of releasable and mobilized hormone. In this context, one can allow for some (1–3%) stochastic variability in the dose-responsive coupling of signals within an axis (3,5,8,9,144,145).

Figure 8 summarizes the foregoing perspective of composite stochastic variability within the GnRH–LH–Te axis: experimental uncertainties in data collection, variability in GnRH pulse generator outputs, and nonuniformity of (idealized) feedback.

Secretion and Elimination Properties

Figure 9 highlights the concepts of distinct underlying secretory bursts giving rise to pulsatile serum hormone concentration profiles. For LH, GnRH is the unobserved proximate stimulus, which corresponds virtually one-to-one with LH-secretory bursts in the rat, monkey, sheep, and human (128,129,150–152). Thus, one can model observed serum LH pulse times as inherited from unseen GnRH signals with a finite time delay. Uncoupling of this GnRH–LH interface is a possible mechanism of hypogonadotropism, as demonstrated recently in the uremic male rat (149).

Hormone release typically occurs as a variable admixture of basal and pulsatile secretory modes. Basal release represents a time-invariant (and presumptively

less regulated) release process, which is minimal in some normal neuroendocrine systems (5,8,9). Pulsatile LH output reflects the stimulus-dependent rapid exocytotic discharge of prestored hormone granules, which output commingles with a slower rise and delayed fall in the rates of cellular gene transcription, de novo hormone biosynthesis, posttranslational protein processing and packaging into secretory granules, and vectorial movement and subsequent extrusion of new granular contents (5,6,25,26). In gonadotrope cells, GnRH acutely stimulates LH synthesis and secretion by activating plasma-membrane adenylyl cyclase and phospholipase C, initiating calcium fluxes, driving protein kinase A- and C–dependent protein phosphorylation and initiating gene transcription, while concurrently discharging immediately releasable (membrane-associated) LH-secretory granules (2,4, 127,153). Although the entire cascade of signaling responses underlying granule exocytosis and LH biosynthesis is not known (2), on modeling grounds, the authors approximate the aggregate process as a summed exponential (Fig. 9) (9). Thus, the resultant LH-secretory burst is expected to exhibit some asymmetry over time (3,5,6,9).

Elimination of LH

Empirical data for a wide variety of neurohormones suggest a nominally (multi-) exponential elimination process in vivo (1,3,154). This inference has been corroborated for LH by using direct intravenous injection of highly purified or rh LH in hypopituitary men (34,154) and leuprolide-downregulated normal volunteers (Fig. 10) (125). Accordingly, to represent the joint

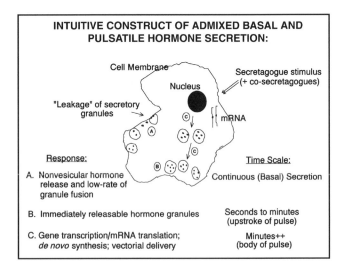

Figure 9 Mechanisms driving an LH-secretory burst: Prompt exocytosis of membrane-docked granules containing gonadotropins achieves immediate release of presynthesized LH molecules. Delayed granule mobilization and new granule formation via de novo glycoprotein–hormone biosynthesis serve to generate a delayed but confluent waveform of more prolonged and asymmetric LH secretion. *Abbreviation*: LH, luteinizing hormone.

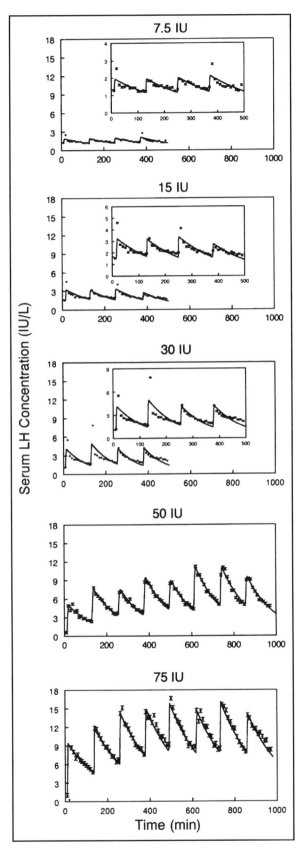

kinetics of hormone distribution and removal, one can use a simple biexponential algebraic function. In the hypopituitary human, mean half-lives of plasma-immunoreactive LH calculated following a bolus intravenous injection of highly purified pituitary extracts approximate 18 and 90 minutes, with a fractional (rapid) contribution of 0.37 of the total decay amplitude (154). Comparable estimates are obtained in GnRH-agonist pretreated healthy men infused with rh LH (125). The apparent half-life of LH appears to be age independent, but increases at higher serum LH concentrations (6,8,9,125,144,154), possibly reflecting partial saturation of tissue removal and/or degradative mechanisms.

Feedback Signal Integration

The coupling between hormones (e.g., Te acting negatively on GnRH output) is inferentially mediated via integral (time-averaged) and/or differential (rate-sensitive) signal processing. Whereas the stress-responsive ACTH–cortisol axis exhibits both integral and differential feedback (126,155), rapid (rate-sensitive) negative feedback has not been observed for Te on GnRH or LH secretion. Thus, one can visualize a time-averaged Te concentration as the negative-feedback signal on GnRH and LH synthesis and release. The exact time delays for these feedback loops are not yet established. Indirect estimates by cross-correlation analyses approximate 60 to 110 minutes for the time-delayed negative-feedback linkage between blood Te and LH concentrations in normal young men (156). By analogous calculations, the feedforward of LH on Te secretions requires 20 to 60 minutes (52,57,156,157). Hypophyseal portal-vein catheterization studies suggest that GnRH–LH coupling evolves over a few minutes (1,2,128, 129,150–152).

Indirect (cross-correlation) analyses suggest that both the feedforward of LH concentrations on Te secretion and the feedback of Te concentrations on LH secretion are altered in the aging male (156). In particular, feedforward of LH on Te appears to be attenuated (albeit of normal latency) and feedback of Te on LH is blunted but more rapid in older men.

Coupling System Components

The output of key regulatory loci (GnRH, LH, and Te), time delays, dose–response interface properties, and hormone-elimination features can be embedded in a set of relevant coupled stochastic differential equations (5,6,8,144,145). Statistical considerations establish that the foregoing system is mathematically consistent, and that mean, variance, and covariance estimates are asymptotically realizable by maximum-likelihood procedures (6). Thereby, one may calculate not only biexponential kinetics, but also basal, pulsatile, and total secretion in mass units normalized per unit distribution volume (see below).

Figure 10 Decay properties of rh LH injected intravenously as a square-wave pulse over six minutes in five leuprolide-downregulated healthy men given varying doses of rh LH (7.5, 15, 30, 50 and 75 IU) every two hours. The slower half-life component shows some concentration dependency. *Abbreviations*: LH, luteinizing hormone; rh, recombinant human. *Source*: From Ref. 9.

Application of Dynamic Concepts to the Appraisal of LH Release in Healthy Young and Older Men

Univariate LH Analysis

To quantitate LH secretion and elimination, the authors studied healthy young (n=13) and older (n=13) men by sampling blood at 10-minute intervals for 24 hours (0800 to 0800 hours) (9,42,52). Sera were submitted to a robotics-assisted monoclonal two-site immunoradiometric assay in duplicate (median within-assay CV 5.2%). Since basal (nonpulsatile) LH-secretion rates are of unknown magnitude in the human, the authors tested three implicit algebraic constructs of basal release: (*i*) zero basal; (*ii*) a fixed percentage basal [11%, based on GnRH antagonist studies (39)]; and (*iii*) model-variable (analytically estimated) basal LH-secretion rate. For each representation of basal release, the estimated secretory burst mass was reduced significantly in older men. Calculated endogenous LH kinetics (rapid and slower half-lives of elimination) and basal LH secretion were independent of age. Irregular LH-release patterns were visually evident in older men, which impression is quantifiable by ApEn analysis (Fig. 4A). Mean daily LH pulse frequency was elevated in aging individuals (p<0.01). Thus, older and young men secrete and eliminate an equivalent amount of LH daily, but older men do so in a more disorderly, high-frequency, and low-amplitude manner.

Irregularity (Pattern-Sensitive) Analysis

The irregularity of 24-hour serum LH concentration profiles in young and older men can be assessed by the regularity statistic, ApEn. ApEn is a family of three-parameter metrics (29,31,32,94,158). It quantitates the degree of sample-by-sample pattern regularity in time series, based on r (threshold for subpattern recurrence), m (pattern length), and N (series length). ApEn is applied to the observed (untransformed) or derivative (e.g., secretion-based) LH-release profiles. For example, deconvolution analyses of serum-hormone concentration values may be used to create sample secretion rates, which are free of autocorrelation due to elimination and are typically stationary (i.e., show little drift of baseline). Data can be stationarized also by application of the heat equation (144). As noted in Figure 4A, LH ApEn values exhibit a vivid age contrast, with higher mean ApEn signifying greater irregularity in the older male. Based on analyses of simpler reductionistic mathematical systems and empirically based feedback experiments, ApEn serves as a barometer of changing strength and complexity of control signals in an interlinked axis (30–32,94,159).

To assess the mechanism(s) underlying more disorderly LH release in the older male, one can also apply ApEn to the short reconstructed sequences of LH pulse mass and interpulse-interval values obtained by deconvolving a serum LH concentration profile (144,145). To normalize ApEn for unequal series lengths, the authors computed LH ApEn *ratios* (mean ratio of an observed

ApEn value to that of 1000 randomly shuffled cognate series) (94). Ratios of unity therefore denote essentially random data. ApEn ratios of successive LH interpulse–interval series are nonunitary and statistically indistinguishable in the two age groups. Mean ApEn ratios of ad seriatim LH pulse-mass estimates are significantly higher in older men (p<0.01). This contrast persists when sequential LH pulse-mass values are normalized to the preceding or following interpulse-interval length (144). Thus, the time evolution of amplitudes (mass) of LH-secretory bursts is more irregular or disorderly in older men, independently of their higher mean pulse frequency.

Bivariate LH–Te Analysis

Figure 11 illustrates synchrony assessment of paired serum LH and Te concentration profiles by cross-ApEn analysis (31). Elevated cross-ApEn values in older men denote the disruption of bidirectional linkages between the corresponding hormones. Moreover, cross-ApEn analysis also reveals age-related loss of coordinate oscillations in LH release and NPT (Fig. 4A), LH and FSH secretion (Fig. 4B), and sleep-stage transitions and Te output (Fig. 12). Such data collectively point to erosion of CNS-dependent control of neurohormone outflow in the aging male.

Trivariate GnRH–LH–Te Analysis

A model of the interlinked (unobserved) output of GnRH and the (observed) secretion of LH and Te could also be evaluated via a modified Bayesian approach (5,6,8,9,144). This statistical tool imposes relevant prior probability constraints on the primary variables; for example, probabilistic half-lives based on the published kinetics of LH and Te (and their variances) (34,154,160–162). In addition, one could implement a statistically based (maximum-likelihood estimation)

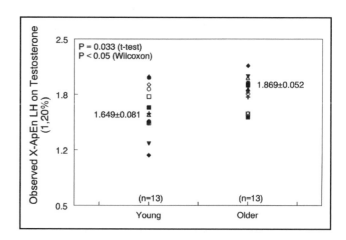

Figure 11   Illustrative cross-ApEn analyses of paired 24-hour serum LH and testosterone concentration time series collected in 13 young and 13 older men. Cross-ApEn (X, ApEn) was calculated for feedforward and feedback coupling. NS denotes P>0.05. *Abbreviation*: ApEn, approximate entropy. *Source*: From Ref. 39.

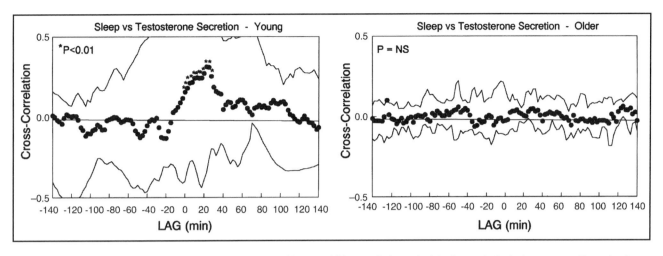

Figure 12 Cross-correlation plot relating sleep-stage transitions and (deconvolution-calculated) sample testosterone secretion rates in young (*top*) and older (*bottom*) men monitored simultaneously by electroencephalogram (EEG) and 2.5-minute blood sampling overnight. Deeper sleep correlates with greater testosterone secretion immediately and up to 22.5 minutes later in young, but not older, men.

iterative peak identification algorithm to appraise the positions and numbers of putative GnRH- or LH-secretory bursts iteratively, while computing basal and pulsatile neurohormone secretion and endogenous biexponential kinetic values simultaneously (Keenan D, Veldhuis JD, unpublished observation). Validation of such methodologies will require both computer-assisted simulations and direct in vivo experiments.

□ PARADIGMS OF THE GnRH–LH–TE FEEDBACK SYSTEM CONTROL

The mechanisms that mediate a reduction in LH pulse mass, an elevation in LH pulse frequency, and more irregular LH release in aging men are not known. Several clinical hypotheses of altered within-axis dynamics can be considered and tested provisionally using a computer-assisted feedback ensemble model (144). Feedback strength is modulated in an interactive biomathematical construct by adjusting the half-maximally effective and/or maximal value(s) of the corresponding interface (dose–response) function, corresponding to the sensitivity (potency) and/or efficacy of the interaction. For example, simulations of random LH pulse trains followed by ApEn analyses can be implemented to appraise different postulates of reproductive aging in the male: (*i*) augmented Te negative feedback on GnRH/LH; (*ii*) blunted LH feedforward on Te (reduced maximum of LH–Te interface); (*iii*) elevated mean GnRH pulse-generator rate; (*iv*) attenuated Te feedback on LH; and (*v*) heightened Te–GnRH/LH feedback along with simultaneously impaired LH–Te feedforward (Fig. 13) (144). Among the foregoing constructs, only the models of restricted LH–Te feedforward and impeded Te–GnRH/LH feedback mimic the observed elevation of LH and Te ApEn and LH–Te cross-ApEn in older men (31,52).

Accentuated or blunted feedback inhibition of LH secretion by Te may operate in aging men, as inferred from the effects of pharmacological delivery of single doses of Te or its 5 alpha-reduced metabolite (2,156,163,164,172,173). Dose-responsive feedback analyses, however, are lacking. Plasma total, free, and bioavailable Te concentrations fall progressively in the older male (52,61,64,165–169). The fall would reduce effectual androgen-dependent negative feedback on GnRH/LH release. Androgen-receptor activity may also change with aging in a tissue-specific manner (170). Model predictions are that LH ApEn and LH–Te cross-ApEn rise in the androgen-withdrawn context (36,144). This forecast is supported by experiments in eugonadal young men, in whom acute blockade of Leydig cell and adrenal steroidogenesis increases LH ApEn (33,34). Withdrawal of negative feedback in the renin–angiotensin and growth hormone insulin–like growth factor–I axes also evokes greater secretory irregularity of the cognate hormones (29,97). Therefore, further studies will be required to appraise the role of hypoandrogenemia in healthy older men in mediating more irregular LH release.

□ UNRESOLVED NEUROENDOCRINE MODELING ISSUES

Table 2 highlights selected unresolved issues in the dynamic control of the male GnRH/LH/Te and GnRH/FSH/inhibin B axes. More refined constructs will be required to explore pathophysiological feedforward/feedback activities in the joint systems; to define the nature of their interactions; and to predict the impact of possible age-related drift in dose–response parameters on the pulsatile, entropic, and 24-hour rhythmic control of GnRH, LH, and Te secretion.

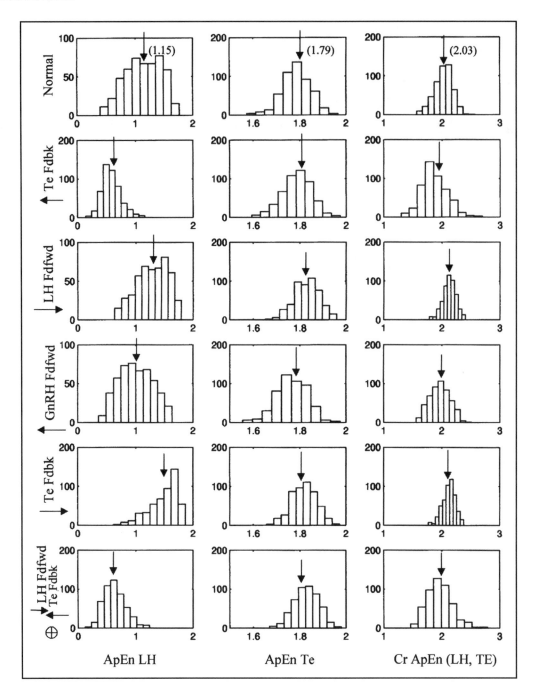

Figure 13   Impact of putative age-related network perturbations on ApEn and cross-ApEn measures of LH- and Te-secretory profiles. Computer-simulated pulse trains were driven by a dynamic feedback- and feedforward-coupled construct of the interactive GnRH–LH–Te axis (Fig. 8). Columns denote LH ApEn, Te ApEn, and LH–Te cross-ApEn. Each row of panels depicts frequency histograms for 300 independent simulations. The respective hypotheses tested include (*topmost to bottom rows*): basal (control, default parameter) conditions; increased testosterone feedback on GnRH/LH (↑ Te); reduced LH feedforward on testosterone (↓ LH); accelerated GnRH pulse frequency (↑ GnRH); decreased testosterone feedback on GnRH/LH (↓ Te); and jointly heightened testosterone feedback on GnRH/LH and blunted LH feedforward on Te. Reduced feedback of Te on GnRH/LH and/or impaired LH feedforward on Te predict elevated LH ApEn, Te ApEn, and LH–Te cross-ApEn. *Abbreviations*: ApEn, approximate entropy; GnRH, gonadotropin-releasing hormone; LH, luteinizing hormone; Te, testosterone. *Source:* From Ref. 144.

□ SUMMARY

Neuroendocrine systems maintain physiological homeostasis by intermittent signaling to remote glandular sites (1,3,36,171). According to this thesis, the pathophysiology of the male gonadotropic axis as a whole cannot be understood by appraising its individual components in isolation. The present chapter illustrates the foregoing interactive concept for the dynamic ensemble of hypothalamic GnRH-secreting neurons, anterior-pituitary gonadotropes, systemic negative feedback by Te on GnRH and LH, and feedforward by LH on Leydig cells. Specific dose-responsive interfaces and time delays couple the foregoing

Table 2 Selected Unresolved Neuroendocrine Modeling Issues in the Male

What are the time delays for GnRH, LH, and/or testosterone feedforward and feedback?
What is the magnitude of "system noise" (or unexplained biological variability) for selected feedforward and feedback interfaces?
What are the stochastic properties of the pulse-generator mechanism?
What is the ensemble time profile generated by the "cascade" of target-tissue responses elicited by an input (feedforward or feedback) signal?
What are the consequences of simultaneous changes in feedforward and feedback signaling?
What is the mechanistic basis for the (multi-) exponential form of LH (or GnRH and testosterone) disappearance from plasma?

Abbreviations: GnRH, gonadotropin-releasing hormone; LH, luteinizing hormone.

primary neuroregulatory loci. This emerging perspective should help to direct new pathophysiological hypotheses, explore potential interventional effects, and stimulate further basic science and clinical experiments.

☐ ACKNOWLEDGMENTS

The authors thank Arthur Chapin for his excellent editorial assistance and Paula P. Azimi for the graphics. This work was supported in part by the General Clinical Research Center of the University of Virginia and NIH RO1 AG14799. This focused report necessarily omits many primary references because of editorial constraints.

☐ REFERENCES

1. Urban RJ, Evans WS, Rogol AD, et al. Contemporary aspects of discrete peak detection algorithms. I. The paradigm of the luteinizing hormone pulse signal in men. Endocr Rev 1988; 9(1):3–37.

2. Veldhuis JD, Yen SSC, Jaffe RB, et al. Male hypothalamic-pituitary-gonadal axis. In: Yen SSC, Jaffe RB, Barbieri RL, eds. Reproductive Endocrinology. 4th ed. 1999; 622–631.

3. Veldhuis JD. Recent insights into neuroendocrine mechanisms of aging of the human male hypothalamo-pituitary-gonadal axis. J Androl 1999; 20:1–17.

4. Marshall JC, Kelch RP. Gonadotropin-releasing hormone: role of pulsatile secretion in the regulation of reproduction. N Engl J Med 1986; 315(23):1459–1467.

5. Keenan DM, Veldhuis JD. A biomathematical model of time-delayed feedback in the human male hypothalamic-pituitary-Leydig cell axis. Am J Physiol 1998; 275(1 Pt 1):E157–E176.

6. Keenan DM, Veldhuis JD, Yang R. Joint recovery of pulsatile and basal hormone secretion by stochastic nonlinear random-effects analysis. Am J Physiol 1998; 275(6 Pt 2): R1939– R1949.

7. Keenan DM, Veldhuis JD. Stochastic model of admixed basal and pulsatile hormone secretion as modulated by a deterministic oscillator. Am J Physiol 1997; 273(3): R1182–R1192.

8. Keenan DM, Sun W, Veldhuis JD. A stochastic biomathematical model of the male reproductive hormone system. SIAM J Appl Math 2000; 61:934–965.

9. Keenan DM, Veldhuis JD. Explicating hypergonadotropism in postmenopausal women: a statistical model. Am J Physiol 2000; 278(5):R1247–R1257.

10. Veldhuis JD, Evans WS, Rogol AD, et al. Intensified rates of venous sampling unmask the presence of spontaneous high-frequency pulsations of luteinizing hormone in man. J Clin Endocrinol Metab 1984; 59(1):96–102.

11. Veldhuis JD, Evans WS, Rogol AD, et al. Performance of LH pulse detection algorithms at rapid rates of venous sampling in humans. Am J Physiol 1984; 247(4 Pt 1):554E–563E.

12. Veldhuis JD, Evans WS, Johnson ML, et al. Physiological properties of the luteinizing hormone pulse signal: impact of intensive and extended venous sampling paradigms on their characterization in healthy men and women. J Clin Endocrinol Metab 1986; 62(5):881–891.

13. Veldhuis JD, Lassiter AB, Johnson ML. Operating behavior of dual or multiple endocrine pulse generators. Am J Physiol 1990; 259(3 Pt 1):E351–E361.

14. Evans WS, Sollenberger MJ, Booth RA Jr, et al. Contemporary aspects of discrete peak detection algorithms. II. The paradigm of the luteinizing hormone pulse signal in women. Endocr Rev 1992; 13(1):81–104.

15. Mulligan T, Delemarre-van de Waal HA, Johnson ML, et al. Validation of deconvolution analysis of LH secretion and half-life. Am J Physiol 1994; 267(1 Pt 2): R202–R211.

16. Wang C, Berman N, Veldhuis JD, et al. Graded testosterone infusions distinguish gonadotropin negative-feedback responsiveness in Asians and white men—a clinical research center study. J Clin Endocrinol Metab 1998; 83(3):870–876.

17. Wu FCW, Butler GE, Kelnar CJH, et al. Patterns of pulsatile luteinizing hormone secretion from childhood to adulthood in the human male: a study using deconvolution analysis and an ultrasensitive immunofluorometric assay. J Clin Endocrinol Metab 1996; 81(5):1798–1805.

18. Veldhuis JD, Urban RJ, Lizarralde G, et al. Attenuation of luteinizing hormone secretory burst amplitude is a

proximate basis for the hypoandrogenism of healthy aging in men. J Clin Endocrinol Metab 1992; 75(3):52–58.

19. Tang LK, Martellock AC, Horiuchi JK. Estradiol stimulation of LH response to LHRH and LHRH binding in pituitary cultures. Am J Physiol 1982; 242(6): E392–E397.

20. Veldhuis JD, Johnson ML. Cluster analysis: a simple, versatile and robust algorithm for endocrine pulse detection. Am J Physiol 1986; 250(4 Pt 1):E486–E493.

21. Partsch C-J, Abrahams S, Herholz N, et al. Variability of pulsatile LH secretion in young male volunteers. Eur J Endocrinol 1994; 131(3):263–272.

22. Veldhuis JD, Moorman J, Johnson ML. Deconvolution analysis of neuroendocrine data: waveform-specific and waveform-independent methods and applications. Methods Neurosci 1994; 20:279–325.

23. Veldhuis JD, Johnson ML. Specific methodological approaches to selected contemporary issues in deconvolution analysis of pulsatile neuroendocrine data. Methods Neurosci 1995; 28:25–92.

24. Veldhuis JD, Evans WS, Johnson ML. Complicating effects of highly correlated model variables on nonlinear least-squares estimates of unique parameter values and their statistical confidence intervals: estimating basal secretion and neurohormone half-life by deconvolution analysis. Methods Neurosci 1995; 28:130–138.

25. Veldhuis JD, Carlson ML, Johnson ML. The pituitary gland secretes in bursts: appraising the nature of glandular secretory impulses by simultaneous multiple-parameter deconvolution of plasma hormone concentrations. Proc Natl Acad Sci USA 1987; 84(21):7686–7690.

26. Veldhuis JD, Johnson ML. Deconvolution analysis of hormone data. Methods Enzymol 1992; 210:539–575.

27. Johnson ML, Veldhuis JD. Evolution of deconvolution analysis as a hormone pulse detection method. Methods Neurosci 1995; 28:1–24.

28. Veldhuis JD, Johnson ML, Faunt LM, et al. Assessing temporal coupling between two, or among three or more, neuroendocrine pulse trains: cross-correlation analysis, simulation methods, and conditional probability testing. Methods Neurosci 1994; 20:336–376.

29. Veldhuis JD, Pincus SM. Orderliness of hormone release patterns: a complementary measure to conventional pulsatile and circadian analyses. Eur J Endocrinol 1998; 138(4):358–362.

30. Pincus SM, Hartman ML, Roelfsema F, et al. Hormone pulsatility discrimination via coarse and short time sampling. Am J Physiol 1999; 277(5):E948–E957.

31. Pincus SM, Mulligan T, Iranmanesh A, et al. Older males secrete luteinizing hormone and testosterone more irregularly, and jointly more asynchronously, than younger males. Proc Natl Acad Sci USA 1996; 93(24):14100–14105.

32. Pincus SM, Keefe DL. Quantification of hormone pulsatility via an approximate entropy algorithm. Am J Physiol 1992; 262(5 Pt 1):E741–E754.

33. Veldhuis JD, Zwart AD, Iranmanesh A. Neuroendocrine mechanisms by which selective Leydig-cell castration unleashes increased pulsatile LH release in the human: an experimental paradigm of short-term ketoconazole-induced hypoandrogenemia and deconvolution-estimated LH secretory enhancement. Am J Physiol 1997; 272(2 Pt 2):R464–R474.

34. Zwart A, Iranmanesh A, Veldhuis JD. Disparate serum free testosterone concentrations and degrees of hypothalamo-pituitary-LH suppression are achieved by continuous versus pulsatile intravenous androgen replacement in men: a clinical experimental model of ketoconazole-induced reversible hypoandrogenemia with controlled testosterone add-back. J Clin Endocrinol Metab 1997; 82(7):2062–2069.

35. Giusti M, Marini G, Traverso L, et al. Effect of pulsatile luteinizing hormone-releasing hormone administration on pituitary-gonadal function in elderly man. J Endocrinol Invest 1990; 13(2):127–132.

36. Giustina A, Veldhuis JD. Pathophysiology of the neuroregulation of GH secretion in experimental animals and the human. Endocr Rev 1998; 19(6):717–797.

37. Aloi JA, Bergendahl M, Iranmanesh A, et al. Pulsatile intravenous gonadotropin-releasing hormone administration averts fasting-induced hypogonadotropism and hypoandrogenemia in healthy, normal-weight men. J Clin Endocrinol Metab 1997; 82(5):1543–1548.

38. Mulligan T, Iranmanesh A, Veldhuis JD. Failed restitution of Leydig cell testosterone secretion despite full normalization of pulsatile release by two weeks of exogenous pulsatile GnRH pump/infusion therapy in older men. 80th Endocrine Society Annual Meeting, New Orleans, LA, June 24–27, 1998.

39. Veldhuis JD, Iranmanesh A, Godschalk M, et al. Older men manifest multifold synchrony disruption of reproductive neurohormone outflow. J Clin Endocrinol Metab 2000; 85:1477–1486.

40. Zwart AD, Urban RJ, Odell WD, et al. Contrasts in the gonadotropin-releasing dose–response relationships for luteinizing hormone, follicle-stimulating hormone, and alpha-subunit release in young versus older men: appraisal with high-specificity immunoradiometric assay and deconvolution analysis. Eur J Endocrinol 1996; 135(4):399–406.

41. Dufau ML, Veldhuis JD, Fraioli F, et al. Mode of secretion of bioactive luteinizing hormone in man. J Clin Endocrinol Metab 1983; 57(5):993–1000.

42. Reyes-Fuentes A, Chavarria ME, Aguilera G, et al. Deconvolution analysis of bioassayable LH secretion and half-life in idopathic oligoasthenospermic men. Int J Androl 1997; 20(2): 118–125.

43. Jaakkola T, Ding Y-Q, Kellokumpu-Lehtinen P, et al. The ratios of serum bioactive/immunoreactive luteinizing hormone and follicle-stimulating hormone in various clinical conditions with increased and decreased gonadotropin secretion: reevaluation by a highly sensitive immunometric assay. J Clin Endocrinol Metab 1990; 70(6):1496–1505.

44. Marrama P, Montanini V, Celani MF, et al. Decrease in luteinizing hormone biological activity/immunoreactivity ratio in elderly men. Maturitas 1984; 5(4):223–231.

45. Dufau ML, Pock R, Newbaner A, et al. In vitro bioassay of LH in human serum: the rat interstitial cell testosterone (RICT) assay. J Clin Endocrinol Metab 1976; 42(5):958–968.

46. Dufau ML, Veldhuis JD, Burger HG. Pathophysiological relationships between the biological and immunological activities of luteinizing hormone. In: Burger HG, ed. Balliere's Clinical Endocrinology and Metabolism. Philadelphia: WB Saunders, 1987:153–176.

47. Matikainen T, Haavisto A-M, Permi J, et al. Effects of oestrogen treatment on serum gonadotropin bioactivity, immunoreactivity and isohormone distribution, and on immunoreactive inhibin levels in prostatic cancer patients. Clin Endocrinol (Oxf) 1994; 40(6):743–750.

48. Burgon PG, Stanton PG, Robertson DM. In vivo bioactivities and clearance patterns of highly purified luteinizing hormone isoforms. Endocrinology 1996; 137(11):4827–4836.

49. Belchetz PE, Plant TM, Nakai Y, et al. Hypophysial responses to continuous and intermittent delivery of hypothalamic gonadotropin-releasing hormone. Science 1978; 202(4368):631–633.

50. Shupnik MA. Effects of gonadotropin-releasing hormone on rat gonadotropin gene transcription in vitro: requirement for pulsatile administration for luteinizing hormone-beta gene stimulation. Mol Endocrinol 1990; 4(10):1444–1450.

51. Veldhuis JD. Pulsatile hormone release as a window into the brain's control of the anterior pituitary gland in health and disease: implications and consequences of pulsatile luteinizing hormone secretion. Endocrinologist 1995; 5:454–469.

52. Mulligan T, Iranmanesh A, Kerzner R, et al. Two-week pulsatile gonadotropin releasing hormone infusion unmasks dual (hypothalamic and Leydig-cell) defects in the healthy aging male gonadotropic axis. Eur J Endocrinol 1999; 141(3):257–266.

53. Mulligan T, Iranmanesh A, Gheorghiu S, et al. Amplified nocturnal luteinizing hormone (LH) secretory burst frequency with selective attenuation of pulsatile (but not basal) testosterone secretion in healthy aged men: possible Leydig cell desensitization to endogenous LH signaling–a clinical research center study. J Clin Endocrinol Metab 1995; 80(10):3025–3031.

54. Veldhuis JD, Iranmanesh A, Demers LM, et al. Joint basal and pulsatile hypersecretory mechanisms drive the monotropic follicle-stimulating hormone (FSH) elevation in healthy older men: concurrent preservation of the orderliness of the FSH release process. J Clin Endocrinol Metab 1999; 84(10):3506–3514.

55. Deslypere JP, Vermeulen A. Leydig cell function in normal men: effect of age, lifestyle, residence, diet and activity. J Clin Endocrinol Metab 1984; 59(5):955–962.

56. Vermeulen A. The male climacterium. Ann Med 1993; 25(6):531–534.

57. Foresta C, Bordon P, Rossato M, et al. Specific linkages among luteinizing hormone, follicle stimulating hormone, and testosterone release in the peripheral blood and human spermatic vein: evidence for both positive (feed-forward) and negative (feedback) within-axis regulation. J Clin Endocrinol Metab 1997; 82(9):3040–3046.

58. Bonavera JJ, Swerdloff RS, Leung A, et al. In the male Brown-Norway (BN) male rat reproductive aging is associated with decreased LH-pulse amplitude and area. J Androl 1997; 18(4):359–365.

59. Gruenewald DA, Naai MA, Hess DL, et al. The Brown Norway rat as a model of male reproductive aging: evidence for both primary and secondary testicular failure. J Gerontol 1994; 49(2):B42–B50.

60. Veldhuis JD, Iranmanesh A, Mulligan T. Age and testosterone feedback jointly control the dose-department actions of gonadotropin-releasing hormone in healthy men. J Clin Endocrinol Metab. 2005; 90:302–309.

61. Baker HWG, Burger HG, de Kretser DM, et al. Changes in the pituitary-testicular system with age. Clin Endocrinol 1976; 5(4):349–372.

62. Tilbrook AJ, de Kretser DM, Cummins TJ, et al. The negative feedback effects of testicular steroids are predominantly at the hypothalamus in the ram. Endocrinology 1991; 129(6):3080–3092.

63. Karpas AE, Bremner WJ, Clifton DK, et al. Diminished luteinizing hormone pulse frequency and amplitude with aging in the male rat. Endocrinology 1983; 112(3):788–791.

64. Desleypere JP, Vermeulen A. Aging and tissue androgens. J Clin Endocrinol Metab 1981; 53(2):530–534.

65. Vigersky RA, Easley RB, Loriaux LD. Effect of fluoxymesterone on the pituitary-gonadal axis: the role of testosterone-estradiol-binding globulin. J Clin Endocrinol Metab 1976; 43(1):1–9.

66. Bagatell CJ, Dahl KD, Bremner WJ. The direct pituitary effect of testosterone to inhibit gonadotropin secretion in men is partially mediated by aromatization to estradiol. J Androl 1994; 15(1):15–21.

67. Santen RJ, Bardin CW. Episodic luteinizing hormone secretion in man. Pulse analysis, clinical interpretation, physiologic mechanisms. J Clin Invest 1973; 52(10):2616–2618.

68. Veldhuis JD, Rogol AD, Samojlik E, et al. Role of endogenous opiates in the expression of negative feedback actions of estrogen and androgen on pulsatile properties of luteinizing hormone secretion in man. J Clin Invest 1984; 74(1):47–55.

69. Urban RJ, Davis MR, Rogol AD, et al. Acute androgen receptor blockade increases luteinizing-hormone secretory activity in men. J Clin Endocrinol Metab 1988; 67(6):1149–1155.

70. Kerrigan JR, Veldhuis JD, Rogol AD. Androgen-receptor blockade enhances pulsatile luteinizing hormone production in late pubertal males: evidence for a

hypothalamic site of physiological androgen feedback action. Pediatr Res 1994; 35(1):102–106.

71. Veldhuis JD, Conn PM, Freeman M. The neuroendocrine control of ultradian rhythms. In: Conn PM, Freeman M, eds. Neuroendocrinology in Physiology and Medicine. Totowa, NJ: Humana Press, 1999: 453–472.

72. Vermeulen A, Deslypere JP. Testicular endocrine function in the ageing male. Maturitas 1985; 7(3):273–279.

73. Vermeulen A, Deslypere JP, De Meirleir K. A new look to the andropause: altered function of the gonadotrophs. J Ster Biochem 1989; 32(1B):163–165.

74. Harman SM, Tsitouras PD. Reproductive hormones in aging men. I. Measurement of sex steroids, basal luteinizing hormone, and Leydig cell response to human chorionic gonadotropin. J Clin Endocrinol Metab 1980; 51(1):35–40.

75. Haavisto AM, Dunkel L, Pettersson K, et al. LH measurements by in vitro bioassay and a highly sensitive immunofluorometric assay improve the distinction between boys with constitutional delay of puberty and hypogonadotropic hypogonadism. Ped Res 1990; 27(3):211–214.

76. Urban RJ, Veldhuis JD, Dufau ML. Estrogen regulates the gonadotropin-releasing-hormone stimulated secretion of biologically active luteinizing hormone in man. J Clin Endocrinol Metab 1991; 72(3): 660–668.

77. Clark PA, Iranmanesh A, Veldhuis JD, et al. Comparison of pulsatile luteinizing hormone secretion between prepubertal children and young adults: evidence for a mass/amplitude-dependent difference without gender or day/night contrasts. 79th Endocrine Society Annual Meeting, Minneapolis, MN, June 11–14, 1997, [abstr # P2-513).

78. Clark PA, Iranmanesh A, Veldhuis JD, et al. Comparison of pulsatile luteinizing hormone secretion between prepubertal children and young adults: evidence for a mass/amplitude-dependent difference without gender or day/night contrasts. J Clin Endocrinol Metab 1997; 82(9):2950–2955.

79. Straume M, Johnson ML, Veldhuis JD. Statistically accurate estimation of hormone concentrations and associated uncertainties: methodology, validation, and applications. Clin Chem 1998; 44(1):116–123.

80. Straume M, Veldhuis JD, Johnson ML. Model-independent quantification of measurement error: empirical estimation of discrete variance function profiles based on standard curves. Methods Enzymol 1994; 240:121–150.

81. Straume M, Johnson ML. Monte Carlo method for determining complete confidence probability distributions of estimated model parameters. Methods Enzymol 1992; 210:117–129.

82. Jia XC, Perlas E, Su JG, et al. Luminescence luteinizing hormone/choriogonadotropin (LH/CG) bioassay: measurement of serum bioactive LH/CG during early pregnancy in human and macaque. Biol Reprod 1993; 49(6):1310–1316.

83. Veldhuis JD, Rogol AD, Johnson ML. Minimizing false-positive errors in hormonal pulse detection. Am J Physiol 1985; 248(4 Pt 1):E475–E481.

84. Veldhuis JD, Weiss J, Mauras N, et al. Appraising endocrine pulse signals at low circulating hormone concentrations: Use of regional coefficients of variation in the experimental series to analyze pulsatile luteinizing hormone release. Pediatr Res 1986; 20(7):632–637.

85. De Nicolao G, Liberati D, Veldhuis JD, et al. LH and FSH secretory responses to GnRH in normal individuals: a nonparametric deconvolution approach. Eur J Endocrinol 1999; 141(3):246–256.

86. De Nicolao G, Liberati D. Linear and nonlinear techniques for the deconvolution of hormone time-series. IEEE Trans Biomed Eng 1993; 40(5):440–445.

87. Schweizer MWF, Walter-Sack I, Rabe TN, et al. Basal and pulsatile secretion of human luteinizing hormone–new methods for the analysis of endocrine secretion processes. Endocrinol Diabetes 1996; 104:235–242.

88. Van Cauter E. Method for characterization of 24-hour temporal variation of blood components. Am J Physiol 1979; 237: E255–E264.

89. McIntosh RP, McIntosh JEA, Lazarus L. A comparison of the dynamics of secretion of human growth hormone and LH pulses. J Endocrinol 1988; 118(2):339–345.

90. Genazzani AD, Rodbard D, Forti G, et al. Estimation of instantaneous secretory rate of luteinizing hormone in women during the menstrual cycle and in men. Clin Endocrinol 1990; 32(5):573–581.

91. Laurentie MP, Garcia-Villar R, Toutain PL, et al. Pulsatile secretion of LH in the ram: a re-evaluation using a discrete deconvolution analysis. J Endocrinol 1992; 133(1):75–85.

92. O'Sullivan F, O'Sullivan J. Deconvolution of episodic hormone data: an analysis of the role of season on the onset of puberty in cows. Biometrics 1988; 44(2):339–353.

93. Rebar R, Perlman D, Naftolin F, et al. The estimation of pituitary luteinizing hormone secretion. J Clin Endocrinol Metab 1973; 37(6):917–927.

94. Veldhuis JD, Straume M, Iranmanesh A, et al. Secretory process regularity monitors neuroendocrine feedback and feedforward signaling strength in humans. Am J Physiol 2001; 280(3):R721–R729.

95. Pincus SM. Quantifying complexity and regularity of neurobiological systems. Methods Neurosci 1995; 28:336–363.

96. Pincus SM, Veldhuis JD, Mulligan T, et al. Effects of age on the irregularity of LH and FSH serum concentrations in women and men. Am J Physiol 1997; 273(5): E989–E995.

97. Hartman ML, Pincus SM, Johnson ML, et al. Enhanced basal and disorderly growth hormone secretion distinguish acromegalic from normal pulsatile growth hormone release. J Clin Invest 1994; 94(3):1277–1288.

98. Roelfsema F, Pincus SM, Veldhuis JD. Patients with Cushing's disease secrete adrenocorticotropin and cortisol jointly more asynchronously than healthy subjects. J Clin Endocrinol Metab 1998; 83(2):688–692.

99. Iranmanesh A, South S, Liem AY, et al. Unequal impact of age, percentage body fat, and serum testosterone concentrations on the somatotropic, IGF-I, and IGF-binding protein responses to a three-day intravenous growth-hormone-releasing-hormone (GHRH) pulsatile infusion. Eur J Endocrinol 1998; 139(1):59–71.

100. Bergendahl M, Aloi JA, Iranmanesh A, et al. Fasting suppresses pulsatile luteinizing hormone (LH) secretion and enhances the orderliness of LH release in young but not older men. J Clin Endocrinol Metab 1998; 83(6):1967–1975.

101. Pincus SM, Gevers E, Robinson ICAF, et al. Females secrete growth hormone with more process irregularity than males in both human and rat. Am J Physiol 1996; 270(1 Pt 1):E107–E115.

102. Veldhuis JD, Liem AY, South S, et al. Differential impact of age, sex-steroid hormones, and obesity on basal versus pulsatile growth hormone secretion in men as assessed in an ultrasensitive chemiluminescence assay. J Clin Endocrinol Metab 1995; 80(11):3209–3222.

103. Meneilly GS, Veldhuis JD, Elahi D. Disruption of the pulsatile and entropic modes of insulin release during an unvarying glucose stimulus in elderly individuals. J Clin Endocrinol Metab 1999; 84(6):1938–1943.

104. Meneilly GS, Ryan AS, Veldhuis JD, et al. Increased disorderliness of basal insulin release, attenuated insulin secretory burst mass, and reduced ultradian rhythmicity of insulin secretion in older individuals. J Clin Endocrinol Metab 1997; 82(12):4088–4093.

105. van den Berg G, Pincus SM, Veldhuis JD, et al. Greater disorderliness of ACTH and cortisol release accompanies pituitary-dependent Cushing's Disease. Eur J Endocrinol 1997; 136(4):394–400.

106. Veldhuis JD, Zwart A, Mulligan T, et al. Muting of androgen negative feedback unveils impoverished gonadotropin-releasing hormone/luteinizing hormone (GnRH/LH) secretory reactivity in healthy older men. J Clin Endocrinol Metab 2001; 86(2):529–535.

107. Veldhuis JD, Iranmanesh A, Godschalk M, et al. Older men manifest multifold synchrony disruption of reproductive neurohormone outflow. J Clin Endocrinol Metab 2000; 85(4):1477–1486.

108. Winters SJ, Troen P. Episodic luteinizing hormone (LH) secretion and the response of LH and follicle-stimulating hormone to LH-releasing hormone in aged men: evidence for coexistent primary testicular insufficiency and an impairment in gonadotropin secretion. J Clin Endocrinol Metab 1982; 55(3):560–565.

109. Harman SM, Tsitouras PD, Costa PT, et al. Reproductive hormones in aging men. II. Basal pituitary gonadotropins and gonadotropin responses to luteinizing hormone-releasing hormone. J Clin Endocrinol Metab 1982; 54(3):547–551.

110. Snyder PJ, Reitano JF, Utiger RD. Serum LH and FSH responses to synthetic gonadotropin releasing hormone in normal men. J Clin Endocrinol Metab 1975; 41(5):938–945.

111. Hall JE, Whitcomb RW, Rivier JE, et al. Differential regulation of luteinizing hormone, follicle-stimulating hormone, and free α-subunit secretion from the gonadotrope by gonadotropin-releasing hormone (GnRH); evidence from the use of two GnRH antagonists. J Clin Endocrinol Metab 1990; 70(2):328–335.

112. Pepperell RJ, de Kretser DM, Burger HG. Studies on the metabolic clearance rate and production rate of human luteinizing hormone and on the initial half-life of its subunits in man. J Clin Invest 1975; 56(1):118–126.

113. Gross KM, Matsumoto AM, Bremner WJ. Differential control of luteinizing hormone and follicle stimulating hormone secretion by luteinizing hormone-releasing hormone pulse frequency in man. J Clin Endocrinol Metab 1987; 64(4):675–680.

114. Schnorr JA, Bray MJ, Veldhuis JD. Aromatization mediates testosterone's short-term feedback restraint of 24-hour endogenously driven and acute exogenous GnRH-stimulated LH and FSH secretion in young men. J Clin Endocrinol Metab 2001; 86(6):2600–2606.

115. Schnorr J, Santen RJ, Veldhuis JD. Role of endogenous aromatase in testosterone's short-term feedback regulation of 24-hour LH, FSH, and GH release in young men. Society for Gynecologic Investigation Annual Meeting, Atlanta, GA, March 11, 1999.

116. Santen RJ, Van den Bossche H, Symoens J, et al. Site of action of low dose ketoconazole on androgen biosynthesis in men. J Clin Endocrinol Metab 1983; 57(4):732–736.

117. Trachtenberg J, Zadra J. Steroid synthesis inhibition by ketoconazole: sites of action. Clin Invest Med 1988; 11(1):1–5.

118. Rotstein DM, Kertesz DJ, Walker KA, et al. Stereoisomers of ketoconazole: preparation and biological activity. J Med Chem 1992; 35(15):2818–2825.

119. Mulligan T, Kuno H, Clore J, et al. Pulsatile infusions of recombinant human LH in leuprolide-downregulated older vs. young men unmask an impoverished Leydig-cell secretory response in aging to mid-physiological LH stimuli. 82nd Endocrine Society Annual Meeting, Toronto, Canada, June 21–24, 2000, [abstr # 249].

120. Brown TJ, MacLusky NJ, Shanabrough M, et al. Comparison of age- and sex-related changes in cell nuclear estrogen-binding capacity and progestin receptor induction in the rat brain. Endocrinology 1990; 126(6):2965–2972.

121. Davis MR, Veldhuis JD, Rogol AD, et al. Sustained inhibitory actions of a potent antagonist of gonadotropin-releasing hormone in postmenopausal women. J Clin Endocrinol Metab 1987; 64(6):1268–1274.

122. Urban RJ, Pavlou SN, Rivier JE, et al. Suppressive actions of a gonadotropin-releasing hormone (GnRH)

antagonist on LH, FSH, and prolactin release in estrogen-deficient postmenopausal women. Am J Obstet Gynecol 1990; 162:1255–1260.

123. Kolp LA, Pavlou SN, Urban RJ, et al. Abrogation by a potent GnRH antagonist of the estrogen/progesterone-stimulated surge-like release of LH and FSH in postmenopausal women. J Clin Endocrinol Metab 1992; 75(4):993–997.

124. Tenover JS, Dahl KD, Vale WW, et al. Hormonal responses to a potent gonadotropin hormone-releasing hormone antagonist in ormal elderly men. J Clin Endocrinol Metab 1990; 71(4):881–888.

125. Mulligan T, Iranmanesh A, Veldhuis JD. Pulsatile intravenous infusion of recombinant human luteinizing hormone (LH) in leuprolide-suppressed men unmasks impoverished Leydig-cell secretory responses to mid-physiological LH drive in the aging male. J Clin Endocrinol Metab 2001; 86(11):5547–5553.

126. Yates FE. Analysis of endocrine signals: the engineering and physics of biochemical communication systems. Biol Reprod 1981; 24(1):73–94.

127. Weiss J, Jameson JL, Burrin JL, et al. Divergent responses of gonadotropin subunit mRNAs to continuous versus pulsatile GnRH in vitro. Mol Endocrinol 1990; 4(4):557–564.

128. Clarke IJ, Cummins JT. The temporal relationship between gonadotropin-releasing hormone (GnRH) and luteinizing hormone (LH) secretion in ovariectomized ewes. Endocrinology 1982; 111(5):1737–1739.

129. Dluzen DE, Ramirez VD. In vivo activity of the LHRH pulse generator as determined with push-pull perfusion of the anterior pituitary gland of unrestrained intact and castrate male rats. Neuroendocrinology 1987; 45(4):328–332.

130. van den Berg G, Veldhuis JD, Frolich M, et al. An amplitude-specific divergence in the pulsatile mode of GH secretion underlies the gender difference in mean GH concentrations in men and premenopausal women. J Clin Endocrinol Metab 1996; 81(7):2460–2466.

131. Davies TF, Platzer M. The perifused Leydig cell: system characterization and rapid gonadotropin-induced desensitization. Endocrinology 1981; 108(5):1757–1762.

132. Ellis GB, Desjardins C. Orchidectomy unleashes pulsatile luteinizing hormone secretion in the rat. Biol Reprod 1984; 30(3):619–627.

133. Boyar M, Finkelstein J, Kapen S, et al. Simultaneous episodic secretion of luteinizing hormone and testosterone during sleep in puberty. J Clin Invest 1973; 52:11–12.

134. Hanker JP, Nieschlag E, Schneider HPG. Hypothalamic site of progesterone action on gonadotropin release. Horm Metabol Res 1985; 17(12):679–682.

135. D'Occhio MJ, Schanbacher B, Kinder JE. Relationship between serum testosterone concentration and patterns of luteinizing hormone secretion in male sheep. Endocrinology 1982; 110(5):1547–1554.

136. Rowe PH, Racey PA, Lincoln GA, et al. The temporal relationship between the secretion of luteinizing hormone and testosterone in man. J Endocrinol 1975; 64(1):17–25.

137. Gordon D, Gray CE, Beastall GH, et al. The effects of pulsatile GnRH infusion upon the diurnal variations in serum LH and testosterone in pre-pubertal and pubertal boys. Acta Endocrinol (Copenh) 1989; 121(2):241–245.

138. Sarberia JM, Giner J, Cortes-Gallegos V. Diurnal variations of plasma testosterone in men. Steroids 1973; 22(5):615–623.

139. Piro C, Frailoi F, Sciarra F, et al. Circadian rhythm of plasma testosterone, cortisol and gonadotropins in normal male subjects. J Ster Biochem 1974; 4(3):321–329.

140. Tenover JS, Matsumoto AM, Clifton DK, et al. Age-related alterations in the circadian rhythms of pulsatile luteinizing hormone and testosterone secretion in healthy men. J Gerontol 1988; 43(6):M163–M169.

141. Butler JP, Spratt DI, O'Dea, et al. Interpulse interval sequence of LH in normal men essentially constitutes a renewal process. Am J Physiol 1986; 250(3 Pt 1):E338–E340.

142. Veldhuis JD, Johnson ML, Dufau ML. Physiological attributes of endogenous bioactive luteinizing hormone secretory bursts in man: assessment by deconvolution analysis and in vitro bioassay of LH. Am J Physiol 1989; 256(2 Pt 1):E199–E207.

143. Veldhuis JD, Johnson ML. In vivo dynamics of luteinizing hormone secretion and clearance in man: assessment by deconvolution mechanics. J Clin Endocrinol Metab 1988; 66(6):1291–1300.

144. Keenan DM, Veldhuis JD. Hypothesis testing of the aging male gonadal axis via a biomathematical construct. Am J Physiol Regul Integr Comp Physiol 2001; 280(6):R1755–R1771.

145. Keenan DM, Veldhuis JD. Disruption of the hypothalamic luteinizing-hormone pulsing mechanism in aging men. Am J Physiol 2001; 281(6):R1917–R1924.

146. Manasco PK, Umbach DM, Muly SM, et al. Ontogeny of gonadotropin, testosterone, and inhibin secretion in normal boys through puberty based on overnight serial sampling. J Clin Endocrinol Metab 1995; 80(7):2046–2052.

147. Kapen S, Boyar RM, Finkelstein JW, et al. Effect of sleep-wake cycle reversal on luteinizing hormone secretory pattern in puberty. J Clin Endocrinol Metab 1974; 39(2):293–300.

148. Albertsson-Wikland K, Rosberg S, Lannering B, et al. Twenty-four hour profiles of luteinizing hormone, follicle-stimulating hormone, testosterone, and estradiol levels: a semilongitudinal study throughout puberty in healthy boys. J Clin Endocrinol Metab 1997; 82(2):541–549.

149. Schaefer F, Daschner M, Veldhuis JD, et al. In vivo alterations in the gonadotropin releasing hormone (GnRH) pulse generator and the secretion and clearance of

luteinizing hormone in the uremic castrate rat. Neuroendocrinology 1994; 59(3):285–296.

150. Clarke IJ, Cummins JT. GnRH pulse frequency determines LH pulse amplitude by altering the amount of releasable LH in the pituitary glands of ewes. J Reprod Fertil 1985; 73(2):425–431.

151. Levine JE, Pau K-Y, Ramirez VD, et al. Simultaneous measurement of luteinizing hormone-releasing and luteinizing hormone release in unanesthetized, ovariectomized sheep. Endocrinology 1982; 111(5): 1449–1455.

152. Claypool LE, Watanabe G, Terasawa E. Effects of electrical stimulation of the medial basal hypothalamus on the in vivo release of luteinizing hormone-releasing hormone in the prepubertal and peripubertal female monkey. Endocrinology 1990; 127(6):3014–3022.

153. Conn PM, Crowley WF Jr. Gonadotropin-releasing hormone and its analogs. Annu Rev Med 1994; 45:391–405.

154. Veldhuis JD, Fraioli F, Rogol AD, et al. Metabolic clearance of biologically active luteinizing hormone in man. J Clin Invest 1986; 77(4):1122–1128.

155. Yates FE. Stimulation and inhibition of adrenocorticotropin release. In: DeGroot LJ, ed. Endocrinology. Vol 4. New York: Grune and Stratton, 1980:367–404.

156. Mulligan T, Iranmanesh A, Johnson ML, et al. Aging alters feedforward and feedback linkages between LH and testosterone in healthy men. Am J Physiol 1997; 273(4 Pt 2):R1407–R1413.

157. Veldhuis JD, King JC, Urban RJ, et al. Operating characteristics of the male hypothalamo-pituitary-gonadal axis: pulsatile release of testosterone and follicle-stimulating hormone and their temporal coupling with luteinizing hormone. J Clin Endocrinol Metab 1987; 65(5):929–941.

158. Pincus SM. Approximate entropy as a measure of system complexity. Proc Natl Acad Sci USA 1991; 88(6):2297–2301.

159. Greenspan S, Klibanski A, Chester Ridgway E. Pulsatile secretion of thyrotropin in normal subjects and in patients with thyroid disease. Serono Symposium from Raven Press 1988; 52:267–278.

160. Evans WS, Bowers CY, Hull LT, et al. Effects of estradiol and of continuous 24-hour GHRH- and GHRP-2 stimulation in women on pulsatile and entropic GH secretion. 82nd Endocrine Society Annual Meeting, Toronto, Canada, June 21–24, 2000, [abstr # 2016].

161. Horton R, Shinsako J, Forsham PH. Testosterone production and metabolic clearance rates with volumes of distribution in normal adult men and women. Acta Endocrinol (Copenh) 1965; 48:446–458.

162. Mauras N, Rogol AD, Veldhuis JD. Appraising the instantaneous secretory rates of luteinizing hormone and testosterone in response to selective mu opiate receptor blockade in late pubertal boys. J Androl 1987; 8(4):201–207.

163. Winters SJ, Sherins RJ, Troen P. The gonadotropin-suppressive activity of androgen is increased in elderly men. Metabolism 1984; 33(11):1052–1059.

164. Deslypere JP, Kaufman JM, Vermeulen T, et al. Influence of age on pulsatile luteinizing hormone release and responsiveness of the gonadotrophs to sex hormone feedback in men. J Clin Endocrinol Metab 1987; 64(1):68–73.

165. Bremner WJ, Vitiello MV, Prinz PN. Loss of circadian rhythmicity in blood testosterone levels with aging in normal men. J Clin Endocrinol Metab 1983; 56(6): 1278–1281.

166. Morley JE, Kaiser FE, Perry HM III, et al. Longitudinal changes in testosterone, luteinizing hormone, and follicle-stimulating hormone in healthy older men. Metab Clin Exp 1997; 46(4):410–413.

167. Morley JE, Kaiser F, Raum WJ, et al. Potentially predictive and manipulable blood serum correlates of aging in the healthy human male: progressive decreases in bioavailable testosterone, dehydroepiandrosterone sulfate, and the ratio of insulin-like growth factor I to growth hormone. Proc Natl Acad Sci USA 1997; 94(14): 7537–7542.

168. Gray A, Feldman HS, McKinlay JB, et al. Age, disease, and changing sex hormone levels in middle-aged men: results of the Massachusetts Male Aging Study. J Clin Endocrinol Metab 1991; 73(5): 1016–1025.

169. Tenover JS. Testosterone in the aging male. J Androl 1997; 18(2):103–106.

170. Roth GS. Hormone receptor changes during adulthood and senescence: significance for aging research. Federation Proc 1979; 38(5):1910–1914.

171. Keenan DM, Licinio J, Veldhuius JD. A feedback-controlled ensemble model of the stress-responsive hypothalamo-pituitary-adrenal axis. Proc Natl Acad Sci USA 2001; 98(7):4028–4033.

172. Muta K, Kato K, Akamine Y, et al. Age-related changes in the feedback regulation of gonadotrophin secretion by sex steroids in men. Acta Endocrinol (Copenh) 1981; 96(2):154–162.

173. Gentili A, Mulligan T, Godschalk M, et al. Unequal impact of short-term testosterone repletion on the somatotropic axis of young and older men. J Clin Endocrinol Metab 2002; 87:825–834.

☐ APPENDIX

Below, we present a summary of our biomathematical model of the hypothalamo–pituitary–testicular axis: the core model structure discussed in "Core Model Structure," p. 40. The full details are given in Ref. (4,8). In the schematic diagram of the axis given in Figure 6, the arrows denote the various feedback (–) and feedforward (+) interactions, enumerated as (1)–(7). The basic formulation of a feedback/feedforward signal is as a time-delayed, time-averaged concentration, with the time delay interval being denoted by (l_1, l_2):

$$\int_{t-l_2}^{t-l_1} Y(r)dr = \frac{1}{l_2-l_1}\int_{t-l_2}^{t-l_1} Y(r)dr \quad \begin{array}{l}\text{(feedback or feedforward}\\ \text{signal at time } t)\end{array}$$

where $Y(r)$ is a hormone concentration at time r. We will denote a given concentration at time t as $X(t)$, in particular, $X_G(t)$, $X_L(t)$, $X_{Te}(t)$ are the concentrations of GnRH (G), LH (L), and testosterone (Te). Similarly, a secretion rate at time t will be denoted by $Z(t)$, for example, $Z_G(t)$, $Z_L(t)$, and $Z_{Te}(t)$ are the the corresponding secretion rates.

We consider the feedback/feedforward effects (discussed in "Deterministic Interfaces," p. 40) to be exerted via dose-response functions [denoted by $H(\cdot)$'s]. Subscripts (e.g., $H_{1,2}$) correspond to the feedback/feedforward relationships [(1)–(7)] given in Figure 6, and the time-delays (see "Time Delays" p. 41) for the j-th relationship are denoted as $(l_{j,1}, l_{j,2})$. We allow four major feedback/feedforward dose–response functions: $H_{1,2}(\cdot)$, which describes the GnRH pulse firing rate as a joint function of Te feedback and GnRH auto-feedback; $H_3(\cdot)$, which gives the rate of GnRH pulse-mass accumulation as a function of Te feedback; $H_4(\cdot)$, which defines the rate of Te secretion as a function of LH feedforward; and, $H_{5,6}(\cdot, \cdot)$ for the rate of accumulation of the LH pulse mass as a function of Te feedback and GnRH feedforward. Interaction (7), not described by a dose-response function, denotes a refractory period for LH pulsing, described below.

We model the above feedback interactions [except for (7)] using empirically determined logistic dose-response functions ("Deterministic Interfaces," p. 40):

$$H(x_1) = \frac{C}{1+\exp\{-(A+B_1x_1)\}}+D, \quad \text{for interactions (3) and (4)}$$

$$H(x_1, x_2) = \frac{C}{1+\exp\{-(A+B_1x_1+B_2x_2)\}}+D, \quad \text{for interaction (5,6)}$$

or where the coefficients themselves are described by logistic functions, for example,

$$H(x_1, x_2) = \frac{C(x_2)}{1+\exp\{-(A+B_1x_1)\}}+D(x_2), \quad \text{for interaction (1,2)}$$

If $B_j > 0$, the feedback is positive (i.e., feedforward effect); if $B_j < 0$, the feedback is negative.

Pulse Generator (See "Stochastic Elements," p. 41)

We assume that GnRH signaling dictates the pulse times for LH after a finite time delay τ_L, reflecting hypothalamo-pituitary portal blood transit, and a post-stimulus refractory interval, r_L, when further GnRH inputs are ignored. Thus, there will be two corresponding sets of pulse times: $T_G^0, T_G^1, T_G^2, \ldots$ and $T_L^0, T_L^1, T_L^2, \ldots$ Let in vivo $T_L^0 = T_G^0 + \tau_L$ and define recursively

$$T_L^k = \left[\underset{j}{\text{Min}}\{T_G^j \mid T_G^j \geq T_L^{k-1}\}\right] + \tau_L.$$

One model for the pulsing mechanism, is that the conditional probability density for T_G^k, given T_G^{k-1}, is a Weibull distribution:

$$p(s \mid T_G^{k-1}) = \gamma \times \lambda^r(s-T_G^{k-1})^{\gamma-1}\exp^{-\lambda^\gamma(s-T_G^{k-1})^\gamma}$$

The parameter λ is a rate, expressing expected number of pulses/day, and γ a scale parameter. The pulse times form a Weibull renewal process. The homogeneous Poisson process is the special case of $\gamma = 1$. For $\gamma > 1$ in the Weibull distribution, variability is less than that for the Poisson process. Thus, γ inversely defines the degree of variability of the inter-pulse interval lengths. If one wishes to allow for Te and GnRH feedback modulation of the "pulsing intensity," then the constant λ, above, needs to be replaced by $\lambda(\cdot)$, now a (random) process, which implements such modulation:

$$\lambda(t) = H_{1,2}\left(\int_{(t-l_{1,2})}^{(t-l_{1,1})} X_{Te}(r)\,dr, \int_{(t-l_{2,2})}^{(t-l_{2,1})} X_G(r)\,dr\right)$$

and the conditional probability density for T_G^k given T_G^{k-1} will then be given by:

$$p\left(s \mid T_G^{k-1}, \lambda(\cdot)\right) = \gamma \times \lambda(s)\left(\int_{T_G^{k-1}}^{s}\lambda(r)dr\right)^{\gamma-1}\exp^{-\left(\int_{T_G^{k-1}}^{s}\lambda(r)dr\right)^\gamma}$$

with associated counting processes:

$$N_G(t) = \sum_{j=0}^{\infty} 1_{\{T_G^j \leq t\}} \quad \text{and} \quad N_L(t) = \sum_{j=0}^{\infty} 1_{\{T_L^j \leq t\}}$$

In [4,8], this formulation of the pulse generator is fully developed and discussed.

Pulsatile (GnRH, LH) and Continuous (Te) Secretion

We assume that for each hormone that there are both basal and nonbasal rates of hormone synthesis. The basal rate β is assumed to be constant. The nonbasal rate of synthesis $S(\cdot)$, however, will be feedback/feedforward modulated, and can be released continuously, or accumulated and released in a pulsatile manner. The gonad cells do not accumulate hormone granules, but always allow newly synthesized unencapsulated hormone to pass directly through the membrane with only diffusion delays, resulting in a continuous release of non-basal synthesis. GnRH (G) and LH (L) mass, however, are released in a pulsatile manner. We will represent a pulse at time t, having started at pulse time T^j, by a function $M^j \times \psi(t - T^j)$, where M^j is the pulse mass, and the pulse shape, $\psi(\cdot)$, represents the instaneous rate of secretion per unit mass per distributional volume:

$$\psi_i(s) = \frac{\beta_i^{(3)}}{\Gamma\left(\beta_i^{(1)}\right)\left(\beta_i^{(2)}\right)^{\left(\beta_i^{(1)}\beta_i^{(3)}\right)}} s^{\left(\beta_i^{(1)}\beta_i^{(3)}\right) - 1} e^{-\left(s/\beta_i^{(2)}\right)^{\beta_i^{(3)}}} \quad [i = G, L]$$

In [8], we show that the mathematical effect of cascadingtarget-tissue reactions to a signal input is (approximately) the multiplication of the initial feedback/feedforward signal by a linear combination of exponential functions, which allows ongoing glandular responses after the signal is withdrawn. In particular, we denoted cascading effect due to the GnRH feedforward on LH, by $\Gamma_G(\cdot)$. Hence, synthesis (S) for GnRH and LH are represented by:

Synthesis (S)

The "average" or expected synthesis: $[H(\cdot)]$, for given feedback/feedforward strengths, plus allowable variation (ξ) (see "Stochastic Elements," p. 41).

$$S_L(t) = H_{5,6}\left(\int_{T_L^{N_L(t)} - l_{5,2}}^{T_L^{N_L(t)} - l_{5,1}} X_G(s)ds \times \Gamma_G\left(t - T_L^{N_L(t)}\right), \int_{t - l_{6,2}}^{t - l_{6,1}} X_{Te}(s)ds\right)$$

$$+ \xi_l(t) \quad [\text{LH synthesis}]$$

$$S_G(t) = H_3\left(\int_{t - l_{3,2}}^{t - l_{3,1}} X_{Te}(s)ds\right) + \xi_G(t) \quad [\text{GnRH synthesis}]$$

An important component of the above model is the allowance for variation (ξ) in LH and GnRH synthesis, which results in allowable variation in the pulse masses (A, below).

j-th Pulse Mass

Accumulation of Mass (Q), Fraction Remaining of Previous Pulse Mass (Ψ), and resulting next Pulse Mass (M), and i = G, L:

$$Q_i^j = \int_{T_i^{j-1}}^{T_i^j} S_i(t)dt \quad [\text{accum. of newly synthesized hormone granules}]$$

$$\Psi_i(T_i^{j-1}, T_i^j) = 1 - \int_{T_i^{j-1}}^{T_i^j} \psi_i(s - T_i^{j-1})ds \quad \text{(fraction of mass remaining for later secretion)}$$

$$M_G^j = \Psi_G(T_G^{j-1}, T_G^j)M_G^{j-1} + Q_G^j \quad \text{(j-th GnRH pulse mass)}$$

$$M_L^j = \Psi_L(T_L^{j-1}, T_L^j)M_L^{j-1} + Q_L^j \quad \text{(j-th LH pulse mass)}$$

Te Synthesis:

$$S_{Te(t)} = H_4\left(\int_{t - l_{4,2}}^{t - l_{4,1}} X_L(s)ds\right)$$

The resulting hormone secretion rates are then given by:

$$Z_G(t) = \beta_G + M_G^j \psi_G(t - T_G^j) \quad \text{for } T_G^j \leq t < T_G^{j+1}$$

$$Z_L(t) = \beta_L + M_L^j \psi_L(t - T_L^j) \quad \text{for } T_L^j \leq t < T_L^{j+1}$$

$$Z_{Te}(t) = \beta_{Te} + H_4\left(\int_{t - l_{4,2}}^{t - l_{4,1}} X_L(s)ds\right)$$

Secreted molecules undergo combined diffusion and advection in the bloodstream at very rapid rates (short half-life component, α_1), and are removed more slowly but irreversibly (long half-life component, α_2), resulting in the following biexponential elimination model for hormone concentrations: $i = G, L, Te$

$$X_i(t) = \left(a_i^{(1)}e^{-\alpha_i^{(1)}t} + a_i^{(2)}e^{-\alpha_i^{(2)}t}\right)X_i(0) + \int_0^t \left(a_i^{(1)}e^{-\alpha_i^1(t-r)}\right.$$
$$\left. + a_i^{(2)}e^{-\alpha_i^2(t-r)}\right)Z_i(r)dr$$

What one then observes is a discrete-time samplingof these processes, plus joint uncertainty due to blood withdrawal, sample processingand hormone measurement errors, $\epsilon_i(k)$:

$$Y_i(k) \overset{\text{def}}{=} X_i(t_k) + \epsilon_i(k), \quad k = 1, \ldots, n, \quad i = G, L, Te.$$

Application of the Model to Pulsatile Data

Without going into detail, in (6,7,9,144) the authors have developed methods to estimate, from observed concentration pulsatile data, the above described pulse times and the various LH secretory and kinetic parameters (see "Application of Dynamic Concepts," p. 44). Similarly, if GnRH concentrations were observed, the GnRH secretion and elimination parameters could be estimated. In this approach, the pulse times are first estimated, and the LH secretion and elimination parameters are then estimated, conditioned on the pulse times. The following linear approximation to the LH secretion rate is the basis for the procedure:

$$Z_L(t) = \beta_L + \sum_{T_L^j \leq t}(\eta_{0,L} + \eta_{1,L} \times (T_L^j - T_L^{j-1}) + A_L^j)\psi_L(t - T_L^j)$$

The j-th pulse mass is assumed to be a linear function of the interpulse length, plus allowable variation in pulse mass: A_L^j.

At present, the authors are developing methods for jointly estimating the LH and testosterone secretory and kinetic parameters, in particular the modulation of testostrone secretion by the LH feedforward signal.

5

Normal Spermatogenesis

Jeffrey B. Kerr
Department of Anatomy and Cell Biology, Monash University, Victoria, Australia

☐ OVERVIEW

Commencing at the early phase of puberty and continuing throughout life into old age (1–3), spermatogenesis is a dynamic, complex process of germ-cell proliferation and maturation that is dependent upon extrinsic hormone support and local cellular interactions—many of which, thus far, remain to be defined.

In histologic sections of the seminiferous tubules in man, the seminiferous epithelium is a tall, stratified epithelium up to 80 μm in depth, and its total volume occupies about half the volume of the entire testis. The stratified appearance is attributable to the layered arrangement of germ cells, commencing with those resting on the basement membrane (spermatogonia) followed by several layers of growing spermatocytes and spermatids, and toward the apical regions of the epithelium, the elongated spermatids and fully formed spermatozoa.

Support for this elaborate stratification is provided by the tall, columnar Sertoli cells that extend from the base of the epithelium and terminate at the luminal margin (Fig. 1). It is the function of the Sertoli cells not only to provide physical support to the germ cells as they ascend apically through the seminiferous epithelium, but also to provide crucial functional support to spermatogenesis through their metabolic secretory activities. Regulation of spermatogenesis occurs via the actions of gonadotropins and steroids, but this is, in a sense, merely the first of many other mechanisms operating within the seminiferous epithelium and is reflected by the intimate association of germ cells with the Sertoli cells (Figs. 2–4). The necessity for local regulatory mechanisms that govern the process of spermatogenesis can be inferred from the synchronous development of the germ cells into six defined histological stages in man (Fig. 5) that are initiated by the controlled proliferation of spermatogonia that eventually produce young spermatocytes. These germ cells are destined to produce spermatozoa over a time period that is fixed for each species (about 10 weeks from spermatogonium to spermatozoa in the human male) (5).

Although the proliferation and morphogenesis of germ cells is dependent upon their own transcriptional and translational activities, the germ cells can only develop in association with the physiological environment that is created within the seminiferous epithelium by the Sertoli cells (4,6). How this is achieved at the cellular and molecular level is not fully understood and is the subject of ongoing investigations into the roles of androgens (7), follicle-stimulating hormone (FSH) (8), the androgen receptor (AR) (9–13), and improved in vitro isolation techniques suitable for molecular studies (14). In keeping with the fact that the germ cells are constantly but slowly changing their morphology in a dynamic, maturing epithelium, the Sertoli cells also show cyclic changes in ultrastructure (15,16) and function (4,17). The question can thus be posed, is it the Sertoli cells or the germ cells that regulate the order and coordination of germ-cell mitosis, meiosis, and sperm formation during spermatogenesis? Recent studies with xenotransplantation of germ cells (rat or hamster testis cells transplanted to mouse testes or mouse testis cells to rat testes) have shown that xenogenic germ cells are capable of populating recipient testes and undergoing normal spermatogenesis, leading to the formation of spermatozoa. The time period required for donor germ cells to complete spermatogenesis appeared to be identical to that associated with the normal in vivo donor germ-cell cycles. This observation indicates that in the environment afforded by the external-recipient Sertoli cells, the donor germ cells control their own fate with passive support from Sertoli cells (18–20).

In summary, it seems that spermatogenesis is a conservative, programmed process that relies on the Sertoli cells as transducers of the hormone signals attributable to the gonadotropins and androgens that are the principal stimulatory agents for normal testicular function.

☐ SPERMATOGONIA: THE SOURCE OF NEW GERM CELLS

Spermatogonia consist of germline stem cells that are self-renewing, as well as a class of spermatogonia that act as differentiating germ cells, further dividing and eventually maturing into spermatozoa. Maintenance and renewal of a stock of spermatogonial stem cells is obviously a prerequisite for the continuity of spermatogenesis. The cytological characteristics and kinetic properties of spermatogonia in mammals and in man have been extensively studied, and several recent

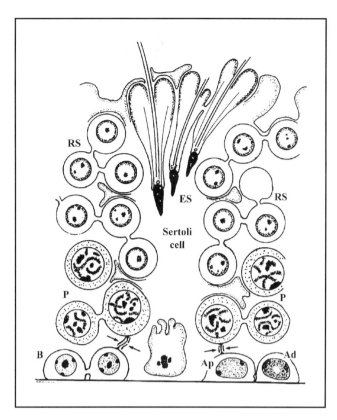

Figure 1 Schematic of a small segment of a human seminiferous tubule showing the germ cells associated with a Sertoli cell at stage I of the cycle of the seminiferous epithelium. The Sertoli cell creates a special physiological environment that simultaneously supports the germ cells as they undergo mitosis (the basal spermatogonia), meiotic maturation (the spermatocytes), and spermiogenesis (round and elongating spermatids). The rate and synchrony of germ-cell development is intrinsic to the germ cells, suggesting that although the germ cells are dependent on Sertoli cells for nutritional and physical support, their patterns of gene expression operate autonomously. Note cytoplasmic bridges that connect B spermatogonia, spermatocytes, and spermatids, indicating synchronous development of conjoined clones of germ cells. Specialized tight junctions (*arrows*) are created in the basal region of Sertoli cells at the sites of apposition of adjacent Sertoli cell plasma membranes. Junctional specializations form the so-called "blood-testis" barrier. *Abbreviations*: Ad, spermatogonia type A dark; Ap, spermatogonia type A pale; B, spermatogonia type B; ES, elongating spermatids; P, pachytene primary spermatocytes; RS, round spermatids. *Source*: From Ref. 4.

reviews are available (21–26). Studies by Clermont of the human seminiferous epithelium and, in particular, the spermatogonia (27,28) provided the first definitive characteristics of their morphology and kinetics of proliferation. Three main types are recognized: two of type A and one of type B. Type A dark (Ad) spermatogonia exhibit dark-staining chromatin in the nucleus with a central pale area. Type A pale (Ap) cells have pale-staining nuclei with one or two nucleoli associated with the nuclear membrane. The type B spermatogonia

that arise by mitosis from the Ap type show a granulated nuclear chromatin and a nucleolus (Fig. 6).

The major functions of the spermatogonia are: (*i*) to act as self-renewing stem cells, (*ii*) to proliferate by mitosis to amplify their numbers, and (*iii*) to differentiate into cells that are committed to supply germ cells that proceed into the meiotic maturation pathway. The last characteristic defines the type B spermatogonia that divide once by mitosis to produce a pair of young primary spermatocytes.

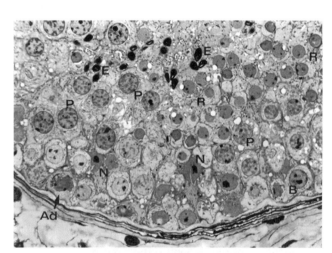

Figure 2 Human seminiferous epithelium at stage I. *Abbreviations*: Ad (*arrow*), type A dark spermatogonium; B, type B spermatogonium; E, elongating spermatids; N, Sertoli cell nuclei; P, pachytene primary spermatocytes; R, round spermatids.

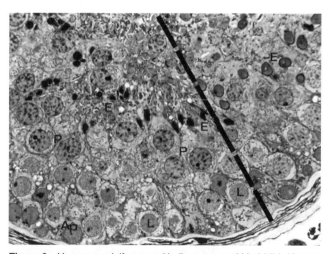

Figure 3 Human seminiferous epithelium at stage V (*middle*). Human seminiferous epithelium at stage IV (*right*). *Abbreviations*: Ap, type A pale spermatogonium; E, spermatocytes, elongating spermatids; L, leptotene; P, pachytene.

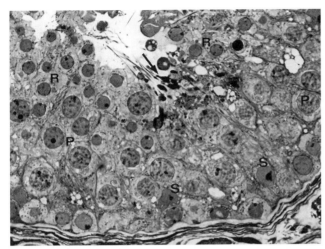

Figure 4   Human seminiferous epithelium at stage II. Mature sperm (*arrows*) to be released into the tubule lumen. *Abbreviations*: P, pachytene primary spermatocytes; R, round spermatids; S, Sertoli cell nuclei.

The role of the type A spermatogonia in relation to the first two functions is not absolutely clear. Various models of spermatogonial proliferation have been proposed (27,28). Based upon the measured proportions of Ad:Ap:B:early-spermatocytes being 1:1:2:4, one such model has proposed that Ad spermatogonia are the stem cells that were once capable of two types of "equivalent" mitoses—that is, they produced either

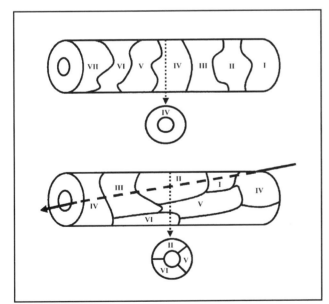

Figure 5   Comparison of the organization of germ-cell associations or stages (*Roman numerals*) in most mammals (*upper*) and in man and some primates (*lower*) when viewed in intact seminiferous tubules. In mammals, the stages usually succeed each other, forming the "wave of the seminiferous epithelium." In man, the stages often are irregularly distributed but occasionally show an ordered pattern along the *broken* line that in three dimensions conforms to a gyrating helical path along the tubule. When viewed in transverse histologic sections, the common mammalian pattern reveals the whole seminiferous epithelium at one of the stages. In contrast, the human seminiferous tubule usually shows two or more stages, giving the impression of an irregular organization of germ-cell stages.

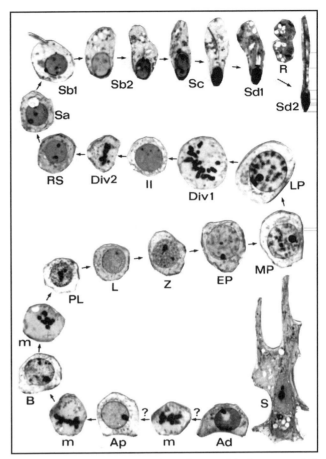

Figure 6   Photomicrographs of the cell types of the human seminiferous epithelium illustrating the sequence of spermatogenesis that requires about 10 weeks for completion. *Abbreviations*: Ad, type A dark spermatogonium; Ap, type A pale spermatogonium; B, type B spermatogonium; Div 1, first maturation division; Div 2, second maturation division; EP, early pachytene spermatocyte; II, secondary spermatocyte; L, leptotene spermatocyte; LP, late pachytene spermatocyte; m, mitosis; MP, mid pachytene spermatocyte; PL, preleptotene spermatocyte; RS, round spermatid; S, Sertoli cell proliferation; Sa, spermatid with acrosomic vesicle (cap to acrosome phase); Sb1, spermatid with developing acrosomic cap; Sb2 and Sc, Spermatids showing elongation, condensing nucleus, and flagellum; Sd1 and Sd2, spermatids with full flagellum and discarded excess residual (R) cytoplasm; Z, zygotene spermatocyte.

a pair of Ad or a pair of Ap spermatogonia. The latter then produced a pair of B spermatogonia by mitosis, which in turn divided to yield a pair of young spermatocytes. With further studies of spermatogonia in primates that also have type A and B cells, the notion that type Ad spermatogonia qualify as stem cells rather than the Ap type has been questioned. Type Ad spermatogonia rarely divide and in fact remain quiescent except, for example, after irradiation of the testis, at which point they resume activity if the numbers of type Ap spermatogonia are depleted (29). The activated Ad cells are reported to transform into Ap type spermatogonia, which then divide further. In man, type Ap spermatogonia (but not Ad cells) persist after radiotherapy, estrogen therapy, and in cryptorchid testes (30,31). In monkeys, type Ap spermatogonia may transform into Ad spermatogonia, suggesting that the latter are set aside as a stock of nonproliferative stem cells (32,33). Current opinion favors type Ad spermatogonia as reserve stem cells.

Studies of the cytological arrangements of spermatogonia in the seminiferous epithelium of mice and rats have shown that the most primitive types of spermatogonia are not randomly dispersed along the basement membrane, but are topographically positioned in niches (34,35). Such niches represent microenvironments in which the cell population and their extracellular matrices consist of a subpopulation of stem cells and their progeny, both of which are regulated with regard to their proliferative activity and maturation. The existence of spermatogonial niches suggests one mechanism for the highly localized control of germ-cell differentiation that leads to the histologically recognizable coordination of spermatogenesis around the circumference and along the axis of the seminiferous tubules. A balance between the renewal of spermatogonial stem cells and their differentiation is required for cyclic waves of spermatogenesis, and an obvious candidate that participates in maintenance of these activities is the Sertoli cell. Recent studies in mice indicate that Sertoli cells express Ets-type transcription factors that are essential for self-renewal of spermatogonial stem cells (36).

When type Ap spermatogonia divide to produce germ cells that are committed to enter the process of spermatogenesis (i.e., cells destined to form sperm), cytokinesis is incomplete, forming two daughter cells that are interconnected by a cytoplasmic bridge. The pair of conjoined spermatogonia remains linked such that when required to divide again to form type B spermatogonia, for example, a chain of germ cells is generated, each connected by intercellular bridges. Exceptions to this arrangement are the stem cells that do not have bridges. Bridges are believed to allow exchange of gene products to produce "clones." The clones further mature and divide during spermatogenesis, but they remain interconnected and therefore develop in synchrony until their morphogenesis is complete and spermatozoa are fully formed, at which point their extremely slender bridges are broken. Individual sperm are then released from the seminiferous epithelium into the lumen of the seminiferous tubule.

In view of the coordination and synchrony of germ-cell clones that proceed through spermatogenesis that explains the arrangement of defined histological stages (Fig. 5), there must be mechanisms that operate to ensure that suitable numbers of germ cells are maintained in the seminiferous epithelium. Significant reduction of their numbers will impact negatively on daily sperm production and fertility, whereas overproduction of germ cells cannot be sustained by a fixed Sertoli-cell population. Cell death during human spermatogenesis is a significant event, contributing to homeostasis within the seminiferous epithelium. In the past, it was believed that germ-cell death accounted for the comparatively poor efficiency of sperm production in man—in contrast to other primates and mammals (37–40). More recent studies have shown that this concept is incorrect. Extensive quantitative analysis of the numbers of germ-cell types and Sertoli cells in rodents, numerous primate species, and in man has shown that the efficiency of spermatogenesis in the human testis is comparable with most other species (41–44). Apoptosis is the mechanism by which abnormal or excessive numbers of germ cells are eliminated from the seminiferous epithelium, with the products of cell degeneration being disposed of by the phagocytic activity of the Sertoli cells. Although apoptosis can occur at any step during spermatogenesis, germ-cell death occurs more frequently at the early phases of cell division and this includes the spermatogonial population (45,46). The impact of apoptosis occurring spontaneously or following experimental induction in spermatogenesis is discussed in several reviews (47–49). The factors responsible for initiating spontaneous apoptosis among spermatogonia or other germ cells remain unknown, but evidence gained from transgenic or gene-knockout studies suggests that many genes encode for cell death or survival. Genes regulating spermatogonial survival include the Bcl-2 family, in which some members favor cell survival and are termed antiapoptotic (Bcl 2, Bcl-x_L, and Bcl-w) while others promote cell death and thus are proapoptotic (Bax, Bak, Bad, and Bim). It is thought that the ratio of these competing proteins determines the susceptibility of spermatogonia to death (49,50). In humans, the incidence of spermatogonial apoptosis is reported to be significantly greater in Asian than in Caucasian subjects (46), and similar trends occur in these groups for spermatocyte and spermatid apoptosis.

In addition to the primary actions of gonadotropins and androgens on spermatogenesis (see below, "Hormone Regulation"), the regulation of spermatogonial kinetics is crucially dependent upon local growth factors and paracrine and autocrine activities. Three such examples are vitamin A, stem-cell factor (SCF), and glial cell line–derived neurotropic factor (GDNF). Exogenous vitamin A or retinoic acid treatment stimulates type A spermatogonial proliferation following mitotic arrest induced by experimental vitamin A deficiency (51). SCF, produced by the Sertoli cells, is a mitogen and survival factor for spermatogonia acting through a membrane receptor termed c-kit; disruption of SCF action prevents spermatogonial mitoses (52,53). GDNF, a member of the TGF-β family, is secreted by Sertoli cells. In transgenic mice with decreased GDNF expression, spermatogonia fail to proliferate, resulting in Sertoli cell-only seminiferous tubules (54).

□ SPERMATOCYTES: THE KEY TO GENETIC DIVERSITY

Mitosis of type B spermatogonia results in the production of two primary spermatocytes that proceed through the process of meiosis, in which each of them divides to produce two secondary spermatocytes, each dividing again to yield four spermatids. Meiosis is fundamentally important for the survival of a species since it allows genetic recombination, thus guaranteeing biological diversity among progeny. Further, meiosis provides a mechanism to create haploid gametes containing a 22,X or 22,Y chromosome complement. Meiotic maturation of spermatocytes is highly conserved in evolution, involving chromosome pairing, exchange of genetic material between homologous chromosomes, and the generation of haploid gametes that occur in single-cell eukaryotes and metazoans.

Preleptotene Stage

The first phase in the life of a primary spermatocyte begins when it loses contact with the basement membrane of the tubule and with subsequent maturation enters the "adluminal" compartment of the seminiferous epithelium; that is, facing the lumen of the seminiferous tubule. This domain is thought to be physiologically distinct from the basal compartment, which is created between the basement membrane and the inter-Sertoli cell tight junctions (blood–testis barrier) that are found on the luminal side of the spermatogonia and the earliest primary spermatocytes (Fig. 1). Designated as preleptotene primary spermatocytes, these germ cells engage in DNA synthesis (for the last time in spermatogenesis), and each chromosome is duplicated to form twin copies termed sister chromatids. Thus, the chromosome number remains diploid (2n), but the DNA content is doubled (4C) compared with the amount found in the spermatogonia. Preleptotene primary spermatocytes have finely granulated chromatin uniformly distributed throughout the nucleus. From the preleptotene stage, the spermatocytes enter the long period (3.5 weeks in man) of meiotic maturation, and each step of their evolution can be distinguished by their distinctive nuclear morphology and gradual increase in size up to the first meiotic division (Figs. 5 and 7).

Leptotene Stage

With the appearance of fine chromatin filaments in the nucleus, the spermatocyte is then classified as a leptotene (thin and thread-like) type, and this marks the commencement of the long prophase of the first meiotic maturation division. Gradual swelling of the nucleus and the thickening of the chromatin threads is characteristic of the zygotene (pairing) step, in which homologous chromosomes become synapsed and remain closely associated by the synaptonemal complexes. The latter are microfibrillar protein complexes (unique to germ cells) that eventually extend the entire length of each male and female homolog in each bivalent.

Pachytene Stage

Increasing in volume again as the zygotene step proceeds into the pachytene (large size) step, the chromosomes

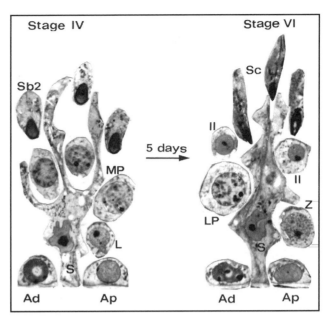

Figure 7 Photomicrographic reconstruction of stage IV and stage VI of the cycle of the seminiferous epithelium in man. As seen in histologic sections, each stage is a "snapshot" of the cell types that make up a defined sequence of cellular associations that may succeed one another in time in a given area of the seminiferous tubule. The postspermatogonial germ cells are constantly but slowly evolving through the process of meiotic maturation, followed by the differentiation of early spermatids into spermatozoa. In stage VI, some late LP can occur in conjunction with secondary spermatocytes (II), reflecting the continuum of germ-cell development that occurs within a cytologically defined stage. Accompanying these cytological changes, the Sertoli cells also show dynamic, cyclic changes in morphology that reflect alterations in their function in response to hormone stimulation and local interactions with the cohorts or families of germ cells that each Sertoli cell supports from the basal lamina to the lumen of the tubule. Stages IV and VI each last for about 24 hours, but it takes around five days for germ cells at stage IV to transform into those recognizable as stage VI. The duration of one series of six stages (I–VI) or of one cycle of the seminiferous epithelium is about 16 days. Completion of spermatogenesis—that is, from the first time that a spermatogonium divides up to the formation of a mature spermatozoon—requires slightly more than four repetitions of the cycle. *Abbreviations*: Ad, type A dark spermatogonium; Ap, type A pale spermatogonium; II, secondary spermatocyte; L, leptotene spermatocyte; LP, late pachytene spermatocyte; MP, mid pachytene spermatocyte; S, Sertoli cell; Sb2 and Sc, spermatids showing elongation, condensing nucleus and flagellum; Z, zygotene spermatocyte.

become characteristically condensed, thickened, and shortened. Crossing over or exchange of genetic material occurs during the long pachytene step (approximately 16 days) to ensure genetic reassessment between male and female homologs in a process termed "genetic recombination." The number of chromosomes in combination with the many recombination sites between them ensures that germ cells emerging from meiosis have many millions of slightly different genotypes, all of which are related.

The process of independent assortment of chromosomes that occurs when each primary spermatocyte divides at the end of meiosis to create two secondary spermatocytes also increases the genetic diversity among the gametes.

DNA Repair

DNA repair is an essential activity during the meiotic recombination process. During homologous recombination, a single DNA strand of one chromatid is paired with one of the two strands of a nonsister chromatid; this paired stretch may contain mismatches that must be recognized and repaired by a mismatch repair system (55). Meiotic recombination in germ cells (crossovers between nonsister chromatids) requires similar mechanisms of breaking and ligation of DNA molecules and proteins that mediate recombination between sister chromatids during double-strand break (DSB) repair in somatic cells. During meiotic prophase, the DSBs are repaired in a controlled manner by specific topoisomerase, an enzyme conserved from yeast to humans that is strongly expressed in meiotic cells (56). The number and location of DSBs in meiosis is strictly controlled, and the crossover sites or foci containing the mismatch protein repair protein can be identified by immunostaining of isolated nuclei. The mouse spermatocyte contains about 23 crossovers, and in humans, more than 50 such foci have been identified (55). If DNA damage is extensive, DNA repair mechanisms may be inadequate, and further cell development will not continue. In mitotically active cells, a control mechanism checks the integrity of the genome during the cell cycle and is capable of blocking the cycle until the DNA damage is repaired. Failure of repair via the cell-cycle checkpoint genes may result in cell apoptosis such as found in pachytene arrest in some mouse models of male infertility. In fact, arrest of spermatogenesis at pachytene is a common finding in testis biopsies taken from infertile men (57–59).

Among the many factors that govern the survival of primary spermatocytes through their long phase of meiotic maturation, local and intracellular levels of steroids certainly play a major role. Although it is not known how steroids—particularly androgens and estrogens—affect the function of germ cells, it is known that withdrawal of endogenous steroids results in extensive germ-cell dysfunction, developmental arrest, and cell death (49,60–63). The key role of the Sertoli cells in supporting meiosis has been emphasized by studies in transgenic mice, in which the overexpression of androgen-binding protein (ABP), a Sertoli cell secretory product, was associated with meiotic arrest (64). The block in spermatogenesis occurs at the pachytene and metaphase I step of meiosis, resulting in germ-cell apoptosis. It is suggested that an excess of intracellular ABP raises bound testosterone but decreases free hormone levels, resulting in disruption of germ-cell function. In short-term cultures of human seminiferous tubules, the addition of testosterone to incubation media significantly suppressed spermatocyte apoptosis that otherwise occurs under serum-free conditions (65). In similar experiments using human seminiferous tubules, estradiol was a potent inhibitor of germ-cell apoptosis, possibly acting via nongenomic mechanisms as the effects on germ-cell survival occurred within four hours of estrogen treatment (66).

With the formation of two secondary spermatocytes at the end of meiosis I, each of them is haploid, containing 22 duplicated autosomes and either a duplicated X or Y chromosome. Secondary spermatocytes are short lived (about one day) and have a spherical nucleus with finely granulated chromatin together with globular chromatin masses. Division II then proceeds without DNA replication to produce two haploid spermatids with 23 single chromosomes.

☐ SPERMATIDS: SPERMIOGENESIS FORMS SPERMATOZOA

The youngest spermatids, about 8 μm in diameter, contain a spherical nucleus with dispersed chromatin and a small nucleolus. Characteristically, the mitochondria tend to cluster near the plasma membrane. Spermiogenesis refers to the morphological and functional transformation of an early spermatid into a fully formed spermatozoon with no cell division. In man, this phase of spermatogenesis requires 24 days. The complex metamorphosis of a round spermatid into a 65-μm spermatozoon is a process that is far from being understood, although studies linking structural changes of the spermatids to changes in their gene expression have been made possible using transgenic and knockout animal models and the availability of appropriate mutations that affect spermiogenesis together with experimental alterations of hormone action and supply (4,57,67–69).

The structural changes to the spermatids as they proceed through spermiogenesis have been extensively studied and documented (5,70–73). Based upon the changing morphology of the spermatid nucleus, as observed in paraffin sections of the human testis (74), six steps in development have been proposed and designated as: Sa, Sb1, Sb2, Sc, Sd1, and Sd2 (Fig. 6). When examined with electron microscopy, these developmental events that shape and transform the spermatids can be conveniently described as four phases, designated as Golgi, cap, acrosomal, and maturation phases. It should be emphasized that these cytological classifications in fact represent a continuously evolving process involving changes that simultaneously occur, to a large degree, in a defined series of structural modifications to the nucleus and the cytoplasm and the development of the sperm tail.

The first two phases are chiefly concerned with the development of the acrosome, a modified secretory granule that originates from the round spermatid Golgi apparatus. Consisting of hydrolytic enzymes and a protein matrix, the biogenesis of the acrosome begins as small granules/vesicles elaborated from the Golgi that are collectively termed "proacrosomic vesicles." These coalesce into a single spherical acrosomic vesicle that attaches to the nucleus.

In the cap phase, the vesicle flattens and expands to cover the surface of the nucleus, eventually covering about 60% of the spermatid nucleus as it transforms from a spherical to a pyriform shape. At the time of sperm–egg fusion during fertilization, the acrosomal hydrolases are released, allowing sperm penetration of the surface of the egg zona pellucida. The formation of the acrosome is dependent upon certain proteins that promote fusion of proacrosomic granules (75), and a failure of this process results in spermatids that have no acrosomes, rendering them incapable of nuclear condensation and elongation—critical for normal sperm development. Such defective spermatozoa have poor motility due to a defective sperm tail that arises because of sperm elongation failure (76). Some of the idiopathic human infertility syndromes associated with reduced sperm count and production of round spermatozoa may be a result of acrosomal dysgenesis of early spermatids (77,78).

While acrosome formation is proceeding at one pole of the nucleus, centrioles at the opposite pole begin to form the primordium of the flagellum or sperm tail. Of the pair of centrioles associated with the nucleus, the proximal component becomes articulated with the nuclear membrane, whereas the distal or longitudinal centriole gives rise to the axial filament, or axoneme of the growing tail, consisting initially of a 9+2 arrangement of microtubules. Both centrioles reside within the sperm neck, a hollow cone consisting of nine cross-striated columns that are continuous with the nine outer dense fibers (ODFs) of the sperm tail. ODFs are the main cytoskeletal structures of the tail and consist of multiple polypeptide molecules (76) that serve to stiffen the tail and run longitudinally with the central axoneme until they disappear at the end of the tail. The 912 arrangement of axoneme microtubules is responsible for sperm motility, since disturbances of the formation of nexin linkages and dynein arms are associated with immotile sperm (79). Initially dispersed in the spermatid cytoplasm, mitochondria external to the ODFs in the middle piece of the tail (approximately 5 μm long) congregate around the ODFs in a helical pattern and serve as a source of energy for motility. Beyond the middle piece is the principal piece of the tail (approximately 45 μm long) that contains seven of the ODFs and long fibrous sheaths that are linked to the ODFs by connecting proteins, termed "transverse ribs." At its termination, the ODFs and fibrous sheaths disappear from the principal piece, and the end piece consists only of a disorganized axoneme.

Genes encoding some ODFs may be transcribed early in primary spermatocytes and other ODFs are transcribed later in early spermatids, whereas translation of the mRNAs for the ODFs commences during spermiogenesis. Thus some of the ODF formation relies upon translational repression until the appropriate development of the sperm tail (80). Temporary storage of mRNAs and their subsequent translation at defined steps in spermiogenesis are a reflection of the fact that transcription in developing spermatids is progressively terminated as the sperm nucleus compacts its chromatin into the condensed spatulate structure of the sperm head.

Once it has acquired a developing acrosome, the spermatid nucleus is reoriented such that it appears to be displaced toward one pole of the cell. At the same time, the spermatid reshapes itself into an oval structure with elongation of the cytoplasm away from the nucleus. The acrosome rotates to face the basal aspect of the seminiferous epithelium, which dictates that the caudal spermatid cytoplasm and the emerging axoneme/flagellum now point toward the tubule lumen. Alignment and positioning of the elongating spermatids are controlled by their interface with the Sertoli cell-plasma membrane. The plasma membrane of the spermatid that covers the acrosome is attached to a unique type of cell–cell junction, termed an "ectoplasmic specialization" (ES). As the spermatid elongates, ESs are formed subjacent to the Sertoli cell-plasma membrane that embraces the developing acrosome and sperm head. ESs facing spermatid nuclei consist of long cisternae of endoplasmic reticulum separated from the spermatid membrane by cytoskeletal proteins that include actin, vinculin, integrins (81), and espin, a protein thought to be an actin-bundling molecule (82). This ES complex provides for adhesion of the sperm heads that are dissembled at the end of spermiogenesis, allowing for release of the spermatozoa into the tubule lumen. Adhesion between Sertoli cells and the spermatid acrosome is both androgen dependent (83,84) and FSH dependent (85).

Remodeling of sperm nuclear architecture accompanied by condensation of the chromatin is associated with a progressive cessation of transcription. As the spermatid nucleus becomes elliptical and then pyriform in shape (Fig. 7), the nuclear chromatin forms many dense aggregations, occasionally interrupted by clear spaces or vacuoles. Eventually, toward the end of the acrosome phase, the nuclear chromatin is highly compacted and forms a homogeneous electron-dense mass. The nuclear histones are replaced by transition proteins (86) and then by protamines (87) that stabilize the DNA. The genes for protamines are transcribed in round and early elongating spermatids that are stored in a translationally repressed state by the binding of protein repressors before being translated into elongated spermatids (88). Compaction of the transcriptionally inert chromatin is associated with a significant reduction in nuclear volume that contributes to the unique and striking differences in head shape unique to each species.

In the maturation phase of spermiogenesis, the long caudal cytoplasm that extends around and along the length of the flagellum is separated from the head and tail. It condenses into several globular components, termed "residual cytoplasmic bodies," that contain a variety of organelles and inclusions together with the redundant nuclear membrane discarded as the sperm nucleus contracts in volume. When the sperm disengage from the ESs of the Sertoli cells, the sperm are released into the tubule lumen, but the residual bodies are retained and are phagocytosed by the Sertoli cells.

☐ GENE EXPRESSION AND SPERMATOGENESIS

In model organisms, many genes have been identified for fertility, and mutations in these genes cause infertility due to developmental defects of the germ cells. Despite the prevalence of human infertility (as many as 1 in 25 men and 15% of couples), few fertility loci have been mapped and about half of all cases of infertility presented by couples can be attributed to the male partners, who are otherwise healthy (89,90). The causes of male infertility or subfertility are far ranging, involving chromosomal aneuploidies, translocations, and point mutations for example in the AR, FSH receptor, and FSH molecule (57,61,91–94).

There is special interest in the genes located on the Y chromosome since there are proven correlations between testicular pathology in infertile men and microdeletions associated with specific regions of the Y chromosome (94–97). In 1976, karyotyping of azoospermic men revealed deletions on the long arm (Yq) of the Y chromosome (98), leading to the azoospermic factor (AZF) hypothesis: the absence of specific fertility genes on the Y chromosome would result in no sperm. Since the microdeletions define these regions, AZFa, AZFb, and AZFc have been named from proximal to distal on Yq (Fig. 8). Most (80%) deletions occur in the AZFc region, with 15% and 5%, respectively, occurring in the AZFb and AZFa regions (99). Deletions occurring across all three AZF regions, although rare, are associated with germ-cell arrest or Sertoli cell–only testes (58). Within the euchromatic segment of the Y chromosome, the male-specific regions occur on both the short

(Yp) and long arms and encode 27 protein-coding genes most of which are mapped to the Yq arm (100).

In the AZFa region, the first gene found to be absent in infertile patients was DFFRY (Drosophila fat facets related Y), recently renamed USP9Y (ubiquitin specific protease 9, Y chromosome). This gene is ubiquitously expressed in a variety of tissues and the testis (101). Deletions of USP9Y have been particularly linked with azoospermia. For the AZFb region, the genes most likely involved in spermatogenesis are those of the RBMY (RNA binding motif on the Y) family. These are expressed only in the germline and their function(s) are not clear. Most deletions in the Y chromosome that are found in severe oligospermia and azoospermia occur in the AZFc region. The *DAZ* gene (deleted in azoospermia) is considered responsible for the AZFc phenotype (58), and it is expressed in primary spermatocytes and spermatogonia (102). The *DAZ* gene family consists of four almost identical copies, but different combinations of partial deletions of these gene copies may result in impaired fertility or may have little or no effect on fertility (59). Partial *DAZ* deletions are infrequently found in cases of cryptorchidism (77). Recent studies report that DAZ proteins are also found in fetal gonocytes (the germline stem cells that give rise to the spermatogonia); this and their persistence in spermatids (103) both suggest that DAZ family proteins may act in multiple cell types at multiple points in spermatogenesis.

There are possibly thousands of genes encoded on both the X and Y chromosomes, as well as the autosomes that influence the process of spermatogenesis (94). Many of these may be expressed not only in the germline but also in the Sertoli cells. Studies of gene inactivations or deletions in knockout mice have shown that more than 200 genes are directly or indirectly involved in male fertility (104). In man, the expression of germ-cell transcripts has suggested that coordinated activities of several thousand genes are linked to full male fertility (105). Genetic screening of testis cDNA arrays and oligonucleotide array probes of genomic DNA are likely to be developed as diagnostic tools in the future evaluation and selection of treatment options for infertile men. A summary of the incidence of microdeletions known to be associated with the Yq chromosome is given in Table 1.

Because testosterone is critical for the maintenance of spermatogenesis, changes to or the absence of a functional AR system will impact androgen signaling and cause moderate-to-severe impairment of germ-cell development. The *AR* gene is located on the X chromosome and point mutations or excessive CAG (polyglutamine) repeats therein are associated with male infertility (106). In healthy populations, the number of CAG repeats ranges between 11 and 31; if greater than 40, however, additional disorders arise, including a variety of neurodegenerative diseases (107). Men with 26 or more CAG repeats in the *AR* gene have a significantly greater chance of being azoospermic compared with those with fewer repeats (108), although a recent study

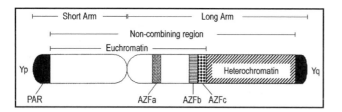

Figure 8 Schematic representation of the Y chromosome. The short arm (Yp) is linked via a centromere to the long arm (Yq). The PAR that pair with the X chromosome during meiosis are located at each end. The nonrecombining region consists of repetitive sequences that may be homologous to parts of the X chromosome or may contain Y-specific regions. The heterochromatin region may be one-half to two-thirds of the Yq. The three loci associated with spermatogenic defects contain gene clusters defined as AZFs and map to AZFa, AZFb, and AZFc. Most infertile men with severe oligospermia or azoospermia have microdeletions in the AZFc locus. Conditions of germ-cell arrest or Sertoli cell-only syndrome commonly have more extensive deletions involving AZFa and AZFb regions. *Abbreviations*: AZF, azoospermic factor; PAR, pseudoautosomal regions; Yp, short arm; Yq, long arm. *Source*: From Refs. 57, 58.

Table 1 Yq Microdeletions in Infertile Men

Category	Total no. studied	% with microdeletions
All patients	4868	8.2
Idiopathic oligospermia	155	11.6
Idiopathic <5 million/mL	35	
Nonobstructive azoospermia	769	10.5
Idiopathic azoospermia	199	18.0
Idiopathic severe hypospermatogenesis	85	24.7
Sertoli cell only	55	34.5
Fertile men	2663	0.4

Source: From Ref. 58.

(109) reported an absence of larger CAG repeat alleles in 30 azoospermic Japanese men. More data are required to define the normal range of *AR* gene CAG repeats in order to clarify male infertility risks as well as to determine if intermediate CAG expansions are benign or silent polymorphisms.

□ HORMONE REGULATION

The primary hormones that act on the testis are luteinizing hormone and FSH. The former stimulates testosterone synthesis and secretion from the Leydig cells, and the latter binds to spermatogonia and Sertoli cells to activate, by largely unknown mechanisms, the proliferation and maturation of the germ cells. Exactly how androgens and FSH initiate the cascade of biochemical activities that causes pubertal maturation of the testis and then maintains adult spermatogenesis is poorly understood. Based upon analyses of the effects of mutations in the human FSH–receptor gene (110) and similar studies of FSH-β and FSH receptor in knockout mice (111,112), it appears that in men, FSH is not essential for spermatogenesis but is required for stimulating quantitatively normal levels of spermatogenesis (113).

With regard to androgens, the cellular sites that respond to testosterone stimulation are beginning to be defined. It is generally accepted that human germ cells do not have ARs; thus, the Sertoli cell ARs are thought to mediate the biological actions of androgens on spermatogenesis (114). In the mouse, spermatogonia lacking functional ARs are capable of undergoing spermatogenesis when introduced into the seminiferous tubules of azoospermic mice with functional AR (115). In vivo, the conversion of round spermatids to spermatozoa is highly dependent on testosterone; in conjunction with FSH, testosterone thus is necessary for the conversion of spermatogonia to spermatocytes (4), but how these events are controlled at the subcellular or molecular level remains unknown. Insights into the role and cellular sites of androgen in spermatogenesis have become available from studies of ubiquitous or conditional (Sertoli cell-specific) AR knockout mice. Ablation of the AR among all cell types results in undescended testes and infertility, whereas Sertoli cell-specific AR knockout models reveal that meiotic maturation of spermatocytes and formation of spermatids is severely impaired and associated with infertility (9–13). These findings show that androgens are an essential requirement for normal spermatogenesis, acting directly via AR in the Sertoli cells. Because Sertoli cell numbers per testis are reduced in ubiquitous AR knockouts but unaffected in Sertoli cell-specific AR knockout mice, it is likely that another cell type, perhaps the androgen-dependent peritubular myoid cells, are required for the normal postnatal proliferation of Sertoli cells that establishes their numbers in the adult testis (12,13). Further studies of AR knockout models may provide opportunities for identification of androgen action on spermatogenesis that are relevant to human fertility.

□ REFERENCES

1. Nielsen CT, Skakkebaek NE, Richardson DW, et al. Onset of the release of spermatozoa (spemarche) in boys in relation to age, testicular growth, pubic hair, and height. J Clin Endocrinol Metab 1986; 62(3): 532–535.

2. Nieschlag E, Lammers U, Freischem CW, et al. Reproductive functions in young fathers and grandfathers. J Clin Endocrinol Metab 1982; 55(4):676–681.

3. Synder PJ. Effects of age on testicular function and consequences of testosterone treatment. J Clin Endocrinol Metab 2001; 86(6):2369–2372.

4. De Kretser DM, Risbridger GP, Kerr JB. Functional morphology. In: DeGroot L, Jameson JL, eds. Endocrinology. 4th ed. Philadelphia: Saunders, 2001: 2209–2231.

5. de Kretser DM, Kerr JB. The cytology of the testis. In: Knobil E, Neill JD, eds. The Physiology of Reproduction. 2nd ed. New York: Raven Press, 1994:1177–1290.

6. Kerr JB. Macro, micro, and molecular research on spermatogenesis: the quest to understand its control. Micros Res Tech 1995; 32(5):364–384.

7. Zhang F, Pakarainen T, Poutanen M, et al. The low gonadotropin-independent constitutive production of testicular testosterone is sufficient to maintain spermatogenesis. Proc Nat Acad Sci USA 2003; 100(23): 13692–13697.

8. Johnston H, Baker PJ, Abel M, et al. Regulation of Sertoli cell number and activity by follicle-stimulating

hormone and androgen during postnatal development in the mouse. Endocrinology 2004; 145(1):318–329.

9. Yeh S, Tsai M, Xu Q, et al. Generation and characterization of androgen receptor knockout (ARKO) mice: an in vivo model for the study of androgen functions in selective tissues. Proc Nat Acad Sci USA 2002; 99(21): 13498–13503.

10. Chang C, Chen Y, Yeh S, et al. Infertility with defective spermatogenesis and hypotestosteronemia in male mice lacking the androgen receptor in Sertoli cells. Proc Nat Acad Sci USA 2004; 101(18):6876–6881.

11. Holdcraft RW, Braun RE. Androgen receptor function is required in Sertoli cells for the terminal differentiation of haploid spermatids. Development 2004; 131(2):459–467.

12. Tan KAL, DeGendt K, Atanassova N, et al. The role of androgens in Sertoli cell proliferation and functional maturation: studies in mice with total or Sertoli cell-selective ablation of the androgen receptor. Endocrinology 2005; 146(6):2674–2683.

13. DeGendt K, Swinnen JV, Saunders PTK, et al. A Sertoli cell-selective knockout of the androgen receptor causes spermatogenic arrest in meiosis. Proc Nat Acad Sci USA 2004; 101(5):1327–1332.

14. Kotaja N, Kimmins S, Brancorsini S, et al. Preparation, isolation and characterization of stage-specific spermatogenic cells for cellular and molecular analysis. Nat Meth 2004; 1(3):249–254.

15. Griswold MD, Russell LD, eds. The Sertoli Cell. Clearwater, FL: Cache River Press, 1993.

16. Kerr JB. An ultrastructural and morphometric analysis of the Sertoli cell during the spermatogenic cycle in the rat. Anat Embryol (Berl) 1988; 179(2):191–203.

17. Sharpe RM. Regulation of spermatogenesis. In: Knobil E, Neill JD, eds. The Physiology of Reproduction. 2nd ed. New York: Raven Press, 1994:1363–1434.

18. Clouthier DE, Avarbock MR, Maika SD, et al. Rat spermatogenesis in mouse testis. Nature 1996; 381(6581): 418–421.

19. Ogawa T, Dobrinski I, Avarbock MR, et al. Xenogenic spermatogenesis following transplantation of hamster germ cells to mouse testes. Biol Reprod 1999; 60(2): 515–521.

20. Ogawa T, Dobrinski I, Brinster RL. Recipient preparation is critical for spermatogonial transplantation in the rat. Tissue Cell 1999; 31(5):461–472.

21. Meachem S, von Schonfeldt V, Schlatt S. Spermatogonia: stem cells with a great perspective. Reproduction 2001; 121(6):825–834.

22. Lin H. The self-renewing mechanism of stem cells in the germline. Curr Opin Cell Biol 1998; 10(6):687–693.

23. de Rooij DG, Grootegoed JA. Spermatogonial stem cells. Curr Opin Cell Biol 1998; 10(6):694–701.

24. de Rooij DG, Russell LD. All you wanted to know about spermatogonia but were afraid to ask. J Androl 2000; 21(6):776–798.

25. Kerr JB, Loveland KL, O'Bryan MK, et al. Cytology of the testis and intrinsic control mechanisms. In Neill JD,

26. ed. Knobil and Neill's Physiology of Reproduction, 3rd ed. Philadelphia, PA: Elsevier, 2006:849–969.

26. Kerr JB, deKretser DM. Functional morphology of the testis. In DeGroot LJ, Jameson JL, eds. Endocrinology, Vol. 3. 5th ed. Philadelphia, PA: Elsevier, 2005: 3089–3120.

27. Clermont Y. Spermatogenesis in man. A study of the spermatogonial population. Fertil Steril 1966; 17(6): 705–721.

28. Clermont Y. Renewal of spermatogonia in man. Am J Anat 1966; 118(2):509–524.

29. van Alphen MM, de Rooij DG. Depletion of the seminiferous epithelium of the rhesus monkey, Macaca mulatta, after X-irradiation. Br J Cancer Suppl 1986; 7:102–104.

30. Schulz C. Morphological characteristics of the spermatogonial stem cells in man. Cell Tissue Res 1979; 198(2): 191–199.

31. Schulz C. Survival of human spermatogonial stem cells in various clinical conditions. Fortschr Der Androl 1981; 7(1):58–68.

32. Fouquet JP, Dadoune JP. Renewal of spermatogonia in the monkey (Macaca fascicularis). Biol Reprod 1986; 35(1):199–207.

33. van Alphen MM, van de Kant HJ, de Rooij DG. Repopulation of the seminiferous epithelium of the rhesus monkey after X irradiation. Radiat Res 1988; 113(3):487–500.

34. Chiarini-Garcia H, Hornick JR, Griswold MD, et al. Disribution of type A spermatogonia in the mouse is not random. Biol Reprod 2001; 65(5):1179–1185.

35. Chiarini-Garcia H, Raymer AM, Russell LD. Nonrandom distribution of spermatogonia in rats: evidence of niches in the seminiferous tubules. Reproduction 2003; 126(4):669–680.

36. Chen C, Ouyang W, Grigura V, et al. ERM is required for transcriptional control of the spermatogonial stem cell niche. Nature 2005; 436(6):1030–1034.

37. Johnson L. Efficiency of spermatogenesis. Microsc Res Tech 1995; 32(5):385–422.

38. Johnson L, Chaturvedi PK, Williams JD. Missing generations of spermatocytes and spermatids in seminiferous epithelium contribute to low efficiency of spermatogenesis in humans. Biol Reprod 1992; 47(6): 1091–1098.

39. Johnson L, Petty CS, Neaves WB. A comparative study of daily sperm production and testicular composition in humans and rats. Biol Reprod 1980; 22(5):1233–1243.

40. Johnson L, Petty CS, Neaves WB. Further quantification of human spermatogenesis: germ cell loss during postprophase of meiosis and its relationship to daily sperm production. Biol Reprod 1983; 29(1):207–215.

41. Wistuba J, Schrod A, Greve B, et al. Organization of seminiferous epithelium in primates: relationship to spermatogenic efficiency, phylogeny, and mating system. Biol Reprod 2003; 69(3):582–591.

42. Luetjens CM, Weinbauer GF, Wistuba J. Primate spermatogenesis: new insights into comparative testicular

organization, spermatogenic efficiency and endocrine control. Biol Rev 2005; 80(4):475–488.

43. Zhengwei Y, McLachlan RI, Bremner WJ, et al. Quantitative (stereological) study of the normal spermatogenesis in the adult monkey (Macaca fascicularis). J Androl 1997; 186:681–687.

44. Zhengwei Y, Wreford NG, Royce P, et al. Stereological evaluation of human spermatogenesis after suppression by testosterone treatment: heterogeneous pattern of spermatogenic impairment. J Clin Endo Metab 1998; 83(6):1284–1291.

45. Heiskanen P, Billig H, Toppari J, et al. Apoptotic cell death in the normal and cryptorchid human testis: the effect of human chorionic gonadotropin on testicular cell survival. Ped Res 1996; 40(2):351–356.

46. Hikim AP, Wang C, Lue Y, et al. Spontaneous germ cell apoptosis in humans: evidence for ethnic differences in the susceptibility of germ cells to programmed cell death. J Clin Endocrinol Metab 1998; 83(1):152–156.

47. Sinha Hikim AP, Lue YH, Wang C, et al. Spermatogenesis and germ cell death. In: Wang C, ed. Male Reproductive Function. Norwell, MA: Kluwer Academic Publishers, 1999:19–39.

48. Blanco-Rodriguez J. A matter of death and life: the significance of germ cell death during spermatogenesis. Int J Androl 1998; 21(5):236–248.

49. Sinha Hikim AP, Swerdloff RS. Hormonal and genetic control of germ cell apoptosis in the testis. Rev Reprod 1999; 4(1):38–47.

50. Adams JM, Cory S. The Bcl-2 protein family: arbiters of cell survival. Science 1998; 281(5381):1322–1326.

51. de Rooij DG, van Dissel-Emiliani FMF. Regulation of proliferation and differentiation of stem cells in the male germ line. In: Potten CS, ed. Stem Cells. London: Academic Press, 1997:283–313.

52. Allard EK, Blanchard KT, Boekelheide K. Exogenous stem cell factor (SCF) compensates for altered endogenous SCF expression in 2,5-hexanedione-induced testicular atrophy in rats. Biol Reprod 1996; 55(1): 185–193.

53. Rossi P, Dolci S, Albanesi C, et al. Follicle-stimulating hormone induction of steel factor (SLF) mRNA in mouse Sertoli cells and stimulation of DNA synthesis in spermatogonia by soluble SLF. Dev Biol 1993; 155(1):68–74.

54. Meng X, Lindahl M, Hyvonen ME, et al. Regulation of cell fate decision of undifferentiated spermatogonia by GDNF. Science 2000; 287(5457):1489–1493.

55. Baarends WM, van der Laan R, Grootegoed JA. DNA repair mechanisms and gametogenesis. Reproduction 2001; 121(1):31–39.

56. Romanienko PJ, Camerini-Otero RD. Cloning, characterization, and localization of mouse and human SPO11. Genomics 1999; 61(2):156–169.

57. McLachlan RI, Mallidis C, Ma K, et al. Genetic disorders and spermatogenesis. Reprod Fertil Dev 1998; 10(1):97–104.

58. Foresta C, Moro E, Ferlin A. Y chromosome microdeletions and alterations of spermatogenesis. Endocr Rev 2001; 22(2):226–239.

59. Ferlin A, Tessari A, Ganz F, et al. Association of partial AZFc regions deletions with spermatogenic impairment and male infertility. J Med Genet 2005; 42(1):209–213.

60. Sharpe RM, Donachie K, Cooper I. Re-evaluation of the intratesticular level of testosterone required for quantitative maintenance of spermatogenesis in the rat. J Endocrinol 1988; 117(1):19–26.

61. Sharpe RM, Maddocks S, Kerr JB. Cell-cell interactions in the control of spermatogenesis as studied using Leydig cell destruction and testosterone replacement. Am J Anat 1990; 188(1):3–20.

62. O'Donnell L, Robertson KM, Jones ME, et al. Estrogen and spermatogenesis. Endocr Rev 2001; 22(3):289–318.

63. Matsumoto AM, Paulsen CA, Bremner WJ. Stimulation of sperm production by human luteinizing hormone in gonadotropin-suppressed normal men. J Clin Endocrinol Metab 1984; 59(5):882–887.

64. Selva DM, Tirado OM, Toran N, et al. Meiotic arrest and germ cell apoptosis in androgen-binding protein transgenic mice. Endocrinology 2000; 141(3):1168–1177.

65. Erkkila K, Henriksen K, Hirvonen V, et al. Testosterone regulates apoptosis in adult human seminiferous tubules in vitro. J Clin Endocrinol Metab 1997; 82(7): 2314–2321.

66. Pentakainen V, Erkkila K, Suomalainen L, et al. Estradiol acts as a germ cell survival factor in the human testis in vitro. J Clin Endocrinol Metab 2000; 85(5):2057–2067.

67. Huhtaniemi I, Bartke A. Perspective: male reproduction. Endocrinology 2001; 142(6):2178–2183.

68. Eidne KA, Henery CC, Aitken RJ. Selection of peptides targeting the human sperm surface using random peptide phage display identity ligands homologous to ZP3. Biol Reprod 2000; 63(5):1396–1402.

69. Kleene KC. A possible meiotic function of the peculiar patterns of gene expression in mammalian spermatogenic cells. Mech Devel 2001; (1061–2):3–23.

70. de Krester DM. Ultrastructural features of human spermiogenesis. Z Zellforsch Mikrosk Anat 1969; 98(4): 477–505.

71. Holstein AF. Ultrastructural observations on the differentiation of spermatids in man. Andrologia 1976; 8(2):157–165.

72. Kerr JB. Ultrastructure of the seminiferous epithelium and intertubular tissue of the human testis. J Electron Microsc Tech 1991; 19(2):215–240.

73. Clermont Y. The cycle of the seminiferous epithelium in man. Am J Anat 1963; 112:35–51.

74. Kang-Decker N, Mantchev GT, Jeneja SC, et al. Lack of acrosome formation in Hrb-deficient mice. Science 2001; 294(5546):1531–1533.

75. Clermont Y, Oko L, Hermo L. Cell biology of mammalian spermiogenesis. In: Desjardins C, Ewing LL, eds. Cell and Molecular Biology of the Testis. Oxford: Oxford University Press, 1993:332–376.

76. Petersen C, Aumuller G, Bahrami M, et al. Molecular cloning of Odf3 encoding a novel coiled-coil protein of sperm tail outer dense fibers. Mol Reprod Dev 2002; 61(1):102–112.

77. Peknicova J, Chladek D, Hozak P. Monoclonal antibodies against sperm intra-acrosomal antigens as markers for male infertility diagnostics and estimation of spermatogenesis. AM J Reprod Immunol 2005; 53(1):42–49.

78. Krausz C, Sassone-Corsi P. Genetic control of spermiogenesis: insights from the CREM gene and implications for human infertility. Reprod Biomed Online 2005; 10(1):64–71.

79. Afzelius BA, Eliasson R. Flagellar mutants in man: on the heterogeneity of the immotile-cilia syndrome. J Ultrastruct Res 1979; 69(1):43–52.

80. Schalles U, Shao X, van der Hoorn FA, et al. Developmental expression of the 84-kDa ODF sperm protein: localization to both the cortex and medulla of outer dense fibers and to the connecting piece. Dev Biol 1998; 199(2):250–260.

81. Mulholland DJ, Dedhar S, Vogl AW. Rat seminiferous (epithelium contains a unique junction ectoplasmic specialization) with signaling properties both of cell/cell and cell/matrix junctions. Biol Reprod 2001; 64(1):396–407.

82. Bartles JR, Zheng L, Wang M, et al. The actin-bundling protein espin and its role in the ectoplasmic specialization. In: Goldberg E, ed. The Testis: from Stem Cell to Sperm Function. New York: Springer, 2000: 151–160.

83. O'Donnell L, McLachlan RI, Wreford NG, et al. Testosterone withdrawal promotes stage-specific detachment of round spermatids from the rat seminiferous epithelium. Biol Reprod 1996; 55(4):895–901.

84. O'Donnell L, Narula A, Balourdos G, et al. Impairment of spermatogonial development and spermiation after testosterone-induced gonadotropin suppression in adult monkeys (Macaca fascicularis). J Clin Endocrinol Metab 2001; 86(4):1814–1822.

85. Cameron DF, Muffly KE, Nazian SJ. Development of Sertoli cell binding competency in the peripubertal rat. J Androl 1998; 19(5):573–579.

86. Meistrich M. Histone and basic nuclear protein transactions in mammalian spermatogenesis. In: Hnilica LS, Stein GS, Stein JL, eds. Histones and Other Basic Nuclear Proteins. Boca Raton, FL: CRC Press, 1989: 165–182.

87. Balhorn R. Mammalian protamines. In: Adolph KW, ed. Molecular Biology of Chromosome Function. New York: Springer Verlag, 1989:366–395.

88. Steger K, Pauls K, Klonisch T, et al. Expression of protamine-1 and -2 mRNA during human spermiogenesis. Mol Human Reprod 2000; 6(3):219–225.

89. Cram DS, Ma K, Bhasin S, et al. Y chromosome analysis of infertile men and their sons conceived through intracytoplasmic sperm injection: vertical transmission of deletions and rarity of de novo deletions. Fert Steril 2000; 74(5):909–915.

90. Clementini E, Palka C, Iezzi I, et al. Prevalence of chromosomal abnormalities in 2078 infertile couples referred for assisted reproductive techniques. Hum Reprod 2005; 20(2):437–442.

91. McPhaul MJ, Griffin JE. Male pseudohermaphroditism caused by mutations of the human androgen receptor. J Clin Endocrinol Metab 1999; 84(10):3435–3441.

92. Amory JK, Bremner W. Endocrine regulation of testicular function in men: implications for contraceptive development. Mol Cell Endocrinol 2001; 182(2): 175–179.

93. von Eckardstein S, Syska A, Gromoll J, et al. Inverse correlation between sperm concentration and number of androgen receptor CAG repeats in normal men. J Clin Endocrinol Metab 2001; 86(6):2585–2590.

94. Cram DS, O'Bryan MK, de Krester DM. Male infertility genetics—the future. J Androl 2001; 22(5):738–746.

95. Cooke HJ. Y chromosome and male infertility. Rev Reprod 1999; 4(1):5–10.

96. Krauz C, Quintana-Murci L, Rajpert-De Meyts E, et al. Identification of a Y chromosome haplogroup associated with reduced sperm counts. Hum Mol Genet 2001; 10(18):1873–1877.

97. Fox MS, Reijo Pera RA. Male infertility, genetic analysis of the DAZ genes on the human Y chromosome and genetic analysis of DNA repair. Mol Cell Endocrinol 2001; 184(1–2):41–49.

98. Tiepolo L, Zuffardi O. Localization of factors controlling spermatogenesis in the nonfluorescent portion of the human Y chromosome long arm. Hum Genet 1976; 34(2):119–124.

99. Ferlin A, Moro E, Rossi A, et al. The human Y chromosome's azoospermia factor b (AZFb) region: sequence, structure, and deletion analysis in infertile men. J Med Genet 2003; 40(1):18–24.

100. Skaletsky H, Kuroda-Kawaguchi T, Minx PJ, et al. The male-specific region of the human Y chromosome is a mosaic of discrete sequence classes. Nature 2003; 423(4):825–837.

101. Brown GM, Furlong RA, Sargent CA, et al. Characterisation of the coding sequence and fine mapping of the human DFFRY gene and comparative expression analysis and mapping to the Sxrb interval of the mouse Y chromosome of the DFFRY gene. Human Mol Genet 1998; 7(1):97–107.

102. Lin YM, Chen CW, Sun HS, et al. Expression patterns and transcript concentrations of the autosomal DAZL gene in testes of azoospermic men. Mol Hum Reprod 2001; 7(11):1015–1022.

103. Reijo RA, Dorfman DM, Slee R, et al. DAZ family proteins exist throughout male germ cell development and transit from nucleus to cytoplasm at meiosis in humans and mice. Biol Reprod 2000; 63(5):1490–1496.

104. Cram D, Lynch M, O'Bryan MK, et al. Genetic screening of infertile men. Reprod Fert Dev 2004; 16(3):573–580.

105. Schultz N, Hamra FK, Garbers D. A multitude of genes expressed solely in meiotic or postmeiotic spematogenic cells offers a myriad of contraceptive targets. Proc Nat Acad Sci USA 2003; 100(11):12201–12206.

106. Dowsing AT, Chen H, Clark M, et al. Linkage between male infertility and trinucleotide repeat expansion in the androgen-receptor gene. Lancet 1999; 354(9179): 640–643.

107. Choong CS, Wilson EM. Trinucleotide repeats in the human androgen receptor: a molecular basis for disease. J Mol Endocrinol 1998; 21(3):235–257.

108. Mifsud A, Sim CK, Boettger-Tong H, et al. Trinucleotide (CAG) repeat polymorphisms in the androgen receptor gene: molecular markers of risk for male fertility. Fertil Steril 2001; 75(2):275–281.

109. Sasagawa I, Suzuki Y, Ashida J, et al. CAG repeat length analysis and mutation screening of the androgen receptor gene in Japanese patients with idiopathic azoospermia. J Androl 2001; 22(5):804–808.

110. Tapanainen JS, Aittomaki K, Min J, et al. Men homozygous for an inactivating mutation of the follicle-stimulating hormone (FSH) receptor gene present variable suppression of spermatogenesis and fertility. Nat Genet 1997; 15(2):205–206.

111. Kumar TR, Wang L, Lu N, et al. Follicle stimulating hormone is required for ovarian follicle maturation but not male fertility. Nat Genet 1997; 15(2): 201–204.

112. Dierich A, Sairam MR, Monaco L, et al. Impairing follicle-stimulating hormone (FSH) signaling in vivo: targeted disruption of the FSH receptor leads to aberrant gametogenesis and hormonal imbalance. Proc Natl Acad Sci USA 1998; 95(23): 13612–13617.

113. Matsumoto AM, Karpas AE, Bremner WJ. Chronic human chorionic gonadotropin administration in normal men: evidence that follicle-stimulating hormone is necessary for the maintenance of quantitatively normal spermatogenesis in man. J Clin Endocrinol Metab 1986; 62(6):1184–1192.

114. Suarez-Quian CA, Martinez-Garcia F, Nistal M, et al. Androgen receptor distribution in adult human testis. J Clin Endocrinol Metab 1999; 84(1):350–358.

115. Johnston DS, Russell LD, Friel PJ, et al. Murine germ cells do not require functional androgen receptors to complete spermatogenesis following spermatogonial stem cell transplantation. Endocrinology 2001; 142(6): 2405–2408.

6

Physiology of the Epididymis

Russell C. Jones
Discipline of Biological Sciences, The University of Newcastle, New South Wales, Australia

Jean-Louis Dacheux
Equipe "Spermatozoides," UMR INRA-CNRS 6073, Institut National de la Recherche Agronomique, Nouzilly, France

☐ INTRODUCTION

It is generally recognized that the mammalian epididymis serves to transport sperm from the testis and then to mature and store them. There has been increasing interest in the epididymis, as its malfunction is recognized as a significant cause of infertility in men, and the recent advent of molecular methods of research has provided new insights into its function. Also, the epididymis now has potential as a target for male contraception. Because few relevant human studies have been performed to date, much of the current knowledge on the epididymis is the result of animal studies, and many of these are discussed this chapter.

☐ STRUCTURE

The extratesticular duct system of mammals consists of a number of units that differ in structure, function, and embryological development. The *rete testis* develops from the rete blastema, the *ductuli efferentes* develop from the mesonephric tubules, and the *ductus epididymidis* and *ductus deferens* develop from the mesonephric (Wolffian) duct. The organ formed by the ductuli efferentes and ductus epididymidis is usually referred to as the epididymis. There are numerous comprehensive descriptions of the structure of the duct system in a variety of mammals (1–3) and two in humans (4,5).

The rete testis is a cavernous region lined by a low epithelium that, in places, folds into the lumen. The intratesticular region receives each end of the seminiferous tubules via terminal regions where the epithelium lacks germinal cells. The ductuli efferentes leave the extratesticular region of the rete. The number of ductuli varies considerably between species: one in a small marsupial, 12 to 18 in humans (each 200–500 cm long) (5), and more than 20 in the elephant. The number is probably determined by the rate of fluid (and sperm) output from the testis. The ductuli are differentiated along their length into an *initial zone* where ductuli are fairly straight and run parallel with one another, and *coni vasculosi* where the ductuli follow a convoluted course and may anastomose. The ductuli may be pigmented brown due to the occurrence of dense bodies in the epithelium, particularly in the coni vasculosi (6). The arrangement of the ductuli in the coni varies between species, from the rat-like model in which pairs successively join together to form a common efferent duct that joins the ductus epididymidis end-to-end, to the human- and elephant-like model in which the caudal ductuli join the ductus end-to-side. In a detailed study of the human caput epididymidis, Yeung et al. (5) described at least seven types of tubules, each characterized by a different epithelium, including ductuli that end blindly and ones that join others together. The main ductuli efferentes of mammals have a tunic of smooth muscle and are lined by a low columnar epithelium composed of nonciliated and ciliated cells. The latter constitutes 15% of the epithelial cells and mainly occurs in groups of one to three cells in the rat (7). Flask-shaped cells have also been noted in human ductuli (4).

The human epididymis is 4 to 5 cm long and it is possible to recognize a caput, corpus, and cauda epididymidis (8), as in other scrotal mammals. The caput is attached to the testis by the superior epididymal ligament, the corpus by the mesoepididymis, and the cauda by the inferior epididymal ligament (9). The ductuli efferentes make up most of the caput epididymidis in humans. The ductus epididymidis, in its connective tissue matrix, makes up the rest of the epididymis. The cauda epididymidis is not as large in humans as in other scrotal mammals, with the exception of cats, gorillas, and some monkeys (10). It is not known why these animals have smaller caudae (which would store relatively fewer sperm).

Unfolded, the human ductus epididymidis is about six meters long, which is much shorter than that of a 3- to 4-kg monotreme (echidna, 12 m), a 6-kg marsupial (wallaby, 35 m), and domestic ungulates such as the ram, boar, and horse (at least 50 m) (11–14). The ductus is narrow proximally and widens toward the ductus deferens. In the rat and most other species, the ductus epididymidis is lined by a pseudostratified epithelium consisting of principal, apical, narrow, clear, basal, and halo (intraepithelial lymphocytes) cells. The epithelium is differentiated along the duct into at least six structurally distinct zones (2), reducing distally in the height and length of its stereocilia and varying in cytology of the principal cells and the occurrence of other cell types. In humans, however, the structural differentiation of the epididymal epithelium is not as distinct (4) as in most species. Yet, even in humans, the expression of genes along the duct is variable, with some genes having gradual changes in expression while others have abrupt changes (15,16).

In all mammals that have been studied, there is an initial segment of the ductus epididymidis that has a characteristic epithelium and microvasculature, and its structure and function is dependent on the luminal fluid flowing from the testis (17,18). The segment has characteristic coarse stereocilia on the principal cells, and narrow cells present in the epithelium and in most eutherian species such as the rat and domestic animals. The epithelium is very tall, with very long stereocilia. The c-ros tyrosine kinase gene is only expressed in the initial segment of the mouse epididymis, and in mice in which this gene has a targeted mutation, the segment is absent and the males are sterile even though spermatogenesis is normal (19). Little is known of the initial segment in the human epididymis: it is short and restricted to the region of the caput epididymidis where the ductuli efferentes join the ductus epididymidis (5). The *c-ros* gene is expressed in the epithelium along the rest of the epididymis but not in the initial segment (20).

The ductus epididymidis has a tunic of smooth muscle that varies along the ductus in thickness, cellular structure, and innervation. From the structural studies on humans (21) and physiological studies on laboratory and domestic animals (22,23), it is interpreted that slender muscle cells coat the length of the ductus, thus continuously moving sperm away from the testis. The effectors involved in ejaculation are an outer layer of thicker cells limited to the cauda epididymidis and ductus deferens. Consequently, repeated ejaculation only recruits sperm from this distal region of the duct system and thus only increases the rate of sperm transport through these regions. About half the number of sperm in the human ejaculate are derived from the distal ductus deferens and ampulla; the remainder come from the proximal ductus deferens and adjacent cauda epididymidis (24).

□ VASCULAR SUPPLY

The epididymis receives blood from two main arteries that anastomose in the corpus epididymidis in scrotal mammals. The epididymal artery branches from the testicular artery just above the spermatic cord and supplies the caput and corpus epididymidis and the deferential artery. The deferential artery branches from the iliac or hypogastric artery and supplies the cauda epididymidis and ductus deferens. The microvasculature is dense and similar along the human epididymis (25) and unlike species like the mouse in which the initial

segment has a dense fenestrated cylindrical network with frequent anastomoses (26).

□ EPITHELIAL FUNCTION AND LUMINAL MILIEU

There are no reports on the changes in composition of luminal fluids along the human epididymis. Early work on the rat indicated that there is a difference in the electrolyte composition of luminal fluids collected from the seminiferous tubules and rete testis of the rat, particularly in the concentration of potassium (27). Subsequent work on Japanese quail, however, indicated that these differences are probably due to contamination of micropuncture samples from the seminiferous tubules (28).

The ductuli efferentes reabsorb 96% of the fluid leaving the testis in the rat (29) and probably a similar proportion in other mammals. This absorptive function is probably essential for male fertility as targeted deletions of the estrogen receptor-α (ERKO) (30) and human epididymis-specific protein 6 (HE6/GPR64) (31) cause dysregulation of fluid reabsorption within the ductuli and infertility (30). In the normal rat, the reabsorption occurs with little net change in the concentration of electrolytes or osmotic pressure of the fluid (2). The epithelium is leaky at the distal end of the initial zone, with the concentration of electrolytes equilibrating between blood and the lumen of the ductuli (29). Acute control of the rate of fluid reabsorption by the ductuli is determined by the rate of flow of fluid into the ductuli and the concentration of sodium chloride in the fluid (32). Although the concentration of protein in fluid leaving the rete testis is low (1 mg/mL) and some protein is secreted by the ductuli, there is a net reabsorption of 80% of the protein entering the ductuli (29).

Whereas the function of the ductuli efferentes is to deliver spermatozoa concentrated in a small volume of luminal fluid, the ductus epididymidis modifies the composition of the fluid. The ductus also concentrates sperm further, mainly in the initial segment; however, the rate of fluid reabsorption is very low in this region compared to the ductuli efferentes (33). The ductus epididymidis maintains the low concentrations of calcium and magnesium that are in the lumen of the rete testis and generates a low pH and bicarbonate concentration. There is a reduction in the concentrations of sodium (and chlorine) and an increase in potassium along the duct so that the ratio of sodium:potassium in the fluid changes from about 10:1 in fluid entering the ductus to no more than 1:1 in the cauda epididymidis (34–36). A number of nonproteinaceous organic substances are secreted into the ductus in all the eutherian mammals that have been studied, particularly inositol (which is present in fluid leaving the testis), carnitine, and glycerophosphocholine. These substances are secreted in specific regions of the epididymis to achieve a luminal concentration higher than in blood and make up a high proportion of the total osmotic pressure of caudal epididymal fluid—about 50% in the rat (34,37,38). This is much higher than in luminal fluid from the ductus deferens of men in which the concentration of each of the organics is less than 6 mM (37). Although the organic compounds have received considerable attention, their role in the epididymis remains uncertain, except that they contribute to making caudal epididymal fluid hyperosmotic compared to blood. It is interpreted that carnitine may transport the acyl group in mitochondria, so that acyl CoA can act as a substrate for producing energy by oxidation (39). Moreover, supplementation with carnitine can significantly improve both sperm concentration and total sperm counts among men with astheno- or oligoasthenozoospermia.

There is considerable secretion and reabsorption of proteins in the epididymis. In the rat, for example, there is a fivefold net increase in protein concentration along the ductus. Two-dimensional electrophoresis of luminal fluids from domestic animals has shown that several hundred different proteins are present in the duct lumen, with some proteins being secreted at one site and reabsorbed a short distance along the epididymis (40–42). Some proteins regulate the function of the duct mucosa, such as basic fibroblast growth factor (43). Some of these are hydrophobes (lipocalines, clusterines, etc.) that may act as steroid-binding proteins for androgens regulating the duct mucosa, or steroids that modify the sperm membrane (44). Some play a role in protecting sperm, for example, against microbes (45), oxidation [glutathione peroxidase (GPX), superoxide dismutase, lactoferrin, etc.], and complement (46). Others, such as proteases and glycosidases and their inhibitors (47,48), are involved in modifying the sperm membrane, whilst others become closely associated with the sperm membrane and have been implicated in gamete fusion (49,50). The human epididymal proteome also contains hundreds of different proteins, and the majority are synthesized and secreted by the epididymal epithelium. The most abundant is clusterin, as in other mammals (51). In humans, however, this protein and others of testicular origin do not seem to be actively reabsorbed as in other species. Also, protein secretion, as well as its composition throughout the epididymis, is not as highly regionalized in humans as in other mammals that have been studied. The secretory activity of certain proteins only varies along the epididymis in amount and not qualitatively as in other species. It is suggested that this may be because human sperm mature more proximally in the epididymis than in other species (51).

□ SPERM TRANSPORT

Sperm spend little time in the ductuli efferentes—about 45 minutes in the rat (52). The rate of transport along the ductus epididymidis varies along its length, slowing considerably distally as the duct widens and sperm are "stored" until removed by ejaculation, as described above. The duration of sperm transit varies from 8 to 13 days in most mammals (Table 1). This process is generally considered to be faster in humans. Mean estimates vary from 4 (53) to 12 days (54), but a period of 2 to 4 days is common for many sperm, and some transit the duct in only 1 day (53,55), indicating that the age of sperm in the cauda epididymidis must vary considerably.

□ SPERM MATURATION

In laboratory and domestic mammals that have been studied, sperm were not found to be capable of fertilizing an ovum when they left the testes, unless they were artificially injected through the zona pellucida of an ovum. They must pass through at least part of the epididymis to achieve the capacity for motility and hyperactivation and to bind to the zona pellucida and undergo the acrosome reaction. Sperm achieve the capacity to fertilize ova more proximally in the epididymis of humans than in other mammals (56,57). They undergo the changes associated with epididymal maturation in other mammals except that there are none of the structural changes that occur in the epididymis of most mammals (8) apart from migration of the cytoplasmic droplet from the neck. Human sperm increase their capacity for motility during epididymal transit (58,59) from an immotile state in the rete testis or just showing slow oscillations of the tail with no forward progression. The percentage of motile sperm increases to almost maximum by the proximal corpus epididymidis, and the rate of forward motility increases until their arrival in the lower corpus epididymidis. Plasmalemma changes involving the loss and gain of specific proteins (58,60,61) occur, and there is a chemical reduction of sulfhydryl groups to form an increased number of disulfide bonds in the nucleus, perinuclear matrix, and tail structures of the sperm (62).

Claims that there is no need for sperm maturation in the mammalian epididymis have been discussed in detail by several authors (8,35,63). The claims based on studies of laboratory or domestic animals are poorly supported and typically have used sperm sampled from the caput epididymidis. These sperm would already have passed through the ductuli efferentes and part of the ductus epididymidis that is involved in sperm maturation. For the studies to be convincing, sperm should be sampled from the testis or rete testis. Nevertheless, in contrast to the results of work on laboratory and domestic animals, there is convincing evidence that posttesticular sperm maturation is not absolutely essential to achieve conception in humans. For example, the elegant epididymovasostomies of Schoysman and Silber have demonstrated conceptions when the ductus epididymidis was bypassed by connecting a seminiferous tubule or the rete testis to the ductus deferens (64,65). It is possible in these studies, however, that following anastomosis, luminal fluids

Table 1 Comparison of Sperm Production in Humans and a Variety of Other Scrotal Mammals

Parameter	Human	Rat	Ram	Rhesus monkey	Tammar wallaby
Body mass (g)	76,400[a]	559[b]	35,000[c]	9200[d]	5800
Testes/body mass (%)	0.06[a]	0.67[b]	0.91[c]	0.5[d]	0.54
Daily sperm production (10^6/g testis)	4.7[a]	23.7[b]	19[d]	23[d]	24
Epididymal transit time (days)	4[a]	8.4[b]	16.4[d]	10.5[d]	13[e]
Number of extragonadal spermatozoa					
$\quad$ 10^6/animal	201[a]	735b	>165,000[d]	6518[d]	9900[f]
$\quad$ 10^6/g body mass	0.003[a]	1.3[b]	4.7[d]	0.7[d]	1.7[f]
Number of ejaculates					
$\quad$ Produced by testes/day	0.8[a,g]	1[b,h]	2[d,i]	1[k]	2[f]
$\quad$ Available in extragonadal ducts[l]	1[a,g]	5[b,h]	28	4[k]	19[f]

[a]Ref. 53 [body mass (108)]; [b]Ref. 107; [c]Ref. 113; [d]Ref. 55; [e]Ref. 114; [f]Ref. 115; [g]Ref. 109; [h]Ref. 111; [i]Ref. 112; [j]Ref. 113; [k]Ref. 116. [l]The number of spermatozoa in the cauda epididymides/number of spermatozoa in an ejaculate of a sexually rested male; Ref.110.

from the testis modify the function of the ductus deferens. Further, it is unlikely that the probability of conception following a single intercourse in case of patients with epididymovasostomies is as high as for men with a normal epididymis. Also, it is perhaps noteworthy that in a study of men with obstructive azoospermia, the use of testicular and epididymal sperm for intracytoplasmic sperm injection (ICSI) produced similar conception rates, but the miscarriage rate was significantly higher when testicular sperm were used (66).

□ SPERM STORAGE

Sperm storage in the epididymis is important for normal male fertility because the period required for mammalian testes to produce sperm is much longer than the duration of coitus. The testes of laboratory and domestic mammals produce sperm equivalent to the number in one (rat) to two (ram) normal ejaculations per day (Table 1), and the cauda epididymidis contains between 5 (rat) and 28 (ram) times the number of sperm produced per testis per day (Table 1). In humans, the rate of sperm production is lower than in other mammals, and the number of sperm stored in the epididymis is relatively less. Humans require between one and two days to produce the number of sperm in a normal ejaculate, and the number stored in the cauda epididymides is only one to three times the daily sperm production. Bedford (8) noted unique characteristics of the human cauda epididymidis (relatively small size, lower content of sperm, and poor survival of sperm compared to other mammals) that are like the experimental response to warming the epididymis of laboratory animals to body temperature. He suggested that these characteristics are due to overheating of the epididymides as a consequence of human clothing. The temperature of the cauda epididymidis is normally a few degrees centigrade below testicular temperature in scrotal mammals (67); however, clothing increases the temperature of the cauda epididymidis in men from 29°C to 30°C in the naked state to 33°C to

34°C and higher, depending upon the tightness of the pants worn and the duration spent in a particular posture, such as sitting (8).

Work on laboratory and domestic animals has shown that sperm isolated in the cauda epididymidis between ligatures can maintain the capacity to fertilize an ovum for three weeks or more, and motility is retained nearly twice as long as the capacity to fertilize an ovum (8,68–72). It is generally considered that the human epididymidis is poorly adapted for sperm storage (8) and in some men, such as cancer patients, sperm motility may be lower in the cauda than corpus epididymidis (59). Bedford (8) suggested that this difference is probably due to sperm aging in the epididymis of men who experience a protracted period of abstinence, and he provided evidence that there is an inverse relationship between sperm viability in the cauda epididymidis and the duration of abstinence. Nevertheless, it is noteworthy that the ability to achieve conception may be retained for a considerable period in humans as sperm in the vas deferens can maintain the capacity for motility for as long as nine weeks postvasectomy (73).

Little is known about the mechanism of sperm storage in the epididymis. The duct mucosa must play an important role, as sperm are very concentrated in the cauda epididymidis, with the volume of sperm: epididymal plasma (spermatocrit) ranging from 21% in the rabbit to 68% in the Rhesus monkey (34). Even at a lower concentration, undiluted ejaculated ram sperm lose their viability within 30 minutes, presumably due to lactate production. It is known that the mucosa of the cauda epididymidis has a much greater capacity to transport fluid and solute than is indicated by estimates of net transport (74), and this must be important in maintaining a stable milieu. It is also known that the temperature of the cauda epididymidis is lower than testicular temperature (67), that oxygen tension is relatively low (75), and that there is no metabolizable sugar and relatively little other metabolic substrate in the luminal fluid (34). Further, the activity of sperm is suppressed in the cauda epididymis. Here, they are immotile in most species, and studies of undiluted caudal epididymal semen from the rat and the Tammar wallaby indicate that their metabolic rate is only one-fifth to one-third that of ejaculated sperm (76,77).

☐ REGULATION OF THE EPIDIDYMIS

There is convincing evidence that the epididymis is dependent on androgen and estrogen. Androgen may be transported from the testis via the vascular system or directly via the lumen of the epididymal ducts. Testosterone is the main androgen that leaves the testis by either route, but it is converted in the epididymis to more potent androgens. Dihydrotestosterone is produced by 5-α-reductase. Its activity is much higher in the proximal epididymis (mainly the initial segment) than more distally (3,78,79), except possibly in man (11,80) and cynomolgus monkey (81). Androstanediol is produced by the action of 3-α-hydroxysteroid dehydrogenase, which is present throughout the ductus epididymidis (3,82). The concentration of androgen in the duct lumen is higher than in peripheral blood, and the amount entering the duct via the rete testis of the rat is sufficient to account for the amount throughout the lumen of the duct (83). Consequently, although systemic androgen can play a role in regulating epididymal function (68), it is probably not essential for fertility.

Recent work shows that estrogen receptors are located in the ductuli efferentes and initial segment of the ductus epididymidis (84,85) and are essential for male fertility (30). Estrogen may be transported directly to the ductuli via the luminal route, or it may be produced by P450 aromatase in sperm (86) or the epithelium of human ductuli efferentes and proximal ductus epididymidis (87).

There is convincing evidence of a local (lumicrine) regulation of the epididymal epithelium by nonsteroidal factors transported with sperm from the testis. Withdrawal of this regulation by ligation of the ductuli efferentes, for example, causes dramatic dedifferentiation of the initial segment of the epididymis even when the concentration of systemic androgen is high (17). Transforming growth factor β has been identified (43,88) as a regulator of the initial segment, but there has been little work on luminal regulation for the rest of the ductus epididymidis.

☐ IMMUNOLOGY

As sperm production does not begin until after self-tolerance has been established by the immune system, the postmeiotic germ cells in the testis and epididymis essentially possess foreign antigens. The immune system is not normally exposed to these antigens, however, as the epithelia lining the duct system have well-developed tight junctions that provide a blood–luminal barrier, preventing the free movement of macromolecules in either direction (89).

Little is known of the immunology of the epididymis (90,91). Studies involving transplantation autografts (92) have suggested that mechanisms are present to maintain a state of immune suppression or immune privilege. Intraepithelial lymphocytes occur in the epididymal mucosa of humans and rats at a frequency similar to that seen in intestinal epithelium (93). The concentration of these lymphocytes varies along the epididymis, with CD8+ cells occurring at a greater frequency than CD4+ cells. It is assumed that the former are suppressor cells that serve to prevent the induction of an immune response to luminal antigens. Further, there is evidence that principal cells in the efferent ducts can express MHC class II antigens following immunization and thus may act as antigen-presenting cells. An immunocytochemical study indicates that the basal cells in human epididymal epithelium are macrophages, and the authors suggest that these cells could scavenge any antigenic products that may pass along the epididymis from the testis (94). In addition, epididymal plasma contains significant concentrations of complement inhibitors (95).

Generally, the blood–luminal barrier prevents the entry of antibody into the extragonadal ducts, with the exception of the rete testis, where some immunoglobulin G (IgG) is able to enter; however, the concentration achieved in the rete testis is less than 1% the concentration in blood (91,96). Most of this antibody is reabsorbed by the ductuli efferentes, but as fluid reabsorption by the ductuli is greater than protein reabsorption, the concentration of immunoglobulin increases about 1.5-fold as it passes through the ductuli. There is a further increase in concentration of IgG along the ductus epididymidis, but the concentration in caudal epididymal fluid only reaches 0.17% (rabbit) to 1.4% (rat) the concentration in blood.

☐ PATHOLOGY OF THE EPIDIDYMIS

Obstructive azoospermia is a major cause of infertility in men. It may develop following vasectomy and can persist even after reversal of vasectomy. As vasectomy prevents normal transport of sperm along the epididymis, sperm may accumulate within the duct. This may eventually cause rupture of the duct and granuloma formation, resulting in the development of antisperm antibodies, as seen in the blood of a high proportion of vasectomized men. Infection may also cause blockage of the duct system. Clavert et al. (97) concluded that the epididymis has little capability of protecting itself against infection and that epididymitis among young adults is often secondary to venereal urethritis, with the infection being propagated from the urethra toward the epididymis. The main infectious organisms are *Chlamydia trachomatis* and *Neisseria gonorrhoeae*. In older men, infection is often due to fecal organisms, particularly *Escherichia coli*.

Obstructive azoospermia may also be caused by primary lymphoma in the epididymis, a condition that could be confused with epididymitis (98). Further, an obstruction in the caput epididymidis with bronchiectasis is a hallmark of Young's syndrome (98).

Mutations of the cystic fibrosis transmembrane conductance regulator (CFTR) gene are a relatively frequent cause of male infertility due to obstructive azoospermia (99). They account for up to 2% of all cases of male infertility and up to 25% of all cases of obstructive azoospermia (100). Different mutations may result in congenital bilateral absence of the vas deferens, bilateral ejaculatory duct obstruction, or bilateral obstructions within the epididymis. The absent or severely reduced activity of CFTR protein affects ionic exchange across the epididymal mucosa and thus the composition of the luminal fluid. The viscosity of epididymal fluid may be increased, and the sloughing of epithelial cells expressing CFTR will further reduce the amount of CFTR activity. As a consequence, different parts of the epididymis or vas deferens may be blocked and progressively obliterated. The resultant obstructive azoospermia can be treated successfully, however, using sperm aspiration and ICSI (101). (For further information on ejaculatory duct obstruction and its treatment, see Chapters 18 and 33.)

Recent evidence indicates subfertility in men suffering from congenital chloride diarrhea (CLD), a rare inherited disease caused by mutations in the solute carrier family 26 member 3 (SLC26A3) gene (102). The gene normally expresses the Cl^-/HCO_3^- exchanger in efferent duct epithelium, but the exchanger was not expressed in a patient with CLD.

De Kretser et al. (103) described a condition called epididymal necrospermia, which is recognized on semen analysis with less than 5% of sperm having motility and normal shape. Although ultrastructural studies of ejaculates show marked degeneration of the acrosome and sperm head and loss of definition of the axonemal doublets, the structure of testicular sperm is normal. Frequent ejaculation usually improves semen quality.

Overheating has also been identified as a factor affecting epididymal function. Studies exposing the epididymis to body temperature (104,105) and aging sperm in the human epididymis indicate that overheating may affect the survival of sperm in the epididymis (8). Further, in a study using ram semen for artificial insemination, Mieusset et al. (106) found that a slight, intermittent increase in the subcutaneous scrotal temperature (1.4°C–2.2°C) can induce a significant increase in the embryonic mortality rate that becomes apparent on the fourth day of heating—an effect that must have occurred to sperm in the epididymis.

□ CONCLUSION

The human epididymis is different from that of most, if not all, scrotal mammals in that it is shorter relative to body mass, not so structurally differentiated, and plays a lesser role in posttesticular development and the storage of sperm. Nevertheless, available evidence indicates that it plays a significant role in ensuring a high probability of a man achieving paternity with natural mating. A number of pathologies of the epididymis have been identified that cause subfertility or infertility. Because some of the compounds involved in epididymal function are specific to the epididymis, it has the potential to be a target for achieving male contraception.

□ ACKNOWLEDGMENTS

The authors are grateful for advice from T.G. Cooper of the Institute of Reproductive Medicine, the University of Münster, Germany.

□ REFERENCES

1. Hamilton DW. Structure and function of the epithelium lining the ductuli efferentes, ductus epididymidis, and ductus deferens in the rat. In: Greep RO, Astwood EB, eds. Handbook of Physiology, Sect 7. Vol. 5. Washington DC: American Physiology Society, 1975: 259–301.

2. Jones RC. Evolution of the vertebrate epididymis. J Reprod Fertil 1998; 53:163–182.

3. Robaire B, Hermo L. Efferent ducts, epididymis, and vas deferens: structure, functions, and their regulation. In: Knobil E, Neill J, eds. The Physiology of Reproduction. Vol. 1. 2nd ed. New York: Raven Press Ltd, 1988:999–1080.

4. Holstein A-F. Morphologische Studien am Nebenhoden des Menschen. Stuttgard: Geortge Thieme Verlag, 1969.

5. Yeung CH, Cooper TG, Bergmann M, et al. Organization of tubules in the human caput epididymidis and the ultrastructure of their epithelia. Am J Anat 1991; 191(3):261–279.

6. Jones RC, Jurd KM. Structural differentiation and fluid reabsorption in the ductuli efferentes testis of the rat. Aust J Biol Sci 1987; 40(1):79–90.

7. Wang S, Jones RC, Clulow J. Surface area of apical and basolateral plasmalemma of epithelial cells of the ductuli efferentes testis of the rat. Cell Tiss Res 1994; 276(3):581–586.

8. Bedford JM. The status and the state of the human epididymis. Hum Reprod Update 1994; 9(11):2187–2199.

9. Shafik A. Epididymal ligaments: anatomy and function. Int J Fertil 1987; 32(4):324–330.

10. Moore HDM, Pryor JP. The comparative ultrastructure of the epididymis in monkeys and man: a search for a suitable animal model for studying epididymal physiology in primates. Amer J Primatol 1981; 1(2):241–250.

11. Chaturapanich G, Jones RC. Morphometry of the epididymis of the tammar wallaby Macropus eugenii and estimation of some physiological parameters. Reprod Fertil Devel 1991; 3(6):651–658.

12. Djakiew D, Jones RC. Stereological analysis of the epididymis of the echidna, Tachyglossus aculeatus, and Wistar rat. Aust J Zool 1982; 30:865–875.

13. Ghetie V. Preparation und Lange des Ductus epididymidis beim Pferd und Schwein. Anat Anz 1939; 87:369–374.

14. Maneely RB. Epididymal structure and function. A historical and critical review. Acta Zoologica 1959; 40:1–21.

15. Kirchhoff C. Gene expression in the epididymis. Int Rev Cytol 1999; 188:133–202.

16. Zhang J-S, Liu Q, Li Y-M, et al. Genome-wide profiling of segmental-regulated transcriptomes in human epididymis using oligo microarray. Molec Cell Endocrinol 2006; 250(1–2):169–177.

17. Fawcett DW, Hoffer AP. Failure of exogenous androgen to prevent regression of the initial segments of the rat epididymis after efferent duct ligation or orchidectomy. Biol Reprod 1979; 20(2):162–181.

18. Fox SA, Yang L, Hinton BT. Identifying putative contraceptive targets by dissecting signal transduction networks in the epididymis using an in vivo electroporation (electrotransfer) approach. Mol Cell Endocrinol 2006; 250(1–2):196–200.

19. Sonnenberg-Riethmacher E, Walter B, Riethmacher D, et al. The c-ros tyrosine kinase receptor controls regionalization and differentiation of epithelial cells in the epididymis. Gen Devel 1996; 10(10):1184–1193.

20. Legare C, Sullivan R. Expression and localization of c-ros oncogene along the human excurrent duct. Hum Molec Reprod 2004; 10(9):697–703.

21. Baumgarten HG, Holstein AF, Rosengren E. Arrangement, ultrastructure and adrenergic innervation of smooth musculature of the ductuli efferentes, ductus epididymidis and ductus deferens of man. Z Zellforsch Mikrosk Anat 1971; 120(1):37–79.

22. Kirton KT, Desjardins C, Hafs HD. Distribution of sperm in male rabbits after various ejaculation frequencies. Anat Rec 1967; 158(3):287–292.

23. Pholpramool C, Triphrom N, Din-Udom A. Intraluminal pressures in the seminiferous tubules and in different regions of the epididymis of the rat. J Reprod Fertil 1984; 71(1):173–179.

24. Friend M, Davis JE. Disappearance rate of sperm from the ejaculate following vasectomy. Fertil Steril 1969; 20(1):163–170.

25. Suzuki F, Nagano T. Microvasculature of the human testis and excurrent duct system. Resin-casting and scanning electron-microscopic studies. Cell Tissue Res 1986; 243(1):79–89.

26. Suzuki F. Microvasculature of the mouse testis and excurrent duct system. Am J Anat 1982; 163(4):309–325.

27. Tuck RR, Setchell BP, Waites GMH, et al. The composition of fluid collected by micropuncture and catheterization from the seminiferous tubules and rete testis of rats. Pflugers Archiv 1970; 318(3):225–243.

28. Clulow J, Jones RC. Composition of luminal fluid secreted by the seminiferous tubules, and after reabsorption by the extratesticular ducts of the Japanese quail, Coturnix coturnix japonica. Biol Reprod 2004; 71:1508–1516.

29. Clulow J, Jones RC, Hansen LA. Micropuncture and cannulation studies of fluid composition and transport in the ductuli efferentes testis of the rat: comparisons with the homologous metanephric proximal tubule. Exp Physiol 1994; 79(6):915–928.

30. Hess RA, Bunick D, Lee KH, et al. A role for oestrogens in the male reproductive system. Nature 1997; 390(6659):509–512.

31. Davies B, Baumann C, Kirchhoff C, et al. Targeted deletion of the epididymal receptor HE6 results in fluid dysregulation and male infertility. Mol Cell Biol 2004; 24(19):8642–8648.

32. Hansen LA, Clulow J, Jones RC. The dependence on Na and Cl of fluid transport in the ductuli efferentes of the rat. Biol Reprod 2004; 71(2):410–416.

33. Jones RC. Changes in protein composition of the luminal fluids along the epididymis of the tammar, Macropus eugenii. J Reprod Fertil 1987; 80(1):193–199.

34. Jones R. Comparative biochemistry of mammalian epididymal plasma. Comp Biochem Physiol 1978; 61(3):365–370.

35. Jones R. To store or mature spermatozoa? The primary role of the epididymis. Int J Androl 1999; 22(2):57–67.

36. Jones RC, Clulow J. Regulation of the elemental composition of the epididymal fluids in the tammar, Macropus eugenii. J Reprod Fertil 1987; 81(2):583–590.

37. Hinton BT, Pryor JP, Hirsh AV, et al. The concentration of some inorganic ions and organic compounds in the luminal fluid of the human ductus deferens. Int J Androl 1981; 4(4):457–461.

38. Hinton BT, White RW, Setchell BP. Concentration of myoinositol in the luminal fluid of the mammalian testis and epididymis. J Reprod Fertil 1980; 58(2):395–399.

39. Ng CM, Blackman MR, Wang C, et al. The role of carnitine in the male reproductive system. Ann NY Acad Sci 2004; 1033(1):177–188.

40. Dacheux J-L, Dacheux F, eds. Proteins Secretion in the Epididymis. New York: Kluwer, Academic/Plenum Publishers, 2002.

41. Dacheux J-L, Gatti J-L, Dacheux F, et al., eds. The Epididymal Proteome. Charlottesville, VA: The Van Doren Company, 2003.

42. Dacheux J-L, Druart X, Fouchecourt S, et al. Role of epididymal secretory proteins in sperm maturation with particular reference to the boar. J Reprod Fertil 1998; 53:99–107.

43. Hinton BT, Lan ZJ, Rudolph DB, et al. Testicular regulation of epididymal gene expression. J Reprod Fertil 1998; 53:47–57.

44. Hamil KG, Liu Q, Sivashanmugam P, et al. LCN6, a novel human epididymal lipocalin. Reprod Biol Endo 2003; 1(1):112–126.

45. von Horsten HH, Derr P, Kirchhoff C. Novel antimicrobial peptide of human epididymal duct origin. Biol Reprod 2002; 67(3):804–813.

46. Drevet JR. The antioxidant glutathione peroxidase family and spermatozoa: a complex story. Mol Cell Endocrinol 2006; 250(1–2):70–79.

47. Tulsiani DRP, Orgebin-Crist MC, Skudlarek MD. Role of luminal fluid glycosyltransferases and glycosidases in the modification of rat sperm plasma membrane glycoproteins during epididymal maturation. J Reprod Fertil 1998; 53:85–97.

48. Thomas Jiborn T, Magnus Abrahamson M, Hanna Wallin H, et al. Cystatin C is highly expressed in the human male reproductive system. J Cytol 2004; 25(4):264–272.

49. Jones R. Plasma membrane structure and remodelling during sperm maturation in the epididymis. J Reprod Fertil Suppl 1998; 53:73–78.

50. Ellerman DA, Cohen DJ, Da Ros VG, et al. Sperm protein "DE" mediates gamete fusion through an evolutionarily conserved site of the CRISP family. Dev Biol 2006; 297(1):228–237.

51. Dacheux J-L, Belghazi M, Lanson Y, et al. Human epididymal secretome and proteome. Molec Cell Endocrinol 2006; 250(1–2):36–42.

52. English HF, Dym M. The time required for materials injected into the rete testis to reach points in the caput epididymis of the rat and observations on the absorption of cationic ferritin. Ann N Y Acad Sci 1981; 383:445–446.

53. Johnson L, Varner DD. Effect of daily spermatozoan production but not age on transit time of spermatozoa through the human epididymis. Biol Reprod 1988; 39(4):812–817.

54. Rowley MJ, Teshima F, Heller GG. Duration of transit of spermatozoa through the human male ductular system. Fertil Steril 1970; 21(5):390–396.

55. Amann RP, Johnson L, Thompson DL, et al. Daily spermatozoal production, epididymal spermatozoal reserves and transit time of spermatozoa through the epididymis of the Rhesus monkey. Biol Reprod 1976; 15(5):586–592.

56. Schoysman R, Bedford JM. The role of the human epididymis in sperm maturation and sperm storage as reflected in the consequences of epididymovasostomy. Fertil Steril 1986; 46(2):293–299.

57. Silber S. Role of epididymis in sperm maturation. J Urol 1989; 33(1):47–51.

58. Dacheux J-L, Chevrier C, Lanson Y. Motility and surface transformation of human spermatozoa during epididymal transit. Ann NY Acad Sci 1987; 513:560–563.

59. Yeung CH, Cooper TG, Oberpenning F, et al. Changes in movement characteristics of human spermatozoa along the length of the epididymis. Biol Reprod 1993; 49(2):274–280.

60. Osterhoff C, Kirchhoff C, Krull N, et al. Molecular cloning and characterization of a novel human sperm antigen (HE2) specifically expressed in the proximal epididymis. Biol Reprod 1994; 50(3):516–525.

61. Tezon TG, Ramella R, Cameo MS, et al. Immunochemical localization of secretory antigens in the human epididymis and their association with spermatozoa. Biol Reprod 1985; 32(3):591–597.

62. Bedford JM, Calvin HI, Cooper GW. The maturation of spermatozoa in the human epididymis. J Reprod Fertil 1973; 18:199–213.

63. Cooper TG. In defence of a function for the human epididymis. Fertil Steril 1990; 54(6):965–975.

64. Schoysman R. Clinical situations challenging the established concept of epididymal physiology in the human. Acta Eur Fertil 1993; 24(2):55–60.

65. Silber SJ. Pregnancy caused by sperm from vasa efferentia. Fertil Steril 1988; 49(2):373–375.

66. Buffat C, Patrat C, Merlet F, et al. ICSI outcomes in obstructive azoospermia: influence of the origin of surgically retrieved spermatozoa and the cause of obstruction. Hum Reprod 2006; 21(4):1018–1024.

67. Brooks DE. Epididymal and testicular temperature in the unrestrained conscious rat. J Reprod Fertil 1973; 35(1):157–160.

68. Chaturapanich G, Jones RC, Clulow J. Role of androgens in survival of spermatozoa in epididymis of the tammar wallaby, Macropus eugenii. J Reprod Fertil 1992; 95(2):421–429.

69. Lubricz-Nawrocki CM, Lau NF, Chang MG. The fertilizing life of spermatozoa in the cauda epididymidis of mice and hamsters. J Reprod Fert 1973; 35(1):165–168.

70. Paufler SK, Foote RH. Morphology, motility and fertility of spermatozoa recovered from different areas of ligated rabbit epididymides. J Reprod Fertil 1968; 17(1):125–137.

71. White WE. The duration of fertility and the histological changes in the reproductive organs after ligation of the vasa efferentia of the rat. Proc Roy Soc London (Biol) 1933; 113:544–553.

72. Young WC. A study of the function of the epididymis. J Exp Biol 1931; 8(2):151–162.

73. Edwards IS. Earlier testing after vasectomy, based on the absence of motile sperm. Fertil Steril 1993; 59(2):431–436.

74. Jones RC, Clulow J. Fluid absorption and sperm maturation and storage in the mammalian epididymis. Proc 1st Asian and Oceanian Physiol Soc Bangkok 1987:229–240.

75. Cross BA, Silver IA. Neurovascular control of oxygen tension in the testis and epididymis. J Reprod Fertil 1962; 3:377–395.

76. Murdoch RN, Armstrong VA, Clulow J, et al. Relationship between motility and oxygen consumption of sperm from the cauda epididymides of the rat. Reprod Fertil Devel 1999; 11(2):87–94.

77. Murdoch R, Jones R. The metabolic properties of spermatozoa from the epididymis of the tammar wallaby, Macropus eugenii. Molec Reprod Devel 1997; 49(1):92–99.

78. Jones RC, Stone GM, Hinds LA, et al. Distribution of 5-alpha-reductase in the epididymis of the tammar wallaby (Macropus eugenii) and dependence of the epididymis on systemic testosterone and luminal fluids from the testis. J Reprod Fertil 1988; 83(2): 779–783.

79. Jones RC, Stone GM, Zupp J. Reproduction in the male echidna. In: Augee ML, ed. Platypus and Echidnas. Sydney, Australia: Royal Society of New South Wales, 1992:115–126.

80. Mahony M, Swanlund D, Billeter M, et al. Regional distribution of 5alpha reductase type 1 and type 2 mRNA along the human epididymis. Fert Steril 1998; 69(6):1116–1121.

81. Mahony MC, Heikinheimo O, Gordon K, et al. Regional distribution of 5alpha-reductase type 1 and type 2 mRNA along the nonhuman primate (Macaca fascicularis) epididymis. J Androl 1997; 18(6):595–601.

82. Robaire B, Ewing LL, Zirkin BR, et al. Steroid delta4-5 alpha-reductase and 3alpha-hydroxysteroid dehydrogenase in the rat epididymis. Endocrinol 1977; 101(5): 1379–1390.

83. Turner TT, Jones CE, Howards SS, et al. On the androgen microenvironment of maturing spermatozoa. Endocrinology 1984; 115(5):1925–1932.

84. Ergun S, Ungefroren H, Holstein AF, et al. Estrogen and progesterone receptors and estrogen receptor-related antigen (ER-D5) in human epididymis. Mol Reprod Dev 1997; 47(4):448–455.

85. Hess RA, Gist DH, Bunick D, et al. Estrogen receptor (alpha and beta) expression in the excurrent ducts of the adult male rat reproductive tract. J Androl 1997; 18(6):602–611.

86. Janulis L, Bahr JM, Hess RA, et al. P450 aromatase messenger ribonucleic acid expression in male rat germ cells: detection by reverse transcription-polymerase chain reaction amplification. J Androl 1996; 17(6): 651–658.

87. Carpino A, Romeo F, Rago V. Aromatase immunolocalization in human ductuli efferentes and proximal ductus epididymis. J Anat 2004; 204(Pt 3):217–220.

88. Yang L, Fox SA, Kirby JL, et al. Putative regulation of expression of members of the Ets variant 4 transcription factor family and their downstream targets in the rat epididymis. Biol Reprod 2006; 74(4):714–720.

89. Friend DS, Gilula NB. Variations in tight and gap junctions in mammalian tissues. J Cell Biol 1972; 53(3): 758–776.

90. Pollanen P, Cooper TG. Immunology of the testicular excurrent ducts. J Reprod Immunol 1994; 26(3):167–216.

91. Pomering M, Jones RC, Holland MK, et al. Restricted entry of IgG into male and female rabbit reproductive ducts following immunization with recombinant rabbit PH-20. Am J Reprod Immunol 2002; 47(3): 174–182.

92. Kazeem AA. A critical consideration of the rat epididymis as an immunologically privileged site. Scand J Immunol 1988; 27(2):149–156.

93. el-Demiry MI, Hargreave TB, Busuttil A, et al. Lymphocyte sub-populations in the male genital tract. Brit J Urol 1985; 57(6):769–774.

94. Yeung CH, Nashan D, Sorg C, et al. Basal cells of the human epididymis--antigenic and ultrastructural similarities to tissue-fixed macrophages. Biol Reprod 1994; 50(4):917–926.

95. Simpson KL, Holmes CH. Differential expression of complement regulatory proteins decay-accelerating factor (CD55), membrane cofactor protein (CD46) and CD59 during human spermatogenesis. Immunol 1994; 81(3):452–461.

96. Knee RA, Hickey DK, Beagley KW, et al. Transport of IgG across the blood-luminal barrier of the male reproductive tract of the rat and the effect of estradiol administration on reabsorption of fluid and IgG by the epididymal ducts. Biol Reprod 2005; 73: 688–694.

97. Clavert A, Cranz CI, Tardieu J, eds. Epididymis and Genital Infection. Rome: Ares Serono Symposia Publications; 1995.

98. Novella G, Porcaro AB, Righetti R, et al. Primary lymphoma of the epididymis: case report and review of the literature. Urol Int 2001; 67(1):97–99.

99. Patrizio P, Salameh WA. Expression of the cystic fibrosis transmembrane conductance regulator (CFTR) mRNA in normal and pathological adult human epididymis. J Reprod Fertil 1998; 53:261–270.

100. Jequier AM, Ansell ID, Bullimore NJ. Congenital absence of the vasa deferentia presenting with infertility. J Androl 1985; 6(1):15–19.

101. McCallum TJ, Milunsky JM, Cunningham DL, et al. Fertility in men with cystic fibrosis: an update on current surgical practices and outcomes. Chest 2000; 118(4): 1059–1062.

102. Hihnala S, Kujala M, Toppari J, et al. Expression of SLC26A3, CFTR and NHE3 in the human male reproductive tract: role in male subfertility caused by congenital chloride diarrhoea. Mol Hum Reprod 2006; 12:107–111.

103. de Kretser DM, Huidobro C, Southwick GJ, et al. The role of the epididymis in human fertility. J Reprod Fertil 1998; 53:271–275.

104. Bedford JM. Influence of abdominal temperature on epididymal function in the rat and rabbit. Am J Anat 1978; 152(4):509–521.

105. Foldesy RG, Bedford JM. Biology of the scrotum. I. Temperature and androgen as determinants of the sperm storage capacity of the rat cauda epididymidis. Biol Reprod 1982; 26(4):673–682.

106. Mieusset R, Quintana Casares P, Sanchez Partida LG, et al. Effects of heating the testes and epididymides of rams by scrotal insulation on fertility and embryonic mortality in ewes inseminated with frozen semen. J Reprod Fertil 1992; 94(2):337–343.

107. Clulow J, Jones R. Production, transport, maturation, storage and survival of spermatozoa in the male Japanese quail, Coturnix coturnix. J Reprod Fertil 1982; 64(2):259–266.

108. Johnson L, Nguyen HB, Petty CS, et al. Quantification of human spermatogenesis: germ cell degeneration during spermatocytogenesis and meiosis in testes from younger and older adult men. Biol Reprod 1987; 37(3): 739–747.

109. Jensen TK, Andersson A-M, Hjollund NHI, et al. Inhibin B as a serum marker of spermatogenesis: correlation to differences in sperm concentration and follicle-stimulating hormone levels. J Clin Endocrin Metab 1997; 82(12):4059–4063.

110. Wentworth BC, Mellen J. Egg production and fertility following various methods of insemination in Japanese quail. J Reprod Fertil 1963; 6:215–220.

111. Bedford JM, ed. Sperm Dynamics in The Epididymis. Norwell, Mass: Serono Symposia, 1990.

112. Salamon S, Morant AJ. Comparison of two methods of artificial breeding in sheep. Aus J Exp Agric Animl Husb 1963; 3:72–77.

113. Kenagy GJ, Trombulak SC. Size and function of mammalian testes in relation to body size. J Mammal 1986; 67:1–22.

114. Setchell BP, Carrick FN. Spermatogenesis in some Australian marsupials. Aust J Zool 1973; 21(4): 491–499.

115. Setchell BP. Fluid secretion by the testes of an Australian marsupial Macropus eugenii. Comp Biochem Physiol 1970; 36:411–414.

116. Valerio DA, Leverage WE, Munster JH. Semen evaluation in Macaques. Lab Anim Care 1970; 20(4 Pt 1):734–740.

7

Physiology of the Prostate

Helen D. Nicholson
Department of Anatomy and Structural Biology, Otago School of Medical Sciences, University of Otago, Dunedin, New Zealand

Stephen J. Assinder
Discipline of Physiology, School of Medical Sciences, University of Sydney, New South Wales, Australia

☐ INTRODUCTION

Of all the male accessory sex glands, the human prostate is probably better known for its pathological conditions rather than its normal function. It is responsible for the production and secretion of various components of seminal fluid, which are discharged from the gland at the time of ejaculation. Prostate diseases such as benign prostatic hyperplasia (BPH) and carcinoma of the prostate are common afflictions in the older male. With an increase in the lifespan of men, the demands on health care related to prostate disease will also rise. This has resulted in a growing awareness of prostatic disease and a requirement for a clearer understanding of the physiology and pathophysiology of the prostate. This chapter will describe the anatomy, development, and normal physiology of the prostate. (Pathophysiologic conditions of the prostate, including BPH, prostate cancer, and prostatitis, are described in Chapter 41.)

☐ ANATOMY OF THE PROSTATE

The human prostate gland is shaped like an inverted cone. It lies at the base of the bladder and completely encircles the urethra. Also entering the prostate are the ejaculatory ducts. These run through the cranial part of the gland and open into the urethra at the verumontanum (Fig. 1). In the young man, the prostate weighs between 15 and 20 g. It consists of glandular tissue, which is responsible for secreting fluid (contributing to approximately 12% of the normal ejaculatory volume), and nonglandular tissue, which forms the prostatic sphincters and fibromuscular capsule.

Early anatomists described the prostate as consisting of five lobes: an anterior, middle or median, posterior, and two lateral lobes. This division of the gland was based on the presence in the embryo of five sets of ducts draining five groups of acini into the embryonic urethra (1). In the absence of BPH, however, the outer surface of the adult prostate does not have any obvious lobes and the cut surface appears homogeneous (2). Division of the gland into four zones, peripheral, central, transition, and periurethral, with each zone related

to a segment of the urethra (3), provides a more clinically relevant and accurate description that has superseded the lobar classification. The urethra enters the prostate at the bladder neck and exits at the apex (Fig. 1). It does not run in a straight line but bends at an approximate angle of 35° midway along its course. This angulation occurs at the level of the verumontanum and divides the urethra into proximal and distal segments (Fig. 2). The peripheral zone comprises around 70% of the total glandular tissue of the normal prostate and surrounds the distal portion of the urethra. Its ducts drain in a double row into the prostatic urethra. The central zone occupies the area around the ejaculatory ducts and consists of 25% of the prostatic glandular tissue (5). The transition and periurethral zones lie around the proximal urethral segment and resemble the shape of an inverted lollipop (4). The transition zone is the larger of theses two areas, comprising approximately 5% of the glandular tissue in young men. This division of the gland into zones is important clinically as the peripheral zone is the main site of carcinoma of the prostate and prostatitis (1,6), although some carcinomas may arise in the transition zone. Benign hyperplasia, however, occurs predominantly in the transition and periurethral zones of the prostate (5). With progression of BPH, the transition zone enlarges significantly and compresses the surrounding central zone to form a pseudocapsule between it and the peripheral zone. This pseudocapsule provides a line of cleavage, allowing nucleation of the hyperplastic tissue.

Surrounding most of the external surface of the prostate is a fibromuscular capsule. Anteriorly, this is augmented by a thickened layer of smooth muscle and fibrous tissue called the anterior fibromuscular stroma (7). Muscular sphincters are also present within the prostate. The preprostatic sphincter is a sleeve of smooth muscle running down from the bladder neck and surrounding the proximal urethra and periurethral zone. Its contraction at ejaculation is thought to prevent retrograde flow of seminal fluid into the bladder (8). A second sphincter is found around the distal urethra. This consists of semicircular loops of striated muscle fibers that are continuous with the external urethral sphincter (7).

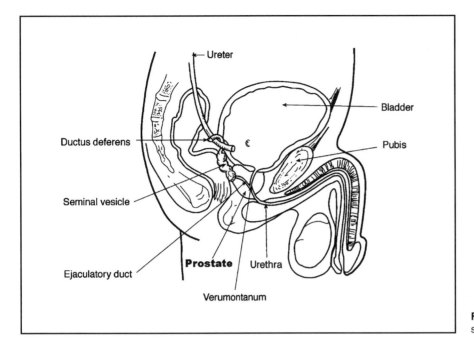

Figure 1 Sagittal view of the male pelvis showing the position of the prostate.

Innervation

The prostate receives both sympathetic and parasympathetic innervation. Sympathetic fibers pass from the sympathetic chain via the hypogastric nerves. Fibers then run along the capsule and innervate the smooth muscle surrounding the prostatic ducts (9). Activation of the sympathetic system produces contraction of the smooth muscle of the capsule and ducts and results in expulsion of prostatic secretions at ejaculation. Parasympathetic fibers enter the pelvic parasympathetic nerves and terminate close to the epithelial cells of the acini (10,11). The arrangement of these fibers suggests that they have a secretomotor function. The identification of several neuropeptides such as neuropeptide Y, enkephalins, and vasoactive intestinal peptide in prostatic neurons suggests that these peptides may also play a role in regulating prostatic activity. As in other parts of the male reproductive tract, there is also evidence that spontaneous contractions of the prostatic smooth muscle occur (12). These contractions presumably allow emptying of the acini and movement of the prostatic secretions, which are constantly being produced.

Blood Supply and Lymphatic Drainage

There is some variation in the origin of the blood supply of the prostate, with branches extending from the inferior vesical and middle rectal arteries. The prostatic arteries enter the prostate laterally at the junction with the bladder. Within the capsule of the prostate, the arteries divide into capsular and urethral branches. The prostatic veins drain into the prostatic plexus, a network of thin-walled veins, which lie between the prostatic fascia and fibromuscular capsule. This venous plexus receives the deep dorsal vein of the penis and the venous flow from the base of the bladder and drains across the pelvic floor into the

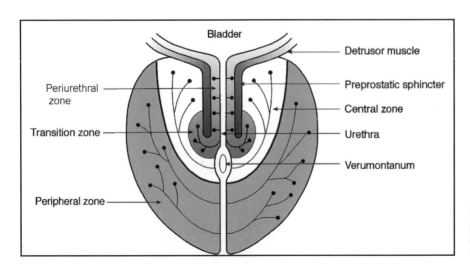

Figure 2 Coronal section of the human prostate showing the positions of the central, peripheral, transition, and periurethral zones. *Source*: Adapted from Ref. 4.

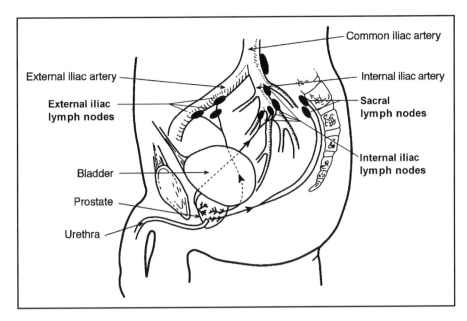

Figure 3 Pathways of lymphatic drainage from the prostate.

internal iliac vein. Lymph from the prostate passes to nodes along both the external and internal iliac arteries (Fig. 3). The superior part of the prostate drains into nodes in the external iliac chain. The inferior and anterior prostate drain into nodes around the origin of the internal iliac artery and the posterior part of the gland drains into nodes in the region of the sacral promontory (13).

Microscopic Anatomy

The structure of the prostate is adapted so that it can gradually accumulate secretions and then rapidly discharge small volumes of fluid at the time of ejaculation. It consists of a series of distensible acini and ducts surrounded by fibromuscular stroma (Fig. 4). The glandular tissue is arranged in a series of acini that drain via collecting ducts into the prostatic urethra. The epithelium of the acini consists of three main cell types. The predominant cell type is the columnar secretory cell. These are 10 to 12 μm tall and contain a large number of secretory granules. They are responsible for secreting various proteins including prostate-specific antigen (PSA) and prostatic acid phosphatase (PAP) and are dependent on androgens for maintenance of their morphology and function (14). Neuroendocrine cells are present throughout the epithelia. They contain a variety of neuropeptides, including serotonin, thyroid-stimulating hormone (TSH), and somatostatin, and probably play a paracrine role in the regulation of secretory activity and growth (15,16). In the rat, basal cells account for less than 10% of the cells within the epithelium, but these are present in a much larger proportion of the epithelial compartment in humans. In the normal human prostate, these cuboidal cells form a complete layer, which rests on the basement membrane (17). These cells contain little secretory product and were thought to act as precursors for the luminal cells (18). However, recent work challenges this idea

by showing that differentiated luminal epithelial cells are capable of mitotic activity (19). Other studies suggest that the basal cells may form a blood–prostate barrier. As such, they may play an important part in the development of benign and malignant prostatic disease.

A basement membrane lies between the epithelium of the acini and the stromal tissue. The stroma consists of extracellular matrix and a variety of cells, including fibroblasts, smooth-muscle cells, blood and lymphatic vessels, and autonomic nerve fibers.

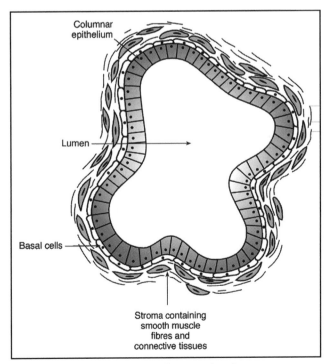

Figure 4 Histological structure of a prostatic acinus.

Differences in the histological appearance of the different zones of the prostate have been described (7) and suggest that they may have differing functions. In the peripheral and transition zones, the acini are small and round and are surrounded by loosely arranged smooth-muscle fibers. The epithelial cells contain clear cytoplasm and small, dark nuclei situated near the basal surface of the cell. In the central zone, the acini are larger and irregular in shape. They contain epithelial cells with granular cytoplasm and large nuclei located at varying positions within the cells. The smooth-muscle fibers of the central zone stroma are denser and have a regular arrangement.

☐ DEVELOPMENT OF THE PROSTATE

The human prostate is thought to develop from the urogenital sinus, while the ejaculatory duct is formed from the Wolffian duct. At 10 weeks of gestation, a series of paired buds begin to emerge from the urogenital sinus (1,20). Under the influence of androgens, especially dihydrotestosterone (DHT), the mesenchyme of the urogenital sinus stimulates the buds to proliferate and differentiate into an epithelial ductal system (21). Meanwhile, the urogenital sinus mesenchyme differentiates into smooth muscle and fibroblasts to form the stromal tissue. Elegant studies by Hayward and Cunha (22) have demonstrated that interactions between the mesenchymal and epithelial cells mediate the androgen-induced development of the prostate and may also be important in the regulation of prostate growth in the adult. Thus, epithelial growth and differentiation requires the presence of functional androgen receptors within the mesenchymal tissue, which, when activated, promote epithelial growth. Similarly, the epithelium induces the mesenchyme to differentiate into smooth muscle.

At birth the prostate is small (approximately 2 g) and the acini may be lined by a metaplastic squamous epithelium induced by maternal estrogens (23,24). Surges of serum testosterone occur during the first year of life and induce changes to produce a pseudostratified epithelium. In the rat, exposure to steroids in the neonatal and prepubertal periods appears to be critical in determining the maximum size that the prostate can attain in later life (25).

The prostate remains small until puberty when, in response to rising androgens, a significant increase in weight occurs. The increase in size is accompanied by an increase in the diameter of the ducts and the formation of large mature acini.

☐ PHYSIOLOGY OF THE PROSTATE

The primary role of the prostate is the production of secretions to augment the seminal fluid. Prostate secretions make up about 15% of the seminal fluid and are involved in insemination and optimizing fertility. They also have a bactericidal effect in the prostate and reproductive tract. The secretory activity of the prostate is controlled by neural and endocrine mechanisms.

Prostate Secretions

The prostate secretes a variety of substances including zinc, magnesium, citrate, nitrogenous compounds such as phosphorylcholine and polyamines, and a collection of proteolytic enzymes.

Citric Acid

The human prostate is one of the major sources of citrate. Tissue levels of citrate are approximately 100 times higher in the prostate than in other soft tissues. The secretory epithelial cells of the prostate produce citrate from aspartic acid and glucose, resulting in concentrations in the seminal fluid of above 52 pmol/L. Citrate acts to bind divalent cations, and in the semen, chelates calcium, thus reducing the rate of calcium-dependent coagulation (14).

Zinc

High levels of zinc are found in human seminal plasma, most of which appears to originate from the prostate. Zinc acts as a cofactor for several metalloenzymes present within the prostate. Zinc has also been implicated in having an antibacterial role in the prostate. Indeed the concentrations of zinc in prostatic secretions from men with chronic bacterial prostatitis are significantly reduced compared to those of normal men (26). Prostatic secretion of zinc is also altered in other pathological conditions, being elevated in some patients with BPH and reduced in men with carcinoma of the prostate (27).

Polyamines

Polyamines are small organic molecules that are basic and positively charged. The precise function of these molecules is unclear, but in vitro polyamines can act as growth factors and enzyme inhibitors. One of the major polyamines produced by the prostate is spermine. Spermine may be involved in regulating the coagulation and liquefaction of semen. Oxidation of spermine and other polyamines results in the formation of reactive aldehyde compounds, which are toxic to both bacteria and sperm (28). It has been suggested that these compounds may have an antibacterial function and may also alter sperm function and motility.

Phosphorylcholine

Another group of positively charged amines present in the seminal fluid is that of the choline compounds. Of these, phosphorylcholine is the most prevalent in the human prostate. PAP in the semen acts on phosphorylcholine to produce free choline (29). The precise function of choline in seminal fluid, however, remains unknown.

Prostatic Secretory Proteins

The prostate produces a variety of proteins of which PSA and PAP are probably the most well known. However, the prostate also produces other proteins such as glycoproteins and small peptides (e.g., thyroid releasing hormone-like peptide, oxytocin, and growth factors). Secretion of these prostatic proteins is regulated by androgens, particularly 5α-reduced androgens such as DHT.

Prostate-Specific Antigen

PSA was first isolated in 1971 (30). It is a 33-kDa glycoprotein that is found exclusively in the epithelial cells of the prostate. PSA is a serine protease, a member of the kallikrein family. It acts to cleave the major seminal vesicle protein present in the seminal coagulate and is thought to be important for the liquefaction of the semen (31,32). Under normal conditions, the basement membrane of the prostatic acini and blood-prostate barrier prevents passage of PSA into the circulation and the protein is released into the lumen of the acini and thus into the ejaculate. These barriers may be breached with the development of prostate cancer, causing PSA to pass out of the acini and into the general circulation producing elevated levels of PSA (see Chapter 41).

Prostatic Acid Phosphatase

PAP is a glycoprotein dimer with a molecular weight of 102 kDa (32). While acid phosphatase is found in other body tissues, activity of this enzyme is more than 100 times higher in the prostate. Prostatic secretion of PAP is the major source of the high levels of this enzyme found in seminal fluid. Phosphatase enzymes hydrolyse organic monophosphate esters to release inorganic phosphate ions. Although the exact biological function of PAP is unclear, its natural substrate is probably phosphorylcholine, which is present in the seminal fluid (29). PAP has also been shown to act on protein tyrosine esters, which are the products of many oncogene protein tyrosine kinases (34). Before the identification of PSA, PAP was used as a marker for metastatic prostate cancer. However, with the advent of more specific and sensitive PSA assays, interest in PAP has declined.

Prostatic Growth and Regulation

Regulation of prostatic growth is a complex process involving the effects of endocrine, paracrine, and autocrine factors as well as interactions between individual cells and the extracellular matrix. The maintenance of the size and structure of the prostate depends, at all times, on a balance between cell growth and regulated cell death (apoptosis). The mechanisms involved are complicated and our current understanding is far from complete. Much of our knowledge at present relies, in part, on animal studies and in vitro experiments that have examined the effects of individual factors. The challenge for the future is to understand how all these parts of the puzzle fit together in man.

The major factors known to be involved in prostate growth are summarized below. Mechanisms involved in the development and progression of disorders of prostate growth, such as BPH and prostate cancer, are discussed in Chapter 41.

Androgens

Androgens were the first factors shown to be important in the development of the prostate and regulation of prostatic growth. Early experiments showed that castration resulted in atrophy of the prostate but that these changes could be prevented by administering exogenous testosterone (35). Although testosterone is the most abundant androgen in the circulation, it is the 5α-reduced steroid DHT that is the biologically active androgen. Testosterone is converted to DHT by the action of the enzyme 5-α-reductase (36). This enzyme exists in two isoforms, types I and II. Although both isoforms are present in the human prostate, type II is the predominant form. Conversion of testosterone to DHT occurs predominantly in the stromal tissue, with only approximately 10% of prostatic DHT being produced in the epithelium (37). DHT is essential for both the development and maintenance of prostatic growth. Males who are deficient in 5-α-reductase exhibit a rare form of pseudohermaphroditism that results in feminization of the external genitalia and either a rudimentary or absent prostate (38).

Within the prostatic cells, DHT binds to the hormone-binding domain of specific androgen receptors located within the nucleus. Androgen binding promotes a conformational change in the receptor that allows it to bind to DNA and activate gene transcription, resulting in the formation of new proteins. The androgen receptor gene is situated on the X chromosome. Although it is a large gene (54 kb), only 17% of its nucleotides form message that is translated into protein. The remaining parts are involved in gene regulation and protein processing. In the normal prostate, androgen receptor is expressed in the stromal cells, some luminal cells, and endothelial cells (39).

Much of our understanding of the actions of androgens comes from animal studies, particularly experiments using castrated rats. Castration results in atrophy of the ventral prostate with a decrease of 90% of the epithelial cells and 40% of stromal cells (40). Similar effects are seen after treatment of men with BPH by orchidectomy, although the predominant decrease in epithelial cells may not provide symptomatic relief (41). In addition to decreased prostate size, castration also results in a reduction in the secretory function of the gland. Administration of androgen results in an increase in the synthesis and secretion of prostatic proteins as well as an increase in DNA synthesis. In the rat, this increase in DNA synthesis is maintained until cell numbers reach the precastrate level (42). Thus, it appears that androgens may act via androgen receptors in the stroma to promote growth in the developing prostate and on epithelial cells to stimulate secretory activity in the adult. As in the developing prostate (21), the interaction between the stromal and epithelial compartments of the gland play an important part in the actions of hormones and their effects on growth (Fig. 5).

Estrogens

Estrogens are produced in the male from conversion of testosterone by the aromatase enzyme. Conversion of testosterone occurs in the adipose tissue, the liver, and tissues of the male reproductive tract, including the prostate. While circulating concentrations of androgens decrease with age, those of estradiol increase. It has been postulated that the change in the ratio of androgen to estrogen may be important in the development of BPH. In the normal prostate, estrogens act synergistically with androgens. In the dog, treatment with estradiol plus 5α-reduced androgens results in an increase in size of the gland and the development of glandular hyperplasia compared with treatment with androgens alone (43). Recent studies have reported a dose-dependent increase in prostate size in castrated dogs treated with exogenous estradiol alone (44). There does seem to be some species specificity in this effect, with less dramatic changes seen in the rat (45). The mechanism of the synergistic action is unclear,

although estrogens have been shown to increase concentrations of the androgen receptor (46) and modify DHT formation.

Estrogens also have a direct effect on stromal growth causing an increase in fibromuscular tissue. At high concentrations such as those seen around the time of birth, estrogen can induce squamous metaplasia of the epithelial cells. More recent studies have also suggested that there is an imprinting effect. Exposure to estrogens during the development of the prostate may regulate the maximal growth that the gland can achieve (47).

Both α and β forms of the estrogen receptor have been identified in the prostate and their expression appears to vary in the normal and diseased prostate. For example, while only the β form is present on epithelial cells in the normal human prostate, both forms are seen in BPH and carcinoma of the gland (48).

Other Hormones

A variety of other hormones have also been implicated in the regulation of prostatic growth. Prolactin (49), for example, is thought to act by potentiating the effects of androgens by increasing androgen-receptor density. Prolactin also has direct actions on the prostate, stimulating production of insulin-like growth factor (IGF)-1 and its receptor (50). Furthermore, transgenic mice that overexpress the prolactin gene develop dramatic enlargement of the prostate with an increase in both cell number and secretory products (51). More recently, prolactin has been shown to be produced locally within the epithelial cells of the rat and human prostate (52,53)

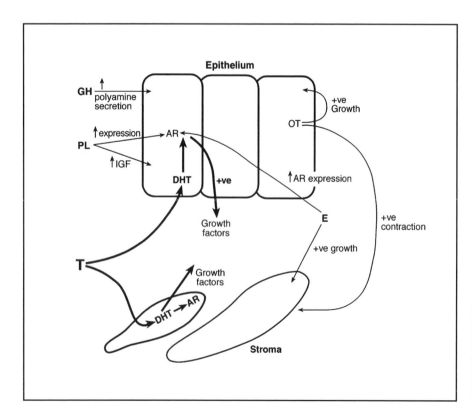

Figure 5 Possible interactions of hormones on the epithelial and stromal compartments of the prostate. *Abbreviations*: –ve, negative effect; +ve, positive effect; AR, androgen receptor; DHT, dihydrotestosterone; E, estrogen; GH, growth hormone; IGF, insulin-like growth factor; OT, oxytocin; PL, prolactin; T, testosterone.

and the presence of prolactin receptors have been identified (54).

Growth hormone has also been implicated in regulating prostatic function. Transgenic mice that overexpress growth hormone have moderately enlarged prostates (55). The hormone has also been shown to stimulate secretion of polyamines such as spermine. Although growth hormone receptors have been identified on epithelial and stromal cells from patients with BPH or carcinoma, they have not been seen in normal human tissue (56). Thyroid hormones have been demonstrated to modulate prostate weight and structure in the rat, and indeed the presence of a prostate–thyroid axis has been postulated with prostatic secretion, stimulating thyroid function (57). Another hormone implicated in prostatic function is oxytocin. Oxytocin is synthesized locally within the rat and human prostate (58) and receptors for the peptide have been demonstrated on the epithelial and stromal cells (59). Oxytocin has been shown to stimulate epithelial growth in the rat (60) and may also affect muscle tone (61).

Growth Factors

Androgens have profound effects on prostate growth, but evidence suggests that their actions may be indirect and mediated by growth factors. Growth factors act by binding to specific receptors and activating kinase enzymes (tyrosine kinase, cyclic AMP protein kinase A, and protein kinase C). Activation of these enzymes results in a cascade of phosphorylation of regulatory proteins that may be accompanied by intracellular release of calcium. These changes switch on the expression of specific growth factor–activated genes, which may promote or inhibit cell replication and growth. Many types of growth factors and their receptors have been identified in the prostate. How these factors interact together to regulate growth is beginning to be understood.

Fibroblast Growth Factors

The fibroblast growth factor (FGF) family, also known as heparin-binding growth factors, consists of more than 10 members, including acidic FGF (aFGF/FGF1), basic FGF (bFGF/FGF2), and keratinocyte growth factor. These growth factors appear to act through common receptors and are regulated by androgens (62). They act as mitogens in both epithelial and cells of mesenchymal origin. In the rat and man, FGF1 and FGF7 appear to be involved in prostate development (63), whereas FGF9 may regulate growth in the adult (64). In the adult, levels of FGF1 are undetectable and other FGFs such as FGF2 are more highly expressed (65).

Epidermal Growth Factor

Epidermal growth factor (EGF) is part of a family of growth factors that includes transforming growth factor α (TGFα). Both EGF and TGFα signal through the EGF receptor, a tyrosine kinase, and promote cell proliferation. EGF is necessary for human prostate cells to grow in vitro. Expression of EGF and TGFα is modulated by androgens and varies in the normal and diseased prostate. In the normal prostate, EGF, TGFα, and the EGF receptor are localized to the basal cells with some staining for TGFα also in smooth-muscle cells (66,67). In BPH and prostatic carcinoma, expression of both growth factors and receptor is increased and is present in luminal epithelial cells.

Transforming Growth Factor β

Transforming growth factor β (TGFβ) is related to the proteins inhibin and Mullerian-inhibiting substance. TGFβ exists as five isoforms, three of which (TGFβ_{1-3}) are found in mammals. TGFβ is an inhibitor of normal prostate epithelial growth and has been shown to block androgen-induced development of the ductal system in the neonatal rat (68). TGFβ is regulated by androgens and its secretion may also be modified by estrogen (69). While TGFβ inhibits epithelial growth, there is evidence that it may also stimulate stromal growth, which may account for the increased expression of TGFβ_2 observed in BPH (70).

Insulin-Like Growth Factors

The insulin growth factor family consists of IGF-I and -II and their respective receptors. The system is complicated further by the presence of a family of IGF binding proteins (IGF-BPs). Thus, IGF action can be regulated at the level of the growth factor, receptor, or BP. For example, recent studies have established that PSA can cleave IGF-BP3 in vitro, thus increasing the concentrations of biologically available IGF-I (71). In the rodent, IGF promotes prostatic growth, but its role in the normal human prostate is unclear. Both IGF-I and -II receptors have been identified in prostatic cells, and IGF-I has been identified in the stromal cells of BPH tissues (72). Men with elevated circulating IGF-I levels are also at higher risk of developing carcinoma of the prostate (73).

Understanding how these various factors interact together remains a challenge. Current evidence suggests that FGFs, EGF, TGFα, and IGFs may act to promote epithelial and stromal growth, with TGFβ acting as an inhibitor to balance these effects on epithelial growth (Fig. 6). The factors involved in preventing hyperproliferation of stromal cells remains unclear at the present time.

Nervous Regulation

There is growing evidence that neural input is involved in controlling prostatic growth. Catecholamines have been shown to have mitogenic effects on stromal cells (74). This effect may result directly from activation of adrenergic receptors or indirectly by inducing the production of other growth factors such as EGF.

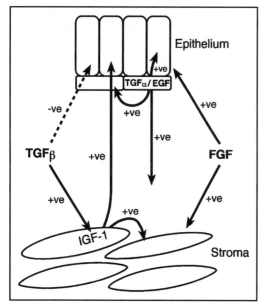

Figure 6 Possible interactions of growth factors on the epithelial and stromal compartments of the prostate. *Abbreviations*: –ve, negative effect; +ve, positive effect; EGF, epidermal growth factor; FGF, fibroblast growth factor; IGF, insulin-like growth factor; TGF, transforming growth factor.

Recent studies have also shown that alpha-1 adrenergic inhibitors may inhibit growth of both epithelial and stromal cells by stimulating apoptosis (75). Denervation of the rat prostate results in morphological changes involving a decrease in the height and a reduction of microvilli on epithelial cells (76). Furthermore, results from experiments where either the sympathetic or the parasympathetic innervation of the prostate is ablated suggest that the two parts of the autonomic nervous system may have opposing effects on prostatic growth (77). Loss of the sympathetic supply results in atrophy, while parasympathectomy promotes hyperplasia of the rat ventral prostate. Although these effects are less dramatic than those seen with androgens, they suggest that an intact nerve supply is necessary to obtain maximal prostatic growth in the rat.

☐ CONCLUSION

The prostate is one of the male accessory sex glands. It lies at the base of the bladder and completely encircles the urethra. The ejaculatory ducts carrying spermatozoa and secretions from the seminal vesicles pass through the prostate and open into the prostatic urethra. The prostate consists of glandular tissue that produces various components of the seminal fluid. The gland can be divided into several zones that differ in their histological appearance and their propensity to develop benign and malignant disease.

Regulation of prostate growth and secretion are important in both health and disease. Androgens, particularly 5α-reduced steroids such as DHT, are important in the stimulation of both prostate growth and secretion. Other hormones such as prolactin, growth hormone, oxytocin, and estrogen are also involved in these processes. Estrogen stimulates growth of the stromal tissue and changes in the ratio of estrogen to androgen with aging have been implicated in the development of benign prostate disease. Recent studies have also shown that, as well as having a direct effect on cell growth, androgens may act indirectly by modulating growth factor production. Several growth factors have been identified within the human prostate and have been shown to have physiological effects on cell growth. Understanding how these various hormones and growth factors interact should provide insight into the regulation of prostate growth and function in health and disease.

☐ REFERENCES

1. Lowsley OS. The development of the human prostate gland with reference to the development of other structures at the neck of the urinary bladder. Am J Anat 1912; 13:299–312.

2. Myers RP. Structure of the adult prostate from a clinician's standpoint. Clin Anat 2000; 13(3):214–215.

3. McNeal JE. Regional morphology and pathology of the prostate. Am J Clin Pathol 1968; 49(3):347–357.

4. McNeal JE. Origin and evolution of benign prostatic enlargement. Invest Urol 1978; 15(4):340–345.

5. Coakley FV, Hricak H. Radiologic anatomy of the prostate gland: a clinical approach. Radiol Clin North Am 2000; 38(1):15–30.

6. McNeal JE. Origin and development of carcinoma of the prostate. Cancer 1969; 23(1):24–34.

7. McNeal JE. Anatomy and normal histology of the human prostate. In: Foster CS, Bostwick DG, eds. Pathology of the Prostate. Philadelphia: WB Saunders, 1998:19–34.

8. Blacklock NJ. Anatomical factors in prostatitis. Br J Urol 1947; 46(1):47–54.

9. Vaalasti A, Hervonen A. Autonomic innervation of the human prostate. Invest Urol 1980; 17(4):293–297.

10. Gosling JA. Autonomic innervation of the prostate. In: Hinman F Jr, ed. Benign prostatic hypertrophy. New York: Springer Verlag, 1983:349–360.

11. Wang JM, McKenna KE, Lee C. Determination of prostatic secretion in rats: effects of neurotransmitters and testosterone. Prostate 1991; 18(4):289–301.

12. Watanabe H, Shima M, Kojima M, et al. Dynamic study of nervous control on prostatic contraction and fluid excretion in the dog. J Urol 1988; 140(6): 1567–1570.

13. Krongrad A, Droller MJ. Anatomy of the prostate. In: Lepor H, Lawson RK, eds. Prostate Diseases. Philadelphia: WB Saunders, 1993:17–27.

14. Luke MC, Coffey DS. The male sex accessory tissues. Structure, androgen action and physiology. In: Knobil E, Neill JD, eds. The Physiology of Reproduction. New York: Raven Press Ltd, 1994:1435–1487.

15. Abrahamsson PA, Lilja H. Partial characterization of a thyroid-stimulating hormone-like peptide in neuroendocrine cells of the human prostate gland. Prostate 1989; 14(1):71–81.

16. di Sant'Agnese PA. Calcitonin-like immunoreactive and bombesin-like immunoreactive endocrine-paracrine cells of the human prostate. Arch Pathol Lab Med 1986; 110(5):412–415.

17. El-Alfy M, Pelletier G, Hermo LS, et al. Unique features of the basal cells of human prostate epithelium. Microsc Res Tech 2000; 51(5):436–446.

18. Robinson EJ, Neal DE, Collins AT. Basal cells are progenitors of luminal cells in primary cultures of differentiating human prostatic epithelium. Prostate 1998; 37(3):149–160.

19. van der Kwast TH, Tetu B, Suburu ER, et al. Cycling activity of benign prostatic epithelial cells during long-term androgen blockade: evidence for self-renewal of the luminal cells. J Pathol 1998; 186(4):406–409.

20. Kellokumpu-Lehtinen P, Santti R, Pelliniemi LJ. Correlation of early cytodifferentiation of the human fetal prostate and Leydig cells. Anat Rec 1980; 196(3): 263–273.

21. Cunha GR, Donjacour AA, Cooke PS, et al. The endocrinology and developmental biology of the prostate. Endocr Rev 1987; 8(3):338–362.

22. Hayward SW, Cunha GR. The prostate: development and physiology. Radiol Clin North Am 2000; 38(1): 1–14.

23. Swyer GIM. Postnatal growth changes in the human prostate. J Anat 1944; 78:130–145.

24. Andrews GS. The histology of the human foetal and prepubertal prostates. J Anat 1951; 85(1):44–54.

25. Naslund MJ, Coffey DS. The differential effects of neonatal androgen, estrogen and progesterone on adult rat prostate growth. J Urol 1986; 136(5):1136–1140.

26. Fair WR, Wehner N. The prostatic antibacterial factor: identity and significance. In: Marberger H, ed. Prostatic Disease. Vol. 6. New York: AR Liss, 1976.

27. Picurelli L, Olcina PV, Roig MD, et al. Determination of Fe, Mg, Cu, and Zn in normal and pathological prostatic tissue. (Article in Spanish). Actas Urologicas Espanolas 1991; 15(4):344–350.

28. Stamey TA, Fair WR, Timothy MM, et al. Antibacterial nature of prostatic fluid. Nature 1968; 218(140): 444–447.

29. Seligman AM, Sternberger NJ, Paul BD, et al. Design of spindle poisons activated specifically by prostatic acid phosphatase (PAP) and new methods for PAP cytochemistry. Cancer Chemother Rep 1975; 59(1): 233–242.

30. Hara M, Inorre T, Fukuyama T. Some physico-chemical characterisations of gamma seminoprotein, an antigenic component specific for human seminal plasma. Jap J Legal Med 1971; 25:322–324.

31. Lilja H. A kallikrein-like serine protease in prostatic fluid cleaves the predominant seminal vesicle protein. J Clin Invest 1985; 76(5):1899–1903.

32. Bilhartz DL, Tindall DJ, Oesterling JE. Prostate-specific antigen and prostatic acid phosphatase: biomolecular and physiologic characteristics. Urology 1991; 38(2): 95–102.

33. Chu TM, Wang MC, Kuciel L, et al. Enzyme markers in human prostatic carcinoma. Cancer Treat Rep 1977; 61(2):193–200.

34. Lin MF, Clinton GM. Human prostatic acid phosphatase has phosphotyrosyl protein phosphatase activity. Biochem J 1986; 235(2):351–357.

35. Huggins C, Hodges CV. Studies on prostatic cancer. I. The effect of castration, of estrogen and of androgen injection on serum phosphatases in metastatic carcinoma of the prostate. 1941. J Urol 2002; 168(1):9–12.

36. Bruchovsky N, Wilson JD. The conversion of testosterone to 5-alpha-androstan-17-beta-ol-3-one by rat prostate in vivo and in vitro. J Biol Chem 1968; 243(8): 2012–2021.

37. Russell DW, Wilson JD. Steroid 5 alpha-reductase: two genes/two enzymes. Annu Rev Biochem 1994; 63: 25–61.

38. Imperato-McGinley J, Guerrero L, Gautier T, et al. Steroid 5alpha-reductase deficiency in man: an inherited form of pseudohermaphroditism. Science 1974; 186(4170):1213–1215.

39. El-Alfy M, Luu-The V, Huang XF, et al. Localization of type 5 17β-hydroxysteroid dehydrogenase, 3β-hydroxysteroid dehydrognase, and androgen receptor in the human prostate by in situ hybridization and immunocytochemistry. Endocrinology 1999; 140(3): 1481–1491.

40. Berry SJ, Isaacs JT. Comparative aspects of prostatic growth and androgen metabolism with aging in the dog versus the rat. Endocrinology 1984; 114(2):511–520.

41. Wendel EF, Brannen GE, Putong PB, et al. The effect of orchiectomy and estrogens on benign prostatic hyperplasia. J Urol 1972; 108(1):116–119.

42. Bruchovsky N, Lesser B, van Doorn E, et al. Hormonal effects on cell proliferation in rat prostate. Vitam Horm 1975; 33:61–102.

43. Walsh PC, Wilson JD. The induction of prostatic hypertrophy in the dog with androstanediol. J Clin Invest 1976; 57(4):1093–1097.

44. Rhodes L, Ding VD, Kemp RK, et al. Estradiol causes a dose-dependent stimulation of prostate growth in castrated beagle dogs. Prostate 2000; 44(1):8–18.

45. Ehrlichman RJ, Isaacs JT, Coffey DS. Differences in the effects of estradiol on dihydrotestosterone induced prostatic growth of the castrate dog and rat. Invest Urol 1981; 18(8):466–470.

46. Trachtenberg J, Hicks LL, Walsh PC. Methods for the determination of androgen receptor content in human prostatic tissue. Invest Urol 1981; 18(5):349–354.

47. Jarred RA, Cancilla B, Prins GS, et al. Evidence that estrogens directly alter androgen-regulated prostate development. Endocrinology 2000; 141(9):3471–3477.

48. Lau KM, LaSpina M, Long J, et al. Expression of estrogen receptor (ER)-alpha and ER-beta in normal and malignant prostatic epithelial cells: regulation by methylation and involvement in growth regulation. Cancer Res 2000; 60(12):3175–3182.

49. Walvoord DJ, Resnick MI, Grayhack JT. Effect of testosterone, dihydrotestosterone, estradiol, and prolactin on the weight and citric acid content of the lateral lobe of the rat prostate. Invest Urol 1976; 14(1): 60–65.

50. Reiter E, Bonnet P, Sente B, et al. Growth hormone and prolactin stimulate androgen receptor, insulin-like growth factor-I (IGF-I) and IGF-I receptor levels in the prostate of immature rats. Mol Cell Endocrinol 1992; 88(1–3):77–87.

51. Wennbo H, Kindblom J, Isaksson OG, et al. Transgenic mice overexpressing the prolactin gene develop dramatic enlargement of the prostate gland. Endocrinology 1997; 138(10):4410–4415.

52. Nevalainen MT, Valve EM, Makela SI, et al. Estrogen and prolactin regulation of rat dorsal and lateral prostate in organ culture. Endocrinology 1991; 129(2): 612–622.

53. Nevalainen MT, Valve EM, Ahonen T, et al. Androgen-dependent expression of prolactin in rat prostate epithelium in vivo and in organ culture. FASEB J 1997; 11(14):1297–1307.

54. Nevalainen MT, Valve EM, Ingleton PM, et al. Prolactin and prolactin receptors are expressed and functioning in human prostate. J Clin Invest 1997; 99(4):618–627.

55. Ghosh PK, Bartke A. Effects of the expression of bovine growth hormone on the testes and male accessory reproductive glands in transgenic mice. Transgenic Res 1993; 2(2):79–83.

56. Kolle S, Sinowatz F, Boie G, et al. Expression of growth hormone receptor in human prostatic carcinoma and hyperplasia. Int J Oncology 1999; 14(5):911–916.

57. Mani Maran RR, Subramanian S, Rajendiran G, et al. Prostate-thyroid axis: stimulatory effects of ventral prostate secretions on thyroid function. Prostate 1998; 36(1):8–13.

58. Ivell R, Balvers M, Rust W, et al. Oxytocin and male reproductive function. Adv Exp Med Biol 1997; 424: 253–264.

59. Frayne J, Nicholson HD. Localization of oxytocin receptors in the human and macaque monkey male reproductive tracts: evidence for a physiological role of oxytocin in the male. Mol Hum Reprod 1998; 4(6): 527–532.

60. Popovic A, Jovovic D, Hristic M, et al. The effect of oxytocin in anterior pituitary gonadotropic function in male rats. Iugoslav Physiol Pharmacol Acta 1982; 18: 95–106.

61. Bodanszky M, Sharaf H, Roy JB, et al. Contractile activity of vasotocin, oxytocin and vasopressin on mammalian prostate. Eur J Pharmacol 1992; 216(2): 311–313.

62. Story MT. Regulation of prostate growth by fibroblast growth factors. World J Urol 1995; 13(5):297–305.

63. Ittman M, Mansukhani A. Expression of fibroblast growth factors (FGFs) and FGF receptors in human prostate. J Urol 1997; 157(1):351–356.

64. Giri D, Ropiquet F, Ittmann M. FGF9 is an autocrine and paracrine prostatic growth factor expressed by prostatic stromal cells. J Cell Physiol 1999; 180(1): 53–60.

65. Mansson PE, Adams P, Kan M, et al. Heparin-binding growth factor gene expression and receptor characteristics in normal rat prostate and two transplantable rat prostate tumors. Cancer Res 1989; 49(9): 2485–2494.

66. Leav I, McNeal JE, Ziar J, et al. The localization of transforming growth factor alpha and epidermal growth factor receptor in stromal and epithelial compartments of developing human prostate and hyperplastic, dysplastic, and carcinomatous lesions. Hum Pathol 1998; 29(7):668–675.

67. De Miguel P, Royuela M, Bethencourt R, et al. Immunohistochemical comparative analysis of transforming growth factor alpha, epidermal growth factor, and epidermal growth factor receptor in normal, hyperplastic and neoplastic human prostates. Cytokine 1999; 11(9):722–727.

68. Massague J. The TGF-beta family of growth and differentiation factors. Cell 1987; 49(4):437–438.

69. Hong JH, Song C, Shin Y, et al. Estrogen induction of smooth muscle differentiation of human prostatic stromal cells is mediated by transforming growth factor-beta. J Urol 2004; 171(5):1965–1969.

70. Moses HL, Yang EY, Pietenpol JA. TGF–beta stimulation and inhibition of cell proliferation: new mechanistic insights. Cell 1990; 63(2):245–247.

71. Cohen P, Graves HC, Peehl DM, et al. Prostate-specific antigen (PSA) is an insulin-like growth factor binding protein-3 protease found in seminal plasma. J Clin Endocrinol Metab 1992; 75(4):1046–1053.

72. Cohen P, Peehl DM, Baker B, et al. Insulin-like growth factor axis abnormalities in prostatic stromal cells from patients with benign prostatic hyperplasia. J Clin Endocinol Metab 1994; 79(5):1410–1415.

73. Chan JM, Stampfer MJ, Giovannucci E, et al. Plasma insulin-like growth factor-I and prostate cancer risk: a prospective study. Science 1998; 279(5350):563–566.

74. Thompson TC, Zhau H, Chung LWK. Catecholamines are involved in the growth and expression of prostate

binding protein by rat ventral prostatic tissues. In: Coffey DS, Bruchovsky N, Gardner WA Jr, et al., eds. Current Concepts and Approaches to the Study of Prostate Cancer. New York: Allan R Liss, Inc., 1987: 239–248.

75. Chon JK, Borkowski A, Partin AW, et al. Alpha 1-adrenoceptor antagonists terazosin and doxazosin induce prostate apoptosis without affecting cell proliferation in patients with benign prostatic hyperplasia. J Urol 1999; 161(6):2002–2008.

76. Wang JM, McKenna KE, McVary KT, et al. Requirement of innervation for maintenance of structural and functional integrity in the rat prostate. Biol Reprod 1991; 44(6):1171–1176.

77. McVary KT, McKenna KE, Lee C. Prostate innervation. Prostate Suppl 1998; 8:2–13.

8

Testosterone and Aging

Horace M. Perry III

Department of Internal Medicine–Geriatrics, St. Louis University School of Medicine, St. Louis, Missouri, U.S.A.

John E. Morley

Department of Medicine, Adelaide University, Australia and Division of Geriatric Medicine, St. Louis University School of Medicine and GRECC, St. Louis VA Medical Center, St. Louis, Missouri, U.S.A.

Gary A. Wittert

School of Medicine, Discipline of Medicine, University of Adelaide; Hanson Research Institute; and Discipline of Medicine, Royal Adelaide Hospital, Adelaide, Australia

☐ INTRODUCTION

In the sixteenth century, the Chinese Textbook of Internal Medicine was the first to suggest the existence of a period of male menopause that began in the fifth decade of life (1). Toward the end of the nineteenth century, Brown-Sequard, the French neurologist, tried to rejuvenate himself by injecting an aqueous extract of animal testes. This led Victor DeLespinase in Chicago to undertake the first human testicular transplant in an attempt to delay the aging process. The shortage of available human testis donors led to Serge Voronoff introducing the concept of chimpanzee testicular transplants for the rich in search of the fountain of youth. This approach was highly utilized in the first part of the twentieth century. It was not until the 1930s, however, that testosterone was isolated from bull testes, enabling its synthetic manufacture.

In the 1940s, testosterone replacement began to be utilized for this male "climacteric," which was defined by Werner (2) in 1946 as having the following symptoms: nervousness (90%), decreased potency (90%), decreased libido (80%), irritability (80%), fatigue (80%), depression (77%), memory problems (76%), sleep disturbances (59%), numbness and tingling (44%), and hot flashes (29%). Even the great author Ernest Hemmingway took testosterone replacement for the last 10 years of his life in an effort to minimize this vast constellation of symptoms. Unfortunately, despite these auspicious beginnings, numerous physicians began to treat all symptoms in older males with testosterone, leading to the fall of the male climacteric into disrepute for the next 40 years.

Since that time, numerous names have been used for the syndrome seen in symptomatic older males as a result of testosterone decline. At present, neither "male menopause" nor "climacteric" is considered to be a politically correct term. At present, the most acceptable terms are "andropause" and "androgen deficiency

in aging males" (ADAM). A more colloquial term is "machopause."

This chapter explores the effects of aging on testosterone, the role of the various available assays in measuring testosterone in older men, the pathogenesis of the fall in testosterone levels with aging, and the effects of testosterone deficiency and replacement in aging men.

☐ AGING AND TESTOSTERONE

It is now well established that testosterone levels decline with aging. This has been demonstrated in both cross-sectional and longitudinal studies (3–7). The rate of fall of testosterone is approximately 10% per decade (7) and occurs with a concurrent increase in sex hormone–binding globulin (SHBG) levels.

The increase in SHBG levels makes total testosterone a poor measure of bioavailable or tissue-available testosterone in older males (8–12). For this reason, some measurement of either bioavailable testosterone (BT) utilizing the ammonium sulfate stripping technique or a calculated BT (cBT) is preferred. Alternatively, a free-testosterone level obtained by dialysis, ultracentrifugation, or calculated free-testosterone can be used. Table 1 demonstrates the studies showing a significant relationship between BT and symptoms of androgen deficiency. Because BT is not always available, the authors have developed a cBT that utilizes total testosterone and SHBG:

$$cBT = \frac{1}{2}(T - SHBG - K_D + \sqrt{(T - SHBG - K_D)^2 + 4 \times K_D \times SHBG}), \text{ where } K_D = 5.88 \times 10^{-9} M.$$

Older persons tend to have an equilibrium dissociation constant (K_D) for the BT assay that is twice that of younger persons, and this value should be used for persons over 60 years of age.

The reason for the decline in testosterone with aging is multifactorial. While there is a decrease in

Table 1 Studies Demonstrating a Relationship Between Bioavailable Testosterone and the Symptoms of Androgen Deficiency

Symptom	Author
Libido	Schiavi et al. (13)
Quality of life	Haren et al. (14)
Mood	Barrett-Conner et al. (15)
Memory	Morley et al. (16), Barrett-Conner et al. (17)
Coronary artery disease	English et al. (18)
Bone mineral density	Kenny et al. (19)
Muscle strength	Miller et al. (20), Haren et al. (21)
Function	Miller et al. (20)

Table 2 Changes of Sex Hormones and Anatomy Seen with Aging in Males

Hormones
Decreased total testosterone (1% per yr) and "free" testosterone
Increased sex hormone-binding globulin
Markedly decreased bioavailable testosterone
Normal estradiol
Decreased bioavailable estradiol
Normal or mild decrease dihydrotestosterone
Decreased androstanedione (1.3% per yr)
Decreased dehydroepiandrosterone (3.1% per yr) and its sulfate (2.2% per yr)
Decreased pregnenolone and its sulfate
Normal LH increasing over 80 yr
Decreased bioactive to immunoactive LH
Increased follicle-stimulating hormone
Decreased inhibin
Increased activin

Anatomy
Decreased testicular size and weight
Decreased number of Leydig cells with intracellular vacuolizations and lipofuscin
Decreased Sertoli cell number
Patchy seminiferous tubule degeneration
Impaired sperm maturation and morphology

Abbreviation: LH, luteinizing hormone.

testosterone production from the testes when human chorionic gonadotropin is administered (21–24), in most older men, the major changes appear to take place within the hypothalamic–pituitary unit. There is a decline in pituitary responsiveness to low dose of gonadotropin-releasing hormone (GnRH) (10). In addition, the secretion of GnRH becomes more chaotic with aging, resulting in altered pulsatility of luteinizing hormone (LH) production (25). LH levels, while increasing slightly, tend to remain in the normal range except in the very old, in whom marked increases in LH levels have been observed (7). Typically, LH pulse amplitude is reduced and the pulse frequency tends to be inappropriately normal (26). LH secretion is also more disorderly.

With aging, there is a decrease in seminiferous tubules and a decrease in sperm production (27). This results in a fall in inhibin (28) and an increase in activin (29) levels. Follicle-stimulating hormone (FSH) levels increase monotonically throughout the lifespan after the age of 40 years. There is an increase in FSH pulse amplitude, and the secretion of FSH remains orderly.

Adrenal androgens decline with aging (16). Estradiol shows minimal changes, but bioavailable estradiol declines with aging (30). Table 2 summarizes the changes in sex hormones seen with aging in males.

☐ EFFECTS OF TESTOSTERONE IN OLDER MALES
Sexual Life

The decline in BT with aging is strongly correlated with libido and male sexuality (13). Numerous studies have demonstrated that testosterone replacement in older men increases libido and, to a lesser extent, sexual performance (1,31). Testosterone is necessary for the production of nitric oxide synthase, which plays a pivotal role in penile tumescence. It should be noted that older men will have enhanced responses to sildenafil after testosterone replacement.

Muscle

Low free-testosterone index correlates with a loss of muscle mass (sarcopenia) and strength in older men (20,32). Several studies have demonstrated that testosterone replacement increases lean body mass and upper muscle strength (33–45). The effects on strength, however, are less robust than the effects on muscle mass. The studies that have examined the effect of testosterone on muscle are summarized in Table 3.

Bone Mineral Density

The relationship of testosterone to bone mineral density has been less clear (47,48). One study did demonstrate a relationship of BT to bone mineral density (19). Three studies have shown that the prevalence of minimal trauma hip fracture is related to low testosterone (49–51). Testosterone replacement therapy has been shown to increase bone mineral density in a number of studies (Table 4) (41–43,46,52) and this benefit appears to enhance even the effects of vitamin D and calcium.

The mechanisms by which testosterone increases bone mineral density seem to occur mainly through its conversion to estradiol. Studies in young men with estrogen receptor or aromatase deficiencies suggest that bone growth mainly depends on estrogen (53). Bioavailable estradiol correlates better with bone mineral density than does BT (54,55). In older men, when testosterone is inhibited and either estrogen or testosterone is replaced, estrogen inhibits osteoclastic activity and stimulates osteoblastic activity while testosterone only has a small effect on the stimulation of osteoblastic activity (56).

Function

Testosterone and BT have been demonstrated to correlate with function in older males (45). A small study has shown that testosterone replacement following

Table 3 The Effect of Testosterone Replacement on Muscle in Older Men

Author (Ref.)	No.	Length of treatment	Type of trial	Lean mass	Upper limb strength	Lower limb strength
Tenover (37)	13	3 mo	Placebo	↑	NC	—
Morley et al. (33)	8	3 mo	Uncontrolled	—	↑	—
Marin et al. (38)	31	9 mo	Uncontrolled	NC	—	—
Urban et al. (35)	6	1 mo	Uncontrolled	↑	NC	↑
Katznelson et al. (36)	27	18 mo	Uncontrolled	↑	—	—
Reid et al. (46)	15	12 mo	Controlled	↑	—	—
Sih et al. (34)	17	12 mo	Placebo, blind	NC	↑	—
Snyder et al. (40)	54	36 mo	Placebo, blind	↑	NC	—
Kenny et al. (42)	34	12 mo	Placebo, blind	↑	—	NC
Bebb et al. (43)[a]	?	12 mo	Placebo, blind	↑	—	NC
Blackman et al. (39)[a]	17	6 mo	Placebo, blind	↑	↑	NC
Tenover et al. (41)[a]	?	36 mo	Placebo, blind	↑	↑	—
Clague et al. (45)	7	3 mo	Uncontrolled	NC	NC	—
Bakhshi et al. (44)	9	2 mo	Uncontrolled	—	↑	—

[a]Abstracts only.
Abbreviation: NC, no change.

hospitalization in men undergoing rehabilitation improved the functional index measure as a rehabilitation outcome (44).

Cognition

It has been demonstrated that BT is correlated with some cognitive functions (16,17). Testosterone replacement in the SAMP8, an animal model of Alzheimer's, reversed the memory defect by reducing the overproduction of amyloid precursor protein (57,58). Studies in humans suggest that testosterone replacement in older hypogonadal males improves visuospatial memory (59–61). (Further information on this topic can be found in Chapter 10.)

Fat and Leptin

Testosterone replacement reduced body fat in older males (62). Both cross-sectionally (63,64) and longitudinally (65,66), it has been shown that leptin increases with age when expressed per unit of adipose tissue. This increase was strongly related to the fall in testosterone. Testosterone replacement decreased leptin levels (34,66).

Leptin has been postulated to play a role in the physiological anorexia of aging (67). Figure 1 illustrates the postulated mechanism by which testosterone

Table 4 Effects of Testosterone Replacement on Bone Mineral Density in Older Males

Author (Ref.)	Length of study (mo)	Calcium + vitamin D	Effect
Reid (46)	12	No	↑
Snyder (40)	36	In some	↑[a]
Kenny (42)	12	Yes	↑
Tenover (41)	36	No	↑
Bebb (43)	12	Yes	↑
Katznelson (36)	18	No	↑

[a]Only in those with low bone mineral density.

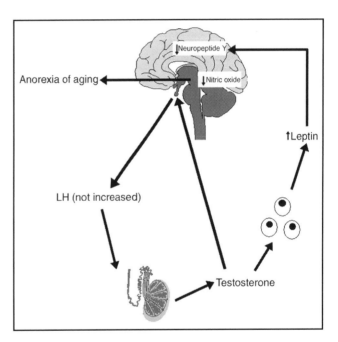

Figure 1 Role of decreased testosterone in the pathogenesis of the anorexia of aging. *Abbreviation:* LH, luteinizing hormone.

decline leads to an increase in leptin and a decrease in Neuropeptide Y and nitric oxide, resulting in anorexia.

Atherosclerosis

Numerous epidemiological studies have found that low testosterone levels are associated with coronary artery disease (68). Interestingly, atherosclerotic plaques in the coronary arteries are more numerous in persons with low testosterone levels (69). Acute administration of testosterone, however, produced coronary artery vasodilation (70,71).

A number of studies have shown that testosterone replacement will reduce angina (Table 5) (18,72–74). Testosterone replacement also reduced ST depression during a stress test in men who had experienced a previous myocardial infarction (75).

Table 5 Effect of Testosterone Replacement on Angina

Author (Ref.)	No.	Effect
Walker (73)	9	Decrease in severity of pain in 7 patients
Hamm (74)	7	Relief from angina
Wu (72)	31	Angina was relieved in 77.4% and myocardial ischemia on Holter improved
English et al. (18)	23	Decreased pain perception role limitation and an increase in time to 1 mm ST-segment depression

Table 6 Major Side Effects of Testosterone Replacement in Older Men

Elevated hematocrit → stroke
Increased symptoms with prostate cancer
Edema (water retention)
Hypertension worsens
Gynecomastia
Worsened sleep apnea
Decreased HDL-cholesterol
Liver dysfunction

Abbreviation: HDL, high-density lipoprotein.

Insulin Growth Factor

Testosterone increased serum insulin growth factor 1 (IGF I) (39) and mRNA for IGF I in muscle (34).

□ SCREENING FOR ADAM

Two screening tests have been developed to detect ADAM. The first test is based on data from 1660 men participating in the Massachusetts Aging Male Study, with ages from 40 to 79 years. Predominantly screening for risk factors, elements of this test include treated diabetes, body mass index, age, headaches, current nonsmoking, treated asthma, low dominance, and sleeplessness (76). While initial results were determined to have a sensitivity of 71% and a specificity of 53%, retesting of 382 of these males in an outpatient setting produced a sensitivity of 76% and a specificity of 49%.

The other screening test is known as the ADAM questionnaire and is based on a 10-point forced yes-or-no style (see the Appendix at the end of this chapter) (77). Developed initially in a sample of 316 males aged 40 to 82 years, it demonstrated a sensitivity of 88% and a specificity of 60%. When patients with low testosterone levels and a positive ADAM questionnaire were treated, they had a marked reduction in their ADAM scores. The major reason for a false positive on the ADAM questionnaire is severe dysphoria.

□ TESTOSTERONE REPLACEMENT

For further information on this topic, please refer to Chapter 29 entitled "Androgen Replacement Therapy."

□ SIDE EFFECTS OF TESTOSTERONE REPLACEMENT IN OLDER MALES

Testosterone replacement is known to cause a number of significant side effects in men (Table 6). For example,

testosterone has been shown to increase hematocrit through an erythropoietin-independent mechanism. When the hematocrit rises above 55%, there is an increased risk of stroke.

In severely hypogonadal older males, there is a small increase in the prostate-specific antigen (PSA) when testosterone is replaced. In most older males, there is no change in PSA with testosterone replacement (1). Testosterone therapy does not appear to increase prostate growth in most older persons with benign prostate hypertrophy (78,79).

It is important to note that testosterone replacement accelerates the growth of established prostate cancer (80). There has been no evidence, however, that testosterone causes growth of prostate cancer in situ. Prostate cancer is associated with very low testosterone levels in epidemiological studies (81,82). More studies are necessary to determine the relationship of testosterone and dihydrotestosterone to the pathogenesis of prostate cancer.

No definitive evidence has been found of the long-term effects of testosterone replacement on men. In one long-term study, Gooren (83) followed eight men over 50 years, who had received testosterone replacement for a 10-year term. No discernible adverse effects, however, were detected.

The effects of testosterone replacement on sleep apnea appear to be unclear, as one study has demonstrated a worsening of sleep apnea with testosterone treatment (84) while another did not (52).

□ CONCLUSION

There is a continuous decline in BT with aging. This decline is associated with a variety of symptoms, many of which may be reversed by the use of testosterone replacement therapy in testosterone-deficient older males. The ADAM questionnaire is considered to be an adequate screening test for the presence of andropause during the initial evaluation of symptomatic patients. There is no adequate data on the long-term safety of testosterone replacement. A greater understanding about the effects of testosterone replacement is needed.

☐ REFERENCES

1. Morley JE, Perry HM III. Androgen deficiency in aging men: role of testosterone replacement therapy. J Lab Clin Med 2000; 135:370–378.

2. Werner AA. The male climacteric: report of two hundred and seventy-three cases. JAMA 1946; 132(4):188–194.

3. Vermeulen A. Androgens in the aging male. J Clin Endocrinol Metab 1991; 73:221.

4. Bhasin S. Clinical review 34: androgen treatment of hypogonadal men. J Clin Endocrinol Metab 1992; 74:1221.

5. Pirke KM, Doerr P. Age related changes in free plasma testosterone, dihydrotestosterone and oestradiol. Acta Endocrinol (Copenh) 1975; 80(1):171.

6. Gray A, Feldman HA, McKinlay JB, et al. Age, disease, and changing sex hormone levels in middle-aged men: results of the Massachusetts male aging study. J Clin Endocrinol Metab 1991; 73(5):1016–1025.

7. Morley JE, Kaiser FE, Perry HM, et al. Longitudinal changes in testosterone, luteinizing hormone, and follicle-stimulating hormone in healthy older men. Metabolism 1997; 46(4):410.

8. Haji M, Tanaka S, Nishi Y, et al. Sertoli cell function decline earlier than Leydig cell function in aging Japanese men. Maturitas 1994; 18(2):143–153.

9. Kaiser FE, Viosca SP, Morley JE, et al. Impotence and aging: clinical and hormonal factors. J Am Geratr Soc 1988; 3:511–519.

10. Korenman SG, Morley JE, Mooradian AD, et al. Secondary hypogonadism in older men: its relation to impotence. J Clin Endocrinol Metab 1990; 71(4):963–969.

11. Nankin HR, Calkins JH. Decreased bioavailable testosterone in aging normal and impotent men. J Clin Endocrinol Metab 1986; 63(6):1418–1420.

12. Leifke E, Forenoi V, Wichers C, et al. Age-related changes of serum sex hormones, insulin-like growth factor-1 and sex-hormone binding globulin levels in men: cross-sectional data from a healthy male cohort. Clin Endocrinol (Oxf) 2000; 53(6):689–695.

13. Schiavi RC, Schreiner-Engel P, White D, et al. The relationship between pituitary-gonadal function and sexual behavior in healthy aging men. Psychosomatic Med 1991; 53(4):363–374.

14. Haren M, Nordin BEC, Pearce CEM, et al. The calculation of bioavailable testosterone. Andrology in the 21st Century (short communication). In: Robaire B, Chemes H, Morales C (eds.), Proceedings of the VII International Congress of Andrology. Medimond: Englewood, NJ pp.209–213.

15. Barrett-Conner E, Von Muhlen DG, Kritz-Silverstein D. Bioavailable testosterone and depressed mood in older men: the Rancho Bernardo Study. J Clin Endocrinol Metab 1999; 84(2):573–577.

16. Morley JE, Kaiser F, Raum WJ, et al. Potentially predictive and manipulable blood serum correlates of aging in the healthy human male–progressive decreases in bioavailable testosterone, dehydroepiandrosterone sulfate, and the ratio of insulin-like growth factor 1 to growth hormone. Proc Nat Acad Sci USA 1997; 94(14):7537–7542.

17. Barrett-Connor E, Goodman-Gruen D, Patay B. Endogenous sex hormones and cognitive function in older men. J Clin Endocrinol Metab 1999; 84(10):3681–3685.

18. English DM, Steeds RP, Jones Th, et al. Low-dose transdermal testosterone therapy improves angina threshold in men with chronic stable angina: A randomized, double-blind, placebo-controlled study. Circulation 2000; 102(16):1906–1911.

19. Kenny AM, Prestwood KM, Marcello KM, et al. Determinants of bone density in healthy older men with low testosterone levels. J Geron 2000; 55A(9): M492–M497.

20. Miller DK, Lui LY, Perry HM III, et al. Reported and measured physical functioning in older inner-city diabetic African Americans. J Geron 1999; 54A(5): M230–M236.

21. Rubens R, Dhont M, Vermeulen A. Further studies on Leydig cell function in old age. J Clin Endocrinol Metab 1974; 39(1):40–45.

22. Harman SM, Tsitouras PD. Reproductive hormones in aging men. I. Measurement of sex steroids, basal luteinizing hormone, and Leydig cell response to human chorionic gonadotropin. J Clin Endocrinol Metab 1980; 51(1):35–40.

23. Longcope E. The effect of human chorionic gonadotropin on plasma steroid levels in young and old men. Steroids 1973; 21(4):583–592.

24. Hammar M. Impaired in vitro testicular endocrine function in elderly men. Andrologia 1985; 17(5):444–449.

25. Keenan DM, Veldhuis JD. Hypothesis testing of the aging male gonadal axis via a biomathematical construct. Am J Physiol Regul Integr Comp Physiol 2001; 280(6):R1755–R1771.

26. Veldhuis JD. Recent neuroendocrine facets of male reproductive aging. Exp Gerontol 2000; 35(9–10): 1281–1308.

27. Neaves SB, Johnson L, Petty CS. Seminiferous tubules and daily sperm production in older men with varied numbers of Leydig cells. Biol Reprod 1987; 36: 301–308.

28. Tenover JS, Matsumoto AM, Plymate SR, et al. The effects of aging in normal men on bioavailable testosterone and luteinizing hormone secretion: response to

clomiphene citrate. J Clin Endocrinol Metab 1987; 65(6):1118–1126.

29. Lona P, Petraglia F, Concari M, et al. Influence of age and sex on serum concentrations of total dimeric activin A. Eur J Endocrinol 1998; 139(5):487–492.

30. Szulc P, Munoz F, Claustrat B, et al. Bioavailable estradiol may be an important determinant of osteoporosis in men: the MINOS study. J Clin Endocrinol Metab 2001; 86(1):192–199.

31. Morales A, Johnston B, Heaton JP, et al. Testosterone supplementation for hypogonadal impotence: assessment of biochemical measures and therapeutic outcome. J Urol 1997; 157(3):849–854.

32. Baumgartner RN, Waters DL, Gallagher D, et al. Predictors of skeletal muscle mass in elderly men and women. Mech Ageing Dev 1999; 107(2):123–136.

33. Morley JE, Perry HM III, Kaiser FE, et al. Effects of testosterone replacement therapy in old hypogonadal males: a preliminary study. J Am Geriatr Soc 1993; 41(2):149–152.

34. Sih R, Morley JE, Kaiser Fe, et al. Testosterone replacement in older hypogonadal men: a 12-month randomized controlled trial. J Clin Endocrinol Metab 1997; 82(6): 1661–1667.

35. Urban RJ, Bodenburg YH, Gilkison C, et al. Testosterone replacement doses of testosterone on muscle size and strength in normal men. N Engl J Med 1996; 335:1–7.

36. Katznelson L, Finkelstein JS, Schoenfeld DA, et al. Increase in bone density and lean body mass during testosterone administration in men with acquired hypogonadism. J Clin Endocrinol Metab 1996; 81(12): 4358–4365.

37. Tenover JS. Effects of testosterone supplementation in the aging male. J Clin Endocrinol Metab 1992; 75:1092–1098.

38. Marin P. Testosterone and regional fat distribution. Obes Res 1995; 3(suppl 4):609S–612S.

39. Blackman MR, Chrisman C, O'Connor KG, et al. Effects of growth hormone and/or sex steroid administration on body composition in healthy elderly men and women. Proc Endoc Soc 81st Annual Meeting, San Diego, CA, 1999 (abstr:392–523).

40. Snyder PJ, Peachey H, Hannoush P, et al. Effect of testosterone treatment on body composition and muscle strength in men over 65 years of age. J Clin Endocrinol Metab 1999; 84(8):2647–2653.

41. Tenover JS. Testosterone for all? Proc Endoc Soc 80th annual meeting, New Orleans, LA, 1998, 24 (abstr #528).

42. Kenny AM, Prestwood KM, Gruman CA, et al. Effects of transdermal testosterone on bone and muscle in older men with low bioavailable testosterone levels. J Geron 2001; 56A(5):M266–M272.

43. Bebb RA, Unawalt BA, Wade J, et al. A randomized placebo controlled trial of testosterone undeconotate administration in aging hypogonadal men. Proc Endoc Soc 83th Annual Meeting 2001, 100 (abstr, OR124–105).

44. Bakhshi V, Elliott M, Gentili A, et al. Testosterone improves rehabilitation outcomes in ill older men. J Am Ger Soc 2000; 48(5):550–553.

45. Clague SE, Wu FC, Horan MA. Difficulties in measuring the effect of testosterone replacement therapy on muscle function in older men. J Androl 1999; 22(4):261–265.

46. Reid IR, Wattie DJ, Evans MC, et al. Testosterone therapy in glucocorticoid-treated men. Arch Intern Med 1996; 156(11):1173–1177.

47. Foresta C, Ruzza G, Mioni R, et al. Testosterone and bone loss in Klinefelter syndrome. Horm Metab Res 1983; 15:56–57.

48. Ongphiphadhanakul B, Rajatanavin R, Chailurkit L, et al. Serum testosterone and its relation to bone mineral density and body composition in normal males. Clin Endocrinol (Oxf) 1995; 43(6):727–733.

49. Stanley HL, Schmitt BP, Poses RM, et al. Does hypogonadism contribute to the occurrence of a minimal trauma hip fracture in elderly men? J Am Geriatr Soc 1991; 39(8):760–771.

50. Abbasi AA, Rudman D, Wilson CR, et al. Observations on nursing home residents with a history of hip fracture. Am J Med Sci 1995; 310(6):229–234.

51. Jackson JA, Riggs MW, Spiekerman AM. Testosterone deficiency as a risk factor for hip fractures in men: a case-control study. Am J Med Sci 1992; 304(1):4–8.

52. Snyder PJ, Peachey H, Hennoush P, et al. Effect of testosterone treatment on bone mineral density in men over 65 years of age. J Clin Endocrinol Metab 1999; 84(6):1966–1972.

53. Katz MS. Geriatrics grand rounds: Eve's rib, or a revisionist view of osteoporosis in men. J Geron 2000; 55A(10):M560–M569.

54. Amin S, Zhang YQ, Sawin DT, et al. Association of hypogonadism and estradiol levels with bone mineral density in elderly men from the Framingham study. Ann Inter Med 2000; 133(12):951–963.

55. Khosla S, Melton LJ III, Atkinson EJ, et al. Relationship of serum sex steroid levels and bone turnover markers with bone mineral density in men and women: a key role for bioavailable estrogen. J Clin Endocrinol Metab 1998; 83(7):2266–2274.

56. Falahati-Nini A, Riggs BL, Atkinson EJ, et al. Relative contributions of testosterone and estrogen in regulating bone resorption and formation in normal elderly men. J Clin Invest 2000; 106(12):1553–1560.

57. Flood JF, Morley JE. Learning and memory in the SAMP8 mouse. Neurosci Biobehav Rev 1998; 22(1):1–20.

58. Flood JF, Farr SA, Kaiser FE, et al. Age-related decrease in plasma testosterone in SAMP8 mice: replacement improves age-related impairment of learning and memory. Physi Beh 1995; 57(4):669–673.

59. Jankowsky JS, Oviatt SK, Orwall ES. Testosterone influences spatial cognition in older men. Behav Neurosci 1994; 108(2):325–332.

60. Cherrier MM, Asthana S, Plymate S, et al. Testosterone supplementation improves spatial and verbal memory in healthy older men. Neurology 2001; 57(1):80–88.

61. Janowsky JS, Chavez B, Orwell E. Sex steroids modify working memory. J Cognitive Neurosci 2000; 12(3): 407–414.

62. Marin P, Krotkiewski M, Bjorntorp P. Androgen treatment of middle-aged, obese men: effects on metabolism, muscle and adipose tissues. Europ J Med 1992; 1(6):329–336.

63. Baumgartner RN, Ross RR, Waters DL, et al. Serum leptin in elderly people: associations with sex hormones, insulin, and adipose tissue volumes. Obesity Res 1999; 7(2):141–149.

64. Luukkaa V, Pesonen U, Huhtaniemi I, et al. Inverse correlation between serum testosterone and leptin in men. J Clin Endocrinol Metab 1998; 83(9):3243–3246.

65. Baumgartner RN, Waters DL, Morley JE, et al. Age-related changes in sex hormones affect the sex difference in serum leptin independently of changes in body fat. Metabolism 1999; 48(3):378–384.

66. Hislop MS, Ratanjee BD, Soule SG, et al. Effects of anabolic-androgenic steroid use of gonadal testosterone suppression on serum leptin concentration in men. Euro J Endocrin 1999; 141(1):40–46.

67. Morley JE, Thomas DR. Anorexia and aging: pathophysiology. (Rev) Nutrition 1999; 15(6):499–503.

68. Barrett-Connor EL. Testosterone and risk factors for cardiovascular disease in men. Diabetes Metab 1995; 21(3):156–161.

69. Phillips GB, Pinkernell BH, Jing TY. The association of hypotestosteronemia with coronary artery disease in men. Arterioscler Thromb 1994; 14(5):701–706.

70. Rosano GM, Leonardo F, Pagnotta P, et al. Acute anti-ischemic effect of testosterone in men with coronary artery disease. Circulation 1999; 99(13):1666–1670.

71. Webb CM, McNeill JG, Hayward CS, de Zeigler D, Collins P. Effects of testosterone on coronary vasomotor regulation in men with coronary heart disease. Circulation 1999; 10(16):1690–1696.

72. Wu SZ, Weng XZ. Therapeutic effects of an androgenic preparation on myocardial ischemia and cardiac function in 62 elderly male coronary heart disease patients. Chin Med J 1993; 106(6):415–418.

73. Walker TC. Use of testosterone propionate and estrogenic substance in treatment of essential hypertension, angina pectoris and peripheral vascular disease. J Clin Endocrinol Metab 1942; 2:560–568.

74. Hamm L. Testosterone propionate in the treatment of angina pectoris. J Clin Endocrinol Metab 1942; 2:325–328.

75. Jaffe MD. Effect of testosterone cypionate on postexercise ST segment depression. Br Heart J 1977; 39(11):1217–1222.

76. Smith KW, Feldman HA, McKinlay JB. Construction and field validation of a self-administered screener for testosterone deficiency (hypogonadism) in ageing men. Clin Endocrinol 2000; 53(6):703–711.

77. Morley JE, Charlton E, Patrick P, et al. Validation of a screening questionnaire for androgen deficiency in aging males. Metabolism 2000; 49(9):1239–1242.

78. Hajjar RR, Kaiser FE, Morley JE. Outcomes of long-term testosterone replacement in older hypogonadal males: a retrospective analysis. J Clin Endocrinol Metab 1997; 82(11):3793–3796.

79. Hartnell J, Korenman SG, Viosca SP. Results of testosterone enanthate therapy in older men. Proc Endoc Soc 72nd Annual Meeting 1990, 428.

80. Fowler JE Jr, Whitmore WF Jr. The response of metastatic adenocarcinoma of the prostate to exogenous testosterone. J Urol 1981; 126(3):372–375.

81. Carter HB, Pearson JD, Metter EJ, et al. Longitudinal evaluation of serum androgen levels in men with or without prostate cancer. Prostate 1995; 27(1):25–31.

82. Ribeiro M, Ruff P, Falkson G. Low serum testosterone and a younger age predict a poor outcome in metastatic prostate cancer. Am J Clin Oncol 1997; 20(6): 605–608.

83. Gooren LJG. A ten-year safety study of the oral androgen testosterone undecanoate. J Andrology 1994; 15(3):212–215.

84. Sandblom RE, Matsumoto AM, Schoene RB, et al. Obstructive sleep apnea syndrome induced by testosterone administration. New Engl J Med 1983; 308(9):508–510.

☐ APPENDIX
Androgen Deficiency in the Aging Male (ADAM) Questionnaire

The ADAM questionnaire is a simple, one-time, yes-or-no self-quiz that can assist a patient in deciding whether or not to talk with his doctor about his symptoms.

1. Do you have a decrease in libido (sex drive)? _____
2. Do you have a lack of energy? _____
3. Do you have a decrease in strength and/or endurance? _____
4. Have you lost height? _____
5. Have you noticed a decreased "enjoyment of life"? _____
6. Are you sad and/or grumpy? _____
7. Are your erections less strong? _____
8. Have you noted a recent deterioration in your ability to play sports? _____
9. Are you falling asleep after dinner? _____
10. Has there been a recent deterioration in your work performance? _____

Source: St. Louis University, ADAM Questionnaire; this questionnaire was developed by John E. Morley, M.B., B.Ch. It is to be used solely as a screening tool to assist your physician in diagnosing androgen deficiency.

Effects of Aging on Spermatogenesis and Sperm Function

Bernard Robaire, Christopher C. Oakes, and Ekaterina V. Zubkova

Departments of Pharmacology and Therapeutics, and Obstetrics and Gynecology, McGill University, Montreal, Quebec, Canada

☐ INTRODUCTION

The highly coordinated process by which very large numbers of spermatozoa are produced on a daily basis from puberty onward has been well described for a variety of species (1,2). The kinetics of spermatogenesis reveals that, once established, the process does not accelerate or decelerate (1). New generations of spermatozoa are continuously initiated in the seminiferous epithelium of the adult; hence, germ cells leaving the testis on an ongoing basis have been dividing and differentiating for a relatively short period of time, in the range of 35 to 64 days, depending on the mammalian species. As a consequence, a common conclusion has been that, unlike female germ cells, male germ cells are always freshly made and hence do not age. Yet, the cells from which male germ cells arise, the pale spermatogonia, act as stem cells and are present throughout the lifespan of the male.

Very few studies have investigated how sperm quality is affected by advancing age, that is, whether the spermatogonia that divide to produce subsequent generations of germ cells accumulate damage that results in spermatozoa of diminished quality as individuals age; however, several clinical studies as well as studies using models of animal aging indicate that there are significant changes that occur in spermatozoa as males enter advanced age and that such changes have consequences for the progeny.

This chapter discusses the effects of aging: on semen properties, in animal models to study the aging of male germ cells, on the quality and structure of chromatin and DNA in sperm nuclei, on the epidemiological aspects of male-mediated genetic defects, and finally on potential factors that could influence the quality of spermatozoa.

☐ CHANGES IN SEMEN CHARACTERISTICS WITH AGE

There have been many studies aimed at shedding light on the effects of aging on semen quality, a key indicator of male fertility. The results of these studies, however, should be interpreted with caution, as there are several common factors that render the interpretation difficult. These factors include: (*i*) duration of abstinence, which has been shown to increase significantly with age (3), (*ii*) age of the female partner, (*iii*) appropriate selection criteria, (*iv*) appropriate controls, and (*v*) a sufficiently large study population. Taking into account these confounding factors, several detailed analyses of existing clinical data were made recently of the impact of age on various semen parameters as well as on fertility (3–5).

Semen Volume

In most studies (4,6), semen volume was one of the parameters that changed consistently with age, with decreases ranging from 3% to 22%. Plas et al. (5) also found semen volume to have a decreasing trend with age, from 1% (for 30-year-old men) to 40% (for 50-year-old men). Although not all studies showed statistically significant effects, overall they demonstrated a strong trend for decreased semen volume with age.

There may be several reasons for this decrease. The well-established decrease in serum androgens during aging (7–9) may certainly be a contributing factor; this would result in decreased secretions from sex accessory glands (e.g., seminal vesicles and prostate) and hence in a reduced semen volume. Another possible explanation is decreased daily sperm production/gram of testicular parenchyma: it has been shown to be decreased by about 30% in men aged 51 to 80 years, compared to men aged 21 to 50 years (10).

Concentration of Spermatozoa

There appears to be a similar number of studies of comparable quality that report increased, decreased, or unchanged spermatozoa concentrations (3–5). Therefore, the evidence regarding this parameter is inconclusive and is possibly indicative of no change associated with age.

Sperm Motility

The parameter that showed the greatest and consistent change with age was the motility of spermatozoa, where decreases of 2% to 37% were reported with age (3,4). This decrease in motility was usually assessed by using standard parameters, as recommended in the WHO guidelines; however, detailed analyses of the effects of age on the characteristics of sperm motility using computerized tracking of sperm motion have not yet been done in humans, although animal studies suggest that such parameters may be affected by age (11).

Sperm Morphology

There appears to be a consistent increase in the incidence of abnormal spermatozoa with advancing age, but the nature of the observed abnormalities is poorly defined (3,4). More commonly reported defects in spermatozoa of older males are increased incidences of sperm-tail defects such as coiling or bending of tails (5). Detailed examinations of these defects using more powerful tools such as electron microscopy or specific markers for structural proteins have yet to be done.

Fertility

Several studies indicate that there is a decrease in fertility with advancing paternal age (3,12,13). While some studies that examine the male factor in age-dependent changes in infertility take into account the age of the female partner, others do not; this has resulted in some reports indicating exceedingly longer time to pregnancy (TTP). Another problem with most studies that seek to examine the impact of the father's age on fertility is that the subject population is often selected from infertility and assisted-conception clinics; this can potentially bias the studies because the subjects are more likely to be prone to fertility problems. Additionally, the problem with studying TTP is that it does not take into account failed attempts at conception. Therefore, it is difficult at this time to extend findings of age-related declines in fertility to the general population of males without preexisting fertility problems.

Hassan and Killick (14) conducted a particularly well-controlled analysis of the relationship between TTP and male age in a large study population, which recruited participants without predetermined fertility problems and controlled for the age of the female partner. They found that increasing male age was associated with a significant decline in fertility, with men over 45 years of age having a fivefold longer TTP than younger men. To establish a firm footing for concluding that fertility is affected by aging of the male partner, additional studies taking a similar approach are necessary.

□ ANIMAL MODELS USED TO STUDY AGING OF MALE GERM CELLS

The intrinsic difficulty associated with conducting aging studies with human subjects to investigate reproduction has prompted investigators to search for animal models of male reproductive aging that would provide results that could be translated to humans. Although several strains of mice have been found to show premature aging [e.g., klotho, senescence accelerated mouse (SAM) (15,16)], remarkable differences exist between these strains. The reproductive system was not extensively studied in any of the strains of mice, nor were there changes that suggest they would be good models for human male reproductive aging. The Brown Norway rat, however, has been established as a highly robust model for the study of male reproductive aging (17–21). This strain of rat has a long lifespan (up to 40 months), does not exhibit many of the age-related pathologies found in other rat strains, such as pituitary and Leydig cell tumors, and does not become obese. There are striking changes in the testis of these animals even though no disease is apparent. Aging of the testis in the Brown Norway rat is marked by a gradual decrease in the percentage of normal seminiferous tubules, total sperm count, and the ability of Leydig cells to produce testosterone as well as several genes and enzymes associated with testosterone production (17–24). Importantly, the decreases seen with age in spermatogenesis and steroidogenesis in the Brown Norway rat have been reported to occur also in aging men (25,26). Additionally, there are dramatic changes in the epididymal epithelial architecture (27–29) and gene expression (30) as Brown Norway rats age. Few studies, however, have been designed to test directly the effects of advancing age on the quality of spermatozoa (11,31,32).

The authors of this chapter conducted a study in which male rats of increasing age (3–24 months) were mated with young females; pregnancy outcome was assessed by counting the numbers of corpora lutea, resorptions, and live fetuses on day 20 of gestation (32). To evaluate progeny outcome, pups were examined for external malformations and weighed daily for two months. There were no significant changes in the numbers of resorptions and live offspring or in the incidence of external malformations. There was, however, more than a threefold increase in the percent of preimplantation loss (corpora lutea minus implantation sites) in litters fathered by old as compared to young males (Fig. 1, top left). Surprisingly, there was a significant decrease in the average fetal weight that was directly associated with increasing paternal age (Fig. 1, top right). In addition, a greater than threefold increase in neonatal deaths was found for progeny fathered by older males (Fig. 1, bottom right). These results clearly indicate that the quality of spermatozoa decreases as males age.

Based on this demonstration that progeny outcome is altered by paternal aging (32) and the observations that there is age-dependent deterioration of the seminiferous tubules (19,33) and epididymal epithelia (27), the authors hypothesized that formation of spermatozoa in the testis and maturation of spermatozoa in the epididymis (i.e., acquisition of motility and loss of the cytoplasmic droplet) may be altered during aging (11). A marked increase was found in the number

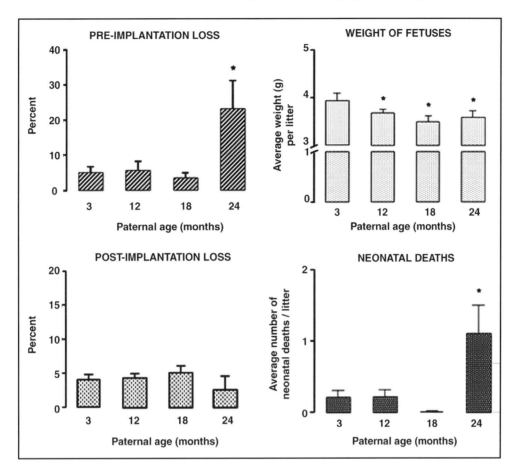

Figure 1 Effect of increasing age on fertility parameters of male Brown Norway rats. All studies were done using male Brown Norway rats aged 3, 12, 18, and 24 months mated with young female Sprague Dawley rats. (*Top left*) Percent preimplantation loss, defined as the number of corpora lutea minus the number of implantation sites. (*Bottom left*) Percent postimplantation loss, defined as the number of implantation sites minus the number of fetuses on day 20 of gestation. (*Top right*) Mean fetal weight per liter on day 20 of gestation. (*Bottom right*) Neonatal death rate of pups during the first four days after birth. Bars represent mean ± SEM, $n = 6$.*$p \leq 0.05$, by ANOVA and Tukey's test. *Abbreviations*: ANOVA, analysis of variance; SEM, standard error of the mean. *Source*: From Ref. 32.

of abnormal flagellar midpieces of spermatozoa with age, suggesting that the formation of spermatozoa in the testes of older males is defective (Fig. 2). In the caput epididymidis, the percentage of motile sperm was similar in young and old rats. In contrast, the percentage of motile spermatozoa was significantly decreased in the cauda epididymidis of old rats. Furthermore, the proportion of spermatozoa that retained their cytoplasmic droplet was markedly elevated. Some of these effects are likely to be due to changes taking place in spermatozoa during the process of spermatogenesis (e.g., formation of the flagellum), while others

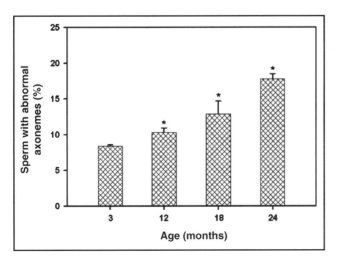

Figure 2 Percentage of cauda epididymal spermatozoa showing an abnormal flagellar midpiece or the presence of several tails surrounded by the same membrane in rats aged 3, 12, 18, and 24 months. Bars represent mean ± SEM, *values differ significantly from three-month-old BN rat by Student's *t* test, $p < 0.05$. *Abbreviations*: BN, Brown Norway; SEM, standard error of the mean. *Source*: From Ref. 11.

could occur during sperm maturation in the epididymis (e.g., acquisition of motility). The multiple effects of aging on sperm morphology, the acquisition of motility, and the shedding of the cytoplasmic droplet further indicate that the quality of spermatozoa is affected by aging.

☐ EFFECTS OF AGE ON THE SPERM GENOME

Epidemiological Considerations

The impact of age on the chromatin quality of sperm is most dramatically evidenced by human diseases that exhibit a "paternal age effect." This is defined by an increase in the age of the father correlating with an increased risk of parenting abnormal offspring or offspring that are more likely to acquire diseases. The father donates only DNA to his offspring; hence, the cause of this effect must be genetic in origin. In 1955, Penrose (34) was the first to recognize that the increased frequency of certain disorders in children born to older parents could primarily be attributed to advanced paternal age. Achondroplasia, the most common form of dwarfism, occurs as a result of an autosomal-dominant mutation in the fibroblast growth factor 3 (FGF3) gene. After controlling for the age of the mother, Penrose demonstrated that children born with the disease were more likely to have older fathers.

Autosomal-dominant mutations that are completely penetrant in the heterozygote are the easiest diseases in which to discern a paternal age effect. Several other diseases of this type also have been shown to possess a strong paternal age effect (35). More recently, several diseases of complex etiology have been associated with a paternal age effect; these include schizophrenia and general psychosis (36,37), Alzheimer's disease (38), cardiac defects (39), and some cancers (40), all of which exhibit increased relative risk for children born to older fathers. In addition, daughters born to older fathers exhibit decreased longevity (41). Although the absolute cause(s) of these diseases are unknown, the paternal age effect underlines the presence of a genetic component.

There was a controversy regarding the effect of paternal age on reproductive success in humans. A study by Selvin and Garfinkel (42) showed that the proportion of abortions in or after the 20th week of gestation increased with paternal age (independent of maternal age), although a later study did not observe this effect (43). A large study of approximately nine million pregnancies in the United States demonstrated that offspring of fathers who were more than 10 years older than their partners were generally at increased risk of fetal death, decreased birth weight, and preterm delivery (44). These findings have recently been supported by others (45,46), although an increase in general birth defects was not found (47). It is interesting to note the similarity between these reports and the results described for the Brown Norway rat above.

Genetic Evidence for Aging of Male Germ Cells

There are many types of genetic insults that can occur in sperm chromatin, and diseases that exhibit a paternal age effect are caused by various types of mutations. Diseases that show such an effect are most commonly the result of single base substitutions (48). The types and frequencies of mutations that occur in normal and aged sperm, however, cannot be directly linked to the causes or frequency of de novo germline genetic disease in the progeny. Genetic abnormalities in sperm are assumed to be much greater, because many mutations are neutral or recessive, and mutations in genes essential for gametogenesis or embryogenesis might not result in fertilization or a live birth. Knowledge of the effects of age on sperm chromatin quality is important for understanding many aspects of reproductive function, including infertility, abnormal fetal development, and perinatal outcomes, as well as de novo genetic diseases.

Very little experimental data are available on the age-dependent genetic integrity of sperm. Studies in mice detected an elevated mutation frequency in the germ cells and sperm from old animals (49,50). These studies clearly demonstrated that the genetic integrity of mature sperm was affected by the age of the animal. A direct measurement of mutation rates in germ cells of men has yet to be done. Using the sperm chromatin structure assay, Evensong and Wyrobek (personal communication, 2003) found a direct correlation between the DNA fragmentation index and increasing age of men. In a large population study, this index rose above 0.3 (the threshold associated with lower fertility) in men older than 50.

Chromosomal nondisjunction during gametic meiotic division results in numerical chromosomal abnormalities and causes the most common congenital anomalies observed in humans. The prevalence of Down's syndrome in natural births is approximately 1/100 (51), and its relationship to maternal age is well established. Nondisjunction in male germ cells accounts for only 7% to 10% of Down's syndrome births (52), yet accounts for 50% of Klinefelter patients (53), which occurs in 1/500 male births (54). The absolute rate of chromosomal aberrations in the sperm of healthy men is much higher than what would be expected from the rates of congenital disease observed in the population. In a recent study by Fisch et al. (55), it was shown that advanced paternal age is a significant contributor to the increased incidence of Down's syndrome found in children of older parents. Increased paternal age doubled the frequency of Down's syndrome when the maternal age was greater than 30. Based on cross-sectional studies in man, Martin and Rademaker (56) reported an increasing incidence of structural chromosomal aberrations in spermatozoa with aging and a higher risk for the development of autosomal-dominant diseases in newborns with increasing paternal age.

Base substitutions appear to be the most common type of age-dependent mutation that occurs in sperm.

Many autosomal-dominant disorders that exhibit paternal-age effects are the result of a base substitution in a gene that produces an observable phenotype. The analysis of achondroplasia and five other syndromes that demonstrate a striking effect of paternal age reveals that in 154 patients, all the mutations were single-base substitutions of paternal origin (48). A strong male bias is found for several other diseases that exhibit weaker but observable paternal-age effects. Based upon the strong male mutation bias and the age-dependent increase in mutation frequency for achondroplasia, it has been estimated that the risk of fathering a child with an autosomal-dominant mutation for men over 40 years is similar to the risk of mothering a child with Down's syndrome for women who are 35 to 40 years (57). This calculation may be an overestimation, as all of the estimated 1000 autosomal-dominant diseases would not be expected to have the same age-dependent increase or be completely penetrant.

Together, many of the above studies have prompted the American Society of Reproductive Medicine (previously the American Fertility Society) to introduce a guideline in 1990, which states that the maximum age of sperm donors should be set at 50 years, which was subsequently reduced to 40 in 1998. Analysis of certain disease rates has led one expert to state, "the greatest mutational health hazard in the human population at present is fertile old males" (58), and another to advise that, "both men and women complete their family before age 40 if possible" (57).

Basis for Decreased Sperm Chromatin Quality

The underlying processes that cause mature sperm from older males to harbor genetic defects are unclear. One of the most obvious explanations is the continuous spermatogonial stem-cell replication process that is required for perpetual sperm production. Prior to puberty, approximately 30 chromosomal replications produce a pool of undifferentiated spermatogonia. Thereafter, spermatogonial stem cells undergo 23 replications every year. Thus, a 20-year-old man generates sperm that are the product of approximately 150 replications (48). This number increases to 840 by the age of 50 and to 1530 by the age of 80. If the fidelity of replication is imperfect, mutations would be expected to accumulate in the spermatogonial stem-cell population.

There are, however, several other processes that could contribute to reduced genetic quality in the sperm of aged individuals. Apoptosis occurs naturally in the testis of young individuals and is required for spermatogenesis to proceed normally (59). Culling of the spermatogonial germ-cell population controls the volume of germ-cell production and prevents overburdening of the testicular resources. It has been suggested that this may also serve as a mechanism to eliminate or reduce damaged germ cells (59,60). A reduced apoptotic rate or a loss of proper recognition of damaged cells could also lead to paternal age effects without a

change in the mutation rate. Indeed, in humans, reduced apoptosis of spermatogonia in aged testes is observed and may reflect decreased spermatogonial proliferation (61). Communication between germ and Sertoli cells in aged rat testis is also reduced (62). For apoptosis to serve as a mechanism to eliminate damaged germ cells, it would be necessary to demonstrate that the Sertoli cells and/or the germ cells themselves are able to recognize specific genetic damage. In young mice, as cells progress from mitotic spermatogonia to meiotic spermatocytes, a decrease in the mutation frequency is observed, suggesting that damage-specific recognition may occur (49).

Another mechanism that may allow for sperm quality control at the level of the epididymis via cell-surface ubiquitination and subsequent phagocytosis of abnormal sperm has recently been suggested (63). Large-scale phagocytosis of sperm by the epididymal epithelium, however, is not observed in young or old animals (64). To date, it has not been clearly demonstrated that genetic damage-specific apoptosis or phagocytosis occurs or that there is an age-dependent increase in epididymal spermiophagy.

A third possible mechanism is that the loss of function of cellular protective factors is indigenous to the germ cell itself, thus leading to an increase in the mutation rate. Cellular proteins that are involved in genomic maintenance and repair of spontaneous damage and/or stress response may be abnormal in germ cells of old individuals. Altered expression of some stress-response proteins is observed in germ cells from old rats (Syntin P, Robaire B; unpublished data, 2002). Proteins involved in certain DNA-repair pathways are highly expressed in young germ cells (65), and these levels are reduced in the germ cells of the aging mouse (66). Germ-cell transcription ceases during the nuclear condensation stage; thus transcripts and proteins expressed in earlier germ-cell types sustain later stages of germ-cell development. Altered expression of protective factors may leave later germ-cell types vulnerable to genetic insults. Consistent with this hypothesis is the observation that the mutation frequency and the spectra of mutational challenge increase in later germ-cell types in the old mouse testis while remaining unchanged in the young (49,50).

Modern understanding of the information carried by DNA has progressed beyond sequence-based information to include epigenetic-based information, which is most commonly involved in the control of gene expression. Epigenetic phenomena have been shown to play significant roles in the processes of genetic imprinting (67), development (68), and in many diseases including cancer (69). The two primary epigenetic mechanisms that have been demonstrated to be involved in the control of mammalian transcription are histone modification and DNA methylation.

The possibility of age-dependent modification of the germ-cell epigenome remains uninvestigated in humans. The fact that sperm DNA is primarily complexed with protamine instead of histone protein largely negates the possibility of histone-based transmission of epigenetic information. Patterns of DNA methylation, however, are preserved during spermatogenesis. The total content and the pattern of gene-specific DNA methylation are altered in the aged somatic tissues of many mammalian species, including humans (70). Studies in the authors' laboratory using the Brown Norway rat model have shown that specific DNA sequences exhibit age-dependent modification of their methylation status, while other sequences do not (71). These modifications may influence gene expression during embryogenesis and may explain some of the paternal age effects previously demonstrated in the Brown Norway model (32).

Epigenetic reprogramming in the early embryo has been demonstrated (72), and aberrantly, methylated gametic sequences may be repaired. Although global demethylation and remethylation events have been described (73), the methylation patterns of imprinted genes and some repetitive DNA sequences endure embryonic reprogramming (74,75). An important focus of future experimentation will be to determine if paternal age-dependent methylation alterations persist into the progeny and to what extent methylation state may be a predictor of paternal age-induced variation in progeny fitness.

It is expected that all these processes would not act in a mutually exclusive manner. For example, if the mutation rate were the result of replication errors alone, the increase in the incidence of disease demonstrating a paternal age effect would be expected to be linear. This is not the case, however, as most diseases studied show an exponential increase with paternal age (35). Thus, multiple mechanisms are expected to contribute to the paternal age effect for most diseases. A recent paper has evaluated the frequency of the achondroplasia mutation in human sperm from donors of various ages and determined, surprisingly, that the age-dependent increase in the mutation rate is much lower than what would be required to explain the paternal age effect (76). This interesting result suggests that the paternal age effect may not be directly due to an age-dependent loss of sperm genetic integrity. Clearly, more work needs to be done to determine the types and frequencies of mutations that occur in sperm and how genetic quality may relate to fertility and progeny health.

☐ FACTORS AFFECTING THE QUALITY OF AGING SPERMATOZOA
Oxidative Stress

Oxidative stress is defined by excessive production of reactive oxidative species (ROS) such as the hydroxide (OH^-) and superoxide (O_2^-) free radicals. Several studies have suggested that there is a correlation between increased ROS production and aging in a range of cell and animal models (77–79). A number of factors can lead to increased production of ROS. These include compromised function and integrity of mitochondria over time causing them to "leak" ROS into the cell (80), waning of the cell's antioxidant abilities with age (73), and increased steroidogenic activity (81). Although many studies exist on the effect of aging on antioxidant enzymes such as catalase, superoxide dismutase, glutathione peroxidase, and glutathione reductase, the results of these studies are controversial and a consensus has not yet been established in this field.

ROS cause damage to the cell's DNA, proteins, and lipids, thus endangering normal function. Spermatozoa are subjected to relatively high levels of oxidative stress because they generate ROS to control capacitation by redox regulation of tyrosine phosphorylation (82). In addition, the presence of leukocytes in human semen results in an increased ROS load since these cells have a high rate of spontaneous production of ROS. Thus, accumulation of ROS over time is likely to render spermatozoa of older men susceptible to particularly elevated levels of oxidative stress. The authors have found that the motility of spermatozoa in older rats becomes significantly more compromised after oxidative challenge when compared to that of young rats (83).

ROS decrease spermatozoa quality through several mechanisms including damaging lipids, DNA, and proteins. The lipid membrane, which is rich in unsaturated fatty acids, is particularly susceptible to oxidative damage. The consequences of membrane perturbation include changes in transport processes, ion channels, metabolite gradients, and receptor-mediated signal transduction, which can decrease the sperm's motility, viability, and ability to undergo capacitation and the acrosome reaction (84). Furthermore, oxidative stress can induce DNA damage in spermatozoa, which can affect fertility of the male and endanger offspring outcome (82). Although spermatozoa with extremely damaged DNA will not be able to fertilize an egg, sperm with less-extensive damage can still successfully fertilize, thus endangering the outcome of the pregnancy (85). Oxidative stress might also increase with age due to the compounding effect of a poor lifestyle, where diet and other factors such as smoking and alcohol consumption may play a particularly important role.

Lifestyle

Several aspects of a man's lifestyle can play a role in the quality of germ cells and are likely to be cumulative with advancing age. Although poor diet, smoking, and excessive drinking can occur in men of all ages, the adverse effects become more evident with increased duration of exposure.

Diet

It has been well documented that a diet rich in antioxidants such as vitamins A, E, C, selenium, and flavonoids provides the body with a stronger antioxidant defense system (86). Furthermore, a strong correlation between vitamin C levels in semen and spermatozoal DNA quality has been observed (87). In some cases of male factor infertility, glutathione supplementation has been shown to significantly protect spermatozoa from lipid peroxidation and increase motility (88). (For further information on the effect of nutrition on male fertility, see Chapter 22.)

Smoking

It is well established that cigarette smoke contains chemicals with mutagenic and carcinogenic properties, such as polycyclic aromatic hydrocarbons and nicotine-derived nitrosamines (89). These chemicals act as oxidants, causing a range of toxic effects including DNA damage in the form of breaks and bulky adducts. Although some DNA repair occurs in spermatocytes and early spermatids, it is not possible once spermatozoa mature (90–92). Thus, smokers have been shown to have a decreased quality of spermatozoa DNA (93), which has been correlated with adverse affects on the well being of their offspring (94).

In addition to DNA damage, smoking has been associated with reduced semen quality, characterized by significant decreases in sperm density, count, number of motile sperm, and percent morphologically normal sperm (95), most probably due to its effect on depleting tissue antioxidants and increasing semen leukocytes (96). The negative impact, however, is apparently reversible and significant improvements in antioxidant status are observed after smoking cessation (97). Interestingly, smoking by males has been demonstrated to decrease the success rates of assisted reproduction procedures, such as in vitro fertilization and intracytoplasmic sperm injection (98).

Alcohol

Alcohol consumption is common in most populations, and moderate consumption has not been linked to decreased semen parameters (99). Continuous excessive alcohol intake, however, can cause decreased free androgens to the point of inducing complete spermatogenic arrest and hypogonadism (100). Similar to cessation of smoking, the cessation of alcohol consumption has been shown to ameliorate reproductive parameters in a murine model (101) as well as in humans (102).

Exposure to Environmental Chemicals

It has been proposed that extensive exposure to industrial chemicals may contribute to declining sperm quality in the industrial world (103,104). In most cases, exposure levels are low and do not adversely affect health, but situations can exist when individuals come in contact with threatening amounts. Although this happens rarely in the general population, it is more common in people working in chemical plants, farmers, and those living in proximity to landfills. An overview of the effect of some environmental chemicals on sperm quality is provided in the following (see also Chapter 21).

Polychlorinated Biphenyls

Polychlorinated biphenyls (PCBs) were once widely used as coolants and lubricants, but the production and use of PCBs became restricted in the late 1970s due to their extreme stability in the environment, their accumulation in fat tissue, and toxicity to liver, skin, and the nervous system. PCBs continue to be released into the environment, however, from hazardous waste sites, improper disposal, and leaks from old PCB-containing equipment (105). Hauser et al. (106) have shown a clear link between PCBs and semen quality. They found decreased spermatozoa concentration, decreased motility, and more cases of abnormal morphology in men with high blood levels of PCBs compared to men with lower PCB blood levels.

Phthalates

Since being banned, PCBs have largely been replaced by other industrial chemicals such as phthalates. Although less toxic than PCBs, phthalates have been demonstrated to have antiandrogenic activity. In a recent study, it was shown that high levels of urinary phthalates are associated with decreased fertility, the main correlations being with sperm concentration, motility, and poor morphology in humans (107). Increased DNA damage in the sperm of the subjects was reported by the same group using the comet assay (108).

Farmers

Farmers constitute a population that is at particular risk for reproductive problems due to their involvement with pesticides and herbicides (109). As early as 1970, Espir et al. (110) reported reversible impotence in farm workers who applied pesticides. Subsequent studies showed that synthetic organochlorine pesticides such as dichlorodiphenyltrichloroethane (DDT) act as endocrine disruptors (111). Some of these chemicals can act as antiandrogens (112), thus causing impotence and decreased sperm count and sperm concentration in farmers. DDT is no longer registered for use in the United States, although it is still used in other (primarily tropical) countries.

Another chemical that is a threat to spermatozoa quality is the phenoxy herbicide 2,4-dichlorophenoxyacetic acid (2,4-D). This chemical is widely used throughout the world and has been shown to be associated with increased asthenozoospermia, necrozoospermia, and teratozoospermia (113). Therefore, it is alarming that up to 50% of Ontario farmers were found to have detectable levels of 2,4-D in their semen (114).

Traffic Pollutants

Another potential threat to the male reproductive system is pollution. As environmental chemical pollution increases, studies addressing its effect on health become crucial. It was found, for example, that men continuously exposed to high levels of traffic pollution had high blood lead levels, high methemoglobin (a marker of nitric oxide exposure), and significant adverse effects on all sperm parameters except for sperm count and semen volume (115). Sperm motility, viability, membrane function, nuclear DNA integrity, and TTP were all dramatically decreased (115). These effects could have been mediated in part by the nitric oxide and lead found in traffic pollution. Controlled amounts of nitric oxide play an important role in spermatozoa capacitation, but this free radical has been shown to inhibit motility when present in large quantities (116). Lead accumulates in male reproductive organs where it can replace zinc in human protamines, causing a conformational change in the protein, and thus, adversely affecting sperm chromatin condensation. Zinc supplementation can help ameliorate these problems (117).

□ CONCLUSION

The existence of a paternal age effect on semen parameters, fertility, and anomalies in children demonstrates that the genetic integrity of otherwise healthy sperm is not immune to the effects of time. Genetic diseases that exhibit a paternal age effect and are of known etiology are commonly the result of single-base substitutions, and, in the absence of much needed experimental data, this implies that these are the most common type of age-dependent genetic alteration found in aging sperm. The cause of increased mutation frequency in sperm from aged males is most likely a combination of an accumulation of replication errors, epigenetic mechanisms, alterations in apoptotic events, and compromised genetic defense. In addition to well-designed epidemiological studies, the more extensive use of animal models is likely to help resolve the nature and range of effects that paternal age can cause in altered progeny outcome. The specific mechanisms during aging that result in DNA/chromatin damage and the degree to which drugs and environmental chemicals exacerbate or protect from such damage is a matter of central concern as our population ages.

□ REFERENCES

1. Clermont Y. Kinetics of spermatogenesis in mammals: seminiferous epithelium cycle and spermatogonial renewal. Physiol Rev 1972; 52(1):198–236.

2. De Rooij DJ. Regulation of the proliferation of spermatogonial stem cells. J Cell Sci 1988; Suppl 10:181–194.

3. Jung A, Schuppe HC, Schill WB. Comparison of semen quality in older and younger men attending an andrology clinic. Andrologia 2002; 34(2):116–122.

4. Kidd SA, Eskenazi B, Wyrobeck AJ. Effects of male age on semen quality and fertility: a review of the literature. Fertil Steril 2001; 75(2):237–248.

5. Plas E, Berger P, Hermann M, et al. Effect of aging on male fertility? Exp Gerontol 2000; 35(5):543–551.

6. Eskenazi B, Wyrobek AJ, Sloter E, et al. The association of age and semen quality in healthy men. Hum Reprod 2003; 18:447–454.

7. Matsumoto AM. Andropause: clinical implications of the decline in serum testosterone levels with aging in men. J Gerontol A Biol Sci Med Sci 2002; 57(2): M76–M99.

8. Swerdloff RS, Wang C. Androgens and aging in men. Exp Gerontol 1993; 28(4–5):435–446.

9. Vermeulen A. Clinical review 24: androgens in the aging male. J Clin Endocrinol Metab 1991; 73(2): 221–224.

10. Johnson L, Petty CS, Neaves WB. Influence of age on sperm production and testicular weights in men. J Reprod Fertil 1984; 70(1):211–218.

11. Syntin P, Robaire B. Sperm structural and motility changes during aging in the Brown Norway rat. J Androl 2001; 22(2):235–244.

12. Abramsson L. On the investigation of men from infertile relations. A clinical study with special regard to anamnesis, physical examination, semen-, hormone- and chromosome analyses, from men with non-"normal" semen. Scand J Urol Nephro Suppl 1988; 113:1–47.

13. Mathieu C, Ecochard R, Bied V, et al. Cumulative conception rate following intrauterine artificial insemination with husband's spermatozoa: influence of husband's age. Hum Reprod 1995; 10(5): 1090–1097.

14. Hassan MA, Killick SR. Effect of male age on fertility: evidence for the decline in male fertility with increasing age. Fertil Steril 2003; 79(suppl 3): 1520–1527.

15. Nagai R, Saito Y, Ohyama Y, et al. Endothelial dysfunction in the klotho mouse and downregulation of klotho gene expression in various animal models of vascular and metabolic diseases. Cell Mol Life Sci 2000; 57(5):738–746.

16. Takeda T, Hosokawa M, Higuchi K. Senescence-accelerated mouse (SAM): a novel murine model of senescence. Exp Gerontol 1997; 32(9):105–109.

17. Robaire B, Syntin P, Jervis K. The Coming of Age of the Epididymis. In: Jegou B, Pineau C, Saez JM, eds. Testis, Epididymis and Technologies in the Year 2000. New York: Springer-Verlag, 2000:229–262.

18. Zirkin BR, Santulli R, Strandberg JD, et al. Testicular steroidogenesis in the aging Brown Norway rat. J Androl 1993; 14(2):118–123.

19. Wright WW, Fiore C, Zirkin BR. The effect of aging in the seminiferous epithelium of the brown Norway rat. J Androl 1993; 14(2):110–117.

20. Gruenewald DA, Naai MA, Hess DL, et al. The Brown Norway rat as a model of male reproductive aging: evidence for both primary and secondary testicular failure. J Gerontol 1994; 49(2):B42–B50.

21. Wang C, Hikim AS, Ferrini M, et al. Male reproductive ageing: using the brown Norway rat as a model for man. Novartis Found Symp 2002; 242:82–95.

22. Chen H, Hardy MP, Huhtaniemi I, et al. Age-related decreased Leydig cell testosterone production in the brown Norway rat. J Androl 1994; 15(6):551–557.

23. Zirkin BR, Chen H. Regulation of Leydig cell steroidogenic function during aging. Biol Reprod 2000; 63(4):977–981.

24. Luo L, Chen H, Zirkin BR. Leydig cell aging: steroidogenic acute regulatory protein (StAR) and cholesterol side-chain cleavage enzyme. J Androl 2001; 22(1): 149–156.

25. Neaves WB, Johnson L, Petty CS. Seminiferous tubules and daily sperm production in older adult with varied numbers of Leydig cells. Biol Reprod 1987; 36(2): 301–308.

26. Vermeulen A. Andropause. Maturitas 2000; 34(1):5–15.

27. Serre V, Robaire B. Segment specific morphological changes in the aging Brown Norway rat epididymis. Biol Reprod 1998; 58(2):497–513.

28. Serre V, Robaire B. The distribution of immune cells in the epithelium of the epididymis of the aging brown norway rat is segment-specific and related to the luminal content. Biol Reprod 1999; 61(3):705–714.

29. Robaire B. Aging of the epididymis. In: Robaire B, Hinton BT, eds. The Epididymis: From Molecules to Clinical Practice: A Comprehensive Survey of Efferent Ducts, the Epididymis and the Vas Deferens. New York: Kluwer Academic/Plenum Publishers, 2001: 285–296.

30. Jervis KM, Robaire B. Changes in gene expression during aging in the Brown Norway rat epididymis. Exp Gerontol 2002; 37(2):897–906.

31. Schoenfeld HA, Hall SJ, Boekelheide K. Continuously proliferative stem germ cells partially repopulate the aged, atrophic rat testis after gonadotropin-releasing hormone agonist therapy. Biol Reprod 2001; 64(4): 1273–1282.

32. Serre V, Robaire B. Paternal age affects fertility and progeny outcome in the Brown Norway rat. Fertil Steril 1998; 70(4):625–631.

33. Levy S, Serre V, Hermo L, et al. The effects of aging on the seminiferous epithelium and the blood-testis barrier of the Brown Norway rat. J Androl 1999; 20(3):356–365.

34. Penrose LS. Parental age and mutation. Lancet 1955; 269(6885):312–313.

35. Risch N, Reich EW, Wishnick MM, et al. Spontaneous mutation and parental age in humans. Am J Hum Genet 1987; 41(2):218–248.

36. Dalman C, Allebeck P. Paternal age and schizophrenia: further support for an association. Am J Psychiatry 2002; 159(9):1591–1592.

37. El-Saadi O, Pedersen CB, McNeil TF, et al. Paternal and maternal age as risk factors for psychosis: findings from Denmark, Sweden and Australia. Schizophr Res 2004; 67(2–3):227–236.

38. Bertram L, Busch R, Spiegl M, et al. Paternal age is a risk factor for Alzheimer disease in the absence of a major gene. Neurogenetics 1998; 1(4):277–280.

39. Olshan AF, Schnitzer PG, Baird PA. Paternal age and the risk of congenital heart defects. Teratology 1994; 50(1):80–84.

40. Hemminki K, Kyyronen P. Parental age and risk of sporadic and familial cancer in offspring: implications for germ cell mutagenesis. Epidemiology 1999; 10(6): 747–751.

41. Gavrilov LA, Gavrilova NS, Kroutko VN, et al. Mutation load and human longevity. Mutat Res 1997; 377(1):61–62.

42. Selvin S, Garfinkel J. Paternal age, maternal age and birth order and the risk of a fetal loss. Hum Biol 1976; 48(1):223–230.

43. Hatch M, Kline J, Levin B, et al. Paternal age and trisomy among spontaneous abortions. Hum Genet 1990; 85(3):355–361.

44. Kinzler WL, Ananth CV, Smulian JC, et al. Parental age difference and adverse perinatal outcomes in the United States. Paediatr Perinat Epidemiol 2002; 16(4): 320–327.

45. Nybo Andersen AM, Hansen KD, Andersen PK, et al. Advanced paternal age and risk of fetal death: a cohort study. Am J Epidemiol 2004; 160(12):1214–1222.

46. Zhu JL, Madsen KM, Vestergaard M, et al. Paternal age and preterm birth. Epidemiology 2005; 16(2): 259–262.

47. Kazaura M, Lie RT, Skjaerven R. Paternal age and the risk of birth defects in Norway. Ann Epidemiol 2004; 14(8):566–570.

48. Crow JF. The origins, patterns and implications of human spontaneous mutation. Nat Rev Genet 2000; 1(1):40–47.

49. Walter CA, Intano GW, McCarrey JR, et al. Mutation frequency declines during spermatogenesis in young mice but increases in old mice. Proc Natl Acad Sci USA 1998; 95(17):10015–10019.

50. Walter CA, Intano GW, McMahan CA, et al. Mutation spectral changes in spermatogenic cells obtained from old mice. DNA Repair (Amst) 2004; 3(5):495–504.

51. Cuckle HS, Wald N, Densem J. Estimating risk of Down's syndrome. Br Med J 1991; 303(6797):312.

52. Muller F, Rebiffe M, Taillandier A, et al. Parental origin of the extra chromosome in prenatally diagnosed fetal trisomy 21. Hum Genet 2000; 106(3):340–344.

53. MacDonald M, Hassold T, Harvey J, et al. The origin of 47,XXY and 47,XXX aneuploidy: heterogeneous mechanisms and role of aberrant recombination. Hum Mol Genet 1994; 3(8):1365–1371.

54. Smyth CM, Bremner WJ. Klinefelter syndrome. Arch Intern Med 1998; 158:1309–1314.

55. Fisch H, Hyun G, Golden R, et al. The influence of paternal age on Down syndrome. J Urol 2003; 169(6): 2275–2278.

56. Martin RH, AW Rademaker. The effect of age on the frequency of sperm chromosomal abnormalities in normal men. Am J Hum Genet 1987; 41: 484–492.

57. Friedman JM. Genetic disease in the offspring of older fathers. Obstet Gynecol 1981; 57(6):745–749.

58. Crow JF. The high spontaneous mutation rate: is it a health risk? Proc Natl Acad Sci USA 1997; 94(16): 8380–8386.

59. Kerr JB. Spontaneous degeneration of germ cells in normal rat testis: assessment of cell types and frequency during the spermatogenic cycle. J Reprod Fertil 1992; 95(3):825–830.

60. Sinha Hikim AP, Swerdloff RS. Hormonal and genetic control of germ cell apoptosis in the testis. Rev Reprod 1999; 4(1):38–47.

61. Kimura M, Itoh N, Takagi S, et al. Balance of apoptosis and proliferation of germ cells related to spermatogenesis in aged men. J Androl 2003; 24(2):185–191.

62. Syed V, Hecht NB. Disruption of germ cell-Sertoli cell interactions leads to spermatogenic defects. Mol Cell Endocrinol 2002; 186(2):155–157.

63. Sutovsky P, Moreno R, Ramalho-Santos J, et al. A putative, ubiquitin-dependent mechanism for the recognition and elimination of defective spermatozoa in the mammalian epididymis. J Cell Sci 2001; 114(Pt 9): 1665–1675.

64. Cooper TG, Yeung CH, Jones R, et al. Rebuttal of a role for the epididymis in sperm quality control by phagocytosis of defective sperm. J Cell Sci 2002; 115(Pt 1):5–7.

65. Alcivar AA, Hake LE, Hecht NB. DNA polymerase-beta and poly(ADP)ribose polymerase mRNAs are differentially expressed during the development of male germinal cells. Biol Reprod 1992; 46(2):201–207.

66. Intano GW, McMahan CA, McCarrey JR, et al. Base excision repair is limited by different proteins in male germ cell nuclear extracts prepared from young and old mice. Mol Cell Biol 2002; 22(7):2410–2418.

67. Tycko B, Trasler J, Bestor T. Genomic imprinting: gametic mechanisms and somatic consequences. J Androl 1997; 18(5):480–486.

68. Hashimshony T, Zhang J, Keshet I, et al. The role of DNA methylation in setting up chromatin structure during development. Nat Genet 2003; 34(2):187–192.

69. Plass C. Cancer epigenomics. Hum Mol Genet 2002; 11:2479–2488.

70. Richardson B. Impact of aging on DNA methylation. Aging Res Rev 2003; 2(3):245–261.

71. Oakes CC, Smiraglia DJ, Plass C, et al. Aging results in hypermethylation of ribosomal DNA in sperm and liver of male rats. Proc Natl Acad Sci USA 2003; 100(4):1775–1780.

72. Reik W, Dean W, Walter J. Epigenetic reprogramming in mammalian development. Science 2001; 293(5532): 1089–1093.

73. Kafri T, Ariel M, Brandeis M, et al. Developmental pattern of gene-specific DNA methylation in the mouse embryo and germ line. Genes Dev 1992; 6(5):705–714.

74. Olek A, Walter J. The pre-implantation ontogeny of the H19 methylation imprint. Nat Genet 1997; 17(3): 275–276.

75. Morgan HD, Sutherland HG, Martin DI, et al. Epigenetic inheritance at the agouti locus in the mouse. Nat Genet 1999; 23(3):314–318.

76. Tiemann-Boege I, Navidi W, Grewal R, et al. The observed human sperm mutation frequency cannot explain the achondroplasia paternal age effect. Proc Natl Acad Sci USA 2002; 99(23):14952–14957.

77. Golden TR, Hinerfeld DA, Melov S. Oxidative stress and aging: beyond correlation. Aging Cell 2002; 1(2): 117–123.

78. Wei YH, Lee HC. Oxidative stress, mitochondrial DNA mutation, and impairment of antioxidant enzymes in aging. Exp Biol Med 2002; 227(9):671–682.

79. Sohal RS, Mockett RS, Orr WC. Mechanisms of aging: an appraisal of the oxidative stress hypothesis. Free Radic Biol Med 2002; 33(5):575–586.

80. Finkel T, Holbrook NJ. Oxidants, oxidative stress and the biology of aging. Nature 2000; 408(6809): 239–247.

81. Chen H, Cangello D, Benson S, et al. Age-related increase in mitochondrial superoxide generation in the testosterone-producing cells of Brown Norway rat testes: relationship to reduced steroidogenic function? Exp Gerontol 2001; 36(8):1361–1373.

82. Aitken RJ. The Amoroso Lecture. The human spermatozoon—a cell in crisis? J Reprod Fertil 1999; 115(1):1–7.

83. Zubkova EV, Robaire B. Effect of glutathione depletion on antioxidant enzymes in the epididymis, seminal vesicles, and liver and on spermatozoa motility in the aging brown Norway rat. Biol Reprod 2004; 71(3): 1002–1008.

84. Sikka SC. Oxidative stress and role of antioxidants in normal and abnormal sperm function. Front Biosci 1996; 1:e78–e86.

85. Zenzes MT. Smoking and reproduction: gene damage to human gametes and embryos. Hum Reprod Update 2000; 6(2):122–131.

86. Urso ML, Clarkson PM. Oxidative stress, exercise, and antioxidant supplementation. Toxicology 2003; 189(1–2):41–54.

87. Fraga CG, Motchnik PA, Shigenaga MK, et al. Ascorbic acid protects against endogenous oxidative DNA damage in human sperm. Proc Natl Acad Sci USA 1991; 88(24):11003–11006.

88. Lenzi A, Gandini L, Picardo M, et al. Lipoperoxidation damage of spermatozoa polyunsaturated fatty acids (PUFA): scavenger mechanisms and possible scavenger therapies. Front Biosci 2000; 5:E1–E15.

89. Pfeifer GP, Denissenko MF, Olivier M, et al. Tobacco smoke carcinogens, DNA damage and p53 mutations in smoking-associated cancers. Oncogene 2002; 21(48): 7435–7451.

90. Baarends WM, van der Laan R, Grootegoed JA. DNA repair mechanisms and gametogenesis. Reproduction 2001; 121(1):31–39.

91. Eddy EM, O'Brien DA. Gene expression during mammalian meiosis. Curr Top Dev Biol 1998; 37:141–200.

92. Aguilar-Mahecha A, Hales BF, Robaire B. Chronic cyclophosphamide treatment alters the expression of stress response genes in rat male germ cells. Biol Reprod 2002; 66(4):1024–1032.

93. Horak S, Polanska J, Widlak P. Bulky DNA adducts in human sperm: relationship with fertility, semen quality, smoking and environmental factors. Mutat Res 2003; 537(1):53–65.

94. Sorahan T, Lancashire R, Prior P, et al. Childhood cancer and parental use of alcohol and tobacco. Ann Epidemiol 1995; 5(5):354–359.

95. Kunzle R, Mueller MD, Hanggi W, et al. Semen quality of male smokers and nonsmokers in infertile couples. Fertil Steril 2003; 79(2 Pt 1):287–291.

96. Fraga CG, Motchnik PA, Wyrobek AJ, et al. Smoking and low antioxidant levels PA increase oxidative damage to sperm DNA. Mutat Res 1996; 351(2): 199–203.

97. Lane JD, Opara EC, Rose JE, et al. Quitting smoking raises whole blood glutathione. Physiol Behav 1996; 60(5):1379–1381.

98. Zitzmann M, Rolf C, Nordhoff V, et al. Male smokers have a decreased success rate for in vitro fertilization and intracytoplasmic sperm injection. Fertil Steril 2003; 79(suppl 3):1550–1554.

99. Vine MF, Setzer RW Jr, Everson RB, et al. Human sperm morphometry and smoking, caffeine, and alcohol consumption. Reprod Toxicol 1997; 11(2–3): 179–184.

100. Villalta J, Ballesca JL, Nicolas JM, et al. Testicular function in asymptomatic chronic alcoholics: relation to ethanol intake. Alcohol Clin Exp Res 1997; 21(1): 128–133.

101. Anderson RA Jr, Willis BR, Oswald C. Spontaneous recovery from ethanol-induced male infertility. Alcohol 1985; 2(3):479–484.

102. Vicari E, Arancio A, Giuffrida V, et al. A case of reversible azoospermia following withdrawal from alcohol consumption. J Endocrinol Invest 2002; 25(5):473–476.

103. Auger J, Eustache F, Andersen AG, et al. Sperm morphological defects related to environment, lifestyle and medical history of 1001 male partners of pregnant women from four European cities. Hum Reprod 2001; 16(12):2710–2717.

104. Sonnenschein C, Soto AM. An updated review of environmental estrogen and androgen mimics and antagonists. J Steroid Biochem Mol Biol 1998; 65(1–6): 143–150.

105. http://www.ec.gc.ca/pcb/eng/index_e.htm

106. Hauser R, Altshul L, Chen Z, et al. Environmental organochlorines and semen quality: results of a pilot study. Environ Health Perspec 2002; 110(3): 229–233.

107. Duty SM, Silva MJ, Barr DB, et al. Phthalate exposure and human semen parameters. Epidemiology 2003; 14(3):269–277.

108. Duty SM, Singh NP, Silva MJ, et al. The relationship between environmental exposures to phthalates and DNA damage in human sperm using the neutral comet assay. Environ Health Perspec 2003; 111(9): 1164–1169.

109. Kenkel S, Rolf C, Nieschlag E. Occupational risks for male fertility: an analysis of patients attending a tertiary referral centre. Int J Androl 2001; 24(6): 318–326.

110. Espir ML, Hall JW, Shirreffs JG, et al. Impotence in farm workers using toxic chemicals. Br Med J 1970; 1(693):423–425.

111. Safe SH. Endocrine disruptors and human health—is there a problem? An update. Environ Health Perspect 2000; 108(6):487–493.

112. Brien SE, Heaton JP, Racz WJ, et al. Effects of an environmental anti-androgen on erectile function in an animal penile erection model. J Urol 2000; 163(4): 1315–1321.

113. Lerda D, Rizzi R. Study of reproductive function in persons occupationally exposed to 2,4-dichlorophenoxyacetic acid (2,4–D). Mutat Res 1991; 262(1): 47–50.

114. Arbuckle TE, Schrader SM, Cole D, et al. 2,4-Dichlorophenoxyacetic acid residues in semen of Ontario farmers. Reprod Toxicol 1999; 13(6): 421–429.

115. De Rosa M, Zarrilli S, Paesano L, et al. Traffic pollutants affect fertility in men. Hum Report 2003; 18(5):1055–1061.

116. Zini A, De Lamirande E, Gagnon C. Low levels of nitric oxide promote human sperm capacitation in vitro. J Androl 1995; 16(5):424–431.

117. Quintanilla-Vega B, Hoover D, Bal W, et al. Lead effects on protamine-DNA binding. Am J Ind Med 2000; 38(3):324–329.

10

Androgen Effects on Cognitive Function

Monique M. Cherrier

Department of Psychiatry and Behavioral Sciences, University of Washington School of Medicine and Veterans Administration Puget Sound Health Care System, Seattle, Washington, U.S.A.

□ INTRODUCTION

Androgens and their effects on behavior have been an area of study for over a century. In 1889, Dr. Brown-Sequard injected himself with an extract from crushed animal testicles, reporting that this treatment gave him increased energy, muscular strength, stamina, and mental agility (1). Although crude, this approach led the way to the discovery of androgens. Since then, the focus of most androgen research has been in the area of reproductive function. More recently, the focus of attention has turned to hormone effects on the central nervous system (CNS) and the process of aging, with particular emphasis on the potential antiaging effects of hormone replacement therapy. This chapter will explore the complex relationship between androgens and cognition. First, mechanisms by which hormones exert their effects in the CNS will be described, including organizational and activational effects. Next, the relationship between androgens and cognition in humans will be examined, including endogenous levels as well as studies on hormone manipulation in healthy young and older populations. Finally, the relationship between androgens and cognition will be considered with respect to the endocrine disorders that result in excessive or insufficient hormone levels. This chapter will feature cognition, rather than human behavioral characteristics such as mood or emotion. Readers may refer to Ref. (2) for a review of the relationship between androgens and mood or behavior.

□ EVIDENCE FROM ANIMAL STUDIES
Hormonal Mechanisms of Action

Several CNS functions are regulated by gonadal steroids—particularly testosterone (T). Examples include prenatal sexual differentiation of the brain, adult sexual behavior, gonadotropin secretion, and cognition. The effects of T are mediated through the androgen receptor (AR), which is widely, but selectively, distributed throughout the brain (3–9). Castration rapidly decreases AR expression, and T upregulates neural AR in a dose-dependent manner in both male and female mice (4,10–12). T also acts via rapid, nongenomic methods of action through

G-protein-coupled, agonist-sequestrable T membrane receptors that initiate a transcription-independent signaling pathway affecting calcium channels (13–16). Thus, activational effects of androgens as discussed below may occur through both genomic and nongenomic mechanisms.

Another important aspect of T action is its active metabolism in vivo. In the body, T is converted to estradiol (E_2) by the enzyme cytochrome P450 aromatase, and to dihydrotestosterone (DHT) by the enzymes 5-α-reductase type 1 and 2 (Fig. 1). E_2 formed from T may then act on target organs via intracellular estrogen receptor alpha (ERα) and estrogen receptor beta (ERβ). DHT binds to ARs with greater affinity than T and is a more potent androgen. Both E_2 and DHT are also widely distributed throughout the male brain (7,8,11,17–21); therefore, androgen effects on cognition may occur through T directly or via its active metabolites E_2 and DHT.

Organizational Effects of Androgens

"Organizational effects" of androgens refer to permanent changes in brain structure and function as a result of exposure to androgens during a critical developmental window. For example, male rats castrated neonatally show a spatial ability pattern closer to the typical female rat pattern, whereas ovariectomized female rats treated with T neonatally demonstrate a typical male spatial ability pattern (22). Intact female rats treated neonatally with T perform better on a maze task than male castrates and intact males (23,24). These examples of permanent behavioral changes resulting from hormone manipulations during critical brain development periods are thought to be examples of "organizational" effects of hormones. Therefore, observed sex differences in healthy normal animals are thought to be due to organizational effects of hormones.

Sexual dimorphisms have been shown to occur with regional concentrations of neuropeptides and neurotransmitters, brain physiology, and behavior (21,25,26). For example, perinatal exposure of female rats to T eliminates the natural cyclic expression of gonadotropic secretion (27). Previously identified sexually dimorphic brain regions include the hypothalamus, pituitary, corpus callosum, adrenal cortex,

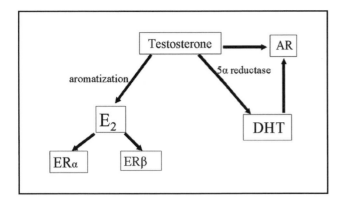

Figure 1 Pathway of androgen metabolism and action in the central nervous system from testosterone through DHT via 5-α-reductase and E_2 via aromatase. *Abbreviations*: AR, androgen receptor; DHT, dihydrotestosterone; E_2, estradiol; ERα, estrogen receptor alpha; ER*β*, estrogen receptor beta.

cerebellum, and prefrontal regions. With regard to cognitive tasks, a common finding in many species is that males outperform females on spatial tasks. This advantage on spatial tasks may be due to a potential sexual dimorphism of brain structures that underlie spatial navigation and spatial memory (e.g., hippocampus and dentate gyrus). Female rats neonatally exposed to T demonstrate more "masculine" or larger hippocampus, dentate gyrus, and corpus callosum (28,29). Thus, the presence of androgens during critical developmental periods may produce sexual dimorphisms or sex differences for cognitive abilities.

Androgen Activational Effects

Androgens modulate cognition and behavior throughout the lifespan. These modulation effects are termed "activational" effects of hormones. For example, postpubertal castrated male rats fail to demonstrate normal sexual behavior; however, sexual behavior can be restored to normal levels with T replacement (30). Thus, certain behaviors are controlled to a large degree by androgens throughout the lifespan. The mechanisms by which androgens exert these effects are likely complex. T replacement in castrated male rats results in decreased dopamine release, increased gamma amino butyric acid (GABA) turnover, and increased choline acetyltransferase levels (2,17,31). Changes in these substances are involved in the regulation of cognition. These effects may occur rapidly, within hours or days, and can remain for years, affecting both brain structure and receptor sensitivity and density (32–34).

ARs and aromatase activity (AA) in mice, rats, and monkeys have been shown to be distributed widely throughout the hypothalamus and limbic system in hormone-sensitive brain circuitry structures that play essential roles in the central regulation of reproductive function and cognition (3,4,35–37). For example, castration in male rats produces androgen-sensitive increases in dopamine axon density in the prefrontal cortex and significant decreases in cholinergic neurons

in the anterior cingulate, posterior parietal cortex, and medial septum compared to animals that underwent sham operations or gonadectomy with T replacement (31,38–41). The prefrontal cortices are involved in cognitive, affective, and memory functions, and gonadectomized rats demonstrate impairments in learning a maze that is restored with T administration (42). These effects appear to be selective for the memory aspects of maze performance, because gonadectomy did not affect performance on a motor task (42).

Studies of T replacement in mice and rats have generally supported a positive relationship between T manipulation and cognitive task performance. Studies of age-accelerated mice and young rats have found beneficial effects of T on avoidance learning and memory tasks (43,44), whereas other studies have failed to find beneficial effects of T on learning and memory (45,46). The differences in these studies may be due to the dose level of T used, because a recent study found a beneficial effect of T on spatial memory at a modest dose and detrimental effects on spatial memory at higher doses (45,47). In addition, the type of memory assessed may also contribute to differences between studies. The recent development of a working-memory water maze task, which separates working memory (a form of scratch pad, or temporary memory) from reference memory (a form of declarative, or long-term memory) found that older male rats given T demonstrate a beneficial increase in working-memory capacity compared to older sham-operated and DHT-treated rats (48). This finding suggests that changes in cognition observed with androgen supplementation or replacement may arise from their selective action on frontal brain regions that underlie working memory and other executive functions. Compared to rats, primates demonstrate a greater expression of aromatase- and AR-containing neurons in the amygdala, which has major output projections to the hippocampus and entorhinal cortices (6,37,49). The amygdala is involved in emotional and reward behavior and the hippocampus is critical for memory formation, which provides good evidence for the involvement of androgen-signaling pathways in emotional behavior and memory formation in addition to executive functions.

The activational effects of DHT on cognition are less well known; however, once formed, DHT is a potent steroid in the CNS. The affinity of DHT for the AR is four times that of T (50). Like T, DHT upregulates neural AR following castration (51). Although both T and DHT upregulate AR after castration, only DHT appears to sustain this effect for a prolonged period (51). Although these findings would suggest that DHT might have stronger effects on cognition than T, animal studies using both T and DHT have not supported greater or differential effects of DHT on cognition despite its greater affinity for the AR (48,52).

The formation of E_2 results from aromatization of T. Brain AA in the male rat occurs primarily in the medial preoptic or anterior hypothalamus region

(37,53). Administration of the AR antagonist flutamide with T or DHT in gonadectomized rats does not induce AA, compared to T or DHT administered alone, suggesting that AA is androgen dependent (37). E_2 treatment in the male rat partially upregulates AR after castration, although the effect is not nearly as strong as that with T or DHT (11). E_2, like T, may act via nongenomic methods, by binding to membrane receptors that are completely distinct from intracellular membrane receptors, causing rapid signaling (54). The functional role of E_2 in males is not well understood. E_2 appears to play an important and sometimes critical role in sexual behavior and social interaction behavior in male rats and other animals (49,55). T and E_2, but not DHT, modulate serotonin receptor mRNA and the density of serotonin receptors in the forebrain (32,33). Tamoxifen, an estrogen receptor agonist, induces changes in catecholamine innervation of the frontal cortex in male mice that mimic the changes produced by castration, whereas flutamide does not (56). Thus, the presence of E_2 secondary to aromatization in the brain may be important with regard to both mood and cognition.

□ EVIDENCE FROM HUMAN STUDIES
Endogenous Androgens

The measurable differences in certain cognitive abilities between men and women may be due to organizational effects of hormones. Hormones present during the development of the CNS may produce structural changes that result in behavioral differences. One area of cognitive ability in which robust differences between men and women are typically observed is spatial ability. The term "spatial" typically refers to information with a geometric or three-dimensional (3D) aspect.

Studies examining the relationship between endogenous androgen levels and cognitive performance have produced inconsistent results. Correlations between endogenous T levels and spatial abilities in men range from near 0 to 0.53 (57,58). In healthy young men, positive relationships have been found between circulating or endogenous T levels and visuo-spatial orientation (57), spatial form comparison (59), and composite visuo-spatial scores (60). Positive relationships have also been found for tactual spatial tasks (61,62). Other studies examining endogenous T levels have failed to find such a relationship between circulating androgen levels and visuo-spatial abilities (63,64). Low T levels have also been found to be associated with better performance on spatial ability tasks and high E_2 levels with better visual memory in men (63,65–67). In contrast, when Gouchie and Kimura (66) studied men and women grouped according to endogenous T levels (high vs. low), they found that high-T women and low-T men demonstrated better spatial abilities than low-T women and high-T men. Examination of young men by a mental rotation test during periods of high and low T levels resulting from

natural diurnal variation revealed a significant positive association of performance with average T levels but not with changes in T levels (i.e., high vs. low); no significant relationships involving T levels were found in other tests (e.g., anagrams and an attention task) (68). These findings have led some to suggest that the beneficial effects of T may be described by a curvilinear relationship such that low-to-moderate T levels improve cognitive abilities but higher levels result in no further improvements or result in even decrements in some abilities (e.g., verbal) (65,66,69).

In a comprehensive review of the literature, Kimura (70) found large gender differences in favor of males on spatial tasks, with the differences sometimes approaching 1 standard deviation for targeting (e.g., throwing darts or catching a ball) and spatial orientation (e.g., imagined spatial rotation). Modest differences were found for spatial visualization (e.g., imagining the result of folding paper in a precut shape), disembedding (finding a simple figure located in a more complex one), and spatial perception (e.g., determining the true vertical among distracting cues). Although some have suggested that experience with spatial tasks (e.g., driving, throwing, and catching) may account for these sex differences, studies controlling for experience continue to find gender differences, and these differences may be present at as early as five years of age (70–72).

The variability of results in the literature may be due to the wide variability in the selection of cognitive tests and their unique task demands. This includes the use of the term "spatial" to describe numerous tests that may tap different cognitive processes or rely upon different brain structures and networks. For example, men tend to outperform women on tasks that require spatial rotation or manipulation. Robust gender differences have been found for spatial rotation tasks (Fig. 2) that require the imaginary rotation of an object (70,73), and the performance of this task correlates with circulating T levels (74). This difference does not appear to be due to the 3D aspect of the task, because these differences are also apparent on two-dimensional (2D) rotation tests (75). Interestingly, in a virtual-reality adaptation of the mental rotation task, in which participants could manipulate a virtual-reality version of the complex design with their hands, these gender

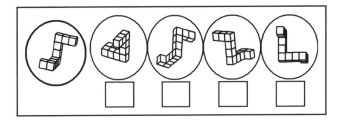

Figure 2 Sample test item from the mental rotations test. The three-dimensional item on the left is the stimulus item. Participants must choose two items on the right that match the stimulus item. Correct items are those that exactly match the stimulus item but have been rotated in three-dimensional space. Incorrect items do not match the stimulus item. *Source*: From Ref. 73.

differences disappeared (76). This latest result indicates a lack of gender differences on nonimagined spatial rotation tasks.

Remembering the location of objects is also considered a spatial task. Although recalling the location of objects clearly has a spatial component to it, several studies have demonstrated that women outperform men at recalling the location and the spatial relationship between objects to be remembered in a spatial array (77,78). Interestingly, this demonstrated difference between men and women on spatial tasks such as mental rotation and memory for spatial array is consistent with findings of gender differences on spatial navigation tasks. For example, on average, men tend to use a Euclidean (distance) or cardinal direction (N, S, E, W) approach to spatial navigation, whereas women, on average, tend to use landmark references. Galea and Kimura (79) found that when young men and women were required to learn a route on a table-top map, men were able to learn the route in fewer attempts, but women remembered more landmarks on the route. Studies comparing men and women on their ability to learn virtual-reality environments tend to support the findings of male advantage in landmark-free or landmark-limited environments (80–82). A tendency to use a nonlandmark or cardinal direction-based route-finding strategy has been found to be positively associated with endogenous T levels (83). Although there is some debate regarding the neural structures that underlie spatial navigation, most studies of humans and animals support a direct role for the hippocampus in spatial navigation and representation of large-scale space and the parahippocampal gyrus in recall of landmarks (84–88). As noted previously, the hippocampus, along with the hypothalamus and other limbic structures, is a target area for gonadal steroids. Male and female rats treated with T demonstrate a larger, or more "masculine-like," hippocampus, characterized by the size and asymmetrical shape of the dentate gyrus (29). Thus, these behavioral tendencies or cognitive styles may reflect differential effects of gonadal hormones on place and landmark systems in the hippocampus (89).

Recent functional magnetic resonance imaging (fMRI) studies provide further evidence that cognitive processing—in particular, the processing of spatial information—activates specific brain regions and neural networks that are unique to the particular task demands. Shelton and Gabrieli (90) found that healthy control participants activated right-sided hippocampus and parahippocampal regions when processing spatial information from a route or navigation perspective. In contrast, when participants view the same information from a survey or aerial perspective, the cuneus, an area associated with processing complex visual information such as objects or faces, demonstrated increased activation. These results are consistent with another fMRI study of human navigation in which selective and distinct brain regions were activated depending on the use

of a spatial versus nonspatial strategy to solve a radial arm maze (91). These results, along with several other recent behavioral and neuroimaging studies, indicate that specific cognitive-task demands will activate unique corresponding brain regions or neural networks. These neural networks have been shown to be gender specific for certain tasks (92). In navigation in a virtual environment, common areas of activation between men and women (e.g., hippocampus, parahippocampus) have been demonstrated (92). Women, however, demonstrate unique activation of right parietal and right prefrontal cortices (92). Thus, evidence from human studies suggests that the organizational and activational effects of hormones interact with task demands and the underlying neural networks associated with those cognitive tasks to produce the outcome of human behavioral performance.

Exogenous Androgens

Cognitive changes due to exogenously manipulated androgen levels have been examined in healthy young men, women, transsexuals, and hypogonadal males (see below). For example, Gordon and Lee (57) examined cognitive performance in response to administration of T enanthate in a group of healthy young men. They administered a low dose of T enanthate (10 mg) to the young men, followed by a battery of cognitive tests both immediately after injection and four hours later. They reported no appreciable effects from hormone administration, because the participants demonstrated the same improvement from baseline to the second test session in the placebo condition as in the T condition; however, no hormone values were reported. Therefore, the relationship between cognition and hormone levels is unknown. In contrast, T administration to a group of female-to-male transsexuals (FMs) demonstrated an improvement in spatial abilities but with decreased verbal abilities (93). In a subsequent study by the same research group, the beneficial effects of androgen treatment on spatial abilities were again confirmed in FMs and remained over a period of one-and-a-half years (94). As expected, untreated male-to-female transsexuals (MFs) had higher scores on visuo-spatial tasks than untreated FMs—group differences that disappeared after three months of cross-sex hormone treatment. The Slabbekoorn et al. (94) study indicates that T had an enhancing—and not quickly reversible—effect on spatial ability performance, but no deleterious effect on verbal fluency in FMs. In contrast, antiandrogen treatment in combination with estrogen therapy had no observable effects on cognition in MFs or men undergoing androgen suppression for prostate cancer (95). Miles et al. (96), however, found that MFs demonstrated improved verbal memory in response to estrogen treatment, with no differences between the treatment and control groups on tests of attention, mental rotation, and verbal fluency. Although it has been suggested that results of transsexual studies may be affected by comorbid psychiatric or mood conditions, no appreciable differences were found between the hormone-treated and wait-list groups on mood measures in the Miles et al. study. Further, Postma et al. (97) found that in a population of healthy nontranssexual young women, short-term T administration (0.5 mg T cyclodextrine) resulted in improved spatial memory compared to placebo on some measures, but not others.

Overall, the results from exogenous manipulation of androgens in healthy young men and women suggest that androgens may have beneficial effects on spatial abilities. Due to study design and lack of documented change in hormone levels, however, findings to date remain inconclusive.

□ AGING EFFECTS ON ANDROGENS

Serum levels of total T and bioavailable T (T that is not bound to sex hormone-binding globulin) decrease in men with age (98–100). Although this decrease is gradual, it can result in decreased muscle mass, osteoporosis, decreased sexual activity, and changes in cognition (98,99,101–106). Androgen replacement therapy in normal older men has demonstrated benefits on bone mass, muscle strength, and sexual functioning (107–110). These benefits, however, may result from direct effects of T or from increased E_2 levels following aromatization of T. Recent evidence from the case of a patient with genetic aromatase deficiency suggests that bone mass changes and other physiological effects in men may in fact be attributable to changes in E_2 levels, rather than to direct T effects (111).

In addition to peripheral physiological effects, age-related declines in T levels may affect cognitive abilities. Two epidemiological studies involving large groups of healthy older males found bioavailable or free T to be significantly and positively correlated with tests of global cognitive functioning (101,102). In a more recent study using sensitive neuropsychological measures that assess specific areas of cognitive functioning rather than global measures, high levels of free T were associated with better performance on visual memory, verbal memory, divided attention, and visuospatial rotation (98). Further, when this large cohort of elderly men was divided according to eugonadal and hypogonadal status, hypogonadal men evidenced significantly poorer performance for visual memory, verbal memory, divided attention, and visuo-spatial rotation compared to eugonadal men. The men were reassessed every two years for up to 30 years in a combination cross-sectional/longitudinal study, and declining T levels over time were significantly associated with declines in visual memory. Although it has been suggested that declines in T levels may be coincident with disease or health decline, these findings remained significant after controlling for variables known to affect cognitive status, such as age, education, and health status. Not all studies, however, have found a positive relationship between cognitive abilities and endogenous T levels (69).

T Replacement in Older and Impaired Men

Studies examining exogenous T administration in older men have produced mixed results; however, carefully designed prospective studies with sensitive neuropsychological batteries tend to show significant effects. Sih et al. (112), using a double-blind, placebo-controlled design, gave older, hypogonadal men biweekly injections of 200 mg of T cypionate for 12 months. Fifteen men were randomly assigned to receive placebo and 17 men were randomly assigned to receive T. The men were in good general health and had a mean age of 68 years. Tests of verbal and visual memory were administered prior to treatment and again after six months. Although grip strength improved, memory measures remained unchanged. The lack of significant findings in this study may be due to nonsignificant changes in T levels from baseline and/or assessment of cognition during periods of minimum T levels. Janowsky et al. (113) found improvements in spatial abilities in a double-blind study using 15 mg T skin patches daily. In this study, 56 healthy older men (mean age 67 years) participated and were randomized to placebo or T treatment for three months. The participants were administered a battery of tests measuring semantic knowledge, constructional ability, verbal memory, fine motor coordination, and divided attention prior to and after the three months of treatment. The treatment group demonstrated improvement on a measure of visuo-constructional ability. In a second study, Janowsky et al. (114) found that weekly injections of T enanthate (150 mg) improved spatial working memory in a group of healthy older males (Fig. 3). These improvements were evident compared to an age-matched placebo group and exceeded practice effects demonstrated by young men (without T treatment). "Working memory" refers to one's ability to maintain information in the mind while simultaneously manipulating or updating the information as needed. It is the mind's scratch pad, and therefore improvements in working memory can affect a number of cognitive and day-to-day tasks.

Consistent with these results, our work reported significant improvements in spatial and verbal memory in a group of healthy older men in response to short-term administration of T enanthate (115). Twenty-five healthy older men (mean age 68 years) were randomized to 100 mg of T enanthate or placebo and received treatment for six weeks followed by six weeks of washout. Participants were administered a comprehensive battery of tests including tests for verbal and spatial memory, spatial abilities, verbal fluency, and selective attention. T-treated participants demonstrated significant improvements in spatial memory (recall of a walking route), spatial ability

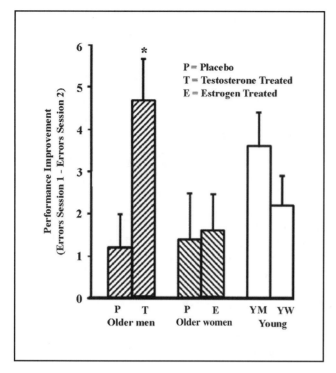

Figure 3 Change in performance after a month of placebo or hormone supplementation (150 mg intramuscular testosterone enanthate weekly for men and 0.625 mg/day conjugated estrogen daily for women) in older subjects (*striped bars*) or after no treatment in younger subjects (*open bars*). Older men on testosterone supplementation showed an improvement in performance (fewer errors; *asterisk*). Younger subjects showed the expected improvement on the task due to practice; older subjects without hormone supplementation or with estrogen supplementation did not. Brackets show standard error of the mean. *Source*: From Ref. 114.

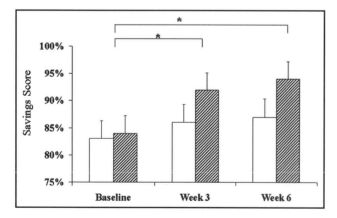

Figure 4 Mean savings score on story recall, measuring verbal memory at baseline and weeks 3 and 6 of treatment for placebo (*open bars*) and T-treated (*cross-hatched bars*) healthy older men (100 mg intramuscular T enanthate weekly). *Savings score* is the number of exact words recalled from a short story after a 20-minute delay divided by the number of words recalled immediately after hearing the story. Therefore, *savings score* represents the percentage of information recalled. Standard error bars represent standard error of measurement. Asterisks and lines above the bars indicate significant changes from baseline in the T-treated group at weeks 3 and 6 as indicated by the lines. *Abbreviation*: T, testosterone. *Source*: From Ref. 115.

(block construction), and verbal memory (recall of a short story) (Fig. 4). Improvements in spatial memory for a task that utilizes navigation in 3D space and verbal memory have not been previously reported. Although improvements were not found for all cognitive measures, changes in measures of verbal fluency or selective attention were not expected.

T Replacement in Older Hypogonadal Men

Several studies have examined androgen supplementation in older men. Kenny et al. (116) assessed a group of 44 older (65–87 years) hypogonadal men randomized to placebo or T patch for one year. Significant improvement associated with T levels was observed on a measure of divided attention in the treatment group. Both the treatment group and the placebo group demonstrated improvement on a measure of complex attention. We have also observed improvement in cognition in a group of older hypogonadal men given T or DHT gel (117). Twelve older (mean age 57 years) hypogonadal men were given T gel and a battery of cognitive tests assessing verbal and spatial memory, language, and attention at baseline (prior to medication) and again at days 90 and 180 of treatment. In addition to robustly raised T and E_2 levels, a significant improvement in verbal memory compared to baseline was evident at day 180 of treatment (Fig. 5a). A beneficial increase in spatial memory was also evident; however, this increase did not reach statistical significance. In a separate study, nine older hypogonadal men (mean age 74 years) were randomized to receive DHT or placebo gel. Participants were given a comprehensive cognitive battery at baseline and at days 30 and 90 of treatment. DHT gel significantly increased DHT and decreased T levels compared to baseline, and a significant improvement in spatial memory was observed (Fig. 5b). The results from these two studies suggest that aromatization of T to E_2 may regulate verbal memory in men whereas nonaromatizable androgens may regulate spatial memory (117).

In addition to brain functional changes measured by psychometric tests, two recent studies provide some evidence that androgen supplementation may optimize brain metabolism. Cerebral perfusion as measured by single-photon emission computed tomography (CT) increased in the superior frontal gyrus and midbrain of seven, older (aged 58–72 years) hypogonadal men treated with T at weeks 3 to 5 of treatment, with further increases in midbrain perfusion at weeks 12 to 14 of treatment (118). Although objective assessment of cognitive function was not included, responses to a questionnaire indicated that the increases in brain perfusion coincided with self-reported increases in cognitive function. These findings are consistent with brain metabolism changes assessed with positron emission tomography (PET) in a group of young hypogonadal men given T replacement (119) (see below, "Isolated Hypogonadotropic Hypogonadism and Kallman's Syndrome").

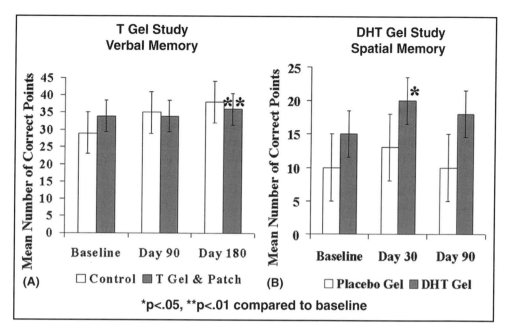

Figure 5 (**A**) T gel study. Mean number of correctly recalled bits of information on story recall, measuring verbal memory at baseline and at days 90 and 180 of treatment for the control group (*open bars*) and T-treated (*gray bars*) hypogonadal men (T gel and T patch together). Standard error bars represent standard error of measurement. Asterisks indicate significant changes from baseline. (**B**) DHT gel study. Mean number of correctly recalled sequence points from the route test, measuring spatial memory at baseline and at days 30 and 90 of treatment for the placebo gel group (*open bars*) and DHT-treated (*gray bars*) hypogonadal men. Standard error bars represent standard error of measurement. Asterisks indicate significant changes from baseline. *Abbreviations*: DHT, dihydrotestosterone; T, testosterone.

T Replacement in Men with Alzheimer's Disease

Hypogonadal men with impairments in memory and cognition may also benefit from androgen supplementation. Tan and Pu (120) treated 10 male patients with Alzheimer's disease (AD) who also met criteria for hypogonadism. The participants were given 200 mg of T every two weeks. A comprehensive cognitive test battery was administered at baseline and at three, six, and nine months of treatment. The AD patients demonstrated a significant

improvement at months 3, 6, and 9 compared to baseline and compared to the placebo group. Although the improvement appeared to wane at month 9 of treatment, it was still greater than for the placebo group (Fig. 6).

In summary, these studies suggest that T administration may have beneficial effects on spatial and verbal memory. These changes in brain function are evident from both performance on psychometric tests and neuroimaging assessments. These findings may be particularly important for older males who may have age-related decreases in endogenous T levels, which is predictive of cognitive loss (98). Unlike studies of estrogen supplementation in women with AD, recent findings of T supplementation appear to be more promising with regard to cognitive benefits. Most studies to date, however, have involved small sample sizes and need replication with larger sample sizes.

☐ ENDOCRINE DISORDERS
Congenital Adrenal Hyperplasia

Congenital adrenal hyperplasia (CAH) is a condition in which the developing fetus is exposed to excessive levels of androgens during gestation. The most common cause of this androgen excess is due to 21-hydroxylase or 11β-hydroxylase deficiency (121). The androgen excess results from the loss of cortisol negative-feedback regulation of adrenocorticotropic hormone secretion. About 75% of children with CAH have an associated

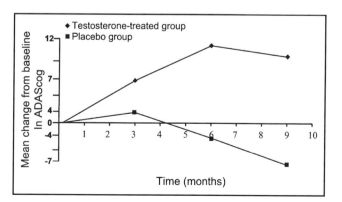

Figure 6 Graph showing the mean change from baseline assessed using the Alzheimer's Disease Assessment Scale—cognitive subscale (ADAScog) with time. *Source*: From Ref. 120.

deficiency in aldosterone production. The salt-wasting variety results in hyponatremia, hyperkalemia, and volume depletion, which is usually present within the first two weeks of life. The condition affects approximately 1 in 5,000 to 1 in 15,000 live births. The clinical presentation in genetic females includes pseudohermaphroditism, whereas affected males tend to have normal or early sexual development. Exposure to excess androgens during early development provides a unique opportunity to examine the organizational effects of hormones in humans.

There is some indication that individuals with CAH may demonstrate greater cerebral lateralization, as evidenced by a higher incidence of sinistrality (left-handedness) (122,123); however, other studies have failed to support this (124). Magnetic resonance imaging (MRI) of CAH patients has revealed mixed findings, with some evidence of atypical lateralization, abnormal white matter distribution, or temporal lobe atrophy in about one-third of patients (125–127); however, these abnormalities do not appear to be related to any detrimental neuropsychological performance or treatment status (125,126). Increased incidence of learning disorders has been found in CAH patients, along with decrements in general intelligence quotient (IQ) level and verbal intelligence quotient (VIQ), suggesting that prenatal exposure to androgens may adversely affect the development of the left hemisphere or hemispheric lateralization, which would adversely affect verbal abilities (125,127–131). For example, female CAH patients demonstrate significantly lower VIQ scores compared to unaffected sisters (123,128,130). Some evidence, however, also supports a higher level of general intelligence in CAH patients (125,132,133). In addition, studies of dichotic listening—a task that is sensitive to hemispheric lateralization—are not supportive of an atypical lateralization pattern in CAH patients (124,134). In a dichotic listening task, different auditory inputs are simultaneously presented to each ear through headphones. In normal individuals with an intact corpus callosum, visual and auditory inputs sent to one hemisphere are quickly shared with the other. This task has been used to discover the typical pattern of left hemisphere dominance for language.

One possible explanation for these findings may be that androgens specifically affect spatial abilities. In particular, if androgens are specific to spatial abilities, one would expect that CAH females would evidence superior spatial abilities compared to matched controls, whereas male CAH patients would evidence modest or no appreciable increase in spatial abilities compared to male controls. A study by Resnick et al. (133) found that CAH adolescent girls performed better than matched familial controls on tests of spatial ability (e.g., the hidden patterns test, card rotations, and mental rotations). A more recent study by Hampson et al. (135) also provides evidence that spatial abilities are specifically increased in CAH girls compared to controls. This study examined a relatively young population of CAH patients (mean age 10 years) matched for IQ level with controls. The participants were administered the perceptual speed test, a task on which females typically outperform males, and the spatial relations test from the primary mental abilities test, a measure of spatial visualization on which males typically outperform females. CAH girls performed less well than controls on the perceptual speed task but outperformed the controls on the spatial test. This effect was large (nearly one standard deviation), and there was no difference between salt wasters versus non–salt wasters. Thus, the atypical advantage of CAH girls on the spatial task and the failure to find a typical advantage on the perceptual speed task represent a double-dissociation effect of androgens in this population. Although other studies have failed to find an advantage in spatial abilities in CAH girls (125,132), evidence of behavioral masculinization has been reported in CAH girls (136–143). Thus, additional carefully designed studies may provide further information regarding the organizational effects of androgens on cognition in this population.

Isolated Hypogonadotropic Hypogonadism and Kallmann's Syndrome

Isolated hypogonadotropic hypogonadism (IHH) results from the deficiency of gonadotropin-releasing hormone (GnRH) from the hypothalamus. When this type of hypogonadism is accompanied by anosmia from agenesis or malformation of the olfactory bulb, sulci, and tracts, the condition is termed "Kallmann's syndrome" (KS). It occurs in about 1 in 10,000 male births, and males predominate at a ratio of 5:1. The syndrome can occur as an inherited or sporadic disorder. X-linked, autosomal dominant, and autosomal recessive modes of inheritance have been described. In one-third or more of patients with KS, the pathology is likely the result of an X-linked form of KS due to a defect in the *KAL* gene. *KAL* encodes a protein called anosmin, which plays a key role in the migration of GnRH neurons and olfactory nerves to the hypothalamus (144). MRI studies have confirmed the absence or aplasia of the olfactory bulb in KS versus IHH patients (145). In IHH without anosmia, a defect in the GnRH receptor (GnRHR) has been reported to be responsible for reproductive function failure, and GnRHR mutations may be more common than previously appreciated in familial cases of normosmic IHH (146). Affected individuals are typically identified during adolescence when they evidence absence of or a delay in puberty. It has been suggested that developmental anomalies arise in the CNS due to a chronic lack of T and E_2. Reported neurologic abnormalities include anosmia, hyposmia, ocular motor abnormalities, pes cavus foot deformities, and impaired smooth pursuit eye movements and mirror movements (any synchronous movement of a corresponding muscle of another extremity occurring with the primary movement) (147). Performance on mirror movements may be impaired due to a lack of inhibitory fibers in the corpus callosum; however, neuroradiology findings have failed to find defects in that area (148).

Men with IHH demonstrate impairments in spatial abilities (149,150) and memory for both verbal and visual information (151). Kertzman et al. (152) found that IHH patients with abnormal mirror movements also demonstrated impairments on a measure of spatial attention. This deficit was not due to motor difficulties, because the IHH patients evidenced faster reaction times than controls. Alexander et al. (153) examined 33 hypogonadal men receiving T replacement therapy, 10 eugonadal men receiving T in a male contraceptive clinical trial, and 19 eugonadal controls for changes in cognition in response to T treatment. Cognitive tests included measures of visuo-spatial ability, verbal fluency, perceptual speed, and verbal memory. Group differences in T levels were unrelated to performance on most cognitive measures, including visuo-spatial ability; however, hypogonadal men were impaired in their verbal fluency compared to eugonadal men at baseline, and showed improved verbal fluency following T treatment. O'Connor et al. (154) also reported poor verbal fluency in a small (*n*=7) group of younger hypogonadal men (age 23–40 years). The hypogonadal group included a combination of IHH and Klinefelter men treated with 200 mg of T enanthate biweekly, which was compared with a group of healthy young men randomized to placebo or 200 mg of T enanthate weekly. A battery of cognitive tests was administered at baseline and again at weeks 4 and 8 of treatment. Eugonadal men declined in performance on supraphysiologic T supplementation. No significant changes were reported for the hypogonadal group. Nonetheless, an examination of the results suggests that the hypogonadal group was impaired on several tasks at baseline and improved on both verbal fluency and block design (spatial ability) to the baseline level of the eugonadal group; however, a comparison of treatment to baseline was not conducted.

The variability in results for androgen treatment in hypogonadal men may be due to the heterogeneity of participants included in the studies. For example, combining participants who are hypogonadal for a variety of etiologies (e.g., IHH, Klinfelter's, and Kallmann's) or who may represent varying time periods of androgen deprivation may mask or wash out actual effects. In addition, there may be small or large individual differences with regard to cognitive changes as there are with other physical symptoms. Zitzmann et al. (119) measured changes in brain metabolism and function in response to androgen treatment in a group of hypogonadal men. Six hypogonadal men were administered a mental rotation task during PET scanning prior to T treatment and again after two months of treatment. The results indicate that four of the six men demonstrated an improvement on the mental rotation task after T treatment and these four men also demonstrated increased brain activation. The men who did not demonstrate an improvement on the task did not show corresponding brain activation changes.

These results suggest that cognitive changes measured by psychometric tests may be observed only in a subset of participants who also demonstrate changes in brain metabolism.

Although the goal of hormonal treatment in male hypogonadism is typically to induce and maintain normal secondary sexual characteristics in adolescents, these studies indicate that changes in cognition may also occur with T treatment and these changes may vary according to individual characteristics and duration of androgen deprivation.

Klinefelter's Syndrome

Klinefelter's syndrome (XXY), or supernumary X, is due to the presence of surplus X chromosomes in phenotypic males (155–157). Klinefelter's syndrome affects approximately 1 in 500 patients and is characterized by testicular failure, impaired spermatogenesis, elevated gonadotropin levels, and androgen deficiency (155–157). Patients appear essentially normal until puberty and adulthood, when these symptoms become apparent. Distinguishing physical characteristics may include long legs and arm span, decreased facial and pubic hair, increased fat deposits in a female pattern, gynecomastia, and small testes and penis. T treatment during adolescence and adulthood is the most common form of treatment, with the goal being to reduce long-term consequences of androgen deficiency, such as osteoporosis.

Cognitive difficulties during childhood and adolescence have been reported, and include lower verbal IQ compared to performance IQ, developmental speech and language delays, learning disabilities (e.g., reading and written expression difficulties), and poor school performance (158–163). Some researchers have reported attentional difficulties (164), while others have found no evidence of attentional difficulties (165,166). Deficits in reasoning have been reported for a nonverbal reasoning test such as the Wisconsin card sorting test (167), although this finding is not consistent across studies (168). Recent evidence of a dissociation between reasoning impairments for verbal versus nonverbal information have led some to suggest that reasoning impairments in Klinefelter's may be restricted to tasks that involve verbal information processing (169). Recently, Patwardhan et al. (170) found that Klinfelter's syndrome (XXY) men demonstrate a reduction in left temporal lobe gray-matter volumes on MRI compared with normal control subjects, and these volumetric changes correlated with deficits in verbal abilities (Fig. 7). Klinefelter's syndrome patients who had never received T treatment evidenced significant reductions in left temporal lobe gray matter compared with those individuals who had received T supplementation.

These results suggest that there may be brain structure changes related to findings of verbal learning disabilities or difficulties with processing verbal information in these patients. In addition, findings of

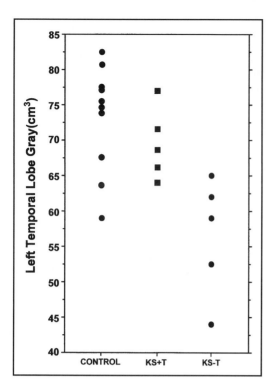

Figure 7   Left temporal lobe gray-matter volumes (cm³) for control subjects, KS subjects with testosterone supplementation (KS+T), and KS subjects without testosterone supplementation (KS-T). *Abbreviation*: KS, Klinefelter's syndrome.

preserved medial temporal lobe structures in patients who received T supplementation suggest that androgens may affect neural structure and integrity throughout the human adult life span.

□ CONCLUSION

Studies reviewed in this chapter demonstrate a relationship between androgens and specific aspects of cognition. Observed effects of androgens on cognition may occur by several mechanisms, including direct effects of T, or via T metabolites such as DHT or E_2. Androgens act via both classic receptor-mediated genomic methods and the more recently characterized nongenomic methods. The temporal relationship of androgen effects was reviewed, including organizational effects that occur due to the presence of androgens during critical neural development periods and result in permanent changes in behavior and cognition, as observed with CAH and Klinefelter's patients. Considerable evidence also suggests that androgens exert modulating effects on cognition throughout the lifespan, as demonstrated by observed cognitive changes in hypogonadal and transsexual individuals undergoing hormone treatment and older adults receiving androgen supplementation, as well as by changes in brain metabolism observed in hypogonadal men receiving T supplementation. Taken together, these data strongly indicate that androgens exert effects on cognition, particularly spatial abilities. Recent evidence from neuroimaging studies have extended our understanding of the complex interactions between androgens and cognition, suggesting that organizational and activational effects of hormones interact with unique cognitive task demands and their associated neural networks. Recent neuroimaging evidence may help explain why androgens appear to have selective rather than widespread effects on cognition and how these effects may differ among individuals. Clearly, more research is needed and future research endeavors will likely further refine the understanding of these complex relationships.

□ ACKNOWLEDGMENTS

Supported by NIA AG00858 and VAPSHCS.

□ REFERENCES

1.   Brown-Sequard CE. The effects produced on man by subcutaneous injections of a liquid obtained from the testicles of animals. Lancet 1889; 2:105–107.
2.   Rubinow DR, Schmidt PJ. Androgens, brain, and behavior. Am J Psychiatr 1996; 153(8):974–984.
3.   Simerly RB, Chang C, Muramatsu M, et al. Distribution of androgen and estrogen receptor mRNA-containing cells in the rat brain: an in situ hybridization study. J Comp Neurol 1990; 294(1):76–95.
4.   Kerr JE, Allore RJ, Beck SG, et al. Distribution and hormonal regulation of androgen receptor (AR) and AR messenger ribonucleic acid in the rathippocampus. Endocrinology 1995; 136(8):3213–3221.
5.   Beyenburg S, Watzka M, Clusmann H, et al. Androgen receptor mRNA expression in the human hippocampus. Neurosci Lett 2000; 294(1):25–28.
6.   Roselli CE, Klosterman S, Resko JA. Anatomic relationships between aromatase and androgen receptor mRNA expression in the hypothalamus and amygdala of adult male cynomolgus monkeys. J Comp Neurol 2001; 439(2):208–223.

7. Ishunina TA, Fisser B, Swaab DF. Sex differences in androgen receptor immunoreactivity in basal forebrain nuclei of elderly and Alzheimer patients. Exp Neurol 2002; 176(1):122–132.

8. Michael RP, Rees HD, Bonsall RW. Sites in the male primate brain at which testosterone acts as an androgen. Brain Res 1989; 502(1):11–20.

9. Janne OA, Palvimo JJ, Kallio P, et al. Androgen receptor and mechanism of androgen action. Ann Med 1993; 25(1):83–89.

10. Brown TJ, Adler GH, Sharma M, et al. Androgen treatment decreases estrogen receptor binding in the ventromedial nucleus of the rat brain: a quantitative in vitro autoradiographic analysis. Mol Cell Neurosci 1994; 5(6):549–555.

11. Lynch CS, Story AJ. Dihydrotestosterone and estrogen regulation of rat brain androgen-receptor immunoreactivity. Physiol Behav 2000; 69(4–5):445–453.

12. Singh R, Pervin S, Shryne J, et al. Castration increases and androgens decrease nitric oxide synthase activity in the brain: physiologic implications. Proc Natl Acad Sci USA 2000; 97(7):3672–3677.

13. Lieberherr M, Grosse B. Androgens increase intracellular calcium concentration and inositol 1,4,5-trisphosphate and diacylglycerol formation via a pertussis toxin-sensitive G-protein. J Biol Chem 1994; 269(10):7217–7223.

14. Benten WP, Lieberherr M, Sekeris CE, et al. Testosterone induces Ca2+ influx via non-genomic surface receptors in activated T cells. FEBS Lett 1997; 407(2):211–214.

15. Benten WP, Lieberherr M, Stamm O, et al. Testosterone signaling through internalizable surface receptors in androgen receptor-free macrophages. Mol Biol Cell 1999; 10(10):3113–3123.

16. Benten WP, Lieberherr M, Giese G, et al. Functional testosterone receptors in plasma membranes of T cells. FASEB J 1999; 13(1):123–133.

17. Cyr M, Calon F, Morissette M, et al. Drugs with estrogen-like potency and brain activity: potential therapeutic application for the CNS. Curr Pharm Des 2000; 6(12):1287–1312.

18. Gundlah C, Kohama SG, Mirkes SJ, et al. Distribution of estrogen receptor beta (ERbeta) mRNA in hypothalamus, midbrain and temporal lobe of spayed macaque: continued expression with hormone replacement. Brain Res Mol Brain Res 2000; 76(2):191–204.

19. Osterlund MK, Gustafsson JA, Keller E, et al. Estrogen receptor beta (ERbeta) messenger ribonucleic acid (mRNA) expression within the human forebrain: distinct distribution pattern to ERalpha mRNA. J Clin Endocrinol Metab 2000; 85(10):3840–3846.

20. Osterlund MK, Grandien K, Keller E, et al. The human brain has distinct regional expression patterns of estrogen receptor alpha mRNA isoforms derived from alternative promoters. J Neurochem 2000; 75(4):1390–1397.

21. de Fougerolles Nunn E, Greenstein B, Khamashta M, et al. Evidence for sexual dimorphism of estrogen receptors in hypothalamus and thymus of neonatal and immature Wistar rats. Int J Immunopharmacol 1999; 21(12):869–877.

22. Dawson JL, Cheung YM, Lau RT. Developmental effects of neonatal sex hormones on spatial and activity skills in the white rat. Biol Psychol 1975; 3(3):213–229.

23. Joseph R, Hess S, Birecree E. Effects of hormone manipulations and exploration on sex differences in maze learning. Behav Biol 1978; 24(3):364–377.

24. Roof RL. Neonatal exogenous testosterone modifies sex difference in radial arm and Morris water maze performance in prepubescent and adult rats. Behav Brain Res 1993; 53(1–2):1–10.

25. Stefanova N, Ovtscharoff W. Sexual dimorphism of the bed nucleus of the stria terminalis and the amygdala. Adv Anat Embryol Cell Biol 2000; 158(III-X):1–78.

26. Kirn J, Lombroso PJ. Development of the cerebral cortex: XI. Sexual dimorphism in the brain. J Am Acad Child Adolesc Psychiatry 1998; 37(11):1228–1230.

27. Gorski RA. Sexual dimorphisms of the brain. J Anim Sci 1985; 61(suppl 3):38–61.

28. Nunez JL, Juraska JM. The size of the splenium of the rat corpus callosum: influence of hormones, sex ratio, and neonatal cryoanesthesia. Dev Psychobiol 1998; 33(4):295–303.

29. Roof RL. The dentate gyrus is sexually dimorphic in prepubescent rats: testosterone plays a significant role. Brain Research 1993; 610(1):148–151.

30. Hamburger-Bar R, Rigter H. Peripheral and central androgenic stimulation of sexual behavior of castrated male rats. Acta Endocrinol (Copenh) 1977; 84(4):813–828.

31. Nakamura N, Fujita H, Kawata M. Effects of gonadectomy on immunoreactivity for choline acetyltransferase in the cortex, hippocampus, and basal forebrain of adult male rats. Neuroscience 2002; 109(3):473–485.

32. McQueen JK, Wilson H, Sumner BE, et al. Serotonin transporter (SERT) mRNA and binding site densities in male rat brain affected by sex steroids. Brain Res Mol Brain Res 1999; 63(2):241–247.

33. Fink G, Sumner B, Rosie R, et al. Androgen actions on central serotonin neurotransmission: relevance for mood, mental state and memory. Behav Brain Res 1999; 105(1):53–68.

34. Sumner BE, Fink G. Testosterone as well as estrogen increases serotonin2A receptor mRNA and binding site densities in the male rat brain. Brain Res Mol Brain Res 1998; 59(2):205–214.

35. Orsini JC. Androgen influence on lateral hypothalamus in the male rat: possible behavioral significance. Physiol Behav 1982; 29(6):979–987.

36. Poletti A, Martini L. Androgen-activating enzymes in the central nervous system. J Steroid Biochem Mol Biol 1999; 69(1–6):117–122.

37. Roselli CE, Resko JA. Androgens regulate brain aromatase activity in adult male rats through a receptor mechanism. Endocrinology 1984; 114(6):2183–2189.

38. Kritzer MF. Long-term gonadectomy affects the density of tyrosine hydroxylase- but not dopamine-beta-hydroxylase-, choline acetyltransferase- or serotonin-immunoreactive axons in the medial prefrontal cortices of adult male rats. Cereb Cortex 2003; 13(3):282–296.

39. Kritzer MF. Effects of acute and chronic gonadectomy on the catecholamine innervation of the cerebral cortex in adult male rats: insensitivity of axons immunoreactive for dopamine-beta-hydroxylase to gonadal steroids, and differential sensitivity of axons immunoreactive for tyrosine hydroxylase to ovarian and testicular hormones. J Comp Neurol 2000; 427(4): 617–633.

40. Kritzer MF, Adler A, Marotta J, et al. Regionally selective effects of gonadectomy on cortical catecholamine innervation in adult male rats are most disruptive to afferents in prefrontal cortex. Cereb Cortex 1999; 9(5):507–518.

41. Kritzer MF. Perinatal gonadectomy exerts regionally selective, lateralized effects on the density of axons immunoreactive for tyrosine hydroxylase in the cerebral cortex of adult male rats. J Neurosci 1998; 18(24): 10735–10748.

42. Kritzer MF, McLaughlin PJ, Smirlis T, et al. Gonadectomy impairs T-maze acquisition in adult male rats. Horm Behav 2001; 39(2):167–174.

43. Vazquez-Pereya F, Rivas-Arancibia S, Loaeza-Del Castillo A, et al. Modulation of short and long term memory by steroid sexual hormones. Life Sci 1995; 56(14):PL255–PL260.

44. Flood JF, Farr SA, Kaiser FE, et al. Age-related decrease of plasma testosterone in SAMP8 mice: replacement improves age-related impairment of learning and memory. Physiol Behav 1995; 57(4):669–673.

45. Naghdi N, Nafisy N, Majlessi N. The effects of intra-hippocampal testosterone and flutamide on spatial localization in the Morris water maze. Brain Res 2001; 897(1–2):44–51.

46. Goudsmit E, Van de Poll NE, Swaab DF. Testosterone fails to reverse spatial memory decline in aged rats and impairs retention in young and middle-aged animals. Behav Neural Biol 1990; 53(1):6–20.

47. Naghdi N, Oryan S, Etemadi R. The study of spatial memory in adult male rats with injection of testosterone enanthate and flutamide into the basolateral nucleus of the amygdala in Morris water maze. Brain Res 2003; 972(1–2):1–8.

48. Bimonte-Nelson HA, Singleton RS, Nelson ME, et al. Testosterone, but not nonaromatizable dihydrotestosterone, improves working memory and alters nerve growth factor levels in aged male rats. Exp Neurol 2003; 181(2):301–312.

49. Roselli CE, Chambers K. Sex differences in male-typical copulatory behaviors in response to androgen and estrogen treatment in rats. Neuroendocrinology 1999; 69(4):290–298.

50. Grino PB, Griffin JE, Wilson JD. Testosterone at high concentrations interacts with the human androgen receptor similarly to dihydrotestosterone. Endocrinology 1990; 126(2):1165–1172.

51. Lu S, Simon NG, Wang Y, et al. Neural androgen receptor regulation: effects of androgen and antiandrogen. J Neurobiol 1999; 41(4):505–512.

52. Frye CA, Lacey EH. Posttraining androgens' enhancement of cognitive performance is temporally distinct from androgens' increases in affective behavior. Cogn Affect Behav Neurosci 2001; 1(2):172–182.

53. Resko JA, Pereyra-Martinez AC, Stadelman HL, et al. Region-specific regulation of cytochrome P450 aromatase messenger ribonucleic acid by androgen in brains of male rhesus monkeys. Biol Reprod 2000; 62(6):1818–1822.

54. Schmidt BM, Gerdes D, Feuring M, et al. Rapid, nongenomic steroid actions: A new age? Front Neuroendocrinol 2000; 21(1):57–94.

55. Kellogg CK, Lundin A. Brain androgen-inducible aromatase is critical for adolescent organization of environment-specific social interaction in male rats. Horm Behav 1999; 35(2):155–162.

56. Kritzer MF, Pugach I. Administration of tamoxifen but not flutamide to hormonally intact, adult male rats mimics the effects of short-term gonadectomy on the catecholamine innervation of the cerebral cortex. J Comp Neurol 2001; 431(4):444–459.

57. Gordon HW, Lee PA. A relationship between gonadotropins and visuospatial function. Neuropsychologia 1986; 24(4):563–576.

58. McKeever WF, Deyo RA. Testosterone, dihydrotestosterone, and spatial task performances of males. Bull Psychon Soc 1990; 28:305–308.

59. Christiansen K, Kussmann R. Androgen levels and components of aggressive behavior in men. Horm Behav 1987; 21(2):170–180.

60. Errico AL, Parsons OA, Kling OR, et al. Investigation of the role of sex hormones in alcoholics' visuospatial deficits. Neuropsychologia 1992; 30(5):417–426.

61. Tan U. The relationship between serum testosterone level and visuomotor learning in right-handed young men. Int J Neurosci 1991; 56(1–4):19–24.

62. Christiansen K. Sex hormone related variations of cognitive performance in Kung San hunter-gathers of Namibia. Neuropsychobiology 1993; 27:97–107.

63. Kampen DL, Sherwin BB. Estradiol is related to visual memory in healthy young men. Behav Neurosci 1996; 110(3):613–617.

64. McKeever WF, Rich DA, Deyo RA, et al. Androgens and spatial ability: Failure to find a relationship between testosterone and ability measures. Bull Psychon Soc 1987; 25:438–440.

65. Moffat SD, Hampson E. A curvilinear relationship between testosterone and spatial cognition in humans: possible influence of hand preference. Psychoneuroendocrinology 1996; 21(3):323–337.

66. Gouchie C, Kimura D. The relationship between testosterone levels and cognitive ability patterns. Psychoneuroendocrinology 1991; 16(4):323–334.

67. Shute VJ, Pellegrino JW, Hubert L, et al. The relationship between androgen levels and human spatial abilities. Bull Psychon Soc 1983; 21:465–468.

68. Silverman JM, Keefe RS, Mohs RC, et al. A study of the reliability of the family history method in genetic studies of Alzheimer disease. Alzheim Dis Assoc Disord 1989; 3(4):218–223.

69. Wolf OT, Kirschbaum C. Endogenous estradiol and testosterone levels are associated with cognitive performance in older women and men. Horm Behav 2002; 41(3):259–266.

70. Kimura D. Sex and Cognition. Cambridge, MA: The MIT Press, 1999.

71. Vederhus L, Krekling S. Sex differences in visual spatial ability in 9-year-old children. Intelligence 1996; 23:33–43.

72. Johnson ES, Meade AC. Developmental patterns of spatial ability: an early sex difference. Child Dev 1987; 58(3):725–740.

73. Vandenberg SG, Kuse AR. Mental rotations, a group test of three-dimensional spatial visualization. Percept Mot Skills 1978; 47(2):599–604.

74. Silverman I, Kastuk D, Choi J, et al. Testosterone levels and spatial ability in men. Psychoneuroendocrinology 1999; 24(8):813–822.

75. Collins DW, Kimura D. A large sex difference on a two-dimensional mental rotation task. Behav Neurosci 1997; 111(4):845–849.

76. Larson P, Rizzo AA, Buckwalter JG, et al. Gender issues in the use of virtual environments. Cyberpsychol Behav 1999; 2:113–123.

77. McBurney DH, Gaulin SJ, Devineni T, et al. Superior spatial memory of women: stronger evidence for the gathering hypothesis. Evol Hum Behav 1997; 18(3):165–174.

78. Eals M, Silverman I. The hunter-gatherer theory of spatial sex differences: proximate factors. Ethol Sociobiol 1994; 15:95–105.

79. Galea LA, Kimura D. Sex differences in route learning. Personality and individual differences 1993; 14(1):53–65.

80. Sandstrom NJ, Kaufman J, Huettel SA. Males and females use different distal cues in a virtual environment navigation task. Brain Res Cogn Brain Res 1998; 6(4):351–360.

81. Moffat SD, Hampson E, Hatzipantelis M. Navigation in a "virtual" maze: sex differences and correlation with psychometric measures of spatial ability in humans. Evol Hum Behav 1998; 19:73–88.

82. Astur RS, Ortiz ML, Sutherland RJ. A characterization of performance by men and women in a virtual Morris water task: a large and reliable sex difference. Behav Brain Res 1998; 93(1–2):185–190.

83. Choi J, Silverman I. The relationship between testosterone and route-learning strategies in humans. Brain Cogn 2002; 50(1):116–120.

84. Maguire EA, Frackowiak RS, Frith CD. Recalling routes around london: activation of the right hippocampus in taxi drivers. J Neurosci 1997; 17(18): 7103–7110.

85. Maguire EA, Frith CD, Burgess N, et al. Knowing where things are parahippocampal involvement in encoding object locations in virtual large-scale space. J Cogn Neurosci 1998; 10(1):61–76.

86. Epstein R, Kanwisher N. A cortical representation of the local visual environment. Nature 1998; 392(6676): 598–601.

87. Aguirre GK, D'Esposito M. Environmental knowledge is subserved by separable dorsal/ventral neural areas. J Neurosci 1997; 17(7):2512–2518.

88. Aguirre GK, Zarahn E, D'Esposito M. An area within human ventral cortex sensitive to "building" stimuli: evidence and implications. Neuron 1998; 21(2): 373–383.

89. Wilson FA, Riches IP, Brown MW. Hippocampus and medial temporal cortex: neuronal activity related to behavioral responses during the performance of memory tasks by primates. Behav Brain Res 1990; 40(1):7–28.

90. Shelton AL, Gabrieli JD. Neural correlates of encoding space from route and survey perspectives. J Neurosci 2002; 22(7):2711–2717.

91. Iaria G, Petrides M, Dagher A, et al. Cognitive strategies dependent on the hippocampus and caudate nucleus in human navigation: variability and change with practice. J Neurosci 2003; 23(13):5945–5952.

92. Gron G, Wunderlich AP, Spitzer M, et al. Brain activation during human navigation: gender-different neural networks as substrate of performance. Nat Neurosci 2000; 3(4):404–408.

93. Van Goozen SH, Cohen-Kettenis PT, Gooren LJ, et al. Activating effects of androgens on cognitive performance: causal evidence in a group of female-to-male transsexuals. Neuropsychologia 1994; 32(10):1153–1157.

94. Slabbekoorn D, van Goozen SH, Megens J, et al. Activating effects of cross-sex hormones on cognitive functioning: a study of short-term and long-term hormone effects in transsexuals. Psychoneuroendocrinology 1999; 24(4):423–447.

95. Baker LD, Sambamurti K, Craft S, et al. 17beta-estradiol reduces plasma Abeta40 for HRT-naive postmenopausal women with Alzheimer disease: a preliminary study. Am J Geriatr Psychiatry 2003; 11(2):239–244.

96. Miles C, Green R, Sanders G, et al. Estrogen and memory in a transsexual population. Horm Behav 1998; 34(2):199–208.

97. Postma A, Meyer G, Tuiten A, et al. Effects of testosterone administration on selective aspects of object-location memory in healthy young women. Psychoneuroendocrinology 2000; 25(6):563–575.

98. Moffat SD, Zonderman AB, Metter EJ, et al. Longitudinal assessment of serum free testosterone concentration predicts memory performance and cognitive status in elderly men. J Clin Endocrinol Metab 2002; 87(11):5001–5007.

99. Tenover JS, Matsumoto AM, Plymate SR, et al. The effects of aging in normal men on bioavailable testosterone and luteinizing hormone secretion: response

to clomiphene citrate. J Clin Endocrinol Metab 1987; 65(6):1118–1126.

100. Tenover JS. Effects of testosterone supplementation in the aging male. J Clin Endocrinol 1992; 75(4):1092–1098.

101. Yaffe K, Lui LY, Zmuda J, et al. Sex hormones and cognitive function in older men. J Am Geriatr Soc 2002; 50:707–712.

102. Barrett-Connor E, Goodman-Gruen D, Patay B. Endogenous sex hormones and cognitive function in older men. J Clin Endocrinol Metab 1999; 84(10):3681–3685.

103. Morley JE. Testosterone replacement and the physiologic aspects of aging in men. Mayo Clin Proc 2000; 75(suppl):S83–S87.

104. Morley JE, Perry HM III. Androgen deficiency in aging men: role of testosterone replacement therapy. J Lab Clin Med 2000; 135(5):370–378.

105. Ravaglia G, Forti P, Maioli F, et al. Body composition, sex steroids, IGF-1, and bone mineral status in aging men. J Gerontol A Biol Sci Med Sci 2000; 55(9): M516–M521.

106. Matsumoto AM. "Andropause"—are reduced androgen levels in aging men physiologically important? West J Med 1993; 159(5):618–620.

107. Swerdloff RS, Wang C, Cunningham G, et al. Long-term pharmacokinetics of transdermal testosterone gel in hypogonadal men. J Clin Endocrinol Metab 2000; 85(12):4500–4510.

108. Swerdloff RS, Wang C. Androgens, estrogens, and bone in men. Ann Intern Med 2000; 133(12):1002–1004.

109. Tenover JS. Androgen administration to aging men. Endocrinol Metab Clin North Am 1994; 23(4):877–892.

110. Lund BC, Bever-Stille KA, Perry PJ. Testosterone and andropause: the feasibility of testosterone replacement therapy in elderly men. Pharmacotherapy 1999; 19(8):951–956.

111. Carani C, Qin K, Simoni M, et al. Effect of testosterone and estradiol in a man with aromatase deficiency. N Engl J Med 1997; 337(2):91–95.

112. Sih R, Morley JE, Kaiser FE, et al. Testosterone replacement in older hypogonadal men: a 12-month randomized controlled trial. J Clin Endocrinol Metab 1997; 82(6):1661–1667.

113. Janowsky JS, Oviatt SK, Orwoll ES. Testosterone influences spatial cognition in older men. Behav Neurosci 1994; 108(2):325–332.

114. Janowsky JS, Chavez B, Orowoll E. Sex steroids modify working memory. J Cogn Neurosci 2000; 12(3):407–414.

115. Cherrier MM, Asthana S, Plymate S, et al. Testosterone supplementation improves spatial and verbal memory in healthy older men. Neurology 2001; 57(1):80–88.

116. Kenny AM, Bellantonio S, Gruman CA, et al. Effects of transdermal testosterone on cognitive function and health perception in older men with low bioavailable testosterone levels. J Gerontol A Biol Sci Med Sci 2002; 57(5):M321–M325.

117. Cherrier MM, Craft S, Matsumoto AH. Cognitive changes associated with supplementation of testoster-

one or dihydrotestosterone in mildly hypogonadal men: a preliminary report. J Androl 2003; 24(4):568–576.

118. Azad N, Pitale S, Barnes WE, et al. Testosterone treatment enhances regional brain perfusion in hypogonadal men. J Clin Endocrinol Metab 2003; 88(7):3064–3068.

119. Zitzmann M, Weckesser M, Schober O, et al. Changes in cerebral glucose metabolism and visuospatial capability in hypogonadal males under testosterone substitution therapy. Exp Clin Endocrinol Diabetes 2001; 109(5):302–304.

120. Tan RS, Pu SJ. A pilot study on the effects of testosterone in hypogonadal aging male patients with Alzheimer's disease. Aging Male 2003; 6(1):13–17.

121. Orth DN, Kovacs WJ, Debold CR. The adrenal cortex. In: Wilson JD, Foster DW, eds. Williams Textbook of Endocrinology, 8th ed. Philadelphia: W.B. Saunders Company, 1992:489–619.

122. Nass R, Baker S, Speiser P, et al. Hormones and handedness: left-hand bias in female congenital adrenal hyperplasia patients. Neurology 1987; 37(4): 711–715.

123. Kelso WM, Nicholls ME, Warne GL. Effects of prenatal and rogen exposure on cerebral lateralization in patients with congenital adrenal hyperplasia (CAH). Brain Cogn 1999; 40:153–156.

124. Helleday J, Siwers B, Ritzen EM, et al. Normal lateralization for handedness and ear advantage in a verbal dichotic listening task in women with congenital adrenal hyperplasia (CAH). Neuropsychologia 1994; 32(7):875–880.

125. Sinforiani E, Livieri C, Mauri M, et al. Cognitive and neuroradiological findings in congenital adrenal hyperplasia. Psychoneuroendocrinology 1994; 19(1): 55–64.

126. Nass R, Heier L, Moshang T, et al. Magnetic resonance imaging in the congenital adrenal hyperplasia population: increased frequency of white-matter abnormalities and temporal lobe atrophy. J Child Neurol 1997; 12(3):181–186.

127. Plante E, Boliek C, Binkiewicz A, et al. Elevated androgen, brain development and language/learning disabilities in children with congenital adrenal hyperplasia. Dev Med Child Neurol 1996; 38(5):423–437.

128. Dittmann RW, Kappes MH, Kappes ME. Cognitive functioning in female patients with 21-hydroxylase deficiency. Eur Child Adolesc Psychiatry 1993; 2:34–43.

129. Nass R, Baker S. Androgen effects on cognition: congenital adrenal hyperplasia. Psychoneuroendocrinology 1991; 16(1–3):189–201.

130. Nass R, Baker S. Learning disabilities in children with congenital adrenal hyperplasia. J Child Neurol 1991; 6(4):306–312.

131. Berenbaum SA, Korman K, Leveroni C. Early hormones and sex differences in cognitive abilities. Learn Individ Dif 1995; 7:303–321.

132. Helleday J, Bartfai A, Ritzen EM, et al. General intelligence and cognitive profile in women with con-

genital adrenal hyperplasia (CAH). Psychoneuroen docrinology 1994; 19(4):343–356.

133. Resnick SM, Berenbaum SA, Gottesman II, et al. Early hormonal influences on cognitive functioning in congenital adrenal hyperplasia. Dev Psychol 1986; 22(2):191–198.

134. Kelso WM, Nicholls ME, Warne GL, et al. Cerebral lateralization and cognitive functioning in patients with congenital adrenal hyperplasia. Neuropsychology 2000; 14(3):370–378.

135. Hampson E, Rovet JF, Altmann D. Spatial reasoning in children with congenital adrenal hyperplasia due to 21-hydroxylase deficiency. Dev Neuropsychol 1998; 14:299–320.

136. Berenbaum SA, Resnick SM. Early androgen effects on aggression in children and adults with congenital adrenal hyperplasia. Psychoneuroendocrinology 1997; 22(7):505–515.

137. Berenbaum SA, Snyder E. Early hormonal influences on childhood sex-typed activity and playmate preferences: Implications for the development of sexual orientation. Dev Psychol 1995; 31:31–42.

138. Dittmann RW, Kappes MH, Kappes ME, et al. Congenital adrenal hyperplasia. II. Gender-related behavior and attitudes in female salt-wasting and simple-virilizing patients. Psychoneuroendocrinology 1990; 15(5–6):421–434.

139. Dittmann RW, Kappes MH, Kappes ME, et al. Congenital adrenal hyperplasia: I. Gender-related behavior and attitudes in female patients and sisters. Psychoneuroendocrinology 1990; 15(5–6): 401–420.

140. Berenbaum SA, Hines M. Early androgens are related to childhood sex-typed toy preferences. Psychol Sci 1992; 3:203–206.

141. Hines M, Kaufman FR. Androgen and the development of human sex-typical behavior: rough-and-tumble play and sex of preferred playmates in children with congenital adrenal hyperplasia (CAH). Child Dev 1994; 65:1042–1053.

142. Zucker KJ, Bradley SJ, Oliver G, et al. Psychosexual development of women with congenital adrenal hyperplasia. Horm and Behav 1996; 30(4):300–318.

143. Dittmann RW. Sexual behavior in adolescent and adult females with congenital adrenal hyperplasia. Psychoneuroendocrinology 1991; 17(2–3):153–170.

144. Oliveira LM, Seminara SB, Beranova M, et al. The importance of autosomal genes in Kallmann syndrome: genotype-phenotype correlations and neuroendocrine characteristics. J Clin Endocrinol Metab 2001; 86(4): 1532–1538.

145. Vogl TJ, Stemmler J, Heye B, et al. Kallman syndrome versus idiopathic hypogonadotropic hypogonadism at MR imaging. Radiology 1994; 191(1):53–57.

146. Beranova M, Oliveira LM, Bedecarrats GY, et al. Prevalence, phenotypic spectrum, and modes of inheritance of gonadotropin-releasing hormone receptor mutations in idiopathic hypogonadotropic hypogonadism. J Clin Endocrinol Metab 2001; 86(4): 1580–1588.

147. Schwankhaus JD, Currie J, Jaffe M, et al. Neurologic findings in men with isolated hypogonadotropic hypogonadism. Neurology 1989; 39(2 Pt 1):223–226.

148. Quinton R, Duke VM, de Zoysa PA, et al. The neuroradiology of Kallmann's syndrome: a genotypic and phenotypic analysis. J Clin Endocrinol Metab 1996; 81(8):3010–3017.

149. Hier DB, Crowley WF Jr. Spatial ability in androgen-deficient men. N Engl J Med 1982; 306(20):1202–1205.

150. Buchsbaum MS, Henkin RI. Perceptual abnormalities in patients with chromatin negative gonadal dysgenesis and hypogonadotropic hypogonadism. Int J Neurosci 1980; 11(3):201–209.

151. Cappa SF, Guariglia C, Papagno C, et al. Patterns of lateralization and performance levels for verbal and spatial tasks in congenital androgen deficiency. Behav Brain Res 1988; 31(2):177–183.

152. Kertzman C, Robinson DL, Sherins RJ, et al. Abnormalities in visual spatial attention in men with mirror movements associated with isolated hypogonadotropic hypogonadism. Neurology 1990; 40(7):1057–1063.

153. Alexander GM, Swerdloff RS, Wang C, et al. Androgen-behavior correlations in hypogonadal men and eugonadal men. II. Cognitive abilities. Horm Behav 1998; 33(2):85–94.

154. O'Connor DB, Archer J, Hair WM, et al. Activational effects of testosterone on cognitive function in men. Neuropsychologia 2001; 39(13):1385–1394.

155. Amory JK, Anawalt BD, Paulsen CA, et al. Klinefelter's syndrome. Lancet 2000; 356(9226):333–335.

156. Smyth CM. Diagnosis and treatment of Klinefelter syndrome. Hosp Pract (Off Ed) 1999; 34(10):111–112, 115–116, 119–120.

157. Smyth CM, Bremner WJ. Klinefelter syndrome. Arch Intern Med 1998; 158:1309–1314.

158. Ratcliffe S. Long-term outcome in children of sex chromosome abnormalities. Arch Dis Child 1999; 80(2): 192–195.

159. Money J. Specific neuro-cognitive impairments associated with Turner (45,X) and Klinefelter (47,XXY) syndromes: a review. Soc Biol 1993; 40(1–2):147–151.

160. Mandoki MW, Sumner GS, Hoffman RP, et al. A review of Klinefelter's syndrome in children and adolescents. J Am Acad Child Adolesc Psychiatry 1991; 30(2):167–172.

161. Walzer S, Bashir AS, Silbert AR. Cognitive and behavioral factors in the learning disabilities of 47,XXY and 47,XYY boys. Birth Defects Orig Artic Ser 1990; 26(4):45–58.

162. Geschwind DH, Boone KB, Miller BL, et al. Neurobehavioral phenotype of Klinefelter syndrome. Ment Retard Dev Disabil Res Rev 2000; 6(2):107–116.

163. Boone KB, Swerdloff RS, Miller BL, et al. Neuropsychological profiles of adults with Klinefelter

syndrome. J Int Neuropsychol Soc 2001; 7(4): 446–456.

164. Rovet J, Netley C, Keenan M, et al. The psychoeducational profile of boys with Klinefelter syndrome. J Learn Disabil 1996; 29(2):180–196.

165. Nielsen J. Sex chromosome abnormalities in adults (author's transl). (Article in German). Nervenarzt 1977; 48(10):517–527.

166. Sorensen K, Nielsen J, Froland A, et al. Psychiatric examination of all eight adult males with the karyotype 46,XX diagnosed in Denmark till 1976. Acta Psychiatrica Scandinavica 1979; 59(2):153–163.

167. Stuss DT, Levine B, Alexander MP, et al. Wisconsin card sorting test performance in patients with focal frontal and posterior brain damage: effects of lesion location and test structure on separable cognitive processes. Neuropsychologia 2000; 38(4):388–402.

168. Bender BJ, Linden M, Robinson A. Cognitive and academic skills in children with sex chromosome abnormalities. Reading and Writing 1991; 3(3–4): 315–327.

169. Fales CL, Knowlton BJ, Holyoak KJ, et al. Working memory and relational reasoning in Klinefelter syndrome. J Int Neuropsychol Soc 2003; 9(6):839–846.

170. Patwardhan AJ, Eliez S, Bender B, et al. Brain morphology in Klinefelter syndrome: extra X chromosome and testosterone supplementation. Neurology 2000; 54(12):2218–2223.

11

Social and Psychological Influences on Male Reproductive Function

William Marsiglio and Ramon Hinojosa
Department of Sociology, University of Florida, Gainesville, Florida, U.S.A.

□ INTRODUCTION

The ability of men to produce viable sperm and achieve biological paternity through intercourse is fundamentally linked to physiological processes associated with puberty and the proper functioning of the sexual and reproductive systems. As persons capable of creating human life, however, men are also influenced by various social, cultural, and psychological factors. Moreover, relatively recent advancements in reproductive technology have radically altered the landscape for infertile men, as well as for those involved with infertile partners. This technology, and the organizations that have been created to employ it, accentuate distinctions between and debates about the relative significance of biological paternity and social fatherhood. Not surprisingly, the procreative realm has become increasingly complex (1).

A broad analysis of male fertility considers how men's procreative lives are intertwined with life experiences embedded in a multilayered, socially constructed world. This type of approach also reveals how the gendered nature of reproductive physiology shapes several aspects of men's procreative experience including their ability to report their fertility experiences accurately, the connection between their sexual and reproductive functioning, their level of control over the gestation process, and possible options for receiving infertility treatments.

Men's intrapsychic experiences represent the most immediate or personal level of this multilayered world. Although it is technically not necessary for men to procreate, the cognitive and emotional dimensions to men's lives as procreative beings shape their decisions relevant to the procreative realm. The awareness of and reaction to the ability or inability to procreate is expressed at this intimate level. Research has shown that the process of becoming aware of one's ability to procreate is largely an unremarkable experience for many young men, but it is highly significant for some (2). Once young men become aware that they presumably can procreate—usually between the ages of 12 and 15—they tend to take this knowledge for granted. Ironically, a relatively small proportion of young

men procreate prior to becoming fully aware of their capacity to do so, and some adult men procreate even though they had assumed they were sterile. Thus, men's perceptions about their fecundity, though important and potentially consequential, may or may not reflect objective, physiological reality.

Men's conscious fertility desires and intentions are expressed within this intrapsychic world as men contemplate their immediate and long-term life goals. Although unconscious phenomena conceivably may be relevant to this intrapsychic domain, theorists tend to distinguish between conscious and unconscious "wants," "desires," or "motivations" (3,4). For most men, this inner world is filtered through their interactions with casual sexual partners, girlfriends, or spouses. The varied nature of these negotiated, interpersonal encounters offers men avenues for thinking about, developing feelings toward, and experiencing their procreative identity and ability in relation to the mother—or potential mother—of their child. Men's awareness of their procreative ability can either be heightened or dampened by their experiences with particular partners. Women's repeated invitations to produce a child most likely sharpen men's attentiveness to their procreative abilities, irrespective of their own desires. Similarly, unsuccessful attempts at reproduction with a partner can lead men to internalize the socially constructed, symbolic meanings they—and perhaps others—associate with their infertility. The likelihood that men will discover their infertility and ponder its personal significance increases when a female partner encourages them to consult a fertility specialist.

The intrapsychic and interpersonal domains are both influenced by cultural forces that represent a third and more illusive layer of social life. For example, the United States' cultural landscape is characterized by pervasive pronatalistic values and norms and guidelines about romantic relationships and family. Adults, particularly those who are married, are encouraged to have children. Although the stigma of voluntary or involuntary childlessness has probably lessened in recent years, and expectations of the ideal number of children have declined (5), the cultural climate reinforces the virtues of adults having and caring for children. Traditional gender ideology plays a role in the United States by accentuating the image that reproducing children can help both men and women fulfill their masculine and feminine desires. Although men are still less likely than women to be bombarded with explicit cultural messages about procreation, they encounter subtle as well as direct messages that they can and should reinforce their adult status as a man by becoming a father and family man. Religious ideologies also continue to promote the idea of men creating families that include children.

Obviously, social support for particular males having children is often contingent on their life course position and personal circumstances. In most circles, males are discouraged from having children if they are either too young, too old, single, homosexual, mentally or emotionally disabled, or poorly prepared to assume the associated financial or care-taking responsibilities. Although financial considerations continue to outweigh care-taking concerns, the potential rise in time and energy demands for fathers stemming from women's increased labor force participation may eventually affect the criteria for evaluating some men's social fitness for fatherhood.

Viewing the three integrated layers (personal fertility beliefs and intentions, negotiations with a partner, and cultural influences) collectively reveals that individuals engage in varying levels of intrapsychic activity by drawing upon the general cultural scenarios that define how certain types of men should think, feel, and express themselves in the procreative realm. These messages, however, are only guidelines at best; men may accept or modify them to varying degrees as they make personal decisions and suggest options for their partner to consider. Thus, the cultural scenarios often provide men with a crude set of borders for constructing their procreative self-image by allowing them to ask and answer questions such as: "Do I want to be a father? Do I want this woman to be the mother of my child? What do I want from the paternal experience?" To the extent that men are influenced at all by cultural guidelines regarding family and procreation, they are likely to modify them to suit their own needs and wishes while interacting with female partners (and gay male companions, too).

Based on this gendered and multilayered conceptual framework, this chapter (*i*) provides a portrait of the social demography of men's fertility attitudes and behaviors, (*ii*) explores selective aspects of the social–psychological context for procreation, and (*iii*) discusses the key social and psychological issues associated with male infertility. Commentary initially focuses on the technological advances altering the context for understanding the relationship between genetic, social, and legal fatherhood (1,6); then, several emerging social and psychological issues that will likely influence men's procreative lives significantly in the future are highlighted.

□ SOCIAL DEMOGRAPHIC PROFILE OF MALE FERTILITY AND INFERTILITY

Summarizing primarily national data using a life stages framework, the Alan Guttmacher Institute's (AGI) 2002 report presents a sociodemographic portrait of the sexual, contraceptive, fertility, marriage/cohabiting, and reproductive health patterns for men aged 15 to 49 in the United States (7,8). This report is supported by more recent unpublished data from the newly released male National Survey of Family Growth (NSFG) conducted in 2002 (9). According to the AGI report, the median ages for men's spermarche, first intercourse, first marriage, and first paternity experience are 14.0, 16.9, 26.7, and 28.5, respectively (7). Table 1 presents NSFG data documenting sexually experienced males' reports of having impregnated someone, irrespective of the outcome of the pregnancy (9). Among the youngest age category of 15- to 19-year-olds, 5.8% acknowledge that they had been told by someone that they had impregnated her, with blacks and Hispanics (11.9% and 11.0%) being more likely to experience this event than whites (3.4%). About 95% of Hispanics aged 40 to 45 have impregnated someone, whereas about 86% and 82% of blacks and whites (respectively) in this age category have done so. Obviously, these figures are likely to be conservative estimates, as some males will be unaware that they have impregnated someone. In addition, some males may have been falsely claimed to be the progenitor (10).

In Table 2, additional NSFG data indicate that 4.8% of males aged 15 to 19 and 79.5% of men aged 40 to 45 report having fathered a biological child (9). Among teenage males, blacks and Hispanics are more likely to have fathered a child (7.7% and 7.8%), compared to non-Hispanic whites (2.8%). Whereas the percentages of black and white men aged 40 to 45 who have fathered a child are relatively close (79.6% and 77.0%), the percentage of Hispanic men in their early 40s who have fathered a child is higher (91.5%). Among men aged 40 to 45 who have had children, 26% have had one child, 33% have had two, 21% have had three, and 19% have had four or more.

Table 1 Percentage of Men Who Have Had Sexual Intercourse and Report Ever Having Impregnated Someone, by Age and Race/Ethnicity (Male National Survey of Family Growth, 2002); Weighted Data

Age (yr)	Total	Blacks	Hispanics	Non-Hispanic whites	Others
15–19	5.8	11.9	11.0	3.4	2.7
20–24	28.1	35.4	44.5	21.7	24.6
25–29	55.4	65.5	69.5	50.4	41.0
30–34	71.3	81.0	79.7	67.7	68.8
35–39	77.6	84.8	83.1	75.4	75.0
40–45	83.9	85.9	95.4	81.6	86.9

Table 2 Percentage of Men Reporting Ever Having a Biological Child by Age and Race/Ethnicity (Male National Survey of Family Growth, 2002); Weighted Data

Age (yr)	Total	Blacks	Hispanics	Non-Hispanic whites	Others
15–19	4.8	7.7	7.8	2.8	3.0
20–24	20.2	29.0	35.7	13.0	17.4
25–29	47.1	52.1	65.2	40.8	39.2
30–34	65.2	73.3	74.7	61.3	63.7
35–39	71.7	79.9	76.8	69.5	69.1
40–45	79.5	79.6	91.5	77.0	86.2

Finally, the AGI reports that about 33% of births to men in their 30s and 40s are unintended (7).

The AGI report (Table 3) also indicates that the men most likely to have had a child by their mid-20s tend to have limited financial resources or have little education (7). Whereas 35% of men (aged 30 to 34 at the time of the interview in the early 1990s) classified as "poor" or "low-income" report having had a child prior to age 25, only 17% of those labeled "better-off" have done so. Similarly, 53% of high-school dropouts and 32% of high-school graduates with no college experience have had a child by age 25, but only 7% of college graduates were fathers by that age. By age 30, 77% of low-income men, 75% of high-school dropouts, 36% of better-off men, and 27% of college graduates have experienced paternity.

Profiling men according to their fertility status is far easier than developing a sociodemographic profile of infertile men because the proportion of men who are infertile but do not seek fertility treatments is unknown. Thus, distinguishing between men who have chosen not to have children intentionally and those who have experienced primary infertility (no paternity during lifetime) or secondary infertility (unable to procreate after having done so in the past) is challenging.

In the United States, approximately 8% (2.4 million) to 15% (5.3 million) of couples including a female is of childbearing age are functionally infertile (11,12). In 30% to 50% of these cases, it is male-factor infertility, and in another 30% to 50% of the cases, it is the female

Table 3 Percentage of Men (Aged 30 to 34 in the Early 1990s) Experiencing Paternity by Age (25 and 30) and Human Capital Measures (Alan Guttmacher Institute Report)

	Financial resources		Education	
	Poor or low-income	Better-off	High-school dropout	High-school graduate
Paternity by age 25	35%	17%	53%	32%
Paternity by age 30	77%	36%	75%	27%

who is infertile. In roughly 5% to 10%, the cause is undetermined or unknown (12–15).

The wide range of estimates reflects the general scholarly consensus on infertility that "true" rates of male and female infertility are difficult to identify. Unfortunately, much of the available data on infertility is based on the white middle-class that seeks fertility treatment (16). Many infertile men, along with their partners, choose not to utilize the services of fertility clinics. About 50% of infertile couples are estimated to not seek fertility treatment (16), in part, because siring a child is not yet an immediate concern. Men in these couples have not yet realized they may be subfecund, so they have no reason to undergo a fertility test. Consequently, no accurate demographic portrait exists for the "typical" infertile male. Some research suggests that non-whites and those with lower incomes are more likely to be infertile; however, these men are also the most likely to not seek fertility treatment, so this population remains virtually unstudied (11,16).

Finally, a subset of men will seek this condition intentionally by opting for a vasectomy. National data from the early 1990s indicated that among all men aged 30 to 34 and 35 to 39 who had had intercourse in the past month, 81% and 84% used some form of contraception. The percentages of men in these two age categories who reported that they relied on a vasectomy were 5% and 20%. Recently published national data from the Male NSFG reveal that 5.8%, 9.6%, and 18.9% of males in the age categories 30 to 34, 35 to 39, and 40 to 45 report having had a vasectomy or other male-sterilizing operation (9). Additional evidence for this pattern is found in women's reports. In 2002, among women using a contraceptive method, male sterilization was used by 9.2%, 14.2%, and 18.4% of the women in the 30 to 34, 35 to 39, and 40 to 44 age categories (17). Women's higher percentages reflects their involvement with older men. The subset of sterilized men may be relevant to medical professionals to the extent that some men may look to have their vasectomy reversed if they change their mind about having (additional) children.

☐ SOCIAL–PSYCHOLOGICAL CONTEXT OF MALE FERTILITY AND INFERTILITY

Male fertility and infertility issues are not solely the intellectual property of medical science. For example, demographers and social psychologists are interested in measuring and studying aspects of men's fertility motivations and experiences. Findings of several national surveys indicate that roughly 92% of the never-married male respondents aged 17 to 25 (surveyed in 1982) and 89% of never-married male respondents aged 15 to 19 (surveyed in 1988) expected to father a child at some point in their life (from the National Longitudinal Survey of Labor Market Experience and National Survey of Adolescent Males, respectively) (1). About 62% of the 2002 male NSFG sample of teenagers indicate they "definitely" intend to have a (another) child, and 36% report "probably." Of those teenagers reporting the number of children they intended to have, 13% indicated one, about 59% said two, and about 20% reported three (9). Another national survey found that 87% of childless married men and 81% of single men intended to have a child at some future point [National Survey of Families and Households (NSFH), 1987 and 1988] (1). One important reason cited is love. Furthermore, although the common assumption is that women are more likely than men to seek a child in an effort to solidify a relationship, research on teenagers reveals that some young men also feel the urge to have a child with someone whom they care about in order to secure their involvement with the person (18).

Studying men's procreative ability using a social–psychological lens allows fertility specialists to understand more fully the interconnection between cultural context, interpersonal issues, and men's reproductive physiology. Previous research highlights the link between socially induced stress (e.g., work or interpersonal) and physiological disruption in erectile ability (14,19,20), which can complicate men's ability to deliver viable sperm to the ovum. While men with erectile dysfunction (ED) represent a relatively small number of cases involving sexual dysfunction and fertility, other research link psychological stress more directly. In a study of 158 males, researchers found stress to be the cause of decreased sperm quality in roughly 44% (21).

To be sure, many texts and articles dealing with male procreative ability address the impact of infertility and infertility treatment on the male psyche (11,14,19–25); however, aside from stating that fertility is an important aspect of male identity (26) and that infertility is psychologically distressful (11,22,23), much of the literature fails to bridge the gap between the social (e.g., expectations of male fecundity), psychological, and physiological experiences of men. For example, explaining why some men (and not others) experience ED under socially induced psychological stress requires an understanding of the intrapsychic processes of identity. The key elements of identity theory will be briefly described in order to bridge the gap between the social and physiological aspects of male fertility.

Identity Theory, Fatherhood, and Masculinity

Sociologists have long assumed that individuals occupy positions in society, or have statuses, that allow them to interact with others in a way that is meaningful to the self and to others (27–29). Statuses are defined by roles, general groupings of behavioral enactments, that allow onlookers to interpret the behavior as being consistent with the status claim being made (28,29). Identities, the internalized social role designations of statuses, are the outcomes of social expectations,

individual agency (individuals choose some identities over others), and cognitive perceptions (how individuals assess an identity's value in constructing the self). In general, identity theory posits that individuals have multiple selves (29), and helps explain how and why social expectations are interpreted and enacted (to varying degrees) by individuals in society.

In a pronatalist society such as the United States, a man is most likely to develop a father identity if he does at least some of the things people expect fathers to do (30); this includes reproductive functioning for the purpose of siring progeny. Identity theory is relevant to understanding male fertility by showing why some men are more likely to be concerned with fecundity issues, more likely to become involved in fertility treatment, and more or less involved in those treatments. Men's fertility treatment decisions often hinge on their perceptions of their own masculine identity and how salient issues of procreation are to them.

Fatherhood represents an important marker of masculine identity, one that symbolizes the male transition into adulthood (1,12,26,31). Our primary interest in fatherhood accentuates how it is tied to male fecundity (procreation requires the production of viable sperm) and masculine identity. Most societies highly value fatherhood, and while being virile is linked to a male's ability to impregnate a woman (26,31), it is also associated with masculinity (1,2,26). Research finds that infertile males or those with some sort of sexual dysfunction tend to report a sense of grief, anger, loss, isolation, foreboding, inadequacy, and the tendency to view the self as unmasculine (12,14,16,26,32,33).

For those whose sexual dysfunction or infertility is due to illness or injury, considerations of identity are especially important. Being able to perform sexually is as important to masculine identity as is able-bodiedness, defined as the lack of disease or physical handicap (34,35). When unexpected medical events such as illness or injury (e.g., cancer or spinal cord injury) are confounding factors in decreased sexual function, males may be especially prone to negative feelings (36,37), particularly when biological fatherhood is a salient issue for them (38). Clinicians have successfully used assisted reproductive technology (ART) to help male cancer patients achieve procreation through cryopreservation of sperm prior to undergoing cancer treatments (39,40). Other techniques to overcome infertility have been used, such as sperm extraction, for those with spinal cord injuries (41,42). Reproductive dysfunction in this population of males, however, needs special consideration due to the complexity surrounding masculine identity, disease, physical handicap, and reproductive capability. Males with salient father identities who find that biological fathering is not an option, because of illness or injury and despite ART, may attempt to reconstruct their identity in other meaningful ways (37,38,43).

A male's "fatherhood readiness" is his subjective sense of how ready he is to take on a father identity and responsibilities (2), and is related to procreative abilities. If a male has a low sense of fatherhood readiness, being infertile may be irrelevant (38). Also relevant is the issue of identity salience—the idea that individuals are more likely to draw on some identities than others (29). A male who is mindful of his current or future father identity is more likely to be concerned with his fertility than a male who is not (44,45). A male may also have a high sense of fatherhood readiness, but not necessarily have a salient father identity. In other words, he may feel he would make a good father, but he is not immediately concerned with becoming one. For this reason, he may not be concerned with his own subfecundity, and would have a diminished desire to seek fertility treatment (38) or stay involved with fertility treatment (11).

A related but separate concept is identity commitment, which describes an individual's investment of time and energy into an identity of personal value. Identity commitment also takes into account the degree to which relationships with others depend on a particular identity (29). It can be expected that a male who has a salient father identity, and is in a relationship contingent upon his procreative future (assuming a father identity), would be more concerned about infertility and more likely to utilize clinical services than a male who does not have a salient father identity or relationships built on a future father identity.

Conversely, a male with a salient masculine identity may attempt to distance himself from a procreative identity if he experiences reproductive dysfunction. Of course, this is feasible as long as his interpersonal relationships do not depend on his procreative ability. If they are contingent upon his procreative identity and he retreats from it, relationship discord may ensue. In practice, couples whose relationships are built upon expectations of sharing future parent identities may encounter difficulties in their relationship when male-factor infertility threatens the ability to realize those identities (23). The relationship may suffer when the man withdraws his involvement in fertility treatments in an effort to avoid what he may view as a threat to his masculine identity. As noted above, some males attempt to reconstruct their masculine identity by committing to identities other than procreative or father identities after numerous unsuccessful attempts at impregnating their partners (12,38). Clinicians should be mindful of these complexities when treating couples for male-factor infertility.

Men's procreative identity (their sense of self as a procreative being) has been greatly affected by new ARTs, including in-vitro fertilization (IVF), microepididymal sperm aspiration (MESA), and direct testicular aspiration [testicular sperm extraction (TESE)]. These technologies make infertility less problematic for men, and may help men overcome the social stigma associated with infertility (26), but again, only those men with salient procreative and father identities are likely to use them (assuming they are able to afford them). Of course, men can experience paternity in ways that do not involve their biological progeny, such as foster parenting or adoption; however, social expectations regarding men's fecundity, men's sense of self, and the interconnection between masculinity and virility (fertility) may lead many men to choose medical paths to paternity over social ones (46).

☐ PSYCHOSOCIAL INFLUENCES ON MALE INFERTILITY

Once young men develop their procreative consciousness during their teen years, most assume they are capable of procreating throughout their lives. In most cases, men's perceptions match their realities. It appears, however, that a growing proportion of adult U.S. men are faced with the stark reality that their ability to procreate is compromised. Some estimate that the proportion of men who are functionally sterile (having sperm counts below 20 million per milliliter of semen) has increased 15-fold since 1938, from one-half of 1% to somewhere between 8% and 12% (47). Evidence suggests that there has been an overall decline in human semen quality over the last 50 years (48–50), but there is no widespread agreement in the academic community and this is still a hotly debated topic (51,52).

The complexity of male infertility goes far beyond the difficulties of estimating the number of men affected as mentioned previously. Male infertility has important and interrelated physiological, social–psychological, and social/cultural dimensions. Fertility is generally thought of as a potential physiological outcome of vaginal intercourse, especially when contraception is not practiced. To be sure, men's opportunities for having a biological child are typically linked to their ability to sustain an erection sufficient for vaginal intercourse. Thus, if men experience some form of sexual dysfunction, whether from psychological distress (21) or illness (37,53), their ability to produce a child biologically related to them is greatly diminished. Similarly, men's chances of producing biological progeny will be adversely affected if they have a high number of impaired sperm parameters (low sperm count, low sperm motility, high sperm morphology, etc.) (54).

Social Class and Male Infertility

Although men's infertility status may be viewed frequently as an individual attribute or as an aspect of a couple's shared experience or identity, sociological factors structure men's experiences as well. For example, social class appears to be a relevant factor affecting the infertility context. One study found that the duration of infertility was six months less for those whose income fell within the upper quartile of family income compared to those with the lowest incomes (55). This difference may reflect affluent couples' ability to pay for the more sophisticated fertility treatments. A more direct link between social class and infertility can be shown by noting that working-class and blue-collar men are more likely to be exposed to occupational hazards such as heat, toxins, and chemicals that are known to decrease sperm counts and increase sperm morphology (56–62). Exposure to hazardous materials on the job affects more than men's ability to procreate. Men who have been exposed to chemicals such as lead and mercury have an increased risk of siring a child with a congenital defect (63). (For further information on this topic, refer to Chapter 21.)

Although impregnating a woman and having children is one visible way for men to demonstrate their masculinity, fulfilling the breadwinner role is another. Ironically, as some men express their masculine identity by fulfilling cultural expectations about the family man as breadwinner, they also place themselves at an increased risk of infertility through exposure to occupational hazards. In other words, the two important routes for working-class males to demonstrate masculine identity are sometimes at odds, as some may be forced to sacrifice one for the other.

Cigarette, Alcohol, and Substance Abuse Behaviors and Male Infertility

A gender lens also highlights how cultural forces affect fertility outcomes for men indirectly by encouraging them to engage in various risk-taking behaviors beyond the work place. Until recently, problems with fertility, childbirth, and child health outcomes have been the province of women/mothers. Males have traditionally escaped the blame for complications with birth outcomes because of how fertility has been socially constructed in practical terms by highlighting women's visible gestation experience over a period of months (15,26,30). Evidence is mounting, however, that men's risk-taking behaviors (e.g., cigarette smoking, alcohol use, and drug use) are linked to infertility and birth outcomes for their offspring.

The masculinity themes captured by the smoking James Dean renegade image of the mid-1900s, the autonomous "Marlboro man," and the blue-collar laborer or military man bonding with their peers while sharing a smoke, have no doubt inspired some boys and men to smoke. Men's quest for this masculine image has compromised the procreative abilities for some. For more than two decades, researchers have identified a link between cigarette smoking and male infertility (64), although the exact relationship remains unclear (65–67). Tobacco smoke is known to have some 4000 chemical compounds, among which are nicotine (and cotinine, its major metabolite), polycyclic aromatic hydrocarbons [benzo(a)pyrene], ammonia, cadmium, and carbon monoxide (68). Cadmium, cotinine, and benzo[a]pyrene are genotoxic, mutagenic, and carcinogenic compounds that are linked with DNA damage in spermatozoa (67–69). Male cigarette smoking is associated with increased sperm-parameter impairment (lowered sperm counts, lowered sperm motility, higher sperm morphology, etc.) and longer time to conception (47,65,66,69). Evidence suggests that cigarette smoking is detrimental to males' procreative ability, although the effects of smoking on men's fecundity are believed to be temporary and reversible (66). The consequences of men's social behavior, however, go beyond their ability to procreate. Paternal smoking is also linked with assisted reproductive complications (70), spontaneous abortion, and childhood diseases—very real consequences for their children's health outcomes (67,69).

Other substances such as marijuana, alcohol, and cocaine are of importance in male sexual reproductive function because males are more likely than females to engage in risky behaviors such as substance use or abuse. Although the magnitude of the effect these substances have on male sexual reproductive function is unclear, it is known that they depress fertility in various ways. Marijuana smoke is linked to depressed sperm counts and abnormal sperm motility in chronic users (71,72). Alcohol is linked indirectly to reproductive function by its adverse effect on the hypothalamus and anterior pituitary glands, and thus the regulatory systems that control sexual function (73). Chronic alcoholism impacts testosterone production and testosterone blood levels, and can lead to testicular atrophy (73). In general, alcohol has little impact unless there is liver damage (42). Cocaine does not directly affect reproductive function or fertility, but can bind to sperm in vitro (74).

Marijuana, alcohol, and cocaine use and/or abuse extend beyond a male's reproductive capabilities by adversely influencing the fetal development of his offspring. Spontaneous abortion, low birth weight, and physical and mental developmental retardation are consequences of men's social behaviors (63,67, 75–78), although the extent to which this is true is unknown (47,69).

☐ PSYCHOSOCIAL IMPACT OF INFERTILITY TREATMENT

As mentioned earlier, medical science has developed several sophisticated procedures such as MESA and TESE that can assist men in overcoming sexual dysfunction and abnormal sperm by retrieving viable sperm to be used later for IVF or intracytoplasmic sperm injection (14). Although these procedures can help individual men overcome the physiological aspects of male infertility; they are costly, so only those with the financial resources to pay for them have access.

In general, females are more likely to initiate the fertility treatment process, and are also much more likely to be involved intimately in it (16,23,54). This may lead clinicians to view men as less interested in the process, and thus, less invested in the fertility treatment outcome. Questions have been raised, however, about the validity of the instruments used to measure women's and men's responses to fertility treatments, as many of these measures are more sensitive to how women experience the fertility treatment process (12,22).

As noted above, paternity is often viewed from a cultural perspective as an important marker of masculine identity (1,26,31). Because most societies highly value paternity, and being virile is linked to being able to procreate, male virility is often associated with masculinity (26). Consequently, males may feel socially stigmatized by their subfecundity and therefore reluctant to undergo fertility treatments. Previous research finds that infertile males tend to have lower self-esteem and exhibit a greater likelihood of mild (nonclinically significant) depression compared to fertile males. As with men experiencing sexual dysfunction, infertile males also tend to report a sense of grief, anger, loss, isolation, foreboding, and inadequacy (12,14,16, 26,32,33). Socially, men are expected to be emotionally reserved in the face of emotional distress (79), and in an effort to minimize that distress, some men withdraw from the treatment process in order to protect their masculine sense of self. That said, men's responses are largely dependent on how salient the father role (and fertility) is to them individually (41).

Donor Insemination

So strong is the desire to avoid the social stigma of infertility that when sophisticated fertility treatments are unsuccessful (or financially unavailable), some men and their partners opt for the products of sperm donation clinics. Donor insemination (DI) became popular shortly after WWII, and since the 1950s, an estimated 1 million children have been born using DI (80,81). Some 30,000 children are born annually from DI, with over 400 sperm banks helping couples overcome male-factor infertility (80). Although DI offers an alternative route to parenthood and allows for a genetic link to at least one parent, it is still shrouded in secrecy to help subfecund men avoid social stigma and shame (80).

DI's popularity has given rise to a commercial industry in which virile semen is commodified, bought, and sold to those willing to pay (82). The commodification of semen brings two important issues to light. First, men recruited to donate sperm may be motivated more by the monetary payment than altruism (81). "The issue of payment as an incentive cannot be separated from the types of men targeted by recruitment methods, and this must be borne in mind when discussing the need for payments" (82). Interestingly, those who donate sperm place themselves in the position of having their fecundity status evaluated, for better or worse. Compared to men who do not donate regularly—especially those who have not yet fathered a child—sperm donors may define themselves in unique ways and be more conscious of their ability to procreate. Second, the recruitment and screening of semen donors means clinicians act as gatekeepers.

In a sense, clinicians control the outcomes of the DI recipient's family because the decision to accept some men as donors and reject others means they control the genetic origins of the resulting offspring (82).

Research on Israeli DI recipients illustrates how societal norms of beauty influence the recruitment of sperm donors and the selection of the sperm sample to be used in the DI procedure. When recipients have a role in the decision-making process, and when physical characteristics of the donor are known, recipients tend to choose semen samples that are congruent with cultural ideals of physical health and beauty (83).

□ FRAMING THE CONTEXT FOR FUTURE RESEARCH

Because the social, demographic, cultural, and technological landscapes of the United States and elsewhere are changing, compelling social science questions related to men's fertility perceptions and behaviors continue to emerge. Several of these developments are highlighted here, and avenues for future research are noted by drawing on the gendered and multilayered framework used to review men's lives within the procreative realm. This perspective accentuates the interrelated nature of the genetic, social, and legal aspects of paternity and social fatherhood.

Evaluating the Impact of Changes in Family Structure

Given recent changes in family demography—most importantly, the growth in stepfamilies—understanding the social–psychological context of fertility decisions made within nontraditional families is becoming increasingly important. Compared to recent cohorts, men today are more likely to form relationships with women who have given birth to another man's child. Thus, scholars and clinicians are faced with unique challenges in studying and working with stepfathers as they consider natural as well as noncoital forms of procreation.

For those men living in stepfamilies who have not yet had biological children, the motivations to have them may be similar to those of first-time fathers in many respects. At the same time, stepfathers with or without biological children may feel that having a child with their partner who is already a mother may help integrate them into and expand their household family. Although little is known about stepfathers' fertility motivations, some qualitative work reveals men's wide-ranging perceptions. Some men report that loving a stepchild satisfies their paternal desires and that they are reluctant to have a biological child because they fear that doing so would limit what they could do with and for their stepchild (84).

An analysis based on two waves of data from the NSFH (1987–1988, 1992–1994) found that spouses think about each other's children when they develop their own fertility intentions. Having a spouse with children influences intentions as much as having children of one's own. For men, a spouse's children are actually more important predictors of intentions (85). Other research using national data shows that men with lower socioeconomic status who become stepfathers gain a "fertility benefit" because their partner is more likely to have a child with them (86).

The presence or absence of men's own children in stepfamily households may be an important factor shaping stepfathers' fertility desires. Some research suggests that stepfathers who also have children of their own, compared to those who do not, "feel more companionship with their stepchildren, experience more intimate stepfather–stepchild interactions, are more involved with their stepchildren's friends, feel fewer negative feelings about stepchildren, and have fewer desires to escape" (18).

In a similar vein, the first author, using national data from 1987 to 1988, found that stepfathers who lived with both stepchildren and biological children compared to their counterparts who only lived with stepchildren were more likely to report perceptions consistent with having a father-like identity (87).

Although issues associated with stepfathers' fertility motivations often involve men who are in a coupled relationship in which fertility is possible through natural means, some stepfathers may confront dilemmas as part of an infertile couple. In some cases, these men will experience a male-factor form of infertility. Irrespective of the infertility source, fertility specialists and support staff should be sensitive to the potentially unique interpersonal dynamics between stepfathers and their partners. Women who have already given birth to another man's child may approach the fertility treatment process and the more general mission to become a social parent differently from those who have never given birth to another man's child. Likewise, stepfathers who have their own biological children from a previous relationship may manage the infertility treatment process differently from nonfathers. Although it does not seem that any study addresses this hypothesis, the authors suspect that stepfathers who have experienced biological fatherhood may be less motivated to pursue/continue fertility treatment while being less supportive of their partner as well. Stepfathers who explore fertility treatment options, however, may be a self-selected, highly motivated sample, as stepfathers with biological children (and the birth mothers with whom they are involved) may be less inclined to seek out the assistance of a fertility specialist in the first place.

As these comments about stepfathers suggest, in contemporary U.S. society, the complexity and fluid nature of relationship formation and family/household structures (88) provide researchers a plethora of opportunities to study the intersection between the social demographic and social–psychological aspects of men's fertility. For example, men increasingly are having children with multiple partners both within and outside of a committed relationship/marriage. In addition, men who forge new romantic relationships after they have fathered a child with someone else often get involved with a woman who is in the twilight of her reproductive years and/or has already given birth. The familial context for fertility decision making in this situation may be quite different from that found among partners in which neither has had a child. Men who have multiple opportunities to develop co-parental roles with different women may tend to have experiences dissimilar to men who restrict their fertility and fathering events to one woman. Researchers need to ask:

- How do men manage their fertility decision-making and fathering in this type of climate?
- How do fertility and parenting experiences with previous partners (both for men and for women) influence men's motivations for future fertility with their current partner?
- How are men's fertility intentions affected when they become stepfathers first, then leave that relationship and face an opportunity to become a biological father with someone else?

Understanding the Impact of Female Partner's Identity and Fertility Goals

In recent decades, it has become increasingly clear that men's lives in the procreative realm are often interconnected with their partners' life experiences and goals, including their growing participation in the work force. Consequently, researchers need to examine more closely how men's fertility desires, intentions, and experiences are related to the types of women they seek to have relationships with, or are in unions with already:

- What types of men are willing to limit or forgo becoming fathers in order to be involved romantically with a particular career-oriented woman?
- How do professional women's decisions to postpone fertility affect men's orientations toward their own procreative desires?
- What types of bargains are negotiated?
- To what extent do men partnered with professional women support their partner or feel disappointed when fertility is postponed or avoided?

Of course, women's increased participation in the labor-force does not directly affect men's physiological capacity to procreate, but women's professional ascendance can influence the social circumstances for men's procreation (89). Being aware of these patterns may enhance the medical professional's chances of addressing men's and couples' therapeutic and reproductive treatment needs in a holistic manner.

Assessing the Impact of New Developments in ART

Technological developments will continue to shape the cultural and social context within which men experience different aspects of the procreative realm. For example, because delayed childbearing has become more prevalent in recent decades, in part due to later ages for first marriages, high rates of relationship and marital dissolution, and strong work-related commitments (90), research questions focusing on men's perception of and involvement with ARTs are timely. As noted earlier, some research has explored men's experiences with ART, but there is much to learn about how men deal with noncoital forms of reproduction. Techniques dependent on donor semen are of particular interest because they potentially raise issues for men about their sense of procreative adequacy, concerns that may be related to or confounded with sexual dysfunction. Research that generates a deeper understanding of men's individual concerns about ART as well as their interactions with their partner can provide fertility specialists and staff useful insights for assisting men and their partners in coping with their stressful attempts to deal with infertility.

Just as modern technology has heightened awareness of the multiple categories of motherhood (ovum, gestation, social legal) (90), the development of DNA fingerprinting technology has fostered efforts to distinguish a man's genetic contribution to paternity from the legal and social dimensions of fatherhood (91). Although relatively few people use this form of testing, the technology's accessibility alters the larger cultural and legal context within which paternity is interpreted and negotiated (92). The technology challenges the simplicity of how paternity typically has been defined in Western countries, prompting a more sensitive approach to the nuances of paternity confirmation (10). On a personal level, a man can now know with certainty if he is a child's genetic father. Even children conceived through ART technologies may be affected if this technology provides them more incentive to identify and verify a sperm donor as being their genetic father.

In the area of contraception, recent advances in surgical techniques for vasectomy (93) that improve this method's reversibility are likely to alter men's experiences (see Chapter 34). Typically, men and their partners have perceived vasectomy to be a permanent form of birth control. As new technologies improve the probability of regaining fecundity (94), vasectomies can provide an alternative temporary birth control strategy. Readily reversible vasectomies will allow men to have sex more freely without the fear of impregnating their partner while being more confident that they can regain their procreative abilities should they choose to pursue that option with their current or future partner.

□ CONCLUSION

As the previous discussion underscores, understanding men as procreative beings in a comprehensive fashion requires that men's lives be interpreted using a gendered and multidisciplinary perspective. Obviously, a wide range of interrelated and emerging conditions associated with culture, social structure, interpersonal relations, psychology, and physiology come into play. Thus, scholarly and clinical approaches that focus on men's desires and abilities/inabilities to create human life must continually consider how social demographic patterns and technological advances can affect men's personal and procreative lives in new ways.

□ REFERENCES

1. Marsiglio W. Procreative Man. New York: New York University Press, 1998:276.
2. Marsiglio W, Hutchinson S. Sex, Men, and Babies: Stories of Awareness and Responsibility. New York: New York University Press, 2002:280.
3. Jacobs MJG. The wish to become a father: how do men decide in favour of parenthood? In: van Dongen MCP, Frinking GAB, Jacobs MJG, eds. Changing Fatherhood: An Interdisciplinary Perspective. Amsterdam: Thesis Publishers, 1995:67–83.
4. Miller WB. Personality traits and developmental experiences as antecedents of childbearing motivation. Demography 1992; 29(2):265–285.
5. Thornton A, Young-DeMarco L. Four decades of trends in attitudes toward family issues in the United States: the 1960s through the 1990s. J Marriage Fam 2001; 63: 1009–1037.
6. Dowd N. Redefining Fatherhood. New York: New York University Press, 2000.
7. Alan Guttmacher Institute. In Their Own Right: Addressing the Sexual and Reproductive Health of American Men. New York: AGI, 2002:88.
8. Bachu A. Fertility of American men. Population Division Working Paper No. 14. Fertility Statistics Branch. Washington, D.C.: U.S. Bureau of the Census, 1996:32.
9. Authors' estimates based on public-use file National Survey of Family Growth. 2002. CD-ROM Series 23, Number 4a. U.S. Department of Health and Human Services, Centers for Disease Control and Prevention, National Center for Health Statistics: Cycle 6. These estimates were generated with the assistance of Melanie Sberna, M.A.
10. Marsiglio W. Qualitative insights for studying male fertility. In: Hofferth S, Casper L, eds. Handbook of Measurement Issues in Family Research. Mahwah, NJ: Lawrence Erlbaum; 2007:303–324.

11. Pasch LA, Christensen A. Couples facing fertility problems. In: Hammer Burns L, Covington SN, eds. Infertility Counseling: A Comprehensive Handbook for Clinicians. New York: CRC Press-Parthenon Publishers Group, 2000:241–267.

12. Webb RE, Daniluk JC. The end of the line: infertile men's experiences of being unable to produce a child. Men Masculinities 1999; 2(1):6–25.

13. De la Rochebrochard E. Sterility and fertility: the role of males. (Article in French). Popul Soc (Paris) 2001; 371:1–4.

14. Elliot S. The relationship between fertility issues and sexual problems in men. Canadian J Hum Sexuality 1998; 7:295–303.

15. Lorber J. In vitro fertilization and gender politics. Women Health 1987; 13(1–2):117–133.

16. Greil AL. Infertility and psychological distress: a critical review of the literature. Soc Sci Med 1997; 45(11): 1679–1704.

17. Mosher WD, Martinez GM, Chandra A, et al. Use of contraception and use of family planning services in the United States, 1982–2002. Advance data from vital and health statistics; no. 350. Hyattsville, Maryland: National Center for Health Statistics, 2004.

18. Sugland BW, Wilder KJ, Chandra A. Sex, pregnancy, and contraception: a report of focus group discussions with adolescents. Washington, D.C.: Child Trends, 1997.

19. Ackerman MD, Carey MP. Psychology's role in the assessment of erectile dysfunction: historical precedents, current knowledge, and methods. J Consult Clin Psychol 1995; 63:862–876.

20. Seidman SN. Exploring the relationship between depression and erectile dysfunction in aging men. J Clin Psychiatry 2002; 63(suppl 5):5–12.

21. Pook M, Rohrle B, Krause W. Individual prognosis for changes in sperm quality on the basis of perceived stress. Psychother Psychosom 1999; 68(2):95–101.

22. Abbey A, Andrews FM, Halman LJ. Gender's role in responses to infertility. Psychol Women Q 1991; 15:295–316.

23. Peterson BD, Newton CR, Rosen KH. Examining congruence between partners' perceived infertility-related stress and its relationship to marital adjustment and depression in infertile couples. Fam Proc 2003; 42(1): 59–70.

24. Pook M, Krause W, Drescher S. Distress of infertile males after fertility workup: a longitudinal study. J Pscyhosom Res 2002; 53(6):1147–1152.

25. Rosen RC, Leiblum SR. Treatment of sexual disorders in the 1990s: an integrated approach. J Consult Clin Psych 1995; 63(6):877–890.

26. Inhorn M. Sexuality, masculinity, and infertility in Egypt: potent troubles in the marital and medical encounters. J Men Stud 2002; 10:343–359.

27. Mead GH. Mind, Self, and Society from the Standpoint of a Social Behaviorist. Chicago: University of Chicago Press, 1934:401.

28. Goffman E. The Presentation of Self in Everyday Life. New York, NY: Doubleday Anchor, 1959:259.

29. Stryker S. Symbolic Interactionism: A Social Structural Version. Menlo Park: Benjamin/Cummings, 1980:161.

30. Larossa R. The Modernization Of Fatherhood: A Social and Political History. Chicago: University of Chicago Press, 1997:287.

31. Dudgeon MR, Inhorn MC. Gender, masculinity, and reproduction: anthropological perspectives. Int J Men's Health 2003; 2(1):31–56.

32. Morawski JG. Imaginings of parenthood: artificial insemination, experts, gender relations, and paternity. In: de Rivera J, Sarbin TR, eds. Believed-In Imaginings: The Narrative Construction of Reality. Washington D. C.: American Psychological Association, 1998:229–246.

33. Potts A. The essence of the hard on; hegemonic masculinity and the cultural construction of erectile dysfunction. Men Masculinities 2000; 3(1):85–103.

34. Gerschick TJ, Miller AS. Coming to terms: masculinity and physical disability. In: Kimmel M, Messner M, eds. Men's Lives. 5th ed. Boston: Allyn and Bacon, 2001:313–326.

35. Kimmel M. Manhood in America: A Cultural History. New York: The Free Press, 1996:544.

36. Herer E, Holzapfel S. The medical causes of infertility and their effects on sexuality. Canadian J Hum Sexual 1993; 2:113–120.

37. Tan G, Waldman K, Bostick R. Psychosocial issues, sexuality, and cancer. Sex Disabil 2002; 20:297–318.

38. Green D, Galvin H, Horne B. The psycho-social impact of infertility on young male cancer survivors: a qualitative investigation. Psychooncology 2003; 12(2): 141–152.

39. Khalifa E, Oehninger S, Acosta AA, et al. Successful fertilization and pregnancy outcome in in-vitro fertilization using cryopreserved/thawed spermatozoa from patients with malignant diseases. Hum Reprod 1992; 7(1):105–108.

40. Lass A, Akagbosu F, Brinsden P. Sperm banking and assisted reproduction treatment for couples following cancer treatment of the male partner. Hum Reprod Update 2001; 7(4):370–377.

41. Heruti RJ, Katz H, Menashe Y, et al. Treatment of male infertility due to spinal cord injury using rectal probe electroejaculation: the Israeli experience. Spinal Cord 2001; 39(3):168–175.

42. Taylor Z, Molloy D, Hill V, et al. Contribution of the assisted reproductive technologies to fertility in males suffering spinal cord injury. Aust N Z J Obstet Gynaecol 1999; 39:84–87.

43. Exley C, Letherby G. Managing a disrupted lifecourse: issues of identity and emotion work. Health 2001; 5(1):112–132.

44. Miller WB, Pasta DJ. Behavioral intentions: which ones predict fertility behavior in married couples? J App Soc Psych 1995; 25(6):530–555.

45. Schoen R, Astone NM, Kim YJ, et al. Do fertility intentions affect fertility behavior? J Marr Fam 1999; 61(3):790–799.

46. van Balen F, Verdurmen J, Ketting E. Choices and motivations of infertile couples. Patient Educ Couns 1997; 31(1):19–27.

47. Environmental Causes of Infertility. http://www.chem-tox.com/infertility. 2003.

48. Carlsen E, Giwercman A, Keiding N, et al. Evidence for decreasing quality of semen during past 50 years. BMJ 1992; 305:609–613.

49. Swan SH, Elkin EP, Fenster L. Have sperm densities declined? A reanalysis of global trend data. Environ Health Perspect 1997; 105(11):1228–1232.

50. Jensen TK, Carlsen E, Jorgensen N, et al. Poor semen quality may contribute to recent decline in fertility rates. Hum Reprod 2002; 17(6):1437–1440.

51. Hauser R, Altshul L, Chen Z, et al. Environmental organochlorines and semen quality: results of a pilot study. Environ Health Perspect 2002; 110(3):229–233.

52. Becker S, Berhane K. Re "Have sperm densities declined? A reanalysis of global trend data." Environ Health Perspect 1998; 106(9):A420–A421.

53. Kao J, Mantz C, Garofalo M, et al. Treatment-related sexual dysfunction in male nonprostate pelvic malignancies. Sex Disabil 2003; 21:3–20.

54. Pook M, Rohrle B, Tuschen-Caffier B, et al. Why do infertile males use psychological couple counselling? Patient Educ Couns 2001; 42(3):239–245.

55. Collins JA, Burrows EA, Willan AR. Occupation and the clinical characteristics of infertile couples. Can J Public Health 1994; 85(1):28–32.

56. Apostoli P, Porru S, Bisanti L. Critical aspects of male fertility in the assessment of exposure to lead. Scand J Work Environ Health 1999; 25(suppl 1):40–43.

57. Figa-Talamanca I, Traina ME, Urbani E. Occupational exposures to metals, solvents and pesticides: recent evidence on male reproductive effects and biological markers. Occup Med (Lond) 2001; 51(3):174–188.

58. De Rosa M, Zarrilli S, Paesano L, et al. Traffic pollutants affect fertility in men. Hum Reprod 2003; 18(5): 1055–1061.

59. Figa-Talamanca I, Cini C, Varricchio GC, et al. Effects of prolonged autovehicle driving on male reproductive function: a study among taxi drivers. Am J Ind Med 1996; 30(6):750–758.

60. Fredricsson B, Moller L, Pousette A, et al. Human sperm motility is affected by plasticizers and diesel particulate extracts. Pharmacol Toxicol 1993; 72(2):128–133.

61. Sheiner EK, Sheiner E, Hammel RD, et al. Effect of occupational exposures on male fertility: literature review. Ind Health 2003; 41(2):55–62.

62. Tielemans E, Burdorf A, te Velde ER, et al. Occupationally related exposures and reduced semen quality: a case-control study. Fertil Steril 1999; 71(4):690–696.

63. Daniels CR. Between fathers and fetuses: the social construction of male reproduction and politics of fetal harm. SIGNS: J Women Cult Soc 1997; 22:579–616.

64. Osser S, Liedholm P, Ransam J. Depressed semen quality: a study over two decades. Arch Androl 1984; 12(1):113–116.

65. Kunzle R, Mueller MD, Hanggi W, et al. Semen quality of male smokers and nonsmokers in infertile couples. Fertil Steril 2003; 79(2):287–291.

66. Wong WY, Thomas CM, Merkus HM, et al. Cigarette smoking and the risk of male factor subfertility: minor association between cotinine in seminal plasma and semen morphology. Fertil Steril 2000; 74(5): 930–935.

67. Robbins W, Vine M, Truong KY, et al. Uses of fluorescence in situ hybridization (FISH) to assess effects of smoking, caffeine, and alcohol on aneuploidy load in sperm of healthy men. Environ Mol Mutagen 1997; 30:175–183.

68. International Agency for Research on Cancer. Tobacco smoking. IARC Monogr Eval Carcinog Risk Chem Hum 1986; 38:47–81.

69. Vine MF, Setzer RW Jr, Everson RB, et al. Human sperm morphometry and smoking, caffeine, and alcohol consumption. Reprod Toxicol 1997; 11(2–3):179–184.

70. Zitzmann M, Rolf C, Nordhoff V, et al. Male smokers have a decreased success rate for in vitro fertilization and intracytoplasmic sperm injection. Fertil Steril 2003; 79(suppl 3):1550–1554.

71. Ehrenkranz JR, Hembree WC. Effects of marijuana on reproductive function. Psychiatr Ann 1986; 16: 243–248.

72. Pardo G, Legua J, Remohi V, et al. Review and update: marijuana and reproduction. (Article in Spanish). Acta Ginecol (Madr) 1985; 42(7):420–429.

73. Emanuele MA, Emanuele NV. Alcohol's effects on male reproduction. Alcohol Health Res World 1998; 22:195–201.

74. Yazigi RA, Odem RR, Polakoski KL. Demonstration of specific binding of cocaine to human spermatozoa. JAMA 1991; 266(14):1956–1959.

75. Asch RH, Smith CG. Effects of delta 9-THC, the principal psychoactive component of marijuana, during pregnancy in the rhesus monkey. J Reprod Med 1986; 31(12):1071–1081.

76. Klonoff-Cohen H, Lam-Kruglick P, Gonzalez C. Effects of maternal and paternal alcohol consumption of the success rates of in vitro fertilization and gamete intrafallopian transfer. Fertil Steril 2003; 79(2):330–339.

77. Schuel H, Burkman LJ, Lippes J, et al. N-acylethanolamines in human reproductive fluids. Chem Phys Lipids 2002; 121(1–2):211–227.

78. Smith CG, Asch RH. Drug abuse and reproduction. Fertil Steril 1987; 48(3):355–373.

79. Kaufman M. The construction of masculinity and the triad of men's violence. In: Kimmel M, Messner M, eds. Men's Lives. 5th ed. Boston: Allyn and Bacon, 2001:4–16.

80. Zolbrod AP, Covington SN. Recipient counseling for donor insemination. In: Schmaling KB and Goldman Sher T, eds. The Psychology of Couples and Illness: Theory, Research, & Practice. Washington, D.C.: American Psychological Association, 2000: 325–343.

81. Emond M, Scheib JE. Why not donate sperm? A study of potential donors. Evol Hum Behav 1998; 19(5): 313–319.

82. Daniels KR, Lewis GM. Donor insemination: the gifting and selling of semen. Soc Sci Med 1996; 42(11): 1152–1536.

83. Birenbaum-Carmeli D, Carmeli YS, Madjar Y, et al. Hegemony and homogeneity: donor choices of Israeli recipients of donor insemination. J Mater Cult 2002; 7(1):73–95.

84. Marsiglio W. Stepdads: Stories of Love, Hope, and Repair. Lanham, MD: Rowman & Littlefield, 2004.

85. Stewart SD. The effect of stepchildren on childbearing intentions and births. Demography 2002; 39(1): 181–197.

86. Anderson KG. The life histories of American stepfathers in evolutionary perspective. Hum Nature 2000; 11(4):307–333.

87. Marsiglio W. Stepfathers with minor children living at home: Parenting perceptions and relationship quality. In: Marsiglio W, ed. Fatherhood: Contemporary Theory, Research, and Social Policy. Thousand Oaks, CA: Sage, 1995:211–229.

88. Cherlin A. Recent changes in American fertility, marriage, and divorce. Ann Am Acad Soc Sci 1990; 510:145–154.

89. Hewlett SA. Creating a Life: Professional Women and the Quest for Children. New York: Miramax Books, 2002:334.

90. Rothman BK. Recreating Motherhood: Ideology and Technology in a Patriarchal Society. New York: Norton, 1989:282.

91. Howe RAW. Legal rights and obligations: an uneven evolution. In: Lerman RI, Ooms TJ, eds. Young Unwed Fathers: Changing Roles and Emerging Policies. Philadelphia: Temple University Press, 1993:141–169.

92. Hubin DC. Daddy dilemmas: untangling the puzzles of paternity. Cornell J Law Public Policy 2003; 13(1): 29–80.

93. Waites GM. Male fertility regulation: the challenges for the year 2000. Br Med Bull 1993; 49(1):210–221.

Part II

Pathophysiology of Male Reproductive Dysfunction

Infertility is defined as a couple's inability to achieve pregnancy following one year of appropriately timed and unprotected intercourse. "Male-factor infertility" is a general term that describes couples in whom an inability to conceive is associated with a problem identified in the male partner, which may be classified into the following etiologies: low sperm production (oligospermia), poor sperm motility (asthenospermia), abnormal sperm morphology (teratospermia), and a combination thereof (oligoasthenoteratozoospermia). Male-factor infertility also describes men who may have normal sperm production, but also exhibit conditions that prevent sperm transport to the vagina during intercourse (e.g., reproductive tract obstruction or ejaculatory dysfunction). Although the fact of male reproductive dysfunction assumes that the male patient in question is of mature, reproductive age, it must be remembered that developmental disorders such as cryptorchidism, testicular torsion, constitutional delay of growth and puberty, hypogonadotropic hypogonadism for any number of reasons, genetic defects such as Klinefelter's syndrome or sickle-cell anemia, and congenital defects such as bilateral absence of the vas deferens, may affect the future fertility of an individual even prior to his own birth. Similarly, events that may have occurred during past sexually active years, such as a remote history of genital infection, and chronic environmental issues such as exposure to hazardous materials or malnutrition, should not be discounted. A current medical history of concomitant systemic disease, such as diabetes or cardiovascular problems, may also be significant contributing factors to infertility. The chapters in Part II of this volume describe each of these conditions in detail.

Male Hypogonadism

Ronald S. Swerdloff

Division of Endocrinology and Metabolism, Harbor-UCLA Medical Center, Torrance, California and Department of Medicine, David Geffen School of Medicine, University of California, Los Angeles, California, U.S.A.

Christina Wang

General Clinical Research Center, Harbor-UCLA Medical Center, Torrance, California and Department of Medicine, David Geffen School of Medicine, University of California, Los Angeles, California, U.S.A.

□ INTRODUCTION

Hypogonadism refers to a deficiency in androgen secretion and/or sperm production. Most androgen-deficient patients are infertile, while most infertile patients have serum testosterone levels within the normal range. Defects of steroid secretion by the Leydig cell may be either primary or secondary. The clinician must be able to distinguish one condition from the other in order to plan appropriate treatment, and the basic scientist focusing on andrology should understand the clinical implications of dysregulation of the reproductive axis.

Patients with androgen undersecretion are traditionally classified as having either primary testicular dysfunction or a hypothalamic–pituitary disorder; however, combinations of the two may occur during aging, or as in hepatic cirrhosis, type 2 diabetes, and sickle-cell disease, and many other chronic diseases (Table 1). A decreased-androgen effect mimicking true hypogonadism may be seen in patients with androgen receptor (AR) abnormalities, postreceptor signaling abnormalities, and failure to convert testosterone to dihydrotestosterone (DHT) (5α-reductase deficiency). The most useful laboratory tests in the management of a patient with hypogonadism are the measurement of plasma follicle-stimulating hormone (FSH), luteinizing hormone (LH), and testosterone concentrations (Fig. 1). If these hormone measurements are borderline and the patient has clinical symptoms or signs of hypogonadism, the free or bioavailable testosterone can be measured to diagnose hypogonadism in patients with low free testosterone and elevated sex hormone-binding globulin (SHBG), as in the case of elderly men.

With the basal concentrations of FSH, LH, and testosterone, a clinician can usually determine the anatomical level of the reproductive disorder (1,2). Low concentrations of testosterone, FSH, and LH are indicative of hypogonadotropic hypogonadism (HH); prepubertal onset is usually indicative of a congenital defect, pituitary or hypothalamic neoplasm, or inflammatory disorder. Prolactin concentrations should be checked to identify patients with hyperprolactinemia.

Anterior pituitary hormone function should be assessed and a magnetic resonance imaging (MRI) scan performed to exclude hypothalamic–pituitary mass lesions. Elevated FSH and LH concentrations in the presence of low testosterone indicate primary pantesticular failure. A karyotype could be performed to exclude Klinefelter's syndrome (KS). Isolated elevations of FSH in the presence of normal LH and testosterone indicate isolated germinal epithelium damage as is commonly seen in azoospermic infertile men. Elevated LH concentrations in the presence of elevated testosterone and estradiol levels suggest androgen resistance; genital skin fibroblast studies or gene analysis will define the abnormality of the AR.

□ TYPES
Primary Gonadal Failure

Primary hypogonadism is a more frequent cause of low serum testosterone in younger men than hypothalamic–pituitary disease. The list of specific etiological causes is long (Table 1) but often definable by careful history, physical examination, and laboratory tests.

Klinefelter's Syndrome

This most common form of congenitally induced primary male hypogonadism (500–1000 male births) was described by Klinefelter (3) in nine men who had small testes with androgen deficiency, azoospermia, bilateral gynecomastia, and increased urinary gonadotropin excretion. Subsequently, eight of the nine men were shown to be positive for a Barr body, indicating an extra X chromosome.

Klinefelter's males are usually shown to have an XXY karyotype (4). There are several genetic mechanisms that can lead to this karyotype. Most are due to nondisjunction of a maternal or paternal sex chromosome during the first meiotic division (5). Although hypogonadism and infertility are the most common clinical signs that identify this disorder, other nonreproductive defects can also occur. These include

Table 1   Common Causes of Male Hypogonadism

Hypothalamic–pituitary disorders (secondary Leydig cell
  dysfunction)
  Idiopathic GnRH deficiency, Kallmann's syndrome,
    Prader–Willi, Laurence–Moon–Biedl syndromes, multiple
    hypothalamic deficiency, pituitary hypoplasia
  Trauma, postsurgical, postirradiation
  Tumor (adenoma, craniopharyngioma, others)
  Vascular (pituitary infarction, carotid aneurysm)
  Infiltrative (sarcoidosis, histiocytosis, tuberculosis,
    fungal infection, hemochromatosis)
  Systemic illness, malnutrition, anorexia nervosa,
    obesity, diabetes mellitus
  Autoimmune hypophysitis
  Drugs (drug-induced hyperprolactinemia, sex steroids)
Testicular disorders (primary Leydig cell dysfunction)
  Chromosomal (Klinefelter's syndrome and variants, XX male
    gonadal dysgenesis)
  Defects in androgen biosynthesis
  Orchitis (mumps, other viral, HIV, leprosy)
  Autoimmune orchitis
  Cryptorchidism
  Myotonia dystrophica
Toxins (alcohol, opiates, fungicides, insecticides, heavy metals,
  cotton seed oil)
Drugs (cytotoxic drugs, ketoconazole, cimetidine, spironolactone)
Systemic illness (uremia, liver failure)
End-organ disorder (impaired androgen action)
Androgen receptor defects
Postreceptor transduction abnormalities
5α-Reductase deficiency

cognitive disabilities, behavioral dysfunction, abnormalities of tooth structure, and atypical findings of relatively longer lower extremities when compared to upper extremities.

The phenotypic manifestations of KS are most classical in men with a 47, XXY karyotype. Some men with the clinical picture of KS have a mosaic pattern where some of the cells are XXY and others are normal XY. In other, less common situations, greater supernumerary X chromosomes may occur, producing a spectrum of XXY, XXXY, and mosaics of these two variants.

Diagnosis of KS prior to puberty is often difficult, although learning disabilities, attention deficits, and behavioral dysfunction may raise a suspicion of KS in early life. The testes are usually small in the neonatal period, failing to increase in size at puberty and remaining less than 1.5 mL in volume (6,7) due to absence of germ cells in the seminiferous tubules. Interestingly, the few testicular biopsies available from prepubertal KS patients show either normal or minimal evidence of germ-cell loss (8–10). LH and FSH levels tend to be normal prior to puberty but rise above the normal range at the age of physiologic pubertal increases in reproductive hormones. Gynecomastia occurs in varying degrees during the postpubertal period, probably due to a relative increase in estradiol secretion from the hyperstimulated testes and decreased ratios of

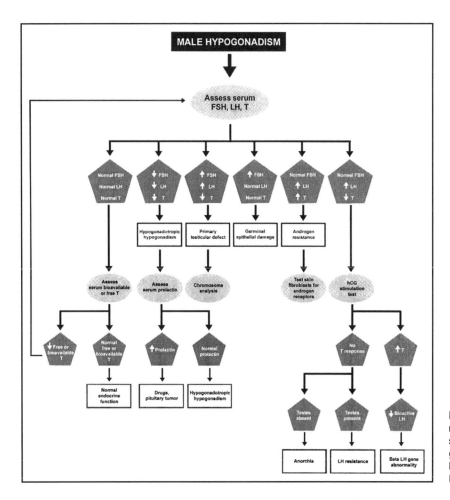

Figure 1   Diagnostic approach to a patient with male hypogonadism. *Abbreviations*: FSH, follicle-stimulating hormone; HCG, human chorionic gonadotropin; LH, luteinizing hormone; MIF, mullerian inhibiting factor; T, testosterone. *Source*: From Ref. 103.

testosterone to estradiol. In KS, muscle mass may appear to be normal but is usually diminished and strength is decreased. Beard and body hair are reflective of the testosterone levels in the patient. The prostate is prepubertal and does not increase in size until androgen treatment is begun. Taurodontism (enlargement of the molar teeth by extension of the pulp) is said to be present in 40% of KS patients when compared to 1% with the general XY population. Other dental abnormalities including increased caries have been frequently seen in the authors' experience.

Serum testosterone levels are usually low or low-normal (11), with free testosterone levels more predictably decreased due to increased SHBG levels (12,13). In many instances, a temporary state of compensated hypogonadism may be present (elevated serum, LH, and FSH with normal serum testosterone), but testosterone levels fall as the patient ages. Serum LH and FSH levels are uniformly elevated in adult KS patients even when serum testosterone falls within the low-normal range. Azoospermic infertility is the rule in KS, with typical testicular biopsies revealing Leydig cell hyperplasia, loss of germ cells, sclerosis of the germ-cell compartment, and thickened tubular basement membranes (4). Mosaic forms may have some degree of immature germ cells on biopsy, but almost all are azoospermic. The reasons for delayed Leydig cell failure and the relationship of spermatogenic failure to the Leydig cell abnormalities are unknown.

Lowered verbal IQ is commonly reported by age seven (14). The reasons for the cognitive dysfunction in KS are not known, but the selective learning (dyslexia) and behavioral difficulties suggest an integrative disorder of the central nervous system (CNS) reminiscent of other frontal–temporal lobe disorders (15). An autopsy study of dyslexic brains with cognitive phenotypes similar to those seen in KS patients has revealed a loss of the typical leftward asymmetry seen in right-handed control subjects, particularly in the area of the first temporal gyri (16). This finding has been corroborated by functional neuroimaging (17), which showed anomalous cerebrum laterally, and by MRI, which showed significant reduction in the total left temporal gray matter volume in KS adults (18). Despite typical histories of poor school advancement and work habits, many KS patients perform well on global IQ testing, with some scoring in the superior range.

The reasons why extra X chromosomes produce this clinical spectrum of events are unknown, but it may be related to the overexpression of genes that are not susceptible to inactivation in the supernumerary X chromosomes. This possibility seems to be supported by the observation that cognitive–behavioral dysfunctions are increased as the number of X chromosomes increases, for example, XXXY (11). The typical hypogonadal manifestations in patients with KS respond favorably to testosterone replacement, while the cognitive dysfunction seems to be immutable, or, at best, variable in its response. Many parents of adolescents with KS claim improved attention span and behavior after testosterone treatment, while others complain of worsening of these manifestations. (For further information on testosterone treatment, please refer to Chapter 29.) Several mouse models of XXY aneuploidy have been developed (19–21) that show reproductive and cognitive deficits. These models may allow more insight into the molecular basis of the various phenotypic manifestations of KS.

XX Males

This chromosome disorder is much rarer than KS (1:10,000 births) (11). Patients with this karyotype constitution and a male phenotype usually have a Y to X translocation, with a portion of the Y chromosome present on one of the X chromosomes (22). They may have partial defects in external genitalia development (i.e., hypospadias, an abnormal opening at the urethra on the ventral shaft of the penis or perineum), are androgen deficient, have small testes, and are infertile. Unlike KS patients, they tend to have short stature, and taurodontism is not present.

XX/XO individuals are a mixed variant of XX males with gonadal dysgenesis and a spectrum of hermaphroditic characteristics. They differ from XX males in that they have a higher incidence of dysgenetic testes and an increased susceptibility to testicular malignancy (20%).

XYY syndrome is another sex chromosomal disorder resulting from paternal meiotic nondisjunction or mitotic nondisjunction of the fertilized egg. These phenotypic men have decreased to low-normal testosterone levels, elevated gonadotropins, azoospermia with hyalinized seminiferous tubules, and increased height compared to the general male population, with a mean height of six feet four inches. The phenotypic similarities of XYY to XXY men are intriguing, perhaps suggesting overexpression of genes common to both the X and Y chromosomes.

Myotonic Dystrophy

This disorder presents later in life (after age 30), is often passed on from father to son, and is characterized by an inability to relax the striated muscles after recent contraction. It is associated with testicular atrophy, decreased fertility, and hypergonadotropic hypogonadism (23). Brain dysfunction of the frontal–temporal lobes may be present. The relationship of testicular dysfunction to the causative mutation is unknown (23,24).

Diabetes Mellitus and Obesity

Both obesity and diabetes mellitus are risks factors for low testosterone levels (25–31). The degree of suppression seems to correlate with the increase of blood sugar (hemoglobin A1C levels) and the severity of obesity.

Mumps Orchitis, Leprosy, Hematochromatosis, and HIV Disease

Following puberty, mumps will be associated with clinical orchitis in 25% of cases; 60% of men with clinically induced mumps orchitis will become infertile (32). Spermatogenic changes occur more often and earlier than Leydig cell dysfunction. Thus, patients with infertility may have normal testosterone and LH values with increased serum FSH. With increasing time, elevations in LH and lowered serum testosterone levels may appear.

Leprosy also produces orchitis (33), but with an apparent tendency to damage either the Leydig cells or spermatogenic tubules selectively, resulting in monotropic increases of LH or FSH (34). HIV infection is often associated with hypogonadism, which can be either hypogonadotropic or hypergonadotropic in classification. The pathogenesis of hypogonadism in this disorder is complicated since gonadal and hypothalamic infection with the HIV virus, infection by other organisms, stress, malnutrition, and malignancies may all coexist (35–37).

Cryptorchidism

Although the incidence of incomplete or undescended testes at birth is high (10%), most testes will descend to the appropriate scrotal location in early childhood. The incidence of bilateral undescended testes is 0.3% to 0.4% following puberty (38). Undescended testes may occur in many congenital syndromes, resulting in HH (see below) (38,39). Bilateral cryptorchidism is associated with infertility 70% of the time (40). This is believed to be the result of heat-induced damage to the germinal tissues due to the absence of the normal cooling effect of the scrotal site for the testes. Unilateral cryptorchidism is associated with infertility to a lesser degree than bilateral cases. The reason(s) why unilateral cryptorchidism is associated with infertility is unclear; perhaps it reflects preexisting dysgenetic testes. Androgen deficiency (Leydig cell dysfunction) is less common but does occur (41). Cryptorchidism should be treated by bringing the testes into the scrotum in early childhood (before age five), thus decreasing the chances of permanent infertility and the testicular malignancies (8%) associated with abdominal testes.

Autoimmune Testicular Failure

Antibodies against the microsomal fraction of the Leydig cells may occur either as an isolated disorder or as part of a multiglandular disorder involving, to variable degrees, the thyroid, pituitary, adrenals, pancreas, and other organs (42).

Testicular Irradiation, Chemotherapy, and Toxins

Irradiation of the testes due to accidental exposure in the treatment of associated malignant disease will produce testicular damage. A dose as low as 15 rad will cause transient decreases in the sperm count; 50 rad exposure may cause azoospermia. After 500 rad, the infertility is usually irreversible. Doses above 800 rad can produce combined spermatogenic and Leydig cell failure characterized by low serum testosterone levels, oligozoospermia, and elevated serum LH and FSH (34). Chemotherapy for malignant disorders has a high association of irreversible germ-cell damage (24). (For further information on the effects of cancer treatment on fertility, see Chapter 20.)

Toxins may also directly damage the testes. Many agents such as fungicides and insecticides (e.g., 1,2-dibromo-3-chloropropane), heavy metals (lead and cadmium), and cottonseed oil (gossypol) produce damage to the germ cells. Leydig cell function is relatively less susceptible to most chemotherapeutic drugs and toxins than the Sertoli germ cells, with serum testosterone levels usually normal despite infertility in the exposed men. Some medications interfere with testosterone biosynthesis (e.g., ketoconazole and spironolactone), thus producing Leydig cell underproduction of testosterone. (For further information on the impact of environmental factors on male fertility, see Chapter 21.)

Trauma, torsion of the testes, and vascular injury may produce hypogonadism (see Chapter 13). Of interest is the observation that unilateral torsion may be associated with subsequent infertility. Trauma during scrotal surgery can result in vascular insults and panhypogonadism (Leydig cell and germ-cell abnormalities).

Androgen End-Organ Failure

Certain conditions have clinical phenotypes mimicking Leydig cell dysfunction (androgen deficiency) in the absence of lowered testosterone secretion and serum concentrations (43–46). These are usually congenital due to decreased end-organ responsiveness to circulating testosterone. This category includes AR defects, postreceptor signal transduction defects, and 5α-reductase deficiency.

Androgens Receptor Defects

Androgens normally induce their effects either directly on their target organs or after conversion to a 5α-reduced metabolite, DHT. Both androgens bind to the C-terminal portion of an intranuclear AR (member of the steroid receptor family). Subsequently, androgen actions are generated by the transcription of specific genes initiated by the binding of the DNA binding domain of the testosterone (or DHT) AR complex to the androgen response element of the target gene. A number of AR defects have been reported, producing a spectrum of clinical manifestations (described below), from "complete" forms (testicular feminization) to "incomplete" forms (Reifenstein's syndrome) and to "minimal" forms (hypospadias) (47).

In testicular feminization, there is essentially no binding of testosterone and DHT to a mutant AR (48). The patients are phenotypically female, with normal-appearing breasts and external genitalia but have blind vaginal pouches; the absence of the uterus results in amenorrhea. The testes are present in the labial canal or intra-abdominally. Serum testosterone levels are normal to elevated, and serum LH and FSH levels may be elevated due to the lack of normal feedback of testosterone on the hypothalamic–pituitary axis. Breast development and female fat distribution reflects increased estradiol levels and unimpeded estrogen effects (49). The testes should be removed because of increased risk of malignancy, and estrogen replacement therapy will be needed, as these patients should be treated as though they were hypogonadal women (50).

Reifenstein's syndrome is a form of partial androgen resistance (47). The receptor defects appear to be heterogenous, with variable inheritance, including X-linked and autosomal recessive forms. Decreased receptor number, decreased receptor stability, and postreceptor response defects are responsible for the hypogonadal state and varying degrees of defective external genitalia differentiation (including bifid scrotum and hypospadias) due to incomplete midline fusion of the urethra and labial folds. Gynecomastia frequently occurs at puberty when LH, testosterone, and estradiol levels rise. More subtle defects, limited to hypospadias and/or impaired spermatogenesis, have also been described. Despite their pseudohermaphroditism, these patients are phenotypically assigned to the male gender. Treatment of incomplete AR deficiency with testosterone has been only partially successful.

AR polymorphisms involving differences in the length of CAG repeats (CAGn) is inversely associated with androgen action. There is a racial distribution with Asian men having longer CAGn and African–American men having shorter CAGn (51). Studies of phenotype (social and physical defects, genotype) and CAGn showed that XXY men (KS) with longer CAGn had more clinical manifestations of testosterone deficiency and were less responsive to testosterone therapy (52).

5α-Reductase Deficiency

5α-reductase deficiency is a fascinating disorder characterized by diminished levels of the enzyme responsible for conversions of testosterone to DHT (Fig. 2) (53). Since DHT is required in males for the normal development of the external genitalia, including growth of the phallus and prostate, these patients have severe pseudohermaphroditism at birth. Because the defect is incomplete, the patients undergo partial masculinization due to the high levels of testosterone secreted at puberty. At that time, muscle mass increases, body fat decreases, and phallic growth occurs, while the rudimentary prostate and severe hypospadias, small testes, and infertility persist (54). LH, FSH, and testosterone levels are normal in these patients, but the ratio of DHT to testosterone is decidedly low (55). Since the disorder is variable in severity and age at detection, management depends on the gender assignment given. Intra-abdominal testes are usually

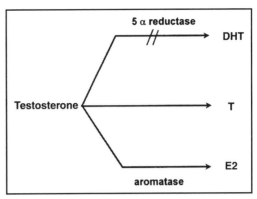

Figure 2 T action is either direct as T or indirect after conversion to DHT by 5α-reductase or to E₂ by aromatase enzyme. In 5α-reductase deficiency DHT levels are low. *Abbreviations*: DHT, dihydrotestosterone; E₂, estradiol; T, testosterone.

removed, and androgen or estrogen treatment will be given depending on the assigned gender management of the hypogonadal genetic male.

Hypogonadotropic Hypogonadism

HH is a deficiency in the secretion of gonadotropins (LH and FSH) due to an intrinsic or functional abnormality in the hypothalamus or pituitary gland. Such disorders result in secondary Leydig cell dysfunction. The clinical manifestations will depend on the age of onset. Since many patients with HH have a congenital deficiency in gonadotropin-releasing hormone (GnRH) secretion, the manifestations include a small phallus, failure to undergo secondary sexual development at the time of puberty, diminished sexual drive (libido), and decreased metabolic effects of testosterone (decreased muscle and bone mass). Acquired loss of gonadotropin secretion such as that occurring after trauma, pituitary tumors, and hypothalamic or pituitary inflammatory disease may present due to the local effects of the CNS disorder (i.e., visual field impairment, hypopituitarism, and headaches) or be clinically indistinguishable from primary gonadal failure. In the latter case, suspicion of a central defect (hypothalamic hypogonadism) comes from the laboratory pattern of low serum testosterone and low or inappropriately normal serum LH and FSH levels. The distinction between central and tubular causes of hypogonadism is important because secondary hypogonadism may imply a progressive and/or specifically treatable disorder; the unintended effect of drugs that inhibit the hypothalamic–pituitary axis, such as tranquilizers, antidepressants and estrogens; systemic illness; and malnutrition, or anorexia nervosa. The infertility associated with HH may be treatable with gonadotropin or GnRH replacement therapy. (For further information on these treatments, see Chapter 29.)

The site of the hypothalamic or pituitary lesion should be localized, if possible, by MRI. A serum prolactin must be measured to exclude the presence of hyperprolactinemia. A single test dose of GnRH (usually 100 µg intravenously) does not distinguish hypothalamic from pituitary disease. A GnRH test preceded by a period of "priming" the pituitary gonadotrophs with repeated low-dose stimulation has been used to diagnose hypothalamic disorders. With prior priming, the GnRH test can demonstrate that low or absent LH responses to a single dose of GnRH in hypothalamic disorders can be augmented to give normal LH levels, whereas priming has no effect in pituitary disorders (56). Difficulty also exists in separating delayed sexual maturation from incomplete HH, because basal LH and FSH levels may be similarly low in both circumstances (57). GnRH testing may be of potential value but is limited by the smaller LH response in normal prepubertal children that can overlap with the response of patients with incomplete HH. Newborns with HH may be identified by measuring the testicular volume sequentially during the first three months of life. Normal children double the testicular volume during this period (58).

Kallmann's Syndrome and Idiopathic HH

A syndrome characterized by delayed or arrested sexual development and anosmia was first described in 1944 (59). All the data available to date point to selective gonadotropin deficiency resulting from an isolated defect in GnRH secretion in this disorder (60–62). Thus, the primary pathogenetic defect in these patients is hypothalamic, and the impaired gonadotropin secretion is secondary to the hypothalamic abnormality (62). The evidence of this disorder is approximately 1 in 10,000 male births (63). Although anosmia and hyposmia are the first described and most well-known associations of this syndrome, a large number of other somatic abnormalities have been recorded (64). The more common associations include color blindness, cleft lip and palate, and cranial nerve defects (including eighth nerve deafness). Horseshoe-shaped kidneys, cryptorchidism, and optic atrophy have also been described. In the molecular pathogenesis of idiopathic HH (IHH), abnormalities of the gonadotropin-releasing hormone receptor (GnRH-R) and associated proteins have explained some of the defects.

GnRH germ-like mutations with associated impaired GnRH binding and ligand-induced signal transduction have been identified (65). Schwanzel-Fukuda and Pfaff (66) have studied the migration of the GnRH neurons in the mouse embryo. These first appear in the epithelium of the olfactory placode in the mouse embryo and then migrate with the olfactory nerves to the forebrain and finally to their ultimate hypothalamic location. Such observations have led to speculation that IHH may be a developmental defect resulting from an abnormal migration of the luteinizing hormone-releasing hormone or GnRH neurons. IHH associated with impaired olfactory function may be caused by mutations of the X chromosomal *Kal 1* gene (encoding anosmia) or the fibroblast growth factor (FGFR1), both leading to agenesis of olfactory ad GnRH secretory neurons (65). Further support for this hypothesis comes from MRI studies that show that olfactory bulbs and sulci are poorly developed in patients with IHH and anosmia/hyposmia (67). Recent studies have demonstrated that familial IHH patients are deficient in the *KAL* gene, which controls the production of an adhesion protein possibly responsible for the co-migration of the olfactory and GnRH neurons.

IHH occurs both in sporadic (nonfamilial) and familial forms, although there are no differences in the clinical presentations of the two subgroups. Earlier studies had suggested that a positive family history is present in about 50% of patients (64,68). In over 120 patients comprehensively studied by Crowley's laboratory (62), however, the majority of cases were sporadic. Hundreds of cases with both an autosomal-dominant and autosomal-recessive mode of inheritance have been described (64,68). Overall, the data are most consistent with an autosomal-dominant inheritance with variable penetrance.

There is significant heterogeneity in the clinical presentation of IHH (69). The phenotype, to a large degree, is determined by the severity of GnRH deficiency. Those with the most severe deficiency may present with complete absence of pubertal development and sexual infantilism. Male patients may have complete absence of secondary sex characteristics, infantile testes, and azoospermia, while female patients have primary amenorrhea. At least 10% of the patients have partial GnRH deficiency and varying degrees of delay in sexual development in proportion to the severity of gonadotropin deficiency (70).

Two variants of IHH (fertile eunuch syndrome and isolated FSH deficiency) are particularly interesting. The term "fertile eunuch syndrome" has been used to describe patients with eunuchoidal proportions and delayed sexual development but with normal-sized testes (71,72). Such individuals appear to have sufficient gonadotropins to stimulate high intratesticular levels to initiate spermatogenesis but not enough testosterone secretion into the blood to adequately virilize the peripheral tissues; they are, in fact, partially gonadotropin deficient. Another variant with predominantly FSH deficiency has also been described (73), although these patients are extremely rare. These men are normally androgenized but have decreased or absent sperm in their ejaculate without concomitant increases in FSH.

The secretory profiles of LH and FSH in men and women with IHH are quite heterogenous in their LH secretory patterns (69). The largest subset comprises patients who display no pulsatile LH secretion at all. This apulsatile group probably represents one extreme characterized by perhaps the most severe GnRH deficiency. A smaller subset displays low-amplitude pulses. Another subset of patient has LH pulses at a markedly reduced frequency. A third subset is characterized by "sleep-entrained" pulses reminiscent of the pattern seen in early stages of puberty. This subset can thus be considered to suffer from a "developmental arrest."

Congenital Syndromes (Non-IHH and Kallmann's)

A number of congenital syndromes have hypogonadotropic hypogonadism as part of the syndrome complex. Most of these syndromes are associated with neurologic damage and mental retardation (34,74). A few of these are described below.

Prader–Willi Syndrome

Prader–Willi syndrome (PWS) has been well described and is a syndrome consisting of obesity, hypotonic musculature, mental retardation, hypogonadism, short stature, and small hands and feet. Hypogonadism, cryptorchidism, and micropenis are common (75). Testicular histology shows that the testis is immature without germinal cells but with Sertoli cells and diminutive tubules (76). The degree of gonadotropin deficiency in these patients is variable (36). A few patients with hypergonadotropic hypogonadism have also been described. Pauli et al. recently described the 15q chromosome in a boy with PWS (77). Subsequent studies have shown that chromosome-15 abnormalities are found in approximately 70% of the patients with PWS (78,79), and maternal disomy of 15 accounts for 25% of cases. The remaining cases result either from genomic imprinting defects (microdeletions or epimutations) of the imprinting center of the 15q11-q13 region or from chromosome 15 translocations. Clomiphene has been shown to "turn on" the pituitary–gonadal axis of individuals of either sex with PWS to secrete gonadotropins and gonadal steroids.

Other Congenital Causes of Secondary Leydig Cell Dysfunction

Laurence–Moon–Biedl (80,81), basal encephalocele, multiple lentigines (82), Rud (74), and cerebellar ataxia (83) are all complex syndromes associated with HH (Table 1).

Acquired Hypogonadotropic Disorders and Functional Disorders

Anorexia nervosa and weight loss are examples of functional defects resulting in low serum testosterone levels. Anorexia nervosa is predominantly a disorder of adolescent girls characterized by excessive weight loss as the result of voluntary dietary restriction (84,85). Occasionally, the disorder is seen in men but usually implies a more severe variant of the psychiatric disorder (86,87). Both women and men may present with the manifestation of HH. Although all investigators agree that anorexia nervosa is associated with profound psychological dysfunction, the nature of the primary pathophysiologic abnormality remains controversial. The anorexic patient is usually born to older, middle- to upper-class Caucasian parents (88) in a

female-dominated family. Typical family values emphasize outward appearance, proper behavior, and achievement more than self-realization and close interpersonal relationships. Poor self-esteem and a sense of ineffectiveness are often described. The onset of illness around the time of puberty suggests that an inability to cope with developing sexuality and a widening social circle plays a role in the pathogenesis of this disorder.

Starvation from other, nonpsychological causes may also reduce gonadotropin secretion (89). Females also seem to be more susceptible to this disorder (90,91).

Strenuous exercise has minimal effects on testicular function in men (92); this contrasts greatly with the well-known phenomenon of dysfunctional reproduction in female long-distance runners and dancers (93–96).

Severe stress and systemic illnesses will also lower gonadotropin and testosterone levels (97,98). Many severe systemic illnesses may result in hypogonadism (24). The pathogenic mechanisms include suppression of the hypothalamic–pituitary secretion of GnRH and LH. Chronic hepatic and renal disease, cancer, and HIV infection are commonly associated with low testosterone levels. Hepatic cirrhosis, sickle-cell disease, hemochromatosis (disorder of iron storage), and severe obesity are disorders in which a combined hypothalamic–pituitary and primary gonadal dysfunction may coexist (34). (For further information on the effects of systemic diseases on fertility, see Chapter 19.)

Organic Hypothalamic–Pituitary Disorders

Neoplastic and nonneoplastic lesions in the region of the hypothalamus and pituitary can directly or indirectly affect gonadotrope function. Lesions involving the hypothalamus may arise in the hypothalamus, suprasellar structures, or within the sella itself and extend upwards.

Pituitary Tumors/Prolactinomas

Prolactinomas present differently in men and women. In women, prolactinomas are common and usually small (microadenomas) when detected because of the symptoms of amenorrhea and galactorrhea. In men, however, these tumors are usually large, being greater than 1 cm in diameter (macroadenomas) at the time of detection. It is unclear whether the large tumor size in the male presentation is due to a late diagnosis caused by the failure of patients and physicians to appreciate the early signs of this disorder or if men experience more rapid growth of these tumors (99–101). The patients usually present with hypogonadism, erectile dysfunction, and manifestations of supersellar mass lesions (Table 2). Visual field cuts are common due to compression of the optic chiasm by the tumor. Hyperprolactinemia is present, with levels above 350 ng/mL being highly diagnostic for a prolactin-secreting tumor. Serum testosterone levels are usually low,

Table 2 Presenting Symptoms in Men with Prolactinomas

Symptoms	Patients (%)
Impotence	75
Visual field d efects	37
Hypopituitarism	35
Headaches	19
Galactorrhea	12

Source: Adapted from Ref. 102.

with low or inappropriately normal serum LH and FSH concentrations (see Fig. 1), and FSH levels are decreased either because of prolactin suppression of GnRH secretion (104) or because of pressure effects on the normal gonadotroph cells. A functional disorder is more common, as evidenced, in many cases, by LH responsiveness to administered GnRH and reversal of both the hypogonadotropic state and Leydig cell dysfunction after the reduction of prolactin with dopamine agonists (102). Patients presenting with large tumors resulting in multiple pituitary hormone deficiencies are more likely to require testosterone or gonadotropin therapy to correct the low testosterone levels. Surgery is not often considered to be a treatment option for this problem.

Nonprolactin-Secreting Tumors

Tumors that secrete growth hormone (GH) present with excess GH levels (acromegaly). GH- and nonsecreting pituitary adenomas are usually large tumors (macroadenomas) with symptoms and signs due to mass effects and acquired HH. Adrenocorticotrophin (ACTH) secretory tumors are usually small, and abnormalities of reproductive function may be associated with cortisol-induced dysfunction of the hypothalamic–pituitary axis.

Glycopeptide secretory adenomas were not appreciated until recently because they tend to be inefficient secretors of hormonal products (TSH, LH, FSH, and their subunits) or because elevated gonadotropins tend not to produce recognizable clinical syndromes. Consequently, these types of adenomas tend to present late as large mass lesions, with visual and other neurologic manifestations. Gonadotroph adenomas often produce increased basal concentrations of FSH but rarely of LH (105). As with other large pituitary tumors, the mass effects can lead to compression of the normal gonadotrophs, decreased LH, and testosterone levels. Occasionally, an elevation of serum LH and Leydig cell dysfunction [lowered testosterone level(s)] may be seen; this is believed to be due to the secretion of a less bioactive form of LH or free α-subunit that is detected in the assay. Elevated LH levels and overstimulation of the Leydig cells with increased testosterone concentrations may also occur. In some cases, the diagnosis of a gonadotroph adenoma can be made by demonstrating paradoxical stimulation of FSH or the LH β-subunit by thyrotropin-releasing hormone (TRH) (106).

☐ CLINICAL MANIFESTATIONS OF HYPOGONADISM
Clinical History and Physical Examination

For general information on the clinical history, physical examination, and laboratory tests involved in a male presenting with infertility, please refer to Chapter 23. Here we review those points specifically relevant to the diagnosis of hypogonadism.

The evaluation of a patient with suspected hypogonadism begins with a detailed and complete history and a physical examination. The medical history should focus on pubertal development, testicular descent, loss of body hair, decrease in shaving frequency, and past and current chronic medical illnesses. In patients presenting with infertility, information should be obtained on previous mumps orchitis, sinopulmonary complaints, sexually transmitted diseases, genitourinary tract infections, and previous surgical procedures such as vasectomy, orchiectomy, and surgery around the vas deferens. Social history should include tobacco and alcohol intake, exposure to toxic chemicals, hot baths and saunas, irradiation, anabolic steroids, cytotoxic chemotherapy, and drugs that may cause hyperprolactinemia. A detailed sexual history should be obtained, including questions on libido, frequency of intercourse, and erectile and ejaculatory functions. In addition, the fertility status of the female partner, and the type and extent of past investigations of the female partner and the patient himself should be ascertained.

The physical examination includes a general medical examination. The clinical manifestation of androgen deficiency depends on the age of onset, with different clinical findings at different ages:

- Early fetal life: ambiguous genitalia (testicular agenesis, androgen biosynthetic defects, or androgen resistance)
- Late fetal development and in the neonate: micropenis
- Adolescence: delayed pubertal development with eunuchoid features
- Adulthood: loss of secondary sex characteristics, decreased sexual function, and infertility

Height, extremity span, and the ratio of upper to lower body segments will determine if a patient is eunuchoidal. Androgen deficiency may lead to increased body fat and decreased muscle mass. Obesity itself will lead to lowered testosterone levels. Loss of pubic, axillary, and facial hair, decreased acne and oiliness of skin, and fine facial wrinkling are features suggestive of low androgen concentrations. Gynecomastia may be present when there is a decreased androgen-to-estrogen ratio. During the physical examination, the stage of development (Tanner's classification) of the gonads and phallus is ascertained. Examination of the scrotum should include palpation of the vas deferens and epididymis and the identification of other scrotal

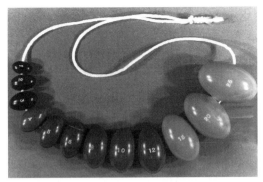

Figure 3 Prader orchidometer for measuring of testicular size.

abnormalities such as varicocele, hydrocele, and hernia. Testis size can be measured by either the Prader or Takihara orchidometers, which consist of a series of plastic ellipsoids with a volume from 1 to 30–35 mL (Fig. 3). A testis volume of less than 15 mL in an adult Caucasian man is regarded as small; testicular size may be slightly less in normal Asian populations. A decreased testis volume usually indicates a decreased mass of the seminiferous tubules since they account for 80% of the mass of normal-sized testes. Alternatively, testis size can be measured by calipers. The length of the testis in eugonadal men ranges between 3.6 and 5.5 cm and the width between 2.1 and 3.2 cm.

Endocrine Tests for Hypogonadism

The laboratory assessment of a patient with suspected hypogonadism includes measurements of the serum concentrations of FSH, LH, and testosterone. In most circumstances, this will be adequate to confirm whether the patient has androgen deficiency, and if so, whether the problem lies in the testes or in the hypothalamic–pituitary areas. In some patients, measurements of other testicular hormones and dynamic tests of the hypothalamic–pituitary–testicular axis may be required (Table 3) (103).

Table 3 Endocrine Tests in Male Reproductive Disorders

Basal hormones
Testosterone, FSH, and LH
Other hormones, binding proteins, and subunits
Free or bioavailable testosterone
Sex hormone binding globulin
Dihydrotestosterone
3α-androstanediol glucuronide
Estradiol
Prolactin
α- and β-subunits of FSH and LH
hCG
Dynamic tests
GnRH stimulation test
Clomiphene stimulation test
hCG stimulation test
Thyrotropin-releasing hormone (TRH) test

Abbreviations: FSH, follicle-stimulating hormone; hCG, human chorionic gonadotropin; LH, luteinizing hormone.
Source: From Ref. 103.

Testosterone (Total and Free or Bioavailable)

Testosterone concentrations are measured by radioimmunoassays (RIA), immunometric assays, or immunofluorometric assays (IFMA). Testosterone secretion has a circadian rhythm in man, with higher levels in the morning than evening. Since the normal ranges are based on morning values, blood samples for testosterone measurements should be drawn between 7 A.M. and 10 A.M. Automated assays for testosterone are frequently utilized by clinical laboratories. In general, these assays have variable and often poor levels of accuracy in the female and severely hypogonadal ranges (107). Liquid chromatography and tandem mass spectroscopy are part of the emerging technology for the most precise and accurate testosterone measurements (107). In most instances, measurement of total plasma testosterone will identify patients with androgen deficiency; however, since testosterone is bound to SHBG in the plasma, changes in SHBG concentrations will lead to changes in total testosterone concentrations. Increases in SHBG occur with hyperestrogenemia and hyperthyroidism, phenytoin treatment, aging, anorexia nervosa, and prolonged stress. Decreases in SHBG are present with androgen treatment, GH excess, obesity, and hypothyroidism. SHBG–binding capacity in the plasma can be assessed by testing the binding of labeled androgens to SHBG after separation from other proteins (i.e., ligand displacement assays) or by RIA. In disorders with abnormal SHBG concentrations, the measurement of total testosterone may be misleading. For example, a patient with gross obesity may have low total testosterone concentrations, reflecting the low SHBG concentrations associated with obesity. To separate true hypogonadism from binding protein defects, it may be necessary to determine the free or bioavailable testosterone concentrations. Free testosterone concentrations are usually measured after equilibrium dialysis of a serum sample. About 3% of testosterone in blood is free, with the rest bound to SHBG (30%) or to albumin and other proteins (67%). The non–SHBG bound testosterone (i.e., free and albumin bound) is the bioavailable portion of circulating testosterone. Bioavailable testosterone can be estimated in the serum by RIA after removal of SHBG by ammonium sulfate or Concanavalin A-Sepharose. Salivary testosterone can also be used as an indicator of free testosterone since SHBG and other proteins are present in very low concentrations in the saliva.

Other Androgen Metabolites

The measurement of plasma DHT is generally not useful in the evaluation of testicular disorders other than 5α-reductase deficiency. In this disorder, usually presenting with ambiguous genitalia in infancy and varying degrees of virilization at puberty, measurement of serum DHT and testosterone will show an abnormally high testosterone-to-DHT ratio especially

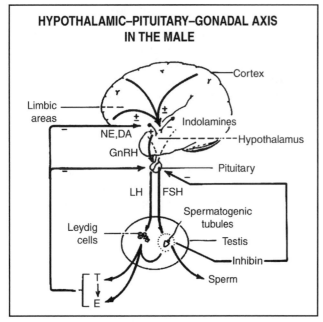

Figure 4 Hypothalamic–pituitary gonadal axis in men (see also Fig. 5). *Abbreviations*: DA, dopamine; E, estrogen; FSH, follicle-stimulating hormone; GnRH, gonadotropin-releasing hormone; LH, luteinizing hormone; NE, norepinephrine; T, testosterone.

after the administration of human chorionic gonadotropins (hCGs).

Estradiol measurements are usually not necessary in the assessment of male reproductive disorders. Estradiol concentrations are elevated in patients with androgen resistance, estrogen-secreting neoplasms, KS, and hypogonadism associated with chronic liver disease and some cases of gynecomastia.

LH and FSH

Measurements of plasma LH and FSH are important in classifying the anatomical level of the defect in hypogonadal patients (discussed further in Chapters 3 and 4) (Figs. 1, 4, and 5). Since both gonadotropins are

secreted in a pulsatile pattern, the collection of three samples, 15 to 20 minutes apart, may give more accurate assessment of the mean LH and FSH concentrations. Primary gonadal defects are characterized by low testosterone and high LH and FSH concentrations, whereas hypothalamic or pituitary disorders have low testosterone, LH, and FSH concentrations. The traditional RIA methods can distinguish clearly high FSH and LH (hypergonadotropic states) from normal concentrations but cannot clearly demarcate between normal and subnormal concentrations (i.e., hypogonadotropic states). The recently developed IFMA provide increased assay sensitivity from 0.5 to 0.05 IU/L for both gonadotropins (108). These new, sensitive gonadotropin assays allow the clinician to distinguish the low gonadotropin concentrations commonly observed in HH, delayed puberty, and after GnRH analog treatment (109). Bioassays of both LH and FSH are also available but generally do not add more information to the sensitive immunoassays. In the rare patient with genetic mutations of the β-LH gene, however, determination of LH by bioassay will show low bioactive LH concentrations in the presence of elevated immunoreactive LH concentrations (110). Rare patients with infertility have biologically inactive but immunoreactive FSH.

Other Pituitary Hormones

Plasma prolactin concentrations should be measured in patients with low testosterone and normal-to-low FSH and LH concentrations to exclude hyperprolactinemia. Measurements of the α- and β-subunits of the gonadotropins may be useful in patients with pituitary tumors, with or without hypogonadism. Many pituitary tumors previously thought to be nonfunctioning secrete large amounts of α- and β-subunits of LH and FSH (111). Moreover, plasma concentrations of α- and β-subunits of the gonadotropins rise in response to TRH administration. In patients with

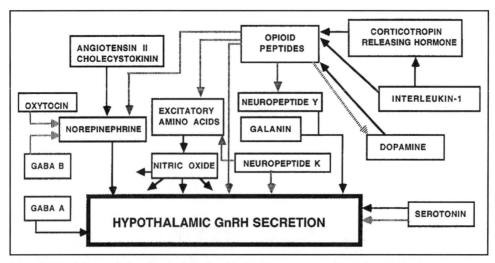

Figure 5 Detailed description of the regulation of gonadotropin-releasing hormone secretion by hypothalamic neurotransmitters. *Solid arrows* represent stimulatory effects; *dashed arrows* represent inhibitory effect. *Abbreviation*: GABA, gamma aminobutyric acid.

germinomas, teratomas, and chorioepitheliomas, β-hCG subunits may also be secreted and can serve as a tumor marker. Since β-hCG cross-reacts with most conventional LH RIA, an elevated LH in a child with a germinoma may be due to cross-reaction from β-hCG in the assay system. β-hCG is usually not detected by the more specific two-site LH immunoassays.

Dynamic Tests of the Hypothalamic–Pituitary–Testicular Axis

Before the development of sensitive assays for the gonadotropins, dynamic tests to evaluate the hypothalamic–pituitary axis were developed. With the use of the more sensitive assays, these dynamic tests are reserved for occasional and unusual diagnostic problems.

Administration of the antiestrogen, clomiphene citrate (100 mg for seven days) causes a rise in plasma LH, FSH, and testosterone concentrations. Clomiphene citrate blocks the negative feedback of estrogens and may have a direct stimulatory action on the gonadotropins. This test has limited practical value in the clinical assessment of male reproductive disorders, however, and does not add information to the measurement of the basal concentrations of gonadotropins and testosterone.

The availability of GnRH gave rise to the hope that the GnRH test (administered as a 100 μg bolus to adults or 50 μg/m² to children) would allow hypothalamic disorders to be distinguished from pituitary disorders; however, the gonadotropin response to a single dose of GnRH is frequently suppressed in patients with hypothalamic disorders. Priming the gonadotrophs with repeated low dose GnRH administration for a week followed by a bolus GnRH injection has been shown to enhance the gonadotropin responsiveness in patients with hypothalamic disorders but not in those with pituitary disorders. In general, information obtained from GnRH tests does not help in the diagnosis of testicular disorders. It is sometimes used in patients with central precocious puberty in whom an exaggerated LH to FSH response is characteristic. Leydig cell function can be stimulated by a single injection of hCG (2000–5000 IU), resulting in peak increases in plasma testosterone concentrations after 72 to 96 hours. The hCG test is useful in infants or children with cryptorchidism. A rise in testosterone in response to hCG indicates the presence of the testes and excludes anorchia. In patients with hypogonadism, elevated LH and low testosterone concentrations and the absence of a testosterone response to hCG suggest resistance to LH associated with Leydig cell hypoplasia or agenesis. A positive response to hCG indicates an abnormality of the endogenously secreted LH molecule. Bioassays of LH followed by molecular biology techniques to identify mutations of the *LH* gene may pinpoint the exact abnormality.

Multiple and frequent samplings for LH and FSH concentrations have been used to delineate the defect in GnRH secretion in patients with IHH (112) and aged men (113,114). Disorders of LH pulsatility, including absence of pulse, sleep-entrained pulses, and decreased frequency of amplitude of pulses have been defined. Sleep-entrained pulsatile secretion of LH is a hallmark of the onset of puberty and can be used to distinguish patients with early puberty from those with HH. Multiple blood samples, however, have to be taken at 10-minute intervals for a minimum of eight total hours to yield meaningful analyses of the pulsatile secretion of the gonadotropins. Because of the frequency and intensity of sampling, these investigative procedures are used mainly in clinical research studies.

Endocrine Tests in the Evaluation of Ambiguous Genitalia

In a neonate presenting with ambiguous genitalia, the chromosomal sex should be determined. In this section, the endocrine tests relevant to male pseudohermaphroditism (46,XY males with testis and with abnormal external and/or internal genitalia) are briefly discussed.

Phenotypically male patients with 46,XX may appear as normal males with varying degrees of hypogonadism and pseudohermaphroditism and can be true hermaphrodites. These sex-reversed patients have a portion of the Y chromosome (i.e., *SRY* gene) located on the X chromosome (115,116). The common causes and key laboratory tests of male pseudohermaphroditism are listed in Table 4 (103). For the diagnosis of the rare defect in infants with 3β-hydroxy steroid dehydrogenase/17α-hydroxylase, 17,20 lyase deficiency, plasma measurements of the C21 steroid precursors such as dihydrogen androsterone, 17α-hydroxyprogesterone, and 17α-hydroxy pregnenolone before and after ACTH or hCG stimulation will confirm the diagnosis. Plasma C19 steroids (testosterone and androstenedione) will be low. XY patients with 17β-hydroxysteroid oxireductase deficiency usually have female or mildly virilized external genitalia at birth and present with some degree of virilization at puberty. Since the defect lies in the conversions of androstenedione to testosterone and estrone to estradiol, the diagnosis is confirmed by finding low ratios of plasma testosterone to plasma androstenedione and estradiol to estrone, both at baseline and after hCG stimulation of Leydig cells.

The laboratory diagnosis of androgen resistance syndrome is made by measuring AR binding and function in genital fibroblast cultures. In patients with this disorder, AR binding may be low, undetectable, or unstable. Other variations in these disorders include abnormal ARs and postreceptor abnormalities. Using molecular biology techniques, single point mutations, multiple mutations, deletion, or premature stop codon defects have been identified to cause absent, quantitatively, or qualitatively abnormal ARs (117,118).

5α-reductase deficiency can be diagnosed by the measurement of the ratio of testosterone to DHT in

Table 4 Laboratory Tests for the Diagnosis of Male Pseudohermaphroditism

Cause	Tests
Testosterone biosynthesis defects	
P450 SCC: cholesterol side chain cleavage	↓ Basal and ACTH stimulated and mineralocorticoids ↓ Testosterone ↑ FSH ↑ LH
3β-Hydroxysteroid dehydrogenase	↑ Basal and ACTH stimulated 17α-pregnenolone, dehydroepiandrosterone, and dehydroepiandrosterone sulphate
P450 c17/17α-hydroxylase/17,20-lyase	↓ Testosterone ↑ FSH ↑ LH ↑ Deoxycorticosterone ↑ Corticosterone ↑ Progesterone ↓ Renin ↑ Basal, ACTH and hCG stimulated 17α-pregnenolone and 17α-progesterone
17β-Hydroxysteroid oxidoreductase	↓ Testosterone ↓ Estradiol ↑ Basal and hCG-stimulated androstenedione and estrone ↑ FSH ↑ LH
Androgen resistance syndromes	↑ LH ↑ Testosterone ↑ Estradiol Normal or ↑ FSH Skin fibroblasts for androgen receptors: low or undetectable, unstable, abnormal receptor; abnormal androgen receptor gene
Defects in testosterone metabolism 5α-Reductase deficiency	↑ Basal and hCG-stimulated testosterone to dihydrotestosterone ratio ↓ Skin fibroblasts conversion of testosterone to dihydrotestosterone
Leydig cell hypoplasia or aplasia	↓ Testosterone Absent testosterone response to hCG
Dysgenetic male pseudohermaphroditism Gonadal dysgenesis, incomplete gonadal dysgenesis	Chromosomal analysis
Vanishing testes (congenital anorchia)	↑ FSH ↑ LH ↓ Mullerian inhibiting factor Absent testosterone response to hCG

Abbreviations: ACTH, adrenocorticotrophin; FSH, follicle-stimulating hormone; hCG, human chorionic gonadotropins; LH, luteinizing hormone.
Source: From Ref. 103.

plasma before and after hCG stimulation. Patients with this metabolic defect of testosterone cannot convert testosterone to DHT, thus resulting in high testosterone-to-DHT ratios (Fig. 1).

In Leydig cell hypoplasia or aplasia, the Leydig cells are resistant to LH and hCG (119). The plasma testosterone concentrations are low and do not respond to exogenously administered hCG; the testes are small and atrophic, and testicular biopsy shows hypoplasia or absence of Leydig cells. In the vanishing testes syndrome, endocrine tests yield the same findings as in Leydig cell hypoplasia. Imaging by ultrasound, computed tomography scan, or magnetic resonance, however, fails to demonstrate the presence of testes.

Recently, assays of mullerian-inhibiting substance have been introduced, and these levels have been found to be very low or undetectable in patients with anorchia. In testicular hypoplasia and genital anorchia, varying differentiation and development of the Mullerian and Wolffian duct structures and external genitalia are present, depending on the date of onset of the testicular regression.

The diagnosis of patients with mixed gonadal dysgenesis [45, X0/46 XY; 45, X0/47, XXY; 46, XYpi (partial loss of short arm of Y chromosome) and variants] depends on detailed chromosomal studies. The diagnosis of the persistence of Mullerian duct structures is typically made when a uterus or Fallopian tubes are found incidentally during laparotomy or surgery for the correction of a hernia in a phenotypic male who may also have a cryptorchid testis. The use of urethrograms or sonograms can help to visualize internal genitalia but are generally more useful in female pseudohermaphroditism presenting as ambiguous genitalia.

Semen Tests

Testicular dysfunction is usually associated with impaired spermatogenesis, whether the primary defect is hypothalamic, pituitary, Leydig cell, Sertoli cell, or germ cell in origin. Such men often present to the physician with the complaint of infertility. The basic investigation of a male patient presenting with infertility is a semen analysis (Table 5) (see Chapters 23 and 24). Sperm antibodies and semen biochemistry are included in the basic tests but should be performed only when indicated. In general, the determination of semen volume, sperm count, motility, and morphology would be sufficient for the investigation of a patient with severe oligozoospermia (fewer than 5 million spermatozoa per mL semen) or asthenozoospermia (fewer than 10% motile) or teratozoospermia (fewer than 10% normal). In patients with normal or moderate impairment of semen parameters, further evaluation with specialized tests may be helpful to delineate specific defects of sperm function. Some of these tests may help to predict the success of assisted reproductive technologies such as in vitro fertilization. It is now known that approximately 20% of men with azoospermia or severe oligospermia harbor microdeletions in the long arm of the Y chromosome, most frequently in the AZF region (120,121).

Routine Semen Analysis

Because of the marked inherent variability of semen parameters, at least two semen analyses at one- to two-week intervals should be assessed in the laboratory. The semen sample should be collected by masturbation. The procedures and methods for routine semen analyses should follow the World Health Organization Laboratory Manual for Human Semen and Sperm Cervical Mucus Interaction (122). Using such standardized methods

Table 5 Laboratory Tests on Semen

Basic
Semen volume
Sperm count, motility, morphology
Sperm antibodies
Semen biochemistry
Specialized
Sperm cervical mucus interaction tests
Sperm motion analysis, assessment of hyperactivated motility
Sperm acrosomal reactivity
Zona-free hamster oocyte sperm penetration test
Zona pellucida-binding tests (in vitro fertilization)
Sperm biochemistry

Source: From Ref. 103.

allows comparison from laboratory to laboratory and quality control within the laboratory. If a sample shows no spermatozoa, it should be centrifuged and the pellet reexamined for the presence of spermatozoa before the diagnosis of azoospermia is given. The semen volume is usually between 2 mL and 5 mL. A low semen volume together with an acidic pH and azoospermia suggests genital tract obstruction caused by congenital bilateral absence of the vas deferens and seminal vesicles. The sperm count is assessed visually under a phase microscope with a white cell–counting chamber. Sperm motility is assessed visually and graded according to whether the spermatozoa has rapid progression, slow progression, no progression, or is nonmotile. A normal semen sample should have a sperm concentration of more than 20 million/mL or total sperm count of more than 40 million and 50% or more spermatozoa with progressive motility (122). A moderate decrease in sperm concentration to between 10 and 20 million/mL is compatible with fertility, provided sperm motility and morphology are normal. Although doubts have been raised about the value of routine semen analysis to distinguish between fertile and infertile men, studies have shown that concentration and morphology are variables capable of predicting fertility status especially in men with grossly abnormal semen parameters (123). In patients with unexplained infertility in whom routine semen analysis is normal, specialized tests of sperm function should be considered (124).

Until recently, sperm morphology has been classified using lenient criteria, with the lower limit for normal morphology being set at 50%. More recently, studies have indicated that by using more strict criteria, taking into consideration not only the shape of the spermatozoa but also the morphometric measurements (length, width, and length-to-width ratio) and the area occupied by the acrosome, sperm morphology was highly predictive of results of in vitro fertilization (125). Moreover, a multiple anomalies index wherein all abnormalities present in spermatozoa were scored (including midpiece and tail defects) showed a correlation with in vivo fertility (126). These studies suggest that stricter criteria with the inclusion of midpiece and tail morphology assessments may be more helpful for the diagnosis of male infertility (122).

The significance of the occurrence of leukocytes in semen is not clear and no direct relationship has been documented between the presence of leukocytes and genital infections. Semen cultures are usually performed if significant numbers of leukocytes (more than 1 million/mL) are present in the semen.

Sperm vitality can be assessed by supravital stains such as eosin-nigrosin (122). Measurement of sperm vitality should be performed in patients with very low sperm motility. This will help to identify whether the nonmotile spermatozoa are living. The hypo-osmotic swelling test (127) assesses the fluidity of the plasma membrane. Although not useful as a test of sperm fertilizing capacity, this test can assess sperm vitality (122).

Specialized Tests of Sperm Function

Specialized tests of sperm function are of great value in assessing patients with unexplained infertility (103). Assessment of sperm motion characteristics, sperm vitality, sperm autoantibodies, and sperm–cervical menses interaction, and human zona pellucida binding tests, zona-free hamster oocyte penetration tests, and the acrosome reaction tests are part of the highly specialized assessment of difficult cases of male factor infertility.

□ CONCLUSION

Hypogonadism may consist of testosterone deficiency, testosterone resistance, or impaired spermatogenesis.

Testosterone deficiency in men encompasses disorders involving the testes (primary), the hypothalamus or pituitary (secondary), or combinations of the two hormonal sites. Impaired spermatogenesis may be seen in association with testosterone deficiency or as an isolated problem. The clinical manifestations of testosterone deficiency depend on the age of onset and the severity of the disorder. The classical symptoms of decreased male phenotype and decreased sexuality may be coupled with decreased muscle and bone mass and increased fat mass. Infertility due to decreased sperm production or function is the result of multiple mechanisms, but these are still not very well understood. Testing for hypogonadism is described in this chapter.

□ REFERENCES

1. Swerdloff RS, Wang C, Kandeel FR. Evaluation of the infertile couple. Endocrinol Metab Clin North Am 1988; 17(2):301–337.
2. Wang C, Swerdloff RS. Evaluation of testicular function. Baillieres Clin Endocrinol Metab 1992; 6(2):405–434.
3. Klinfelter HFJ, Reifenstien EC J, Albright F. Syndrome characterized by gynecomastia, aspermatogenesis without a-Leydigism, and increased exertion of follicle-stimulating hormone. J Clin Endocrinol 1942; 2:615–627.
4. Paulsen CA, Plymate SR. Klinefelter's syndrome. In: King RA, Rotter JI, Motulsky A, eds. The Genetic Basis of Common Diseases. New York, NY: Oxford University Press, 1992: 876–894.
5. Jacobs PA, Hassold TJ, Whittington E, et al. Klinefelter's syndrome: an analysis of the origin of the additional sex chromosome using molecular probes. Ann Hum Genet 1988; 52(Pt 2):93–109.
6. Laron Z, Hochman IH. Small testes in prepubertal boys with Klinefelter's syndrome. J Clin Endocrinol Metab 1971; 32(5):671–672.
7. Ratcliffe SG, Bancroft J, Axworthy D, et al. Klinefelter's syndrome in adolescence. Arch Dis Child 1982; 57(1):6–12.
8. Cohen FL, Durham JD. Sex chromosome variations in school-age children. J Sch Health 1985; 55(3):99–102.
9. Laron Z. Klinefelter's syndrome: early diagnosis and social aspects. Hosp Practice 1972; 7:135–139.
10. Santen RJ, Kulin RE. The male reproductive system. In: Kelly VC, ed. Practice of Pediatrics. Hagerstown, MD: Harper and Row. Vol. 1. 1976:1–43.
11. Plymate SR, Paulsen CA. Klinefelter's syndrome. In: King RA, Motulsky A, ed. The Genetic Basis of Common Disease. New York, NY: Oxford University Press, 1989:876–894.

12. Plymate SR, Leonard JM, Paulsen CA, et al. Sex hormone-binding globulin changes with androgen replacement. J Clin Endocrinol Metab 1983; 57(3):645–648.
13. Wieland RG, Zorn EM, Johnson MW. Elevated testosterone-binding globulin in Klinefelter's syndrome. J Clin Endocrinol Metab 1980; 51(5):1199–1200.
14. Ratcliffe SG. Klinefelter's syndrome in children: a longitudinal study of 47 XXY boys identified by population screening in Klinefelter's syndrome. In: Bandmann HJ, Briet R, Perwin E, ed. Klinefelter's Syndrome. New York: Springer-Verlag, 1984:38.
15. Boone KB, Swerdloff RS, Miller BL, et al. Neuropsychological profiles of adults with Klinefelter syndrome. J Int Neuropsychol Soc 2001; 7(4):446–456.
16. Galaburda AM. Neuroanatomic basis of developmental dyslexia. Neurol Clin 1993; 11(1):161–173.
17. Itti E, Gaw G, I, Boone KB, et al. Functional neuroimaging provides evidence of anomalous cerebral laterality in adults with Klinefelter's syndrome. Ann Neurol 2003; 54(5):669–673.
18. Patwardhan AJ, Eliez S, Bender B, et al. Brain morphology in Klinefelter syndrome: extra X chromosome and testosterone supplementation. Neurology 2000; 54(12):2218–2223.
19. Hunt PA, Worthman C, Levinson H, et al. Germ cell loss in the XXY male mouse: altered X-chromosome dosage affects prenatal development. Mol Reprod Dev 1998; 49(2):101–111.
20. Lue Y, Jentsch JD, Wang C, et al. XXY mice exhibit gonadal and behavioral phenotypes similar to Klinefelter syndrome. Endocrinology 2005; 146(9):4148–4154.
21. Lue Y, Rao PN, Sinha Hikim AP, et al. XXY male mice: an experimental model for Klinefelter syndrome. Endocrinology 2001; 142(4):1461–1470.
22. Andersson M, Page DC, de la Chapelle A. Chromosome Y-specific DNA is transferred to the short arm of X chromosome in human XX males. Science 1986; 233(4765):786–788.

23. Vazquez JA, Pinies JA, Martul P, et al. Hypothalamic-pituitary-testicular function in 70 patients with myotonic dystrophy. J Endocrinol Invest 1990; 13(5): 375–379.

24. Handelsman DJ. Testicular dysfunction in systemic disease. Endocrinol Metab Clin North Am 1994; 23(4): 839–856.

25. Allen NE, Appleby PN, Davey GK, et al. Lifestyle and nutritional determinants of bioavailable androgens and related hormones in British men. Cancer Causes Control 2002; 13(4):353–363.

26. Barrett-Connor E. Lower endogenous androgen levels and dyslipidemia in men with non-insulin-dependent diabetes mellitus (see comments). Ann Intern Med 1992; 117(10):807–811.

27. Feldman HA, Longcope C, Derby CA, et al. Age trends in the level of serum testosterone and other hormones in middle-aged men: longitudinal results from the Massachusetts male aging study. J Clin Endocrinol Metab 2002; 87(2):589–598.

28. Field AE, Colditz GA, Willett WC, et al. The relation of smoking, age, relative weight, and dietary intake to serum adrenal steroids, sex hormones, and sex hormone-binding globulin in middle-aged men. J Clin Endocrinol Metab 1994; 79(5):1310–1316.

29. Glass AR, Swerdloff RS, Bray GA, et al. Low serum testosterone and sex-hormone-binding-globulin in massively obese men. J Clin Endocrinol Metab 1977; 45(6):1211–1219.

30. Gray A, Feldman HA, McKinlay JB, et al. Age, disease, and changing sex hormone levels in middle-aged men: results of the Massachusetts Male Aging Study. J Clin Endocrinol Metab 1991; 73(5):1016–1025.

31. McKinlay JB, Longcope C, Gray A. The questionable physiologic and epidemiologic basis for a male climacteric syndrome: preliminary results from the Massachusetts Male Aging Study. Maturitas 1989; 11(2):103–115.

32. Ballew JW, Masters WH. Mumps; a cause of infertility. I. Present considerations. Fertil Steril 1954; 5(6):536–543.

33. Shilo S, Livshin Y, Sheskin J, et al. Gonadal function in lepromatous leprosy. Lepr Rev 1981; 52(2):127–134.

34. Plymate S. Hypogonadism. Endocrinol Metab Clin North Am 1994; 23(4):749–772.

35. Croxson TS, Chapman WE, Miller LK, et al. Changes in the hypothalamic-pituitary-gonadal axis in human immunodeficiency virus-infected homosexual men. J Clin Endocrinol Metab 1989; 68(2):317–321.

36. Grinspoon SK, Donovan DS Jr, Bilezikian JP. Aetiology and pathogenesis of hormonal and metabolic disorders in HIV infection. Baillieres Clin Endocrinol Metab 1994; 8(4):735–755.

37. Lefrere JJ, Laplanche JL, Vittecoq D, et al. Hypogonadism in AIDS. AIDS 1988; 2(2):135–136.

38. Roth DR, Lipshultz LI. Overview of cryptorchidism with emphasis on the human. In: Abney TO, Keel BA, eds. The Cryptorchidism Testes. Boca Raton, FL: CRC Press, 1989:1–15.

39. Rajfer J, Walsh PC. Testicular descent. Normal and abnormal. Urol Clin North Am 1978; 5(1):223–235.

40. Albescu JZ, Bergada C, Cullen M. Male fertility in patients treated for cryptorchidism before puberty 19. Fertil Steril 1971; 22(12):829–833.

41. Jockenhovel F, Swerdloff RS. Alterations in steroidogenic capacity of Leydig cells in cryptorchid testis. In: Abney TO, Keel BA, eds. The Cryptorchid Testis. Boca Raton, FL: CRC Press, 1989:35–54.

42. Elder M, Maclaren N, Riley W. Gonadal autoantibodies in patients with hypogonadism and/or Addison's disease. J Clin Endocrinol Metab 1981; 52(6):1137–1142.

43. Eil C. Familial incomplete male pseudohermaphroditism associated with impaired nuclear androgen retention. Studies in cultured skin fibroblasts. J Clin Invest 1983; 71(4):850–858.

44. Griffin JE, Punyashthiti K, Wilson JD. Dihydrotestosterone binding by cultured human fibroblasts. Comparison of cells from control subjects and from patients with hereditary male pseudohermaphroditism due to androgen resistance. J Clin Invest 1976; 57(5):1342–1351.

45. Gyorki S, Warne GL, Khalid BA, et al. Defective nuclear accumulation of androgen receptors in disorders of sexual differentiation. J Clin Invest 1983; 72(3): 819–825.

46. Wilson JD, Harrod MJ, Goldstein JL, et al. Familial incomplete male pseudohermaphroditism, type 1. Evidence for androgen resistance and variable clinical manifestations in a family with the Reifenstein syndrome. N Engl J Med 1974; 290(20):1097–1103.

47. McPhaul MJ, Marcelli M, Zoppi S, et al. Genetic basis of endocrine disease. 4. The spectrum of mutations in the androgen receptor gene that causes androgen resistance. J Clin Endocrinol Metab 1993; 76(1):17–23.

48. Kovacs WJ, Griffin JE, Weaver DD, et al. A mutation that causes lability of the androgen receptor under conditions that normally promote transformation to the DNA-binding state. J Clin Invest 1984; 73(4): 1095–1104.

49. MacDonald PC, Madden JD, Brenner PF, et al. Origin of estrogen in normal men and in women with testicular feminization. J Clin Endocrinol Metab 1979; 49(6):905–916.

50. O'Leary JA. Comparative studies of the gonad in testicular feminization and cryptorchidism. Fertil Steril 1965; 16(6):813–819.

51. Irvine RA, Yu MC, Ross RK, et al. The CAG and GGC microsatellites of the androgen receptor gene are in linkage disequilibrium in men with prostate cancer. Cancer Res 1995; 55(9):1937–1940.

52. Zitzmann M, Depenbusch M, Gromoll J, et al. X-chromosome inactivation patterns and androgen receptor functionality influence phenotype and social characteristics as well as pharmacogenetics of testosterone therapy in Klinefelter patients. J Clin Endocrinol Metab 2004; 89(12):6208–6217.

53. Imperato-McGinley J, Guerrero L, Gautier T, et al. Steroid 5alpha-reductase deficiency in man: an inherited

form of male pseudohermaphroditism. Science 1974; 186(4170):1213–1215.

54. Imperato-McGinley J, Peterson RE. Male pseudohermaphroditism: the complexities of male phenotypic development. Am J Med 1976; 61(2):251–272.

55. Peterson RE, Imperato-McGinley J, Gautier T, et al. Male pseudohermaphroditism due to steroid 5-alpha-reductase deficiency. Am J Med 1977; 62(2):170–191.

56. Snyder PJ, Rudenstein RS, Gardner DF, et al. Repetitive infusion of gonadotropin-releasing hormone distinguishes hypothalamic from pituitary hypogonadism. J Clin Endocrinol Metab 1979; 48(5):864–868.

57. Boyar RM, Finkelstein JW, Witkin M, et al. Studies of endocrine function in "isolated" gonadotropin deficiency. J Clin Endocrinol Metab 1973; 36(1):64–72.

58. Cassorla FG, Golden SM, Johnsonbaugh RE, et al. Testicular volume during early infancy. J Pediatr 1981; 99(5):742–743.

59. Kallman FJ, Schonfeld WA, Barrera W. The genetic aspects of primary eunuchoidism. Am J Ment Def 1944; 48:203–236.

60. Lieblich JM, Rogol AD, White BJ, et al. Syndrome of anosmia with hypogonadotropic hypogonadism (Kallmann syndrome): clinical and laboratory studies in 23 cases. Am J Med 1982; 73(4):506–519.

61. Santen RJ, Paulsen CA. Hypogonadotropic eunuchoidism. I. Clinical study of the mode of inheritance. J Clin Endocrinol Metab 1973; 36(1):47–54.

62. Whitcomb RW, Crowley WF Jr. Clinical review 4: diagnosis and treatment of isolated gonadotropin-releasing hormone deficiency in men. J Clin Endocrinol Metab 1990; 70(1):3–7.

63. Jameson JL, Deutsch PJ, Chatterjee KK, et al. Regulation of alpha ad CG beta gene expression. In: Chin WW, Boime I, eds. Glycoprotein Hormones. Norwell: Serono Symposia, 1990:269–278.

64. Santen RJ, Bardin CW. Episodic luteinizing hormone secretion in man. Pulse analysis, clinical interpretation, physiologic mechanisms. J Clin Invest 1973; 52(10):2617–2628.

65. Karges B, de Roux N. Molecular genetics of isolated hypogonadotropic hypogonadism and Kallmann syndrome. Endocr Dev 2005; 8:67–80.

66. Schwanzel-Fukuda M, Pfaff DW. Origin of luteinizing hormone-releasing hormone neurons. Nature 1989; 338(6211):161–164.

67. Klingmuller D, Dewes W, Krahe T, et al. Magnetic resonance imaging of the brain in patients with anosmia and hypothalamic hypogonadism (Kallmann's syndrome). J Clin Endocrinol Metab 1987; 65(3):581–584.

68. White BJ, Rogol AD, Brown KS, et al. The syndrome of anosmia with hypogonadotropic hypogonadism: a genetic study of 18 new families and a review. Am J Med Genet 1983; 15(3):417–435.

69. Whitcomb RW, Crowley WF Jr. Male hypogonadotropic hypogonadism. Endocrinol Metab Clin North Am 1993; 22(1):125–143.

70. Merriam GR, Beitins IZ, Bode HH. Father-to-son transmission of hypogonadism with anosmia: Kallmann's syndrome. Am J Dis Child 1977; 131(11):1216–1219.

71. Faiman C, Hoffman DL, Ryan RJ, et al. The "fertile eunuch" syndrome: demonstration of isolated luteinizing hormone deficiency by radioimmunoassay technique. Mayo Clin Proc 1968; 43(9):661–667.

72. Pasqualini RQ, Bur G. Hypoandrogenic syndrome with spermatogenesis. Fertil Steril 1955; 6(2):144–157.

73. Mozaffarian GA, Higley M, Paulsen CA. Clinical studies in an adult male patient with "isolated follicle stimulating hormone (FSH) deficiency". J Androl 1983; 4(6):393–398.

74. Rimoin DL, Schimke RN. The gonads. In: Rimoin DL, Schimke RN, eds. Genetic Disorders of the Endocrine Glands. St. Louis: Mosby, 1971:258–356.

75. Bray GA, Dahms WT, Swerdloff RS, et al. The Prader-Willi syndrome: a study of 40 patients and a review of the literature. Medicine (Baltimore) 1983; 62(2):59–80.

76. Hamilton CR Jr. Scully RE, Kliman B. Hypogonadotropinism in Prader-Willi syndrome. Induction of puberty and sperm altogenesis by clomiphene citrate. Am J Med 1972; 52(3):322–329.

77. Pauli RM, Meisner LF, Szmanda RJ. "Expanded" Prader-Willi syndrome in a boy with an unusual 15q chromosome deletion. Am J Dis Child 1983; 137(11): 1087–1089.

78. Bittel DC, Butler MG. Prader-Willi syndrome: clinical genetics, cytogenetics and molecular biology. Expert Rev Mol Med 2005; 7(14):1–20.

79. Ledbetter DH, Mascarello JT, Riccardi VM, et al. Chromosome 15 abnormalities and the Prader-Willi syndrome: a follow-up report of 40 cases. Am J Hum Genet 1982; 34(2):278–285.

80. Green JS, Parfrey PS, Harnett JD, et al. The cardinal manifestations of Bardet-Biedl syndrome, a form of Laurence-Moon-Biedl syndrome. N Engl J Med 1989; 321(15):1002–1009.

81. Perez-Palacios G, Uribe M, Scaglia H, et al. Pituitary and gonadal function in patients with the Laurence-Moon-Biedl syndrome. Acta Endocrinol (Copenh) 1977; 84(1):191–199.

82. Gorlin RJ, Anderson RC, Blaw M. Multiple lentigenes syndrome. Am J Dis Child 1969; 117(6):652–662.

83. Volpe R, Metzler WS, Johnston MW. Familial hypogonadotropic eunuchoidism with cerebellar ataxia. J Clin Endocrinol Metab 1963; 23:107–115.

84. Boyar RM. Endocrine changes in anorexia nervosa. Med Clin North Am 1978; 62(2):297–303.

85. Drossman DA. Anorexia nervosa: a comprehensive approach. Adv Intern Med 1983; 28:339–361.

86. Buvat J, Lemaire A, Ardaens K, et al. Profile of gonadal hormones in 8 cases of male anorexia nervosa studied before and during weight gain. Ann Endocrinol (Paris) 1983; 44(4):229–234.

87. Wheeler MJ, Crisp AH, Hsu LK, et al. Reproductive hormone changes during weight gain in male anorectics. Clin Endocrinol (Oxf) 1983; 18(4):423–429.

88. Crisp AH, Harding B, McGuiness B. Anorexia nervosa. Psychoneurotic characteristics of parents: relationship to prognosis. A quantitative study. J Psychosom Res 1974; 18(3):167–173.

89. Chlebowski RT, Heber D. Hypogonadism in male patients with metastatic cancer prior to chemotherapy. Cancer Res 1982; 42(6):2495–2498.

90. Truswell AS, Hansen JD. Medical and nutritional studies of Kung Bushmen in north-west Botswana: a preliminary report. S Afr Med J 1968; 42(49):1338–1339.

91. van der Walt LA, Wilmsen EN, Jenkins T. Unusual sex hormone patterns among desert-dwelling hunter-gatherers. J Clin Endocrinol Metab 1978; 46(4):658–663.

92. Bagatell CJ, Bremner WJ. Sperm counts and reproductive hormones in male marathoners and lean controls. Fertil Steril 1990; 53(4):688–692.

93. Baker ER, Mathur RS, Kirk RF, et al. Female runners and secondary amenorrhea: correlation with age, parity, mileage, and plasma hormonal and sex-hormone-binding globulin concentrations. Fertil Steril 1981; 36(2):183–187.

94. Frisch RE, Wyshak G, Vincent L. Delayed menarche and amenorrhea in ballet dancers. N Engl J Med 1980; 303(1):17–19.

95. Shangold MM. Exercise and amenorrhea. Semin Reprod Endocrinol 1985; 3:35–50.

96. Warren MP. The effects of exercise on pubertal progression and reproductive function in girls. J Clin Endocrinol Metab 1980; 51(5):1150–1157.

97. Dolecek R, Dvoracek C, Jezek M, et al. Very low serum testosterone levels and severe impairment of spermatogenesis in burned male patients. Correlations with basal levels and levels of FSH, LH and PRL after LHRH + TRH. Endocrinol Exp 1983; 17(1):33–45.

98. Plymate SR, Vaughan GM, Mason AD, et al. Central hypogonadism in burned men. Horm Res 1987; 27(3):152–158.

99. Kudlow JE, Gerrie BM. Production of growth factor activity by cultured bovine calf anterior pituitary cells. Endocrinology 1983; 113(1):104–110.

100. Prysor-Jones RA, Silverlight JJ, Jenkins JS. Oestradiol, vasoactive intestinal peptide and fibroblast growth factor in the growth of human pituitary tumour cells in vitro. J Endocrinol 1989; 120(1):171–177.

101. Vance ML, Thorner MO. Prolactinomas. Endocrinol Metab Clin North Am 1987; 16(3):731–753.

102. Molitch M. Prolactinoma. In: Melmed S, ed. The Pituitary. Cambridge, MA: Blackwell Science, 1995:443–477.

103. Wang C, Swerdloff RS. Male reproductive disorders. In: Rock RC, Noe D, eds. Laboratory Medicine. The selection and interpretation of clinical laboratory studies. Williams and Wilkens, 1993:838–857.

104. Fine SA, Frohman LA. Loss of central nervous system component of dopaminergic inhibition of prolactin secretion in patients with prolactin-secreting pituitary tumors. J Clin Invest 1978; 61(4):973–980.

105. Snyder PJ. Gonadotroph adenomas. In: Melmed S, ed. The Pituitary. Cambridge, MA: Blackwell Science, 1975:559–575.

106. Trouillas J, Girod C, Sassolas G, et al. The human gonadotropic adenoma: pathologic diagnosis and hormonal correlations in 26 tumors. Semin Diagn Pathol 1986; 3(1):42–57.

107. Wang C, Catlin DH, Demers LM, et al. Measurement of total serum testosterone in adult men: comparison of current laboratory methods versus liquid chromatography-tandem mass spectrometry. J Clin Endocrinol Metab 2004; 89(2):534–543.

108. Jaakkola T, Ding YQ, Kellokumpu-Lehtinen P, et al. The ratios of serum bioactive/immunoreactive luteinizing hormone and follicle-stimulating hormone in various clinical conditions with increased and decreased gonadotropin secretion: reevaluation by a highly sensitive immunometric assay. J Clin Endocrinol Metab 1990; 70(6):1496–1505.

109. Salameh W, Bhasin S, Steiner BS, et al. Effect of improved assay sensitivity on luteinizing hormone pulse detection after gonadotropin-releasing hormone antagonist treatment in man. J Clin Endocrinol Metab 1992; 75(6):1479–1483.

110. Weiss J, Axelrod L, Whitcomb RW, et al. Hypogonadism caused by a single amino acid substitution in the beta subunit of luteinizing hormone. N Engl J Med 1992; 326(3):179–183.

111. Snyder PJ. Gonadotroph cell adenomas of the pituitary. Endocr Rev 1985; 6(4):552–563.

112. Crowley WFJ, Filicori M, Spratt DI, et al. The physiology of gonadotropin-releasing hormone (GnRH) secretion in men and women. Recent Prog Horm Res 1985; 41:473–531.

113. Veldhuis JD, Iranmanesh A, Mulligan T. Age and testosterone feedback jointly control the dose-dependent actions of gonadotropin-releasing hormone in healthy men. J Clin Endocrinol Metab 2005; 90(1):302–309.

114. Veldhuis JD, Zwart A, Mulligan T, et al. Muting of androgen negative feedback unveils impoverished gonadotropin-releasing hormone/luteinizing hormone secretory reactivity in healthy older men. J Clin Endocrinol Metab 2001; 86(2):529–535.

115. Page DC, Brown LG, de la Chapelle A. Exchange of terminal portions of X- and Y-chromosomal short arms in human XX males. Nature 1987; 328(6129): 437–440.

116. Page DC, de la Chapelle A, Weissenbach J. Chromosome Y-specific DNA in related human XX males. Nature 1985; 315(6016):224–226.

117. Brown TR, Lubahn DB, Wilson EM, et al. Deletion of the steroid-binding domain of the human androgen receptor gene in one family with complete androgen insensitivity syndrome: evidence for further genetic heterogeneity in this syndrome. Proc Natl Acad Sci USA 1988; 85(21):8151–8155.

118. Marcelli M, Tilley WD, Zoppi S, et al. Androgen resistance associated with a mutation of the androgen

receptor at amino acid 772 (Arg—Cys) results from a combination of decreased messenger ribonucleic acid levels and impairment of receptor function. J Clin Endocrinol Metab 1991; 73(2):318–325.

119. David R, Yoon DJ, Landin L, et al. A syndrome of gonadotropin resistance possibly due to a luteinizing hormone receptor defect. J Clin Endocrinol Metab 1984; 59(1):156–160.

120. Simoni M. Molecular diagnosis of Y chromosome microdeletions in Europe: state-of-the-art and quality control. Hum Reprod 2001; 16(3):402–409.

121. Vogt PH. Genomic heterogeneity and instability of the AZF locus on the human Y chromosome. Mol Cell Endocrinol 2004; 224(1–2):1–9.

122. World Health Organization. Laboratory Manual for the Examination of Human Semen and Sperm Cervical Mucus Interaction. 4th ed. Cambridge University Press, 1999.

123. Wang C. Bioassays of follicle stimulating hormone. Endocr Rev 1988; 9(3):374–377.

124. Aitken RJ, Best FS, Warner P, et al. A prospective study of the relationship between semen quality and fertility in cases of unexplained infertility 18. J Androl 1984; 5(4):297–303.

125. Kruger TF, Acosta AA, Simmons KF, et al. Predictive value of abnormal sperm morphology in in vitro fertilization. Fertil Steril 1988; 49(1):112–117.

126. Jouannet P, Ducot B, Feneux D, et al. Male factors and the likelihood of pregnancy in infertile couples. I. Study of sperm characteristics. Int J Androl 1988; 11(5):379–394.

127. Jeyendran RS, van der Ven HH, Perez-Pelaez M, et al. Development of an assay to assess the functional integrity of the human sperm membrane and its relationship to other semen characteristics. J Reprod Fertil 1984; 70(1):219–228.

13

Cryptorchidism, Testicular Torsion, and Torsion of the Testicular Appendages

Bartley G. Cilento, Jr.

Department of Urology, Children's Hospital and Department of Surgery, Harvard Medical School, Boston, Massachusetts, U.S.A.

Anthony Atala

Department of Urology, Wake Forest University School of Medicine, Wake Forest Institute for Regenerative Medicine, Winston-Salem, North Carolina, U.S.A.

□ CRYPTORCHIDISM
Incidence

In 1950, Scorer followed 1499 male newborns and reported an overall incidence of undescended testis (cryptorchidism) in 2.7% at birth and 0.8% at three months of age (1). Subsequent reports (2) have demonstrated an increasing number of cases—5.9% at birth and 1.6% at three months of age. An increased rate of up to 9% was reported in premature and low birth weight neonates. The incidence of cryptorchidism also increases in neural tube defect disorders, myelomeningocele, omphalocele, anencephaly, abnormalities of testosterone biosynthesis defects, 5-α-reductase deficiency, peripheral androgen-receptor abnormalities, and in disorders of gonadotropin deficiencies such as Kallmann's syndrome, Prader–Willi syndrome, and Lawrence–Moon–Biedl syndrome. Genetic predisposition seems to play a role in cryptorchidism, with similar manifestations noted in 1% to 4% of siblings and 6% of fathers with cryptorchidism (3). There also appears to be an increased incidence of intersexuality (ambiguous genitalia) in children with cryptorchidism and hypospadias. An intersexual individual is one who is born with genitalia and/or secondary sex characteristics determined as neither exclusively male nor female, or who exhibits combined features of the male and female sexes. The incidence of intersexuality increases with the severity of cryptorchidism and the degree of hypospadias (4).

Embryology

The fetal gonad is indeterminate until six to eight weeks of gestation. In the presence of the *SRY* gene, on the short arm of the Y chromosome, and as a result of the developmentally regulated program of gene expression, the undifferentiated gonad develops into a testis. During this period, the Sertoli cells release a mullerian-inhibiting substance (MIS), which causes the regression of the mullerian structures. Testosterone is produced in as early as the eighth week of gestation. Under the influence of testosterone, the Wolffian system develops into the epididymis, seminal vesicles, and vas deferens. The external genitalia develop at 10 to 15 weeks of gestation by the peripheral conversion of testosterone to dihydrotestosterone by the enzyme 5-α-reductase. During the same period (approximately 11 to 12 weeks), the processus vaginalis is located at the level of the internal inguinal ring. At this stage, the most distal aspect of the processus vaginalis is abutted by the gelatinous material destined to be the gubernaculum. (For further information on the embryology of the male gonads, see Chapter 2.)

The descent of the testis takes place in two different stages. The first stage is called the "transabdominal descent," in which the testis moves from the urogenital ridge to the level of the internal inguinal ring. The transabdominal migration is thought to be the result of differential somatic growth of the developing fetus (5). By the 17th week of gestation, the testis is located at the internal inguinal ring (6). Studies suggest that transabdominal descent is androgen independent (7).

The testis remains at the internal inguinal ring until the 20th week of gestation, when it begins the descent into the scrotum. The second stage of descent is called the "inguinal scrotal stage," and is normally complete by 40 weeks of gestation. The second stage is believed to be secondary to gubernacular regression (8). Hormonal factors may also be involved. Research suggests the involvement of a low-molecular-weight fraction of the fetal testicular extract called descendin, which is a stimulatory to the gubernacular cells (8). Testosterone may also have a role in the initiation of gubernacular regression (8). Other studies have suggested that MIS may have a role as a promoter of testicular descent (7). Several studies have also implicated a role for estrogen in testicular descent. Estrogens act by increasing the resistance of the mullerian duct to MIS (9,10). Additionally, estrogens may induce atrophy of the gubernacular tissue. Indirect evidence suggests that

MIS initiates descent by stimulating the growth and shortening of the gubernaculum (7). Nevertheless, these studies have failed to show that MIS directly controls any phase of testicular descent.

Transection of the genital femoral nerve prevents the inguinal scrotal stage of testicular descent in experimental animal models (7). The genital femoral nerve courses down the psoas muscle, through the inguinal canal to the scrotum, and then ascends to meet the gubernaculum. After transection of the genitofemoral nerve, the gubernaculum is insensitive to hormonal control. The gubernaculum is thought to be androgen sensitive, despite an inability to demonstrate androgen receptors on the gubernaculum (11). Hutson and Beasley believe that the receptors for the androgens are located in the central nervous system (CNS), and that the genitofemoral nerve acts as a mediator of testosterone on the gubernaculum, enabling testicular descent (7). In support of this hypothesis, it has been shown that disorders of the CNS affecting the genitofemoral nerve would result in cryptorchidism. Meningomyelocele causes segmental paralysis of the spinal nerves, and is associated with a higher incidence of cryptorchidism. The genitofemoral nerve spinal nucleus is located in the first and second lumbar segments.

Other proposed theories for testicular descent involve changes in intra-abdominal pressure (12). Because the mechanism of normal testicular descent has not been fully elucidated, the exact causes of cryptorchidism are still unknown.

Endocrine Aspect

Cryptorchidism was previously thought to be a disorder of primarily mechanical or anatomic origin. A hormonal cause or mechanism, however, has long been suspected. Many clinical syndromes are characterized by deficiencies in gonadal hormone synthesis, androgen-receptor defects, or deficiencies in gonadotropin production, and such conditions can be associated with cryptorchidism (Kallmann's syndrome, encephalia, and penoscrotal hypospadias due to deficiency of 5-α-reductase) (11,13). Many studies cite an abnormality in the pituitary–gonadal axis under both static and stimulated conditions (14). Maternal antibodies also have been implicated (15). In support of the pituitary–gonadal axis abnormality, Job et al. reported that cryptorchid infants demonstrate decreased mean levels of testosterone and luteinizing hormone (LH) between 30 and 120 days of age (16). They also found a 50% incidence of antigonadotropic autoantibodies in cryptorchid children, as measured by immunofluorescent techniques, suggesting that a partial gonadotropin deficiency in the pituitary may hamper testicular descent. This group also showed a diminished LH peak after stimulation with luteinizing hormone-releasing hormone (LHRH), also known as gonadotropin-releasing hormone (GnRH), in cryptorchid versus normal infants.

Other studies, however, have shown normal hormonal conditions in all of these areas. Walsh et al. were unable to demonstrate any difference in basal plasma testosterone levels between normal and cryptorchid children (17). Cacciari et al. found no difference in pituitary LH and follicle-stimulating hormone (FSH) secretion in normal and cryptorchid boys after stimulating the hypothalamic pituitary axis with growth hormone-releasing hormone (18). Thus, the inconclusive studies presented suggest that current knowledge of the hormonal regulation of testicular descent remains limited.

Investigations

No standard classification exists for describing the cryptorchid testis. The best method is to describe the location of the testis on physical examination. The child should be placed on the examination table in a warm room with abdomen and genitalia exposed. Visual inspection of the abdomen and scrotum is performed first. The ipsilateral hemiscrotum is often underdeveloped in the cryptorchid patient. Frequently, a retractile testis is visible in the hemiscrotum, and this could become cryptorchid. A testicle is considered retractile if it is located high in the scrotum or up near the groin. An abdominal examination is performed, and then gentle pressure is placed just medial to the iliac crest (level of the internal inguinal ring). The examining hand is gently advanced down the inguinal crease as the other hand palpates the ipsilateral hemiscrotum. The ipsilateral hemiscrotum is gently inverted to meet the advancing upper hand. The testis is often corralled in this fashion. An attempt is made to bring the testis down into the most dependent portion of the hemiscrotum. Care should be taken not to mistake a low cryptorchid testis for a fully descended testis; the scrotal tissue should be brought up around the testis. If the testis is not located, the child should be placed in the Tailor's position (seated with legs crossed) and the scrotum reexamined. This maneuver usually abolishes the cremasteric reflex. A hot compress applied to the inguinal region may also relax the cremasteric muscle. The cremasteric muscle reflex, which pulls up the scrotum and testis on the side that is lightly stroked on the superior and medial part of the thigh, is not reliably present until 30 months of age; therefore, the neonatal period is the ideal time to examine the genitalia (19). If one is not afforded this opportunity, then records of the neonatal examination should be reviewed. This may clarify the diagnosis if retractile testes are suspected. If the newborn examination report documents a fully descended testis that subsequently became cryptorchid, then this most certainly is a retractile testis.

There is a clinical entity called testicular ascent; however, controversy surrounds its cause. This may represent ascent of a previously descended testicle or an unrecognized retractile testis (20).

The position of the testis should be described as either palpable or nonpalpable. If palpable, its location on examination should be described: internal inguinal ring, external inguinal ring, scrotal inlet, or ectopic

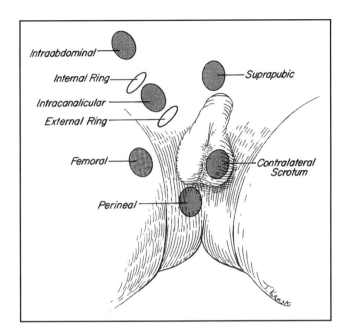

Figure 1 Location of undescended testis. Location of the testes along the normal course of descent: intra-abdominal and intracanalicular. Location of the ectopic positions outside the normal course of descent: suprapubic, femoral, perineal, and contralateral scrotum.

(Fig. 1). Ectopic locations are outside the normal course of descent. Ectopic positions may include the perineal, femoral, or penile location.

In patients with bilateral nonpalpable testes, a human chorionic gonadotropin (hCG) stimulation test should be performed to determine the presence of testicular tissue. If there is no corresponding rise of testosterone to hCG, and the basal level of the FSH is high, testicular absence can be diagnosed, and surgical exploration may not be necessary (21). Some authors have also proposed that hCG is preoperatively efficacious in causing the nonpalpable, undescended testis to become palpable in 39% of patients (22).

MIS is produced by the prepubertal testis, and it is responsible for the regression of the mullerian structures in males, which is necessary for normal sexual development. In children with virilization and impalpable gonads, only those children with testicular tissue should have detectable serum concentrations of MIS. MIS was studied in 65 children with nonpalpable testes. The sensitivity and specificity of the MIS assay for detecting the absence of testicular tissue were 92% and 98%, respectively, compared with 69% and 83% for the measurement of testosterone after the administration of hCG or during the normal physiologic increase of testosterone in male infants (23). Additionally, MIS assays may be able to discern children with abnormal and normal testes based on the serum concentrations of MIS. MIS can further be used to determine testicular status in children with nonpalpable testes, thereby differentiating bilateral cryptorchidism from anorchia.

Ultrasonography and magnetic resonance imaging (MRI) may demonstrate the position of the nonpalpable testis; however, nonvisualization by these techniques does not exclude the presence of testicular tissue. Therefore, if the testis is nonpalpable on examination, the authors do not recommend that any imaging techniques be pursued.

Hormonal Treatment

Hormonal treatment for cryptorchidism dates back to the 1930s, when Ascheim and Zondek observed stimulation of the sex glands by urinary substances from pregnant women (24). During the same period, others demonstrated genital growth and stimulation with anterior pituitary extract (25,26). In 1937, Thompson et al. reviewed the treatment of undescended testes with anterior pituitary-like substances and found variable success rates (25–100%) (27). In the 1950s, Deming reviewed the treatment of cryptorchidism with urinary hCG and noted a wide variation in success (0–90%) (28).

In the United States, hormonal treatment is primarily performed with hCG, which consists mainly of LH. Other agents have also been used, such as human menopausal gonadotropin (hMG), which consists mainly of FSH. Subsequent studies have shown that hMG works equally as well or in combination with hCG, as compared with hCG alone (29). Scheduled dosages of hCG injection vary, and there is presently no consensus. Some investigators propose injections on alternate days; however, others believe that hCG injections at intervals of less than four days are unnecessary (30). Forest et al. randomized 183 cryptorchid boys to two protocols: one group receiving 1500 IU every other day, and the other group receiving 100 IU/kg at four- to five-day intervals (30). Testosterone rose to normal levels, and the success of treatment was similar between the groups. Several studies demonstrated a continued rise in plasma testosterone after a single injection of hCG, which peaked at four days. Further hCG injections within this period have little additional stimulatory effect. The frequency of injections also does not seem to be significant (30–32). Hesse and Ficher showed that the same total dose given in three injections of hCG was as effective as 10 smaller dose injections of hCG in the treatment of cryptorchidism (33).

Age seems to be significant in the response rate: response rates are reportedly the least successful prior to the first year of life (26). The descent was 15% at two to five years, versus 44% at 10 to 14 years (34). Garagorri et al. found only a 9% success rate in patients aged 6 to 35 months (35). The position of the testicle at the time of treatment seems to be important: the lower the testicle, the higher the reported success rate. Canlorbe et al. reported a success rate of 47.6% in testes located in the inguinal area, but only a 20% success rate with abdominal testes (36). A retractile testis is likely to be a confounding factor. After treatment, return of the testis to its pretreatment condition has been reported; therefore, follow-up of these cryptorchid patients is required (37). Some authors have advocated a second course of hCG, quoting some partial success, although others believe that a second course is useless (37–39).

In Europe, the effects of GnRH via nasal spray in cryptorchid children have been studied. Gonadotropin response to GnRH given intranasally was studied in the 1970s (40,41). Those studies demonstrated a maximum LH response with 2.5 mg of GnRH, but also showed a significant LH response with as little as 200 μg of GnRH (34). The results with this form of treatment, however, vary widely. In a double-blind placebo-controlled study of GnRH nasal spray, 237 cryptorchid children were evaluated by two examiners in an attempt to isolate patients with retractile testes. Children with obviously ectopic (penile, perineal, or femoral) testes were also excluded, as were children with an inguinal hernia or chromosomal or dysmorphic syndromes. There was no statistical difference in the success rate of testicular descent between the placebo group (8%) and the GnRH treatment group (9%) (42).

There are several points to consider regarding the present status of hormonal treatment in cryptorchid children. Nearly all investigators agree that hormonal manipulation works best in older children (high success rate in children more than seven years old) (13). There is histologic evidence that germ cell damage is well established by the age of two, with 40% of testes demonstrating azoospermia (43–45). In addition, several double-blind hormonal treatment studies show little or no benefit in the treatment of truly cryptorchid testes. Perhaps the main role of hormonal treatment is to identify the retractile testis from the truly undescended testis (26,46,47). Some authors have studied the effects of early hormonal treatment on germinal epithelium and have shown a detrimental effect (48).

Surgical Treatment

Surgical therapy is successful in 90% of patients with nonpalpable testes and in over 90% of patients with palpable testes (49). Most authors recommend surgical treatment after the age of 6 months but before 18 months (13). Surgery affords the best chance of germinal epithelium preservation, yet only 30% of pediatricians and 14% of family practitioners recommend orchiopexy between 6 and 12 months of age (50). It may be, however, that the cryptorchid testis follows a predetermined course of germinal atrophy secondary to an embryologic abnormality. The results of current early surgical interventions will not be seen until these children are beyond puberty. Nevertheless, surgery obviates the need for a series of injections and long-term or frequent follow-up to evaluate for possible testicular ascent after successful hormonal therapy.

At the time of surgery and just after the administration of general anesthesia, the child should be reexamined to detect a truly retractile testis. If the cryptorchid testis (testes) is palpable, a horizontal inguinal incision is made along Langer's line. The testicle and its vascular supply are carefully identified. Usually, there is an associated patent processus vaginalis that is dissected free, and a high ligation of the hernia sac is performed at the level of the internal inguinal ring. Many inguinally located cryptorchid testes will have sufficient length to reach the scrotum at this point. A subdartos pouch is made with a small scrotal incision. The testicle is then brought down to the scrotum and placed into this pocket just beneath the scrotal skin. Careful inspection of the spermatic cord should be performed to ensure that it is not twisted. If the length of the spermatic cord is inadequate to reach the scrotum, an additional 1 to 2 cm may be obtained by mobilizing the spermatic cord from the transversalis fascia. This is performed by mobilizing the testicular artery and vein beyond the internal inguinal ring. Occasionally, a Prentice maneuver is performed, in which the testicle and spermatic cord are rerouted in a more direct path of descent. This is done by bringing the testicle around the inferior epigastric vessels and through the floor of Hasselbach's triangle at the level of the pubic tubercle. This maneuver can gain an additional 1 to 2 cm of length.

If the preoperative examination demonstrates a unilateral impalpable testis, then the possibility of gonadal absence should be discussed with the parents. The use of a testicular prosthesis should also be discussed. Because of the recent leakage problems occurring with similar breast prostheses, a moratorium was placed on the implantation of gel-filled silicone testicular prostheses in the United States; these are no longer being manufactured. Presently, solid or saline-jelled silicone prosthetic devices are being used.

Laparoscopy continues to have a greater role in the diagnosis and treatment of the nonpalpable testis. In the case of a unilateral nonpalpable testis, laparoscopy will demonstrate its position, and may be helpful in planning therapy. If a testis is located at the level of or just proximal to the internal inguinal ring, two options are available to the surgeon. A standard laparoscopic-assisted one-stage orchiopexy may be performed. If the testicle appears to have insufficient length for obtaining a good intrascrotal position, or appears higher in the abdomen, a two-stage orchiopexy, termed the Fowler–Stephens procedure (in which the testicular vessels are ligated and the testicle is mobilized on a peritoneal flap with collateral blood supply from the deferential artery), or a microvascular reanastomosis may be planned. In many instances, an intra-abdominal testis can be brought down into the scrotum in one stage by dissecting the vas deferens and vessels retroperitoneally. This procedure can be performed either with a standard open surgery technique or laparoscopically. Both authors currently are performing these surgeries laparoscopically. Atrophied intra-abdominal testes may be removed at the time of initial laparoscopy. Over the past several years, the authors have favored the two-stage orchiopexy for intra-abdominal testes. It is their belief that an excellent scrotal position can be uniformly obtained during the second stage without compromising testicular survival. The one-stage orchiopexy procedure for intra-abdominal testes is often associated with an insufficient length to obtain a tension-free position in the dependent portion of the hemiscrotum. Other authors have reported similar experiences using the two-stage procedure, with good testicular survival (51–53).

In 1975, Martin and Menck addressed the issue of the risk of surgery for postpubertal cryptorchid testis and the relationship to the risk of testicular cancer (54). Farrer et al. reexamined this issue in 1985 by using germ cell testis tumor mortality data (55). It was recommended that postpubertal men less than 32 years of age should undergo orchiectomy, whereas men more than 32 years of age should be observed with frequent examinations.

Surgical complications include a high-riding testis, bleeding, hematoma, infections, and an injury to either the vasculature or the vas deferens. Long-term findings include tunica albuginea calcifications and hypoechogenic cysts (56).

Complications of Cryptorchidism

The naturally acquired complications of cryptorchidism are infertility and testicular cancer. Infertility tends to have a more pronounced effect in cryptorchid patients because it is so much more prevalent in this population compared with testicular cancer. Elder et al. found oligospermia in 31% of both unilateral and bilateral cryptorchid patients (57). They reported azoospermia in 14% of patients with unilateral cryptorchidism and in 42% of patients with bilateral cryptorchidism. A 65% to 89% pregnancy rate was noted in patients with unilateral cryptorchidism, compared with a 50% to 60% pregnancy rate in those with bilateral cryptorchidism (58). Some evidence is beginning to accumulate that early orchiopexy may preserve fertility. Ludwig and Potempa studied patients who underwent orchiopexy between the ages of 1 and 13 years (59). Patients who underwent surgery between the ages of one and two years had a fertility rate of 87.5%. The fertility rate of the children operated on between the ages of three and four years was 44%. Puri and O'Donnell noted normal sperm counts in 74% of boys with unilateral cryptorchidism and in 30% with bilateral cryptorchidism, all treated between the ages of 7 and 14 years (60).

Testicular cancer is the other major sequela of cryptorchidism. Of all patients diagnosed with testicular cancer, 7.3% have a history of cryptorchidism (52). In addition, a man with cryptorchidism has a 9.7 times greater chance of dying from testicular cancer. In unilateral cryptorchidism, testicular cancer will arise in the contralateral and normally descended testis in 20% of cases (25). The prevalence of carcinoma in situ in men with a history of cryptorchidism is 2% to 3% (61). Orchiopexy does not appear to affect the incidence of

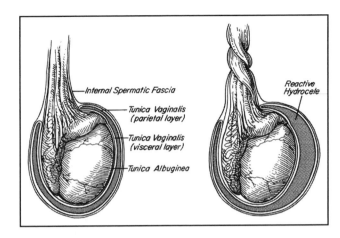

Figure 2 Extravaginal torsion. The testicle twists upon the spermatic cord outside the attachments of the tunica vaginalis. This occurs primarily in the neonatal period.

subsequent testicular cancer. The risk of cancer correlates with the degree of cryptorchidism; therefore, patients with an intra-abdominal testis carry the highest risk of developing testicular malignancy.

☐ TESTICULAR TORSION
Introduction

Testicular torsion, which leads to vascular compromise of the testicular parenchyma, may be due to two different mechanisms. In extravaginal torsion, which occurs mainly in the neonatal setting, the testicle twists upon the spermatic cord or outside the investing tunica vaginalis (Fig. 2). In intravaginal torsion (Fig. 3), which occurs mainly in the pubertal period, the testicle twists upon its vasculature within the investing tunica vaginalis.

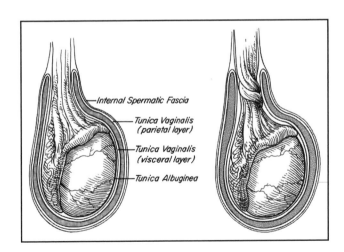

Figure 3 Intravaginal torsion. The testicle twists upon its vasculature within the investing tunica vaginalis. This occurs primarily in the pubertal age group and is often associated with a bell-clapper deformity.

Incidence

A bimodal frequency of occurrence of testicular torsion is evident, with one peak in the perinatal period and the other at puberty (62). Some authors have reported an increase in the incidence of testicular torsion. Anderson and Williamson reviewed 670 patients with torsion of the spermatic cord who presented between 1960 and 1984 (63). They found that the diagnosis of testicular torsion in patients presenting with testicular pain increased fourfold from 11.2% between 1960 and 1964 to 42.8% between 1980 and 1984, probably secondary to an increased awareness of this condition by general practitioners. The testicular salvage rate improved from 17% between 1960 and 1964 to 67% between 1980 and 1984, mainly due to earlier recognition and intervention (63). Overall, the risk of developing torsion of the testicle or its appendages by the age of 25 years has been reported to be about 1 in 160 (64).

Testicular torsion may also occur in the undescended testis. The undescended testis may be more prone to torsion secondary to abnormal mesorchial attachments (5). The child with unexplained abdominal pain with no history of urologic surgery and an empty scrotum should be considered to have torsion of an intra-abdominal testis until proven otherwise.

Neonatal Torsion

Neonatal torsion is well recognized, and accounts for approximately 12% of all cases of testicular torsion. The term "neonatal torsion" has been used to describe both prenatal and postnatal torsion. Some of these may account for the entity known as testicular agenesis (vanishing testis) in the older child. Neonatal torsion does not seem to correlate with birth weight, prematurity, perinatal trauma, or the method of delivery, and is nearly always asymptomatic (65,66). Generally, the examination demonstrates an edematous, ecchymotic hemiscrotum that does not transilluminate. A simultaneous rectal examination and abdominal examination should be performed to exclude an incarcerated inguinal hernia. Nuclear scans show decreased perfusion and decreased radio-isotope uptake on the affected side in more than 95% of cases (67). The affected testis appears unhomogeneously hypoechoic, with a surrounding brightly echogenic rim (68). Nevertheless, these studies may be technically inadequate in the neonate due to the small testicular size (69). (For further details of imaging of the male reproductive tract, see Chapter 28.)

The cause of neonatal torsion is believed to be, in part, secondary to the hypermobility and elasticity of the perinatal testicular tissue, which is not fixed in the scrotum until the first several days of life (70). Therefore, most cases of postnatal torsion occur within the first 10 days after birth (65).

If the newborn has a normal scrotal examination at birth and later develops signs of testicular torsion, he should be treated as a surgical emergency in the hope of maximizing testicular salvage (69). Surgical exploration in a neonate with prenatal torsion is recommended on an elective basis. This recommendation is based on findings that irreversible testicular damage has already occurred at the time of presentation (18). Controversy remains over the management of the contralateral testes in babies with prenatal torsion. Some believe that contralateral fixation is not necessary, whereas others believe that it needs to be undertaken promptly (71). Bilateral testicular torsion has been reported in both synchronous (without delay) and asynchronous (delayed) fashions (72–74). At Children's Hospital in Boston, Massachusetts, the authors have observed three patients with asynchronous bilateral testicular torsion (69,74). One nine-hour-old baby with prenatal unilateral torsion was rendered anorchid when the contralateral testis torsed (71). Therefore, prompt but elective exploration is recommended to perform a contralateral orchiopexy, which may protect the remaining testicular tissue. In addition, prompt exploration removes the torsed testicle, which potentially may alter future fertility by immunologic means. The surgical approach should be inguinal if a testicular malignancy is suspected.

Pubertal Torsion

As the term implies, this condition occurs around puberty, and the incidence declines from puberty to childhood. Only 50 cases have been reported after the age of 30 years (75). The diagnosis is associated with the horizontal lie of the testicle, also known as the bell-clapper deformity (76,77). Failure of the normal posterior anchoring of the gubernaculum epididymis and testis is called a bell-clapper deformity because it leaves the testis free to swing and rotate within the tunica vaginalis of the scrotum much like the clapper of a bell. The incidence of the bell-clapper deformity was as high as 12% of all men in one autopsy series (78). There is a statistically significant increased incidence of torsion in the colder months, presumably secondary to cremasteric contractions.

The differential diagnosis of a child with testicular torsion includes appendiceal torsion, epididymitis, testicular trauma, tumor, polyorchidism, incarcerated inguinal hernia, Henoch–Schonlein purpura, acute hydronephrosis, funiculitis, and idiopathic scrotal edema. Henoch–Schonlein purpura is a vasculitis that may involve the scrotum and may mimic testicular torsion (79).

The most important aspect in discerning the correct diagnosis is the history and physical examination. Information such as the duration of symptoms, character and quality of pain, associated nausea or vomiting, time of onset of symptoms, activity at the time of initial symptoms, and the patient response to symptoms are all important. A history of trauma is important, but does not rule out torsion (80). A history of prior testicular surgery decreases the chance of acute torsion. There have been reported cases of testicular torsion, however, despite prior orchiopexy, even if nonabsorbable sutures were used (81–83). A history of prior episodes of scrotal pain that occurs suddenly but rapidly resolves is suggestive of intermittent torsion. Up to 50% of patients with acute torsion have experienced previous episodes of acute testicular pain. The family history of torsion may be helpful because familial torsion of the testicle has been reported (84).

Pubertal torsion presents in stark contrast to neonatal torsion. The patient experiences hemiscrotal pain, abdominal pain, or both. Nausea is common. The symptoms are usually sudden in onset. Physical examination usually shows an elevated hemiscrotum. Palpation of the upper scrotum or inguinal canal may demonstrate a thickened or twisted spermatic cord. Next, an attempt to elicit the cremasteric reflex should be made by gently stroking the inner thigh, which should cause the ipsilateral hemiscrotum to contract. In a series spanning seven years and involving 245 boys with acute scrotal swelling, a 100% correlation between the presence of the ipsilateral cremasteric reflex and the absence of testicular torsion was noted (85). The absence of the cremasteric reflex, however, was not diagnostic of torsion, because other conditions that cause absence of the reflex may be present (acute hernia, hydrocele, testicular tumor, and testicular leukemia). The scrotum should be observed for a "blue-dot sign," an aid to diagnosis of a torsed or necrotic appendage of the testis. The blue-dot sign is a blue to purple discoloration of the scrotum caused by a torsed and ischemic appendix testis or appendix epididymis. The blue-dot sign is most easily visible during the first few hours following the torsion and particularly in fair skinned boys. If the blue-dot sign is seen and the testis is palpably normal, the patient has torsion of an appendix. Analgesics usually are sufficient treatment. Laboratory examination should include a complete blood count and urinalysis. Leukocytosis and pyuria suggest an infectious cause, such as epididymitis or epididymo-orchitis.

Manual detorsion may be attempted. The torsed testicle twists in a lateral to medial fashion. The physician may completely or partially relieve the torsion by rotating the testis from medial to lateral within the scrotal sac. This rotation does not obviate emergent or urgent surgery, but may help in testicular salvage (86).

There is currently no diagnostic test to establish the diagnosis of torsion unequivocally. The criticism of imaging studies lies in their time consumption and subsequent delay in surgery, which can cause decreased testicular salvage rates. Good imaging studies, however, can certainly be helpful in diagnosis. Color Doppler sonography is a good imaging modality, particularly in those cases in which the physical examination and history are equivocal. Burks et al. reported that color Doppler was 86% sensitive, 100% specific, and 97% accurate in the diagnosis of torsion (87). Nevertheless, false-negative Doppler examinations have been reported in patients with testicular torsion, and the study is operator-dependent (88). With nuclear scans, the scintigraphic pattern in torsion varies depending on the degree of torsion (89). In spite of these limitations, scrotal imaging is relatively accurate (90,91). Nuclear MRI has also been used to diagnose torsion and to differentiate torsion from epididymitis (92). Its use, however, is limited, because of the need for sedation in young children and the fact that other, less expensive imaging modalities are available.

Treatment of the torsed testicle is surgical exploration. The viability of the testicle at the time of surgery will dictate whether orchiopexy or orchiectomy is performed. This is determined by gross inspection of the testicle before and after detorsion. After manual detorsion, the testicle is wrapped in a warm saline-soaked sponge while fixation of the contralateral testis is performed. Contralateral scrotal exploration and fixation are essential, particularly because torsion of the contralateral testis as high as 40% has been reported in one series (15). There have been no reports of testicular loss as a result of septopexy, a type of surgery to keep the testis placed well down in the scrotum without tension. After the contralateral orchiopexy has been performed, the testicle is unwrapped. If the degree of viability is still questionable, a small incision is made in the tunica albuginea to observe for bleeding. If there is no bleeding, most surgeons will remove the testicle.

Prognosis

It is well established that the ratio of ischemia determines testicular salvage. Testicular size correlates primarily with germinal epithelial mass. The supporting cells (Sertoli and Leydig) account for a small percentage of the testicular volume and are more resistant to ischemic damage than the germinal epithelium (93). Four hours of ischemia time causes irreversible damage to dog spermatogonia (germinal epithelium), whereas 8 to 10 hours of ischemia may cause irreversible damage to the Sertoli and Leydig cells (94). Testicular salvage rates decreased to less than 20% in patients explored 12 hours after the onset of symptoms (15,95).

There is a reported age delay in the presentation of testicular torsion, and a subsequent decline in the rate of testicular salvage. Berada et al. noted that male patients less than 18 years of age presented 20 hours (median time) after the onset of symptoms (96). Male patients older than 18 years presented four hours (median time) after the onset of symptoms. The incidence of orchiectomy in the two groups was considerably higher in the younger age group (44% vs. 8%). This difference may be related to the younger age group's dependency on adults for access to medical care. Therefore, this group should be targeted for improved health education regarding the early evaluation of scrotal pain.

Assuming that the testicle is viable at the time of surgery, what is the effect on fertility from its ischemic episode? Endocrine function (testosterone production from the Leydig cells) appears to be unaffected if the testis remains viable (97). Exocrine function (spermatogenesis) has been reported to be abnormal, however, suggesting that the ischemic event has affected the contralateral testis (97). Antisperm antibodies have been implicated as a result of the exposure of testicular tissue androgens to the bloodstream after the ischemic event (97). Detection of antisperm antibodies after torsion is variable (98–100). Many reports have confirmed abnormal semen analysis after acute testicular torsion (101–103). Anderson and Williamson suggest that there may be a congenital bilateral defect in spermatogenesis associated with the (bell-clapper) deformity in the hypermobile testis. In support of this theory, biopsies of the contralateral testis at the time of orchiopexy have demonstrated histologic abnormalities in as high as 53% of patients (98,104,105). Additional work is being performed in this area to further assess the late effects of testicular torsion.

☐ TORSION OF THE TESTICULAR APPENDAGES
Introduction

The testicular appendages are also subject to torsion. The appendix testis is a remnant from the regressed mullerian duct, and is located at the upper pole of the testis. The appendix epididymis is a remnant of the partially regressed mesonephric duct, and is located at the head of the epididymis. Torsion of these appendages may cause scrotal pain and present as an acute scrotum. The history and physical are important to help distinguish this entity from torsion of the testicle. Tenderness localized to the upper pole of the testis, a necrotic appendage visualized through the scrotal skin, and an assessment of the cremasteric reflex all help to better determine the correct diagnosis.

Treatment

If the diagnosis of torsion of the appendage can be made with confidence, then conservative therapy may be instituted. This includes the use of analgesics for pain control, a decreased level of activity, and an ice pack over the affected area. Prompt surgical exploration is necessary to exclude torsion of the testicle if scrotal swelling obscures the diagnosis and radiologic tests are inconclusive (105).

Prognosis

The prognosis is excellent with no known untoward sequelae.

☐ REFERENCES

1. Scorer CG. The descent of the testis. Arch Dis 1964; 39:605.
2. John Radcliffe Cryptorchidism Study Group. Cryptorchidism: an apparent substantial increase since 1960. Br Med J 1986; 293:1401.
3. Hadziselimovic F. Cryptorchidism: Management and Implications. New York: Springer-Verlag, 1983:20.
4. Kaefer M, Diamond D, Hendren WH, et al. The incidence of intersexuality in children with cryptorchidism and hypospadias: stratification based on gonadal palpability and meatal position. J Urol 1999; 162(3 Pt 2):1003.
5. Johnston JH. The undescended testicle: a review article. Arch Dis Child 1965; 40:113.
6. Wells LJ. Descent of the testis: anatomical and hormonal considerations. Surgery 1943; 14:436.
7. Hutson JM, Beasley SW. Embryologic controversies in testicular descent. Vaughan ED, ed. Semin Urol 1988; 6(2):68.
8. Wensig CJG. The embryology of testicular descent. Horm Res 1988; 30(4–5):144.
9. Hutson JM, Donahue PK, MacLaughlin DT. Steroid modulation of Mullerian duct regression in the chick embryo. Gen Comp Endrocrinol 1985; 57(1):88.
10. MacLauglin DT, Hutson JM, Donahoe PK. Specific estradiol binding in embryonic Mullerian ducts: a potential modulation of regression in the male and female chick. Endocrinology 1983; 113(1):141.
11. Rajfer J. Hormonal regulation of testicular descent. Eur J Pediatr 1987; 146(suppl 2):6.
12. Mininberg DT. The epididymis and testicular descent. Eur J Pediatr 1987; 146(suppl 2):28.
13. Palmer JM. The undescended testis. Endocrinol Metab Clin North Am 1991; 20(1):231.
14. Job JC, Toublanc JE, Chaussain J, et al. The pituitary-gonadal axis in cryptorchid infants and children. Eur J Pediatr 1987; 146:S2.
15. Workman ST, Kogan BA. Old and new aspects of testicular torsion. Semin Urology 1988; 6(2):146.
16. Job JC, Toublanc JE, Chaussain J, et al. Endocrine and immunological findings in cryptorchid infants. Horm Res 1988; 30(4–5):167.
17. Walsh PC, Curry N, Mills RC, et al. Plasma androgen response to hCG stimulation in prepubertal boys with hypospadias and cryptorchidism. J Clin Endocrinol Metab 1976; 42(1):52.
18. Cacciari E, Cicognani A, Pirazoll P, et al. Hypophysogondal function in the cryptorchid child: difference between unilateral and bilateral cryptorchids. Acta Endocrinol (Copenh) 1976; 83(1):182.
19. Caesar RE, Kaplan GW. The incidence of the cremasteric reflex in normal boys. J Urol 1994; 152 (2 Pt 2):779.

20. Rabinowitz R, Hulbert WC Jr. Late presentation of cryptorchidism: the etiology of testicular re-ascent. J Urol 1997; 157(5):1892.

21. Davenport M, Brain C, Vandenberg C, et al. The use of the hCG stimulation test in the endocrine evaluation of cryptorchidism. Brit J Urol 1995; 76(6):790.

22. Polascik TJ, Chan-Tack KM, Jeffs RD, et al. Reappraisal of the role of human chorionic gonadotropin in the diagnosis and treatment of the nonpalpable testis: a 10-year experience. J Urol 1996; 156(2 Pt 2):804.

23. Lee MM, Donahoe PK, Silverman BL, et al. Measurement of serum mullerian inhibiting substance in the evaluation of children with nonpalpable gonads. New Eng J Med 1997; 336(21):1480.

24. Ascheim S, Zondek B. Die schwangerschafts diagnose ausdem harn durch nachweis des hypophysenvorder-lappenhormons. II: praktische und theoretische ergeb-nisse aus den harnuntersuchungen. Klin Wochenschr 1928; 31:1453.

25. Saenger P, Reiter EO. Management of cryptorchidism. Trends Endocrinol Metab 1992; 3(2):249.

26. De Muinck Keizer-Schrama SM, Hazebroek FW. Hormonal treatment of cryptorchidism: role of pitui-tary gonadal axis. Semin Urol 1988; 6(2):84.

27. Thompson WO, Bevan AD, Heckel NJ, et al. The treat-ment of undescended testes with anterior pituitary-like substance. Endocrinology 1937; 21:220.

28. Deming CL. The evaluation of hormonal therapy in cryptorchidism J Urol 1952; 68(1):354.

29. Contafonieri A, DellaMorte E, Gunbacorta M, et al. Treatment of cryptorchidism. A survery of the results in the Department of Urology, Hospital of Deslo (1968–1978). In: Bierich JR, Giarola A, eds. Cryptorchidism. New York/London: Academic Press, 1979:469.

30. Forest MG, David M, David C, et al. Undescended testis in comparison of two protocols of treatment with human chorionic gonadotropin. Horm Res 1988; 30(4–5):198.

31. Dunkel L, Perheentupa J, Apter D. Kinetics of the steri-odongenic response to single versus repeated doses of human chorionic gonadotropin in boys in prepuberty and early puberty. Pediatr Res 1985; 19(1):1.

32. Forest MG, David M, Leconq A, et al. Kinetics of the hCG induced steriodogenic response of the human testis: III. Studies in children of the plasma levels of testosterone and hCG: Rationale for testicular stimula-tion test. Pediatr Res 1980; 14(6):819.

33. Hesse V, Fischer G. Three injections of human chori-onic gonadotropin are as effective as ten injections in the treatment of cryptorchidism. Horm Res 1988; 30(4–5):193.

34. Rajfer J, Darrer JH, Xie HW, et al. Response of pituitary gland to increasing doses of intranasal gonadotropin-releasing hormone. Fertil Steril 1984; 42(2):327.

35. Garagorri JM, Job JC, Canlorbe P, et al. Results in early treatment of cryptorchidism with human chorionic gonadotropin. J Pediatr 1982; 101(6):923.

36. Canlorbe P, La Clyde JP, Toublanc JE, et al. Results of treatment with hCG in cryptorchidism. Pediatric Adolescent Endocrinol 1979; 6:167.

37. Forest MG, David M, Francois R. Treatment of cryp-torchidism, Brussels, Imprimerle des Sciences. 1985; 45.

38. Dickerman Z, Bauman B, Sandovsky U, et al. Human chorionic gonadotropin (hCG) treatment in cryp-torchidism. Andrologia 1983; 15:542.

39. Pagliano Sassi L. Significance and results of medical treatment in cryptorchidism. In: Bierich JR, Giarola A, eds. Cryptorchidism. New York: Academic Press, 1979:435.

40. Bergada C, Mancini RE. Effects of gonadotropins in the induction of spermatogenesis in human prepuber-tal testis. J Clin Endocrinol Metab 1973; 37(6):935.

41. Dahlen HG, Keller E, Schneider HPG. Linear dose dependent LH release following intranasally sprayed LRH. Horm Res 1974; 6(6):510.

42. De Muinck Kelzer-Schrama SM, Hazebroek FW, Matroos AW, et al. Double-blinded, placebo-control-led study of luteinizing hormone-releasing hormone nasal spray in treatment of undescended testis. Lancet 1986; 1(8486):876.

43. Hadziselmovic F. Cryptorchidism. In: Gillenwater JG, Grayhack TT, Howards SS, et al., eds. Adult and Pediatric Urology. Chicago: Yearbook Medical Publishers, 1987.

44. Hadziselmovic F, Girard J, Herzog B. Lack of germ cells and endocrinology in cryptorchid boys from one to six years of life. In: Bierich JR, Giarola A, eds. Cryptorchidism. New York: Academic Press, 1979:129.

45. Mengel W, Heinz HA, Sipe WG, et al. Studies on cryp-torchidism: a comparison of histological findings in the germinative epithelium before and after the second year of life. J Pediatr Surg 1974; 9(4):445.

46. Christiansen P, Muller J, Buhl S. Treatment of cryp-torchidism with human chorionic gonadotropin or gonadotropin releasing hormone. Horm Res 1988; 30(4–5):187.

47. Rajfer J, Handelsman D, Swerdloff R, et al. Hormonal therapy of cryptorchidism: a randomized, double-blinded study comparing human chorionic gonado-tropin and gonadotropin-releasing hormone. N Engl J Med 1986; 314(8):446.

48. Cortes D, Thorup J, Visfeldt J. Hormonal treatment may harm the germ cells in 1 to 3-year-old boys with cryptorchidism. J Urol 2000; 163(4):1290.

49. Kogan SJ, Saenger P. Cryptorchidism. In: Barden W, ed. Current Therapy in Endocrinology and Metabolism. 3rd ed. Philadelphia: BC Decker, 1988:236.

50. Steckler RE, Zaontz MR, Skoog SJ, et al. Cryptorchidism, pediatricians, and family practitioners: patterns of practice and referral. J Pediatrics 1995; 127(6):948.

51. Caldamone AA, Amaral JF. Laparoscopic stage 2 Fowler-Stephens orchiopexy. J Urol 1994; 152(4):1253.

52. Law GS, Perex LM, Joseph DB. Two stage Fowler-Stephens orchiopexy with laparoscopic clipping of the spermatic vessels. J Urol 1997; 158(3 Pt 2):1205.

53. Esposito C, Garipoli V. The value of 2-step laparoscopic Fowler-Stephens orchiopexy for intra-abdominal testes. J Urol 1997; 158(5):152.

54. Martin DC, Menck HR. The undescended testis: management after puberty. J Urol 1975; 114(1):77.

55. Farrer JH, Walker AH, Rajfer J. Management of the postpubertal cryptorchid testis: a statistical review. J Urol 1985; 134(6):1071.

56. Ward JF, Cilento BG Jr, Kaplan GW, et al. The ultrasonic description of postpubertal testicles in men who have undergone prepubertal orchiopexy for cryptorchidism. J Urol 2000; 163(5):1448.

57. Elder JS. The undescended testes: hormonal and surgical management. Surg Clin North Am 1988; 68(5):983.

58. Lee PA, O'leary LA, Songer NJ, et al. Paternity after bilateral cryptorchidism. A controlled study. Arch Pediatr and Adol Med 1997; 151(3):260.

59. Ludwig G, Potempa J. Der optmale zeit punkt der behandlung des kryptochismus. Dstch Med Wochenscher 1975; 100(13):680.

60. Puri P, O'Donnell B. Semen analysis of patients who had orchiopexy at or after seven years of age. Lancet 1988; 2(8619):1051.

61. Giweunan A, Brunn E, Frimoldt-Muller C, et al. Prevalence of carcinoma in situ and other histopathological abnormalities in testes of males with a history of cryptorchidism. J Urol 1989; 142(4):998.

62. Melekos MD, Asbach HW, Markou SA. Etiology of acute scrotum in 100 boys with regard to age distribution. J Urol 1988; 139(5):1023.

63. Anderson JB, Williamson RC. Testicular torsion in Bristol: a 25 year review. Br J Surg 1988; 75(10):988.

64. Williamson RCN. Torsion of the testis and allied conditions. Br J Surg 1976; 63:465(6).

65. Das S, Singer A. Controversies of perinatal torsion of the spermatic cord: a review. Survey and recommendations. J Urol 1990; 143(2):231.

66. Huff DS, WU H, Synder HMN, et al. Evidence in favor of the mechanical (intrauterine) theory over the endocrinopathy (cryptorchidism) theory in the pathogenesis of testicular agenesis. J Urol 1991; 146(2 Pt 2):630.

67. Rodriguez DD, Rodriguez WC, Rivera JJ, et al. Doppler ultrasound versus testicular scanning in the evaluation of the acute scrotum. J Urol 1981; 125(3):343.

68. Zerin JM, DiPetro MA, Grignon A, et al. Testicular infarction in the newborn: ultrasound findings. Pediatr Radiol 1990; 20(5):329.

69. Atala A, Retik AB. The contralateral testis: hazards of management. Dialogues Pediatri Urol 1991; 14(5):5.

70. Campbell MF. The male genital tract and the female urethra. In: Campbell MF, Harrison JH, eds. Urology. 3rd ed. Philadelphia: WB Saunders, 1970:1834.

71. Feins NR. To pex or not to pex. J Pediatr Surg 1983; 18(6):697.

72. Barker K, Raper FP. Torsion of the testis. Br J Urol 1964; 36:35.

73. Kay R, Strong DW, Tank ES. Bilateral spermatic cord torsion in the neonate. J Urol 1980; 123(2):293.

74. LaQuaglia MP, Bauer SB, Eraklis A, et al. Bilateral neonatal torsion. J Urol 1987; 138(4 Pt 2):1051.

75. Perry S, Hoopinger D, Askins D. Testicular torsion in the older patient. Ann Emerg Med 1983; 12(5):319.

76. Coulere J. Horizontal lie of the testicle: a diagnostic sign in torsion of the testis. J Urol 1972; 107(4):616.

77. Schulsinger D, Glassberg K, Strashun A. Intermittent torsion: association with horizontal lie of the testicle. J Urol 1991; 145(5):1053.

78. Caesar RE, Kaplan GW. The incidence of the bell-clapper deformity in an autopsy series. Urology 1994; 44(1):114.

79. Laor T, Atala A, Teele RL. Scrotal sonography in Henoch-Schonlein purpura. Pediatr Radiol 1992; 22(7):505.

80. Cos LR, Rabinowitz R. Trauma-induce testicular torsion in children. J Traum 1982; 22(3):244.

81. Hulecki ST, Crawford JP, Broeker B. Testicular torsion after orchiopexy with nonabsorbable sutures. Urology 1986; 28(2):131.

82. Kossow AS. Torsion following orchiopexy. NY State J Med 1980; 80(7 Pt 1):1136.

83. May RE, Thomas WE. Recurrent torsion of the testis following previous surgical fixation. Br J Surg 1980; 67(2):129.

84. Stewart JO, Maiti AK. Familial torsion of the testicle. Br J Urol 1985; 57(2):190.

85. Rabinowitz R. The importance of the cremasteric reflex in acute scrotal swelling in children. J Urol 1984; 132(1):89.

86. Frazier WJ, Bucy JG. Manipulation of torsion of the testicle. J Urol 1975; 114(3):410.

87. Burks DD, Markey BJ, Burkhard TK, et al. Suspected testicular torsion and ischemia: evaluation with color doppler sonography. Radiology 1990; 175(3):815.

88. Nasrallah PF, Manzone D, King LR. Falsely negative Doppler examinations in testicular torsion. J Urol 1977; 118 (1 Pt 2):194.

89. Majd M. Nuclear medicine in pediatric urology. In: Kelalis PP, King LR, Belman AB, eds. Clinical Pediatric Urology. Philadelphia: W.B. Saunders, 1992:117.

90. Lutzker LG. The fine points of scrotal scintigraphy. Semin Nuc Med 1982; 12(4):387.

91. Paltiel HJ, Connollu LP, Atala A, et al. Acute scrotal symptoms in boys with a indeterminate clinical presentation: comparison of color Doppler sonography and scintigraphy. Radiology 1998; 207(1):223.

92. Trambert MA, Mattrey RF, Levine D, et al. Subacute scrotal pain: evaluation of torsion versus epididymitis with MR imaging. Radiology 1990; 175(1):53.

93. Mikuz G. Testicular torsion: simple grading for histological evaluation of tissue damage. App Path 1985; 3(3):134.

94. Smith GI. Cellular changes from grading testicular ischemia. J Urol 1955; 73(2):355.

95. Donohue RE, Utley WLF. Torsion of spermatic cord. Urology 1978; 11(1):33.

96. Barada JH, Weingarten JL, Cromie WJ. Testicular salvage and age-related delay in the presentation of testicular torsion. J Urol 1989; 142(3):746.

97. Anderson JB, Williamson RCN. Fertility after torsion of the spermatic cord. Br J Urol 1990; 65(3):225.

98. Cerasaro TS, Nachtsheim DA, Otero F, et al. The effect of testicular torsion on contralateral testis and the production of antisperm antibodies in rabbits. J Urol 1984; 132(3):577.

99. Hadziselmovic F, Synder H, Duckett J, et al. Testicular histology in children with unilateral testicular torsion. J Urol 1986; 136(1 Pt 2):208.

100. Ryan PC, Fitzpatrick JM. Experimental testicular torsion: do spermatozoal autoantigens cause immunological activation. World J Urol 1986; 4(4):92.

101. Bartsch G, Frank S, Marberger H, et al. Testicular torsion: late results with special regard to fertility and endocrine function. J Urol 1980; 124(3):375.

102. Mastrogiacomo I, Zanchetta R, Graziotti P, et al. Immunological and clinical study in patients after spermatic cord torsion. Andrologia 1982; 14(1):25.

103. Thomas WEG, Cooper MJ, Crane GA, et al. Testicular exocrine malfunction after torsion. Lancet 1984; 2(8416):1357.

104. Horica CA, Hadziselmovic F, Kreutz G, et al. Ultrastructural studies of the contorted and contralateral testicle in unilateral testicular torsion. Eur Urol 1982; 8(6):358.

105. Holland JM, Graham JB, Ignatoff JM. Conservative management of twisted testicular appendages. J Urol 1981; 125(2):213.

14

Disorders of Male Puberty

Erick J. Richmond
Pediatric Oncology, National Children's Hospital, San Jose, Costa Rica

Alan D. Rogol
Clinical Pediatrics, University of Virginia, Charlottesville, Virginia, U.S.A.

☐ DEFINITION OF PUBERTY

Puberty is the period during which sexual maturity is reached, resulting in the capacity for reproduction. It involves the growth and maturation of the primary sexual characteristics (gonads and genitals) and the appearance of secondary sexual characteristics (including sexual hair and voice change).

A study of more than 17,000 healthy 3- to 12-year-old girls sponsored by the American Academy of Pediatrics suggests that puberty occurs at an earlier age today than in the past (1). Consequently, a change in the lower limit of puberty in girls (from eight to seven years of age in whites, and six years of age in African-Americans) was proposed recently by the Lawson Wilkins Pediatric Endocrine Society (2). On the other hand, two recent studies in boys (3,4) did not show a distinct trend toward earlier maturation, and in one of them (4), the investigators did not find a significant difference in the timing of puberty based on race. Thus, puberty continues to be considered normal in boys if it starts after the age of 9 years and before the age of 13.5 years.

☐ PHYSIOLOGY OF NORMAL PUBERTY
Physical Changes
Secondary Sexual Characteristics

The method described by Tanner (stages 1–5) (5) is the most utilized throughout the world for assessing sexual maturation. The stages are defined by physical measurements of development based on external primary and secondary sexual characteristics, such as the size of the breasts and genitalia, and the development of pubic hair. Although pubic hair is usually the first evidence of puberty in girls, increased testicular size is the first physical evidence of puberty in boys. In general, pubertal testicular enlargement has begun when the longitudinal measurement of a testis is greater than 2.5 cm (excluding the epididymis) or the volume is equal to or greater than 4 mL (6). The right testis is usually larger than the left, and the left testis is located lower in the scrotum than the right.

The phallus is more accurately measured in the stretched, flaccid state. The length of the erectile tissue (excluding the foreskin) increases from an average of 6.2 cm in the prepubertal stage to 12.4±2.7 cm in the white adult; in black men, the mean length is 14.6 cm, and in Asians, 10.6 cm (7).

During puberty, the male larynx, cricothyroid cartilage, and laryngeal muscles enlarge; the voice breaks at approximately 13.9 years and the adult voice is achieved by 15 years of age (8).

Pubertal Growth Spurt

The pubertal growth spurt can be divided into three stages: the stage of minimal growth velocity just before the spurt (takeoff velocity), the stage of most rapid growth, or peak height velocity (PHV), and the stage of decreased velocity and cessation of growth at epiphyseal fusion. Boys reach PHV approximately two years later than girls and are taller at takeoff; PHV occurs at stages three to four of puberty in most boys and is completed by stage five in more than 95% of boys (9,10). The mean takeoff age is 11 years, and the PHV occurs at a mean age of 13.5 years in boys. The total height gain in boys between takeoff and cessation of growth is approximately 31 cm (11). The mean height difference (boys taller than girls) between adult-height men and women is 12.5 cm.

Bone Age and Body Composition

Skeletal maturation is assessed by comparing radiographs of the hand, the knee, or the elbow with standards of maturation in a normal population (12). In normal children, bone age, an index of physiological maturation, does not have a well-defined relationship to the onset of puberty and is as variable as the chronologic age; however, in boys with delayed puberty, bone age correlates better with the onset of secondary sexual characteristics than does chronologic age.

There are dramatic changes during puberty in males, including increases in lean body mass, skeletal mass, bone-mineral density, and body water, and decreases in percentage fat mass (13). In boys, bone-mineral density reaches a peak early in the third decade of life, well after the PHV. The growth spurt at a time well before peak bone mass may be a factor that results in a period of increased fragility and susceptibility to trauma (14).

Hormonal Changes
Gonadotropins

Before puberty, the pulse amplitude of gonadotropin release [luteinizing hormone (LH) and follicle-stimulating hormone (FSH)] is low and occurs infrequently. The onset of pubertal hormonal changes is first evident in dramatic episodes of LH release of short duration that first occurs during sleep. With maturity, this release occurs regularly throughout the day (15). The intermittent release of gonadotropin is reflective of the episodic release of gonadotropin-releasing hormone (GnRH) (16). The increased sex hormone production by the testes (predominantly testosterone) results from increased LH stimulation; FSH stimulates the Sertoli cells, which, in conjunction with testosterone, stimulate maturation of spermatogenesis.

Testosterone

Prepubertal boys have plasma testosterone concentrations of less than 0.3 nmol/L (0.1 ng/mL) (17), except during the first three to five months of life, when pubertal levels are found. Nighttime elevations of serum testosterone are detectable in the male before the onset of physical signs of puberty and during early puberty after the development of sleep-entrained secretion of LH (18). In the daytime, testosterone levels begin to increase at approximately 11 years of age, after the testis volume is at least 4 mL, and continue to increase throughout puberty (19). The steepest increment in testosterone levels occurs between pubertal stages two and three (20).

Estrogens

In the male, approximately 75% or more of estradiol is derived from extraglandular aromatization of testosterone and (indirectly) androstenedione, and the remainder is secreted by the testes (21). Many actions of testosterone on growth, skeletal maturation, and accretion of bone mass are, to a great extent, the result of its aromatization to estrogen (22).

In boys, low levels of estradiol are present before puberty and rise throughout puberty until the pubertal growth spurt occurs, and decrease thereafter (23).

Adrenal Androgens

There is a progressive increase in plasma levels of dehydroepiandrosterone (DHEA) and its sulfated form (DHEAS) in both boys and girls beginning at the age of seven or eight years and continuing throughout early adulthood. The increase in the secretion of adrenal androgens and its precursors is known as "adrenarche." Dissociation of adrenarche and gonadarche (maturation of the gonads) occurs in several disorders of sexual maturation, including premature adrenarche (onset of pubic or axillary hair before the age of eight years) and central precocious puberty (CPP) (24).

Growth Hormone

Serum growth hormone (GH) levels rise during pubertal development in both boys and girls as a result of increased gonadal steroid secretion. Basal GH secretion is evident before puberty; the amplitude and mass of GH secretion, but not secretory episodes, are increased during pubertal development (25). This increase in pubertal GH secretion is characterized by a concomitant rise in plasma insulin-like growth factor-1 (IGF-1) concentration.

The aromatization of testosterone to estradiol accounts for a significant portion of the effect of testosterone on GH secretion (26,27). Treatment of late pubertal boys with the estrogen antagonist tamoxifen leads to smaller GH secretory peaks and, to a lesser degree, fewer GH secretory episodes, supporting the critical role of estrogens in regulating GH secretion (26).

☐ DISORDERS OF PUBERTY
Delayed Puberty
Constitutional Delay of Growth and Puberty

Constitutional delay of growth and puberty (CDGP) is a frequent variant of normal pubertal maturation. It is characterized by a slowing of the growth rate as well as by a delay in the *timing* and *tempo* (rate of progression of the various stages) of puberty (28). Typically, these boys seek medical evaluation in the early teens as they become aware of the discrepancy in sexual development and height between themselves and their peers.

Clinically, these patients have a height age (the age corresponding to the height at which the patient's height is at the 50% percentile) that is delayed with respect to their chronological age but is concordant with their bone age. Sexual development is prepubertal or early pubertal, and is again appropriate for the bone age, but delayed for chronological age. There is often a family history of one parent or a sibling of either sex having also been a "late bloomer."

Height velocity continues at a prepubertal rate or slows slightly as a prepubertal dip, in contrast to peers of the same chronological age, whose height velocities begin to accelerate at the age of 13 to 14 years. When the height is plotted on the standard growth curve, the height gain of these boys appears to be decelerating since the standard growth curve incorporates the pubertal growth spurt at an "average" age. This further accentuates the difference between the delayed boys and their normally developing counterparts. The apparent deceleration in growth compared with chronologically matched peers is usually a compelling concern of the patient and/or his family and brings the adolescent to medical attention.

Biochemically, boys with CDGP resemble normal boys with comparable bone ages. Serum levels of GH, IGF-1, insulin-like growth factor binding protein 3 (IGF-BP3), LH, FSH and testosterone may be low for chronological age, but are normal when compared with levels in boys of the same stage of sexual development (29,30).

The suppressed hypothalamic–pituitary–gonadal axis found in CDGP represents an extension of the physiological hypogonadotropic hypogonadism present since infancy.

Hypogonadotropic Hypogonadism

Insufficient pulsatile secretion of GnRH and the resulting LH and FSH deficiency lead to lack of sexual maturation, or sexual "infantilism." The degree of this deficit varies, and hence the phenotype can vary from complete sexual infantilism to conditions that are difficult to differentiate from CDGP (Table 1).

The GnRH deficiency may be secondary to a genetic or developmental defect that is not detected until the age of the expected puberty, or it may be due to a tumor, an inflammatory process, a vascular lesion, or trauma.

CNS Disorders

Tumors. CNS tumors that delay puberty are usually extrasellar masses that interfere with GnRH synthesis, secretion, or stimulation of pituitary gonadotropes. In this particular condition, virtually all patients have a deficiency of one or more additional pituitary hormones. GH deficiency due to neoplasms is often associated with a relatively late onset of growth failure, in contrast to idiopathic and familial hypopituitary children, who usually have growth failure early in life.

Craniopharyngioma is the most common brain tumor of nonglial origin and the most common brain tumor associated with hypothalamic–pituitary dysfunction and sexual infantilism. These tumors account for 80% to 90% of neoplasms arising in the pituitary region. They originate from squamous rest cells in the remnant of Rathke's pouch between the adenohypophysis and the neurohypophysis. The tumors may

Table 1 Hypogonadotropic Hypogonadism

CNS disorders
Tumors
Other CNS disorders
Isolated gonadotropin deficiency
Kallmann's syndrome
X-linked congenital adrenal hypoplasia
Isolated luteinizing-hormone deficiency
Miscellaneous disorders
Prader–Willi syndrome
Laurence–Moon syndrome
Bardet–Biedl syndrome
Cystic fibrosis
Other chronic diseases

Abbreviation: CNS, central nervous system.

be completely intrasellar (25%), solely extrasellar, or a combination of both (31).

Although histologically benign, craniopharyngiomas can be aggressive, sending papillae that invade surrounding tissues. In addition, they commonly have cystic components that may be multiple and may enlarge, causing compression of adjacent neurological structures. Craniopharyngiomas commonly present with nonendocrine symptoms such as headache and visual disturbance and, less commonly, with manifestations of endocrine deficiency such as delayed growth. Up to 80% of patients have evidence of endocrine dysfunction at diagnosis (32). GH deficiency is the most frequent finding, present in up to 75% of patients, followed by gonadotropin deficiency in 40%, adrenocorticotropic hormone (ACTH) and thyroid-stimulating hormone (TSH) deficiency in 25%, and diabetes insipidus in 9% to 17% (33,34).

Surgery is the treatment of choice for craniopharyngioma and, ideally, total resection of the tumor. In all but small, totally intrasellar or circumscribed tumors, for which total resection is possible, it is clear that surgical management alone carries an unacceptably high rate of recurrence and adjunctive radiotherapy should be given.

The treatment-associated morbidity is dependent on the size and invasiveness of tumor at diagnosis, the experience of the surgeon, and the route of surgical approach. Regardless of the approach, the incidence of endocrine dysfunction is high following surgical treatment (35), although it may be less when a transphenoidal approach is used (36).

Sexual infantilism can be caused by other extrasellar tumors that arise or involve the hypothalamus. Germinomas or other germ cell tumors of the CNS are the extrasellar tumors that most commonly cause sexual infantilism, although, when all primary CNS tumors are considered, germinomas are rare (37). The diagnosis is usually made during the second decade of life. Polydipsia and polyuria are among the most common symptoms, followed by visual difficulties, growth failure, and delayed or precocious puberty. The most common hormonal abnormalities are diabetes insipidus and GH deficiency. Pure germinomas are radiosensitive, and thus, radiation is the preferred treatment. When a mixed germ cell tumor is found, both radiation and chemotherapy may be required (38).

Hypothalamic and optic gliomas or astrocytomas as well as prolactinomas can also cause sexual infantilism.

Other CNS Disorders. Radiation of the head for treatment of CNS tumors, leukemia, or neoplasm may cause hypothalamic–pituitary damage. GH deficiency is the most common endocrine abnormality, followed by gonadotropin deficiency; consequently, delayed puberty and growth failure should always be suspected in children who have received CNS radiation therapy.

Midline malformations of the head and the CNS are associated with a variety of endocrine deficiencies. In septo-optic or optic dysplasia, the optic nerve is usually affected, leading to small, dysplastic, pale optic discs and nystagmus; severely affected patients may be blind. The midline hypothalamic defect may cause GH, TSH, ACTH, and gonadotropin deficiency; short stature and delayed puberty are common (39).

Other rare CNS disorders that can lead to delayed puberty include tuberculous or sarcoid granulomas of the CNS, hydrocephalus, vascular abnormalities, and head trauma (40).

Isolated Gonadotropin Deficiency

In contrast to patients with brain tumors and secondary GH deficiency or CDGP, patients with isolated gonadotropin deficiency are usually of appropriate height for age. Because levels of gonadal steroids are too low to fuse the epiphyses, these children develop eunuchoid body proportions, defined as having an arm span that is 2 cm greater than the total body height, with the lower body being 2 cm longer than the upper body. If not treated, these children will become tall adults, although only rarely is more than 2.5 to 7.5 cm added to the adult height (41).

Kallmann's syndrome is the most common form of isolated hypogonadotropic hypogonadism with delayed puberty; anosmia or hyposmia due to agenesis or hypoplasia of the olfactory lobes and/or sulci is associated with GnRH deficiency. Undescended testes, micropenis, and gynecomastia are frequent findings; other less common defects include cleft lip, cleft palate, seizure disorder, short metacarpals, pes cavus, hearing loss, cerebellar ataxia, ocular motor abnormalities, and renal dysplasia or aplasia (42,43).

Hypogonadotropic hypogonadism can be transmitted by autosomal recessive inheritance with none of the other features of Kallmann's syndrome in patients with X-linked congenital adrenal hypoplasia, which is due to a deletion or mutation of the *DAX1* gene. Affected boys with X-linked congenital adrenal hypoplasia frequently have severe primary adrenal insufficiency, which can be lethal if untreated (44). The testes are undescended in many of the patients, but micropenis is rare. At the age of expected puberty, signs of sexual maturation do not develop, including the lack of development of pubic and axillary hair and testicular enlargement and persistent low levels of serum FSH, LH, and testosterone (45).

Isolated LH deficiency (the fertile eunuch syndrome) is associated with deficient testosterone production and spermatogenesis; in most cases, the isolated gonadotropin deficiency is incomplete. Treatment with human chorionic gonadotropin (hCG) has been shown to increase testosterone secretion and spermatogenesis (46).

Miscellaneous Disorders

Prader–Willi syndrome is a complex, multisystem disorder that includes neonatal hypotonia and failure to thrive, developmental delay and mild cognitive impairment, characteristic facial appearance, early childhood-onset obesity, hypogonadism with genital hypoplasia and incomplete pubertal development, and mildly short stature (47).

This genetic disorder is caused by the lack of expression of normally active paternally inherited genes at chromosome 15q11-q13. Approximately 70% of the patients have a paternal deletion of the 15q11-q13, and 25% have uniparental disomy in which both chromosomes 15 are derived from the mother, possibly by nondisjunction during maternal meiosis (48).

The Laurence–Moon and Bardet–Biedl syndromes are two different entities, although both are autosomal recessive traits, and both feature retinitis pigmentosa and hypogonadism. Many Bardet–Biedl syndrome patients have developmental delay, as do all Laurence–Moon syndrome patients.

Chronic systemic disorders and malnutrition are associated with delayed puberty or failure to progress through the stages of puberty. It is necessary to distinguish the effects of malnutrition, which can lead to functional hypogonadotropic hypogonadism, from the primary effects of the disease. In general, any cause of weight loss to less than 80% of ideal weight for height can lead to gonadotropin deficiency (49); weight gain usually restores hypothalamic–pituitary–gonadal function.

Cystic fibrosis also delays puberty—in large part, through malnutrition (50). Even with normal pubertal progression, however, boys usually have oligospermia caused by obstruction of the spermatic ducts with viscid material unrelated to their nutritional status (51). Further, boys with cystic fibrosis have an autoimmune reaction against sperm that could be detected at the time of appearance of spermatogenesis (52).

Boys with sickle cell anemia often have mild delayed puberty and impaired Leydig cell function, due to ischemia of the testes or gonadotropin deficiency, or both (53). Other chronic conditions, including thalassemia major, hemophilia, Crohn's disease, celiac disease, chronic renal disease, poorly controlled diabetes mellitus, and hypothyroidism are also associated with delayed pubertal development.

Chemotherapy for malignant diseases may also influence the age of puberty and, if administered during puberty, can impair gonadal function and cause primary hypogonadism (54). Radiation to the head may cause hypogonadotropic hypogonadism and/or GH deficiency, and radiation to the abdomen and pelvis and certain types of chemotherapy.

Hypergonadotropic Hypogonadism
Klinefelter's Syndrome and Its Variants

Klinefelter's syndrome, the most frequent cause of hypergonadotropic hypogonadism in phenotypic males (approximately 1 in 600 to 1 in 800 males), does not delay the onset of sexual development. Common features include small, firm testes, impaired spermatogenesis, gynecomastia, and eunuchoid body proportions. Puberty starts at the usual age, but with small testes, the secondary sex characteristics do not attain normal development. The diagnosis is confirmed by the presence of one or more extra X chromosomes in the karyotype. School performance is usually poor, with an average verbal intelligence quotient that is 10 to 20 points below normal controls (55). Hormonal measurements at adolescence usually show high FSH levels, moderately elevated LH levels, and plasma testosterone in the low normal range (56).

Klinefelter variants with more than one extra chromosome include 46, XY/47, XXY; 48, XXYY, and 48, XXXY karyotypes—all associated with more severe genital and mental impairment. The rare 46, XX male also has some features of Klinefelter's syndrome.

Other Forms of Primary Testicular Failure

Other types of primary congenital testicular failure in otherwise normal males include anorchia and "vanishing testes syndrome." The latter condition features an empty scrotum at birth, with evidence of the temporary presence and function of testes in utero (57). Anorchia (total absence of testes) can be differentiated from abdominal cryptorchidism (undescended testes) by the high levels of LH and/or FSH, their elevated responses to a GnRH challenge, and, most importantly, the lack of testosterone response to stimulation with exogenous hCG.

LH resistance caused by an LH receptor abnormality has been reported as a cause of infantilism in a phenotypic male (58).

Acquired bilateral lesions of the testes that occur during childhood and may lead to hypogonadism at adolescence include bilateral testicular torsion, severe scrotal trauma, and orchitis (e.g., mumps).

Treatment

Treatment of delayed puberty depends on the diagnosis (59). Most boys with constitutional delay of growth and adolescence, without intervention, will undergo normal pubertal development spontaneously, and will reach their target height as predicted by parental stature (60). Development may, however, occur several years after that of their peers, and many adolescents will suffer significant emotional distress because they differ in their appearance from their peers during these years. Androgen therapy was initially proposed to alleviate this psychological stress. Recent data have emerged that support androgen therapy in these boys for its beneficial effects on bone-mineral density and body composition, in addition to its psychological benefits (61).

In the authors' practice, testosterone enanthate or cypionate 50 to 100 mg is administered intramuscularly every four weeks for three months. Almost all boys respond to this therapeutic trial by showing some increase in appetite, body weight, and height, and many show early testicular enlargement. An early-morning testosterone level measured at least three weeks after the last injection will reflect the boy's own endogenous testosterone production. If no physiologic changes are apparent after three months, the dose may

be increased by 25 to 50 mg every four weeks. Treatment is continued for another three months, and the boys are then reevaluated: an increase in testicular size indicates gonadotropin release despite exogenous testosterone. It should be noted that boys with permanent hypogonadotropic hypogonadism will not have testicular growth. If growth and development cannot be sustained without therapy after one year of testosterone treatment, the presence of permanent hypogonadotropic hypogonadism is more likely, and further investigation is warranted.

The use of pulsatile GnRH administration is not practical for the routine induction of puberty in adolescent boys, due to high cost, the frequency of administration (every 90–120 minutes), and the route of administration (subcutaneously or intravenously); therefore, long-term testosterone replacement is the treatment of choice for hypothalamic or pituitary gonadotropin deficiency.

Congenital or acquired gonadotropin deficiency due to CNS lesions requires testosterone replacement therapy at the normal age of onset of puberty. An exception may occur when GH deficiency coexists; in this condition, it is generally advisable to initiate testosterone replacement by the age of 14 years to maximize linear growth.

Plasma testosterone and LH levels should be monitored every six months during puberty, and yearly thereafter in patients with Klinefelter's syndrome. If the LH level rises by more than 2.5 SD above the mean value or if the testosterone level decreases below the normal range for age, testosterone replacement therapy is indicated.

Gonadal steroid treatment regimens are the same in both hypogonadotropic hypogonadism and hypergonadotropic hypogonadism. Boys are given testosterone enanthate, 50 to 100 mg every four weeks intramuscularly at the start, and this is increased gradually every two to three weeks to adult replacement doses of 200 mg (62). Skin patches of testosterone (2.5 and 5 mg) may be useful in motivated teenagers.

Precocious Puberty

By definition, precocious puberty is the appearance of any sign of secondary sexual maturation before the age of nine years in boys.

Precocious puberty can be central (GnRH-dependent) or peripheral (GnRH-independent) (Table 2). In both cases, linear growth is accelerated during childhood, often with markedly advanced bone maturation. Paradoxically, a tall boy may become short in adulthood because of the very early epiphyseal closure.

Central Precocious Puberty

CPP is either idiopathic or secondary to a central nervous system abnormality. The definitive diagnostic test for CPP is GnRH stimulation of gonadotropin release. CPP is diagnosed when there is a "pubertal response," that is, when the rise of LH is greater than

Table 2   Precocious Puberty

Central
   Idiopathic
   CNS tumors
   Other CNS disorders
Peripheral
   Congenital adrenal hyperplasia
   Virilizing adrenal tumors
   Leydig cell tumors
   Familial testotoxicosis
   McCune–Albright syndrome
   Longstanding hypothyroidism

Abbreviation: CNS, central nervous system.

the range of response among prepubertal children of the same sex using the same gonadotropin assay.

Idiopathic

In this condition, puberty is physiologically normal, but chronologically early.

In contrast to its occurrence in girls, CPP occurs less frequently in boys, and a larger percentage of boys with CPP have CNS lesions than the idiopathic variety. Therefore, the CNS assessment of boys with early puberty, usually including an MRI scan, should be emphasized.

In boys with idiopathic CPP, the testes usually enlarge under gonadotropin stimulation before other signs of puberty are seen. Progression of sexual maturation is often more rapid than normal. The rapid growth is associated with increased GH secretion and elevation of serum IGF-1 levels because of stimulation of this axis by gonadal steroid hormones (63).

The ratio of bone age to chronological age and the rise of IGF-1 above normal values for age are predictive of outcome: Children with modest clinical signs progress less rapidly and may attain their target heights (64).

CNS Tumors

Optic and hypothalamic glioma, astrocytoma, and, rarely, craniopharyngioma, ependymomas, and germinomas can cause CPP. The prevalence of CPP is increased especially in girls after cranial radiation for local tumors or leukemia. Hamartomas of the tuber cinereum are now detected in many boys previously thought to have idiopathic CPP. These hamartomas are not true neoplasms and should not be approached surgically, except in unusual circumstances (65). Sexual precocity may be the first manifestation of any posterior hypothalamic tumor. In addition, headaches, visual problems, diabetes insipidus, and hydrocephalus may develop due to an enlarging mass.

The location of these tumors usually makes surgical removal difficult. A conservative approach is recommended; the pathologic findings of a biopsy of the neoplasm should direct treatment.

Other CNS Disorders

CNS abnormalities associated with CPP include encephalitis, developmental delay, hydrocephalus,

epilepsy, previous CNS radiation therapy, head trauma, arachnoid cyst, brain abscess, and sarcoid or tuberculous granuloma of the hypothalamus.

Neurofibromatosis type 1 (von Recklinghausen's disease) and septo-optic dysplasia are associated with both precocious puberty and delayed puberty (66).

Chronic Exposure to Sex Steroids

CPP may be secondary to prolonged sex steroid exposure associated with peripheral precocious puberty (PPP). Boys may develop CPP as a consequence of prolonged hyperandrogenic state in inadequately treated congenital virilizing adrenal hyperplasia (67). Patients with this disorder may initially have PPP but later develop CPP after prolonged excessive androgen stimulation.

Peripheral Precocious Puberty

In this disorder, the secretion of testosterone is independent of GnRH. Affected individuals do not have a pubertal response to GnRH stimulation and may have suppressed gonadotropin concentrations. Usually, the testes are smaller than expected from the serum testosterone level.

The causes of PPP include congenital adrenal hyperplasia (CAH), hCG-secreting tumors, virilizing adrenal tumors, testicular tumors, testotoxicosis, McCune–Albright syndrome, and longstanding hypothyroidism.

Congenital Adrenal Hyperplasia

Undiagnosed or undertreated CAH due to 21-hydroxylase deficiency is the most common cause of PPP in boys. Approximately 75% of patients with CAH due to 21-hydroxylase deficiency have salt loss resulting from impaired aldosterone secretion and low serum sodium and high serum potassium levels. Increased plasma concentrations of 17-hydroxyprogesterone, advanced bone age, and rapid growth are characteristic findings (68). One-fourth of patients with CAH are non–salt losers; these boys may escape early diagnosis and present with virilization during childhood.

Germ cell or mixed germ cell tumors, hepatomas, and hepatoblastomas may secrete hCG. Boys with these hCG-secreting neoplasms may have slightly enlarged testes and may be difficult to differentiate from boys with CPP on the basis of physical examination (69). Plasma hCG levels are elevated without an increase in the concentration of FSH or LH (69). The prevalence of mediastinal germ cell tumors is increased 30 to 50 times in boys with Klinefelter's syndrome.

Virilizing Adrenal Tumors

Virilizing adrenal carcinomas and adenomas secrete large amounts of DHEA, DHEAS, and, occasionally, testosterone. Rare adrenal adenomas produce both testosterone and aldosterone, leading to precocious puberty and hypertension with hypokalemia (70).

Adrenal rests, or heterotopic adrenal tissue in the testes, may enlarge with endogenous corticotropin stimulation in boys with undiagnosed or undertreated CAH and may mimic interstitial cell tumors, occasionally leading to massive enlargement of the testes.

Leydig Cell Tumor

This testicular tumor may cause sexual precocity. It causes a unilateral enlargement of the testes. These tumors must be differentiated from testicular adrenal rest cell hyperplasia, which usually occurs bilaterally, and may be seen in patients with poorly controlled CAH. Most of these tumors are benign and present in boys less than six years of age.

Familial Testotoxicosis

Affected boys have penile enlargement, which may be present at birth, and bilateral enlargement of the testes to the early or mid-puberty range. Basal and GnRH-stimulated gonadotropins are prepubertal. Plasma testosterone levels are in the normal pubertal or adult range. If untreated, affected individuals may have superimposed CPP (71). This condition is caused by heterozygous activating mutations of the Gs protein-coupled LH/hCG receptor. It is commonly inherited as a male-limited autosomal dominant trait.

McCune–Albright Syndrome

This syndrome, which occurs far more frequently in females than in males, includes a unique form of PPP in which there is an activating missense mutation in the gene for the α-subunit of the Gs protein—the G protein that stimulates cAMP formation (72). Abnormalities consist of localized osseous lesions (polyostotic fibrous dysplasia), melanotic cutaneous macules (café au lait spots), and endocrinopathy. Endocrinopathies may include sexual precocity, hyperthyroidism, hyperadrenocorticism, pituitary gigantism, and hypophosphatemia.

Longstanding Hypothyroidism

This is an uncommon cause of PPP in boys, in which precocious puberty may occur in association with impaired growth and delayed bone age (73). The signs of sexual maturation are not accompanied by a pubertal growth spurt; rather, growth is impaired. In some cases, there is an enlargement of the sella turcica and pituitary gland, which has led to misdiagnosis of a pituitary neoplasm.

Treatment

Treatment of CPP is indicated to prevent progression of puberty, untimely statural growth, the development of associated psychosocial problems, and foreshortened adult height (74).

Three principal agents have been used in the treatment of CPP, whether idiopathic or neurologic: medroxyprogesterone acetate, cyproterone acetate, and GnRH agonists. The first two drugs have been replaced by GnRH agonists; at present, they are useful as backup agents for occasional patients who develop untoward effects from GnRH agonist therapy.

Chronic administration of GnRH agonists suppresses LH and FSH release, gonadal steroid output, and gametogenesis after an initial, brief stimulation of gonadotropin release (75). Suppression is due to binding of the agonist to the GnRH receptors on gonadotropes and desensitization of the gonadotropes to GnRH. Various agonists are available, but the intramuscular depot formulation of leuprorelin (leuprolide acetate) is the most commonly prescribed; it is safe and effective (76). Careful monitoring of serum gonadotropins and gonadal steroids is necessary for the evaluation of effectiveness of the treatment. Untoward reactions to GnRH agonists include local and systemic allergic reactions, sterile abscess, and weight gain. Changes in secondary sexual characteristics occur within the first six months of therapy: the pubic hair thins, the testes decrease in size, acne and seborrhea regress, penile erections and masturbation become much less frequent, high energy levels and aggressive behavior diminish, and self-esteem improves. From the second year on, height velocity for bone age is usually appropriate.

Treatment of PPP depends on the diagnosis: if there is an underlying cause resulting in early puberty, medical therapy involves treatment of this cause, if possible. Examples of treatment for underlying conditions include surgery and radiation or chemotherapy for tumors of CNS, ectopic gonadotropin-producing, testicular, or adrenal origin.

Treatment with glucocorticoids and mineralocorticoids (when appropriate) suppresses the abnormal androgen secretion and arrests virilization and corrects electrolyte imbalance.

In testotoxicosis and McCune–Albright syndrome, ketoconazole and, recently, the more potent aromatase inhibitors have been used to suppress gonadal and adrenal biosynthesis. Secondary CPP often occurs when the bone age advances to or has already reached the pubertal range, at which time addition of a GnRH agonist is appropriate. Another approach involves the use of the antiandrogen, spironolactone, combined with testolactone, an inhibitor of the conversion of androgens to estrogens. Recently, tamoxifen, a potent antiestrogen agent, has been proposed as an alternative treatment in patients with McCune-Albright syndrome (77).

Treatment with levothyroxine in patients with longstanding hypothyroidism not only corrects the hypothyroid state, but may reverse the incomplete sexual maturation and pituitary enlargement (when associated).

☐ CONCLUSION

During the last decade, intensive basic and clinical research has enhanced the understanding of the normal physiology of puberty. Using this knowledge, it is essential to determine which patients should undergo an in-depth evaluation and which conditions should be considered normal variants.

Most boys with CDGP will undergo normal puberty without intervention; however, androgen therapy may have beneficial effects on bone-mineral density and body composition, in addition to its psychological benefits.

Delayed puberty may be secondary to insufficient pulsatile secretion of GnRH (hypogonadotropic hypogonadism) or testicular failure despite high levels of gonadotropins (hypergonadotropic hypogonad-

ism). In both conditions, testosterone treatment is indicated to induce and/or maintain sexual maturation and to maximize linear growth.

Precocious puberty can be central (Gn RH-dependent) or peripheral (GnRH-independent). GnRH agonist therapy is effective in the treatment of CPP. On the other hand, treatment of PPP is directed toward the specific pathophysiologic process.

□ REFERENCES

1. Herman-Giddens ME, Slora EJ, Wasserman RC, et al. Secondary sexual characteristics and menses in young girls seen in office practice: a study from the Pediatric Research in Office Settings network. Pediatrics 1997; 99(4):505–512.

2. Kaplowitz PB, Oberfield SE. The Drug and Therapeutics and Executive Committees of the Lawson Wilkins Pediatric Endocrine Society. Reexamination of the age limit for defining when puberty is precocious in girls in the United States: implications for evaluation and treatment. Pediatrics 1999; 104(4):936–941.

3. Sonis WA, Comite F, Blue J, et al. Behavior problems and social competence in girls with true precocious puberty. J Pediatr 1985; 106(1):156–160.

4. Biro FM, Lucky AW, Huster GA, et al. Pubertal staging in boys. J Pediatr 1995; 127(1):100–102.

5. Tanner JM. Growth at Adolescence. Springfield, IL: Charles C Thomas, 1962.

6. Zachmann M, Prader A, Kind HP, et al. Testicular volume during adolescence: cross-sectional and longitudinal studies. Helv Pediatr Acta 1974; 29(1): 61–72.

7. Sutherland RS, Kogan BA, Baskin LS, et al. The effect of prepubertal androgen exposure on adult penile length. J Urol 1996; 156(2 Pt 2):783–787.

8. Karlberg P, Taranger J. The somatic development of children in a Swedish urban community. Acta Pediatr Scand Suppl 1976; 258:1–48.

9. Tanner JM, Whitehouse RH, Marubini E, et al. The adolescent growth spurt of boys and girls of the Harpenden growth study. Ann Hum Biol 1976; 3(2):109–126.

10. Largo RH, Gasser T, Prader A, et al. Analysis of the adolescent growth spurt using smoothing spline functions. Ann Hum Biol 1978; 5(5):421–434.

11. Abbassi V. Growth and normal puberty. Pediatrics 1998; 102(2):507–511.

12. Greulich WS, Pyle SI. Radiograph Atlas of Skeletal Development of the Hand and Wrist. Stanford, CA: Stanford University Press, 1959.

13. Roemmich JN, Clark PA, Mai V, et al. Alterations in growth and body composition during puberty: III. Influence of maturation, gender, body composition, fat distribution, aerobic fitness, and energy expenditure on nocturnal growth hormone release. J Clin Endocrinol Metab 1998; 83(5):1440–1447.

14. Bonjour JP, Theintz G, Law F, et al. Peak bone mass. Osteoporos Int 1994; 4(suppl 1):7–13.

15. Delemarre-Van De Waal HA, Wennink JM, Odink RJ. Gonadotrophin and growth hormone secretion throughout puberty. Acta Pediatr Scand Suppl 1991; 372:26–31.

16. Knobil E. The neuroendocrine control of the menstrual cycle. Recent Prog Horm Res 1980; 36:53–88.

17. Albertsson-Wikland K, Rosberg S, Lannering B, et al. Twenty-four-hour profiles of luteinizing hormone, follicle-stimulating hormone, testosterone, and estradiol levels: a semi-longitudinal study throughout puberty in healthy boys. J Clin Endocrinol Metab 1997; 82(2):541–549.

18. Boyar RM, Rosenfeld RS, Kapen S, et al. Human puberty. Simultaneous augmented secretion of luteinizing hormone and testosterone during sleep. J Clin Invest 1974; 54(3):609–618.

19. August GP, Grumbach MM, Kaplan SL. Hormonal changes in puberty. 3. Correlation of plasma testosterone, LH, FSH, testicular size, and bone age with male pubertal development. J Clin Endocrinol Metab 1972; 34(2):319–326.

20. Knorr D, Bidlingmaier F, Butenandt O, et al. Plasma testosterone in male puberty. I. Physiology of plasma testosterone. Acta Endocrinol (Copenh) 1974; 75(1):181–194.

21. Weinstein RL, Kelch RP, Jenner MR, et al. Secretion of unconjugated androgens and estrogens by the normal and abnormal human testis before and after human chorionic gonadotropin. J Clin Invest 1974; 53(1):1–6.

22. Mauras N, O'Brien KO, Welch S, et al. Insulin-like growth factor I and growth hormone (GH) treatment in GH-deficient humans: differential effects on protein, glucose, lipid, and calcium metabolism. J Clin Endocrinol Metab 2000; 85(4):1686–1694.

23. Klein KO, Martha PM Jr, Blizzard RM, et al. A longitudinal assessment of hormonal and physical alterations

during normal puberty in boys. II. Estrogen levels as determined by an ultrasensitive bioassay. J Clin Endocrinol Metab 1996; 81(9):3203–3207.

24. Sklar CA, Kaplan SL, Grumbach MM. Evidence for dissociation between adrenarche and gonadarche: studies in patients with idiopathic precocious puberty, gonadal dysgenesis, isolated gonadotropin deficiency, and constitutionally delayed growth and adolescence. J Clin Endocrinol Metab 1980; 51(3):548–556.

25. Veldhuis JD, Roemmich JN, Rogol AD. Gender and sexual maturation-dependent contrasts in the neuroregulation of growth hormone secretion in prepubertal and late adolescent males and females-a general clinical research center-based study. J Clin Endocrinol Metab 2000; 85(7):2385–2394.

26. Metzger DL, Kerrigan JR. Estrogen receptor blockade with tamoxifen diminishes growth hormone secretion in boys: evidence for a stimulatory role of endogenous estrogens during male adolescence. J Clin Endocrinol Metab 1994; 79(2):513–518.

27. Keenan BS, Richards GE, Ponder SW, et al. Androgen-stimulated pubertal growth: the effects of testosterone and dihydrotestosterone on growth hormone and insulin-like growth factor-I in the treatment of short stature and delayed puberty. J Clin Endocrinol Metab 1993; 76(4):996–1001.

28. Houchin LD, Rogol AD. Androgen replacement in children with constitutional delay of puberty: the case for aggressive therapy. Baillieres Clin Endocrinol Metab 1998; 12(3):427–440.

29. Sanayama K, Noda H, Konda S, et al. Spontaneous growth hormone secretion and plasma somatomedin-C in children of short stature. Endocrinol Jpn 1987; 34(5): 627–633.

30. Kerrigan JR, Martha PM Jr, Blizzard RM, et al. Variations of pulsatile growth hormone release in healthy short prepubertal boys. Pediatr Res 1990; 28(1):11–14.

31. Bunin GR, Surawicz TS, Witman PA, et al. The descriptive epidemiology of craniopharyngioma. J Neurosurg 1998; 89(4):547–551.

32. Sklar CA. Craniopharyngioma: endocrine abnormalities at presentation. Pediatr Neurosurg 1994; 21(suppl 1):18–20.

33. Thomsett MJ, Conte FA, Kaplan SL, et al. Endocrine and neurologic outcome in childhood craniopharyngioma: review of effect of treatment in 42 patients. J Pediatr 1980; 97(5):728–735.

34. Lyen KR, Grant DB. Endocrine function, morbidity, and mortality after surgery for craniopharyngioma. Arch Dis Child 1982; 57(11):837–841.

35. Scott RM, Hetelekidis S, Barnes PD, et al. Surgery, radiation, and combination therapy in the treatment of childhood craniopharyngioma-a 20-year experience. Pediatr Neurosurg 1994; 21(suppl 1):75–81.

36. Fahlbusch R, Honegger J, Paulus W, et al. Surgical treatment of craniopharyngiomas: experience with 168 patients. J Neurosurg 1999; 90(2):237–250.

37. Mootha SL, Barkovich AJ, Grumbach MM, et al. Idiopathic hypothalamic diabetes insipidus, pituitary stalk thickening, and the occult intracranial germinoma in children and adolescents. J Clin Endocrinol Metab 1997; 82(5):1362–1367.

38. Paulino AC, Wen BC, Mohideen MN. Controversies in the management of intracranial germinomas. Oncology 1999; 13(4):513–521.

39. Hanna CE, Mandel SH, LaFranchi SH. Puberty in the syndrome of septo-optic dysplasia. Am J Dis Child 1989; 143(2):186–189.

40. Asherson RA, Jackson WP, Lewis B. Abnormalities of development associated with hypothalamic calcification after tuberculous meningitis. Br Med J 1965; 5466:839–843.

41. Uriarte MM, Baron J, Garcia HB, et al. The effect of pubertal delay on adult height in men with isolated hypogonadotropic hypogonadism. J Clin Endocrinol Metab 1992; 74(2):436–440.

42. Kallmann F, Schonfeld WA, Barrera SW. Genetic aspects of primary eunuchoidism. Am J Ment Defic 1944; 48:203–236.

43. Danek A, Heye B, Schroedter R. Cortically evoked motor responses in patients with Xp22.3-linked Kallmann's syndrome and in female gene carriers. Ann Neurol 1992; 31(3):299–304.

44. Kruse K, Sippell WG, Schnakenburg KV. Hypogonadism in congenital adrenal hypoplasia: evidence for a hypothalamic origin. J Clin Endocrinol Metab 1984; 58(1):12–17.

45. Hay ID, Smail PJ, Forsyth CC. Familial cytomegalic adrenocortical hypoplasia: an X-linked syndrome of pubertal failure. Arch Dis Child 1981; 56(9):715–721.

46. Smals AG, Kloppenborg PW, van Haelst UJ, et al. Fertile eunuch syndrome versus classic hypogonadotrophic hypogonadism. Acta Endocrinol (Copenh) 1978; 87(2):389–399.

47. Cassidy SB. Clinical and laboratory diagnosis of Prader-Willi syndrome. The Endocrinologist 2000; 10:17S–20S.

48. Knoll JH, Nicholls RD, Magenis RE, et al. Angelman and Prader-Willi syndromes share a common chromosome 15 deletion but differ in parental origin of the deletion. Am J Med Genet 1989; 32(2):285–290.

49. Frisch RE, McArthur JW. Menstrual cycles: fatness as a determinant of minimum weight for height necessary for their maintenance or onset. Science 1974; 185(4155):949–951.

50. Reiter EO, Stern RC, Root AW. The reproductive endocrine system in cystic fibrosis. I. Basal gonadotropin and sex steroid levels. Am J Dis Child 1981; 135(5): 422–426.

51. Taussig LM, Lobeck CC, Sant'Agnese PA, et al. Fertility in males with cystic fibrosis. N Engl J Med 1972; 287(12):586–589.

52. Vazquez-Levin MH, Kupchik GS, Torres Y, et al. Cystic fibrosis and congenital agenesis of the vas deferens,

antisperm antibodies and CF-genotype. J Reprod Immunol 1994; 27(3):199–212.

53. Olambiwonnu NO, Penny R, Frasier SD. Sexual maturation in subjects with sickle cell anemia: studies of serum gonadotropin concentration, height, weight, and skeletal age. J Pediatr 1975; 87(3):459–464.

54. Vilska S, Lahteenmaki P, Kaihola HL, et al. Endocrine status and growth after malignancy treated in childhood or adolescence. Int J Fertil 1988; 33(4):283–290.

55. Graham JM Jr, Bashir AS, Stark RE, et al. Oral and written language abilities of XXY boys: implications for anticipatory guidance. Pediatrics 1988; 81(6):795–806.

56. Sasagawa I, Kazama T, Terada T, et al. Hormone profiles in Klinefelter's syndrome with and without testicular epidermoid cyst. Arch Androl 1988; 21(3):205–209.

57. Lustig RH, Conte FA, Kogan BA, et al. Ontogeny of gonadotropin secretion in congenital anorchism: sexual dimorphism versus syndrome of gonadal dysgenesis and diagnostic considerations. J Urol 1987; 138(3): 587–591.

58. David R, Yoon DJ, Landin L, et al. A syndrome of gonadotropin resistance possibly due to a luteinizing hormone receptor defect. J Clin Endocrinol Metab 1984; 59(1):156–160.

59. Rogol AD. New facets of androgen replacement therapy during childhood and adolescence. Expert Opin Pharmacother 2005; 6(8):1319–1336.

60. Crowne EC, Shalet SM, Wallace WH, et al. Final height in boys with untreated constitutional delay in growth and puberty. Arch Dis Child 1990; 65(10):1109–1112.

61. Bertelloni S, Baroncelli GI, Battini R, et al. Short-term effect of testosterone treatment on reduced bone density in boys with constitutional delay of puberty. J Bone Miner Res 1995; 10(10):1488–1495.

62. Bourguignon JP. Linear growth as a function of age at onset of puberty and sex steroid dosage: therapeutic implications. Endocr Rev 1988; 9(4):467–488.

63. Ross JL, Pescovitz OH, Barnes K, et al. Growth hormone secretory dynamics in children with precocious puberty. J Pediatr 1987; 110(3):369–372.

64. Fontoura M, Brauner R, Prevot C, et al. Precocious puberty in girls: early diagnosis of a slowly progressing variant. Arch Dis Child 1989; 64(8):1170–1176.

65. Hochman HI, Judge DM, Reichlin S. Precocious puberty and hypothalamic hamartoma. Pediatrics 1981; 67(2): 236–244.

66. Habiby R, Silverman B, Listernick R, et al. Precocious puberty in children with neurofibromatosis type 1. J Pediatr 1995; 126(3):364–367.

67. Pescovitz OH, Comite F, Cassorla F, et al. True precocious puberty complicating congenital adrenal hyperplasia: treatment with a luteinizing hormone-releasing hormone analog. J Clin Endocrinol Metab 1984; 58(5): 857–861.

68. White PC, Speiser PW. Congenital adrenal hyperplasia due to 21-hydroxylase deficiency. Endocr Rev 2000; 21(3):245–291.

69. Sklar CA, Conte FA, Kaplan SL, et al. Human chorionic gonadotropin-secreting pineal tumor: relation to pathogenesis and sex limitation of sexual precocity. J Clin Endocrinol Metab 1981; 53(3):656–660.

70. Schmitt K, Frisch H, Neuhold N, et al. Aldosterone and testosterone producing adrenal adenoma in childhood. J Endocrinol Invest 1995; 18(1):69–73.

71. Rosenthal IM, Refetoff S, Rich B, et al. Response to challenge with gonadotropin-releasing hormone agonist in a mother and her two sons with a constitutively activating mutation of the luteinizing hormone receptor—a clinical research center study. J Clin Endocrinol Metab 1996; 81(10):3802–3806.

72. Shenker A, Weinstein LS, Moran A, et al. Severe endocrine and non endocrine manifestations of the McCune-Albright syndrome associated with activating mutations of stimulatory G protein GS. J Pediatr 1993; 123(4): 509–518.

73. Anasti JN, Flack MR, Froehlich J, et al. A potential novel mechanism for precocious puberty in juvenile hypothyroidism. J Clin Endocrinol Metab 1995; 80(1): 276–279.

74. Lee PA. Central precocious puberty. An overview of diagnosis, treatment, and outcome. Endocrinol Metab Clin North Am 1999; 28(4):901–918.

75. Marshall JC, Kelch RP. Gonadotropin-releasing hormone: role of pulsatile secretion in the regulation of reproduction. N Engl J Med 1986; 315(23):1459–1468.

76. Conn PM, Crowley WF Jr. Gonadotropin-releasing hormone and its analogs. Annu Rev Med 1994; 45: 391–405.

77. Eugster EA, Shankar R, Feezle LK, et al. Tamoxifen treatment of progressive precocious puberty in a patient with McCune-Albright syndrome. J Pediatr Endocrinol Metab 1999; 12(5):681–686.

15

Male Varicoceles

Benjamin K. Canales, Nissrine Nakib, Ann Lavers, and Jon L. Pryor
Department of Urologic Surgery, University of Minnesota Medical School, Minneapolis, Minnesota, U.S.A.

□ INTRODUCTION

The male varicocele and its association with infertility have been recognized for many centuries. In *De Medicina*, written during the first century A.D., Celsus credits the Greeks with the first description of a varicocele and then remarks on veins that "are swollen and twisted over the testicle, which becomes smaller than its fellow, in as much as its nutrition has become defective" (1). Improvements in semen quality after varicocele repair were first suggested by Barwell in 1885, Bennett in 1889, and Macomber and Sanders in 1929 (2–4). In spite of these reports, surgical repair of the varicocele was virtually forgotten until 1952, when the Edinburgh surgeon Selby Tulloch demonstrated the restoration of fertility following excision of bilateral varicoceles in an azoospermic patient (5). Since then, thousands of studies on the diagnosis and surgical correction of varicoceles have appeared in the literature. Unfortunately, this entire body of experimental evidence has been able to neither identify the mechanism of spermatogenesis impairment nor explain why surgical correction improves semen parameters. This chapter will discuss the diagnosis and consequences of varicoceles, review the etiology and hypothesized mechanisms of gonadal effect, and explore treatment options and complications, with a brief consideration of the adolescent varicocele.

Definition/Prevalence

Defined as an abnormal dilatation of the veins of the pampiniform plexus within the spermatic cord, varicoceles have traditionally been reported predominantly on the left side (77–92%), with isolated right-sided (1%) and bilateral varicoceles (10%, range 7–22%) reported much less commonly (6,7). Varicoceles present almost exclusively after puberty (8) and are often discovered during an infertility evaluation. They are congenital in origin, although acquired lesions have been described in association with renal tumors, retroperitoneal masses, lymphadenopathy, thrombosis or occlusion of the vena cava, and situs inversus (9). While large varicoceles are typically asymptomatic, they may occasionally present as a persistent, aching discomfort often described by patients as a "heavy" sensation. This feeling of heaviness is almost

always relieved on the adoption of a supine position because of varicocele collapse.

The mean incidence of varicocele is between 10% and 15% of the male population (10–12). In men presenting with primary infertility, these figures rise to 35%, with one large, recent prospective study suggesting that bilateral varicoceles may be as common as 80% in this population (13). Men with secondary infertility (i.e., men who were previously fertile) have a varicocele incidence of 69% to 81% (14–16). The increased frequency in cases of secondary infertility suggests that varicoceles progressively harm spermatogenesis and that prior fertility in men with varicocele does not confer resistance to its progressive, deleterious effects (17). Furthermore, since the generally accepted incidence of infertility in males is 5%, it is important to remember that varicoceles are present in many men with normal fertility (18,19). In fact, the largest study of varicoceles to date by the World Health Organization found varicoceles in 25.4% of 3626 men with abnormal semen analyses and in 11.7% of 3468 men with normal semen (20). Interestingly, varicocele incidence is 53% in first-degree relatives of men with varicocele, with no correlations between size or bilaterality (21).

□ ANATOMY AND PATHOPHYSIOLOGY

It is particularly important to consider the testicular vascular anatomy in order to understand proposed pathophysiologic mechanisms of varicoceles and the high frequency of their occurrence on the left side.

Anatomic Etiology

The arterial supply to the testis has three major components: the testicular artery, the cremasteric artery, and the vasal artery. Although most arterial blood in the testis derives from the testicular artery, rich collateral testicular circulation allows adequate perfusion of the testis even if the testicular artery is injured or ligated (22–24). Venous drainage of the testis is provided by the pampiniform plexus, which leads into the testicular (internal spermatic), vasal (deferential), and cremasteric (external spermatic) veins. Since spermatic vein varicocities are discovered almost exclusively around the age of puberty, it is likely that the normal physiologic changes that occur during puberty result in increased testicular blood flow, exposing underlying venous anomalies to overperfusion and, eventually, to clinically evident venous ectasia (25).

Increased Venous Pressure

Differences in the configuration of the right and left internal spermatic veins are thought to contribute to marked left-sided internal spermatic vein tortuosity, dilation, and retrograde blood flow (25). Venous blood from the right testicle drains into the inferior vena cava at an oblique angle (approximately 30°). This angle, coupled with greater inferior vena caval flow (termed the "Venturi effect"), is thought to enhance right-sided drainage (26). Comparatively, the left testicular vein drains perpendicularly into the left renal vein (approximately 90°). The insertion into the left renal vein occurs 8 to 10 cm more craniad than the insertion of the right internal spermatic vein, resulting in a left-sided 8- to 10-cm higher hydrostatic column with increased pressure and a relatively slower flow of blood in the upright position (27). The left renal vein may also be compressed proximally between the superior mesenteric artery and the aorta (0.7% of varicocele cases) as well as distally between the left common iliac artery and vein (0.5% of varicocele cases) (28). This "nutcracker phenomenon" may also result in increased pressure in the left testicular venous system.

Collateral Venous Anastomoses

Detailed anatomic studies have demonstrated a superficial and deep anastomotic drainage system, along with left-to-right venous communications at the ureteric (L3-5), spermatic, scrotal, retropubic, saphenous, sacral, and pampiniform plexi (28–30). The left spermatic vein branches into medial and lateral divisions at the L4 level in almost all men (30)—findings that must be taken into consideration when choosing a treatment for varicocele. In particular, procedures performed above the level of L4 are at higher risk of failure due to the multiple divisions of the spermatic venous system (30).

Incompetent Valves

In 1966, Ahlberg proposed that testicular veins contained valves that were protective against varicoceles, and it was their lack or incompetence on the left side that caused varicoceles (31). In support of his argument, he found an absence of valves in 40% of postmortem left spermatic veins compared with 23% absence on the right. Doubt has been cast on this theory, however, as recent radiographic studies by Braedel et al. (32) found that 26.2% of patients with a competent valve system still had a varicocele present. Some modern anatomists have even proposed that there are no valves in either the right or left spermatic vein system (30,33).

Overall, there are multiple theories to explain varicocele formation. For the clinician, it is beneficial to know this background in order to review anatomy with patients and to explain, at least anatomically, why varicoceles exist. Despite these various etiologies, the larger question still looms: "Why do varicoceles cause detrimental effects on testicular function?"

Pathophysiologic Mechanisms of Varicocele Effect

Several mechanisms have been hypothesized to explain the phenomenon of subfertility found in men with unilateral or bilateral varicocele, including increased intrascrotal temperatures causing bilateral gonadal dysfunction, reflux of renal and adrenal metabolites from the renal vein, hypoxia, and accumulation of gonadotoxins.

Bilateral Dysfunction

Like many other aspects of varicoceles, the cause of bilateral testicular dysfunction in the presence of a unilateral varicocele is still under investigation. Retrograde right-sided venous flow has been demonstrated in men with left-sided varicoceles and has been proposed as a possible mechanism (34). Venographic and pressure studies of the right venous plexus have been explored and have all been found to be normal (35,36). The most likely mechanistic hypothesis was proposed in the early 1970s by Zorgniotti and MacLeod, in which clinical data on oligospermic men with varicoceles revealed intrascrotal temperatures that were 0.6°C higher than in oligospermic patients without varicoceles (37). Saypol et al. (27) and Green et al. (38) both described increased bilateral testicular blood flow and temperature in experimental animal models following artificial production of a unilateral varicocele. Additionally, subsequent repair of the varicocele resulted in the normalization of flow and temperature (27,38). Since then, researchers have demonstrated that DNA polymerase activity and the enzymes of DNA recombination in germ cells are temperature sensitive, with optimal activity at 33°C. Temperature for protein synthesis in round spermatids has been shown to be optimal at 34°C (39,40). Germ-cell proliferation may be affected by the increased temperature from the varicocele due to inhibition of one or more of these important enzymes. Hyperthermic injury is consistent with the reduction in spermatogonal numbers as well as apoptosis observed in testis biopsy samples from patients with a varicocele (41). Despite these findings, not all investigators have found an association between higher intratesticular temperatures and varicoceles (42,43), leading to the development of alternate mechanistic theories.

Reflux of Vasoactive Metabolites

Because the left adrenal and gonadal veins drain in close proximity to each other at the renal vein, MacLeod (44) proposed that metabolites derived from the kidney or adrenals may reflux into the gonadal vein. If these metabolites were vasoactive (such as prostaglandins), he postulated that they could have deleterious effects on testicular function. Results from animal and human studies have not supported this theory, however. Elevated levels of norepinephrine, prostaglandin E and F, and adrenomedullin (a potent vasodilator) have been identified within the spermatic vein of men with varicocele (45–47). Other metabolites such as renin, dehydroepiandrosterone, or cortisol have not been identified (48). Some authors contend that even in the presence of metabolites, reflux does not alter spermatogenesis (49).

Hypoxia

In 1980, Shafik and Bedeir theorized that differences in pressure gradients (and subsequent oxygen gradients) between the renal and gonadal vein may cause hypoxia within the gonadal vein (35). Two other "hypoxia" theories have also been proposed: increased venous pressure with exercise resulting in hypoxia (50) and stasis of blood causing reduced oxygen tension (51). In support of these, Tanji et al. (52) reported that men with varicoceles were more likely to have "atrophy-pattern" cremasteric fibers on histochemical studies, a denervation-type injury thought to be due to hypoxia. Despite these findings, no significant difference between control and varicocele blood gas oxygen patterns in animal models has been proven (53).

Gonadotoxins

Several studies have demonstrated that smoking in the presence of a varicocele has a greater adverse effect than either factor alone (54,55). Smokers have at least a twofold increase in the incidence of varicoceles (56), and those with varicoceles have a tenfold increase in the incidence of oligospermia when compared to non-smokers with varicoceles. Nicotine has been implicated as a cofactor in the pathogenesis of varicoceles in animal studies as well as the chemotherapeutic agent cyclophosphamide (55). Cadmium, a well-recognized gonadotoxin that causes apoptosis, has been found in significantly higher testicular concentrations in men with varicocele and decreased spermatogenesis than in men with varicocele and normal spermatogenesis or obstructive azoospermia (57). Further work in this area continues to generate interest, and perhaps future efforts will elicit the exact mechanism of action.

☐ DIAGNOSIS AND CONSEQUENCE OF VARICOCELE
Diagnosis

Although a multitude of radiologic and physical exam techniques exist for describing varicoceles, the lack of quantitative gold standards for classifying varicoceles has made it difficult to perform comparative studies and outcome analyses (17). Most clinicians agree, however, that a diligent physical examination is the cornerstone for diagnosis.

Physical Examination

The examination is initially performed in a warm room with the patient standing, to accentuate venous dilatation (58). The scrotum should first be carefully observed for a bluish distention of the dilated cord veins. If the varicocele is not visually apparent, the cord structures should then be bilaterally palpated, with Valsalva maneuver (which tends to distend venous cord structures) as well as without Valsalva. A palpable varicocele has been described as feeling like a "bag of worms," although in less obvious cases, there may be simple asymmetry or thickening of the cord (58). The examination should continue with the patient supine, primarily to differentiate a cord lipoma (thickened, fatty cords found while standing that do not disappear when supine) from a varicocele. Palpation and measurement of the testicle using an orchidometer (for consistency and size, respectively) may also give the clinician insight into intragonadal pathology. Classically, if disproportionate testicular lengths or volumes are found, the index of suspicion for a varicocele should increase (59).

Varicoceles have been arbitrarily assigned a clinical grading classification (Table 1). Although this system allows practitioners to clinically follow their own patients more easily (60,61), it is subjective in nature and has developed without validation. In a physical examination study, Hargreave compared the physical findings by two experienced clinicians and found disagreement in 26% of the patients (62). Yet, the authors of this paper feel that the optimal diagnosis of varicocele can still be made by a skilled clinician with an acceptable degree of error despite inherent flaws in both physical examination techniques and the current grading system. In an effort to ameliorate the present inconsistencies in the classification and diagnosis of varicoceles, however, various radiologic modalities including ultrasound, venography, thermography, scintigraphy, and magnetic resonance imaging (MRI) continue to be studied.

Ultrasonography

Color Doppler ultrasound (CDUS) is a simple, inexpensive, noninvasive, objective method that may be used to investigate the scrotum not only for the presence of varicocele but also for other pathologic processes and the documentation of testicular size (63,64). Sensitivities

Table 1 Classification of Varicocele

Grade	Physical examination findings
I	Detectable by palpation with difficulty More prominent with Valsalva
II	Detectable easily by palpation More prominent with Valsalva Not visible through scrotal skin
III	Palpable without Valsalva Visible through scrotal skin

are reportedly as high as 97% (65), with specificities around 94%. Generally, varicoceles are considered present by gray scale evaluation if two or more veins are identified, with at least one vein having a diameter of 3 mm (63–65). Dilated veins that are 5 mm or larger in diameter have been proven to be almost always clinically palpable (66).

In 1991, Petros et al. hypothesized that retrograde flow within the pampiniform plexus detected on color Doppler sonography was diagnostic of varicocele regardless of the dimensions of the veins involved (63). Two small subsequent papers, however, disputed these controversial findings: in 1993, Aydos et al. demonstrated that 59% to 83% of their infertile male patient population had reflux detected by CDUS without clinical evidence of varicocele (67), and Eskew et al. subsequently published that CDUS reflux was relatively insensitive for the detection of venographically confirmed varicoceles in a population of 33 men with possible male-factor infertility (68). In addition to identifying retrograde flow with questionable meaningfulness, ultrasonography sensitivity has also progressed to detecting scrotal varicocities that are too subtle to identify on physical examination, known as "subclinical varicoceles." Studies continue to be published concerning the development of criteria to differentiate pathological from physiologically normal components of testicular vasculature (69). Because of these reasons, scrotal ultrasound is not routinely used in the varicocele evaluation. Further, ultrasound is extremely operator dependent (70), and improper interpretations of flow or subclinical findings of unknown significance may lead to unwarranted surgical procedures.

Venography

Historically, radiologic placement of contrast through a catheter tip into the spermatic vein orifice (venography) is considered the best *diagnostic* test for varicocele (17). Result reproducibility is high, assessment of anatomy and presence of reflux is feasible, and simultaneous, immediate treatment with embolization (detachable coils or balloons) or sclerosing therapy is certainly an option (71). The procedure is invasive, however, and has associated complication rates (see section "Treatment"). Most authors agree that variations in operator technique and the lack of standardization for contrast injection pressures make the assessment of results and outcomes difficult. When used exclusively for diagnostic purposes, venography is recommended only in the subset of patients with recurrent varicoceles post varicocelectomy to aid in the detection of aberrant venous drainage (58).

Thermography, Scintigraphy, and MRI

Originally described in 1979 using scrotal skin contact strips (72), thermography assessment of varicoceles is an infrequent form of varicocele evaluation. Although newer liquid crystal contact strips have been developed,

multiple studies have found these strips to be unreliable during the physical exam (sensitivity 97% and specificity 9%) (65,73). More promising is the development of a fairly sensitive, focal-plane-array thermal imaging camera designed to look for asymmetrical patterns of scrotal temperatures. Small, promising correlation studies between thermography and venography have recently been published and may have some promise for future varicocele diagnosis (74). Published studies on ^{99m}Tc-based compound scintigraphy time-activity curves as well as the use of gadolinium-enhanced magnetic resonance angiography to evaluate varicoceles have not been demonstrated to be clinically reliable and are limited by the need for sophisticated equipment and cost (75,76).

Consequence of Varicocele

Once the diagnosis of varicocele is made, a discussion of its relevance to infertility may be warranted, particularly in the case of male patients presenting with infertility problems.

Semen Analysis

Although studied extensively, there is no consensus on the relationship between varicocele and changes in semen count, motility, or morphology. MacLeod (44) introduced the following varicocele-associated impairments in semen parameters in 1965: a decrease in motility (observed in 85% of study patients), oligospermia (defined as a sperm concentration of less than 20×10^6 and observed in 65% of study patients), as well as the concept of "stress pattern." MacLeod's classic description of stress pattern included the following characteristics: greater than 15% of sperm having a tapered shape (tapered forms), immature cells of the germinal line (typically, early spermatids), and increased amorphous cells. MacLeod did acknowledge that similar morphologic changes were present in infertile patients without varicocele, including those suffering from viral illness, acute allergic reactions, and other environmental insults with antispermatogenic agents (44). Multiple other papers have subsequently affirmed that "stress pattern" is not specific for varicocele and can be found in infertile patients without varicocele (77,78). Fertile men with varicoceles do not, in general, exhibit the stress pattern of tapered spermatozoa (20,79).

Moro (80) discovered that 20% of men with varicocele and severe oligospermia (defined as a sperm concentration less than 5 million/mL) have microdeletions of the Y chromosome. Three recent studies in men with large varicoceles (Grade III) and varicocele-associated testicular atrophy have demonstrated lower sperm counts and motility than men with smaller varicoceles or without atrophy, respectively (81–83). Overall, there is no reliable, predictable relationship between semen parameter changes and varicoceles. While abnormal semen parameters do not confirm nor exclude a varicocele, they do, however, provide insight into abnormal testicular function and may be followed serially when treating men with varicoceles and infertility.

Pathologic and Endocrine Changes

Alterations in testicular tissue and the hypothalamic–pituitary axis in men with varicoceles have repeatedly been proven. Apoptotic germ cells are increased to 10% in men with varicocele compared with 0.1% in normal fertile controls (84). Histologic changes present in both testicles in the presence of unilateral varicocele include tubular thickening, interstitial fibrosis, decreased spermatogenesis in seminiferous tubules, degenerative changes in Leydig and Sertoli cells, and maturation arrest (85). Lastly, multiple adult and adolescent studies have demonstrated that the presence of a unilateral varicocele causes a progressive decline in testicular function over time (14,15,59,86–88) as well as impaired ipsilateral testicular growth (20,89).

Elevations in serum follicle-stimulating hormone (FSH) (90) and abnormal gonadotropin releasing hormone (GnRH) stimulation tests (91) are occasionally present in subfertile men with varicocele, but no causality has been established in most cases. Serum luteinizing hormone and testosterone levels in men with varicoceles are quite variable and not reliably predictive (90–94). Some have speculated that variable serum testosterone findings in men with varicocele may relate to compensatory Leydig cell hyperplasia (17), suggesting that the majority of men with varicoceles are fertile because they start with "high spermatogenic potential" and thus "remain within the fertile range despite the adverse effect of the varicocele" (95).

Overall, it is clear that varicoceles are detrimental to testicular spermatogenesis. They are associated with testicular decline over time and may or may not show systemic endocrine effects. Most importantly, physicians should remember that the presence of a varicocele alone does not necessarily translate into infertility. Other causes of infertility such as the female factor and microdeletion of the Y chromosome should be explored if clinically applicable.

□ TREATMENT

For a young couple faced with infertility, surgery may be one of the most difficult decisions they have faced, as it may produce financial hardship in the form of medical bills or lead to partner frustration, guilt, or blame. Care should be taken to counsel both partners correctly on all potential outcomes of varicocele repair in the presence of infertility. In the following brief review of the literature, each of the following concerns is addressed: predictive factors (i.e., men who have been shown to benefit from varicocele repair), surgical and nonsurgical options and complications, and the expected effects on semen analysis, testicular growth, and fertility rates after repair.

Predictive Factors

When counseling patients on varicocele treatment, it is helpful to consider certain clinical parameters as predictive factors for improved outcome (Table 2). In fact, a key to providing appropriate patient counseling for the treatment for varicoceles involves an understanding of varicocelectomy outcomes data. Three recent series have demonstrated an inverse relationship between preoperative semen values and varicocele size, with greater improvement in semen parameters and pregnancy rates after repair of larger varicoceles (82,96,97). Varicocele repair has been shown to be efficacious in patients with a "total motile sperm count" that is greater than five million (98,99) and in patients with low to normal morphology in the presence of oligospermia (100). As discussed previously, testicular hypotrophy is associated with decreased sperm count, and, in correlation, Yoshida et al. found testicular volume greater than 30 cc to be an independent predictor of fertility following varicocelectomy (97). Repair of subclinical varicoceles remains controversial, as two poorly designed studies suggested a statistical improvement in seminal parameters (7,71) but did not demonstrate a meaningful effect on pregnancy rates (101). A large noncontrolled trial in men with subclinical varicocelectomy showed no change in mean sperm count in over 260 men (102).

Men with Y-chromosome microdeletions or Sertoli-cell-only azoospermia do not typically benefit from a varicocelectomy (100,103). Normal serum FSH levels were shown by Yoshida to be predictive of increased postoperative fertility following repair (97). Strengthening this finding, Schrepferman et al. found that men with varicoceles and elevated FSH levels demonstrated a poor response to varicocelectomy (99).

In all, these outcome data are meant to guide the decision-making process. It is important to note that factors of anatomy, physiology, and endocrinology are often interrelated and, therefore, each patient's infertility evaluation should be treated as a unique continuum of gonadal effects.

Treatment Options

Treatment options include surgical repair or nonsurgical management via transvenous varicocele ablation. Surgical repair of varicoceles may occur by any one of five different approaches: retroperitoneal, laparoscopic, inguinal, subinguinal, or scrotal. Transvenous varicocele ablation includes embolization (using detachable coils or balloons) or sclerosing therapy.

Table 2 Factors Associated with Improved Outcomes Following Varicocelectomy

Grade III varicocele (82,96,97)
Normal testicular exam (>20 cc) (97)
Normal serum follicle-stimulating hormone levels (97)
Total motile sperm count>5×10^6 (98,99)

The advantages and disadvantages to each approach are briefly reviewed here.

The retroperitoneal (also called "high ligation" or "modified Palomo") approach involves splitting the abdominal musculature low along the mid-axillary line and offers easy access to the spermatic vein just above the level of the internal inguinal ring. The vein is freed, anastomosing collaterals are identified, and all veins are ligated as superiorly as possible toward the renal vein. This approach offers a greatly reduced risk of damage to the testicular artery, as it is distinctly separate from the spermatic veins at this level. Most authors, however, report increased postoperative hydrocele formation (7–33% of adults and 15–45% of children) (104) as well as high varicocele recurrence rates in both men and children (up to 15%) (105,106); both of these trends are likely due to the large number of crossing vessels present prior to the confluence of the testicular veins. This procedure may now be performed with laparoscopy, allowing for excellent visualization of the spermatic veins and easy preservation of the lymphatics. While the laparoscopic technique results in a similarly high rate of recurrence, laparoscopic complications are rare (less than 1%) and are related to initial abdominal access (solid organ, bowel, or vascular injury), pneumoperitoneum (ventilation impedence, hypotension secondary to impeded venous return, and gas embolism), tissue dissection, or incisional hernia formation. Even with the possibility of improved technical precision, the significant disadvantages of increased operative time and the associated high equipment costs have caused the laparoscopic approach to fall out of favor (107).

The inguinal approach or modified Ivanissevich procedure is one of the most commonly used techniques today, as it allows for high ligation of both external cremasteric and testicular veins. After induction with general anesthesia or under local anesthesia, access to the spermatic cord is obtained by incising the external oblique aponeurosis, similar to the technique used in performing inguinal hernia repair. Surgical loupes, papaverine, and intraoperative Doppler sonography may aid in the identification of the testicular artery. Preservation of the lymphatics is extremely important in decreasing the risk of postoperative hydrocele formation (100).

Although similar to the inguinal approach, the subinguinal (or low inguinal) approach is performed just below the external oblique fascia, obviating the need to disrupt this aponeurosis (108,109). Intraoperative magnification by use of a microscope is commonly employed (110), and most patients have less postoperative pain and activity restrictions after surgery as a result. The major drawbacks of subinguinal varicocelectomy include a greater risk of damage to the numerous branches of spermatic veins as well as to the testicular artery, which maintains a more intimate relationship with the veins at this level. This procedure is also more technically challenging than the inguinal approach. Yet, subinguinal varicocelectomy

remains ideal for patients with a history of previous inguinal surgery, including hernia repair or previous varicocelectomy.

The oldest technique for varicocelectomy, the scrotal approach, has largely been abandoned by modern urologists. Although somewhat effective, high complication rates include injury to small branches of the testicular artery, testicular atrophy, and hydrocele formation in as many as 40% of the patients (111).

Nonoperative, percutaneous methods of varicocele treatment are offered by the interventional radiologist. Venography is first performed through a jugular, basilic, or femoral vein stick. Varicocele ablation then occurs either by the use of balloon or coil placement or the injection of a sclerosing agent. The success of these procedures is highly operator dependent and cannot always account for anatomic variations. There is also a higher recurrence rate (15–25%) when compared to newer surgical techniques (0–1%). Rare but serious complications include vascular perforation, coil or balloon migration, sclerosis of testicular or renal veins, and allergic contrast reaction (112). As percutaneous interventions may be performed under local anesthesia, this treatment option is often chosen for those patients who cannot tolerate general anesthesia for their varicocelectomy or for men with recurrent varicocele following open varicocelectomy.

Complications

In addition to technique-associated complications and routine postoperative wound infections or hematomas, varicocelectomy is associated with three specific major complications: hydrocele formation, recurrent varicocele, and testicular atrophy secondary to damage of the testicular artery (Table 3).

The most frequent complication of varicocelectomy is hydrocele formation, occurring in as many as 30% of the patients, depending on the technique. The etiology is likely that of lymphatic obstruction, evidenced by the high average protein content of postvaricocelectomy hydroceles compared to that of edematous fluid produced by venous obstruction (104). Formation of hydrocele requires surgical intervention due to scrotal discomfort in at least 50% of the cases. Use of magnification to identify and preserve lymphatics can

Table 3   Complications of Varicocelectomy

Technique	Hydrocele (%)	Failure (%)	Potential for serious morbidity
Retroperitoneal	7	15–25	No
Historical inguinal	3–30	5–15	No
Laparoscopic	12	5–15	Yes
Radiographic/ embolization	0	15–25	Yes
Microscopic or loupe inguinal; subinguinal	<1	1–3	No

Source: From Ref. 113.

virtually eliminate the risk of hydrocele formation after varicocelectomy (100,109,110).

Incidence of vascular compromise via injury or ligation of the testicular artery during varicocelectomy is impossible to measure, but scattered case series have been published. Startzl (114) reported a 14% incidence of frank testicular atrophy when the testicular artery was purposefully ligated during renal transplantation, but Goldstein and coworkers (115) reported neither the development of pain, testicular atrophy, nor a worsening of semen parameters after the inadvertent ligation of the internal spermatic artery in 18 patients during varicocelectomy. In most adults, if intentional or inadvertent testicular artery ligation occurs, collateral circulation will be provided by the cremasteric and vasal arteries. Rare cases of testicular ischemia and even complete testicular loss, however, have been reported in men with a history of previous groin or scrotal surgery, especially vasectomy (116). Care should be taken to forewarn patients of this terrible potential complication.

Recurrent or persistent varicocele after surgical repair varies from 0.6% to 45% depending on the technique. The microsurgical approach using optical loupes lowers the incidence of varicocele recurrence to only 1% to 2% amongst children, adolescents, and adults equally, compared with 9% to 16% using nonmagnified inguinal techniques (100,109,110,117,118). As previously stated, venography is recommended in the case of recurrent or persistent varicocele, as an interventional radiologist may be able to locate and occlude the aberrant venous drainage.

Effect of Repair
Semen Parameters and Testicle Growth

Improvement in seminal parameters has been extensively demonstrated in men after surgical varicocele repair, including motility (70% of patients), sperm density (51% of patients), and morphology (44% of patients) (89,96,110,119–130). Varicocelectomy has also been performed in men with nonobstructive azoospermia, resulting in the induction of spermatogenesis and the successful return of sperm to the ejaculate in approximately 40% of cases (Table 4) (103,131–133). Over 25% of these men were able to father children, including 5% who did so without the help of assisted reproduction interventions.

Varicocelectomy has also been used successfully in other conditions not directly related to a dysfunction in semen parameters. Peterson et al. in 1998 followed up 35 men who underwent varicocelectomy for orchalgia (134). Of these, 30 (86%) had complete resolution of pain, one man had partial resolution, and the remaining four had persistent pain or a worsening of it (134). Further, varicocelectomy has been shown to significantly increase serum testosterone levels in young, infertile men (135), possibly reflecting an improvement in both hormonal and spermatogenic function. Although still under contention, varicocelectomy has

Table 4 Improvements in Motile Sperm and Unassisted Pregnancy

		Motile sperm		Pregnancy[a]	
Study	N	(n)	%	(n)	%
Matthews et al., 1998 (131)	22	12	55	3	14
Kim et al., 1999 (132)	28	12	43	0	0
Kadioglu et al., 2001 (103)	24	5	21	NR	NR
Pasqualotto et al., 2003 (133)[b]	15	7	47	1	7
Totals	89	36	40	4	5

Note: Rates in azoospermic men after varicocelectomy.
[a]Unassisted pregnancies.
[b]Relapses back to azoospermia noted in five patients.
Abbreviations: N, total men in study with complete azoospermia; NR, not reported.

also resulted in significantly increased serum testosterone levels in selected older men, supporting the concept that varicocelectomy may halt or even partially reverse Leydig cell dysfunction and age-related androgen deficiency—a clinical condition increasingly referred to as "andropause" (135). In adolescents, varicocele repair can also result in catch-up growth of the affected ipsilateral testicle (89,136,137), a result that has not been replicated in adults.

Fertility

Perhaps the most controversial issue with respect to varicocelectomy is the effect of repair on pregnancy rates. Most studies examining the effect of varicocele on fertility have been uncontrolled, with average pregnancy rates of 30% to 60% (108,120,124,138–140). In a study designed to compare cost and pregnancy rates between intracytoplasmic sperm injection (ICSI) and varicocelectomy, Schlegel reported an average collated pregnancy rate of 33% in the varicocele repair group (305/928, or 95%, with a CI of 28–39%) compared with 16% in the control group (164/999, or 95%, with a CI of 13–20%) (141). Since 1979, only eight randomized controlled trials have been published (Table 5) (142). The results of these studies are limited by low pregnancy rates in both treatment and nontreatment groups, raising the question of contributing female factors (143), biased nontreatment arms (137), publication bias (151), and the unintentional inclusion of men with normal semen parameters or subclinical varicoceles (143–147,151).

In the three trials of clinically present varicoceles (137,148,151), all are limited by high dropout rates, poor methods of randomization, and significant differences in male selection factors such as age, duration of infertility, and varicocele grade (142). Madgar et al. (148) reported a 60% pregnancy rate after one year in the treatment group (15/25 couples) as opposed to a 10% pregnancy rate in the nontreatment arm (2/20 couples). In this convincing, crossover-design study, the nontreated arm was followed for one year of infertility, at which point varicocele repair was performed.

Table 5 Randomized Controlled Studies of Pregnancy Rate Following Varicocele Repair Vs. Observation[a]

Study	N (tx/control)	Varicocele type	Type of infertility	Duration of infertility (mo)	Treatment type	Follow-up (mo)	Pregnancy rate treatment (%)	Pregnancy rate control (%)	p value
Men with normal semen analysis included									
Nilsson et al., 1979 (143)	51/45	CV	1°	24–96	Open	36–74	4/51 (8)	8/45 (18)	0.16
Breznik et al., 1993 (144)	43/36 (corrected)	SV, CV	NR	NR	Open, embolization, sclerosation	12–48	18/43 (42)	17/36 (47)	0.63
Male subfertility[b] with subclinical varicocele									
Yamamoto et al., 1996 (145)	45/40	SV	NR	12–60	Open	24–60	3/45 (7)	4/40 (10)	0.758
Grasso et al., 2000 (146)	34/34	SV	NR	≥12	Open	12	1/34 (3)	2/34 (6)	0.56
Unal et al., 2001 (147)	21/21	SV	NR	≥12	Open	6	2/21 (13)	1/21 (7)	0.5
Male subfertility with clinical varicocele									
Madgar et al., 1995 (148)	25/20	CV	NR	≥12	Open	12	15/25 (60)	2/20 (10)	<0.001
Hargreave, 1997 (151)	67/68	CV	NR	≥12	Open	12	(35)	(17)	<0.003
Nieschlag et al., 1995/1998 (19,150)	62/63	CV	NR	≥12	Open, embolization w/histacryl	12	18/62 (29)	16/63 (23)	0.65

[a]Unal et al. evaluated patients with surgery versus clomiphene citrate; Nieschlag et al. evaluated patients with surgery versus psychological counseling.
[b]Yamamoto et al. had no subfertility inclusion requirements.
Abbreviations: 1°, primary infertility; CV, clinical varicocele; NR, not reported; SV, subclinical varicocele; mo, month.

Pregnancy rates rose fourfold (44%) in the observation group during the first year after surgical correction. Hargreave (151) published only limited results from a small population observed in a WHO varicocele trial. A larger study by Nieschlag et al. in 1998 (150) showed no relative benefit in 125 couples who received either surgical treatment or psychological counseling. Unfortunately, nonmicrosurgical techniques were used for the repairs, and follow-up was inadequate to determine recurrence, with most of the varicoceles repaired being small or moderate in size. Overall, further randomized, controlled clinical trials in men with clinically apparent varicoceles are necessary as there is as yet no conclusive evidence that varicocele repair alters pregnancy rates.

ADOLESCENT VARICOCELE

The emerging condition of adolescent varicocele deserves mention. Several studies have revealed an incidence of approximately 15%, which is similar to that of adults (12). The mechanism of varicoceles in adolescent males is not well understood, but most population studies suggest a causal relationship between puberty and the formation of adolescent varicoceles (149).

The best clinical indication of significant testicular dysfunction related to the varicocele in adolescents is testicular growth arrest. A size discrepancy of 2 mL or greater between the left and right testis in this population (as determined most accurately by ultrasound) constitutes significant growth arrest in the left testis and should be the main indication for surgery (12). Reversal of hypotrophy by surgical correction has been reported in 53% to 100% of cases (21,152). Other indications for varicocelectomy in adolescents that have been accepted by most pediatric urologists include the following: a decrease in testicular growth by at least two standard deviations from normal growth curves, symptomatic scrotal pain, large varicoceles (Grade III), bilateral varicoceles, or the presence of a solitary testicle (153). As GnRH stimulation studies have yet to be correlated with subsequent infertility and are both expensive and logistically difficult, its use is not currently advocated in the evaluation of a pediatric varicocele.

SUMMARY

Varicoceles are present in a large percentage of the male population. The majority of these men do not encounter any of the aforementioned sequelae, including scrotal pain, loss of testicular mass, testicular failure, or infertility. Despite the many viable hypotheses, the true etiology of varicocele and the mechanism of its effect remain unclear. Pathologic studies of varicoceles and their association with cigarettes have been shown to be detrimental to testicular spermatogenesis over time. For these reasons, ongoing research is required to fully explain the presence of varicocele and its true impact on the male testicle. Infertile men with oligospermia, large varicoceles (Grade III), and normal serum endocrine measurements are most likely to benefit from varicocelectomy. Treatment of varicocele-related scrotal pain has been demonstrated to resolve orchalgia in over 80% of patients. Testicular atrophy in adolescents has repeatedly been demonstrated to result in catch-up

growth of the affected ipsilateral testicle. Varicocelectomy in those presenting for infertility helps to improve conventional semen parameters about two-thirds of the time. Varicocelectomy remains one of the few surgical interventions available for infertility treatment, and couples will likely continue to elect to have this procedure performed if there is any chance that it will improve the possibility of conception. Although difficult to obtain accurately, it is likely that surgical repair improves pregnancy rates by 20% to 30% in the setting of clinical varicocele and subfertility. Ongoing clinic trials, however, continue to identify couples who would have attained pregnancy without intervention. It is for these patients that research on the controversial topic of varicocele is continued.

□ REFERENCES

1. Spencer WG. Celsus de Medicina (With an English Translation). Cambridge: Harvard University Press, 1938.
2. Barwell R. One hundred cases of varicocele treated by the subcutaneous wire loop. Lancet 1885; 1:978.
3. Bennett WH. Varicocele, particularly with reference to its radical cure. Lancet 1889; 1:261.
4. Macomber D, Sanders MB. The spermatozoa count: its value in the diagnosis, prognosis, and treatment of sterility. N Engl J Med 1929; 200:981–984.
5. Tulloch WS. Consideration of sterility: subfertility in the male. Edinb Med J 1952; 59:29.
6. Kursh ED. What is the incidence of varicocele in a fertile population? Fertil Steril 1987; 48(3):510–511.
7. Dubin L, Amelar RD. Etiologic factors in 1294 consecutive cases of male infertility. Fertil Steril 1971; 22(8):469–474.
8. Oster J. Varicocele in children and adolescents. Acta Paediatr Scand Suppl 1970; 206:81.
9. Grillo-Lopez AJ. Primary right varicocele. J Urol 1971; 105(4):540–541.
10. Johnson DE, Pohl DR, Rivera-Correa H. Varicocele: an innocuous condition? South Med J 1970; 63(1):34–36.
11. Saypol DC. Varicocele. J Androl 1981; 2(2):61.
12. Skoog SJ, Roberts KP, Goldstein M, et al. The adolescent varicocele: what's new with an old problem in young patients? Pediatrics 1997; 100(1):112–122.
13. Gat Y, Bachar GN, Zukerman ZV, et al. Varicocele: a bilateral disease. Fertil Steril 2004; 81(2):424–429.
14. Gorelick J, Goldstein M. Loss of fertility in men with varicocele. Fertil Steril 1993; 59(3):613–616.
15. Witt MA, Lipshultz LI. Varicocele: a progressive or static lesion? Urology 1993; 42(5):541–543.
16. Jarow JP, Coburn M, Sigman M. Incidence of varicoceles in men with primary and secondary infertility. Urology 1996; 47(1):73–76.
17. Fretz PC, Sandlow J. Varicocele: current concepts in pathophysiology, diagnosis, and treatment. Urol Clin N Am 2002; 29(4):921–937.
18. Vermeulen A, Vanderweghe M. Improved fertility after varicocele correction: fact or fiction? Fertil Steril 1984; 42(2):249–256.
19. Nieschlag E, Hertle L, Fischedick A, et al. Treatment of varicocele: counselling as effective as occlusion of the vena spermatica. Hum Reprod 1995; 10(2):347–353.
20. World Health Organization. The influence of varicocele on parameters of fertility in a large group of men presenting to infertility clinics. Fertil Steril 1992; 57(6):1289–1293.
21. Walmsley K, Coleman JA, Goldstein M. The inheritance of varicocele. J Urol 2001; 165(5 suppl):334.
22. Mellinger BC. Varicocelectomy. Tech Urol 1995; 1(4):188–196.
23. Parrott TS, Hewatt L. Ligation of the testicular artery and vein in adolescent varicocele. J Urol 1994; 152(2 Pt 2):791–793.
24. Yamamoto M, Tsuji Y, Ohmura M, et al. Comparison of artery-ligating and artery-preserving varicocelectomy: effect on post-operative spermatogenesis. Andrologia 1995; 27(1):37–40.
25. Schneck FX, Bellinger MF. Abnormalities of the testis and scrotum and their surgical management. In: Walsh PC, Retik AB, Vaughan ED Jr, et al., eds. Campbell's Urology. 8th ed. Philadelphia: WB Saunders, 2002:2385–2386.
26. Shafik A, Moftah A, Olfat S, et al. Testicular veins: anatomy and role in varicocelogenesis and other pathologic conditions. Urology 1990; 35(2):175–182.
27. Saypol DC, Howards SS, Turner TT, et al. Influence of surgically induced varicocele on testicular blood flow, temperature, and histology in adult rats and dogs. J Clin Invest 1981; 68(1):39–45.
28. Coolsaet BL. The varicocele syndrome: venography determining the optimal level for surgical management. J Urol 1980; 124(6):833–839.

29. Turek PJ, Lipschultz LI. The varicocele controversies. I. Etiology and pathophysiology. AUA Update Series. Vol. 14, lesson 13. Baltimore: American Urologic Association, 1995:106–111.

30. Wishahi MM. Detailed anatomy of the internal spermatic vein and the ovarian vein. Human cadaver study and operative spermatic venography: clinical aspects. J Urol 1991; 145(4):780–784.

31. Ahlberg NE, Bartley O, Chidekel N. Right and left gonadal veins. An anatomical and statistical study. Acta Radiol Diagn (Stockh) 1966; 4(6):593–601.

32. Braedel HU, Steffens J, Ziegler M, et al. A possible ontogenic etiology for idiopathic left varicocele. J Urol 1994; 151(1):62–66.

33. Dennison AR, Tibbs DJ. Varicocele and varicose veins compared. A basis for logical surgery. Urology 1986; 28(3):211–217.

34. Narayan P, Amplatz K, Gonzalez R. Varicocele and male subfertility. Fertil Steril 1981; 36(1):92–97.

35. Shafik A, Bedeir GAM. Venous tension patterns in cord veins. I. In normal and varicocele individuals. J Urol 1980; 123(3):383–385.

36. Etriby A, Ibrahim A, Mahmoud KZ, et al. Subfertility and varicocele. I. Venogram demonstration of anastomosis sites in subfertile men. Fertil Steril 1975; 26(10):1013–1017.

37. Zorgniotti AW, MacLeod J. Studies in temperature, human semen quality, and varicocele. Fertil Steril 1973; 24(11):854–863.

38. Green KF, Turner TT, Howard SS. Varicocele: reversal of testicular blood flow and temperature effects by varicocele repair. J Urol 1984; 131(6):1208–1211.

39. Fujisawa M, Yoshida S, Matsumoto O, et al. Deoxyribonucleic acid polymerase activity in the testes of infertile men with varicocele. Fertil Steril 1988; 50(5):795–800.

40. Fujisawa M, Yoshida S, Kojima K, et al. Biochemical changes in testicular varicocele. Arch Androl 1989; 22(2):149–159.

41. Heinz HA, Voggenthaler J, Weissbach L. Histological findings in testes with varicocele during childhood and their therapeutic consequences. Eur J Pediatr 1980; 133(2):139–146.

42. Tessler AN, Krahn HP. Varicocele and testicular temperature. Fertil Steril 1966; 17(2):201–203.

43. Stephenson JD, O'Shaughnessy EJ. Hypospermia and its relationship to varicocele and intrascrotal temperature. Fertil Steril 1968; 19(1):110–117.

44. MacLeod J. Seminal cytology in the presence of varicocele. Fertil Steril 1965; 16(6):735–757.

45. Cohen MS, Plainse L, Brown JS. The role of internal spermatic vein plasma catecholamine determinations in subfertile men with varicoceles. Fertil Steril 1975; 26(12):1243–1249.

46. Ito H, Fuse H, Minagawa H, et al. Internal spermatic vein prostaglandins in varicocele patients. Fertil Steril 1982; 37(2):218–222.

47. Ozbek E, Yurekli M, Soylu A, et al. The role of adrenomedullin in varicocele and impotence. BJU Int 2000; 86(6):694–698.

48. Comhaire F, Vermeulen A. Varicocele sterility: cortisol and catecholamines. Fertil Steril 1974; 25(1):88–95.

49. Netto NR Jr, Lerner JS, Paolini RM, et al. Varicocele: the value of reflux in the spermatic vein. Int J Fertil 1980; 25(1):71–74.

50. Di Luigi L, Gentile V, Pigozzi F, et al. Physical activity as a possible aggravating factor for athletes with varicocele: impact on the semen profile. Hum Reprod 2001; 16(6):1180–1184.

51. Chakraborty J, Hikim AP, Jhunjhunwala JS. Stagnation of blood in the microcirculatory vessels in the testes of men with varicocele. J Androl 1985; 6(2):117–126.

52. Tanji N, Tanji K, Hiruma S, et al. Histochemical study of human cremaster in varicocele patients. Arch Androl 2000; 45(3):197–202.

53. Turner TT, Jones CE, Roddy MS. Experimental varicocele does not affect the blood–testis barrier, epididymal electrolyte concentrations, or testicular blood gas concentrations. Biol Reprod 1987; 36(4):926–932.

54. Klaiber EL, Broverman DM, Pokoly TB, et al. Interrelationships of cigarette smoking, testicular varicoceles, and seminal fluid indexes. Fertil Steril 1987; 47(3):481–486.

55. Peng BC, Tomashefsky P, Nagler HM. The cofactor effect: varicocele and infertility. Fertil Steril 1990; 54(1):143–148.

56. Klaiber EL, Broverman DM, Vogel W. Increased incidence of testicular varicoceles in cigarette smokers. Fertil Steril 1980; 34(1):64–65.

57. Benoff S, Gilbert BR. Varicocele and male infertility: part I. Preface. Hum Reprod Update 2001; 7(1):47–54.

58. Pryor JL, Howards SS. Varicocele. Urol Clin N Am 1987; 14(3):499–513.

59. Lipshultz LI, Corriere JN Jr. Progressive testicular atrophy in the varicocele patient. J Urol 1977; 117(2):175–176.

60. Dubin L, Amelar RD. Varicocele size and results of varicocelectomy in selected subfertile men with varicocele. Fertil Steril 1970; 21(8):606–609.

61. Uehling DT. Fertility in men with varicocele. Int J Fertil 1968; 13(1):58–60.

62. Hargreave TB, Liakatas J. Physical examination for varicocele. Br J Urol 1991; 67(3):328.

63. Petros JA, Andriole GL, Middleton WD, et al. Correlation of testicular color Doppler ultrasonography, physical examination and venography in detection of left varicoceles in men with infertility. J Urol 1991; 145(4):785–788.

64. Pierik FH, Dohle GR, van Muiswinkel JM, et al. Is routine scrotal ultrasound advantageous in infertile men? J Urol 1999; 162(5):1618–1620.

65. Trum JW, Gubler FM, Laan R, et al. The value of palpation, varicoscreen contact thermography and colour

Doppler ultrasound in the diagnosis of varicocele. Hum Reprod 1996; 11(6):1232–1235.

66. McClure RD, Hricak H. Scrotal ultrasound in the infertile man: detection of subclinical unilateral and bilateral varicoceles. J Urol 1986; 135(4):711–715.

67. Aydos K, Baltaci S, Salih M, et al. Use of color Doppler sonography in the evaluation of varicoceles. Eur Urol 1993; 24(2):221–225.

68. Eskew LA, Watson NE, Wolfman N, et al. Ultrasonographic diagnosis of varicoceles. Fertil Steril 1993; 60(4):693–697.

69. Meachum RB, Townsend RR, Rademacher D, et al. The incidence of varicoceles in the general population when evaluated by physical examination, gray scale sonography and color Doppler sonography. J Urol 1994; 151(6):1535–1538.

70. World Health Organization. Comparison among different methods for the diagnosis of varicocele. Fertil Steril 1985; 43(4):575–582.

71. Marsman JW. Clinical versus subclinical varicocele: venographic findings and improvement of fertility after embolization. Radiology 1985; 155(3):635–638.

72. Lewis RW, Harrison RM. Contact scrotal thermography: application to problems of infertility. J Urol 1979; 122(1):40–42.

73. Basile-Fasolo C, Izzo PL, Canale D, et al. Doppler sonography, contact scrotal thermography and venography: a comparative study in evaluation of subclinical varicocele. Int J Fertil 1986; 30(4):62–64.

74. Gat Y, Zukerman ZV, Bachar GN, et al. Adolescent varicocele: is it unilateral disease? Urology 2003; 62(4):742–746.

75. Fuse H, Nozaki T, Ohta S, et al. Sequential scrotal scintigraphy for the study of varicocele. Int Urol Nephrol 1999; 31(4):511–517.

76. Von Heijne A. Recurrent varicocele. Demonstration by 3D phase-contrast MR angiography. Acta Radiol 1997; 38(6):1020–1022.

77. Ayodeji O, Baker HW. Is there a specific abnormality of sperm morphology in men with varicoceles? Fertil Steril 1986; 45(6):839–842.

78. Rodriguez-Rigau LJ, Smith KD, Steinberger E. Varicocele and the morphology of spermatozoa. Fertil Steril 1981; 35(1):54–57.

79. Fariss BL, Fenner DK, Plymate SR, et al. Seminal characteristics in the presence of a varicocele as compared with those of expectant fathers and prevasectomy men. Fertil Steril 1981; 35(3):325–327.

80. Moro E, Marin P, Rossi A, et al. Y chromosome microdeletions in infertile men with varicocele. Mol Cell Endocrinol 2000; 161(1–2):67–71.

81. Sigman M, Jarow JP. Ipsilateral testicular hypotrophy is associated with decreased sperm counts in infertile men with varicoceles. J Urol 1997; 158(2):605–607.

82. Steckel J, Dicker AP, Goldstein M. Relationship between varicocele size and response to varicocelectomy. J Urol 1993; 149(4):769–771.

83. Zini A, Buckspan M, Berardinucci D, et al. Loss of left testicular volume in men with clinical left varicocele: correlation with grade of varicocele. Arch Androl 1998; 41(1):37–41.

84. Baccetti B, Collodel G, Piomboni P. Apoptosis in human ejaculated sperm cells (notulae seminologicae 9). J Submicrosc Cytol Pathol 1996; 28(4):587–596.

85. Hadziselimovic F, Leibundgut B, Da Rugna D, et al. The value of testicular biopsy in patients with varicocele. J Urol 1986; 135(4):707–710.

86. Russell JK. Varicocele, age, and fertility. Lancet 1957; 273(6988):222.

87. Nagler HM, Li XZ, Lizza EF, et al. Varicocele: temporal considerations. J Urol 1985; 134(2):411–413.

88. Chehval MJ, Purcell MH. Deterioration of semen parameters over time in men with untreated varicocele: evidence of progressive testicular damage. Fertil Steril 1992; 57(1):174–177.

89. Lyon RP, Marshall S, Scott MP. Varicocele in childhood and adolescence: implication in adulthood fertility? Urology 1982; 19(6):641–644.

90. Swerdloff RS, Walsh PC. Pituitary and gonadal hormones in patients with varicocele. Fertil Steril 1975; 26(10):1006–1012.

91. Hudson RW, Crawford VA, McKay DE. The gonadotropin response of men with varicoceles to a four-hour infusion of gonadotropin-releasing hormone. Fertil Steril 1981; 36(5):633–637.

92. Ando S, Giacchetto C, Beraldi E, et al. Testosterone and dihydrotestosterone seminal plasma levels in varicocele patients. Acta Eur Fertil 1982; 13(3):113–117.

93. Younes AK. Low plasma testosterone in varicocele patients with impotence and male infertility. Arch Androl 2000; 45(3):187–195.

94. Hudson RW, Hayes KA, Crawford VA, et al. Seminal plasma testosterone and dihydrotestosterone levels in men with varicoceles. Int J Androl 1983; 6(2):135–142.

95. Sigman M, Jarow JP. Male infertility. In: Walsh PC, Retik AB, Vaughan ED Jr, et al., eds. Campbell's Urology. 8th ed. Philadelphia: WB Saunders, 2002:1507.

96. Tinga DJ, Jager S, Bruijnen CL, et al. Factors related to semen improvement and fertility after varicocele operation. Fertil Steril 1984; 41(3):404–410.

97. Yoshida K, Kitahara S, Chiba K, et al. Predictive indicators of successful varicocele repair in men with infertility. Int J Fertil Womens Med 2000; 45(4):279–284.

98. Matkov TG, Zenni M, Sandlow J, et al. Preoperative semen analysis as a predictor of seminal improvement following varicocelectomy. Fertil Steril 2001; 75(1):63–68.

99. Schrepferman CG, Ehle J, Sparks AET, et al. Preoperative total motile count (TMC) and follicle-stimulating hormone (FSH) are predictive of response to varicocelectomy. Fertil Steril 2000; 74(3 suppl 1):S240.

100. Cayan S, Kadioglu TC, Tefekli A, et al. Comparison of results and complications of high ligation surgery and microsurgical high inguinal varicocelectomy in the treatment of varicocele. Urology 2000; 55(5):750–754.

101. Yarborough MA, Burns JR, Keller FS. Incidence and clinical significance of subclinical scrotal varicoceles. J Urol 1988; 141(6):1372–1374.

102. Jarow JP, Ogle SR, Eskew LA. Seminal improvement following repair of ultrasound detected subclinical varicoceles. J Urol 1996; 155(4):1287–1290.

103. Kadioglu A, Tefekli A, Cayan S, et al. Microsurgical inguinal varicocele repair in azoospermic men. Urology 2001; 57(2):328–333.

104. Szabo R, Kessler R. Hydrocele following internal spermatic vein ligation: a retrospective study and review of the literature. J Urol 1984; 132(5):924–925.

105. Homonnai ZT, Fainman N, Engelhard Y, et al. Varicocelectomy and male fertility: comparison of semen quality and recurrence of varicocele following varicocelectomy by two techniques. Int J Androl 1980; 3(4):447–458.

106. Kass EJ, Marcol B. Results of varicocele surgery in adolescents: a comparison of techniques. J Urol 1992; 148(2 Pt 2):694–696.

107. Rashid TM, Winfield HN, Lund GO, et al. Comparative financial analysis of laparoscopic versus open varix ligation for men with clinically significant varicoceles. J Urol 1994; 151(331):310A.

108. Marmar JL, DeBenedictis TJ, Praiss D. The management of varicoceles by microdissection of the spermatic cord at the external inguinal ring. Fertil Steril 1985; 43(4):583–588.

109. Marmar JL, Kim Y. Subinguinal microsurgical varicocelectomy: a technical critique and statistical analysis of semen and pregnancy data. J Urol 1994; 152(4): 1127–1132.

110. Goldstein M, Gilbert BR, Dicker AP, et al. Microsurgical inguinal varicocelectomy with delivery of the testis: an artery and lymphatic sparing technique. J Urol 1992; 148(6):1808–1811.

111. Iacono F, Capparelli G, Darmiento M. Bilateral varicocele repair by transscrotal extratunica vaginalis procedure in outpatients: a novel technique. Tech Urol 2000; 6(3):196–200.

112. Riedl P, Lunglmayr G, Stackl W. A new method of transfemoral testicular vein obliteration for varicocele using a balloon catheter. Radiology 1981; 139(2): 323–325.

113. Goldstein M. Surgical management of male infertility and other scrotal disorders. In: Walsh PC, Retik AB, Vaughan ED Jr, eds. Campbell's Urology. 8th ed. Philadelphia: WB Saunders, 2002:1571–1579.

114. Penn I, Mackie G, Halgrimson CG, et al. Testicular complications following renal transplantation. Ann Surg 1972; 176(6):697–699.

115. Chan PT, Wright EJ, Goldstein M. Incidence and post-operative outcomes of accidental ligation of the testicular artery during microsurgical varicocelectomy. J Urol 2005; 173(2):482–484.

116. Amelar RD. Early and late complications of inguinal varicocelectomy. J Urol 2003; 170(2 Pt 1):366–369.

117. Lemack GE, Uzzo RG, Schlegel PN, et al. Microsurgical repair of the adolescent varicocele. J Urol 1998; 160(1):179–181.

118. Minnevich E, Wacksman J, Lewis AG, et al. Inguinal microsurgical varicocelectomy in the adolescent: technique and preliminary results. J Urol 1998; 159(3):1022–1024.

119. Dubin L, Amelar RD. Varicocelectomy: 986 cases in a twelve-year study. Urology 1977; 10(5):446–449.

120. Brown JS. Varicocelectomy in the subfertile male: a ten-year experience with 295 cases. Fertil Steril 1976; 27(9):1046–1053.

121. Charny CW, Baum S. Varicocele and infertility. JAMA 1968; 204(13):1165–1168.

122. MacLeod J. Further observations on the role of varicocele in human male infertility. Fertil Steril 1969; 20(4):545–563.

123. Newton R, Schinfeld JS, Schiff I. The effect of varicocelectomy on sperm count, motility and conception rate. Fertil Steril 1980; 34(3):250–254.

124. Marks JL, McMahon R, Lipshultz LI. Predictive parameters of successful varicocele repair. J Urol 1986; 136(3):609–612.

125. Parsch EM, Schill WB, Erlinger C, et al. Semen parameters and conception rates after surgical treatment and sclerotherapy of varicocele. Andrologia 1990; 22(3):275–278.

126. Sayfan J, Soffer Y, Orda R. Varicocele treatment: prospective randomized trial of 3 methods. J Urol 1992; 148(5):1447–1449.

127. Yavetz H, Levy R, Papo J, et al. Efficacy of varicocele embolization versus ligation of the left internal spermatic vein for improvement of sperm quality. Int J Androl 1992; 15(4): 338–344.

128. Schatte E, Hirshberg SJ, Fallick ML, et al. Varicocelectomy improves sperm strict morphology and motility. J Urol 1998; 160(4):1338–1340.

129. Kamal KM, Jarvi K, Zini A. Microsurgical varicocelectomy in the era of assisted reproductive technology: influence of initial semen quality on pregnancy rates. Fertil Steril 2001; 75(5):1013–1016.

130. Kibar Y, Seckin B, Erduran D. The effects of subinguinal varicocelectomy on Kruger morphology and semen parameters. J Urol 2002; 168(3):1071–1074.

131. Matthews GJ, Matthews ED, Goldstein M. Induction of spermatogenesis and achievement of pregnancy after microsurgical varicocelectomy in men with azoospermia and severe oligoasthenospermia. Fertil Steril 1998; 70(1):71–75.

132. Kim ED, Leibman BB, Grinblat DM, et al. Varicocele repair improves semen parameters in azoospermic men with spermatogenic failure. J Urol 1999; 162 (3 Pt 1):737–740.

133. Pasqualotto FF, Lucon AM, Hallak J, et al. Induction of spermatogenesis in azoospermic men after varicocele repair. Hum Reprod 2003; 18(1):108–112.

134. Peterson AC, Lance RS, Ruiz HE. Outcomes of varicocele ligation done for pain. J Urol 1998; 159(5): 1565–1567.

135. Su LM, Goldstein M, Schlegel PN. The effect of varicocelectomy on serum testosterone levels in infertile men with varicoceles. J Urol 1995; 154(5):1752–1755.

136. Okuyama A, Nakamura M, Namiki M, et al. Surgical repair of varicocele at puberty: preventive treatment for fertility improvement. J Urol 1988; 139(3): 562–564.

137. Kass EJ, Belman AB. Reversal of testicular growth failure by varicocele ligation. J Urol 1987; 137(3): 475–476.

138. Tulloch WS. Varicocele in subfertility. Results of treatment. 1955. J Urol 2002; 167(2 Pt 2):1184–1185.

139. Cockett AT, Urry RL, Dougherty KA. The varicocele and semen characteristics. J Urol 1979; 121(4):435–436.

140. Schlesinger MH, Wilets IF, Nalger HM. Treatment outcome after varicocelectomy: a critical analysis. Urol Clin North Am 1994; 21(3):517–529.

141. Schlegel PN. Is assisted reproduction the optimal treatment for varicocele-associated male infertility? A cost-effectiveness analysis. Urology 1997; 49(1):83–90.

142. Evers JL, Collins JA. Assessment of efficacy of varicocele repair for male subfertility: a systematic review. Lancet 2003; 361(9372):1849–1852.

143. Nilsson S, Edvinsson A, Nilsson B. Improvement of semen and pregnancy rate after ligation and division of the internal spermatic vein: fact or fiction? Br J Urol 1979; 51(6):591–596.

144. Breznik R, Vlaisavljevic V, Borko E. Treatment of varicocele and male fertility. Arch Androl 1993; 30: 157–60.

145. Yamamoto M, Hibi H, Hirata Y, et al. Effect of varicocelectomy on sperm parameters and pregnancy rate in patients with subclinical varicocele: a randomized prospective controlled study. J Urol 1996; 155(5): 1636–1638.

146. Grasso M, Lania M, Castelli M, et al. Low-grade left varicocele in patients over 30 years old: the effect of spermatic vein ligation on fertility. BJU Int 2000; 85(3):305–307.

147. Unal D, Yeni E, Verit A, et al. Clomiphene citrate versus varicocelectomy in treatment of subclinical varicocele: a prospective randomized study. Int J Urol 2001; 8(5):227–230.

148. Madgar I, Weissenberg R, Lunenfeld B, et al. Controlled trial of high spermatic vein ligation for varicocele in infertile men. Fertil Steril 1995; 63(1):120–124.

149. Akbay E, Cayan S, Doruk E, et al. The prevalence of varicocele and the varicocele-related testicular atrophy in Turkish children and adolescents. BJU Int 2000; 86(4):490–493.

150. Nieschlag E, Hertle L, Fischedick A, et al. Update on treatment of varicocele: counselling as effective as occlusion of the vena spermatica. Hum Reprod 1998; 13(8):2147–2150.

151. Hargreave TB. Varicocele: overview and commentary on the results of the World Health Organization varicocele trial. In: Waites G, Frick J, Baker HWG, eds. Current Advances in Andrology. Proceedings of the Sixth International Congress of Andrology, Salzburg, Austria, May 25–29, 1997. Bologna: Monduzzi Editore, 1997:31–44.

152. Yamamoto M, Hibi H, Katsuno S, et al. Effects of varicocelectomy on testis volume and semen parameters in adolescents: a randomized prospective study. Nagoya J Med Sci 1995; 58(3–4):127–132.

153. Diamond DA. Adolescent varicocele: emerging understanding. BJU Int 2003; 92(suppl 1):48–51.

16

Male Genital Tract Infections and Infertility

Durwood E. Neal, Jr.
Department of Urology, University of Missouri Medical School, Columbia, Missouri, U.S.A.

Stephen H. Weinstein
Director of Clinical Skills, University of Missouri Medical School, Columbia, Missouri, U.S.A.

☐ INTRODUCTION

Without a doubt, male genitourinary (GU) tract infections significantly contribute to male-factor infertility. Considering that as many as half of all cases of couple infertility may be attributable to the male (1), it follows that the effect of GU tract infections on seminal quality—and, indirectly, on the female reproductive tract—is substantial.

The effects of GU tract infections on the male may take several different directions. The first is that of direct damage or other noxious effects to the sperm or, secondarily, the seminal fluid (2,3). Fortunately, these are the most easily treatable of the potential deleterious effects. Usually, simple elimination of the offending agent is required for cure. A second effect may be seen on the development of sperm, either by direct or by indirect actions (4–6). The severity of the infectious process may affect the body constitutionally and, as such, may divert the body's metabolic energy toward fighting the infection and away from activity that is less vital to an individual's immediate survival and recovery needs, such as the synthesis or maturation of spermatozoa (7). The adverse effects of systemic illness on fertility (7–9) as well as the anti-infective agents used to treat them (10–13) have been established. It has been demonstrated that while some antibiotics may affect spermatogenesis, others may impact seminal fluid quality.

Over the years, controversy regarding the effects of infectious GU disease and its consequent antibiotic treatment on fertility has emerged, as the specific etiologic agents have not always been positively elucidated (14). On the other hand, the literature also abounds with reports of improvements in seminal quality and even improved pregnancy outcomes following empiric antibiotic treatment of the male (15–17). Unfortunately, many of these reports are not controlled well enough to be able to draw cause-and-effect conclusions. It is possible that the microorganisms that may be causing the infection are not detectable by the usual investigations. Although several studies have focused on organisms such as *Chlamydia, Mycoplasma,* and *Ureaplasma*, among others, the findings, with some

regard to cause and effect, have been inconsistent at best (18). Interestingly, some researchers have detected bacterial deoxyribonucleic acid (DNA) and other bacterial genetic fingerprints in the GU tract of infertile males, but in no way does this prove the causative nature of bacteria in infertility (19).

☐ CLASSIFICATION OF MALE GU TRACT INFECTIONS
Prostatitis

The strict, original definition of prostatitis referred to an infectious or inflammatory process in the prostate gland. This disease entity, however, was typically accompanied by a rather amorphous set of signs and symptoms that were not quantified. Over time, this definition was expanded by the work of Meares and Stamey, which showed that the prostate gland could sequester and thus shield bacteria from the body's host defense mechanisms as well as the actions of antibiotics (20,21). Their data helped to provide a greatly improved understanding of the pathophysiologic mechanism for chronic bacterial prostatitis. Most recently, the definition of prostatitis has been further elaborated to include not only bacterial infections, but also nonbacterial and noninflammatory conditions (22). As most of these conditions involve pain, this symptom has evolved into the defining factor of prostatitis. A symptom score sheet has been developed and validated to assist in the evaluation of the prostatitis patient (22).

The bacterial types of prostatitis (Categories I and II) are easily understood; however, it remains unclear which organisms may be considered pathologic and which commensal. Many cases are self-evident, but others can be confusing. For example, some cases of both A and B category III prostatitis may, in fact, be category II prostatitis, when the results of the cultures are assessed accurately. In the absence of culturable bacteria, fastidious organisms such as *Mycoplasma, Chlamydia,* and *Ureaplasma* can be the inciting organisms. It is still unclear if these agents cause the same symptoms as bacterial infections; however, they have been implicated in male infertility, especially in cases of *Chlamydia* infection (1,18,23,24). In the absence of an etiologic agent, category III prostatitis remains an enigma, and its role in male infertility is not well defined. (For more information on the physiology of the prostate, please refer to Chapter 7.)

Urethritis

Urethral infection/inflammation commonly causes infertility by direct effects of the infectious organisms on sperm. Fortunately, this is uncommon, because symptoms caused by the infection limit continuation of exposure. Tissue scarring subsequent to infection represents the main pathologic mechanism that could interfere with sperm deposition in the female by reducing the count or the volume, or both.

In the past, the most common agent implicated in urethritis was *Neisseria gonorrhea*. This gram-negative diplococcus is sexually transmitted and easily identified on Gram stains of urethral discharge. Even though this organism has become increasingly resistant to many antibiotics, its incidence has diminished in both relative and absolute numbers. *Chlamydia trachomatis* and other species are the typical etiologic agents for most cases of so-called nonspecific urethritis (18,23–25). These pathogens cause more cases of urethritis than does *Neisseria*, but the inflammatory response is not as exuberant and thus the incidence of scarring (urethral stricture disease) is not as common. Urethritis may also be caused by more unusual organisms such as *Trichomonas vaginalis* and *Candida albicans*, but the impact of these organisms on fertility tends to be limited, especially if adequately treated. *Ureaplasma* species are thought to be etiologic in cases of both male and female infertility (25), but because the organism has also been isolated in the urethrae of fertile males, the significance of this finding is not clear.

There are also forms of noninfectious urethritis that may result from irritants such as latex condoms, spermicidal jelly, soaps, fabric softeners, detergents, and others. Allergic responses to these agents may be seen as well. Reiter's syndrome, a constellation of symptoms that is part of a group of collagen vascular diseases, is a relatively unusual cause of urethral inflammation; the corticosteroid treatment of this condition, however, may actually be more deleterious to fertility than the disease itself (1). In all, these forms of urethritis account for a small minority of cases, but should be borne in mind, clinically.

Epididymitis/Orchitis

Infection of the testicle and its appendicular structures can be extremely hazardous to future fertility. The lacy microscopic network of tubules that makes up the epididymis is particularly susceptible to damage from infection or inflammation. (For further information on the physiology of the epididymis, please refer to Chapter 6.) Although most of these infections tend to be sexually transmitted, they also usually occur only

in a well-defined age range. Over the ages of 40 to 50 years, the most common etiologic agents gradually change from *Neisseria*, *Chlamydia*, *Ureaplasma*, and *Mycoplasma* to gram-negative rods, chiefly the *Enterobacteriaceae* (3,25). This alteration occurs not only because of changes in sexual behavior, but also from the increasing age-related incidence of symptomatic benign prostatic hyperplasia and obstructive voiding, both of which predispose men to bacterial urinary tract infections (UTIs). Either type of bacteria will greatly diminish fertility, both acutely and chronically, but in later years, fertility typically becomes less of a concern in men.

Noninfectious epididymoorchitis is probably quite common, although little epidemiologic data are available. Chemical irritation from the reflux of urine into the ejaculatory ducts can cause a condition almost indistinguishable from bacterial epididymitis, often preceded by an episode of straining or vigorous physical activity with a full bladder. There may also be intense inflammation and subsequent drainage, even in the absence of a definable bacterial infection. These symptoms are usually recurring, because the ejaculatory duct may be aberrantly inserted or otherwise more susceptible to urinary reflux than normal.

☐ MECHANISMS OF INFERTILITY
Bacterial Effects

Bacteria may adversely affect fertility in several ways. One mechanism occurs through the direct inhibition of fertilization by the spermatozoa. This situation arises when the bacteria bind to the sperm, preventing motility or even sperm binding to the ovum. When bacteria bind the surface receptors on the spermatozoa, it can result in permanent agglutination and loss of spermatozoal motility. This effectively eliminates access to the ova. Bacterial sperm binding may also prevent fertilization by covering the binding sites needed for the attachment of sperm to the ovum. The bacterial appendages that affect spermatozoan binding are referred to as fimbriae. Most bacteria have many of these on their cell surfaces, and the most well-studied are those of *Escherichia coli* (26–30). Of these, the fimbriae that have been characterized most completely are the P-fimbriae (mannose-resistant) and the Type I fimbriae (mannose-sensitive). Both types of fimbriae are capable of binding to the spermatozoa itself, with the P-fimbriae preferentially binding to the head of the sperm and the Type I fimbriae binding to the tail. The P-fimbriae bind to the α-galanin-like peptide (GALP)-(1-4)-β-GALP-O methyl–binding site on human and primate urothelial cell surfaces. The specific *E. coli* that harbor these fimbriae are the same as those that most commonly cause bladder infections as well as prostatitis and ascending pyelonephritis by avidly binding to the perineum, foreskin, and urethra, as well as to the urothelium (30). It appears, then, that *E. coli* are uniquely suited to their environment in the human GU tract with respect to colonization and invasion.

Also known to affect fertility are the numerous indirect effects of bacterial infections, as well as the host inflammatory and immune responses to these agents. Although bacterial secretions may be locally toxic to sperm, these soluble factors, largely proteins, also elicit an intense inflammatory response that may be even more deleterious than the direct effects of bacterial toxins (5,31). The mere presence of polymorphonuclear (PMN) leukocytes has been shown to affect fertility adversely, and these blood cells are summoned to the site by a number of soluble substances (32). After the initial arrival of these leukocytes, the recruitment process begins as more PMNs are attracted to the site. These chemical attractants are also toxic to sperm and thus may adversely affect seminal quality. Adverse effects of this process on sperm quality are usually demonstrated in sperm penetration assay. Hydrogen peroxide, along with its attendant free radicals, is among the substances involved in the inflammatory cascade that can cause sperm immobilization (33).

Another means by which bacteria may adversely affect fertility is again illustrated by the paradigm of *N. gonorrhea*. This sexually transmitted organism initially causes urethritis, and if not adequately treated at this stage, scarring of the urethra occurs, and by reducing the volume and inhibiting the force of ejaculation, may prevent the placement of sperm in propinquity to the ovum. Furthermore, when urethral stricture disease is present, there is a strong predilection toward recurrent bacterial UTIs; this condition alone may independently diminish fertility. The gram-negative diplococcus may migrate from its port of entry to the prostate and, from there, through the vas deferens to the testis and its adnexal structures. In these areas, it causes acute suppurative PMN inflammation that may permanently damage the delicate network of tubules, cause obstruction, and reduce or eliminate sperm transport (34). Other sexually transmitted organisms that may cause a similar type of infection are *C. trachomatis* and *Ureaplasma urealyticum*, but these cause far fewer symptoms. Infection of the testicular appendicular structures in the adult male is most often a result of the *Enterobacteriaceae*, of which *E. coli* is the most prevalent (35,36). With preexisting benign prostatic hyperplasia or other forms of bladder outlet obstruction, these infections may be particularly severe, resulting in abscess formation and occasionally testicular loss. Most recently, there has been a rise in infections of the male GU tract with the organism *Staphylococcus saprophyticus* (37). In any case, when a man presents with a bacterial UTI, one must also consider the risk of a preexisting congenital (or acquired) anomaly that may be a predisposing factor. Even without infection, these anatomical abnormalities may also cause infertility. (For further information on obstruction of the ejaculatory ducts, please refer to Chapter 18.)

Infection of the prostate gland may result in specific effects on fertility, independent of the infection itself. Since the ejaculatory ducts pass through the parenchyma of the prostate, an acute (or chronic) inflammatory process could cause obstruction of this structure that, with cicatricial formation, could permanently cause obstructive azoospermia (38,39). There have been a number of published reports demonstrating recovered semen quality or fertility after transurethral resection of the ejaculatory ducts. When the ducts are obstructed, the inspissated secretions may serve to contribute to a chronic bacterial infection by reducing normal drainage and thus creating a relatively protected enclave wherein bacteria may thrive, relatively unencumbered by the body's immune response and isolated from antibiotic action. The function of the prostate gland may also be hampered by a prostatic infection, in that the secretory activity of the gland is impaired during infection (40,41). The prostate is then unable to sequester and secrete its complement of divalent cations, the most necessary of which are calcium and zinc (41). The latter element has been shown to be essential for normal sperm motility and activity. The acute inflammatory process decreases zinc levels to near zero, and there is variable recovery with time. In addition, zinc is the active component of prostatic antibacterial factor, which has been shown to assist in the prevention of UTIs in the male (40). When this substance is nonfunctional, infections are presumed to occur with greater facility. This substance is not easily replaced with oral supplementation.

Immunity

UTIs elicit a profound immune response, the degree of which is dependent upon the amount of tissue invasion. For example, isolated bladder infections do not provoke a very intense immune response in most cases, as the bladder mucosa may serve as somewhat of a barrier to tissue invasion. When there is penetration of the local barriers, the immune response is primarily humoral, with an occasional cell-mediated component (42,43). These humoral antibodies are primarily concentrated in the urine but are detectable systemically. Whereas surface immunoglobulin A (sIgA) is perhaps the most important for long-term immunity, the species of immunoglobulin M (IgM) and immunoglobulin G (IgG) are also present (42). The IgM component may have a more important role in clearing the initial infection. There is also a protective effect of humoral immunity after a bladder infection that may be initiated or augmented by immunization. Recently, a vaccine has been developed that confers immunity to many of the more common uropathogens. Prostatic infection usually results in a more intense immune response—primarily humoral—that is at least partially protective of future infections (43). This antibody response includes not only specific antibodies directed against bacterial antigens but also autoantibodies directed against host antigens (44). The most devastating of these are antisperm antibodies, specifically IgG, IgM, and sIgA, found in the prostate gland and seminal plasma (45,46). The immunobead test is currently the assay of choice for the measurement of antisperm antibody concentrations. Some of the antisperm antibodies may actually be cross-reactive antibodies against bacterial antigens, or they may be specific only to sperm. In any case, when the antibodies bind to the spermatozoa, several effects may be seen. The first of these is gross agglutination, which effectively eliminates sperm motility and most other sperm functions. Some antisperm antibodies as well as cross-reacting antibodies against bacterial antigens may bind to the sperm tail, thus decreasing motility. Similarly, some may bind to the head epitopes of the spermatozoa, which may reduce the affinity of sperm binding to the ovum. The effect on fertility is the same. (For further information on antibody assays and immune factors in fertility, please refer to Chapters 26 and 36.)

Leukocytospermia

The finding of white blood cells (WBCs) in the ejaculate is highly predictive of infertility (4,47,48). Infertile men have higher WBC counts in their ejaculates than fertile men. It has been estimated that 10% to 20% of male infertility patients may have leukocytospermia (49,50). Specifically, this condition is defined by the World Health Organization as more than 1×10^6 leukocytes/mL. This may not, however, correlate with infection that is demonstrable by routine culture methods. Upon examination of the subpopulations of WBCs present, there seems to be a preponderance of neutrophils, followed by macrophages and T-lymphocytes. As in the serum, the degree of chronicity may be judged by the relative numbers of each species present. For example, in circumstances where antisperm antibodies are present, there is a predominance of lymphocytes (51). This is an example of a chronic inflammatory process, in that when sperm antigens are involved, there is a concomitant demonstrable lack of granulocytes (51). WBCs, especially PMNs, elaborate a number of enzymes that are deleterious to sperm function. Enzymes that produce reactive oxygen species, such as hydrogen peroxides and superoxide radicals, are associated with the infertile state. Lipid peroxidase has been measured in the semen of infertile patients, and may be correlated with infertility (52). In fact, oxidative stress may be the primary reason for this condition in patients with leukocytospermia. Granulocyte elastase is abundant in the seminal fluid of patients with genital inflammation (53). This enzyme may provide an objective measurement of the degree that inflammation has on infertility. It has even been reported to contribute to female-factor infertility by interfering with fallopian tube function (53). Most of the enzymes elaborated by PMNs are deleterious to other cells and even to whole tissues. Sperm are inactivated by most of these proteases, and the binding to an ovum is prevented by damage to the binding sites. (For further information on semen analysis, please refer to Chapter 24.)

Many cytokines have been implicated in the infertility process. These may be secreted by inflammatory cells, which further harm sperm motility and viability. Most of the proinflammatory cytokines, as would be predicted, reduce fertility status or, at least, are associated with infertility. The most notable of this group are interleukin-6, tumor necrosis factor α, and interleukin-8 (54,55). These cytokines are isolatable from the seminal plasma, vagina, or female serum. Furthermore, those cytokines that are immunosuppressive tend to be higher in the infertile male than in the fertile population. These include prostaglandin E2 and interleukin-10 (56). The roles of transforming growth factor β, interleukin-11, soluble CD23, and others await elucidation (57–59). Similarly, the effects on the endocrinology of sperm fruition are not clear (60).

□ EVALUATION
History

Probably the most important information obtainable in the history is whether or not the patient has ever had a sexually transmitted disease (STD). Because of the multifaceted injury that these diseases may cause, the impact on fertility is dramatic. Questions regarding the sexual history of both partners may also be helpful. Treatment of any STD, either proven or empiric, should be queried as well. Traumatic injuries to the patient, with specific emphasis on the GU tract, should be discussed. Even relatively minor events such as straddle injuries may have important implications. Trauma may take on an even subtler connotation, in that certain repetitive activities, not always considered to be of a traumatic nature, may nonetheless be injurious. Motorcycle or bicycle riding, horseback riding, and any of the contact sports or martial arts may cause this type of problem. A history of prior surgery in the area should be elicited, as hydrocele or hernia surgery may result in injury to the vas deferens. Orchiopexy, either for cryptorchidism or for torsion, is even more obvious as a potential cause of male-factor infertility. Even prior urethral catheterization for surgery unrelated to the GU tract may cause damage. With the improvement and widespread ability of modern immunizations, infection with certain agents, such as mumps, occurs rarely; therefore, a history of postpubertal mumps would be considered highly significant. Lastly, a history of congenital defects as well as cryptorchidism should be elicited. (For further information on the evaluation of the male patient presenting with infertility, please refer to Chapter 23.)

Physical Examination

Clues to the cause of infertility may be obtained from the physical examination, but those that are related to inflammation or infection are relatively few. Prior infection may damage a testicle such that a size discrepancy may be discernable. This is most commonly due to mumps orchitis (61), but bacterial infections may cause the same outcome. Epididymitis may cause palpable scarring or cyst formation. Whereas epididymal cysts are not the exclusive result of infection, the inflammation may cause obliteration of the tubules, resulting in obstruction. If severe enough, the obstruction may cause cystic changes in the proximal tubules. Examination of the prostate may give a few clues to the etiology of infection. Although changes in prostatic consistency, such as the identification of boggy or spongy areas, have been recognized as being consistent with an inflammation, these findings have never been scientifically correlated. Similarly, prostatic tenderness may signal an inflammatory condition, but some patients may be sufficiently apprehensive to be tender even in the absence of infection. Lastly, palpable scarring on the ventrum of the penis or in the perineum may lend clues to the existence of stricture disease.

Laboratory Tests

The most consistent and useful laboratory test is the semen analysis. Infections may cause a host of nonspecific abnormalities in the seminal fluid and may include oligospermia, which results from damage to the germinal epithelium, the epididymis, ejaculatory duct, and prostate, or a combination thereof. Asthenospermia may be a result of stress in the system at some level or may possibly be due to the previously mentioned bacterial products that are toxic to sperm metabolism. Similar effects may be seen in the condition of leukocytospermia, with certain proteins and cytokines elaborated by the WBCs. One of the major concerns is proper identification of the cells present in the ejaculate (61). Specifically, some of the cells that have the appearance of WBCs may actually be immature spermatozoa. These cells are typically round and have a visible nucleus. If not WBCs, they may be spermatids or even spermatocytes. A number of stains are available to assist in determining the cell's origin, such as benzidine–cyanosine or Papanicolaou. More recently, fluorescence-activated cell sorting as well as flow cytometry has been employed to more accurately identify the species of cell present (10,62).

Once a GU tract infection has been documented, some effort should be made to ascertain the etiologic agent. This is especially important, considering the plethora of adverse side effects associated with the use of antibiotics, ranging from life-threatening diarrhea and allergic reactions to negative results on semen quality or even on the germinal epithelium. Culturing the semen has been shown to be an effective means of isolating organisms (63). This material should be obtained fresh, and bacterial cultures should include the more fastidious agents such as *Chlamydia*, *Mycoplasma*, and *Ureaplasma*, as well as obligate intracellular organisms. Newer alginate swab DNA tests for these latter agents are likely to be more sensitive and less labor intensive for the laboratory. The four-glass technique, as described by Meares and Stamey (20), is also an excellent way of confirming the causative agent but is time consuming and expensive. This technique, however, is considered to be the gold standard for localizing infections. It has also been suggested that obtaining a urine sample after prostate massage (VB3) is as accurate an investigation as is necessary, since the precise location of the infection may be less important than the identity and sensitivity pattern of the organism. It is currently advocated that a mid-stream sample and either a semen culture or a VB3 should be obtained.

Molecular Techniques

Most recently, molecular techniques have been developed that are able to detect very small amounts of bacteria by utilizing RT-PCR with primers for 16S ribosomal ribonucleic acid (rRNA) (64). It must be noted, however, that these bacterial "fingerprints" do not necessarily imply that an infection is present, but only that bacteria are present. The genus and species of the bacteria may be determined by sequencing the rRNA and comparing it to banked rRNA information. On occasion, the bacteria cannot be fully identified, as information banks may not be complete. Criteria need to be established with respect to the significance of finding bacterial genetic material in parts of the GU tract, and its relationship to infertility.

☐ TREATMENT
Antibiotics

The treatment of bacterial infection in the GU tract must take into account three principles: bacterial sensitivity, GU penetration, and gonadotoxicity. Most of the time, bacterial sensitivity will have been determined by specific testing. In this case, the other two principles must take precedence. If the clinician has made the decision to treat empirically and if one of the fastidious organisms is suspected, one might choose either the macrolide or the tetracycline group of antibiotics. For *Chlamydia*, doxycycline administered 100 mg twice daily for 10 days or erythromycin 500 mg four times daily are considered to be equally effective. These agents are effective and have fair penetration into tissue (prostatic fluid and ejaculate). Tetracyclines also have an adequate gram-negative spectrum, whereas macrolides are most appropriate to cover gram-positive species. The fluoroquinolone group of antibiotics has several advantages: a very broad spectrum in addition to obligate intracellular organisms coverage, high penetration into the GU tract, and good concentration in the prostatic tissue—all achieved after a single dose (65). Some of the other antibiotic classes have a good spectrum of activity, but the GU penetration is only fair (66). The cephalosporin group is widely utilized because of its spectrum and safety, but the penetration is marginal. Penicillins are similarly concerning, even though both penicillins and cephalosporins are highly excreted in the urine. Of the penicillins, carbenicillin indanyl sodium is specifically indicated for chronic prostatitis. This drug, however, has no coverage for intracellular bacteria, and is dosed four times per day. Aminoglycosides have very little penetration except in the urine and are only rarely appropriate in this scenario. The issue of culture-negative WBC elevations is controversial. Treatment with anti-inflammatory agents is reasonable, but a clear benefit has not been demonstrated.

The gonadotoxicity of agents used in the treatment of male genital infections must also be considered. Nitrofurantoin, commonly used for the treatment of UTI, as well as various tetracyclines (doxycycline, minocycline) that are frequently used for the treatment of STDs, can impair the ability of the sperm to penetrate the zona pellucida of the ovum and further impair fertility (10,67). The sulfas and aminoglycosides have also been shown to have deleterious effects on sperm function and motility (68). The antifungal agent, ketoconazole, has a marked antiandrogen effect and may affect spermatogenesis via that mechanism (2). (For further information on pharmacological effects on fertility, please refer to Chapters 20 to 22.)

Ancillary Treatment

For further information on ancillary treatments, including surgery and assisted reproductive techniques, please refer to Part IV "Treatment of Male Reproductive Function" in the book.

☐ REFERENCES

1. Hellstrom WJG, Neal DE Jr. Diagnosis and therapy of male genital tract infections. Infer Repro Med Clin N Amer 1992; 3(2):399–411.
2. Caldamone AA, Cockett ATK. Infertility and genitourinary infection. Urology 1978; 12(3):304.
3. Fowler JE Jr. Infections of the male reproductive tract and infertility: a selected review. J Androl 1981; 2(3):121–131.
4. Berger RE, Karp LE, Williams RA, et al. The relationship of pyospermia and seminal plasma bacteriology to sperm function as related in the sperm penetration assay. Fertil Steril 1982; 37(4):557.
5. Teague NS, Boyarsky S, Glenn JF. Interference of human spermatozoa motility by Escherichia coli. Fertil Steril 1971; 22(5):281.
6. Witkin SS, Toth A. Relationship between genital tract infections, sperm antibodies in seminal fluid, and infertility. Fertil Steril 1983; 40(6):805.
7. Megory E, Zuckerman H, Schoham Z, et al. Infections and male infertility. Obstet Gynecol Surv 1987; 42(5):283.
8. Lipshultz LI, Howards SS. Evaluation of the subfertile man. Semin Urol 1984; 2(2):73.
9. McConnell JD. The role of infection in male infertility. Probl Urol 1987; 1(3):467.
10. Crotty KL, May R, Kulvicki A, et al. The effect of antimicrobial therapy on testicular aspirate flow cytometry. J Urol 1995; 153(3 Pt 1):835–838.
11. Schlegel PN, Chang TS, Marshall FF. Antibiotics: potential hazards to male infertility. Fertil Steril 1991; 55(2):235.
12. Nelson WO, Bunge RG. The effect of therapeutic dosages of nitrofurantoin (furadantin) upon spermatogenesis in man. J Urol 1957; 77(2):275.
13. Murdia A, Mathur V, Kothari LK, et al. Sulpha-trimethoprim combinations and male fertility. Lancet 1978; 2(8085):375.
14. McGowan MP, Burger HG, Baker HW, et al. The incidence of non-specific infection in the semen in fertile and sub-fertile males. Int J Androl 1981; 4(6):657.
15. Krisp A, Horster S, Skrzypek J, et al. Treatment with levofloxacin does not resolve asymptomatic leucocytospermia-a randomized controlled study. Andrologia 2003; 35(4):244–247.
16. Esfandiari N, Saleh RA, Abdoos M, et al. Positive bacterial culture of semen from infertile men with asymptomatic leukocytospermia. Int J Fertil Womens Med 2002; 47(6):265–270.
17. Weidner W. Which efforts towards conservative treatment of male infertility will be successful? antibiotic therapy. Andrologia 1999; 31(5):297.
18. Krause W, Bohring C. Male infertility and genital chlamydial infection: victim or perpetrator? Andrologia 2003; 35(4):209–216.
19. Toth M, Patton DL, Campbell LA, et al. Detection of chlamydial antigenic material in ovarian, prostatic, ectopic pregnancy and semen samples of culture-negative subjects. Am J Reprod Immunol 2000; 43(4):218–222.
20. Meares EM, Stamey TA. Bacteriologic localization patterns in bacterial prostatitis and urethritis. Invest Urol 1968; 5(5):492–518.
21. Meares EM Jr, Stamey TA. The diagnosis and management of bacterial prostatitis. Br J Urol 1972; 44(2):175–179.
22. Krieger JN, Nyberg L Jr, Nickel JC. NIH consensus definition and classification of prostatitis. JAMA 1999; 282(3):236–237.
23. Swenson CE, Toth A, O'Leary WM. Ureaplasma urealyticum and human infertility: the effect of antibiotic therapy on semen quality. Fertil Steril 1979; 31:660.
24. Poletti F, Medici MC, Alinovi A, et al. Isolation of Chlamydia trachomatis from the prostatic cells in patients affected by nonacute abacterial prostatitis. J Urol 1985; 134(4):691.

25. Hellstrom WJG, Schacter J, Sweet RL, et al. Is there a role for chlamydia trachomatis and genital mycoplasma in male infertility? Fertil Steril 1987; 48(2):337.

26. Roberts JA, Kaack B, Källenius G, et al. Receptors for pyelonephritogenic Escherichia coli in primates. J Urol 1984; 131(1):163.

27. Roberts JA. Pathogenesis of pyelonephritis. J Urol 1983; 129(6):1102.

28. Källenius G, Möllby R, Svenson SB. The pk antigen as receptor for the hemagglutination of pyelonephritogenic E. Coli. FEMS Microbiol Lett 1980; 8:127.

29. Dilworth JP, Neal DE Jr, Fussell EN, et al. Experimental prostatitis in nonhuman primates: I. Bacterial adherence in the urethra. Prostate 1990; 17(3):227–231.

30. Roberts JA. Management of pyelonephritis and upper urinary tract infections. Urol Clin North Am 1999; 26(4):753–763.

31. Huwe P, Diemer T, Ludwig M, et al. Influence of different uropathogenic microorganisms on human sperm motility parameters in an in vitro experiment. Andrologia 1998; 30(1):55–59.

32. Fowler JE Jr, Mariano M. Bacterial infection and male infertility: Absence of immunoglobulin A with specificity for common E. coli O-serotypes in seminal fluid of infertile men. J Urol 1983; 130(1):171.

33. Paulson JD, Polakoski KL. Isolation of spermatozoal immobilization factor from Escherichia coli filtrates. Fertil Steril 1977; 28(2):182.

34. Schwarzer JU, Fiedler K, Hertwig I, et al. Male factors determining the outcome of intracytoplasmic sperm injection with epididymal and testicular spermatozoa. Andrologia 2003; 35(4):220–226.

35. Neal DE Jr. Host defense mechanisms in urinary tract infections. Urol Clin North Am 1999; 26(4):677–686.

36. Vicari E. Effectiveness and limits of antimicrobial treatment on seminal leukocyte concentration and related reactive oxygen species production in patients with male accessory gland infection. Hum Reprod 2000; 15(12):2536–2544.

37. Von Eiff C, Proctor RA, Peters G. Coagulase-negative staphylococci. Pathogens have major role in nosocomial infections. Postgrad Med 2001; 110(4):63–64, 69–70, 73–76.

38. Fisch H, Kang YM, Johnson CW, et al. Ejaculatory duct obstruction. Curr Opin Urol 2002; 12(6):509–515.

39. Paick J, Kim SH, Kim SW. Ejaculatory duct obstruction in infertile men. BJU Int 2000; 85(6):720–724.

40. Fair WR, Couch J, Wehner N. Prostatic antibacterial factor: Identity and significance. Urology 1976; 7(2):169–177.

41. Neal DE Jr, Kaack MB, Fussell EN, et al. Changes in seminal fluid zinc during experimental prostatitis. Urol Res 1993; 21(1):71–74.

42. Neal DE Jr, Kaack MB, Baskin G, et al. Attenuation of antibody response to acute pyelonephritis treatment with antibiotics. Antimicr Agents Chemo 1991; 34(11):2340–2344.

43. Mulholland SG. Lower urinary tract antibacterial defense mechanisms. Invest Urol 1979; 17(2):93–97.

44. Fjallbrandt B, Nilsson S. Decrease of sperm antibody titer in males and conception after treatment of chronic prostatitis. Int J Fertil 1977; 22(4):255.

45. Micic S, Petrovic S, Dotlic R. Seminal antisperm antibodies and genitourinary infection. Urology 1990; 35(1):54.

46. Quesada EM, Dukes CD, Deen CH, et al. Genital infection and sperm agglutinating antibodies in infertile men. J Urol 1968; 99(1):106.

47. Wolff H, Anderson DJ. Immunohistologic characterization and quantification of leukocyte subpopulations in human semen. Fertil Steril 1988; 49:497.

48. Kasfar JV, Holmes RP, Wallen CA, et al. Identification and quantification of seminal leukocytes by flow cytometry. J Urol 1991; 145:327A.

49. Anderson DJ. Cell-mediated immunity and inflammatory processes in male infertility. Arch Immunol Ther Exp (Warsz) 1990; 38(1–2):79.

50. Saleh RA, Agarwal A, Kandirali E, et al. Leukocytospermia is associated with increased reactive oxygen species production by human spermatozoa. Fertil Steril 2002; 78(6):1215–1224.

51. Grygielska B, Fiszer D, Domagala A, et al. Modification of humoral antisperm response. Adv Exp Med Biol 2001; 495:241–244.

52. Dandekar SP, Nadkarni GD, Kulkarni VS, et al. Lipid peroxidation and antioxidant enzymes in male infertility. J Postgrad Med 2002; 48(3):186–189.

53. Zorn B, Sesek-Briski A, Osredkar J, et al. Semen polymorphonuclear neutrophil leukocyte elastase as a diagnostic and prognostic marker of genital tract inflammation—a review. Clin Chem Lab Med 2003; 41(1):2–12.

54. Mulayim N, Palter SF, Selam B, et al. Expression and regulation of interleukin-8 in human fallopian tubal cells. Am J Obstet Gynecol 2003; 188(3):651–656.

55. Kocak I, Yenisey C, Dundar M, et al. Relationship between seminal plasma interleukin-6 and tumor necrosis factor α levels with semen parameters in fertile and infertile men. Urol Res 2002; 30(4):263–267.

56. Camejo MI. Relation between immunosuppressive PGE(2) and IL-10 to proinflammatory IL-6 in seminal plasma of infertile and fertile men. Arch Androl 2003; 49(2):111–116.

57. Matalliotakis I, Arici A, Goumenou A, et al. Distinct expression pattern of cytokines in semen of men with genital infection and oligo-terato-asthenozoospermia. Am J Reprod Immunol 2002; 48(3):170–175.

58. Swatowski D, Jakiel G. The influence of asymptomatic leukocytospermia on interleukin IL-2 and IL-6 levels in male semen plasma. Ginekol Pol 2002; 73(10):841–844.

59. Robertson SA, Ingman WV, O'Leary S, et al. Transforming growth factor β—a mediator of immune

deviation in seminal plasma. J Reprod Immunol 2002; 57(1–2):109–128.

60. Diemer T, Hales DB, Weidner W. Immune-endocrine interactions and Leydig cell function: the role of cytokines. Andrologia 2003; 35(1):55–63.

61. Kaufman DG, Nagler HM. Aspiration flow cytometry of the testes in the evaluation of spermatogenesis of the infertile male. Fertil Steril 1987; 48:287.

62. Hellstrom WJG, Tesluk H, Deitch AD, et al. Comparison of flow cytometry to routine testicular biopsy in male infertility. Urology 1990; 35(4):321.

63. Kumon H. Detection of a local prostatic immune response to bacterial prostatitis. Infection 1992; 20 (suppl 3):S236–S238.

64. Krieger JN, Riley DE, Roberts MC, et al. Prokaryotic DNA sequences in patients with chronic idiopathic prostatitis. J Clin Microbiol 1996; 34(12):3120–3128.

65. Roach MB, George WJ, Figueroa TE, et al. Ciprofloxacin versus gentamicin in prophylaxis against bacteremia in transrectal prostate needle biopsy. Urology 1991; 38(1):84–87.

66. Ruebush TK Jr, McConville JH, Calia FM. A double-blind study of trimethoprim-sulfamethoxazole prophylaxis in patients having transrectal needle biopsy of the prostate. J Urol 1979; 122(4):492.

67. Timmermans L. Influence of antibiotics on spermatogenesis. J Urol 1974; 112(3):348–349.

68. Levi AJ, Fisher Ara, Hughes L, et al. Male infertility due to phasalazine. Lancet 1979; 2(8137):276.

17

HIV and Male Fertility

Timothy B. Hargreave

Department of Oncology, University of Edinburgh, Western General Hospital, Fertility Problems Clinic, Edinburgh, Scotland, U.K.

Chhanda Ghosh

Department of Oncology, University of Edinburgh, Edinburgh, Scotland, U.K.

□ INTRODUCTION

This chapter describes the effect of HIV on the male reproductive system and on the management of male infertility. HIV was not fully recognized by clinicians and scientists until 1981 (1). In the year 2005, it has been estimated that there were 40.3 million people living with HIV. Currently the largest site of the epidemic is in sub-Saharan Africa (Table 1) (2). It is possible that the virulence of the virus may change (3) or mutations may render current testing strategies ineffective; however, new and increasingly effective treatments are being developed. After infection with HIV, there is a latent period of a number of years when the person remains well but the virus can be detected in the blood. At this early stage, treatment with antiviral agents such as zidovudine (AZT) has been shown to delay the progression of the disease. For these reasons, it is important to have a cautious and flexible approach so as to minimize risk to infertile couples and to future children.

□ TRANSMISSION OF HIV BETWEEN PARTNERS
Male-to-Female Sexual Transmission

The overall chance of transmission of HIV from an infected man to his female partner from a single act of unprotected receptive vaginal intercourse is 0.0005 to 0.0015 (4,5). This risk may increase as the disease advances and white cell counts fall. The managing clinician is responsible for ensuring that both partners have full information about risks and strategies to prevent transmission.

Prevention of Sexual Transmission

Currently there is no effective vaccine against HIV, and prospects for a vaccine have been disappointing. At present the AIDS epidemic is out of control and whenever possible spread should be prevented. The only effective strategies are education (particularly of young men), enhancement of the status of women, and the use of barrier methods of contraception. The most effective barrier method is the male condom. The female condom is a slightly less effective barrier. It is common to advocate the use of spermicide with condoms but it is not known whether this reduces the risk of HIV transmission. There is evidence that treatment with AZT in men reduces the cellularity of the ejaculate and presumably reduces the chance of male-to-female transmission (6).

Risk Factors for Sexual Transmission
High-Risk Sexual Behavior

Multiple partners and male homosexuality have both been identified as high-risk behavior with respect to the chance of HIV transmission. Table 2 provides the Center for Disease Control Guidelines for high-risk behavior associated with risk of HIV transmission.

Concurrent Sexually Transmitted Disease

Concurrent sexually transmitted diseases (STDs) can increase the chance of HIV spread either because open genital sores or ulcers provide an entry port for HIV or because an increase in the number of immune cells in the ejaculate associated with urethritis increases the viral load in the ejaculate (8,9). In the context of infertility treatment for the couple where the male partner is HIV positive, STDs should be treated in both the man and his partner(s), and fertility management should be deferred until the conclusion of STD treatment.

Circumcision

Three prospective randomized trials have shown that male circumcision reduces the risk of the man acquiring HIV by approximately 50%. The three studies involved a total of 10,912 men and three studies had to be stopped at interim analysis because it was judged unethical to continue because of the evidence of a significant reduction in risk of the circumcised man acquiring HIV (Table 3). Nevertheless, the role of male

Table 1   Regional HIV/AIDS Statistics and Features, End of 2000

Region	Epidemic started	Adults and children living with HIV/AIDS	Adults and children newly infected with HIV	Adult prevalence rate[a] (%)	Percentage of HIV-positive adults who are women (%)	Main model(s) of transmission for adults living with HIV/AIDS
Sub-Saharan Africa	Late 1970s–early 1980s	25.3 million	3.8 million	8.8	55	Hetero
North Africa and the Middle East	Late 1980s	400,000	80,000	0.2	40	Hetero, IDU
South and Southeast Asia	Late 1980s	5.8 million	780,000	0.56	35	Hetero, IDU
East Asia and the Pacific	Late 1980s	640,000	130,000	0.07	13	IDU, hetero, MSM
Latin America	Late 1970s–early 1980s	1.4 million	150,000	0.5	25	MSM, IDU, hetero
Caribbean	Late 1970s–early 1980s	390,000	60,000	2.3	35	Hetero, MSM
Eastern Europe and Central Asia	Early 1990s	700,000	250,000	0.35	25	IDU
Western Europe	Late 1970s–early 1980s	540,000	30,000	0.24	25	MSM, IDU
North America	Late 1970s–early 1980s	920,000	45,000	0.6	20	MSM, IDU, Hetero
Australia and New Zealand	Late 1970s–early 1980s	15,000	500	0.13	10	MSM
Total		36.1 million	5.3 million	1.1	47	

[a]The proportion of adults (15 to 49 years of age) living with HIV/AIDS in 2000, using 2000 population numbers.
Abbreviations: Hetero, heterosexual transmission; IDU, transmission through injecting drug use; MSM, sexual transmission among men who have sex with men.
Source: From Ref. 2.

circumcision in the context of HIV prevention strategy remains controversial because of concerns that circumcised men may cease to use proven methods of HIV prevention such as using condoms. There is a need for continued research to define the effect of male circumcision on the risk of transmission to the partner (female or male) and on the sexual behavior, condom usage etc. of men who have been circumcised. (Please refer to the chapter entitled "Male Circumcision" for further information on this topic.)

□ VERTICAL TRANSMISSION

HIV transmission to a child may occur at the time of insemination if sperm from the HIV-positive father are used. It may also occur from the mother to the child through the placenta, at birth, or by breastfeeding. Many of these risks are not amenable to prevention but common sense indicates that good antenatal and obstetric care should be given and that situations such

as undiagnosed placenta previa or obstructed labor should be avoided. Several studies indicate that breast-fed infants are at greater risk of acquiring HIV from their infected mothers than bottle-fed infants (11). Thus, breastfeeding is best avoided in this situation unless there is potential for increased infant morbidity and mortality due to unsanitary water conditions.

Prevention of Vertical Transmission with AZT

The European Collaborative study (12) reported transmission rates observed in 600 children born to HIV-positive mothers as of June 1990. The vertical transmission rate based on results in 372 children with at least 18 months follow-up was 12.9% (c.i. 9.5–16.3). At the time of this study, treatment with AZT was not widely used for HIV-positive pregnant women. There is good evidence that the chance of vertical transmission from the HIV-positive mother to the child may be reduced by treating the woman with AZT during the peripartum period and six weeks of AZT for the

Table 2   High-Risk Behavior

Men who have had sex with another man in the preceding 5 yrs
Persons who report nonmedical intravenous, intramuscular, or subcutaneous injection of drugs in the preceding 5 yrs
Persons who have engaged in sex in exchange for money or drugs in the preceding 5 yrs
Persons with hemophilia or related clotting disorders who have received human-derived clotting factor concentrates
Persons who have had sex in the preceding 12 mo with any person described in the above four categories or with a person known or suspected to have HIV infection
Persons who have been exposed in the preceding 12 mo to known or suspected HIV-infected blood through percutaneous inoculation or through contact with an open wound, nonintact skin or mucous membrane
Inmates of correctional systems. (This exclusion is to address issues such as difficulties with informed consent as well as increased prevalence of HIV in this population)

Source: From Ref. 7.

Table 3 Three Prospective Studies in Sub-Saharan Africa of the Effect of Male Circumcision on the Risk of the Man Acquiring HIV

	Orange Farm (South Africa)	Rakai (Uganda)	Kisumu (Kenya)
Population	Semi-urban	Rural	Urban
MC rate	20%	16%	10%
HIV incidence	1.6%	1.3%	1.8%
Age range	18–24 yrs	15–45 yrs	18–24 yrs
No. of men (sample size)	3128	5000	2784
Interim analysis data when trial stopped (planned completion date)	Nov 04 (April 05)	Dec 06 (June 07)	Dec 06 (Sept 07)
No. of infection in circ. group/no. of infection in uncirc. group	20/49	22/43	22/47
Protective effect of circ.	60% (95% CI 34–77%)	48%	53%

Abbreviations: circ., circumcised; uncirc., uncircumcised.

infants (13). This is an expensive treatment approach and is not available in all countries. Furthermore, it may be that shorter courses of AZT will be equally or nearly as effective, which is currently under investigation in clinical trials.

☐ THE EFFECT OF HIV ON MALE REPRODUCTIVE BEHAVIOR

There is concern that in traditional societies, particularly in Africa where fertility is a mark of manhood, knowledge of HIV status may promote more promiscuous behavior because the man knows that he will not live a normal lifespan. In this situation, the problem is made more difficult by the unequal status of women. It is recommended that focused programs of testing and counseling need to target men, particularly those without access to modern media (14).

☐ THE EFFECT OF HIV ON THE MALE REPRODUCTIVE SYSTEM
The Effect of HIV on Spermatogenesis

It is rare for HIV to cause infertility per se, although ill health associated with advanced disease may reduce fertility. In general, men who are seropositive but without AIDS show little or no difference in semen characteristics, whereas those who have AIDS may have pyospermia and abnormal sperm (15).

Within the last five years, the infertility clinic at the Western General Hospital in Edinburgh, Scotland has seen no case where the primary presentation has been a male partner with infertility in association with HIV infection. HIV entered the Edinburgh population in the mid-1980s; the current prevalence is approximately 1 in 100 men under the age of 30. In the same

period, we have seen more than 1000 couples in the infertility clinic. Our experience indicates that HIV is an uncommon cause of male infertility.

Reduced fertility in men with STD may be the result of damage to spermatogenesis following orchitis or abnormal ejaculation in association with urethral stricture. Although both these conditions may occur in patients with HIV, they are not part of the primary disease process. It is worth mentioning that we have seen several young men present with HIV and urethral stricture and three young men who had difficult-to-treat orchitis (16).

The Effect of HIV on Male Sex Hormones

A relatively common autopsy finding in patients who have died of AIDS is adrenal necrosis, and several studies have identified adrenal defects in AIDS patients. Hypogonadotropic hypogonadism was identified in 24 of 63 patients with AIDS and a correlation was noted between this finding and lymphocyte depletion and weight loss (17). It has been postulated that the weight loss may be related to a defect in dihydrotestosterone generation but clinical data does not support this hypothesis (18); however, rather surprisingly, there are also reports of an increase in total and free testosterone in some cases (19). With more effective treatment of HIV, emphasis will shift from cure to quality-of-life issues. Further work will be needed to define androgen status depending on the stage of the illness and the treatment given. In advanced cases, there may be a benefit from androgens to promote weight gain, but any benefit would be from the general anabolic effect of the androgen rather than correction of a specific defect (20).

☐ FERTILITY TREATMENT FOR COUPLES IN WHOM ONE OR BOTH PARTNERS HAVE HIV

If the decision is made that it is reasonable to proceed with treatment, the couple should cooperate to reduce the chance of infection of the uninfected partner, and, most importantly, to reduce the chance of the child becoming infected. In a survey in the United Kingdom in 1995, 9 of 58 in vitro fertilization (IVF) centers were providing treatment for couples in whom the male partner was HIV positive (21). The ethical question of offering fertility treatment is discussed below.

Preventing/Reducing Male-to-Female Transmission in the HIV-Discordant Couple

HIV-discordant couples in this situation have used various approaches to avoid male-to-female transmission. The most common approach is artificial insemination with the sperm after laboratory processing to remove HIV. For those couples who do not have access to laboratory processing, an alternative is to use barrier methods at all times except the woman's fertile period.

Use of this strategy has resulted in the birth of 24 live born children and only one new HIV infection (22).

Couples should receive advice about sexual practices to minimize transmission to the unaffected partner. Advice given should include the use of condoms, proper treatment of any concurrent STDs, and avoidance of sexual intercourse during menstruation and/or until any open genital sores have been treated and healed (23).

Insemination of HIV-Negative Women with Processed Sperm from an HIV-Positive Partner

Results from Milan indicate that the use of gradient centrifugation followed by swim-up effectively removed HIV-1 infected cells from the ejaculate of HIV-positive men. In 29 serodiscordant couples, 17 pregnancies were achieved in 15 women. There were no cases of seroconversion and 10 babies born to these mothers remain seronegative (24); however, centrifugation and swim-up, while reducing HIV-1 infected cells, may not altogether eliminate risk. In another study from Italy, HIV-1 particles have been found incorporated within human spermatozoa and can be introduced into the human oocyte (25).

In Vitro Fertilization and the HIV-Positive Couple

There is little information in the literature about the use of IVF in the presence of HIV, but in principle, the same considerations that apply in other infertility treatments apply here. Special consideration must be given to the staff regarding proper disinfection of all nondisposable equipment.

☐ HIV AND SURGERY OF THE MALE GENITAL TRACT

With the increasing prevalence of HIV, surgical staff have adopted universal precautions for every patient, with no special precautions for the HIV-positive surgical patient. Good practice includes regular review of universal precautions, and whenever possible, adoption of safer surgical practices.

☐ DONOR INSEMINATION
HIV and Gamete Donor Recruitment

The clinician responsible for a donor gamete program has a duty to obtain healthy gametes that pose no risk to the couple or the future child; however, there is also a duty to the gamete donor. In many countries, donation of gametes is voluntary and without payment; hence, it is important to have a clinical practice that is kind to donors. If problems are encountered, there must be adequate facilities to offer donors appropriate advice and treatment. The consequences of discovering HIV

must be discussed with a prospective donor before he or she agrees to participate. Sometimes this may result in a potential donor deciding not to go ahead with screening tests. If unexpected HIV infection or any other infection is discovered, the results have to be communicated to the potential donor and appropriate counseling and treatment must be made available. Lastly, potential gamete donors should sign a consent statement indicating that they have reviewed and understood the information regarding the spread of HIV, and that they will not donate should they be HIV positive or at risk of acquiring HIV.

All donors should be subject to a screening program to reduce the risk of transmitting HIV and other infections. Many of the of these precautions will also apply to donation of other tissues; for example, blood donation and organ donation. The screening program should include:

1. History taking and exclusion of prospective donors based on acknowledged risk behavior (see Table 1). Interviewers should ask direct questions about high-risk behavior.
2. Physical examination and exclusion of those with signs or symptoms of HIV or any other STD, or needle tracks indicating drug abuse.
3. Tests to exclude those who are positive for HIV or any other STD. Samples should be tested for antibody to both HIV1 and HIV2. Current tests rely on the detection of antibodies to HIV, but there is a period between inoculation and the detection of antibodies or antigen in blood samples and, in order to avoid missing infected donors, sperm are stored in liquid nitrogen and quarantined (see below).

☐ STORAGE OF GAMETES IN LIQUID NITROGEN BANKS AND QUARANTINE
Quarantine Time for Stored Gametes in Relation to the Seroconversion Period of HIV

The quarantine period for stored gametes needs to exceed the seroconversion period for HIV; that is, the period from inoculation with the virus to the appearance of antibodies or antigens in the serum (Table 4). It is difficult to obtain precise information about the seroconversion period because there is often doubt about the date of inoculation, except in those situations where there has been a transfusion with infected blood, implantation of an infected organ, or accidental needle stick. An analysis of published data led to an estimated median of 2.1 months from exposure to antibody detection (33). These investigators concluded that 95% of cases would be expected to seroconvert within 5.8 months and that HIV infection for longer than six months without detectable antibody was uncommon. It is also worth noting that with new testing technology, it is possible to detect virus antigen using the p24 enzyme immunoassay test, which can shorten the time from inoculation to virus detection compared with the

Table 4 Quarantine Time for Stored Gametes in Relation to the Seroconversion Period of HIV

Method of inoculation	Date of inoculation		Seroconversion period[a]	Type of test used	References
	Known	Assumed			
Factor VIII to 18 hemophiliac patients	√		30–60 day	ELISA, Western blotting	26
Factor VIII after synovectomy	√		44 day	Antibody to HTLV III	27
Needle stick injury	√		49 day	Antibody to HTLV III	28
Needle sharing with an AIDS patient		√	2 mo	ELISA, Western blotting	29
Needle stick	√		7 mo	"Elavia" (ELISA) confirmed by Western blotting and indirect immunofluorescence	30
Kidney transplant	√		40–50 day	ELISA confirmed by indirect immunofluorescence and Western blotting test	31
Kidney transplant	√		30–56 day	ELISA confirmed by indirect immunofluorescence and Western blotting test	31
Blood transfusion	√		42–56 day	Antibody to p24	32

[a]Seroconversion period is calculated from the time of inoculation to the time of appearance of antibody in the blood.
Abbreviation: HTLV III, human T-cell lymphotropic virus III.

usual seroconversion periods calculated from data obtained using antibody tests. Another important consideration is that HIV is a new disease that is now infecting large numbers of humans; in these circumstances, it is possible that there may be adaptation by the virus to the human host and virulence and incubation periods could change.

The main arguments against the quarantine of sperm have focused on the cost and reported lower success rates when frozen sperm are used compared with fresh sperm. There is variation in practice between countries; in 1987 it was estimated that 80% of donor inseminations in the United States were using fresh semen (34). Since then, with the advent of intracytoplasmic sperm injection (ICSI), the need for donor insemination has diminished and the use of frozen semen has increased. In the United Kingdom, all donor insemination is performed using frozen quarantined sperm according to guidelines issued by the UK Human Fertilisation and Embryology Authority. The recommended quarantine period is six months; however, in our clinic in Edinburgh, for the last six years, we have quarantined all samples for one year because of occasional reports of longer seroconversion periods and to guard against the possibility of virus adaptation with longer seroconversion periods.

Quarantine as Protection Against Problems with Virus Detection

Another reason to quarantine sperm is to guard against virus mutation resulting from difficulties with virus detection. Problems with the detection of HIV are more than theoretical as seen in a study of British Public Health laboratories (35). A new HIV assay was put into use with the advantage of increased sensitivity for outlier HIV variants. However, following the reporting of false negative results, use of the assay was restricted. Out of 20,973 samples tested, there were four false-negative results giving a sensitivity of 99.2%

(497/501). In this case, our one-year quarantine period in Edinburgh would have protected our patients against detection problems.

Prevention of Contamination of Stored Gametes within the Store

There have been no direct examples of HIV cross-contamination of sperm samples stored in a liquid nitrogen sperm bank; however, this must not be a matter for complacency. There has been evidence of cross-contamination of hepatitis B virus from a contaminated cryopreservation tank (36). Thus, there is a potential hazard when untested samples are stored alongside those in quarantine. It is not practical to sterilize the outside of the storage ampoule or straw. If there is contamination of the outside of the straw, then there is the possibility of contamination of the liquid nitrogen and the coating of all other ampoules in the store with virus particles. While not routinely practiced, consideration needs to be given to the use of storage straws or ampoules that are double wrapped.

There is also a risk of lost straws or ampoules or small particles of contaminated material falling to the bottom of a large container. These may remain undiscovered for some time. It is recommended that the storage container be periodically emptied and cleaned, and this cleaning should be recorded in a log. Consideration needs to be given to designing storage straws or ampoules with a second outer wrapping to eliminate the risk of contamination of the outside of the straw by the liquid nitrogen.

HIV Transmission Using Infected Sperm that Have Been Banked in Liquid Nitrogen

In previous years the main form of help for couples with male factor infertility has been insemination with donor sperm. More recently this is used less frquently because of IVF, and, in particular, ICSI has enabled fertilization with a single sperm in situations formerly considered untreatable. As originally practiced, donor insemination involved the use of fresh sperm but with the advent of HIV infection, most clinics in the world have switched to the use of frozen and quarantined sperm.

There is a report of HIV transmission from fresh sperm used for donor insemination (37). Although there is a report of transmission of HIV from cryopreserved semen (38), no details are given about the quarantine period or retesting of the donor.

□ ETHICAL CONSIDERATIONS WHEN TREATING COUPLES IN WHOM ONE PARTNER HAS HIV

The main ethical problems center on risks to the future child and risks of transmission of HIV to the partner.

HIV Transmission to the Child

Most cultures put the interests of the future child ahead of the interests of the infertile couple. Some clinicians would regard any risk of HIV transmission to the child as a contraindication for any fertility treatment that would facilitate conception; however, if the actual risk of HIV positivity in the child is remote, other clinicians would regard help for the couple as acceptable; thus whether to proceed or not is judged according to risk.

HIV Transmission to the Partner

The transmission of HIV to the uninfected partner should be prevented, and clearly both partners need to be informed about HIV. When one partner is not willing to inform the other regarding HIV positivity, the clinician is in a difficult situation and must do everything possible to persuade the patient to change his or her mind. If the patient refuses, it would be very difficult to justify helping with any fertility treatment. Also, a decision has to be made about whether to inform the other partner. If the other partner is also a patient of the clinician, there is a conflict between the duty of confidentiality to patient one and the duty of care to patient two. In these circumstances, the duty of care would seem to override the duty of confidentiality. There can be little doubt about this if the uninfected partner is the woman who wishes to become pregnant.

Is It Right to Deny Fertility Treatment?

If a decision to help a couple with HIV toward fertility is made, it must be remembered that the child has a need for a healthy parent. Thus, it is in the interest of the future child to try to prevent cross-infection to the uninfected partner. For couples who are unable or unwilling to try to minimize transmission of HIV to the uninfected partner or to the child, the attending clinician must consider whether the interests of a future child are best served by helping with fertility treatments.

□ REFERENCES

1. Laurence J. Update: a 25th anniversary and a UN global AIDS summit. AIDS Read 2006; 16(7):331–332.
2. UNAIDS. AIDS Epidemic Update December 2000. 2000; http://data.unaids.org/Publications/IRC-pub05/AIDSEpidemicReport2000_en.pdf.
3. Sinicco A, Fora R, Raiteri R, et al. Is the clinical course of HIV-1 changing? Cohort study. Br Med J 1997; 314(7089): 1232–1237.
4. Wiley JA, Herschkorn SJ, Padian NS. Heterogeneity in the probability of HIV transmission per sexual contact: the case of male-to-female transmission in penile-vaginal intercourse. Stat Med 1989; 8(1):93–102.
5. Downs AM, De Vincenzi I. Probability of heterosexual transmission of HIV: relationship to the number of unprotected sexual contacts. European Study Group in Heterosexual Transmission of HIV. J Acquir Immune Defic Syndr 1996; 11(4):388–395.
6. Politch JA, Mayer KH, Abbott AF, et al. The effects of disease progression and zidovudine therapy on semen quality in human immunodeficiency virus type 1 sero-positive men. Fertil Steril 1994; 61(5):922–928.
7. Rogers MF, Simonds RJ, Lawton KE, et al. CDC Guidelines for Preventing Transmission of Human Immunodeficiency Virus through Transplantation of Human Tissue and Organs, Atlanta, GA, May 20, 1994.
8. Mhalu FS. Inter-relationships between HIV infection and other sexually transmitted diseases. East Afr Med J 1990; 67(7):512–517.
9. van Dam CJ. Sexually transmitted diseases and HIV infection: implications for control and prevention. J Indian Med Assoc 1994; 92(1):8–10.
10. Oliver RT, Oliver J, Ballard RC. Male circumcision and HIV prevention. More studies need to be done before widespread circumcision is implemented. Br Med J 2000; 321(7274):1468–1469.
11. de Martino M, Tovo PA, Tozzi AE, et al. HIV-1 transmission through breast-milk: appraisal of risk according to duration of feeding. Aids 1992; 6(9): 991–997.
12. Ades AE, Newell ML, Peckham CS. Children born to women with HIV-1 infection: natural history and risk of transmission. European Collaborative Study. Lancet 1991; 337(8736):253–260.

13. Roland M. Post-exposure prophylaxis following sexual or injection drug use exposure to HIV: current knowledge and future research strategies. J HIV Therapy 1998; 3(1):17–20.

14. Gregson S, Zhuwau T, Anderson RM, et al. Is there evidence for behaviour change in response to AIDS in rural Zimbabwe? Soc Sci Med 1998; 46(3):321–330.

15. Krieger JN, Coombs RW, Collier AC, et al. Fertility parameters in men infected with human immunodeficiency virus. J Infect Dis 1991; 164(3):464–469.

16. Parr NJ, Prasad BR, Hayhurst V, et al. Suppurative epididymo-orchitis in young "high risk" patients—a new problem? Br J Urol 1993; 72(6):949–951.

17. Dobs AS, Dempsey MA, Ladenson PW, et al. Endocrine disorders in men infected with human immunodeficiency virus. Am J Med 1988; 84(3 Pt 2):611–616.

18. Arver S, Sinha-Hikim I, Beall G, et al. Serum dihydrotestosterone and testosterone concentrations in human immunodeficiency virus-infected men with and without weight loss. J Androl 1999; 20(5):611–618.

19. Merenich JA, McDermott MT, Asp AA, et al. Evidence of endocrine involvement early in the course of human immunodeficiency virus infection. J Clin Endocrinol Metab 1990; 70(3):566–571.

20. Bhasin S, Storer TW, Javanbakht M, et al. Testosterone replacement and resistance exercise in HIV-infected men with weight loss and low testosterone levels. JAMA 2000; 283(6):763–770.

21. Balet R, Lower AM, Wilson C, et al. Attitudes towards routine human immunodeficiency virus (HIV) screening and fertility treatment in HIV-positive patients—a UK survey. Hum Reprod 1998; 13(4): 1085–1087.

22. Ryder RW, Kamenga C, Jingu M, et al. Pregnancy and HIV-1 incidence in 178 married couples with discordant HIV-1 serostatus: additional experience at an HIV-1 counselling centre in the Democratic Republic of the Congo. Trop Med Int Health 2000; 5(7):482–487.

23. Kuznetsova II, Pokrovskii VV. The factors and cofactors affecting the heterosexual transmission of human immunodeficiency virus (HIV) infection. Vopr Virusol 1993; 38(5):207–209.

24. Semprini AE, Levi-Setti P, Bozzo M, et al. Insemination of HIV-negative women with processed semen of HIV–positive partners. Lancet 1992; 340(8831): 1317–1319.

25. Baccetti B, Benedetto A, Collodel G, et al. The debate on the presence of HIV-1 in human gametes. J Reprod Immunol 1998; 41(1–2):41–67.

26. Simmonds P, Lainson FA, Cuthbert R, et al. HIV antigen and antibody detection: variable responses to infection in the Edinburgh haemophiliac cohort. Br Med J (Clin Res Ed) 1988; 296(6622):593–598.

27. Tucker J, Ludlam CA, Craig A, et al. HTLV-III infection associated with glandular-fever-like illness in a haemophiliac. Lancet 1985; 1(8428):585.

28. Needlestick transmission of HTLV-III from a patient infected in Africa. Lancet 1984; 2(8416):1376–1377.

29. Vittecoq D, Autran B, Bourstyn E, et al. Lymphadenopathy syndrome and seroconversion two months after single use of needle shared with an AIDS patient. Lancet 1986; 1(8492):1280.

30. Neisson-Vernant C, Arfi S, Mathez D, et al. Needlestick HIV seroconversion in a nurse. Lancet 1986; 2(8510):814.

31. Schwarz A, Hoffmann F, L'Age-Stehr J, et al. Human immunodeficiency virus transmission by organ donation. Outcome in cornea and kidney recipients. Transplantation 1987; 44(1):21–24.

32. Esteban JI, Shih JW, Tai CC, et al. Importance of western blot analysis in predicting infectivity of anti-HTLV-III/LAV positive blood. Lancet 1985; 2(8464):1083–1086.

33. Horsburgh CR, Jr., Ou CY, Jason J, et al. Duration of human immunodeficiency virus infection before detection of antibody. Lancet 1989; 2(8664):637–640.

34. Sherman JK. Frozen semen: efficiency in artificial insemination and advantage in testing for acquired immune deficiency syndrome. Fertil Steril 1987; 47(1):19–21.

35. Evans BG, Parry JV, Mortimer PP. HIV antibody assay that gave false negative results: multicentre collaborative study. Br Med J 1997; 315(7111):772–774.

36. Tedder RS, Zuckerman MA, Goldstone AH, et al. Hepatitis B transmission from contaminated cryopreservation tank. Lancet 1995; 346(8968):137–140.

37. Chiasson MA, Stoneburner RL, Joseph SC. Human immunodeficiency virus transmission through artificial insemination. J Acquir Immune Defic Syndr 1990; 3(1):69–72.

38. Stewart GJ, Tyler JP, Cunningham AL, et al. Transmission of human T-cell lymphotropic virus type III (HTLV-III) by artificial insemination by donor. Lancet 1985; 2(8455):581–585.

Ejaculatory Duct Obstruction in the Infertile Male

Erik T. Goluboff

College of Physicians and Surgeons, Columbia University and New York-Presbyterian Hospital, New York, New York, U.S.A.

Harry Fisch

College of Physicians and Surgeons, Columbia University and Male Reproductive Center, Columbia-Presbyterian Medical Center, New York, New York, U.S.A.

□ INTRODUCTION

Although obstructions of the epididymis and proximal vas deferens have become well-recognized and readily treated causes of male infertility (1), more distal obstructions have only relatively recently been recognized and treated (2–5). Ejaculatory duct obstruction, although rare, is a surgically correctable cause of male infertility (2,5–11). The use of high-resolution transrectal ultrasound (TRUS) has resulted in an increased incidence of diagnosis of this disorder (3,10,12,13). Treatment of ejaculatory duct obstruction by transurethral resection of the ejaculatory ducts (TURED) has also become more common; there have been several reports of pregnancies following relief of ejaculatory duct obstruction using this technique (2,4,5,9,11,14,15). Although various symptoms, signs, TRUS, radiographic, and cystoscopic findings have been associated with ejaculatory duct obstruction, none is pathognomonic for this disorder (2). Moreover, the pathogenesis of ejaculatory duct obstruction in association with these findings, and how this obstruction impacts on male fertility, is not well understood. By examining the anatomy of the ejaculatory ductal system, and correlating it with symptomatology, semen analyses, TRUS, and pathologic findings in patients with a presumptive diagnosis of ejaculatory duct obstruction, a better understanding of ejaculatory duct obstruction and its impact on male infertility can be gained.

□ ANATOMY

The ejaculatory ducts develop from the distal-most vas (the Wolffian duct system). The seminal vesicles develop as a blind diverticulum at the most terminal end of the vas (16). The ejaculatory ducts are a direct continuation of the seminal vesicles and, anatomically, begin after the ampulla of the vas joins the seminal vesicle duct on its medial aspect at an acute angle (Fig. 1) (6,17,18). The ducts are approximately 1 to 2 cm long and enter the prostate obliquely and posteriorly at its base, course medially and anteriorly through the prostatic glandular tissue, and enter the prostatic urethra at the verumontanum (6,9,17,18). Between the two ejaculatory ducts at the verumontanum sits the prostatic utricle—a Mullerian tubercle remnant of endodermal origin (18). The ejaculatory ducts open, in the majority of cases, anterolateral to the orifice of the utricle (18). In most men, the utricle is less than 6 mm in size but can exceed 10 mm in up to 10% of men (19). The utricle does not communicate with any other structures (6,17,18,20). Injection of methyl methacrylate into the vas deferens of intact autopsy prostate/seminal vesicles/vasa specimens reveals the ejaculatory ducts exiting close to one another at the verumontanum, with a small utricle lying between them. No methyl methacrylate can be seen exiting the utricle (Fig. 2) (21). In sagittal sections, the ejaculatory duct forms an almost straight course from the prostatic base to the verumontanum (Fig. 3). The close relationship of the ejaculatory ducts to the utricle can be seen in the transverse section at the verumontanum of a radical retropubic prostatectomy specimen (Fig. 4) (21). The anatomic structures of the ejaculatory ductal system and their relationships can also be demonstrated using rectal coil magnetic resonance imaging (MRI) (5,22). In sagittal images, the relationships between the bladder, bladder neck, seminal vesicles, prostate, and ejaculatory ducts are demonstrated. In addition, this patient has a midline cyst that divides the ejaculatory ducts laterally (Fig. 5). Also note that the distal ejaculatory duct and cyst are distal and inferior to the bladder neck. Each duct is surrounded by circular lamellar tissue and, in turn, both ducts are surrounded by a communal muscular envelope (17,23). The existence of a sphincter spermaticus has been confirmed, but its role in the pathophysiology of partial or functional ejaculatory duct obstruction remains poorly understood (4,7). The ejaculatory ducts are lined by a yellow pigmented cuboidal to pseudostratified columnar epithelium (Fig. 6) (17,23). (For further details on male anatomy, please refer to Chapter 2.)

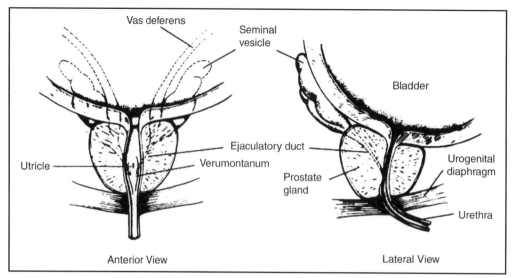

Figure 1   Schematic representation of the distal ejaculatory duct anatomy.

□ ETIOLOGIES OF OBSTRUCTION

Ejaculatory duct obstruction can be either congenital or acquired (9,11). Congenital causes include congenital atresia or stenosis of the ejaculatory ducts, and utricular, Mullerian, and Wolffian duct cysts. Acquired causes may be secondary to trauma, either iatrogenic or otherwise, or may have infectious or inflammatory etiologies (9,11). Calculus formation secondary to infection may also cause obstruction (4). Cyst formation from prior instrumentation or infection may also occur (20). Many times, patients with ejaculatory duct obstruction have no significant antecedent history (6). Several authors have found that patients with congenital or noninfectious causes of ejaculatory duct obstruction do better after treatment than those with infectious causes (9,11). Other authors, however, have not been able to support this (6,24,25).

□ SYMPTOMS

Patient complaints associated with ejaculatory duct obstruction can be quite variable, but may include infertility, decreased force of ejaculate, pain on or after ejaculation, decreased ejaculate volume, hematospermia, perineal or testicular pain, history of prostatitis or epididymitis, low back pain, urinary obstruction, dysuria, or no symptoms at all (2,5,6,7,9,24). Symptoms are generally less pronounced or absent in patients with partial obstructions (4,5). No one symptom or constellation of symptoms can help make a definitive diagnosis of ejaculatory duct obstruction.

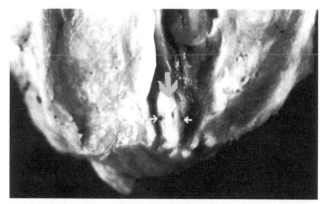

Figure 2   Coronal section of the prostate from an autopsy specimen after injection of methyl methacrylate into the vasa deferentia. Notice methyl methacrylate exiting from distal ejaculatory ducts (*small white arrows*), which sit lateral to the midline utricle (*large grey arrow*).

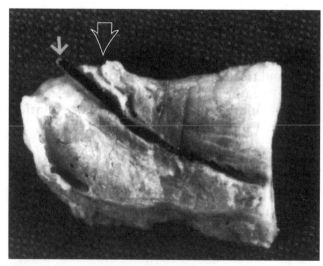

Figure 3   Sagittal section of the prostate from an autopsy specimen after injection of methyl methacrylate into the vasa deferentia. Notice ejaculatory duct (*grey arrow*) exiting distal and inferior to the utricle (*open arrow*). Notice the almost straight course of the ejaculatory duct from the prostate base to the verumontanum.

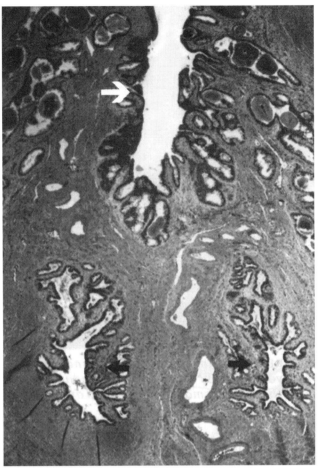

Figure 4 Transverse section through the verumontanum from a radical retropubic prostatectomy specimen showing the close relationship of the ejaculatory ducts (*black arrows*) to each other and to the utricle (*white arrow*).

□ SIGNS

Patients with suspected ejaculatory duct obstruction classically have normal physical examinations,

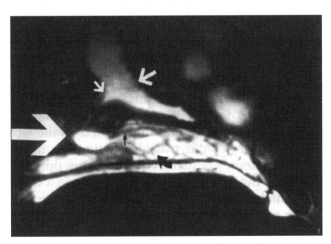

Figure 5 Sagittal image from a rectal coil magnetic resonance image showing the relationships between the bladder (*medium white arrow*), bladder neck (*small white arrow*), seminal vesicles (*curved black arrow*), and ejaculatory ducts (*tiny black arrow*), with a midline cyst (*large white arrow*). Note that the distal ejaculatory duct and midline cyst are quite distal and inferior to the bladder neck.

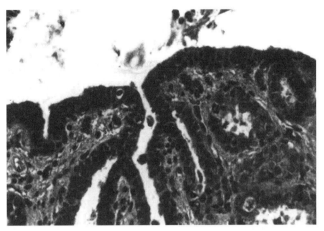

Figure 6 Histologic section of the distal ejaculatory duct epithelium from transurethral resection of the ejaculatory ducts. Specimen shows cuboidal and pseudostratified columnar epithelium. (H&E)

including normal testes, absence of varicoceles, palpable vasa, normal rectal examinations, normal secondary sexual characteristics, and normal hormonal profiles (2,5,6,9,24). Occasionally, there will be a palpable seminal vesicle or mass on rectal examination, or prostatic or epididymal tenderness (2,5,6,9,24). Of course, these patients can, however, have more than one disorder at the same time; i.e., a patient with ejaculatory duct obstruction might also have a varicocele or a patient with testicular failure might also have ejaculatory duct obstruction. Although a patient might seem to demonstrate findings only of ejaculatory duct obstruction, a complete evaluation for other concomitant, possibly treatable, disorders is necessary. (For further information on the physical findings present in ejaculatory duct obstruction, please refer to Chapter 23.)

Semen analysis findings in men with partial ejaculatory duct obstruction include oligospermia or azoospermia, decreased motility, and decreased ejaculate volume (2,6). In some men with only mild, partial obstructions, semen analyses can approach normal parameters, although motility may remain low (4,24). Decreased ejaculate volume, i.e., volumes of less than 1 cc (normal being 1.5–5 cc), may be suggestive of ejaculatory duct obstruction, but it is by no means pathognomonic (2,4,5,6,12). With complete ejaculatory obstruction, seminal fluid should be theoretically fructose negative; however, fructose is often present, implying the presence of only partial obstruction (5). Pryor and Hendry (9) have stated that the finding of a small volume of acidic semen (which does not contain fructose) in a patient with palpable vasa is pathognomonic for ejaculatory duct obstruction. (For further information on semen analysis findings and interpretations, please refer to Chapter 24.)

Historically, vasography was the gold standard for diagnosis of proximal and distal ejaculatory duct obstruction (5,9,10,12). The invasive nature of this study, however, with its significant risks of iatrogenic stricture and vasal occlusion as well as the relative risks of general anesthesia and radiation exposure, has made TRUS a more attractive diagnostic technique (2,10,12–14,26). TRUS is much less invasive and can demonstrate the anatomic relationships of the prostate, seminal vesicles, and ejaculatory ducts with exquisite detail (3,5,10,12,13,18,27,28). Katz et al. (29) reported the use of ultrasound-guided transrectal seminal vesiculography under local anesthesia. Under TRUS guidance, a 22-G needle is advanced into the seminal vesicle, and, after its position is confirmed with aspiration, the contrast medium is injected. Although it has not been generally accepted as yet, this technique eliminates the risks associated with vasography while preserving excellent radiographic visualization of the ejaculatory ducts. Jarow (30) has also shown that TRUS-guided seminal vesicle aspiration was useful in the diagnosis of partial ejaculatory duct obstruction when motile sperm are found in the aspirate. Orhan et al. (31) describe the use of TRUS-guided seminal vesicle aspiration both to diagnose ejaculatory duct obstruction and to collect sperm for assisted reproduction techniques. (For further information on TRUS findings, please refer to Chapter 28.)

TRUS findings in suspected ejaculatory duct obstruction include midline cysts (Fig. 7), dilated seminal vesicles (Fig. 8A) or ejaculatory ducts, and hyperechoic regions suggestive of calcifications (Fig. 8B) (2–6,13,27). Although seminal vesicle dilation has been frequently associated with ejaculatory duct obstruction, it is not always present; conversely, normal fertile men can, at times, have dilated seminal vesicles (18,28,32,33). Jarow (12) showed that seminal vesicle width, length, and area did not differ between fertile and infertile men on TRUS; he also stated, however, that cystic dilation of the seminal vesicles in association with abnormally low ejaculate volume is

pathognomonic for ejaculatory duct obstruction. Recent literature proposes that seminal vesicles larger than 15 mm in transverse diameter are abnormal and suggest ejaculatory duct obstruction (2,12,13); however, this has not been universally accepted.

Midline cysts can be classified into two general categories: those that contain sperm and those that do not (14,20,34,35). These can often be difficult to distinguish (20,26,34). The latter are generally called utricles, or Mullerian duct cysts. The differences between utricular and Mullerian duct cysts include the following: (*i*) their dissimilar embryologic origin, with the utricular cysts being of endodermal and Mullerian duct cysts being of mesodermal origin; (*ii*) location, with utricular cysts being midline near the verumontanum and Mullerian duct cysts nearer the prostate base; and (*iii*) association, with enlarged utricles seen in intersex disorders (12,13,36). In any case, both cystic conditions cause ejaculatory duct obstruction by compressing the ducts, and both can be treated by TURED—albeit Mullerian duct cysts may be more difficult to resect due to their more posterior location (36).

Cysts that contain sperm have been called Wolffian cysts, or ejaculatory duct cysts or diverticula, and are less common than the Mullerian duct cysts (12,20,26,34,35). Confusion as to whether a cyst is Mullerian or Wolffian in origin can be compounded by the fact that secondary epididymal obstruction can occur after long-term ejaculatory duct obstruction, resulting in the possible absence of sperm in a Wolffian structure (25,27). Midline cysts cause obstruction of the ejaculatory ducts by deviating them laterally or compressing them (6). Jarow (12) showed when comparing TRUS findings between fertile and infertile men that infertile men had a significantly greater incidence of midline Mullerian duct cysts (11% vs. 0%), but he could not draw any conclusions concerning the functional significance of this finding. As was true for seminal vesicle dilation, the presence of a midline cyst does not assure the diagnosis of ejaculatory duct obstruction, but certainly suggests it in the correct clinical setting.

Calcifications along the course of ejaculatory ducts might be directly involved in obstruction, but those in the prostate itself are associated with prior inflammation—although not necessarily with symptomatic prostatitis (3,4,6). How prostate inflammation leads to ejaculatory duct obstruction has not been well characterized; the inflammatory involvement of the ducts themselves leading to stenosis or obstruction could play a role, whereas changes in compliance of the ejaculatory duct walls or of the adjacent prostatic tissue could also cause a functional obstruction (9,11,13). Calcifications at the junction of the ejaculatory ducts and the urethra have been described in normal individuals, on TRUS (3,12). Prostate or ejaculatory duct calcifications are associated with ejaculatory duct obstruction but are not a reliable indicator of it. Jarow (12) found that hyperechoic lesions on TRUS were present in a similar proportion of fertile and infertile men.

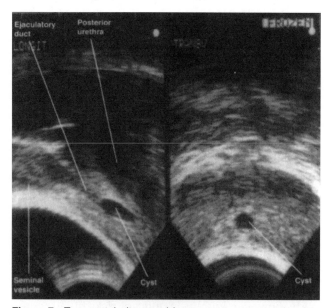

Figure 7 Transrectal ultrasound images, transverse on the right and longitudinal on the left, showing a small midline cyst at the distal ejaculatory duct.

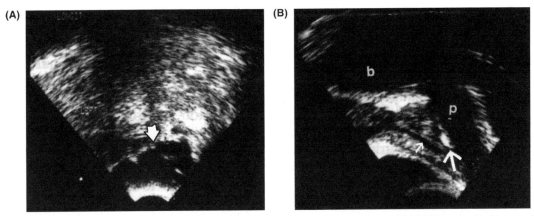

Figure 8   (**A**) TRUS longitudinal image of a dilated fluid-filled vesicle (*arrow*) measuring 21.8 mm. (**B**) TRUS longitudinal image showing highly echogenic areas (*large white arrow*) in the region of the distal ejaculatory duct (*small white arrow*). *Abbreviations*: b, bladder; p, posterior urethra; TRUS, transrectal ultrasound.

□ TREATMENT

In patients with suspected ejaculatory duct obstruction, TURED has become the standard procedure (2,4,6,13). It was originally described by Farley and Barnes in 1973 (7), and several reports have documented its efficacy (2–9,11,15).

TURED requires a setup similar to that of transurethral resection of the prostate (6). An O'Connor drape is used. Cystourethroscopy is performed to rule out strictures in the anterior and bulbar urethra, as well as for evaluation of the posterior urethra. Cystoscopic findings include distorted verumontanum anatomy, splaying of the ejaculatory ducts, bulbous or bilobed verumontana, midline cysts, and inflammatory calcifications (6). Once this is done, the resectoscope is inserted. The proximal verumontanum, which may be enlarged, is resected in the midline (Fig. 9). TURED is performed using pure cutting current without coagulation. Commonly, one or two chips are resected, removing the proximal verumontanum only. Although, historically, lateral Colling's knife incisions

were made (13), resection lateral to the verumontanum is not necessary because the ejaculatory ducts are midline structures in this region (6).

With the bladder filled with irrigation fluid, palpation of the seminal vesicles is made easier. Mild pressure is exerted on the seminal vesicles, resulting in fluid being expressed from the respective ejaculatory ducts. If no fluid is expressed, another small bite can be taken from the verumontanum and seminal vesicle pressure applied again. In the authors' experience, operative success for TURED is defined as fluid expression from both ejaculatory ducts at the termination of the procedure. If bleeding is encountered, gentle coagulation is recommended, taking care to avoid the ejaculatory ducts. A catheter is inserted into the bladder and may be left in place for 24 to 48 hours. Postoperative urinary retention can occur after catheter removal, particularly in patients with prior voiding dysfunction. In these cases, reinsertion of the catheter for an additional 24 to 48 hours may be necessary (6).

Complications due to TURED are rare if the procedure is done carefully and with expertise. Obviously, if resection is performed too proximally, damage to the bladder neck can result in retrograde ejaculation postoperatively. Resection too distally can cause damage to the external sphincter, with subsequent urinary incontinence. Excessive postoperative fibrosis may result in scarring and subsequent azoospermia, implying reocclusion of the ejaculatory ducts. If this occurs, a repeat TURED may be necessary (6). Reflux of urine into the seminal vesicles, resulting in contamination of the ejaculate with urine, has also been reported (37,38), although the clinical significance of this has not been elucidated. The authors have reported on a patient with seminal vesicle urinary reflux following TURED, causing significant postvoid dribbling (39). Secondary epididymal obstruction can occur after long-term ejaculatory duct obstruction, necessitating scrotal exploration and vaso-epididymostomy for patients who fail to improve after TURED and in whom this is suspected (25,27).

The patient is asked to refrain from sexual activity for 7 to 10 days. When sexual activity is resumed,

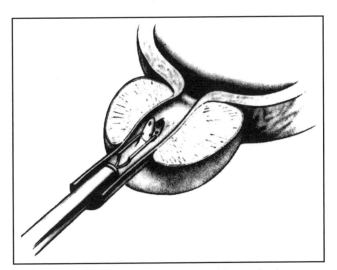

Figure 9   Schematic diagram of resection of the proximal verumontanum. *Source*: From Ref. 6.

hematospermia may be evident but is self-limited; the patient should be warned of this occurrence and reassured. A semen analysis is obtained one month following the resection.

Weintraub et al. (5) reported on eight patients with ejaculatory duct obstruction diagnosed by TRUS, rectal coil MRI, and vasography. Of these, 80% were improved symptomatically after TURED, with the majority having improvements in sperm density or volume, or both; 25% were able to impregnate their wives (5). Hellerstein et al. (4) reported on two patients with infertility: one with a large midline cyst and one with dilated seminal vesicles, both of whom underwent TURED for presumed ejaculatory duct obstruction. Both had significant improvements in semen parameters and both were able to impregnate their wives. Finally, Meacham et al. (2) reported on 24 patients with clinical profiles consistent with ejaculatory duct obstruction—all of whom underwent TURED. Fifty percent had an increase in sperm density or motility, and 29% had an increase in ejaculate volume only. Of the 24, seven (29%) were able to impregnate their wives (2). Again, none of these studies report on the long-term effects of this procedure. Turek et al. (40) showed a greater than 50% improvement in semen parameters in 65% of patients after TURED. Twenty percent were able to initiate a pregnancy; there was a 20% overall complication rate, with the most common being a watery ejaculate. Netto et al. (41) showed that the etiology of the ejaculatory duct obstruction was a significant predictor of success after TURED. In those patients with a congenital cause to the obstruction, success rates were excellent, with 100% improvement in semen parameters (motility, volume), 83% improvement in sperm count, and 66% pregnancy rate. In those patients with an acquired cause to the obstruction, only 37.5% had improved semen parameters and 12.5% pregnancy rate. Furthermore, although 33% of each group had complications, those in the congenital group were more minor in nature.

Aside from TURED, Colpi et al. (42) described antegrade seminal tract washout to relive ejaculatory obstruction. The vasa were exposed scrotally and saline was injected antegrade to the seminal vesicles until the obstruction was relieved. Fertility was restored in this patient.

□ CONCLUSION

With the advent and increased use of high-resolution TRUS, abnormalities of the distal ejaculatory ducts related to infertility have been well documented (2–6,12). Although there are no pathognomonic findings associated with ejaculatory duct obstruction, several clinical findings are highly suggestive. In an infertile male with oligospermia or azoospermia with low ejaculate volume, normal secondary sex characteristics, testes, and hormonal profile, and dilated seminal vesicles, midline cyst, or calcifications on TRUS, the diagnosis of ejaculatory duct obstruction is suggested (2,6,12,13). Of course, other causes of infertility may be concomitantly present, and these need to be sought and treated as well. In select cases, TURED has resulted in marked improvement in semen parameters, and pregnancies have been achieved (2–6,12). As is the case with all surgical procedures, proper patient selection and surgical experience are necessary to obtain optimal results. In patients with evidence of testicular dysfunction, chances of success are minimal. In addition, extended follow-up periods are needed after TURED to examine the long-term effects of this procedure. Better understanding of the anatomy and pathology of the ejaculatory ducts will help refine diagnostic and therapeutic procedures for this disorder.

□ REFERENCES

1. Belker AM, Bennett AH. Applications of microsurgery in urology. Surg Clin North Am 1988; 68(5): 1157–1178.
2. Meacham RB, Hellerstein DK, Lipshultz LI. Evaluation and treatment of ejaculatory duct obstruction in the infertile male. Fertil Steril 1993; 59(2):393–397.
3. Carter SS, Shinohara K, Lipshultz LI. Transrectal ultrasonography in disorders of the seminal vesicles and ejaculatory ducts. Urol Clin North Am 1989; 16(4): 773–790.
4. Hellerstein DK, Meacham RB, Lipshultz LI. Transrectal ultrasound and partial ejaculatory duct obstruction in male infertility. Urology 1992; 39(5):449–452.
5. Weintraub MP, De Mouy E, Hellstrom WJ. Newer modalities in the diagnosis and treatment of ejaculatory duct obstruction. J Urol 1993; 150(4):1150–1154.
6. Fisch H. Transurethral resection of the ejaculatory ducts. Curr Surg Techn Urol 1992; 5(5):2–7.
7. Farley S, Barnes R. Stenosis of ejaculatory ducts treated by endoscopic resection. J Urol 1973; 109(4):664–666.
8. Carson CC. Transurethral resection for ejaculatory duct stenosis and oligospermia. Fertil Steril 1984; 41(3):482–484.
9. Pryor JP, Hendry WF. Ejaculatory duct obstruction in subfertile males: analysis of 87 patients. Fertil Steril 1991; 56(4):725–730.
10. Belker AM, Steinbock GS. Transrectal prostate ultrasonography as a diagnostic and therapeutic aid for

ejaculatory duct obstruction. J Urol 1990; 144(2 Pt 1): 356–358.

11. Goldwasser BZ, Weinerth JL, Carson CC III. Ejaculatory duct obstruction: the case for aggressive diagnosis and treatment. J Urol 1985; 134(5):964–966.

12. Jarow JP. Transrectal ultrasonography of infertile men. Fertil Steril 1993; 60(6):1035–1039.

13. Worischeck JH, Parra RO. Transrectal ultrasound in the evaluation of men with low volume azoospermia. J Urol 1993; 149(5 Pt 2):1341–1344.

14. Shabsigh R, Lerner S, Fishman IJ, et al. The role of transrectal ultrasonography in the diagnosis and management of prostatic and seminal vesicle cysts. J Urol 1989; 141(5):1206–1209.

15. Porch PP Jr. Aspermia owing to obstruction of distal ejaculatory duct and treatment by transurethral resection. J Urol 1978; 119(1):141–142.

16. Sadler TW. Langman's Medical Embryology. Baltimore: Williams & Wilkins, 1985:247–280.

17. McCarthy JF, Ritter S, Klemperer P. Anatomical and histological study of the verumontanum with especial reference to the ejaculatory ducts. J Urol 1924; 17:1–16.

18. McMahon S. An anatomical study by injection technique of the ejaculatory ducts and their relations. J Urol 1938; 39:422–443.

19. Morgan RJ, Williams DI, Pryor JL. Mullerian duct remnants in the male. Br J Urol 1979; 51(6):488–492.

20. Mayersak JS. Urogenital sinus-ejaculatory duct cyst: a case report with a proposed clinical classification and review of the literature. J Urol 1989; 142(5):1330–1332.

21. Stifelman MD, Tanaka K, Jones JG, et al. Transurethral resection of ejaculatory ducts: anatomy and pathology (abstr O-117). Fertil Steril 1993; 60:S55–S56.

22. Schnall MD, Pollack HM, Van Arsdalen K, et al. The seminal tract in patients with ejaculatory dysfunction: MR imaging with an endorectal surface coil. Am J Roentgenol 1992; 159(2):337–341.

23. Jirasek JE. Normal development of the male accessory glands. In: Spring-Mills E, Hafez ESE, eds. Male Accessory Sex Glands. New York: Elsevier/North-Holland, 1980:3–16.

24. Weintraub CM. Transurethral drainage of the seminal tract for obstruction, infection and infertility. Br J Urol 1980; 52(3):220–225.

25. Silber SJ. Ejaculatory duct obstruction. J Urol 1980; 124(2):294–297.

26. Takatera H, Sugao H, Sakurai T. Ejaculatory duct cyst: the case for effective use of transrectal longitudinal ultrasonography. J Urol 1987; 137(6):1241–1242.

27. Patterson L, Jarow JP. Transrectal ultrasonography in the evaluation of the infertile man: a report of three cases. J Urol 1990; 144(6):1469–1471.

28. Fuse H, Okumura A, Satomi S, et al. Evaluation of seminal-vesicle characteristics by ultrasonography before and after ejaculation. Urol Int 1992; 49(2):110–113.

29. Katz D, Mieza M, Nagler HM. Ultrasound guided transrectal seminal vesiculography: a new approach to the diagnosis of male reproductive tract abnormalities (abstr 330). J Urol 1994; 151:310A.

30. Jarow JP. Seminal vesicle aspiration in the management of patients with ejaculatory duct obstruction. J Urol 1994; 152(3):899–901.

31. Orhan I, Onur R, Cayan S, et al. Seminal vesicle sperm aspiration in the diagnosis of ejaculatory duct obstruction. BJU International 1999; 84(9):1050–1053.

32. Littrup PJ, Lee F, McLeary RD, et al. Transrectal US of the seminal vesicles and ejaculatory ducts: clinical correlation. Radiology 1988; 168(3):625–628.

33. Wessels EC, Ohori M, Grantmyre JE, et al. The prevalence of cystic dilatation of the ejaculatory ducts detected by transrectal ultrasound (TRUS) in a self-referred (screening) group of men (abstr 973). J Urol 1992; 147:456A.

34. Kirkali Z, Yigitbasi O, Diren B, et al. Cysts of the prostate, seminal vesicles and diverticulum of the ejaculatory ducts. Eur Urol 1991; 20(1):77–80.

35. Elder JS, Mostwin JL. Cyst of the ejaculatory duct/urogenital sinus. J Urol 1984; 132(4):768–771.

36. Van Poppel H, Vereecken R, De Geeter P, et al. Hemospermia owing to utricular cyst: embryological summary and surgical review. J Urol 1983; 129(3): 608–609.

37. Malkevich DA, Mieza M, Nagler HM. Patency of ejaculatory ducts after transurethral resection of ejaculatory ducts verified by reflux seen on voiding cystourethrogram (abstr 295). J Urol 1994; 151:301A.

38. Nagler HM, Vazquez-Levin MH, Dressler KP. Urine contamination of seminal fluid after transurethral resection of the ejaculatory ducts (abstr 297). J Urol 1994; 151:302A.

39. Goluboff ET, Kaplan SA, Fisch H. Seminal vesicle urinary reflux as a complication of transurethral resection of the ejaculatory ducts. J Urol 1995; 153(4):1234–1235.

40. Turek PJ, Magana JO, Lipshultz LI. Semen parameters before and after transurethral surgery for ejaculatory duct obstruction. J Urol 1996; 155(4):1291–1293.

41. Netto NR, Esteves SC, Neves PA. Transurethral resection of partially obstructed ejaculatory ducts: seminal parameters and pregnancy outcomes according to the etiology of obstruction. J Urol 1998; 159(6): 2048–2053.

42. Colpi GM, Negri L, Patrizio P, et al. Fertility restoration by seminal tract washout in ejaculatory obstruction. J Urol 1995; 153(6):1948–1950.

19

Male Hormones and Systemic Disease

John E. Morley

Department of Medicine, Adelaide University, Australia and Division of Geriatric Medicine, St. Louis University School of Medicine and GRECC, St. Louis VA Medical Center, St. Louis, Missouri, U.S.A.

Gary A. Wittert

School of Medicine, Discipline of Medicine, University of Adelaide; Hanson Research Institute; and Discipline of Medicine, Royal Adelaide Hospital, Adelaide, Australia

☐ INTRODUCTION

Numerous systemic diseases alter gonadal function in males, either by inhibiting testosterone synthesis in the testes or by altering the release of luteinizing hormone (LH) and follicle-stimulating hormone (FSH) from the pituitary. Severe systemic illness results in the marked inhibition of LH and FSH release, thereby causing subsequent hypotestosteronemia (1–5). LH pulsatility is likewise decreased during critical illness (6). Administration of dopamine during the period of critical illness further decreases gonadotropin secretion (7). Table 1 summarizes the changes in the hypothalamic–pituitary–testicular axis that occur in a variety of chronic diseases. Unfortunately, these are limited studies that examine the effect of testosterone replacement in disease states, making it nearly impossible to conclude whether or not the testosterone decrease observed in disease processes is protective or harmful.

This chapter will review literature involving several of the most common systemic disease states that alter gonadal function, detailing the specific hormonal changes observed in each condition and what is known about their resultant effects on male sexual function.

☐ RENAL FAILURE

Patients with chronic renal failure commonly have a poor libido, decreased potency, and diminished testicular size. Testicular biopsy of renal failure patients shows diminished Leydig cells and a thickened basement membrane with maturation arrest of the germinal epithelium (8). The majority of patients with end-stage renal failure have severe oligospermia or azoospermia (9).

Numerous studies have found low testosterone levels in patients with chronic renal failure (10–13), which may be explained by increased metabolic break down of testosterone (14). Although there is preservation of the testosterone circadian rhythm (10) as well as the response to human chorionic gonadotropin

(hCG) in renal failure patients (10,15), there is no uniformity in the reports on sex hormone–binding globulin (SHBG) (14,16,17).

Renal failure produces almost a universal increase in gonadotropin levels, including bioactive and immunoactive LH (15,18–21) and FSH levels (9,15,18,22), and gonadotropin response to gonadotropin-releasing hormone (GnRH) is exaggerated in most cases (19). Levels of estradiol (23) and inhibin (12,24) are similarly increased. Erythropoietin increased testosterone and SHBG but did not lower prolactin levels (25–27).

In some renal failure patients, low zinc levels may also be associated with the low testosterone levels (28,29). In one study, zinc replacement was shown to increase testosterone in patients on dialysis (30). Renal transplantation improves gonadal function in some, but not all patients (9,31–35). Some of the continued deterioration appears to be due to immunosuppressive therapy. Uncontrolled trials have suggested that anabolic steroids improve anemia, malnutrition, and sexual dysfunction in uremic patients (36). This was confirmed in a control study utilizing nandrolone (37).

☐ CIRRHOSIS

Testicular atrophy, decreased libido, and gynecomastia are common manifestations in patients with cirrhosis of the liver (38). In addition, there is a reduction in prostate size and decreased incidence of benign prostatic hypertrophy (38,39).

In some studies, both the production rates and the plasma levels of total and free testosterone are reduced in patients with cirrhosis (40), whereas, in others, total plasma testosterone levels are not significantly different from that measured in controls (41,42). Discrepancies in studies may relate to differences in the severity of liver disease, since testosterone decreases in proportion to the severity of the liver disease (43) or the cause of the cirrhosis.

Particularly in the case of alcohol-induced cirrhosis, plasma SHBG concentrations are typically increased,

Table 1 Alternations in the Hypothalamic–Pituitary–Gonadal Axis in Male Patients with Systemic Disorders

	Testosterone	Sex hormone-binding globulin	Estradiol	FSH	LH	Prolactin
Renal failure	↓	↓	N or ↑	N or ↑	↑	N or ↑
Cirrhosis	↓	↑	↑	N	N or ↓	N or ↑
Hemochromatosis	↓	—	—	↓	↓	↓
Thalassemia	↓	—	—	↓	↓	—
Sickle cell anemia	↓	—	—	↑ or N	↑ or N	N
Hansen's disease (lepromatous)	↓	—	↓ or ↑	↑	↑	↑
Hansen's disease (tuberculoid)	N or ↑	—	↑	N or ↓	N or ↑	↑
Myotonia dystrophica	↓	—	—	↑	↑	—
Paraplegia	↑ or N	N	N or ↑	↑	↑	N or ↑
Hyperthyroidism	↑		↑	↑	↑	—
Hypothyroidism	↓		—	—	—	↑
Diabetes	↓	↑ or ↓	↑	N or ↓	N or ↓	N or ↑
Cushing's syndrome	↓		—	↓	↓	—
Protein-calorie malnutrition[a]	↓	↓	↓	↓	↓	—
Obesity[a]	↓		↑	N	N	—
Sleep apnea	↓	↓				
Chronic obstructive pulmonary disease	↓	↑	—		↑↓[b]	—
Rheumatoid arthritis	↑	—	—	↑	↑	↑

[a]Not discussed in the text.
[b]In persons receiving glucocorticoids.
Abbreviations: FSH, follicle-stimulating hormone; LH, luteinizing hormone.

at least partly as a consequence of increased plasma estrone and estradiol (40,41), and, therefore, bioavailable testosterone is usually decreased. This increase in SHBG could explain why total testosterone levels are not always decreased in patients with cirrhosis compared to controls.

In cirrhosis due to idiopathic hemochromatosis, SHBG concentrations and the peripheral conversion of androgens to estrogens are similar to the levels of healthy men (44). The peripheral conversion of androgens to estrogens (i.e., androstenedione to estrone and testosterone to estradiol) is increased in alcohol-induced cirrhosis (45–49). The function of the hypothalamus and pituitary is essentially normal in alcohol-induced cirrhosis.

Basal LH and FSH levels are often slightly elevated, and the primary abnormality appears to be the function of the testes. The gonadotropin response to GnRH is mostly normal, but hyper-responsiveness is seen in some patients and can be suppressed in end-stage disease (40,50,51).

In male patients with viral cirrhosis, significant alterations in plasma estradiol and testosterone levels either do not occur (52) or mimic those changes seen as the result of alcohol-induced cirrhosis (53). Patients with nonalcoholic liver disease have low total and free testosterone levels and increased levels of SHBG (54). Gonadal function improved, but was not normalized, one year after liver transplantation, and the gonadotropin response to GnRH suggested the presence of a hypothalamic defect.

Plasma prolactin levels have been found to be normal or increased in males with cirrhosis (55–57). Although there is a normal prolactin response to thyrotropin-releasing hormone in most patients, an exaggerated response occurs in some (58–60). The

prolactin circadian rhythm becomes lost in cirrhosis (61,62). Elevated prolactin levels correlate with elevated "free" tryptophan levels (59). The increased prolactin levels present in some cirrhotics appear to be due to the elevated estrogen levels and delayed prolactin clearance by the liver.

The altered hormonal changes seen in patients with cirrhosis are summarized in Figure 1. The mechanism of the gonadal hormonal changes would appear to be due to increased estrogen production, secondary to increased peripheral conversion of androgens (63). The elevated estrogens lead to an increase in SHBG with a resultant decrease in free testosterone. The increased prolactin levels may be secondary to the increase in estrogen levels. Testicular damage may also

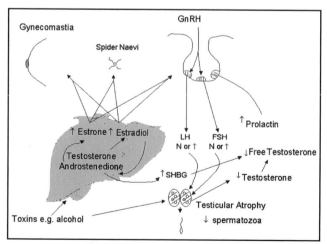

Figure 1 Hormonal changes and their results in men with cirrhosis. *Abbreviations*: FSH, follicle-stimulating hormone; GnRH, gonadotropin-releasing hormone; LH, luteinizing hormone; SHBG, sex hormone–binding globulin.

occur, particularly in cases when the cirrhosis is secondary to known testicular toxins such as alcohol.

Testosterone supplementation in men with alcoholic cirrhosis is of minimal benefit. It should be noted, however, that in men with hypogonadism due to hemochromatosis, the administration of testosterone treatment produces an almost immediate recovery in well-being, libido, and potency, with no adverse effects on liver function (64).

☐ BLOOD DYSCRASIAS
Hemochromatosis

Testicular atrophy was first recognized in patients with hemochromatosis in the 1930s (65,66). A later study of 1000 patients with hemochromatosis revealed an incidence of testicular atrophy approaching 17% (67). Most studies have suggested that patients with hemochromatosis have low LH levels and an impaired response to GnRH (68–70). Long-term treatment with hCG serves to elevate testosterone levels (71). These findings are compatible with the finding that iron deposits are prominent in the pituitary (71) but scanty in the testes (70). Venesection has produced partial reversal of the hypogonadotropic hypogonadism seen in hemochromatosis, but only in persons less than 40 years of age (72). Patients with hypogonadism from hemochromatosis have symptomatic improvement when treated with testosterone (73).

In conclusion, hemochromatosis produces a secondary hypogonadism. Liver disease plays little-to-no role in the pathogenesis of the hypogonadism.

Thalassemia

Patients with beta-thalassemia receive frequent blood transfusions that often lead to secondary hemosiderosis. This condition may be responsible for delayed puberty, hypogonadism, and short stature. Thalassemic patients have a poor responsiveness of LH and FSH to GnRH (74). Some children with delayed puberty, however, have been shown to respond to pulsatile GnRH administration, suggesting an actual problem of impaired hypothalamic GnRH release (75). Testosterone therapy given at the time of puberty typically produces a growth spurt, with an increase in nocturnal growth hormone levels and insulin-like growth factor-I and insulin growth-like factor binding protein 3 (IGFBP-3) (74).

Sickle Cell Anemia

Sickle cell anemia is similarly associated with delayed puberty. In a large series of sickle cell patients, one-third were found to be hypogonadal, exhibiting testicular atrophy (76). In this study, the patients also had low levels of androstenedione and dihydrotestosterone. LH and FSH levels were elevated basally and there was an exaggerated response to GnRH with a diminished testosterone response. Other researchers have reported a similar hormonal profile suggestive of primary hypogonadism in sickle cell disease (77–79). The low serum testosterone levels in sickle cell disease are associated with low erythrocyte zinc levels (76). As in the case of renal failure mentioned previously, Prasad et al. (80) found that zinc replacement in persons with sickle cell disease increased testosterone levels.

Other studies have suggested that testosterone deficiency in sickle cell disease is due to pituitary infarction secondary to intravascular thrombosis (81,82). Modebe and Ezeh (83) reported normal FSH, LH, and prolactin levels in patients with sickle cell disease and low testosterone levels. Landefeld et al. (84) reported the case of a 19-year-old male with sickle cell disease, who demonstrated an increase in testosterone, LH, and FSH levels when treated with oral clomiphene. One major complication of testosterone therapy in hypogonadal males with sickle cell disease is the possibility of priapism (85,86).

Overall, it would appear that most cases of hypogonadism in patients with sickle cell disease are due to testicular failure. Some patients, however, clearly develop a secondary hypogonadism. The role of zinc deficiency in patients with hypogonadism due to sickle cell disease deserves further investigation.

☐ HANSEN'S DISEASE (LEPROSY)

Low testosterone levels have been identified in 43% of patients with lepromatous leprosy and 5% of those patients with borderline lepromatous leprosy (87). Low testosterone levels were originally reported in patients with lepromatous leprosy in 1968 by Martin et al. (88) and have since been confirmed by a number of other studies (89–94). The testosterone response to hCG was attenuated in patients with lepromatous leprosy (93). This is in keeping with the 1952 report by Grabstald and Swann (95) that the testes are invaded in 90% of males with lepromatous leprosy. Destruction of the Leydig cells occurs after destruction of the seminiferous tubules. Histopathologic examination of lepromatous testes showed inflammatory, degenerative, and fibrotic changes (94). Although reduced testicular size has been observed in up to half of lepromatous leprosy patients (90), this is not a universal finding, particularly in early disease (89). Additionally, some patients develop Leydig cell hyperplasia (96).

In view of the testicular atrophy, it is not surprising that both urinary gonadotropins (95) and serum LH and FSH levels have been reported to be elevated in lepromatous leprosy (87,89,91–93). The gonadotropin response to GnRH is exaggerated in patients with lepromatous leprosy compared to those with tuberculoid leprosy and normal controls (89).

Estradiol levels have been found to be either low (89) or elevated (90,91,93) in patients with lepromatous leprosy. Prolactin levels are typically increased (93). In one study, 12 out of 16 patients with lepromatous leprosy had oligospermia or azoospermia (90).

The situation in the tuberculoid form of Hansen's disease is less certain. Some authors have reported no effect of tuberculoid leprosy on gonadal function (89,91,92). Two studies, however, have suggested that testosterone levels were low, with normal or reduced LH and FSH levels suggestive of secondary hypogonadism. Prolactin and estradiol levels were elevated (93,97). In addition, patients with the tuberculoid type of Hansen's disease were found to have a reduction in sperm count and motility and an increase in abnormal forms of spermatozoa (97). Because these studies utilized healthy young men as controls, however, it is possible that the physiological hypogonadotropic hypogonadism associated with aging was a predominant factor that clouded their results. Alternatively, these findings could be explained by the presence of granulomatous disease of the meninges affecting the hypothalamic–pituitary stalk.

In conclusion, patients with Hansen's disease of the lepromatous type have primary hypogonadism due to testicular invasion by the *lepra* bacilli. It is possible that patients with the tuberculoid form of leprosy develop a secondary hypogonadism secondary to granulomatous disease involving the hypothalamus or pituitary.

Myotonic Dystrophy

Myotonic Dystrophy is a genetic disorder caused by multiple CTG repeats lying upstream of a gene that encodes a novel protein kinase. This disease is characterized by muscle weakness, baldness, cataracts, and abnormal regulation of adrenocorticotrophic hormone and cytokine production. Metabolic disturbances, peripheral insulin insensitivity, and cognitive dysfunction are common features, including the failure of testicular and adrenal testosterone production (98–100). Testicular atrophy was first reported in 1909 in patients with myotonic dystrophy (101). Approximately 80% of patients with myotonia will develop hypogonadism, although this typically occurs later in life, where many patients could have completed their families earlier in life (102). On testicular biopsy, tubular fibrosis and abnormal spermatogenesis are the most common findings (103,104). LH and FSH levels are elevated, and the response to GnRH is exaggerated (101,104–106). A poor testicular response to hCG has been reported in one patient (104). The hypogonadism in myotonic dystrophy is of the primary type. Although testosterone treatment increases muscle mass in patients with myotonic dystrophy, it does not increase muscle strength (107).

Paraplegia

Patients with paraplegia have decreased skeletal muscle and a relative increase in adiposity (108). They also develop osteoporosis, particularly of the pelvis and lower limbs. Gynecomastia is not an uncommon finding in patients with paraplegia (109,110). Early studies suggest that evidence of testicular dysfunction could be found in up to half of men who become paraplegic following trauma (111,112).

Testicular biopsies are abnormal in approximately 40% of persons with paraplegia (113,114). In these patients, there is generalized hypoplasia of the germinal epithelium associated with spermatogenetic arrest. Leydig cells are usually normal, but nodular hyperplasia is seen in some subjects. Interestingly, the higher the level of the spinal cord lesion, the greater the degree of seminiferous tubule damage (115). Sperm counts have been reported to be greater than 20 million in just over 60% of subjects (114). Motility, however, was low, with 77% of patients exhibiting less than 20% motility, which may be related to elevated FSH levels. Perkash et al. (114) have suggested that the minimization of urinary tract infections and the prevention of sperm stagnation in the lower storage areas by periodic rectal probe electrostimulation may improve spermatozoa motility.

Plasma testosterone levels tend to be below normal for the first two to three months following the acute trauma before rising into the normal range (116,117). This increase is thought to be due to an earlier posttraumatic increase in circulating epinephrine levels, which occurs very soon after the acute trauma has taken place. In quadriplegics, testosterone levels remain low for a longer period of time (118,119). Interestingly, some paraplegic patients demonstrate slightly higher long-term testosterone levels than in nonparaplegics (108), but another study has suggested that other patients might develop lower than normal levels (120). One study reported that the majority of free androgen indices (testosterone/SHBG) in persons with paraplegia were within the normal range (121). In another study with small numbers of patients, adequate testosterone response to hCG was found (113).

In contrast to the normal testosterone levels, elevated LH and FSH levels associated with an exaggerated gonadotropin response to GnRH have been reported in many patients with paraplegia (113,116,120,122,123). This suggests that many of these patients have, in fact, compensated primary hypogonadism. In quadriplegics, however, LH levels appear to be low, particularly in the acute period following the traumatic injury (117,119), suggesting that these patients, who often also have low testosterone, have secondary hypogonadism. Plasma prolactin levels are elevated in a number of paraplegics (116,123).

☐ ENDOCRINE DISORDERS

The autoimmune underpinnings of many endocrine failure disorders lead to hypogonadism being associated with a variety of other endocrine disorders. Both Type I and Type II polyglandular autoimmune syndromes are associated with hypogonadism (124–126). Antisperm antibodies have been reported to be present in Type I polyglandular failure (127). POEMS syndrome consists of plasma cell dyscrasias with polyneuropathy, organomegaly, endocrinopathy (diabetes mellitus and primary gonadal failure), M protein in plasma, and skin changes (hyperpigmentation) (128). The Kearns–Sayre syndrome is a rare syndrome characterized by myopathic abnormalities leading to ophthalmoplegia and progressive weakness associated with hypoparathyroidism, primary gonadal failure, diabetes mellitus, and hypopituitarism (129). Patients with Down's syndrome often develop hypogonadism (130). Adrenoleukodystrophy is a genetic paroxysmal disorder associated with progressive antral demyelination, primary adrenal insufficiency, and primary hypogonadism (131).

One in five patients with hyperthyroidism develop gynecomastia (132–134). This is associated with increased total (135,136) and free (134,137) estradiol levels. Ridgway et al. (138) showed that the decreased plasma clearance rate of estradiol was due to increased binding of estradiol to SHBG. Hyperthyroidism had minimal effects on estradiol production rate. Serum estradiol levels decline after treatment of hyperthyroidism (124,135).

In hyperthyroidism, total testosterone and SHBG levels are increased (135–137,139–143) and free or bioavailable testosterone is decreased (137,142,143). Androstenedione (139) and 17-hydroxyprogesterone (144) levels are also elevated. The testicular response to hCG has been found to be impaired (142,144–146). Prolactin levels are unchanged in hyperthyroidism (142).

Gonadotropin levels are increased in hyperthyroidism (135,136,141,146). There is no change in the pulsatility of LH and FSH secretion in hyperthyroidism (142). Patients with hyperthyroidism had an exaggerated response to GnRH (142,145,147).

Zinc deficiency occurs in hyperthyroidism, and, as with other conditions previously mentioned, this has been demonstrated to be associated with a decline in testosterone production (148). The changes in the hormonal milieu in hyperthyroidism appear to be predominantly due to the increased SHBG levels associated with a mild defect in gonadal testosterone production.

Hypothyroid patients have abnormalities in spermatogenesis and Leydig cell function (149). Androgen secretion declines in hypothyroidism and the metabolic transformation of testosterone is shifted toward etiocholanolone rather than androsterone (150). The low testosterone levels in hypothyroidism are associated with low gonadotropin levels; thus, these patients have secondary hypogonadism (151,152). SHBG levels are decreased in hypothyroid patients (152). Prolactin levels are elevated in some, but not all, patients with hypothyroidism (151). Thyroxin replacement reverts the hypothalamic–pituitary–gonadal axis to normal in patients with hypothyroidism (151,152).

Men with Addison's disease have dehydroepiandrosterone (DHEA) levels that are one-tenth of those seen in normal men (153). They also have a decreased response of testosterone to hCG.

Persons with Cushing's syndrome have decreased libido, impotence, oligospermia, and histological changes in the testes (154–157). Testosterone levels are reduced in males with Cushing's syndrome (158–160). Steroids have an antigonadotropic action on the Leydig cell membrane (161).

Testosterone decreases and LH increases when dexamethasone is administered acutely (162). It would appear, however, that the ability of steroids to inhibit LH at the pituitary level leading to secondary hypogonadism is the major reason for hypogonadism in patients with Cushing's syndrome.

Diabetes Mellitus

Plasma total and free testosterone levels are reduced in men with diabetes mellitus, independent of age and body mass index (163). Furthermore, a stepwise decrease in mean testosterone levels per categorical increase in fasting plasma glucose is apparent in both diabetics and nondiabetics (164). In men with Type 1 diabetes mellitus, plasma testosterone is lowest when control is very poor (165), but there is no relationship between the severity of retinopathy (166) or other complications (167) and the level of plasma testosterone. Levels of SHBG have been reported to be either increased (168,169) or decreased (170,171) in diabetics. There is a mild impairment of the testosterone response to hCG in diabetics (168). Basal gonadotropin levels are normal in diabetics (171–174), but the LH and FSH response to GnRH is impaired, particularly in the presence of hyperglycemia (175). Dihydrotestosterone (164,173), DHEA (176), and DHEA-sulfate (164,176,177) have all been found to be lower in patients with diabetes, whereas estradiol levels were found to be slightly increased in one study (178). Young men with diabetes exhibit prolactin secretion that has a normal pulse frequency, but a decline in maximal peak amplitude and peak area (179), whereas older persons with Type II diabetes were reported to have elevated prolactin levels (180).

Excessive visceral adiposity results in decreased plasma testosterone and insulin resistance and substantially increases the risk of diabetes mellitus. Administration of testosterone under these circumstances may decrease visceral fat and improve glucose tolerance (181). Type II diabetes mellitus is, however, associated with lowered plasma testosterone levels independent of obesity in both Melanesian and Caucasian men (182,183). In older diabetic men, there is a relationship between the presence of diabetic dyslipidemia and the decrease in plasma testosterone (183).

Total testosterone and SHBG have been associated with defects in nonoxidative glucose disposal and upper body adiposity in normoglycemic men (184). Insulin has been shown to stimulate testosterone production (and suppress SHBG production) in both normal and obese men (185). Administration of testosterone to centrally obese, hypogonadal, middle-aged men has improved insulin sensitivity.

Leptin is produced from fat cells, and while women have higher leptin levels than men when corrected for adipose cell mass (186,187), leptin levels are independently associated with testosterone level (188); testosterone replacement in hypogonadal males serves to reduce leptin levels (189,190).

Data from the Massachusetts Male Aging Study showed that after controlling for potential confounders, diabetes at follow-up was predicted jointly and independently by lower baseline levels of free testosterone and SHBG (191).

In conclusion, persons with diabetes have low testosterone levels secondary to both gonadal and hypothalamic–pituitary defects. Testosterone replacement improves sexual performance in diabetes (172).

☐ PULMONARY DISEASE
Obstructive Sleep Apnea

Sleep apnea results in decreased plasma testosterone and SHBG levels in proportion to the severity of the sleep apnea (192). Gonadotropin levels are normal (192). Men with obstructive sleep apnea have lower plasma testosterone levels than those men who only snore, even when matched for body mass index. Furthermore, successful treatment of sleep apnea results in an improvement in both plasma testosterone levels and sexual function (192,193). Conversely, testosterone administration has been demonstrated to depress ventilatory drive and increase sleep apnea in adult men by affecting the neuromuscular control of upper airway patency during sleep (194,195). This would appear to be an effect of exogenously administered testosterone, since one week of androgen blockade using flutamide had no clinically significant effect on sleep, sleep-disordered breathing, or chemosensitivity in patients with moderate-to-severe sleep apnea (196). Snyder et al. (197) demonstrated no deleterious effects of testosterone in patients with sleep apnea when the testosterone was administered by patch resulting in physiologic levels of testosterone.

Chronic Obstructive Pulmonary Disease

In 1979, Semple et al. (198) reported that persons with chronic obstructive pulmonary disease (COPD) had very low testosterone levels. The decrease in circulating testosterone levels was related to the severity of hypoxia (199), and was associated with a marked decline in sexual activity in men with COPD (200). Oral glucocorticoid treatment produces a marked decrease in testosterone due to a direct effect on the hypothalamic–pituitary axis (201–203). Similar effects on testosterone are not seen with inhaled corticosteroids (201). The low testosterone levels are reversed by oxygen therapy (204–206). Overall, the cause of the low testosterone levels appears to involve both testicular and hypothalamic–pituitary defects (207,208).

☐ RHEUMATOID ARTHRITIS

In 1986, Gordon et al. (209) reported that males with rheumatoid arthritis had low testosterone and a free testosterone index associated with an increase in LH and FSH compared to age-matched controls. Subsequently, others have confirmed the low testosterone levels in patients with rheumatoid arthritis (210–215). These patients have low testosterone response to hCG when compared to normal subjects (211). Testosterone levels decrease during rheumatoid arthritis flares and increase slowly after the flare settles (212). LH and FSH levels are elevated in patients with rheumatoid arthritis who are not taking glucocorticoids (216). Salivary testosterone, androstenedione, and DHEA-sulfate are also decreased in patients with rheumatoid arthritis (217). Serum prolactin levels are also elevated in these patients (218).

A pilot study suggested that testosterone replacement may increase the CD8+ T cells and decrease immunoglobulin M rheumatoid factor levels (219). This was associated with an improvement in clinical correlates of rheumatoid arthritis. A randomized clinical trial of testosterone for nine months failed to show a positive effect of testosterone on disease activity in males with rheumatoid arthritis (220).

☐ REFERENCES

1. Nierman DM, Mechanick JI. Hypotestosteronemia in chronically ill men. Critical Care Med 1999; 27(11): 2418–2421.

2. Spratt DI, Cox P, Orav J, et al. Reproductive axis suppression in acute illness is related to disease severity. J Clin Endocrinol Metab 1993; 76(6):1548–1554.

3. Woolf PD, Hamill RW, McDonald JV, et al. Transient hypogonadotropic hypogonadism caused by critical illness. J Clin Endocrinol Metab 1985; 60(3):444–450.

4. Goussis OS, Pardridge WM, Judd HL. Critical illness and low testosterone: effects of human serum on testosterone transport into rat brain and liver. J Clin Endocrinol Metab 1983; 56(4):710–714.

5. Quint AR, Kaiser FE. Gonadotropin determinations and thyrotropin-releasing hormone and luteinizing hormone-releasing hormone testing in critically ill postmenopausal women with hypothyroxinemia. J Clin Endocrinol Metab 1985; 60(3):464–471.

6. van den Berghe G, Weekers F, Baxter RC, et al. Five-day pulsatile gonadotropin-releasing hormone administration unveils combined hypothalamic-pituitary-gonadal defects underlying profound hypoandrogenism in men with prolonged critical illness. J Clin Endocrinol Metab 2001; 86(7): 3217–3226.

7. van den Berghe G, de Zegher F, Lauwers P, et al. Luteinizing hormone secretion and hypoandrogenaemia in critically ill men: effect of dopamine. Clin Endocrinol 1994; 41(5):563–569.

8. Schmitt WG, Shehadeh I, Sawin CT. Transient gynecomastia in chronic renal failure during chronic intermittent hemodialysis. Ann Intern Med 1968; 69(1): 73–79.

9. Lim VS, Fang VS. Gonadal dysfunction in uremic men: a study of the hypothalamo-pituitary-testicular axis before and after transplantation. Am J Med 1975; 58(5): 655–662.

10. Rager K, Bundschu H, Gupta D. The effect of HCG on testicular androgen production in adult men with chronic renal failure. J Reprod Fertil 1975; 42(1): 113–120.

11. Zadeh JA, Koutsaimanis KG, Roberts AP, et al. The effect of maintenance haemodialysis and renal transplantation on the plasma testosterone levels of male patients in chronic renal failure. Acta Endocrinol 1975; 80(3):577–582.

12. Sasagawa I, Tateno T, Suzuki Y, et al. Circulating levels of inhibin in hemodialysis males. Arch Androl 1998; 41(3):167–171.

13. Prem AR, Punekar SV, Kalpana M, et al. Male reproductive function in uraemia-efficacy of haemodialysis and renal transplantation. Br J Urol 1996; 78(4): 635–638.

14. Van Kammen E, Thijssen JHM, Schwarz F. Sex hormones in male patients with chronic renal failure. The production of testosterone and androstenedione. Clin Endocrinol (Oxf) 1978; 8(1):7–14.

15. Holdsworth S, Atkins RC, deKretser DM. The pituitary-testicular axis in men with chronic renal failure. N Engl J Med 1977; 296(22):1245–1249.

16. Chen JC, Vidt DG, Zorn EM, et al. Pituitary-Leydig cell function in uremic males. J Clin Endocrinol Metab 1970; 31(1):14–17.

17. Gupta D, Bundschu HD. Testosterone and its binding in the plasma of male subjects with chronic renal failure. Clin Chim Acta 1972; 36(2):479–484.

18. Stewart-Bentley M, Gans D, Horton R. Regulation of gonadal function in uremia. Metabolism 1974; 23(11): 1065–1072.

19. Distiller LA, Morley JE, Sagel J, et al. Pituitary-gonadal function in chronic renal failure: the effect of luteinizing hormone-releasing hormone and its influence of dialysis. Metabolism 1975; 24(6):711–720.

20. Guevara A, Vidt D, Halbert MC, et al. Serum gonadotropin and testosterone levels in uremic males. Metabolism 1969; 18(12):1062–1066.

21. Handelsman DJ, Spaliviero JA, Turtle JR. Bioactive luteinizing hormone in plasma of uraemic men and men with primary testicular damage. Clin Endocrinol 1986; 24(3):259–266.

22. Sawin CT, Longcope C, Schmitt GW, et al. Blood levels of gonadotrophins and gonadal hormones in gynecomastia associated with chronic hemodialysis. J Clin Endocrinol Metab 1973; 36:988–990.

23. Franchimont P. Pituitary gonadotrophins. Clin Endocrinol Metab 1977; 6(1):101–116.

24. Phocas I, Sarandakou A, Rizos D, et al. Serum alpha-immunoreactive inhibin in males with renal failure, under haemodialysis and after successful renal transplantation. Andrologia 1995; 27(5):253–258.

25. Lawrence IG, Price DE, Howlett TA, et al. Erythropoietin and sexual dysfunction. Nephrol Dialysis Transplant 1997; 12(4):741–747.

26. Foresta C, Mioni R, Bordon P, et al. Erythropoietin stimulates testosterone production in man. J Clin Endocrinol Metab 1994; 78(3):753–756.

27. Wu SC, Lin SL, Jeng FR. Influence of erythropoietin treatment on gonadotropic hormone levels and sexual function in male uremic patients. Scand J Urol Nephrol 2001; 35(2):136–140.

28. Antoniou LD, Shalhoub RJ, Sudhaker T, et al. Reversal of uraemic impotence by zinc. Lancet 1977; 2(8044): 895–898.

29. Swaminathan S, Kanagasabapathy AS, Selvakumar R, et al. Zinc and testicular hormone profiles before and after renal transplantation. Nephrol 1997; 3: 289–291.

30. Mahajan SK, Prasad AS, McDonald FD. Sexual dysfunction in uremic male: improvement following oral zinc supplementation. Contributions Nephrol 1984; 38: 103–111.

31. Phadke AG, MacKinnon KJ, Dossetor JB. Male fertility in uremia. Restoration by renal allografts. Can Med Assoc J 1970; 102(6):607–608.

32. Baumgarten SR, Lindsay GK, Wise GJ. Fertility problems in the renal transplant patient. J Urol 1977; 118(6):991–993.

33. Morley JE, Distiller LA, Unterhalter S, et al. Effect of renal transplantation on pituitary-gonadal function. Metabolism 1978; 27(7):781–785.

34. Chopp RT, Mendez R. Sexual function and hormonal abnormalities in uremic men on chronic dialysis and after renal transplantation. Fertil Steril 1978; 29(6): 661–666.

35. Handelsman DJ, Ralec VL, Tiller DJ, et al. Testicular function after renal transplantation. Clin Endocrinol (Oxf) 1981; 14(5):527–538.

36. Soliman G, Oreopoulos DG. Anabolic steroids and malnutrition in chronic renal failure. Perit Dial Int 1994; 14(4):362–365.

37. Johansen KL, Mulligan K, Schambelan M. Anabolic effects of nandrolone decanoate in patients receiving dialysis: a randomized controlled trial. JAMA 1999; 281(14):1275–1281.

38. Paulsen CA. Gynecomastia. In: Williams RH, ed. Textbook of Endocrinology. Philadelphia: Saunders, 1968:443.

39. Van Thiel DH, Lester R, Sherins RJ. Hypogonadism in alcoholic liver disease: evidence for a double defect. Gastroenterology 1974; 67(6):1188–1199.

40. Baker HW, Burger HG, de Kretser KD, et al. A study of the endocrine manifestations of hepatic cirrhosis. Q J Med 1976; 45(177):145–178.

41. Bahnsen M, Gluud C, Johnsen SG, et al. Pituitary-testicular function in patients with alcoholic cirrhosis of the liver. Eur J Clin Invest 1981; 11(6):473–479.

42. Gluud C, Bahnsen M, Bennett P, et al. Hypothalamic-pituitary-gonadal function in relation to liver function in men with alcoholic cirrhosis. Scand J Gastroentrol 1983; 18(7):939–944.

43. Gluud C. Testosterone and alcoholic cirrhosis. Epidemiologic, pathophysiologic and therapeutic studies in men. Dan Med Bull 1988; 35(6):564–575.

44. Kley HK, Niederau C, Stremmel W, et al. Conversion of androgens to estrogens in idiopathic hemochromatosis: comparison with alcoholic liver cirrhosis. J Clin Endocrinol Metab 1985; 61(1):1–6.

45. Elewaut A, Barbier F, Vermeulen A. Testosterone metabolism in normal males and male cirrhotics. J Gastroenterol 1979; 17(7):402–405.

46. Vermeulen A, Mussche M, Verdonck L. Testosterone and estradiol production rates and interconversion in normal males and male cirrhotics. Proceedings of the Fourth International Congress of Endocrinology, Abstract 305, Amsterdam, Excerpta Medica, 1971, p. 123.

47. Thijssen JHH, Lourens J, Donker GH, et al. The role of the liver in the biogenesis of oestrogens in cirrhosis of the liver. Acta Endocrinol (suppl) (Kbh) 1975; 199:234.

48. Edman CD, MacDonald PC, Combes D. Extraglandular production of estrogen in subjects with liver disease. Gastroenterology 1975; 69:1-19/819.

49. Thijssen JHH, Lurens J, Donker GH. Increased oestrogen production by peripheral conversion of androgens in male patients with cirrhosis of the liver. J Endocrinol 1973; 57:49.

50. Mowat NA, Edwards CRW, Fisher R, et al. Hypothalamic-pituitary-gonadal function in men with cirrhosis of the liver. Gut 1976; 17(5):345–350.

51. Distiller LA, Sagel J, Dubowitz B, et al. Pituitary-gonadal function in men with alcoholic cirrhosis of the liver. Horm Metab Res 1976; 8(6):461–465.

52. Pignata S, Daniele B, Galati MG, et al. Oestradiol and testosterone blood levels in patients with viral cirrhosis and hepatocellular carcinoma. Eur J Gastroenterol Hepatol 1997; 9(3):283–286.

53. Wang YJ, Wu JC, Lee SD, et al. Gonadal dysfunction and changes in sex hormones in postnecrotic cirrhotic men: a matched study with alcoholic cirrhotic men. Hepatogastroenterology 1991; 38(6):531–534.

54. Handelsman DJ, Strasser S, McDonald JA, et al. Hypothalamic-pituitary-testicular function in end-stage non-alcoholic liver disease before and after liver transplantation. Clin Endocrinol 1995; 43(3): 331–337.

55. Van Thiel DH, Gavaler JS, Lester R, et al. Plasma estrone, prolactin, neurophysin and sex steroid-binding globulin in chronic alcoholic men. Metabolism 1975; 24(9):1015–1019.

56. Turkington RW. Serum prolactin levels in patients with gynecomastia. J Clin Endocrinol Metab 1972; 34(1):62–66.

57. Horrobin DF, Manku MS, Nassar BA. Letter: hepatorenal syndrome and prolactin. N Engl J Med 1974; 290(7):408.

58. Green JRB. Mechanism of hypogonadism in cirrhotic males. Gut 1977; 18(10):843–853.

59. Panerai AE, Salerno F, Manneschi M, et al. Growth hormone and prolactin responses to thyrotropin-releasing hormone in patients with severe liver disease. J Clin Endocrinol Metab 1977; 45(1):134–139.

60. Zanoboni A, Zanoboni-Muciaccia W. Gynecomastia in alcoholic cirrhosis. Lancet 1975; 2:876.

61. Van Thiel DH, McClain CJ, Elson MK, et al. Evidence for autonomous secretion of prolactin in some alcoholic men with cirrhosis and gynecomastia. Metabolism 1978; 27(12):1778–1784.

62. Tarquini B, Gheri R, Anichini P, et al. Circadian study of immunoreactive prolactin in patients with cirrhosis of the liver. Gastroenterology 1977; 73(1):116–119.

63. Olivo J, Gordon GG, Rafi F, et al. Estrogen metabolism in hyperthyroidism and cirrhosis of the liver. Steroids 1975; 26(1):47–56.

64. Kley HK, Stremmel W, Kley JB, et al. Testosterone treatment of men with idiopathic hemochromatosis. Clin Investig 1992; 70(7):566–572.

65. Sheldon JH. Haemochromatosis. London: Oxford University Press, 1935.

66. Althausen TL, Kerr WJ. Hemochromatosis II: a report of three cases with endocrine disturbances and notes on a previously reported case. Discussion of etiology. Endocrinol 1933; 17:621–628.

67. Finch SC, Finch CA. Idiopathic hemochromatosis: an iron storage disease. Medicine (Baltimore) 1955; 34(4): 381–412.

68. Stocks AE, Powell LW. Pituitary function in idiopathic hemochromatosis and cirrhosis of the liver. Lancet 1972; 2:298–299.

69. Bezwoda WR, Bothwell TH, van der Walt LA, et al. An investigation into gonadal dysfunction in patients with idiopathic haemochromatosis. Clin Endocrinol 1977; 6(5):377–385.

70. Gilbert-Dreyfus M. La fonction testiculaire dans l'hemachromatoses idiopathique. Rev Fr Endocrinol Clin Nutr Metab 1977; 10:191–203.

71. McDonald RA, Mallory GK. Hemochromatosis and hemosiderosis: study of 211 autopsied cases. Arch Intern Med 1970; 105:686–700.

72. Cundy T, Butler J, Bomford A, et al. Reversibility of hypogonadotrophic hypogonadism associated with genetic haemochromatosis. Clin Endocrinol 1993; 38(6):617–620.

73. Berent R, Allinger S, Hobling W, et al. Loss of libido and erectile dysfunction as initial symptoms of haemochromatosis in a 24 year old man [German]. Deutsche Medizinische Wochenschrift 2000; 125:1466–1468.

74. Roth C, Pekrun A, Bartz M, et al. Short stature and failure of pubertal development in thalassaemia major: evidence for hypothalamic neurosecretory dysfunction of growth hormone secretion and defective pituitary gonadotropin secretion. Europ J Pediat 1997; 156(10):777–783.

75. Valenti S, Giusti M, Mcguinness D, et al. Delayed puberty in males with beta-thalassemia major: pulsatile gonadotropin-releasing hormone administration induces changes in gonadotropin isoform profiles and an increase in sex steroids. Europ J Endocrinol 1995; 133(1):48–56.

76. Abbasi AA, Prasad AS, Ortega T, et al. Gonadal function abnormalities in sickle cell anemia. Studies in adult male patients. Ann Intern Med 1976; 85(5):601–605.

77. Singhal A, Gabay L, Serjeant GR. Testosterone deficiency and extreme retardation of puberty in homozygous sickle-cell disease. West Indian Med J 1995; 44(1):20–23.

78. Parshad O, Stevens MC, Preece MA, et al. The mechanism of low testosterone levels in homozygous sickle cell disease. West Indian Med J 1994; 43(1):12–14.

79. Osegbe DN, Akinyanju OO. Testicular dysfunction in men with sickle cell disease. Postgrad Med J 1987; 63(736):95–98.

80. Prasad AS, Abbasi AA, Rabbani P, et al. Effect of zinc supplementation on serum testosterone level in adult male sickle cell anemia subjects. Am J Hematol 1981; 10(2):119–127.

81. Wintrobe MM. Sickle cell disease, thalassemia and abnormal hemoglobin syndromes. In: Wintrobe MM, ed. Clinical Hematology. Philadelphia: Lea & Febiger, 1967:687–735.

82. Daughaday WH. The Adenohypophysis. In: Williams RH, ed. Textbook of Endocrinology. Philadelphia: Saunders, 1974:55.

83. Modebe O, Ezeh UO. Effect of age on testicular function in adult males with sickle cell anemia. Fertil Steril 1995; 63(4):907–912.

84. Landefeld CS, Schambelan M, Kaplan SL, et al. Clomiphene-responsive hypogonadism in sickle cell anemia. Ann Int Med 1983; 99(4):480–483.

85. Kachhi PN, Henderson SO. Priapism after androstenedione intake for athletic performance enhancement. Ann Emerg Med 2000; 35(4):391–393.

86. Slayton W, Kedar A, Schatz D. Testosterone induced priapism in two adolescents with sickle cell disease. J Pediat Endocrinol Metab 1995; 8(3):199–203.

87. Rea TH. A comparative study of testicular involvement in lepromatous and borderline lepromatous leprosy. Int J Lepr Other Mycrobact Dis 1988; 56(3):383–388.

88. Martin FI, Maddocks I, Brown JB, et al. Leprous endocrinopathy. Lancet 1968; 2(7582):1320–1321.

89. Morley JE, Distiller LA, Sage J, et al. Hormonal changes associated with testicular atrophy and gynaecomastia in patients with leprosy. Clin Endocrinol 1977; 6(4): 299–303.

90. Saporta L, Yuksel A. Androgenic status in patients with lepromatous leprosy. Brit J Urology 1994; 74(2): 221–224.

91. Garg R, Agarwal JK, Singh G, et al. Hormone profile in leprosy. Indian J Leprosy 1989; 61(4):428–431.

92. Levis WR, Lanza AP, Swersie S, et al. Testicular dysfunction in leprosy: relationships of FSH, LH and testosterone to disease classification, activity and duration. Leprosy Rev 1989; 60:94–101.

93. Kannan V, Vijaya G. Endocrine testicular functions in leprosy. Horm Metab Res 1984; 16(3):146–150.

94. Dass J, Murugesan K, Laumas KR, et al. Androgenic status of lepromatous leprosy patients with gynecomastia. Int J Lepr Other Mycobact Dis 1976; 44(4): 469–474.

95. Grabstald H, Swann LL. Genitourinary lesions in leprosy with special reference to atrophy of testes. JAMA 1952; 119(14):1287–1291.

96. Ishikawa S, Mizushima M, Furuta M, et al. Leydig cell hyperplasia and the maintenance of bone volume: bone histomorphometry and testicular histopathology in 29 male leprosy autopsy cases. Int J Lepr Other Mycobact Dis 2000; 68(3):258–266.

97. Sultan Sheriff D. Endocrine profile and seminal plasma composition in Hansen's disease. Transactions Royal Soc Tropical Med Hygiene 1984; 78(3):311–313.

98. Johansson A, Henriksson A, Olofsson BO, et al. Adrenal steroid dysregulation in dystrophia myotonica. J Intern Med 1999; 245(4):345–351.

99. Mastrogiacoma I, Bonanni G, Menegazzo E, et al. Clinical and hormonal aspects of male hypogonadism in myotonic dystrophy. Ital J Neurol Sci 1996; 17(1): 59–65.

100. Marinkovic Z, Prelevic G, Wurzburger M, et al. Gonadal dysfunction in patients with myotonic dystrophy. Exp Clin Endocrinol 1990; 96(1):37–44.

101. Sagel J, Distiller LA, Morley JE, et al. Myotonia dystrophica: studies on gonadal dysfunction using luteinizing hormone-releasing hormone. J Clin Endocrinol Metab 1975; 40:1110–1113.

102. Morley JE, Melmed S. Gonadal dysfunction in systemic disorders. Metabolism 1979; 28(10):1051–1073.

103. Drucker WD, Rowland LP, Sterling K, et al. On the function of the endocrine glands in myotonic muscular dystrophy. Am J Med 1961; 31:941–950.

104. Febres F, Scaglia H, Lisker R, et al. Hypothalamic-pituitary-gonadal function in patients with myotonic dystrophy. J Clin Endocrinol Metab 1975; 41(5): 833–839.

105. Takeda R, Ueda M. Pituitary-gonadal function in male patients with myotonic dystrophy. Serum luteinizing hormone, follicle stimulating hormone and testosterone levels and histological damage of the testis. Acta Endocrinol 1977; 84(2):382–389.

106. Heymsfield SB, Bethel RA, Rudman D. Hyper-responsiveness of patients with clinical and premyopathic myotonic dystrophy to human growth hormone. J Clin Endocrinol Metab 1977; 45:147–158.

107. Griggs RC, Pandya S, Florence JM, et al. Randomized controlled trial of testosterone in myotonic dystrophy. Neurology 1989; 39(2 Pt 1):219–222.

108. Bauman WA, Spungen AM. Metabolic changes in persons after spinal cord injury. Phys Med Rehab Clinic NA 2000; 11:109–140.

109. Guttman C. Spinal Cord Injuries. Blackwell Scientific: Oxford, 1973:456.

110. Cooper IS, Horn TI. Gynecomastia in paraplegic males. J Clin Endocrinol Metab 1949; 9:457–461.

111. Munro D, Horne HW, Pauli DP. The effect of injury to the spinal cord and cauda equina on the sexual potency of men. New Engl J Med 1948; 239:903–911.

112. Copper IS, Rynearson EH, MacCarty CS, et al. Metabolic consequences of spinal cord injury. J Clin Endocrinol Metab 1950; 10(8):858–870.

113. Morley JE, Distiller LA, Lissoos I, et al. Testicular function in patients with spinal cord damage. Hormone Metabolic Res 1979; 11(12):679–682.

114. Perkash I, Martin DE, Warner H, et al. Reproductive biology of paraplegics: results of semen collection, testicular biopsy and serum hormone evaluation. J Urology 1985; 134(2):284–288.

115. Bors E, Engle E, Rosenquist R. Fertility in paraplegic males; a preliminary report of endocrine studies. J Clin Endocrinol Metab 1950; 10(4):381–398.

116. Cortes-Gallegos V, Castaneda G, Alonso R, et al. Diurnal variations of pituitary and testicular hormones in paraplegic men. Arch Androl 1982; 8(3):221–226.

117. Naftchi NE, Viau AT, Sell GH, et al. Pituitary-testicular axis dysfunction in spinal cord injury. Arch Phys Med Rehab 1980; 61(9):402–405.

118. Claus-Walker J, Scurry M, Carter RE, et al. Steady state hormonal secretion in traumatic quadriplegia. J Clin Endocrinol Metab 1977; 44(3):530–535.

119. Naftchi NE. Alterations of neuroendocrine functions in spinal cord injury. Peptides 1985; 6(suppl 1): 85–94.

120. Hayes PJ, Krishnan KR, Diver MJ, et al. Testicular endocrine function in paraplegic men. Clin Endocrinol 1979; 11(5):549–552.

121. Finsen V, Indredavik B, Fougner KJ. Bone mineral and hormone status in paraplegics. Paraplegia 1992; 30(5): 343–347.

122. Nance PW, Shears AH, Givner ML, et al. Gonadal regulation in men with flaccid paraplegia. Arch Phys Med Rehab 1985; 66(11):757–759.

123. Young RJ, Strachan RK, Seth J, et al. Is testicular endocrine function abnormal in young men with spinal cord injuries? Clin Endocrinol 1982; 17(3):303–306.

124. Hoffman WH, Kovacs KT, Gala RR, et al. Macroorchidism and testicular fibrosis associated with autoimmune thyroiditis. J Endocrinol Invest 1991; 14(7):609–616.

125. Smith BR, Furmaniak J. Adrenal and gonadal autoimmune diseases. J Clin Endocrinol Metab 1995; 80(5): 1502–1505.

126. Turkington RV, Lebowitz HE. Extra-adrenal endocrine deficiencies in Addison's disease. Am J Med 1967; 43:499–507.

127. Tsatsoulis A, Shalet SM. Antisperm antibodies in the polyglandular autoimmune (PGS) syndrome Type I: response to cyclical steroid therapy. Clin Endocrinol (Oxf) 1991; 35(4):299–303.

128. Intragumtornchai T, Phanthumchinda K, Lerdlum S, et al. POEMS syndrome: a case with proliferative vasculopathy and a review of cases Thailand. J Med Assoc Thai 1993; 76(10):585–590.

129. Harvey JN, Barnett D. Endocrine dysfunction in Kearns-Sayre syndrome. Clin Endocrinol 1992; 37(1):97–103.

130. Fialkow PJ, Thuline HC, Hecht F, et al. Familial predisposition to thyroid disease in Down's syndrome: controlled immunoclinical studies. Am J Hum Genet 1971; 23(1):67–86.

131. Aversa A, Palleschi S, Cruccu G, et al. Rapid decline of fertility in a case of adrenoleukodystrophy. Hum Reprod 1998; 13(9):2474–2479.

132. Ashkar FS, Smoak WM, Gilson AJ, et al. Gynecomastia and mastoplasia in Graves' disease. Metab 1970; 19(11): 946–951.

133. Becher KL, Winnacker JL, Matthews MT, et al. Gynecomastia and hyperthyroidism: an endocrine

and histological investigation. J Clin Endocrinol Metab 1968; 28(2):277–285.

134. Chopra IJ. Gonadal steroids and gonadotropins in hyperthyroidism. Med Clin North Am 1975; 59(5): 1109–1121.

135. Chopra IJ, Abraham GE, Chopra U, et al. Alterations in circulating estradiol-17 in male patients with Graves' disease. New Engl J Med 1972; 286(3): 124–129.

136. Chopra IJ, Tulchinsky D. Status of estrogen-androgen balance in hyperthyroid men with Graves' disease. J Clin Endocrinol Metab 1974; 38(2):269–277.

137. Hudson RW, Edwards AL. Testicular function in hyperthyroidism. J Androl 1992; 13(2):117–124.

138. Ridgway EC, Longcope C, Maloof F. Metabolic clearance and blood production rates of estradiol in hyperthyroidism. J Clin Endocrinol Metab 1975; 41(3): 491–497.

139. Southren AL, Olivo J, Gordon GG, et al. The conversion of androgens to estrogens in hyperthyroidism. J Clin Endocrinol Metab 1974; 38(2):207–214.

140. Mowszowicz I, Dray F. Taux plasmatique de la production de la testosterone dans la thyrotoxicose masculine. Ann Biol Clin (Paris) 1967; 25(7):879–888.

141. Ruder H, Corval P, Mahoudeau JA, et al. Effects of induced hyperthyroidism on steroid metabolism in man. J Clin Endocrinol Metab 1971; 33(3):382–387.

142. Zahringer S, Tomova A, vonWerder KI, et al. The influence of hyperthyroidism on the hypothalamic-pituitary-gonadal axis. Exp Clin Endocrinol Diabetes 2000; 108(4):282–289.

143. Ford HC, Cooke RR, Keightley EA, et al. Serum levels of free and bound testosterone in hyperthyroidism. Clin Endocrinol 1992; 36(2):187–192.

144. Velazquez EM, Arata GB. Effects of thyroid status on pituitary gonadotropin and testicular reserve in men. Arch Androl 1997; 38(1):85–92.

145. Foldes J, Banos C, Feher T, et al. Functional relationships of the hypothalamic-pituitary-testicular system in Graves' disease. Acta Med Acad Sci Hung 1982; 39(3–4):109–116.

146. Jaya Kumar B, Khurana ML, Ammini AC, et al. Reproductive endocrine functions in men with primary hypothyroidism: effect of thyroxine replacement. Hormone Res 1990; 34(5–6):215–218.

147. Rojdmark S, Berg A, Kallner G. Hypothalamic-pituitary-testicular axis in patients with hyperthyroidism. Hormone Res 1988; 29(5–6):185–190.

148. Yoshida K, Kiso Y, Watanabe TK, et al. Erythrocyte zinc in hyperthyroidism: reflection of integrated thyroid hormone levels over the previous few months. Metab Clin Exp 1990; 39(2):182–186.

149. Huff TA, Lebovitz HE. Dynamics of insulin secretion in myotonic dystrophy. J Clin Endocrinol Metab 1968; 28(7):992–998.

150. Hellman L, Bradlow HL, Zumoff B. Recent advances in human steroid metabolism. Adv Clin Chem 1970; 13:1–35.

151. Donnelly P, White C. Testicular dysfunction in men with primary hypothyroidism; eversal of hypogonadotropic hypogonadism with replacement thyroxine. Clin Endocrinol 2000; 52(2):197–201.

152. Cavaliere H, Abelin N, Medeiros-Neto G. Serum levels of total testosterone and sex hormone binding globulin in hypothyroid patients and normal subjects treated with incremental doses of L-T4 or L-T3. l J Androl 1988; 9(3):215–219.

153. Nieschlag E, Kley HK. Possibility of adrenal-testicular interaction as indicated by plasma androgens in response to HCG in men with normal, suppressed and impaired adrenal function. Horm Metab Res 1975; 7(4):326–330.

154. Cope O, Raker JW. Cushing's disease: the surgical experience in the care of 46 cases. N Engl J Med 1955; 253:119–124.

155. Welbourn RB, Montgomery DA, Kennedy TL. The natural history of treated Cushing's syndrome. Br J Surg 1971; 58:1–16.

156. Milcou SM, Stoica T. Testicular function in Cushing's syndrome. Rev Rome Endocrinol 1966; 3:3–7.

157. Gabrilove JL, Nicolis GL, Shoval AR. The testis in Cushing's syndrome. J Urol 1974; 112:95–99.

158. Gandy HM, Peterson RE. Measurement of testosterone and 17 ketosteroids in plasma by the double isotope dilution-derivative technique. J Clin Endocrinol Metab 1968; 28(7):949–977.

159. Luton JP, Thieblot P, Valcke JC, et al. Reversible gonadotrophin deficiency in male Cushing's disease. J Clin Endocrinol Metab 1977; 45:488–495.

160. Smals AGH, Kloppenborg PWC, Benraad TJ. Plasma testosterone profiles in Cushing's syndrome. J Clin Endocrinol Metab 1977; 45(2):240–245.

161. Evain D, Morera AM, Seaz JM. Recepteurs de glucocorticoides dans le testicule de rat. Ann Endocrinol (Paris) 1976; 37:101–102.

162. Doerr P, Pirke KM. Glucocorticoid-induced suppression of testosterone in men. Proceedings of the Fifth International Congress of Endocrinology, Hamburg, 1976, A452.

163. Morley JE. Sex hormones and diabetes. Diabetes Rev 1998; 6:6–15.

164. Barrett CE, Khaw KT, Yen SS. Endogenous sex hormone levels in older adult men with diabetes mellitus. Am J Epidemiol 1990; 132(5):895–901.

165. Valimaki M, Liewendahl K, Nikkanen P, et al. Hormonal changes in severely uncontrolled type 1 (insulin-dependent) diabetes mellitus. Scand J Clin Lab Invest 1991; 51(4):385–393.

166. Haffner SM, Klein R, Moss SE, et al. Sex hormones and the incidence of severe retinopathy in male subjects with type I diabetes. Opthalmology 1993; 100(12): 1782–1786.

167. Fushimi H, Horie H, Inoue T, et al. Low testosterone levels in diabetic men and animals: a possible role in testicular impotence. Diabetes Res Clin Pract 1989; 6(4):297–301.

168. Geisthovel W, Niedergerke U, Morgner KD, et al. Androgen status of male diabetics: total testosterone before and following stimulation with HCG, free testosterone, and testosterone binding capacity of patients with and without potency disorders. Med Klin 1975; 70(36):1417–1423.

169. Ando S, Rubens R, Rottiers R. Androgen plasma levels in male diabetics. J Endocrinol Invest 1984; 7(1): 21–24.

170. Andersson B, Marin P, Lissner L, et al. Testosterone concentrations in women and men with NIDDM. Diabetes Care 1994; 17(5):405–411.

171. Tibblin G, Adlerberth A, Likndstedt G, et al. The pituitary-gonadal axis and health in elderly men: a study of men born in 1913. Diabetes 1996; 45(11):1605–1609.

172. Murray FT, Wyss HU, Thomas RG, et al. Gonadal dysfunction in diabetic men with organic impotence. J Clin Endocrinol Metab 1987; 65(1):127–135.

173. Arreola F, Paniagua R, Herrera J, et al. Low plasma zinc and androgen in insulin-dependent diabetes mellitus. Arch Androl 1986; 16:151–154.

174. Cailleba A, Moinade S, Gaillard G, et al. Pituitary-gonadal function in male diabetic patients (author's transl). (Article in French). Nouvelle Presse Medicale 1982; 11(18):1375–1377.

175. Distiller LA, Sagel J, Morley JE, et al. Pituitary responsiveness to luteinizing hormone-releasing hormone in insulin-dependent diabetes mellitus. Diabetes 1975; 24(4):378–380.

176. Yamauchi A, Takei I, Kasuga A, et al. Depression of dehydroepiandrosterone in Japanese diabetic men: comparison between non-insulin-dependent diabetes mellitus and impaired glucose tolerance. Eur J Endocrinol 1996; 135(1):101–104.

177. Cohen HN, Paterson KR, Wallace AM, et al. Dissociation of adrenarche and gonadarche in diabetes mellitus. Clin Endocrinol (Oxf) 1984; 20(6): 717–724.

178. Small M, MacRury S, Beastall GH, et al. Oestradiol levels in diabetic men with and without a previous myocardial infarction. Q J Med 1987; 64(243):617–623.

179. Iranmanesh A, Veldhuis JD, Carlsen EC, et al. Attenuated pulsatile release of prolactin in men with insulin-dependent diabetes mellitus. J Clin Endocrinol Metab 1990; 71(1):73–78.

180. Mooradian AD, Morley JE, Billington CJ, et al. Hyperprolactinemia in male diabetics. Postgrad Med J 1985; 61:11–14.

181. Marin P, Arver S. Androgens and abdominal obesity. Baillieres Clin Endocrinol Metab 1998; 12(3):441–451.

182. Defay R, Papoz L, Barny S, et al. Hormonal status and NIDDM in the European and Melanesian populations of New Caldonia: a case-control study. The CALedonia DIAbetes Mellitus (CALDIA) Study Group. Int J Obes Relat Metab Disord 1998; 22:927–934.

183. Barrett-Connor E. Lower endogenous androgen levels and dyslipidemia in men with non-insulin-dependent diabetes mellitus. Ann Intern Med 1992; 117(10): 807–811.

184. Ebeling P, Stenman UH, Seppala M, et al. Androgens and insulin resistance in type 1 diabetic men. Clin Endocrinol 1995; 43(5):601–607.

185. Nestler JE, Jakubowicz DJ, Falcon A, et al. Insulin stimulates testosterone biosynthesis by human thecal cells from women with polycystic ovary syndrome by activating its own receptor and using inositolglycan mediators as the signal transduction system. J Clin Endocrinol Metab 1998; 83(6):2001–2005.

186. Perry HM III, Morley JE, Horowitz M, et al. Body composition and age in African-American and Caucasian women: relationship to plasma leptin levels. Metabolism 1997; 46(12):1399–1405.

187. Rosenbaum M, Nicolson M, Hirsch J, et al. Effects of gender, body composition, and menopause on plasma concentrations of leptin. J Clin Endocrinol Metab 1996; 81(9):3424–3427.

188. Baumgartner RN, Waters DL, Morley JE, et al. Age-related changes in sex hormones affect the sex difference in serum leptin independently of changes in body fat. Metab Clin Exp 1999; 48(3):378–384.

189. Sih R, Morley JE, Kaiser FE, et al. Testosterone replacement in older hypogonadal men: a 12-month randomized controlled trial. J Clin Endocrinol Metab 1997; 82(6):1661–1667.

190. Jockenhovel F, Blum WF, Vogel E, et al. Testosterone substitution normalizes elevated serum leptin levels in hypogonadal men. J Clin Endocrinol Metab 1997; 82(8):2510–2513.

191. Stellato RK, Feldman HA, Hamdy O, et al. Testosterone, sex hormone-binding globulin, and the development of type 2 diabetes in middle-aged men: prospective results from the Massachusetts male aging study. Diabetes Care 2000; 23(4):490–494.

192. Grunstein RR, Handelsman DJ, Lawrence SJ, et al. Neuroendocrine dysfunction in sleep apnea: reversal by continuous positive airways pressure therapy. J Clin Endocrinol Metab 1989; 68(2):352–358.

193. Santamaria JD, Prior JC, Fleetham JA. Reversible reproductive dysfunction in men with obstructive sleep apnoea. Clin Endocrinol 1988; 28:461–470.

194. Cistulli PA, Grunstein RR, Sullivan CE. Effect of testosterone administration on upper airway collapsibility during sleep. Am J Respir Crit Care Med 1994; 149(2): 531–532.

195. Matsumoto AM, Sandblom RE, Schoene RB, et al. Testosterone replacement in hypogonadal men: effects on obstructive sleep apnoea, respiratory drives, and sleep. Clin Endocrinol 1985; 22(6):713–721.

196. Stewart DA, Grunstein RR, Berthon-Jones M, et al. Androgen blockade does not affect sleep-disordered breathing or chemosensitivity in men with obstructive sleep apnea. Am Rev Respir Dis 1992; 146(6): 1389–1393.

197. Snyder PJ, Peachey H, Hannoush P, et al. Effect of testosterone treatment 203.on bone mineral density in men over 65 years of age. J Clin Endocrinol Metab 1999; 84(6):1966–1972.

198. Semple PD, Watson WS, Beastall GH, et al. Diet, absorption, and hormone studies in relation to body weight in obstructive airways disease. Thorax 1979; 34(6):783–788.

199. Semple PD, Beastall GH, Watson WS, et al. Serum testosterone depression associated with hypoxia in respiratory failure. Clin Sci 1980; 58(1):105–106.

200. Fletcher EC, Martin RJ. Sexual dysfunction and erectile impotence in chronic obstructive pulmonary disease. Chest 1982; 81(4):413–421.

201. MacAdams MR, White RH, Chipps BE. Reduction of serum testosterone levels during chronic glucocorticoid therapy. Ann Int Med 1986; 104(5):648–651.

202. Morrison D, Capewell S, Reynolds SP, et al. Testosterone levels during systemic and inhaled corticosteroid therapy. Resp Med 1994; 88(9):659–663.

203. Kamischke A, Kemper DE, Castel MA, et al. Testosterone levels in men with chronic obstructive pulmonary disease with or without glucocorticoid therapy. Europ Resp J 1998; 11(1):41–45.

204. Aasebo U, Gyltnes A, Bremnes RM, et al. Reversal of sexual impotence in male patients with chronic obstructive pulmonary disease and hypoxemia with long-term oxygen therapy. J Steroid Biochem Mol Biol 1993; 46(6):799–803.

205. Banks WA, Cooper JA. Hypoxia and hypercarbia of chronic lung disease: minimal effects on anterior pituitary function. South Med J 1990; 83(3):290–293.

206. Bratel T, Wennlund A, Carlstrom K. Impact of hypoxaemia on neuroendocrine function and catecholamine secretion in chronic obstructive pulmonary disease (COPD). Effects of long-term oxygen treatment. Resp Med 2000; 94(12):1221–1228.

207. Gow SM, Seth J, Beckett GJ, et al. Thyroid function and endocrine abnormalities in elderly patients with severe chronic obstructive lung disease. Thorax 1987; 42(7): 520–525.

208. Semple PD, Beastall GH, Watson WS, et al. Hypothalamic-pituitary dysfunction in respiratory hypoxia. Thorax 1981; 36(8):605–609.

209. Gordon D, Beastall GH, Thomson, et al. Androgenic status and sexual function in males with rheumatoid arthritis and ankylosing spondylitis. Q J Med 1986; 60(231):671–679.

210. Spector TD, Perry LA, Tubb G, et al. Low free testosterone levels in rheumatoid arthritis. Ann Rheumatic Dis 1988; 47(1):65–68.

211. Cutolo M, Balleari E, Giusti M, et al. Sex hormone status of male patients with rheumatoid arthritis: evidence of low serum concentrations of testosterone at baseline and after human chorionic gonadotropin stimulation. Arthritis Rheum 1988; 31(10): 1314–1317.

212. Gordon D, Beastall GH, Thomson JA, et al. Prolonged hypogonadism in male patients with rheumatoid arthritis during flares in disease activity. Br J Rheumatol 1998; 27(6):440–444.

213. Spector TD, Ollier W, Perry LA, et al. Free and serum testosterone levels in 276 males: a comparative study of rheumatoid arthritis, ankylosing spondylitis and healthy controls. Clin Rheumatol 1989; 8(1):37–41.

214. Ollier W, Spector T, Silman A, et al. Are certain HLA haplotypes responsible for low testosterone levels in males? Dis Markers 1989; 7(3):139–143.

215. Stafford L, Bleasel J, Giles A, et al. Androgen deficiency and bone mineral density in men with rheumatoid arthritis. J Rheumatol 2000; 27:2786–2790.

216. Martens HF, Sheets PK, Tenover JS, et al. Decreased testosterone levels in men with rheumatoid arthritis: effect of low dose prednisone therapy. J Rheumatol 1994; 21:1427–1431.

217. Mateo L, Nolla JM, Bonnin MR, et al. Sex hormones status and bone mineral density in men with rheumatoid arthritis. J Rheumatol 1995; 22(8): 1455–1460.

218. Mateo L, Nolla JM, Bonnin MR, et al. High serum prolactin levels in men with rheumatoid arthritis. J Rheumatol 1998; 25:2077–2082.

219. Cutolo M, Balleari E, Giusti M, et al. Androgen replacement therapy in male patients with rheumatoid arthritis. Arthritis Rheum 1991; 34(1):1–5.

220. Hall GM, Larbre JP, Spector TD, et al. A randomized trial of testosterone therapy in males with rheumatoid arthritis. Br J Rheumatol 1996; 35(6):568–573.

20

The Effects of Chemotherapy and Radiotherapy on Testicular Function

Simon J. Howell and Steve M. Shalet

Department of Endocrinology, Christie Hospital NHS Trust, Withington, Manchester, U.K.

☐ INTRODUCTION

It has been recognized for many years that testicular dysfunction is relatively common following treatment with cytotoxic chemotherapy and radiotherapy. The number of malignancies that are potentially treatable has increased over the last few decades. This, coupled with the improving long-term survival rates of many cancers, has meant that the number of surviving patients who have received cytotoxic therapy or radiotherapy is growing rapidly, and cancer treatment is becoming an increasingly common cause of acquired testicular dysfunction.

Germinal epithelial damage resulting in oligo- or azoospermia has long been a recognized consequence of certain chemotherapeutic agents and radiotherapy, and there is also some evidence of Leydig cell dysfunction following treatment. Testicular damage is drug specific and dose related (1–4). The chance of recovery of spermatogenesis following cytotoxic insult and also the extent and speed of recovery are related to the agent used and the dose received. It has also been suggested that the germinal epithelium of the adult testis is more susceptible to damage than that of the prepubertal testis (5), implying that patient age or maturation of the testis at the time of cytotoxic insult may influence the degree of damage. Radiotherapy-induced testicular damage is similarly dose dependent, with speed of onset, chance of reversal, and time to recovery of spermatogenesis all related to the testicular dose of irradiation (6). In contrast, however, the little data available regarding the influence of pubertal status suggest that, unlike the germinal epithelium, Leydig cell function may be more prone to damage from irradiation in prepubertal life compared with in adulthood (7).

☐ CHEMOTHERAPY

Spitz (8) first described testicular damage from cytotoxic drugs in humans in 1948, when he found azoospermia in 27 of 30 men at autopsy following treatment with nitrogen mustard. Many other drugs, particularly alkylating agents, have subsequently been shown to be gonadotoxic, and the agents most commonly implicated are listed in Table 1. The germinal epithelium is far more sensitive to the effects of cytotoxic drugs than the Leydig cells, and whilst complete azoospermia is not uncommon following therapy, evidence of Leydig cell dysfunction is usually limited to raised luteinizing hormone (LH) levels with normal or low-normal testosterone levels. Most research has focused on either cyclophosphamide given alone for immunologically mediated disease or combination chemotherapy used in the treatment of hematological malignancies and testicular cancer.

Cyclophosphamide Alone

Rivkees and Crawford (5) published an analysis of 30 studies that examined gonadal function after various chemotherapy regimens, which included a total of 116 males who had been treated with cyclophosphamide alone. Gonadal function and/or histology were assessed by a number of different methods: semen analysis, basal LH and follicle-stimulating hormone (FSH) levels, and testicular biopsy being the most commonly used. Of the 116 patients, 52 (45%) had evidence of testicular dysfunction following treatment. The incidence of gonadal dysfunction correlated with the total dose of cyclophosphamide, occurring in over 80% of postpubertal patients who received more than 300 mg/kg.

Treatment of Hematological Malignancy

The impact on testicular function of chemotherapy used in the treatment of lymphomas, especially Hodgkin's disease (HD), has been widely reported. Several studies have reported azoospermia with raised FSH levels in over 90% of men following cyclical chemotherapy with mustine, vinblastine, procarbazine, and prednisolone (MVPP) (13,14).

In an attempt to reduce the gonadotoxic effect of MVPP by halving the alkylating drug and reducing the procarbazine dose, a hybrid of chlorambucil, vinblastine, prednisolone, procarbazine, doxorubicin, vincristine, and etoposide (ChlVPP/EVA) has been used. In a direct comparison with MVPP, however, hybrid chemotherapy was found to have the same effect on gonadal function (15). An alternative regime, however,

Table 1 Gonadotoxic Drugs

Group	Definite gonadotoxicity
Alkylating agents	Cyclophosphamide (5)
	Chlorambucil
	Mustine
	Melphalan
	Busulfan (9)
	Carmustine (10)
	Lomustine (10)
Antimetabolites	Cytarabine
Vinca alkaloids	Vinblastine (11)
Others	Procarbazine
	Cisplatin (12)

consisting of adriamycin, bleomycin, vinblastine, and dacarbazine (ABVD) has been shown to be less gonadotoxic. Viviani et al. (16) studied a total of 53 men treated with combination chemotherapy for HD. Of 29 men treated with MOPP (similar to MVPP but with vinblastine replaced by vincristine), 28 were azoospermic at a median time of six months after the completion of therapy. Of these, 21 were retested 18 to 58 months after the initial analysis, and in only three was any recovery of spermatogenesis seen. The impact of ABVD was, however, considerably less, with a normal sperm count in 11 of 24 patients and oligospermia in a further five. Furthermore, full recovery of spermatogenesis occurred within 18 months of the first evaluation in all 13 men in whom the sperm count was repeated.

Other chemotherapy regimens utilized for the treatment of lymphomas have also been investigated. The effect on adult testicular function has been assessed in patients treated for HD during childhood with ChlVPP. Mackie et al. (17) found testicular dysfunction, as indicated by raised gonadotrophin levels, in a significant proportion of a cohort of 46 male patients treated with ChlVPP, with 89% and 24% having raised FSH and LH levels, respectively. The use of cyclophosphamide, vincristine, procarbazine, and prednisolone (COPP), which includes the gonadotoxic agent cyclophosphamide in addition to procarbazine, is associated with even more marked gonadal dysfunction. Charak et al. (18) found azoospermia in all 92 patients following treatment with six or more cycles of COPP, along with significant increases in gonadotrophin levels compared with pretreatment values. Median follow-up in this study was six years, with 17% of patients treated more than 10 years previously, suggesting that germinal epithelial failure is likely to be permanent.

In addition to effects on the germinal epithelium, there is also some evidence of Leydig cell dysfunction following chemotherapy for lymphomas. Howell et al. (19) measured testosterone and LH levels in 135 men treated with either MVPP or ChlVPP/EVA hybrid. They demonstrated a significantly higher LH level in patients compared with a cohort of age-matched controls (mean LH 7.8 IU/L vs. 4.1 IU/L). This group suggested that this raised LH level indicated a reduction in hypothalamopituitary negative feedback consequent

upon a small reduction in testosterone production. This may still result in testosterone levels within the cross-sectional normal range, and thus mild Leydig cell dysfunction was defined as a raised LH in the presence of a testosterone level in the lower half of the normal range or frankly subnormal. This combination was found in 44 men (31%) following chemotherapy, with a further 10 (7%) having a raised LH level alone. This suggests that a significant proportion of men treated with cytotoxic chemotherapy have biochemical abnormalities, suggesting mild testosterone deficiency; the clinical significance of this is discussed later.

Chemotherapy regimens used for the treatment of non-Hodgkin's lymphoma (NHL) are generally less gonadotoxic than those used for HD. Pryzant et al. (1) reported on 71 patients treated with cyclophosphamide, doxorubicin, vincristine, and prednisolone (CHOP)–based chemotherapy. All men were rendered azoospermic during treatment, but by five years, 67% had recovered to normospermic levels, with a further 5% oligospermic. The reduced incidence of permanent infertility in men treated for NHL compared with HD patients is probably related to the absence of procarbazine in the standard regimens used for NHL (20), although the reduction in the dose of alkylating agents may also be important. The absence of procarbazine and alkylating drugs is also the likely explanation for the reduced toxicity of ABVD reported by Viviani et al. (16). Other regimens not containing procarbazine, which have been used for NHL, have also been shown to be less gonadotoxic. Vincristine, doxorubicin, prednisolone, etoposide, cyclophosphamide, and bleomycin (VAPEC-B) (21), vinblastine, doxorubicin, prednisolone, vincristine, cyclophosphamide, and bleomycin (VACOP-B) (22), MACOP-B (mustine in place of vinblastine) (22), and VEEP (vincristine, etoposide, epirubicin, and prednisolone) (23) have all been associated with normal posttreatment fertility in the vast majority of men.

Testicular function following high-dose chemotherapy used as preparation for bone marrow transplantation has also been studied. Sanders et al. (9) reported on 155 men treated with cyclophosphamide (200 mg/kg) or busulphan and cyclophosphamide (busulphan 16 mg/kg and cyclophosphamide 200 mg/kg). After an average of two to three years posttransplant, 67 of 109 who received cyclophosphamide (61%), but only 8 of 46 (17%) patients treated with busulphan and cyclophosphamide, had recovery of testicular function defined by normal LH, FSH, and testosterone levels with evidence of sperm production. The only prospective study to examine testicular function following high-dose treatment reported on 13 men who received either BEAM (BCNU, etoposide, Ara-C, and melphalan) ($n = 11$) or melphalan and single-fraction total body irradiation ($n = 2$) (24). All had previously received multiagent chemotherapy, and four had abnormal semen parameters before transplantation. All patients were azoospermic two to three months posttransplantation, which is associated with raised FSH levels. LH levels increased and testosterone levels decreased after transplantation, indicating that Leydig cell damage was apparent in addition to germ-cell failure.

These findings were also confirmed by Howell et al. (19), who studied 68 patients treated with high-dose chemotherapy (either cyclophosphamide, BCNU and etoposide, busulphan and cyclophosphamide or BCNU, etoposide, doxorubicin, and melphalan) as conditioning for bone marrow transplant. They demonstrated a raised FSH in 60 patients (88%) and a raised LH level in 47 men (69%), 22 of whom (32%) also had a testosterone level in the lower half of the normal range or frankly subnormal.

Treatment for Testicular Cancer

The other group of patients in whom the effects of chemotherapy on testicular function have been widely investigated is those with testicular cancer (25–28). To attempt to delineate which abnormalities are the results of cytotoxic chemotherapy, several of these studies also examined pretreatment testicular function or have compared chemotherapy-treated patients with those who underwent orchiectomy alone. Lampe et al. (27) analyzed data concerning 170 patients with testicular germ cell cancers who underwent treatment with either cisplatin- or carboplatin-based chemotherapy. Of them, 40 (24%) were azoospermic prior to treatment, with a further 41 (24%) oligospermic. A median of 30 months after the completion of chemotherapy, only 64% of those who were normospermic before therapy remained normospermic, while 54 (32%) of the total cohort were azoospermic and 43 (25%) oligospermic. The probability of recovery to a normal sperm count was found to be higher for those men with a normal pretreatment sperm count, those who received carboplatin- rather than cisplatin-based therapy, and in those treated with less than five cycles of chemotherapy. Recovery continued for more than two years, with the calculated chance of spermatogenesis at two years being 48%, and at five years, 80%. Several authors have compared testicular function in patients following chemotherapy with that of patients treated with orchiectomy alone (25,26,28). All have demonstrated greater testicular dysfunction in the cytotoxic-treated groups, with evidence of germinal epithelial damage indicated by raised FSH levels and/or reduced sperm counts. In addition, mild Leydig cell dysfunction, as indicated by raised LH levels in the presence of a normal testosterone level, was found in 59% to 75% of men following chemotherapy, compared with 6% to 45% in those following orchiectomy alone.

Other Malignancies

Similar results have been demonstrated in patients treated with cisplatin-based chemotherapy for osteosarcoma (29) and lung cancer (30). The majority of patients treated with cytotoxic chemotherapy for leukemia, however, do not have persistent gonadal dysfunction. Wallace et al. (31) found long-term germinal epithelial dysfunction in only 6 out of 36 (17%) patients treated during childhood for acute lymphocytic leukemia, although the period of follow-up in this study was considerable and the majority of patients had evidence of germinal epithelial damage on testicular biopsy immediately after chemotherapy (which included cyclophosphamide and cytosine arabinoside) at a median time of 10.7 years earlier.

□ RADIOTHERAPY

The testis is one of the most radiosensitive tissues, with even very low doses of radiation causing significant impairment of function. Damage may be caused during direct irradiation of the testis or, more commonly, from scattered radiation during treatment directed at adjacent tissues.

Single-Dose Irradiation

The effects of relatively low-dose, single-fraction irradiation on spermatogenesis in healthy fertile men have been well documented (6) and are illustrated in Figure 1. The more immature cells are more radiosensitive, with doses as low as 0.1 Gy causing morphological and quantitative changes to spermatogonia. Doses of 2 to 3 Gy result in overt damage to spermatocytes, leading to a reduction in spermatid numbers. At doses of 4 to 6 Gy, numbers of spermatozoa are significantly decreased, implying damage to spermatids. The decline in sperm count following damage to more immature cells, with doses of up to 3 Gy, takes 60 to 70 days, with doses above 0.8 Gy resulting in azoospermia and doses below 0.8 Gy giving rise to oligospermia. A much faster fall in sperm concentration occurs following doses of 4 Gy and above due to damage to spermatids.

Recovery of spermatogenesis takes place from surviving stem cells (type A spermatogonia) and is dependent on the dose of radiation. Complete recovery, as indicated by a return to preirradiation sperm concentrations and germinal cell numbers, takes place within 9 to 18 months for doses of 1 Gy or less, 30 months for doses of 2 to 3 Gy, and five years or more for doses of 4 Gy and above.

Scattered Irradiation

Animal data suggest that fractionation of radiotherapy increases its gonadal toxicity, and the evidence suggests that this is also the case in humans. Speiser et al. (32) studied 10 patients who received a testicular dose of radiation of 1.2 to 3 Gy in 14 to 26 fractions during inverted Y-inguinal field irradiation for HD. All patients were azoospermic following treatment, and recovery was not seen in a single patient despite follow-up of over 15 months in four patients and up to 40 months in one. An update of these data published in 1994 (33) revealed no recovery of spermatogenesis in patients receiving doses of 1.4 to 2.6 Gy after 17 to 43 months of follow-up, but a return of fertility occurred

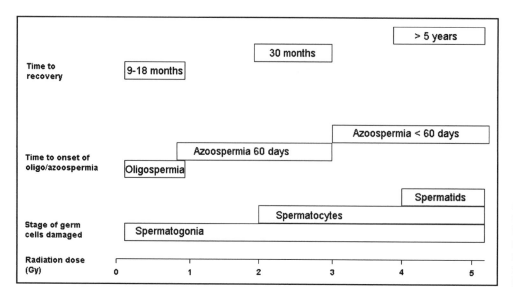

Figure 1 Impairment of spermatogenesis following single-dose irradiation: the effect of radiation dose on stage of germ-cell damage and time to onset and recovery from germ-cell damage. Source: From Ref. 6.

in the two patients with testicular radiation doses of 1.2 Gy, suggesting that this may represent a threshold for permanent testicular damage. Hahn et al. (34) carried out serial semen analysis on 11 cancer patients who had received large pelvic field irradiation or interstitial ^{125}I seeds implanted in the prostate gland. The dose of radiation to the testis was 1.18 to 2.28 Gy delivered in 24 to 34 fractions. All patients became azoospermic and recovery to oligospermia (three men) or normospermia (two men) was only seen in five patients. The other six remained azoospermic during a follow-up period of 35 to 107 weeks.

Lower doses of radiation to the testes are, however, associated with better recovery rates for spermatogenesis. Centola et al. (33) reported a return of spermatogenesis in all eight patients who received radiation doses of 0.28 to 0.9 Gy for testicular seminoma, with four out of five reviewed at 12 months having normal sperm counts. Kinsella et al. (35) published data concerning 17 patients who had received low-dose, scattered irradiation during treatment of HD. Testicular doses of less than 0.2 Gy had no significant effect on FSH levels or sperm counts, while doses between 0.2 and 0.7 Gy caused a transient dose-dependent increase in FSH and reduction in sperm concentration, with a return to normal values within 12 to 24 months.

Leydig Cell Function

Leydig cells are more resistant to damage from radiotherapy than the germinal epithelium. Significant rises in LH have been demonstrated with single-dose radiation doses of above 0.75 Gy (6) and fractionated doses of above 2 Gy (36). No change in testosterone level, however, was seen at these doses, and LH values showed a gradual return to normal levels over 30 months. Higher testicular radiation doses do, however, result in more marked Leydig cell insufficiency. Giwercman et al. (37) studied 20 men previously treated with unilateral orchiectomy for testicular

cancer, who received direct testicular irradiation at a dose of 20 Gy in 10 fractions for carcinoma in situ in the remaining testis. A significant increase in mean LH levels was observed within the first three months (10.4–15.6 IU/L), with a decrease in mean serum testosterone level (13.3 nmol/L). Similar results were observed by Shalet et al. (7) in adults treated with high-dose (30 Gy) testicular irradiation following unilateral orchiectomy. Serum testosterone levels were significantly reduced (12.5 nmol/L vs. 16.0 nmol/L), and LH levels significantly increased (16 IU/L vs. 6 IU/L) compared with a control group who had undergone unilateral orchiectomy without subsequent radiotherapy. In addition, more marked abnormalities were observed in a group of five adult men treated with the same testicular dose of irradiation during childhood. Median LH level was greater than 32 IU/L, median testosterone level less than 2.5 nmol/L, and there was no response to a human chorionic gonadotrophin stimulation test, suggesting that the prepubertal testis is much more vulnerable to radiation-induced Leydig cell damage.

Clinical Impact of Leydig Cell Dysfunction

A significant proportion of men have evidence of impairment of Leydig cell function following high-dose chemotherapy, procarbazine-containing chemotherapy, or radiation involving the testis. The biochemical abnormalities are usually mild and consist of a raised LH level associated with a low/normal testosterone level. The deleterious impact of overt testosterone deficiency and the clear, subsequent benefits of androgen replacement in such patients on bone density, body composition, and quality of life have been well demonstrated. There are few data, however, concerning the impact of milder forms of testosterone deficiency.

Howell et al. (19) investigated a cohort of men treated with MVPP, ChlVPP/EVA hybrid, or high-dose chemotherapy for a variety of malignancies. They identified a cohort of 35 men with biochemical evidence of mild Leydig cell insufficiency as defined by a raised LH level and a testosterone level in the lower half of the normal range or frankly subnormal. Significantly reduced bone mineral density at the hip as well as some evidence of altered body composition, reduced sexual activity, and alterations in mood were demonstrated in these men when compared with a similarly treated cohort with normal hormone levels (38,39). The LH-insufficient men were then enrolled into a 12-month randomized, single-blind, placebo-controlled trial of testosterone replacement (40). During the 12-month study period, however, there were no significant improvements in bone density, body composition, sexual function, energy levels, or mood in the testosterone-treated group compared with the controls.

Thus, it seems likely that the mild biochemical abnormalities (raised LH, low/normal testosterone) observed in many men following cytotoxic chemotherapy are not of clinical importance in the vast majority of patients and that androgen replacement cannot be routinely indicated for such patients. It remains possible, however, that a minority of men with more marked biochemical abnormalities may benefit from androgen therapy.

☐ GENETIC DAMAGE FOLLOWING CYTOTOXIC TREATMENT

In addition to impairment of steroidogenesis and sperm production, there has been concern that cytotoxic chemotherapy may also result in transmissible genetic damage. Animal studies have demonstrated untoward effects in the offspring of animals treated with cytotoxic agents, but no clear evidence of this has been reported in humans. Increased aneuploid frequency has been observed in human sperm following chemotherapy for HD (41,42), and an increase in chromosomal abnormalities has been demonstrated several years after treatment for testicular cancer (43). Data concerning the outcome of pregnancies, however, have not shown any increase in genetically mediated birth defects, altered sex ratios, or birthweight effects in the offspring of cancer survivors (44)—possibly as a result of selection bias against genetically abnormal sperm. With the available evidence thus far, it is therefore reasonable to conclude that patients treated with cytotoxic chemotherapy who remain fertile are not at increased risk of fathering children with genetic abnormalities.

☐ PROTECTION OF TESTICULAR FUNCTION DURING CANCER TREATMENT

The deleterious effect of chemotherapy and radiotherapy on germinal epithelial function has initiated a search for possible strategies to preserve fertility in men undergoing therapy.

Semen Cryopreservation and Assisted Reproduction

Cryostorage of semen has become standard practice and should be offered to all men before they undergo potentially sterilizing therapy. Improvements in the techniques used to store semen (45) and advances in the field of assisted reproduction, such as intra-cytoplasmic sperm injection (ICSI), have increased the chance of successful pregnancies using cryopreserved sperm. There are, however, some limitations to this method of preserving fertility. Firstly, it is not a feasible option for prepubertal patients. Furthermore, testicular function in adult males with malignant disease is often impaired before treatment (46), resulting in poor sperm quality or difficulty providing semen for storage. Oligospermia is found in one-third to one-half of patients with HD, NHL, and testicular cancer pretreatment and also occurs in men with leukemia and soft-tissue cancer (47). Sperm motility is also impaired in these patients and the process of freezing and thawing semen further reduces the sperm quality. Although successful fertilization may be achieved with only a few viable sperm using ICSI, pregnancy rates using this method are lower with abnormal semen than with normal semen (48). As a result, methods for protecting or enhancing the recovery of normal spermatogenesis following gonadotoxic therapy have been pursued (see Chapters 33 and 38).

Hormonal Manipulation

The belief that prepubertal boys have a lower rate of permanent chemotherapy-induced gonadal damage (5) has led many investigators to propose that suppression of testicular function in adult men (i.e., inducing a prepubertal state) will provide a degree of protection against cytotoxic therapy. Irrespective of the validity of the hypothesis, data derived from animal models have been encouraging, but there is at present no convincing evidence of similar success in humans. Ward et al. (49) demonstrated enhanced recovery of spermatogenesis in procarbazine-treated rats by the administration of the GnRH analogue Zoladex for two weeks before chemotherapy and during chemotherapy. Increased stem-cell survival was evident by 50 days, and at 90 days, sperm count was close to normal values and significantly higher than procarbazine-only–treated rats. Similar protective effects of hormonal treatment have been described following the use of testosterone (50), testosterone and estradiol (51), GnRH and testosterone (52), and GnRH and the antiandrogen flutamide (53,54) following gonadal insult with procarbazine, cyclophosphamide, or radiotherapy. Pogach et al. (52) suggested that testosterone administered after treatment with procarbazine enhanced the recovery of spermatogenesis. More recently, Meistrich and Kangasniemi (55) have confirmed that treatment with either testosterone or Zoladex following irradiation with 3.5 Gy markedly improves the recovery of spermatogenesis, even if treatment is delayed for 10 weeks after irradiation. The same group had previously shown that spermatogenesis did not occur after a similar dose of irradiation despite the presence of type A spermatogonia in the seminiferous tubules (56); they postulated that the role of hormonal treatments in the "protection" of germinal epithelial function may be to enhance the recovery of surviving type A spermatogonia and to facilitate their differentiation to more mature cells rather than to protect them from damage during cytotoxic therapy or radiotherapy. They suggested that a reduction in intratesticular testosterone or one of its metabolites is the mechanism by which hormone therapy stimulates recovery of spermatogenesis (56).

In humans, attempts to reproduce the protective effects seen in animals have been unsuccessful. Several groups have used GnRH analogues, with and without testosterone, to suppress testicular function during MOPP (57) or MVPP (58) chemotherapy for lymphoma, cisplatin-based chemotherapy for teratoma (59), and testicular irradiation for seminoma (60). None has demonstrated any significant protective effect of these therapies in terms of maintenance of spermatogenesis or increasing the rate of recovery; however, none of the studies involved the continuation of gonadal-suppressive therapy for a significant period of time after the completion of chemotherapy or radiotherapy. The most recent animal data suggest that hormonal treatment may enhance recovery of spermatogenesis from surviving stem cells rather than protect them from damage during cytotoxic or radiation insult. Thus, suppression of gonadal function with a GnRH agonist or testosterone for a fixed time after the completion of irradiation or chemotherapy may prove more successful in reducing the impact of these treatments on fertility.

This approach relies on enhancing the recovery of sperm production, and, therefore, a prerequisite for its success is the survival of stem cells during the gonadotoxic insult. There are, however, few data regarding testicular histology after chemotherapy or radiotherapy. Following cisplatin-based chemotherapy and low-dose radiation, spontaneous recovery of spermatogenesis occurs in most patients, although there is often a latent period of azoospermia that may last several years. The eventual recovery of spermatogenesis, however, implies the survival of type A spermatogonia. Following chemotherapy for HD with procarbazine-containing regimens and high-dose radiotherapy, recovery to oligo- or normospermia is much less common. Testicular biopsies taken after standard chemotherapy (MVPP and COPP) for HD have shown complete germinal aplasia with a Sertoli-cell-only pattern (13,18,46,61,62), and this is also the case in men treated with 20 Gy radiotherapy (37). There have been some recent reports of the isolation of mature sperm in the testicular parenchyma of some men with biopsy evidence of Sertoli-cell-only, suggesting that even in this situation there may be small foci of spermatogenesis (63). In addition, recovery of spermatogenesis occurs in a minority of these patients, indicating that some germ cells survive in some

patients; however, the absence of histological evidence of any spermatogenesis at biopsy in many men suggests that all spermatogonia may be eradicated during chemotherapy.

Hormonal manipulation after treatment to enhance the recovery of spermatogenesis is therefore likely to be of most benefit in those patients in whom the testicular insult is less severe, as it is these patients in whom there is significant preservation of type A spermatogonia. The success of this approach in those patients who have undergone more gonadotoxic therapy will depend on whether any stem cells remain. Complete ablation of the germinal epithelium may occur in many men following treatment with procarbazine-based chemotherapy regimens for HD, and this will clearly be irreversible.

Stem-Cell Cryopreservation

Results from recent animal experiments have also indicated another possible method of preserving testicular function during gonadotoxic therapy. In 1994, Brinster and Zimmermann (64) demonstrated that stem cells isolated from a donor mouse could be injected into the seminiferous tubules of a sterile recipient mouse and result in the initiation of spermatogenesis. Later, the same group was able to demonstrate that spermatogenesis can be achieved in previously sterile mice following cryopreservation, with subsequent injection of donor stem cells into the testis. Potentially, therefore, stem cells could be harvested from the human testis before the start of sterilizing therapy, freeze-stored, and reimplanted at a later date, with a subsequent return of spermatogenesis.

A clinical trial testing this hypothesis is currently underway in adults: 16 men have had testicular tissue harvested shortly before commencing treatment with sterilizing chemotherapy for HD or non-Hodgkin's lymphoma. In each case, a 0.5-cm cube of testicular tissue is enzymatically digested to produce a single-cell suspension that, following equilibration in cryo-protectant, is stored in liquid nitrogen (65). Seven men have now successfully completed chemotherapy, and thawed testicular suspension has been reinjected into the donor testis. Semen analysis has demonstrated a return of spermatogenesis in one man at the time of writing; however, this may simply represent spontaneous recovery of spermatogenesis—as is seen in a small proportion of men following treatment—rather than repopulation from cryopreserved stem cells. The lack of greater success may relate to problems in reinjecting the testicular suspension. The seminiferous tubules in adult men are too fibrous to allow direct injection, and therefore the indirect approach of injecting into the rete testes and relying on retrograde flow to fill the tubules was necessary. This may not occur to a sufficient extent to allow repopulation and a return of spermatogenesis. Further studies are currently being undertaken using nondisaggregated testicular tissue and the results are awaited with interest.

□ SUMMARY

Treatments with cytotoxic chemotherapy and radiotherapy are associated with significant gonadal damage in men. Alkylating agents such as cyclophosphamide and procarbazine are the most common agents implicated. The vast majority of men receiving procarbazine-containing regimens for the treatment of lymphomas are rendered permanently infertile. Treatment with ABVD appears to have a significant advantage in terms of testicular function, with a return to normal fertility in the vast majority of patients. Cisplatin-based chemotherapy for testicular cancer results in temporary azoospermia in most men, with a recovery of spermatogenesis in about 50% after two years and 80% after five years. There is also evidence of Leydig-cell impairment in a proportion of these men, although this appears to be of no clinical significance in the majority of patients. The germinal epithelium is very sensitive to radiation-induced damage, with changes to spermatogonia occurring after as little as 0.1 Gy and permanent infertility after fractionated doses of 2 Gy and above.

All men should be counseled regarding the possible effects of treatment on testicular function, and sperm banking should be offered to all patients undergoing potentially sterilizing therapy. Hormonal manipulation to enhance the recovery of spermatogenesis and cryopreservation of testicular tissue are possible future methods of preserving fertility but are as yet unproven. Regular semen analyses should be offered to men following cytotoxic treatment to allow appropriate family planning. Measurement of testosterone and LH levels is appropriate for men with symptoms consistent with testosterone deficiency who have received significant doses of irradiation to the testes, procarbazine-containing chemotherapy, or high-dose chemotherapy. Mild elevations of LH accompanied by testosterone levels within the normal range (the most common abnormality) do not require treatment, but patients with subnormal testosterone levels and markedly elevated LH levels may benefit from androgen replacement.

□ REFERENCES

1. Pryzant RM, Meistrich ML, Wilson G, et al. Long-term reduction in sperm count after chemotherapy with and without radiation therapy for non-Hodgkin's lymphomas. J Clin Oncol 1993; 11(2):239–247.

2. Meistrich ML, Chawla SP, Da Cunha MF, et al. Recovery of sperm production after chemotherapy for osteosarcoma. Cancer 1989; 63(11):2115–2123.

3. da Cunha MF, Meistrich ML, Fuller LM, et al. Recovery of spermatogenesis after treatment for Hodgkin's disease: limiting dose of MOPP chemotherapy. J Clin Oncol 1984; 2(6):571–577.

4. Watson AR, Rance CP, Bain J. Long term effects of cyclophosphamide on testicular function. Br Med J Clin Res Ed 1985; 291(6507):1457–1460.

5. Rivkees SA, Crawford JD. The relationship of gonadal activity and chemotherapy-induced gonadal damage. JAMA 1988; 259(14):2123–2125.

6. Rowley MJ, Leach DR, Warner GA, et al. Effect of graded doses of ionizing radiation on the human testis. Radiat Res 1974; 59(3):665–678.

7. Shalet SM, Tsatsoulis A, Whitehead E, et al. Vulnerability of the human Leydig cell to radiation damage is dependent upon age. J Endocrinol 1989; 120(1): 161–165.

8. Spitz S. The histological effects of nitrogen mustard on human tumours and tissues. Cancer 1948; 1:383–398.

9. Sanders JE, Hawley J, Levy W, et al. Pregnancies following high-dose cyclophosphamide with or without high-dose busulfan or total-body irradiation and bone marrow transplantation. Blood 1996; 87(7): 3045–3052.

10. Clayton PE, Shalet SM, Price DA, et al. Testicular damage after chemotherapy for childhood brain tumors. J Pediatr 1988; 112(6):922–926.

11. Vilar O. Effect of cytostatic drugs on human testicular function. In: Mancini RE, Martini L, ed. Male fertility and sterility. Vol. 5. London: Academic Press. 1974: 423–440.

12. Wallace WH, Shalet SM, Crowne EC, et al. Gonadal dysfunction due to cis-platinum. Med Pediatr Oncol 1989; 17(5):409–413.

13. Chapman RM, Sutcliffe SB, Rees LH, et al. Cyclical combination chemotherapy and gonadal function. Retrospective study in males. Lancet 1979; 1(8111): 285–289.

14. Whitehead E, Shalet SM, Blackledge G, et al. The effects of Hodgkin's disease and combination chemotherapy on gonadal function in the adult male. Cancer 1982; 49(3):418–422.

15. Clark ST, Radford JA, Crowther D, et al. Gonadal function following chemotherapy for Hodgkin's disease: a comparative study of MVPP and a seven-drug hybrid regimen. J Clin Oncol 1995; 13(1): 134–139.

16. Viviani S, Santoro A, Ragni G, et al. Gonadal toxicity after combination chemotherapy for Hodgkin's disease. Comparative results of MOPP vs ABVD. Eur J Cancer Clin Oncol 1985; 21(5):601–605.

17. Mackie EJ, Radford M, Shalet SM. Gonadal function following chemotherapy for childhood Hodgkin's disease. Med Pediatr Oncol 1996; 27(2):74–78.

18. Charak BS, Gupta R, Mandrekar P, et al. Testicular dysfunction after cyclophosphamide-vincristine-procarbazine-prednisolone chemotherapy for advanced Hodgkin's disease. A long-term follow-up study. Cancer 1990; 65(9):1903–1906.

19. Howell SJ, Radford JA, Ryder WDJ, et al. Testicular function after cytotoxic chemotherapy: evidence of Leydig cell insufficiency. J Clin Oncol 1999; 17(5): 1493–1498.

20. Bokemeyer C, Schmoll HJ, van Rhee J, et al. Long-term gonadal toxicity after therapy for Hodgkin's and non-Hodgkin's lymphoma. Ann Hematol 1994; 68(3): 105–110.

21. Radford JA, Clark S, Crowther D, et al. Male fertility after VAPEC-B chemotherapy for Hodgkin's disease and non-Hodgkin's lymphoma. Br J Cancer 1994; 69(2):379–381.

22. Muller U, Stahel RA. Gonadal function after MACOP-B or VACOP-B with or without dose intensification and ABMT in young patients with aggressive non-Hodgkin's lymphoma. Ann Oncol 1993; 4(5):399–402.

23. Hill M, Milan S, Cunningham D, et al. Evaluation of the efficacy of the VEEP regimen in adult Hodgkin's disease with assessment of gonadal and cardiac toxicity. J Clin Oncol 1995; 13(2):387–395.

24. Chatterjee R, Mills W, Katz M, et al. Germ cell failure and Leydig cell insufficiency in post-pubertal males after autologous bone marrow transplantation with BEAM for lymphoma. Bone Marrow Transplant 1994; 13(5):519–522.

25. Hansen SW, Berthelsen JG, von der Maase H. Long-term fertility and Leydig cell function in patients treated for germ cell cancer with cisplatin, vinblastine, and bleomycin versus surveillance. J Clin Oncol 1990; 8(10): 1695–1698.

26. Stuart NS, Woodroffe CM, Grundy R, et al. Long-term toxicity of chemotherapy for testicular cancer—the cost of cure. Br J Cancer 1990; 61(3):479–484.

27. Lampe H, Horwich A, Norman A, et al. Fertility after chemotherapy for testicular germ cell cancers. J Clin Oncol 1997; 15(1):239–245.

28. Palmieri G, Lotrecchiano G, Ricci G, et al. Gonadal function after multimodality treatment in men with testicular germ cell cancer. Eur J Endocrinol 1996; 134(4): 431–436.

29. Siimes MA, Elomaa I, Koskimies A. Testicular function after chemotherapy for osteosarcoma. Eur J Cancer 1990; 26(9):973–975.

30. Aasebo U, Slordal L, Aanderud S, et al. Chemotherapy and endocrine function in lung cancer. Acta Oncol 1989; 28(5):667–669.

31. Wallace WH, Shalet SM, Lendon M, et al. Male fertility in long-term survivors of childhood acute lymphoblastic leukaemia. Int J Androl 1991; 14(5): 312–319.

32. Speiser B, Rubin P, Casarett G. Aspermia following lower truncal irradiation in Hodgkin's disease. Cancer 1973; 32(3):692–698.

33. Centola GM, Keller JW, Henzler M, et al. Effect of low-dose testicular irradiation on sperm count and fertility in patients with testicular seminoma. J Androl 1994; 15(6):608–613.

34. Hahn EW, Feingold SM, Nisce L. Aspermia and recovery of spermatogenesis in cancer patients following incidental gonadal irradiation during treatment: a progress report. Radiology 1976; 119(1):223–225.

35. Kinsella TJ, Trivette G, Rowland J, et al. Long-term follow-up of testicular function following radiation therapy for early-stage Hodgkin's disease. J Clin Oncol 1989; 7(6):718–724.

36. Shapiro E, Kinsella TJ, Makuch RW, et al. Effects of fractionated irradiation of endocrine aspects of testicular function. J Clin Oncol 1985; 3(9):1232–1239.

37. Giwercman A, von der Maase H, Berthelsen JG, et al. Localized irradiation of testes with carcinoma in situ: effects on Leydig cell function and eradication of malignant germ cells in 20 patients. J Clin Endocrinol Metab 1991; 73(3):596–603.

38. Howell SJ, Radford JA, Adams JE, et al. The impact of mild Leydig cell dysfunction following cytotoxic chemotherapy on bone mineral density (BMD) and body composition. Clin Enocrinol (Oxf) 2000; 52(5):609–616.

39. Howell SJ, Radford JA, Smets EMA, et al. Fatigue, sexual function and mood following treatment for haematological malignancy—the impact of mild Leydig cell dysfunction. Br J Cancer 2000; 82(4):789–793.

40. Howell S, Radford J, Adams J, et al. Randomised placebo controlled trial of testosterone replacement in men with mild Leydig cell insufficiency following cytotoxic chemotherapy. Clin Endocrinol (Oxf) 2001; 55(3): 315–324.

41. Monteil M, Rousseaux S, Chevret E, et al. Increased aneuploid frequency in spermatozoa from a Hodgkin's disease patient after chemotherapy and radiotherapy. Cytogenet Cell Genet 1997; 76(3–4): 134–138.

42. Robbins WA, Meistrich ML, Moore D, et al. Chemotherapy induces transient sex chromosomal and autosomal aneuploidy in human sperm. Nat Genet 1997; 16(1):74–78.

43. Genesca A, Benet J, Caballin MR, et al. Significance of structural chromosome aberrations in human sperm: analysis of induced aberrations. Hum Genet 1990; 85(5):495–499.

44. Robbins WA. Cytogenetic damage measured in human sperm following cancer chemotherapy. Mutat Res 1996; 355(1–2):235–252.

45. Royere D, Barthelemy C, Hamamah S, et al. Cryopreservation of spermatozoa: a 1996 review. Hum Reprod Update 1996; 2(6):553–559.

46. Chapman RM, Sutcliffe SB, Malpas JS. Male gonadal dysfunction in Hodgkin's disease. A prospective study. JAMA 1981; 245(13):1323–1328.

47. Padron OF, Sharma RK, Thomas AJ Jr, et al. Effects of cancer on spermatozoa quality after cryopreservation: a 12-year experience. Fertil Steril 1997; 67(2):326–331.

48. Aboulghar MA, Mansour RT, Serour GI, et al. Fertilization and pregnancy rates after intracytoplasmic sperm injection using ejaculate semen and surgically retrieved sperm. Fertil Steril 1997; 68(1):108–111.

49. Ward JA, Robinson J, Furr BJ, et al. Protection of spermatogenesis in rats from the cytotoxic procarbazine by the depot formulation of Zoladex, a gonadotropin-releasing hormone agonist. Cancer Res 1990; 50(3): 568–574.

50. Delic JI, Bush C, Peckham MJ. Protection from procarbazine-induced damage of spermatogenesis in the rat by androgen. Cancer Res 1986; 46(4 Pt 2):1909–1914.

51. Kurdoglu B, Wilson G, Parchuri N, et al. Protection from radiation-induced damage to spermatogenesis by hormone treatment. Radiat Res 1994; 139(1):97–102.

52. Pogach LM, Lee Y, Gould S, et al. Partial prevention of procarbazine induced germinal cell aplasia in rats by sequential GnRH antagonist and testosterone administration. Cancer Res 1988; 48(15): 4354–4360.

53. Meistrich ML, Parchuri N, Wilson G, et al. Hormonal protection from cyclophosphamide-induced inactivation of rat stem spermatogonia. J Androl 1995; 16(4):334–341.

54. Kangasniemi M, Wilson G, Huhtaniemi I, et al. Protection against procarbazine-induced testicular damage by GnRH-agonist and antiandrogen treatment in the rat. Endocrinology 1995; 136(8):3677–3680.

55. Meistrich ML, Kangasniemi M. Hormone treatment after irradiation stimulates recovery of rat spermatogenesis from surviving spermatogonia. J Androl 1997; 18(1):80–87.

56. Kangasniemi M, Huhtaniemi I, Meistrich ML. Failure of spermatogenesis to recover despite the presence of a spermatogonia in the irradiated LBNF1 rat. Biol Reprod 1996; 54(6):1200–1208.

57. Johnson DH, Linde R, Hainsworth JD, et al. Effect of a luteinizing hormone releasing hormone agonist given during combination chemotherapy on posttherapy fertility in male patients with lymphoma: preliminary observations. Blood 1985; 65(4):832–836.

58. Waxman JH, Ahmed R, Smith D, et al. Failure to preserve fertility in patients with Hodgkin's disease. Cancer Chemother Pharmacol 1987; 19(2):159–162.

59. Kreuser ED, Hetzel WD, Hautmann R, et al. Reproductive toxicity with and without LHRHA administration during adjuvant chemotherapy in patients with germ cell tumors. Horm Metab Res 1990; 22(9):494–498.

60. Brennemann W, Brensing KA, Leipner N, et al. Attempted protection of spermatogenesis from irradiation in patients with seminoma by D-Tryptophan-6 luteinizing hormone releasing hormone. Clin Investig 1994; 72(11):838–842.

61. Ortin TT, Shostak CA, Donaldson SS. Gonadal status and reproductive function following treatment for Hodgkin's disease in childhood: the Stanford experience. Int J Radiat Oncol Biol Phys 1990; 19(4): 873–880.

62. Das PK, Das BK, Sahu DC, et al. Male gonadal function in Hodgkin's disease before and after treatment. J Assoc Physicians India 1994; 42(8): 604–605.

63. Mulhall JP, Burgess CM, Cunningham D, et al. Presence of mature sperm in testicular parenchyma of men with nonobstructive azoospermia: prevalence and predictive factors. Urology 1997; 49(1):91–95.

64. Brinster RL, Zimmermann JW. Spermatogenesis following male germ-cell transplantation. Proc Natl Acad Sci USA 1994; 91(24):11298–11302.

65. Brook P, Radford J, Shalet S, et al. Isolation of germ cells from human testicular tissue for low temperature storage and autotransplantation. Fertil Steril 2001; 75(2):269–274.

21

Environmental Toxins and Male Fertility

Rebecca Z. Sokol

Keck School of Medicine, University of Southern California, Los Angeles, California, U.S.A.

☐ INTRODUCTION

The potential hazard of toxicants to the male reproductive system is well established (Table 1) (1–3). A toxicant, whether a chemical, physical, or biological agent, acts by interrupting biological processes either by a direct chemical action or indirectly via metabolic products by altering physiological control systems (4). In the male reproductive system, such an interruption can occur at any level of the hypothalamic–pituitary–testicular axis, or alternatively, by altering posttesticular events such as sperm motility and/or function. Any disruption of these events by toxicants may lead to hypogonadism and/or infertility (3).

The most extensively studied toxicants are the chemotherapeutic agents and radiation therapies used to treat malignancies (5–7). Of the thousands of chemicals used in the workplace, relatively few have been examined for their effects on reproductive function (8). Recent interest has focused on the contribution of environmental toxic exposure to changes in male reproductive function (9,10).

☐ ENVIRONMENTAL AND OCCUPATIONAL CHEMICAL EXPOSURE

The environmental theory suggests that environmental or occupational exposure to compounds with endocrine-disruptive properties may account for changes in male reproductive health. In support of this hypothesis are the possible global decline in sperm concentration and the recent increase in the incidence of testicular cancer and other disorders of the male reproductive tract, particularly hypospadias and cryptorchidism (11).

The most widely studied evidence of potential environmental reproductive hazards is the report that sperm counts have declined in certain industrialized countries around the world (9–13). The debate was initiated by Carlsen et al. in 1992 (12) when they published a meta-analysis of semen data reported in 61 studies worldwide between 1966 and 1991. These authors concluded that a significant decrease in mean sperm concentration of approximately 50% had occurred in industrialized nations during the time period studied (12). In response to this publication, a number of investigators published data in support of and in conflict with the Carlsen data. Reanalysis of the original Carlsen data by a number of investigators, some of whom expanded the meta-analysis to include studies published through 1996, verified a significant decrease in sperm density in the United States (13–15). Reanalysis of the data by others using a different statistical approach, however, led them to conclude that no significant decrease had occurred in the United States (16,17).

Because of the controversy, a number of European and U.S. investigators researched if similar decreases in sperm counts could be documented in their clinics and laboratories. Variable results were reported. Some groups reported a decline in sperm concentration, whereas others did not (18–23).

In the United States, Paulsen et al. noted no change in sperm parameters amongst healthy men studied between 1972 and 1993 in Seattle (22). Sokol and colleagues (23) recently reported that the semen parameters in a group of 1385 samples collected from men presenting for an initial screening semen analysis in Los Angeles, California, over a three-year period were similar to those reported in studies conducted by MacLeod et al. on a similar population of men in New York in the 1950s and 1970s (24–25): 17% of the men in the 1951 study, 15% of the men in the 1976 study, 18% in the recent Los Angeles study had sperm concentrations less than 20 million sperm/mL, the WHO cut-off for a normal sperm concentration (26). Mean and median sperm concentrations, percentage motility, and percentage normal sperm forms were almost identical amongst the three groups studied.

These variable findings have led most investigators to conclude that if a decline in semen quality actually exists, there may be significant geographic differences. In support of this hypothesis are the published reports suggesting that sperm concentration in the United States is dependant on geographic location (27,28). In one of the first studies to suggest a relationship between semen quality and geographic locale, the highest sperm concentrations were found in samples collected for sperm banks in New York, with intermediate numbers in Minnesota, and the lowest numbers in Los Angeles (27). A recent study reported that men living in an agrarian city had significantly lower sperm concentrations than men living in urban areas (28).

Table 1   Toxicants Documented to Alter Male Reproduction

Metals
  Boron
  Cadmium
  Chromium
  Lead
  Mercury
Industrial chemicals
  Chlorinated hydrocarbons
  Polychlorinated biphenyls
  Organic solvents
  Phthalates
  Polycyclic aromatic hydrocarbons
  Vinyl chloride
Agricultural chemicals
  Dibromochloropropane
  Dichloro-diphenyl-trichloroethane
  Dioxins
  Epichlorohydrin
  Ethylene dibromide
  Kepone (chlordecone)
  Methoxychlor
Antineoplastic agents
Radiation

Theories explaining this geographic phenomenon are based on environmental, socioeconomic, racial, age, and methodological parameters, the latter primarily in methods of semen analysis, selection criteria for subjects, season during which the semen analysis was performed, and abstinence time prior to collection of the semen sample (10,29). Arguing against the racial and socioeconomic theories are the findings of the National Survey of Family Growth, which found no differences in the prevalence of infertility across education levels or racial or ethnic categories in the United States (30). A similar geographic difference in the incidence of testicular cancer and other male reproductive congenital defects has been reported (10).

Although numerous chemicals have been suggested as potential male reproductive toxicants, few have been extensively studied. Identified toxicants leading to reproductive dysfunction in males can be categorized according to their source of exposure and their chemical composition.

Heavy Metals

The adverse reproductive effects of a number of heavy metals have been described in humans and experimental animals (1–3). Of these, the most extensively studied is lead.

The reproductive toxicity of lead was recognized in the days of the Roman Empire (31). Although lead exposure has been dramatically reduced because of the regulation of lead-containing gasoline (31), the environmental exposure to toxic levels of lead occurs in a number of industries, with potential adverse effects on the reproductive capacity of exposed men (32–36). Clinical and animal studies indicate that abnormalities of spermatogenesis result from toxic exposure to lead (36–38). In animals, lead exposure results in a dose–response suppression of serum testosterone and

spermatogenesis (39). Mechanistic studies suggest that lead exposure disrupts all levels of the reproductive axis (36–40). Adverse reproductive effects appear to be dose related, reversible, and age related, with pubertal animals being the most sensitive (36). Clinical studies are less definitive than the animal studies but support the evidence that toxicity occurs at all levels of the reproductive axis. In a pioneering study, Lancranjan et al. (33) evaluated the semen, serum testosterone levels, and urinary gonadotropins of men who worked in a battery plant and were exposed to lead on the production line versus office workers. They found a dose-related suppression of spermatogenesis, normal or decreased serum testosterone, and normal urinary gonadotropins in the exposed workers. Follow-up studies by investigators throughout the world reported variable results, some concluding that the primary site of toxicity is the central nervous system, with others concluding that the gonad is the most sensitive organ. Recent evidence suggests that lead interferes with the ability of spermatozoa to undergo the acrosome reaction, thus leading to infertility (37). Ion-channel polymorphisms may also cause differential sensitivities to lead exposure (37).

Less thorough studies have been reported on the effects of the other heavy metals on male reproduction. Cadmium, another ubiquitous metal, is a testicular toxin. Animal studies suggest direct testicular toxicity (37,41). Clinical studies also associate cadmium exposure with testicular toxicity, altered libido, and infertility (38). Studies similar to those of lead exposure suggest a cadmium-based disruption of the acrosome reaction (37).

Both organic and inorganic mercury can alter spermatogenesis and fertility in experimental animals (41). Workers are primarily exposed to mercury during the manufacture of thermometers, mercury vapor lamps, paint, electrical appliances, and in mining (41).

Boron is extensively used in the manufacture of many products including glass, cements, soaps, carpets, crockery, and leather. Earlier studies conducted using animal models suggested that the major adverse reproductive effect of boron is on the testes (3,42). Exposure of rats to low levels of boric acid induces an inhibition of elongate spermatid release and may interfere with hypothalamic–pituitary control of spermatogenesis (41). Oligospermia and decreased libido were reported in men working in boric acid-producing factories (42). The effects of chromium exposure on male reproduction remain unclear (43,44).

Industrial Chemicals

The most thoroughly studied nonheavy metal industrial chemical is methyl chloride, a colorless gas used primarily as a chemical intermediate in the production of organosilicate compounds and gasoline antiknock additives (3,45). Acute exposure of rats to methyl chloride causes toxicity in both the testis and epididymis. In a series of elegant studies, investigators identified the initial testicular lesion to be caused by delayed release of late-stage spermatids from the seminiferous epithelium, followed by generalized disruption and disorganization of the seminiferous epithelium (45). Further studies have provided evidence to implicate the testicular toxicity of methyl chloride in the induction of the cytotoxic effects on sperm that eventually lead to failure of fertilization and concomitant increased preimplantation loss postexposure (46).

Organic solvents have also been reported to induce deleterious changes in semen quality, testicular size, and gonadotropins (8). Phthalate esters—commonly found in plastics—may affect development and reproduction, including disruption to germ cells, cryptorchidism, and hypospadias in laboratory animals (47) and to sperm motility in human males by acting as estrogen agonists (48). In females, phthalate esters have been proposed as an etiology for premature breast development (49). A number of polycyclic aromatic hydrocarbons, which form during incomplete combustion of organic materials, act as antiandrogens in vitro (50). Polychlorinated biphenyls, ubiquitous chemicals in nature, act as estrogen agonists and are associated with the feminization of fish, reptiles, and mammals (51).

Agricultural Chemicals

Dibromochloropropane (DBCP) is a nematocide that was widely used in agriculture in the United States and Europe until 1977. The initial studies reported by Whorton found a direct relationship between sperm count and duration of DBCP exposure in DBCP production workers in Northern California (52). Animal and human studies confirmed that DBCP is a testicular toxin (53). Exposed workers usually present with elevated follicle-stimulating hormone levels and abnormal semen analyses (54). Recovery of spermatogenesis and fertility by exposed men is variable following removal of the exposure (55,56). Using an animal model, Meistrich et al. reported evidence of stem-cell spermatogonia after DBCP treatment of rats, suggesting the possibility of recovery of spermatogenesis with gonadotropin-releasing hormone agonists (57). Although DBCP use is now prohibited in the United States, well water continues to be contaminated in some states, and DBCP use is still allowed in a number of countries.

Other agricultural chemicals implicated as male reproductive toxicants include epichlorohydrin, dichloro-diphenyl-trichloroethane (DDT), ethylene dibromide, kepone, and the dioxins (3). DDT, a commonly used pesticide, acts as an estrogen antagonist when absorbed, competing with estradiol for estrogen receptors. Thus, DDT can alter the male reproductive system by disrupting the hypothalamic–pituitary–testicular axis. For further information on the hypothalamic–pituitary–testicular axis (see Chapters 3 and 4). Exposure to DDT and its metabolites is proposed as the cause of ambiguous genitalia and lowered testosterone levels in Florida alligators (58) and reproductive disorders in the Florida panther (59).

Similarly, kepone, a chlorinated polycyclic ketone, manifests estrogen-like actions. Low-dose kepone exposure in male rats and quail adversely affects the testes. Abnormal sperm morphology and abnormal testicular biopsies have been reported in kepone production workers (60).

Agent Orange, the most widely used of the herbicides during the Vietnam War, was actually a blend of two herbicides, one of which was 2,4,5-trichlorophenoxyacetic acid—itself widely used in the United States until it was banned in 1979. These herbicides have been investigated as possible male reproductive toxicants. Data published on the toxic effects of Agent Orange continue to elicit controversy. In an epidemiologic study conducted by Townsend et al. (61), no adverse reproductive events were documented in the wives of employees exposed to chlorinated toxins. Most investigators report no alteration in semen characteristics or infertility in men exposed to Agent Orange (62). A more recent study, however, suggests an association between currently used pesticides and reduced semen quality (63). In a case-control study, men in whom all semen parameters were low (cases) were compared to men in whom all semen parameters were within normal limits (controls). The levels of metabolites of pesticides (atrazine and alachlor) in urine samples were higher in the men from an agrarian state (Missouri) than in those from an urban state (Minnesota). This is, however, an association and does not support cause and effect.

Radiation Therapy and Chemotherapeutic Agents

Exposure to X-rays, neutrons, and radioactive material can cause germinal cell destruction (6,64). Radiation effects on spermatogenesis depend on the total dose received and the developmental stage of the germ cell at the time of exposure (65).

The increasingly successful treatment of patients with malignant disease with either chemotherapy or radiation therapy has focused attention on the long-term effects of these therapies on gonadal function and fertility (64,65). Cytotoxic damage to the testicular germinal epithelium by cancer treatment with chemotherapy, with or without radiation, is well documented. A review of the literature suggests that in adults the severity of germ-cell damage and the recovery of spermatogenesis are related to the category of the chemotherapeutic agent prescribed and to the dose and duration of therapy. The effects of radiation and chemotherapy on male reproductive function are discussed further in the Chapters 20 and 38.

□ CONCLUSION

The need to identify reproductive toxicants in the environment and workplace is clear. The evaluation of the infertile man should include a careful history to uncover any exposures that might have compromised fertility. The clinician can and should take an active role in the identification and prevention of reproductive toxicity by taking the following steps (66):

■ Identify the exposure and the potential health effects.
■ Characterize the extent of exposure.
■ Assess the degree of risk to the patient.

■ Initiate a plan to control or prevent the exposure.

The evaluation and treatment of a man presenting with infertility induced by occupational or environmental chemical exposure(s) should proceed in a manner similar to that of any man presenting with infertility.

□ REFERENCES

1. Sokol RZ. The hypothalamic-pituitary-gonadal axis as a target for toxicants. In: Boekelheide K, Chapin RE, Hoyer PB, et al., eds. Reproductive and Endocrine Toxicology. In: Snipes IG, McQueen CA, Gandolfi AJ, eds. Comprehensive Toxicology. New York: Elsevier Science Inc., 1997:87–98.

2. Sokol RZ. Lead neuroendocrine toxicology. In: Korach KS, ed. Reproductive and Developmental Toxicology. New York: Marcel Dekker Inc., 1998:249–258.

3. Sokol RZ. Toxicants and infertility: identification and prevention. In: Whitehead ED, Nagler HM, eds. Management of Impotence and Infertility. Philadelphia: JB Lippincott Company, 1994:380–389.

4. Mattison DR. The mechanisms of action of reproductive toxins. Am J Industr Med 1983; 4(1–2):65–79.

5. Damewood MD, Grochow LB. Prospects for fertility after chemotherapy or radiation for neoplastic disease. Fertil Steril 1986; 45(4):443–459.

6. Costabile RA, Spevak M. Cancer and male factor infertility. Oncology 1998; 12(4):557–568.

7. Howell S, Shalet S. Gonadal damage from chemotherapy and radiotherapy. Endocrinol Metab Clin North Am 1998; 27(4):927–943.

8. Congress of the US. Reproductive hazards in the workplace. Office of Technology Assessment,1985.

9. Safe S. Endocrine disrupters and human health—is there a problem? An update. Environ Health Perspect 2000; 108(6):487–493.

10. Moline JM, Golden AL, Bar-Charma N, et al. Exposure to hazardous substances and male reproductive health: a research framework. Environ Health Perspect 2000; 108(9):803–813.

11. Sharpe RM, Skakkebaek NE. Are oestrogens involved in falling sperm counts and disorders of the male reproductive tract? Lancet 1993; 341(8857):1392–1395.

12. Carlsen E, Giwercman A, Keiding N, et al. Evidence for decreasing quality of semen during the past 50 years. Br Med J 1992; 305:609–613.

13. Swan SH, Elkin EP, Fenster L. The question of declining sperm density revisited: an analysis of 101 studies published 1934–1996. Environ Health Perspect 2000; 108(10):961–966.

14. Becker S, Berhane K. A meta-analysis of 61 sperm count studies revisited. Fertil Steril 1997; 67(6):1103–1108.

15. Swan SH, Elkin EP, Fenster L. Have sperm densities declined? A reanalysis of global trend data. Environ Health Perspect 1997; 105(11):1228–1232.

16. Sherins RJ. Are semen quality and male fertility changing? N Eng J Med 1995; 332(5):327–328.

17. Olsen GW, Bodner KM, Ramlow JM, et al. Have sperm counts been reduced 50 percent in 50 years? A statistical model revisited. Fertil Steril 1995; 63(4):887–893.

18. Rasmussen PE, Erb K, Westergaaud LG, et al. No evidence for decreasing semen quality in four birth cohorts of 1,055 Danish men born between 1950 and 1970. Fertil Steril 1997; 68(6):1059–1064.

19. Auger J, Kunstmann JM, Czyglik F, et al. Decline in sperm quality among fertile men in Paris during the past 20 years. N Engl J Med 1995; 332(5):281–285.

20. Bujan L, Mansat A, Fontonnier F, et al. Time series analysis of sperm concentration in fertile men in Toulouse, France between 1977 and 1992. Br Med J 1996; 312(7029):471–472.

21. Bonde JP, Ernst E, Jensen TK, et al. Relation between semen quality and fertility: a population-based study of 430 first-pregnancy planners. Lancet 1998; 352(9135):1172–1177.

22. Paulsen CA, Berman NG, Wang C. Data from men in greater Seattle areas reveals no downward trend in semen quality: further evidence that deterioration of semen quality is not geographically uniform. Fertil Steril 1996; 65(5):1015–1020.

23. Acacio BD, Gottfried T, Israel R, et al. Evaluation of a large cohort of men presenting for screening semen analysis. Fertil Steril 2000; 73(3):595–597.

24. MacLeod J. Semen quality in one thousand men of known fertility and in eight hundred cases of infertile marriages. Fertil Steril 1951; 2(2):115–139.

25. MacLeod J, Gold RZ. The male factor in fertility and infertility II: an analysis of motility activity in the spermatozoa of 1,000 fertile men and 1,000 men in infertile marriages. Fertil Steril 1951; 2:187–204.

26. World Health Organization. WHO Laboratory Manual for the Examination of Human Sperm and Semen-Cervical Mucus Interaction. 4th ed. Cambridge: Cambridge University Press, 1999:60–61.

27. Fisch H, Goluboff E, Olson J. Semen analyses in 1,283 men from the United States over a 25-year period: no decline in quality. Fertil Steril 1996; 65(5):1009–1014.

28. Swann SH, Brazil C, Drobnis EZ, et al. Geographic differences in semen quality of fertile US males. Environ Health Perspect 111(4):414–420.

29. Handelsman DJ. Sperm output of healthy men in Australia: magnitude of bias due to self-selected volunteers. Hum Reprod 1997; 12(12):2701–2705.

30. Abma JC, Chandra A, Mosher WD, et al. Fertility, family planning, and women's health: new data from the 1995 National Survey of Family Growth. Vital Health Stat 1997; 23(19):1–114.

31. Gilfillan SC. Lead poisoning and the fall of Rome. J Occup Med 1965; 7:53–60.

32. Apostoli P, Kiss P, Porru S, et al. Male reproductive toxicity of lead in animals and humans. ASCLEPIOS Study Group. Occup Environ Med 1998; 55(6):364–374.

33. Lancranjan I, Popescu HI, Gavanescu O, et al. Reproductive ability of workmen occupationally exposed to lead. Arch Environ Health 1975; 30(8):396–401.

34. Cullen MR, Robins JM, Eskenazi B. Adult inorganic lead intoxication: presentation of 31 new cases and a review of recent advances in the literature. Medicine 1983; 62(4):221–247.

35. Winder C. Reproductive and chromosomal effects of occupational exposure to lead in the male. Reprod Toxicol 1989; 3(4):221–233.

36. Sokol RZ. Lead neuroendocrine toxicity. In: Korach K, ed. Reproductive and Development Toxicology. New York: Marcel Dekker, 1999:221–232.

37. Benoff S, Jacob A, Hurley IR. Male infertility and environmental exposure to lead and cadmium. Hum Reprod Update 2000; 6(2):107–121.

38. Telisman S, Cvitkovic P, Jurasovic J, et al. Semen quality and reproductive endocrine function in relation to biomarkers of lead, cadmium, zinc, and copper in men. Environ Health Perspect 2000; 108(1):45–53.

39. Sokol RZ, Madding CE, Swerdloff RS. Lead toxicity and the hypothalamic–pituitary-testicular axis. Biol Reprod 1985; 33(3):722–728.

40. Sokol RZ. Hormonal effects of lead acetate in the male rat: mechanism of action. Biol Reprod 1987; 37(5):1135–1138.

41. Barlow SM, Sullivan FM. Reproductive hazards of industrial chemicals. London: Academic Press, 1982.

42. Weir RJ, Fisher RS. Toxicologic studies on borox and boric acid. Toxicol Appl Pharmacol 1972; 23:351–364.

43. Ku WW, Chapin RE, Wine N, et al. Testicular toxicity of boric acid (BA): relationship of dose to lesion development and recovery in the F344 rat. Reprod Toxicol 1993; 7(4):305–319.

44. Pellerin C, Booker SM. Reflections on hexavalent chromium: health hazards of an industrial heavyweight. Environ Health Perspect 2000; 108(9):A402–A407.

45. Chellman GJ, Hurtt ME, Bus JS, et al. Role of testicular versus epididymal toxicity in the induction of cytotoxic damage in Fischer-344 rat sperm by methyl chloride. Reprod Toxicol 1987; 1(1):25–35.

46. Chapin RE, White RD, Morgan KT, et al. Studies of lesions induced in the testes and epididymis of F-344 rats by inhaled methyl chloride. Toxicol Appl Pharmacol 1984; 76:328–343.

47. Siddiqui A, Srivastava SP. Effect of di(2-ethylhexyl) phthalate administration on rat sperm count and on sperm metabolic enzymes. Bull Environ Contam Toxicol 1992; 48(1):115–119.

48. Fredricsson B, Moller L, Pousette A, et al. Human sperm motility is affected by plasticizers and diesel particle extracts. Pharmacol Toxicol 1993; 72(2):128–133.

49. Colon I, Caro D, Bourdony CJ, et al. Identification of phthalate esters in the serum of young Puerto Rican girls with premature breast development. Environ Health Perspect 2000; 108(9): 895–900.

50. Vinggaard AM, Hnida C, Larsen JC. Environmental polycyclic aromatic hydrocarbons affect androgen receptor activation in vitro. Toxicology 2000; 145(2–3): 173–183.

51. Toppari J, Larsen JC, Christiansen P, et al. Male reproductive health and environmental xenoestrogens. Environ Health Perspect 1996; 104(suppl 4):741–803.

52. Whorton D, Krauss RM, Marshall S, et al. Infertility in male pesticide workers. Lancet 1977; 2(8051):1259–1261.

53. Whorton D, Foliart D. DBCP: eleven years later. Reprod Toxicol 1988; 2(3–4):155–161.

54. Lipshultz LI, Ross CE, Whorton D, et al. Dibromochloropropane and its effects of testicular function in man. J Urol 1980; 124(4):464–468.

55. Lantz GD, Cunningham GR, Huckins C, et al. Recovery from severe oligospermia after exposure to dibromochloropropane. Fertil Steril 1981; 35(1):46–53.

56. Potashnik G, Porath A. Dibromochloropropane (DBCP): a 17-year reassessment of testicular function and reproductive performance. J Occup Environ Med 1995; 37(11):1287–1292.

57. Meistrich ML, Wilson G, Porter K, et al. Restoration of spermatogenesis and fertility in dibromochloropropane (DBCP)-sterilized rats by hormone suppression. Toxicol Sci 76(2): 418–426.

58. Guillette LJ Jr, Gross TS, Masson GR, et al. Developmental abnormalities of the gonad and abnormal sex hormones concentrations in juvenile alligators from contaminated and control lakes in Florida. Environ Health Perspect 1994; 102(8):680–688.

59. Facemire CF, Gross TS, Guillette LJ Jr. Reproductive impairment in the Florida panther: nature or nurture? Environ Health Perspect 1995; 103(suppl 4):79–86.

60. Lione A. Polychlorinated biphenyls and reproduction. Reprod Toxicol 1988; 2(2):83–89.

61. Townsend JC, Bodner KM, Van Pennen PF, et al. Survey of reproductive events of wives of employees exposed

to chlorinated dioxins. Am J Epidemiol 1982; 115(5): 695–713.

62. Suskind RR, Hertzberg VS. Human health effects of 2, 4, 5-T and its toxic contaminants. JAMA 1984; 251(18):2372–2380.

63. Swan SH, Kruse RL, Liu F, et al. Semen quality in relationship to biomarkers of pesticide exposure. Environ Helath Perspect 2003; 111(12):1478–1484.

64. Shalet SM. Effects of cancer chemotherapy on gonadal function of patients. Cancer Treatment Rev 1980; 7(3):141–152.

65. Naysmith TE, Blake DA, Harvey VJ, et al. Do men undergoing sterilizing cancer treatments have a fertile future? Hum Reprod 1998; 13(11):3250–3255.

66. Clegg ED, Sakai CS, Voyteck PE. Assessment of reproductive risks. Biol Reprod 1986; 34(1):5–16.

22

Micronutrients and Male Fertility

Nan B. Oldereid

Department of Obstetrics and Gynecology, Rikshospitalet–Radiumhospitalet Medical Center, Oslo, Norway

☐ INTRODUCTION

The relationship between nutrition and health has been appreciated since antiquity. The Greek physician Hippocrates wrote on this subject around 400 B.C., and prior to that time another Greek physician, Dioscorides, wrote about the medical properties of different plants (1). Only recently, however, has attention been paid to the impact of micronutrients on fertility.

Micronutrients can be defined as elements needed in relatively minute amounts in the diet (<1 ppm) and by the body (<1%) (2) for the maintenance of health and growth in animals and in humans. Vitamins and trace mineral elements are regarded as the major classes of micronutrients in the diet.

Relatively little is known about the impact of micronutrients, nutritional status, and nutritional supplements on human male reproductive function. An improved understanding of the mechanisms of action and effects of micronutrients on male fertility is needed, as both deficiency and excess of these elements can disrupt biological equilibrium and impact fertility. Nutritional abnormalities may be an important and neglected cause of reproductive impairment in man. The recommended dietary reference intakes of major elements and vitamins thought to impact reproductive function for adult men are listed in Table 1 (3).

This chapter will briefly summarize the impact of micronutrients on the fertility of animals and females and review available data on the mechanisms and effects of various trace elements and vitamins on male reproductive function.

☐ MICRONUTRIENTS AND ANIMAL FERTILITY

The reproductive well-being and performance of farm animals are largely dependent on the nutritional status. Animal studies have shown that poor nutrition caused by inadequate, excess, or imbalanced nutrient intake may adversely affect the various stages of the reproductive event (Table 2). Micronutrients are involved in functions such as intracellular detoxification of free radicals, synthesis of reproductive steroids and other hormones, and the metabolism of carbohydrates, proteins, and nucleic acids. Deficiencies and/or excesses of micronutrients can impair spermatogenesis and libido in the male and postpartum recovery and milk production in the female, as well as the in utero and postbirth development and survival of offspring (2).

☐ MICRONUTRIENTS AND FEMALE FERTILITY

In women, micronutrients may also play a necessary role in maintaining normal fertility potential. The importance of amino acids and water-soluble vitamins in optimizing culture media for in vitro fertilization is well documented (4). Furthermore, detectable amounts of homocysteine, vitamins B_{12} and B_6, and folate (folic acid, B_{11}) have been demonstrated in the follicular fluid (5). Therefore, it is reasonable to assume that such micronutrients must be present in sufficient amounts in the female for her to have normal fertility potential.

The relationship between nutritional status and obstetric outcome is well established (6). Impaired maternal nutrition may be related to the intrauterine fetal "programming" of disease expressed in adulthood (7,8). There is, however, a paucity of the literature regarding the impact of nutrition and micronutrients on female fertility. The number of well-documented studies is still very small.

☐ MICRONUTRIENTS AND MALE FERTILITY

A number of antioxidants, trace elements, and vitamins are thought to affect male reproductive function. The following is a review of the relative impact of each of these micronutrient classes.

Antioxidants

The presence of seminal oxidative stress in infertile men suggests its role in the pathophysiology of infertility (9). Reactive oxygen species (ROS) are involved in the peroxidative damage of human spermatozoa seen in many cases of male infertility (10). These free radicals may arise from defective spermatozoa and from leukocytes (11). ROS convert superoxide anions to hydrogen peroxide and initiate a lipid peroxidation cascade. In the terminal stages of sperm differentiation

Table 1 Recommended Daily Intake of Major Micronutrients for Adult Men

Nutrient	Recommended daily allowance	Selected food sources
Trace elements		
Selenium	55 μg	Organ meats, seafood, and plants (depending on selenium content of soil)
Zinc	11 mg	Fortified cereals, red meats, certain seafood
Vitamins		
Vitamin A	900 μg	Enriched cereal grains, dark leafy vegetables, enriched and whole-grain breads and bread products, fortified ready-to-eat cereals
Vitamin C	90 mg	Citrus fruits, tomatoes, tomato juice, potatoes, Brussels sprouts, cauliflower, broccoli, strawberries, cabbage and spinach
Vitamin D	5–15 μg	Fish liver oils, flesh of fatty fish, fortified milk products and fortified cereals
Vitamin E	15 mg	Vegetable oils, unprocessed cereal grains, nuts, fruits, vegetables and meats
Folic acid	400 μg	Enriched cereal grains, dark leafy vegetables, enriched and whole-grain breads and bread products, fortified ready-to-eat cereals

Source: From Ref. 3.

in humans, a considerable portion of the sperm cytoplasm is discarded and the remnants are confined to the mid-piece (10). As a consequence, these cells are not well endowed with the cytoplasmic defensive enzymes that protect most other cell types from peroxidative damage. This developmental event, combined with the presence of high concentrations of unsaturated fatty acids in the plasma membrane, could potentially render the spermatozoa susceptible to oxidative stress (10).

A number of antioxidant systems are present in semen to protect against the damaging effects of ROS (12). Glutathione peroxidase is one such system that is assumed to have a role in protecting cells from the harmful effects of toxic metabolites and free radicals by preventing lipid peroxidation of membranes (13).

The effects of oral antioxidant treatment (*N*-acetyl-cysteine or vitamin A plus E) and essential fatty acids on sperm quality in 27 infertile men were recently reported (14). During treatment, the amount of ROS was reduced and the percentage of induced acrosome reaction increased. Sperm motility and morphology were not improved, but sperm concentration was increased in oligozoospermic men (7.4±1.3–12.5± 1.9 million/mL).

In an in vitro study, antioxidants were shown to reduce the loss of sperm motility caused by ROS generated by polymorphonuclear leukocytes (15). The impairment of sperm motility observed in the presence of activated leukocytes was reduced by the presence of glutathione, *N*-acetyl-cysteine, hypotaurine, and catalase. The authors concluded that these antioxidants can protect against sperm movement damage induced by ROS and may be of clinical value in assisted conception procedures.

Trace Elements
Selenium

Selenium is an essential trace mineral that is of major importance in human biology (16). The effects of selenium in serum and tissues of mammals appear to be mediated by the activation of several selenium-dependent compounds, including glutathione peroxidases (17) and other selenoproteins (18). As an essential component of the enzyme glutathione peroxidase (19), which is present in both animal and human semen (20), the ability of selenium to protect tissues from damage by free radicals may be related to its antioxidation properties (13).

Both low and high seminal plasma selenium levels may be harmful to male fertility (21). A reduction in selenium concentration could theoretically render spermatozoa more vulnerable to oxygen radicals. ROS are involved in the initiation of normal biochemical processes in human spermatozoa, such as hyperactivated motility and the acrosome reaction (10), which occur after the sperm reach the uterus and fallopian tubes. Since a premature induction of these

Table 2 The Importance of Micronutrients on Reproduction in Farm Animals

Micronutrient	Deficiency consequences
Vitamin A	Delayed puberty
	Low conception rate
	High embryonic mortality
	Reduced libido
Vitamin E	Low sperm concentration
	High incidence of cytoplasmic droplets
	Retained fetal membrane
Selenium	Reduced sperm motility
	Reduced uterine contraction
	Cystic ovaries
	Low fertility rate
	Retained fetal membrane
Copper	Low fertility
	Delayed/depressed estrus
	Abortion/fetal resorption
Zinc	Impaired spermatogenesis
	Impaired development of secondary sex organs in males
	Reduced fertility and litter size in multiparous species

Source: From Ref. 2.

processes would be detrimental to the fertilization process, it is likely that mechanisms exist in the semen that hinder this from occurring too early.

In animals, selenium has been shown to be an essential element for normal male reproductive function. The most well-characterized effects of selenium deficiency on mammalian spermatozoa include loss of motility, breakage at the mid-piece level, and an increased incidence of sperm-shape abnormalities, mostly of the sperm head (22,23).

Selenium concentrations in the reproductive organs seem to differ geographically, depending on dietary intake. The concentrations of selenium were found to be generally higher in a Norwegian study (30% and 15% higher in testes and prostate tissues, respectively) compared to the tissue concentrations reported for the same organs in a Finnish study (24,25). This is in accordance with the blood levels of selenium, which also appear to be lower in the Finnish population (26). This discrepancy may be explained by differences in dietary intake.

Selenium has been reported to protect against the toxic effects of heavy metals through undefined mechanisms (27). The tendency of selenium to form complexes with heavy metals may be one way to explain its protective effect (28); its antioxidant properties may be another (29).

The testis is reported to be the reproductive organ with the highest concentration of selenium (Table 3). This high selenium concentration may be important in regulating certain enzymes during spermatogenesis. The selenium concentration in the testis is regulated by a homeostatic mechanism, which ensures a priority in the supply of selenium to the male gonads over other tissues (30). Furthermore, the selenium requirement of the testis is increased during pubertal maturation, in parallel with the beginning of spermatogenesis (31). The high rates of mitosis and the various stages of meiosis in the seminiferous tubules may expose germinal cell chromosomes to the potentially damaging influence of free radicals in the local environment, thus creating a need for an effective antioxidant system such as that offered by selenium.

The role of intracellular selenium in spermatozoa is still poorly understood (32). Selenium appears to be present in spermatozoa (20) and, at least in rats, is incorporated during the secondary spermatocyte or early spermatid stage, where a specific selenoprotein is found in the outer membrane of the sperm mitochondria (33).

Despite the relatively high selenium concentration in the testes described above, selenium concentration in seminal plasma is less than 50% of serum values (25), suggesting a relative barrier at the level of the secretory epithelia in the male reproductive organs. Subsequent studies, however, have shown that selenium supplementation raises the selenium concentration and glutathione peroxidase activities in the seminal fluid of subfertile men (32,34), indicating an equilibrium between the blood and seminal compartments.

The selenium concentrations in the semen of infertile men were not found to be statistically different from a control group (23). Reports on the relationships between sperm quality and selenium in seminal fluid are inconsistent. Some studies reported that selenium concentrations in seminal plasma correlate positively with sperm density (21,24,35,36), while others were unable to show such a relationship (37,38). Selenium proteins can detach from the outer surface of the spermatozoa during centrifugation, which may explain the positive correlation between sperm count and seminal-fluid selenium noted in some studies. On the other hand, approximately 75% to 85% of the total ejaculated content of selenium originates from the seminal plasma (21,35). Indeed, the high values found in vasectomized men have suggested that the majority of semen selenium originates from the accessory sex glands (21). A positive correlation between selenium and zinc concentrations in seminal plasma (24,37) suggests that the prostate plays a significant role in the secretion of selenium, since zinc is an acknowledged marker of prostatic secretion. (For further information on this topic, please refer to Chapter 7.) The presence of selenium in the prostate fraction of ejaculation (the prostate and epididymal secretions are the earlier portions of ejaculatory fluid) ensures its interaction with the spermatozoon before the latter is confronted with the hostile vaginal environment.

The concentrations of selenium in the accessory sex glands and epididymis are approximately 50% of that in the testes (24,25). Despite the fluid resorption capacity of the epididymis (39), it has a selenium concentration less than half of that found in the testes. If the selenium in the testis was solely associated with sperm cells, a higher level would have been expected in the epididymis because of the accumulation of sperm cells in the epididymal tubule. It is therefore more likely that selenium primarily exists in the testis, not only in the spermatozoa, but also in the other tissue compartments. Indeed, evidence suggesting the presence of a specific selenium receptor in the rat testes has been presented (40). Selenium was also found to be concentrated in the Sertoli cells of bulls (41). The significant correlations between the tissue levels of selenium in the reproductive organs suggest that its uptake and/or biochemical activities in these tissues

Table 3 Selenium Concentration (μg/g Dry Weight) in Tissue Samples of Human Reproductive Organs, Kidney, and Liver from 41 Men

Organ	SD	Mean	Median	Range
Testis	2.6	0.8	2.6	1.6–6.3
Epididymis	1.2	0.4	1.1	0.2–1.9
Prostate	1.3	0.4	1.3	0.6–2.1
Seminal vesicle	1.5	0.5	1.5	0.6–2.6
Kidney	4.7	1.7	4.3	2.2–9.7
Liver	1.9	0.6	1.9	0.9–3.7

Source: From Ref. 24.

are controlled by similar mechanism(s). One possibility is that selenium concentrations are regulated by androgen-dependent events.

The need for dietary selenium supplementation is well defined for experimental animals and livestock; however, the optimal need for this trace element in humans is not well characterized, and the intake of selenium in human seems to vary between different geographical regions (42). The recommended daily allowance of selenium for adult men is currently estimated to be 55 μg (Table 1) (3). Supplementation of subfertile men with 100 μg selenium per day for three months significantly increased sperm motility (43). This is in contrast to another study, in which a selenium supplementation of 200 μg improved neither the sperm motility nor other characteristics of spermatozoal quality (32).

In experimental animals and in livestock supplied with selenium in amounts commonly accepted as being adequate, further supplementation was not shown to improve reproductive capacity. In fact, even moderate overdosing was found to have negative effects on the number of spermatozoa and their motility (44).

Zinc

As a constituent of several metalloenzymes, zinc is involved in several different enzymatic reactions associated with carbohydrate metabolism, protein synthesis, and nucleic acid metabolism, rendering this trace element essential for proper cell growth (45).

The zinc concentrations in the normal human prostate gland and seminal plasma are high compared with those in other body tissues and fluids (46). Zinc in semen is secreted almost entirely by the prostate both in its free form and as zinc citrate, and may later bind to high molecular-weight proteins derived from the seminal vesicles (47–49).

Zinc plays an important role in reproduction, and deficiencies may have negative consequences on spermatogenesis. In the human male, zinc deficiency may cause hypogonadism (50). Both Leydig cell synthesis of testosterone and conversion of testosterone into dihydrotestosterone seem to be influenced by dietary zinc intake (51,52). There is evidence that zinc influences metabolic and functional processes in the seminal plasma, including oxygen consumption of the spermatozoa, sperm motility, and acrosin activity (53–56).

During normal ejaculation, the majority of sperm cells are expelled in the first fractions together with the prostatic fluid, which contains a high level of bioavailable zinc. This preserves a high content of chromatin zinc and thereby confers a high degree of chromatin stability (57,58). A low content of chromatin zinc was found to be associated with a low degree of chromatin stability in men with unexplained infertility (58).

Reports indicate that zinc can protect various tissues against the toxic and carcinogenic effects of cadmium. There is evidence that zinc protects against

testicular injury induced by cadmium, at least in the rat (59).

There has been concern that smoking may have adverse effects on male reproduction. The effects of smoking on sperm quality and on male fertility are still controversial, despite a number of recent studies; however, the zinc contents of seminal plasma appear to differ between smoking and nonsmoking men. The total quantity of zinc in the ejaculates of smokers is significantly lower than that found in nonsmokers (60,61). The reduction in zinc secretion into the semen of smoking men is especially interesting when considering the noted zinc deficiency found in the fetuses of smoking mothers (62). The latter observation is thought to be due to zinc entrapment by the placenta. Similarly, the lower prostatic secretion of zinc has been attributed to entrapment by the prostatic epithelium subsequent to a cadmium–zinc interaction. This hypothesis was suggested to explain the marked reduction in seminal zinc noted in the presence of a slight increase in seminal cadmium. As described above, the reduction in seminal zinc concentration may reduce sperm chromatin stability. Reduction in the protective effect of zinc on the sperm chromatin could increase the vulnerability of the sperm DNA to external influences, including heavy metals, and precipitate premature chromatin decondensation prior to fertilization, thus adversely influencing embryonic development.

A significant reduction in the concentration of zinc occurs in the testes with increasing age (63). This could lead to increased vulnerability of the testis with aging.

It is currently unknown whether supplementation with zinc can increase human semen quality. In a recent study, treatment with zinc sulfate alone did not significantly alter semen parameters, while treatment with a combination of both zinc sulfate and folic acid significantly increased both sperm concentration and total normal sperm count, although a significant increase in the percent of abnormal spermatozoa was also observed (64). Whether this improvement will lead to an increased pregnancy rate remains to be elucidated; therefore, a larger, placebo-controlled study is recommended.

Vitamins

Vitamins are organic substances essential to normal health. Each of these vitamins is soluble either in water or in fat. As such, fat-soluble vitamins (A, D, E, and K) are capable of being stored in the body; hence an excessive intake of these vitamins may accumulate to harmful levels. Because water-soluble vitamins (B and C) usually do not accumulate, they are stored only in small quantities. Thus, deficiencies of water-soluble vitamins occur faster than deficiencies of fat-soluble vitamins.

Vitamin A

Vitamin A deficiency is very rare in industrial countries, but it is common in many developing nations.

Vitamin A is mainly stored in the liver, and, as a result, its excessive intake may cause liver damage and other toxicity problems (6). Conversely, in vitamin A-deficient male rats, spermatogenesis becomes arrested, and degeneration and loss of germ cells take place. The seminiferous tubules of vitamin A-deficient rats were found only to contain Sertoli cells, type A spermatogonia, and some spermatocytes. When vitamin A-deficient rats were treated with retinoic acid, the full development of spermatogenic cells into elongated spermatids was observed (65).

Vitamin E

The most active form of vitamin E is alpha-tocopherol. Vitamin E seems to play an important function as a specific lipid-soluble antioxidant in the cell membrane. The role of vitamin E in testis development is not fully clear (66). In a study of nine men with oligo-asthenoteratozoospermia, a condition characterized by low sperm concentration, decreased motility, and abnormal morphology, the combination of selenium and vitamin E supplementation for a period of six months increased sperm motility and the percent live and percent normal spermatozoa. Notably, this was not a placebo-controlled study and the number of subjects was small (34).

Vitamin C

Vitamin C (ascorbic acid) is involved in the synthesis of collagen, protects against oxidation of vitamins A and E and fatty acids, plays a role in the metabolism of amino acids, steroids, catecholamines, and folic acid, and stimulates the absorption of inorganic iron (6). Ascorbic acid is found in high concentrations in seminal fluid compared to the concentration in blood plasma, presumably reflecting a physiological role (67). A study comparing dietary and seminal ascorbic acid with the endogenous levels of oxidative damage using oxo^{8}dG, an oxidative DNA damage product, indicated that dietary ascorbic acid protects human sperm from endogenous oxidative damage to DNA (68). When dietary ascorbic acid was decreased from 250 to 5 mg/day, the seminal fluid ascorbic acid decreased by half and the level of oxo^{8}dG in sperm increased by 91%. Short-term ascorbic acid depletion in eight healthy men did not adversely affect sperm qualities related to fertility. Similarly, moderate supplementation (up to 250 mg/day) did not improve sperm quality (69). This is in contrast to another interventional study reporting that ascorbic acid supplementation in excess of 200 mg/day in heavy smokers resulted in improved sperm quality (70).

Vitamin D

Vitamin D is essential in the homeostasis of calcium and phosphate. The importance of vitamin D and its role in the reproductive cycle has received little attention. Vitamin D and its metabolites were found to be necessary for normal reproductive functions in the male rat (71). In this study, male rats were fed vitamin D-deficient and vitamin D-replete diets until maturity, and then mated to age-matched, vitamin D-replete females. Successful matings by vitamin D-deficient rats were fewer compared to the vitamin D-replete rats. Fertility was also reduced after inseminations by vitamin D-deficient rats compared to inseminations by vitamin D-replete rats.

Folic Acid (Folate)

Another important micronutrient is folic acid (folate). Folate is involved in the synthesis of DNA through interaction with vitamin B$_{12}$. Periconceptional folate supplementation in the female is recommended to prevent neural tube defects in offspring (72). Few published studies were found to describe the impact of folic acid on male reproductive function. In an interventional study, folic acid (10 mg) was administered for 30 days to 40 normo- or oligozoospermic men. Although increased levels of folic acid were determined in the semen, it was found that sperm quality, as judged by sperm counts, motility, and DNA content of spermatozoa, was not affected (73). The interventional period of 30 days in this study may have been too short to be effective, however, because the spermatogenesis process requires approximately 70 days. As mentioned above, a significant increase in sperm concentration and total normal sperm count was observed after supplementation with folic acid and zinc sulfate in subfertile men. Treatment with folic acid alone, however, did not significantly change semen variables except for a slight decrease in percent normal sperm (64). Therefore, the actions of folate and zinc on sperm quality seem to be dependent on one another.

☐ CONCLUSION

The current interest in the potential role of oxidative damage in sperm function has highlighted the importance of natural food substances involved in protecting tissues and cells from free radical damage. In this regard, micronutrients may play important roles in conferring protection in the reproductive organs.

Only sparse information is available, however, regarding the impact of micronutrients on human male fertility, and further studies on these trace elements are needed to define the optimal daily requirements. Studies published on the benefit of oral supplementation may suffer from problems such as a lack of placebo-control, a limited number of participating subjects, and a short duration of study. Some of these studies are indeed presented as pilot observations and, thus, further investigation is recommended. Hopefully, in the future, double-blind, placebo-controlled interventional studies will clarify the impact of micronutrients on male reproductive function so that recommendations for clinical practice will be possible.

☐ REFERENCES

1. Seibel MM. The role of nutrition and nutritional supplements in women's health. Fertil Steril 1999; 72(4): 579–591.

2. Smith OB, Akinbamijo OO. Micronutrients and reproduction in farm animals. Anim Reprod Sci 2000; 60–61:549–560.

3. Committee on Use of Dietary Reference Intakes in Nutrition Labeling (Food and Nutrition Board: Institute of Medicine of the National Academies). Dietary Reference Intakes: Guiding Principles for Nutrition Labeling and Fortification. Washington, D.C.: National Academies Press, 2003.

4. Staessen C, Van den Abbeel E, Janssenswillen C, et al. Controlled comparison of Earle's balanced salt solution with Menezo B2 medium for human in-vitro fertilization performance. Hum Reprod 1994; 10: 1915–1919.

5. Steegers-Theunissen RP, Steegers EA, Thomas CM, et al. Study on the presence of homocysteine in ovarian follicular fluid. Fertil Steril 1993; 60(6):1006–1010.

6. Steegers-Theunissen BP. Maternal nutritional and obstetric outcome. Baillieres Clin Obst Gynaecol 1995; 9(3):431–443.

7. Barker DJ, Bull AR, Osmond C, et al. Fetal and placental size and risk of hypertension in adult life. Br Med J 1990; 301(6746):259–262.

8. Godfrey KM, Forrester T, Barker DJ, et al. Maternal nutritional status in pregnancy and blood pressure in childhood. Br J Obstet Gynaecol 1994; 101(5):398–403.

9. Pasqualotto FF, Sharma RK, Nelson DR, et al. Relationship between oxidative stress, semen characteristics, and clinical diagnosis in men undergoing infertility investigation. Fertil Steril 2000; 73(3):459–464.

10. Aitken RJ. A free radical theory of male infertility. Reprod Fertil Dev 1994; 6(1):19–23.

11. Aitken RJ, West KM. Analysis of the relationship between reactive oxygen species production and leucocyte infiltration in fractions of human semen separated on Percoll gradients. Int J Androl 1990; 13(6):433–451.

12. Kovalski NN, de Lamirande E, Gagnon C. Reactive oxygen species generated by human neutrophils inhibit sperm motility: protective effect of seminal plasma and scavengers. Fertil Steril 1992; 58(4):809–816.

13. Alvarez JG, Storey BT. Role of glutathione peroxidase in protecting mammalian spermatozoa from loss of motility caused by spontaneous lipid peroxidation. Gamete Res 1989; 23(1):77–90.

14. Comhaire FH, Christophe AB, Zalata AA, et al. The effects of combined conventional treatment, oral antioxidants and essential fatty acids on sperm biology in subfertile men. Prostaglandins Leukot Essent Fatty Acids 2000; 63(3):159–165.

15. Baker HW, Brindle J, Irvine DS, et al. Protective effect of antioxidants on the impairment of sperm motility by activated polymorphonuclear leukocytes. Fertil Steril 1996; 65(2):411–419.

16. Rayman MP. The importance of selenium to human health. Lancet 2000; 356(9225):233–241.

17. Behne D, Kyriakopoeulos A, Weiss-Nowak C, et al. Newly found selenium-containing proteins in the tissues of the rat. Biol Trace Elem Res 1996; 55(1–2): 99–110.

18. Hill KE, Xia Y, Åkesson B, et al. Selenoprotein P concentration in plasma is an index of selenium status in selenium-deficient and selenium-supplemented Chinese subjects. J Nutr 1996; 126(1):138–145.

19. Rotruck JT, Pope AL, Ganther HE, et al. Selenium: biochemical role as a component of glutathione peroxidase. Science 1973; 179(73):588–590.

20. Saaranen M, Kantola M, Saarikoski S, et al. Human seminal plasma cadmium: comparison with fertility and smoking habits. Andrologia 1989; 21(2):140–145.

21. Bleau G, Lemarbre J, Faucher G, et al. Semen selenium and human fertility. Fertil Steril 1984; 42(6):890–894.

22. Wallace E, Cooper GW, Calvin HI. Effects of selenium deficiency on the shape and arrangement of rodent sperm mitochondria. Gamete Res 1983; 7(4):389–399.

23. Watanabe T, Endo A. Effects of selenium deficiency on sperm morphology and spermatocyte chromosoms in mice. Mutat Res 1991; 262(2):93–99.

24. Oldereid NB, Thomassen Y, Purvis K. Selenium in human male reproductive organs. Hum Reprod 1998; 13(8):2172–2176.

25. Saaranen M, Suistomaa U, Kantola M, et al. Selenium in reproductive organs, seminal fluid and serum of men and bulls. Hum Reprod 1986; 1(2):61–64.

26. Thomassen Y, Aaseth J. Selenium in human tissues. In: Ihnat M, ed. Occurrence and Distribution of Selenium. Boca Raton, Florida: CRC Press, 1989:169–212.

27. Wahba ZZ, Coogan TP, Rhodes SW, et al. Protective effects of selenium on cadmium toxicity in rats: role of altered toxicokinetics and metallothionein. J Toxicol Environ Health 1993; 38(2):171–182.

28. Diplock AT, Watkins WJ, Hewison M. Selenium and heavy metals. Ann Clin Res 1986; 18(1):55–60.

29. Sugawara N, Sugawara C. Selenium protection against testicular lipid peroxidation from cadmium. J Appl Biochem 1984; 6(4):199–204.

30. Behne D, Höfer T, von Berswordt–Wallrabe R, et al. Selenium in the testis of the rat: studies on its regulation and its importance for the organism. J Nutr 1982; 112(9):1682–1687.

31. Behne D, Duk M, Elger W. Selenium content and glutathione peroxidase activity in the testis of the maturing rat. J Nutr 1986; 116(8):1442–1447.

32. Iwanier K, Zachara BA. Selenium supplementation enhances the element concentration in blood and seminal

fluid but does not change the spermatozoal quality characteristics in subfertile men. J Androl 1995; 16(5): 441–447.

33. Calvin HI, Grosshans K, Musicant-Shikora SR, et al. A developmental study of rat sperm and testis selenoproteins. J Reprod Fertil 1987; 81(1):1–11.

34. Vézina D, Mauffette F, Roberts KD, et al. Selenium-vitamin E supplementation in infertile men. Effects on semen parameters and micronutrient levels and distribution. Biol Trace Elem Res 1996; 53(1–3):65–83.

35. Noack-Füller G, De Beer C, Seibert H. Cadmium, lead, selenium and zinc in semen of occupationally unexposed men. Andrologia 1993; 25(1):7–12.

36. Xu B, Chia SE, Tsakok M, et al. Trace elements in blood and seminal plasma and their relationship to sperm quality. Reprod Toxicol 1993; 7(6):613–618.

37. Behne D, Gessner H, Wolters G, et al. Selenium, rubidium and zinc in human semen and semen fractions. Int J Androl 1988; 11(5):415–423.

38. Roy AC, Karunanithy R, Ratnam SS. Lack of correlation of selenium level in human semen with sperm count/motility. Arch Androl 1990; 25(1):59–62.

39. Levine N, Marsh DJ. Micropuncture studies of the electrochemical aspects of fluid and electrolyte transport in individual seminiferous tubules, the epididymis, and the vas deferens in rats. J Physiol 1971; 213(3):557–570.

40. Gomez B Jr, Tappel AL. Selenoprotein P receptor from rat. Biochim Biophys Acta 1989; 979(1):20–26.

41. Vanha-Perttula T, Remes E. Incorporation of selenium-75 into seminal plasma and spermatozoa of the bull. Andrologia 1990; 22(1):34–41.

42. Fairweather-Tait SJ. Bioavailability of selenium. Eur J Clin Nutr 1997; 51(suppl 1):S20–S23.

43. Scott R, MacPherson A, Yates RW, et al. The effect of oral selenium supplementation on human sperm motility. Br J Urol 1998; 82(1):76–80.

44. Hansen JC, Deguchi Y. Selenium and fertility in animals and man—a review. Acta Vet Scand 1996; 37(1):19–30.

45. Garnica AD, Chan WY, Rennert OM. Trace elements in development and disease. Curr Probl Pediatr 1986; 16(2):45–120.

46. Mann T. The biochemistry of semen and of the male reproductive tract. London: Methuen & Co., Ltd, 1964: 91–96.

47. Arver S. Zinc and zinc ligands in human seminal plasma. III. The principal low molecular weight zinc ligand in prostatic secretion and seminal plasma. Acta Physiol Scand 1982; 116(1):67–73.

48. Björndahl L, Kjellberg S, Kvist U. Ejaculatory sequence in men with low sperm chromatin-zinc. Int J Androl 1991; 14(3):174–178.

49. Arver S, Eliasson R. Zinc and zinc ligands in human seminal plasma. II. Contribution by ligands of different origin to the zinc binding properties of human seminal plasma. Acta Physiol Scand 1982; 115(2): 217–224.

50. Sandstead HH, Prasad AS, Schulert AR, et al. Human zinc deficiency, endocrine manifestations and

51. Hunt CD, Johnson PE, Herbel J, et al. Effects of dietary zinc depletion on seminal volume and zinc loss, serum testosterone concentrations, and sperm morphology in young men. Am J Clin Nutr 1992; 56(1): 148–157.

52. Netter A, Hartoma R, Nahoul K. Effect of zinc administration on plasma testosterone, dihydrotestosterone, and sperm count. Arch Androl 1981; 7(1): 69–73.

53. Takihara H, Cosentino MJ, Cockett AT. Effect of low-dose androgen and zinc sulfate on sperm motility and seminal zinc levels in infertile men. Urology 1983; 22(2):160–164.

54. Roomans GM, Lundevall E, Björndahl L, et al. Removal of zinc from subcellular regions of human spermatozoa by EDTA treatment studied by x-ray microanalysis. Int J Androl 1982; 5(5):478–486.

55. Stevens FS, Griffin MM, Chantler EN. Inhibition of human bovine sperm acrosin by divalent metal ions. Possible role of zinc as a regulator of acrosin activity. Int J Androl 1982; 5(4):401–412.

56. Papadimas J, Bontis J, Ikkos D, et al. Seminal plasma zinc and magnesium in infertile men. Arch Androl 1983; 10(3):261–268.

57. Björndahl L, Kvist U. Influence of seminal vesicular fluid on the zinc content of human sperm chromatin. Int J Androl 1990; 13(3):232–237.

58. Kvist U, Kjellberg S, Björndahl L, et al. Zinc in sperm chromatin and chromatin stability in fertile men and men in barren unions. Scand J Urol Nephrol 1988; 22(1):1–6.

59. Saxena DK, Murthy RC, Singh C, et al. Zinc protects testicular injury induced by concurrent exposure to cadmium and lead in the rats. Res Commun Chem Pathol Pharmacol 1989; 64(2):317–329.

60. Oldereid NB, Thomassen Y, Purvis K. Seminal plasma lead, cadmium and zinc in relation to tobacco consumption. Int J Androl 1994; 17(1):24–28.

61. Pakrashi A, Chatterjee S. Effect of tobacco consumption on the function of male accessory sex glands. Int J Androl 1995; 18(5):232–236.

62. Kuhnert BR, Kuhnert PM, Groh-Wargo SL, et al. Smoking alters the relationship between maternal zinc intake and biochemical indices of fetal zinc status. Am J Clin Nutr 1992; 55(5):981–984.

63. Oldereid NB, Thomassen Y, Attramadal A, et al. Concentrations of lead, cadmium and zinc in the tissues of reproductive organs of men. J Reprod Fert 1993; 99: 421–425.

64. Wong WY, Merkus HM, Thomas CM, et al. Effects of folic acid and zinc sulfate on male factor subfertility: a double-blind, randomized, placebo-controlled trial. Fertil Steril 2002; 77(3):491–498.

65. van Pelt AM, de Rooij DG. Retinoic acid is able to reinitiate spermatogenesis in vitamin A-deficient rats and high replicate doses support the full development

of spermatogenic cells. Endocrinology 1991; 128(2): 697–704.

66. Anonymous. Vitamin E deficiency and male infertility. Nutr Rev 1988; 46(5):200–202.

67. Dawson EB, Harris WA, Rankin WE, et al. Effect of ascorbic acid on male fertility. Ann N Y Acad Sci 1987; 498:312–323.

68. Fraga CG, Motchnik PA, Shigenaga MK, et al. Ascorbic acid protects against endogenous oxidative DNA damage in human sperm. Proc Natl Acad Sci 1991; 88(24):11003–11006.

69. Jacob RA, Pinalto ES, Agee RE. Cellular ascorbate depletion in healthy men. J Nutr 1992; 122(5):1111–1118.

70. Dawson EB, Harris WA, Teter MC, et al. Effect of ascorbic acid supplementation on the sperm quality of smokers. Fertil Steril 1992; 58(5):1034–1039.

71. Kwiecinski GG, Petrie GI, DeLuca HF. Vitamin D is necessary for reproductive functions of the male rat. J Nutr 1989; 119(5):741–744.

72. MRC Vitamin Study Research Group. Prevention of neural tube defects: results of the Medical Research Council Vitamin Study. Lancet 1991; 338(8760): 131–137.

73. Landau B, Singer R, Klein T, et al. Folic acid levels in blood and seminal plasma of normo- and oligospermic patients prior and following folic acid treatment. Experientia 1978; 34(10):1301–1302.

Part III

Investigation of Male Reproductive Dysfunction

Even in this era of state-of-the-art imaging and surgical technology, an accurate impression of the correct diagnosis of male infertility can often be obtained from an initial office visit after the completion of a thorough history, physical examination, and the light microscopic examination of a semen specimen. Thus, the most important parts of the evaluation of the infertile male are the history and physical examination. Therefore, the minimum evaluation for any male patient presenting with a reproductive complaint should include a complete medical history (past medical history, family history, fertility history, sexual history, and ejaculate history), a physical examination (with special interest given to an assessment of body habitus, any evidence of clinical features associated with hypothalamic or pituitary defects, and the genital exam), and at least two semen analyses. Additional procedures and tests (endocrine evaluation, genital tract imaging studies, anti-sperm antibody testing, sperm function testing, detailed biochemical analysis of the semen, and genetic evaluation) may be indicated based on the results of the initial evaluation, and usually serve to confirm the diagnosis and help direct the course of therapy.

Clinical Assessment of the Infertile Male

Chakriya D. Anunta

Department of Diabetes, Endocrinology and Metabolism, City of Hope National Medical Center, Duarte, California, U.S.A.

Fouad R. Kandeel

Department of Diabetes, Endocrinology and Metabolism, City of Hope National Medical Center, Duarte, California, and David Geffen School of Medicine, University of California, Los Angeles, California, U.S.A.

□ INTRODUCTION

Male factor infertility is a general term that describes couples in whom the inability to conceive is associated with a problem identified in the male partner. This problem may be classified into the following etiologies: low sperm production (oligospermia), poor sperm motility (asthenospermia), or abnormal sperm morphology (teratospermia) (1). Male factor infertility also describes men who may have normal sperm production but also exhibit conditions that prevent sperm transport to the vagina during intercourse (e.g., reproductive tract obstruction or ejaculatory dysfunction).

Historically, the approach to the infertile couple has begun with an evaluation of the female, primarily because it is usually the female partner who has initiated a workup by consultation with her gynecologist. It is only within the last 50 years that the importance of the male factor contribution to infertility has been recognized. The social perception that infertility is associated with impotence or decreased masculinity may have aided in the propagation of this theory (2).

An accurate impression of the correct diagnosis can often be obtained even during the initial visit simply by taking a thorough history, physical examination, and the light microscopic examination of a semen specimen. Thus, the most important parts of the evaluation of the infertile male are the history and physical examination. Additional testing usually serves to confirm the diagnosis and help direct the course of therapy. The identification and treatment of reversible conditions may improve the male's fertility; in fact, the majority of couples suffering from infertility may receive sufficient treatment to achieve pregnancy through sexual intercourse. Further, approximately 1% of men who present with reproductive issues will, in fact, have an underlying serious medical problem causing the infertility whose presence was unknown prior to the initiation of the fertility workup; thus, failing to identify these diseases, such as testicular cancer or a pituitary tumor, may jeopardize the man's health or even his life (3,4). On the other hand, detection of

conditions for which there is currently no available treatment will spare couples the distress of attempting ineffective therapies. Similarly, the detection of certain genetic causes of male infertility may inform couples of the potential to transmit chromosomal abnormalities that may affect the health of any offspring. Thus, an appropriate male evaluation may allow the couple to understand the basis of their infertility more fully and to obtain genetic counseling when appropriate.

□ PATHOPHYSIOLOGIC CONSIDERATION

"Infertility" is defined as a couple's inability to achieve pregnancy following one year of appropriately timed and unprotected intercourse. According to this criterion, it has been estimated that approximately one in six couples attempting to conceive are unable to do so. Approximately, 20% to 30% of infertility cases are caused exclusively by a male factor, and another 30% to 40% of cases are the result of both male and female factors (5). Statistically, these data suggest that in more than 50% of couples presenting with infertility, a male factor is contributory. If these numbers were extrapolated to the general population, it is possible that 10% of all men in the United States—or as many as 2.5 million individuals—could potentially benefit from fertility evaluations. This process includes a history and physical examination and at least two semen analyses and is recommended at the time of presentation, even if it has been less than one year of unprotected intercourse, particularly in the case of advanced female age (greater than 35 years), the presence of known male infertility risk factors (such as an undescended testicle), or if a man questions his fertility potential (6).

Table 1 lists causes of infertility in the human male. The most common identifiable physical abnormality in men with infertility is the presence of a varicocele, a dilation of the pampiniform venous plexus and the internal spermatic vein. Although the etiologic role of a varicocele in causing male infertility remains

Table 1 Causes of Male Infertility

Causes	Frequency (approximate %)
Primary testicular disorders	10–13
Klinefelter's syndrome and variants	
Cryptorchidism	
Orchitis	
Irradiation	
Cytotoxic therapy	
Partial androgen resistance	
Hypothalamic–pituitary disease	1
Idiopathic, tumors, hyperprolactinemia	
Genital tract obstruction	8–10
Congenital or acquired obstruction of vas deferens or epididymis	
Previous vasectomy	
Sperm autoimmunity	4–6
Drugs, toxins, stress, illness	?
Coital problems	1
Idiopathic	70–75
Azoospermia, oligospermia, normospermia	
Poor sperm motility, teratospermia (varicocele, chronic prostatitis)	

controversial, its presence may raise the temperature of the testis, thus adversely influencing testicular function. This condition occurs in approximately 15% to 20% of all males and in 40% of infertile males (7,8). (For further information on varicoceles, please refer to Chapter 15.)

Another major cause of infertility in men is obstruction of the male reproductive tract (8). This is particularly true for men with azoospermia. Men with azoospermia can be divided into two broad groups: (*i*) men who have some type of pathology causing physical obstruction of the ejaculatory duct; and (*ii*) men who are unable to produce sperm (nonobstructive azoospermia). The distinction between these groups can be made by performing a testicular biopsy. (For additional information on testicular biopsies, please refer to Chapters 25 and 33.) Frequent causes of obstructive azoospermia include injury to the scrotum or testicles, a current or previous infection, including childhood mumps and sexually transmitted diseases, a physical/structural defect in the vas deferens or other structures, such as congenital bilateral absence of the vas deferens (CBAVD), paralysis, and a history of previous vasectomy. (For further details on these topics, please refer to Chapters 16 to 18.) Erectile dysfunction may be considered, in itself, a type of obstructive condition, as a lack of erections can make it difficult to ejaculate.

Conversely, conditions that can affect hormonal control of sperm production and cause nonobstructive azoospermia include testicular failure, a history of cryptorchidism in childhood or later, diabetes, hypertension, and ongoing or previous cancer radiation therapy and chemotherapy (8). Environmental or work hazards may also lead to nonobstructive azoospermia. (For further information on these topics, please refer to Chapter 13 and Chapters 19–22).

□ EVALUATION OF THE MALE PATIENT WITH INFERTILITY

The minimum full evaluation for male infertility for every patient should include a complete medical history, physical examination by a urologist or other specialist in male reproduction, and at least two semen analyses. Additional procedures and tests, used to elucidate problems discovered by the full evaluation, may be suggested based upon the results of initial testing. An algorithm that summarizes the approach to the diagnosis of the infertile man is depicted in Figures 1 and 2.

Patient History

A thorough history and methodical physical examination will guide the course of choosing any supplemental investigations, with the primary goal of elucidating treatable causes of infertility, the presence of any significant diseases that may be associated with male subfertility, or any conditions that may be transmitted to future offspring.

Fertility History

In some practices, prior to arrival at the office, prospective patients are invited to fill out a detailed fertility questionnaire with their partners (9). The history begins with an assessment of the couple's prior and current fertility status. The age of the partners and the duration of unprotected intercourse are established. The pursuit of a fertility evaluation becomes more appropriate sooner rather than later when the female partner is over the age of 35, if there has been a history of infertility in a prior relationship, or risk factors exist that have led the couple to suspect that a fertility problem exists (e.g., a past history of cryptorchidism, testicular neoplasm, or chemotherapy).

For idiopathic infertility, the chance of ultimate success is inversely related to the duration of infertility. Female age is an important factor, as in vitro fertilization results steadily and inexorably decline after age 34 (9). It should be established as to whether the infertility is primary (no conception has ever occurred) or secondary (children have been born in the past but couple cannot conceive now) for each partner, and, if secondary, the nature and outcome of prior pregnancies with the same or any previous partner. Any previous infertility evaluation or treatment for either partner should be noted as well.

Sexual History

In approximately 5% of couples presenting for infertility evaluation, sexual dysfunction is the root cause (9). Questions to be addressed include: Is the semen ejaculated into the vagina? Does the couple use lubricants, jellies, oils, or saliva, most of which are known to be somewhat spermicidal? If lubrication is necessary, Astroglide, Replens, or mineral oil should be

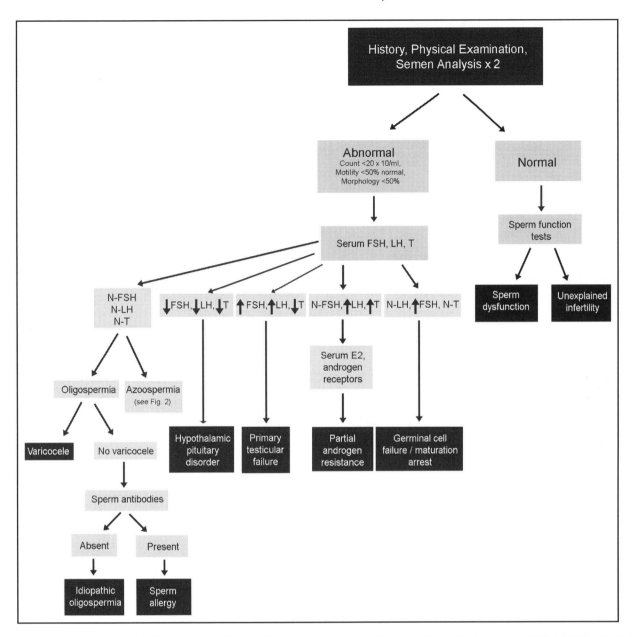

Figure 1 Algorithmic approach to the diagnosis of the infertile man. *Abbreviations*: N, normal; LH, luteinizing hormone; FSH, follicle-stimulating hormone; T, testosterone. *Source*: From Ref. 10. (*Continued on next page*.)

recommended. Because of the limitations imposed by an approximately 48-hour window of viability for sperm within the female reproductive tract, the timing of intercourse is important. Patients should be made aware that too frequent intercourse or compulsive masturbation depletes sperm reserves, decreasing the concentration of viable sperm in the ejaculate and thus lowering the chances of achieving fertilization. The sexual history should also include an assessment of libido, which may reflect the state of androgen production and/or action.

Ejaculate History

The male partner should be questioned regarding the nature and volume of a typical ejaculate. A markedly diminished semen volume may be associated with

hypogonadism. Also, decreased ejaculatory volume and a preponderance of clear, water-like fluid suggest an absence of the seminal vesicle component, and this may be associated with either ejaculatory duct obstruction or CBAVD. Normal orgasm with low or absent semen volume should lead one to suspect retrograde ejaculation, warranting the examination of a postejaculatory urine specimen for the presence of sperm. Semen that fails to liquefy suggests prostatic dysfunction. Proteolytic enzymes present in prostatic secretions cause liquefaction of the protein coagulum derived from the seminal vesicles.

Medical History

Cryptorchidism means a "hidden testis." This condition is present in about 0.8% of newborn or one-year-old

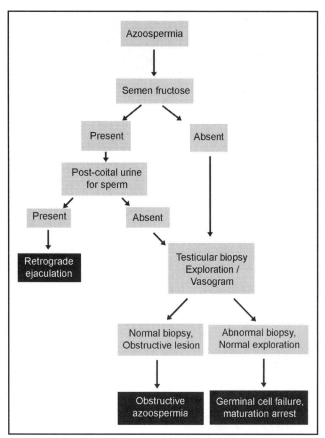

Figure 2 (*Continued*) Algorithmic approach to the diagnosis of the infertile man. *Source*: From Ref. 10.

males and is an important risk factor for infertility. Fifty percent of men with a history of unilateral cryptorchidism and 90% of men with a history of bilateral cryptorchidism are subfertile (9). Hernia repair in infancy or childhood is associated with a 3% to 17% risk of injury to the inguinal or retroperitoneal vas deferens. Postpubescent mumps is associated with a 30% risk of unilateral orchitis and a 10% risk of bilateral orchitis, which may result in severe ipsilateral abnormalities in spermatogenesis. The approximate age of onset of puberty is ascertained. Men will usually remember pubertal landmarks only if they were very early or very late. Precocious puberty suggests an adrenal abnormality such as congenital adrenal hyperplasia. Very delayed or incomplete sexual maturation suggests hypogonadotropic hypogonadism (Kallmann's syndrome, when associated with anosmia) or pantesticular failure such as Klinefelter's syndrome. (For further information on this topic, please refer to Chapter 12.)

Any and all conditions or illnesses for which the patient has been or is currently being treated, including all medications currently or previously taken, should be documented. Many prescription drugs interfere with spermatogenesis, including cimetidine, sulfasalazine, nitrofurantoin, and anabolic steroids. Drugs of abuse such as alcohol, marijuana, and cocaine are directly gonadotoxic. A detailed occupational history is directed toward identifying exposure to any additional gonadotoxic agents such as heat, ionizing radiation,

heavy metals, and pesticides. (Please refer to Chapter 21 for further information.) A family history directed at uncovering fertility problems in parents and siblings may be important. Intrauterine exposure to diethylstilbestrol is also associated with male genitourinary tract anomalies and dysfunction.

Physical Examination
General Examination

The patient should disrobe completely and stand with his arms outstretched. The general body habitus and hair distribution should be observed carefully. Men who are incompletely masculinized will have disproportionately long extremities due to absent or deficient androgen stimulation required for epiphyseal closure at the time of puberty. These features are seen in men with hypogonadotropic hypogonadism (Kallmann's syndrome when associated with absent sense of smell or other midline defects) or Klinefelter's syndrome.

The patient should be assessed for the presence or absence of clinical features associated with hypothalamic or pituitary defects (e.g., eye fundus abnormalities, loss of vision or the ability to smell, the presence of midline defects, and other signs of disease associated with pituitary tumors). The thyroid is palpated and the heart and lungs auscultated. Chronic bronchitis associated with congenital epididymal dysplasia is seen in Young's syndrome. Situs inversus with associated immotile sperm is seen in immotile cilia (Kartagener's) syndrome. The breasts are observed and palpated for gynecomastia, which can be associated with estrogen-secreting testicular neoplasms, adrenal tumors, and liver disease. Nipple discharge or tenderness may be seen with prolactin-secreting pituitary adenomas. The abdomen is palpated and percussed. An enlarged liver suggests hepatic dysfunction, which may be associated with infertility due to altered sex steroid metabolism.

Genital Examination

Physical examination is performed in a warm room by an examiner with warm, gloved hands. Contraction of the dartos muscle is induced by a cold room or cold examining hands, and this makes examination of the scrotum and its contents difficult (9). It should be noted that a proper fertility examination will extend beyond a casual observation of the scrotum and palpation of its contents.

The penis and urethral meatus are examined for congenital or acquired abnormalities, including infections. Severe hypospadias may result in inadequate delivery of semen into the vagina. The urethra is milked for discharge, and the presence or absence of genital ulcers or condylomata is noted. The location of the meatus is noted.

Scrotal examination is first performed with the patient supine. This allows a varicocele, if present, to collapse; testis size and consistency can then be properly assessed by an orchidometer. Normal testicular volume ranges from 15 to 30 cm^3. The testes should be firm in consistency. A change in testicular consistency is indicative of testicular pathology. Small soft testes indicate poor spermatogenesis. Small hard testes suggest postorchitis or posttorsion atrophy or Klinefelter's syndrome. Focal irregularities in consistency raise the suspicion of malignancy. Smooth firm nodules palpated on the surface of the testes usually represent tunica albuginea cysts. Mobile small hard bodies, or corpora amylacea, floating within the tunica vaginalis may be determined by palpation. Transillumination of the scrotum in a darkened room differentiates solid from cystic masses. In general, testes that are normal in size and consistency usually will have normal sperm production, whereas small-volume, soft testes are associated with impaired spermatogenesis. The normal epididymis, posterolateral to the testes, is soft and barely palpable. Induration, modularity, or irregularities are suggestive of epididymal pathology. A full, firm, easily outlined epididymis that is nontender suggests epididymal obstruction. Epididymal cysts are firm, smooth, transilluminate, and almost always located in the caput. The vas deferens should be palpated bilaterally. The vas is approximately the diameter and consistency of a Venetian blind cord and is usually posteromedial and separate from the internal spermatic cord structures. Bilateral CBAVD is observed in approximately 1.3% of patients presenting for infertility evaluation (9). With a relaxed scrotum, the diagnosis of CBAVD can almost always be made by palpation. These men will have azoospermia associated with low seminal volumes and nonclotting, clear ejaculate.

With the patient standing, large varicoceles are readily seen through the relaxed scrotal skin in a warm room. Small varicoceles may be appreciated as a distinct impulse and palpable dilation of the internal spermatic veins during execution of the Valsalva maneuver. The best method to elicit a strong and sustained Valsalva is to tell the patient to bear down as if having a bowel movement. If a varicocele is detected, the patient should then be placed supine. A varicocele should completely collapse when the patient is supine. A large varicocele, which does not collapse in the supine position, leads to suspicion of a retroperitoneal mass, and an abdominal sonogram is indicated.

Digital rectal examination should always be performed. The size and consistency of the prostate is noted. Masses, cysts, irregularities, tenderness, and whether or not the seminal vesicles are palpable are noted. Stool should be tested for occult blood.

☐ LABORATORY EVALUATIONS
Semen Analysis

Male infertility is evaluated primarily with the semen analysis. This is a common, convenient measure of assessing the male and should precede any invasive tests of the female. Characteristics examined include the volume of the semen sample, the contents of the seminal fluid, the number of sperm, and if they are adequately mobile (motility) and normally shaped (morphology), as measured by standardized techniques (Table 2). Ejaculate volumes between 2 and 6 mL and sperm concentrations of greater than 15 to 20 million per mL with more than 50% motile sperm and more than 50% oval forms are considered normal (10).

Semen specimens are obtained by masturbation into a sterile wide-mouth container after two to five days of abstinence and analyzed within two hours of collection. Because of the inherent marked variability in semen parameters from day to day within each individual, at least two, and preferably three, semen analyses should be performed with at least two-week intervals between collections. In the setting of a recent febrile illness or exposure to gonadotoxic agents, a semen analysis should be repeated no sooner than three months later.

General Characteristics: Volume and Concentration

Semen is initially an opalescent coagulum that liquefies within 20 to 25 minutes of ejaculation. Sixty-five percent of the volume is from the seminal vesicles, 30% to 35% from the prostate, and 3% to 5% from the vasa. The coagulation protein derives from the seminal vesicle; seminal fructose also derives from the seminal vesicles. Liquefaction is then secondary to the action of prostatic proteases. Failure of liquefaction is due to abnormalities of the prostate or its ducts. Thus, azoospermia coupled with low ejaculate volume of nonclotting, watery fluids that are fructose-negative (see below "Seminal Fructose") usually implies an obstruction of the ejaculatory duct. If the vasa are palpable, a transrectal ultrasound can diagnose this condition (see below). Patients who are not azoospermic, but oligo- or asthenospermic, with a low semen volume (less than 1 mL, except in patients with bilateral vasal agenesis or clinical signs of hypogonadism), may have partial ejaculatory duct obstruction or retrograde ejaculation. Retrograde ejaculation is seen most commonly in diabetics with autonomic neuropathy, as well as in men who have had transurethral surgery at or near the bladder neck. A postejaculatory urine specimen should then be obtained by having the patient first empty his bladder prior to ejaculation, and then void following ejaculation into a separate container.

Because pregnancy can be achieved with a single sperm, specimens originally read as azoospermic should be centrifuged and the pellet examined for the presence of sperm. Specimens with head-to-head or tail-to-tail agglutination are evaluated for antisperm antibodies or infection. Infection may be inferred from the presence of leukospermia ($>1 \times 10^6$ WBC/mL). Men with agglutination or leukospermia should have their semen cultured for aerobic and anaerobic organisms, as well as for *Chlamydia* and *Mycoplasma*. The penis and scrotum should be washed with an antibacterial scrub prior to culture to avoid inadvertent contamination with skin or fecal flora.

Table 2 Semen Analysis Reference Values

Semen characteristics	Units	WHO (1992)
Volume	mL	≥2.0
pH	pH units	(7.2–8.0)
Sperm concentration	×10⁶/mL	≥20
Total sperm count	×10⁶/ejaculate	≥40
Motility (within 60 min of ejaculation)	% motile	≥50
Progression at 37°C	Scale 0–4	3–4
Morphology	% normal sperm	≥30
Vitality	% live sperm	≥75
White blood cells	×10⁶/mL	<1.0
Immunological tests		
Immunobead test	Fewer than 20% spermatozoa with adherent particles	
MAR test	Fewer than 10% spermatozoa with adherent particles	
Seminal plasma biochemical analysis		
α-Glucosidase	mU	≥20
Carnitine	mmol	0.8–2.9
Zinc (total)	mmol	≥2.4
Citric acid	mmol	≥52
Acid phosphatase (total)	U	≥200
Fructose (total)	mmol	≥13

Abbreviations: MAR, mixed agglutination reaction test; WHO, World Health Organization.
Source: From Ref. 1.

Motility

The flagellar activity of the sperm cell is needed for normal transport through the female reproductive tract and for penetration of the ovum (11). Assessment of sperm motility can therefore provide important information on sperm function (see below). Sperm motility is usually rated in two ways: the percentage of motile cells is determined and the quality of sperm movement (e.g., how fast and how straight the sperm swim) is assessed. Sperm movement has been traditionally rated on a scale of 0 to 4+ (12). Normal values for sperm motility in the semen are at least 50% to 60% motile cells, and normal quality is considered greater than 2+. The subjectivity of this assessment, however, has limited its usefulness: for example, semen specimens with higher sperm concentrations may appear to have greater activity. Yet, manual light microscopic evaluation of sperm concentration, motility, and morphology remains the gold standard for semen analysis; however, more elaborate or automated methods such as time-exposure photomicrography or computer-assisted semen analysis (CASA) are becoming available in many practices and may provide information that could change the course of therapy (10). Some problems may be encountered with mechanization, however. For example, azoospermic specimens may be misread by the computer as being oligospermic, and the interpretation of computerized morphology may be difficult. CASA does, however, provide interesting information on sperm velocity and angularity that has proven to be useful in the research setting.

Morphology

Sperm morphology is usually expressed as a percentage of "normal cells," although the percentages of specific abnormal types (oval, tapered, amorphous) have also been reported (12). Proper interpretation of morphologic parameters requires an understanding of the scoring system and criteria employed by the testing laboratory, the most common being the Kruger criteria (Table 3) (13) and those established by the World Health Organization (WHO, Table 4) (1). The use of Kruger criteria offers a more detailed analysis of sperm morphology, evaluating the shape and size of the head, midpiece, and tail much more stringently than WHO standards. Kruger morphology can assist the clinician in determining the most appropriate reproductive

Table 3 Kruger Criteria

Strict criteria of sperm morphology established by Kruger et al. define normal spermatozoa as having an oval configuration with a smooth contour. The head length is 5–6 μm, the diameter (width) is 2.5–3.5 μm, and the width/length ratio is 1/2–3/5. The acrosome is well defined, comprising 40–70% of the distal part of the head. No abnormalities of the neck, midpiece, or tail and no cytoplasmic droplets of more than half of the sperm head are accepted. Borderline forms are considered abnormal.

The amorphous-head group is divided into two categories:
Slightly amorphous, with a head diameter of 2.0–2.5 μm, with slight abnormalities in the head's shape but with normal acrosome
Severely amorphous, with no acrosome at all and those with an acrosome smaller than 30% or larger than 70% of the sperm head; completely abnormal shapes also are put into this category.

Neck defects are also classified in two categories:
Slightly amorphous, referred to those sperm with debris around the neck or a thickened neck but with a normal-shaped head.
Severely amorphous, referred to those sperm with a bent neck or midpiece of more than 30%, or a severely amorphous head shape, as described.

All other abnormal sperm forms—round, small, large, tapered, double head, double or coiled tail, cytoplasmic droplets—are classified following the WHO classification (Table 4).

Normal and borderline forms grouped together are called "the morphology index." Patients with a morphology index less than 30% will have a severe reduction in fertilization as compared with patients having an index greater than 30%. In Kruger's practice, the normal forms considered alone are called the PIF. A PIF greater as 4% is considered favorable and less than 4% unfavorable. At least 200 cells per slide are to be evaluated. A micrometer in the eyepiece of the microscope is used for routine measurements.

Abbreviation: PIF, percentage of ideal forms.
Source: From Ref. 13.

Table 4 WHO Morphology Criteria for Assessing Normal Sperm Morphology[a]

Head
As an empirical reference value, 30% normal forms and above are considered normal. The head should be oval and smooth. Round, pyriform, pin, double, and amorphous heads are all abnormal. A normal spermatozoon has an oval head shape with regular outline and a well-defined acrosomal region covering 40–70% of head; vacuoles occupy less than 20% of the head area. Dimensions of the head: length: 4–5.5 μm, width: 2.5–3.5 μm, length/width ratio: 1.5–1.75 μm; no cytoplasmic droplets more than 1/3 of the size of a normal sperm head.

Midpiece
The midpiece should be straight and slightly thicker than the tail. No dimensions and no description of a normal midpiece are mentioned. Neck or midpiece defects include its being bent or abnormally thin.

Tail
The tail should be single, unbroken, straight, and without kinks or coils. No dimensions of a normal tail are mentioned. Tail defects include short, multiple hairpin, broken, irregular width or coiled tails, tails with terminal droplets, or any combination of these.

[a]A minimum of 100 sperm must be counted.
Source: From Ref. 1.

technique for the patient. Broadly viewed, profound abnormalities in morphology are associated with poor fertilizing capacity when strict criteria (Kruger) are used (9). Men with fewer than 40% perfectly shaped sperm usually fail to fertilize without micromanipulation. Large numbers of tapered sperms are seen in testes with elevated temperatures, such as varicocele, cryptorchid, or retractile testes, or in the testes of men who take saunas or hot baths.

While reference values are important in standardization, the current trend in using sperm morphology alone in predicting male fertility remains problematic, as overreliance on this characteristic can lead to misdiagnosis and unnecessary invasive treatment with intracytoplasmic sperm injection (ICSI) (14). Light microscopic examination of sperm morphology does not permit the visualization of many of the subcellular components vital for adequate sperm function (10). Consequently, morphologic assessment is subjective, qualitative, nonrepeatable, and difficult to teach to students and technicians. Nallella et al. (15) compared overlapping sperm characteristics among four groups of patients: men undergoing infertility evaluations, patients with established male factor infertility, healthy sperm donors, and men with proven fertility. It was shown that the parameters of sperm motility and concentration were the best discriminators of fertility versus infertility when compared to morphology.

Additional Considerations

It should be noted that even normal results on semen analysis cannot conclusively eliminate the presence of male factor infertility. Infections or sperm antibodies can diminish fertilizing capacity. Subtle biochemical abnormalities can result in defects in the sperm head that can be detected with sperm function tests such as the hamster oocyte penetration assay (see below). A thorough evaluation of the male partner is necessary in all cases of infertility. Reevaluation is important in men with a normal semen analysis when no cause of decreased fertility is apparent or when therapy in the woman fails to result in pregnancy.

Endocrine Evaluation

An initial endocrine evaluation should include checking at least serum testosterone (T) and follicle-stimulating hormone (FSH), but frequently luteinizing hormone (LH) is included as well. This should be performed if there is (i) an abnormally low sperm concentration, especially if less than 10 million/mL; (ii) impaired sexual function; or (iii) other clinical findings suggestive of hypogonadism. T is necessary for the development and maintenance of secondary sexual characteristics and libido, as well as for the initiation and maintenance of spermatogenesis (please refer to the chapters in Part I: Physiology of Male Reproductive Function for further details). Serum FSH crudely reflects the status of the seminiferous epithelium. Genital tract obstruction is suspected in men with azoospermia and/or severe oligospermia with normal serum FSH concentrations and normal-sized testes. Elevated serum FSH results from impaired secretion of inhibin, a Sertoli cell product that normally feeds back at the pituitary and hypothalamus to suppress FSH secretion and suggests abnormalities in the seminiferous epithelium, and, subsequently, spermatogenesis. An FSH level greater than two to three times the upper limits of normal suggests severely impaired seminiferous tubules, but this condition may still be treatable. LH is stimulatory to the Leydig cells and hence T production. Isolated LH abnormalities are very rare. LH levels may be obtained in men with abnormal T levels to determine whether hypogonadism is primary (testicular) or secondary (pituitary/hypothalamic) in origin.

Low levels of FSH, LH, and T are diagnostic of hypogonadotropic hypogonadism. These men have a delay or failure in the onset of puberty, and therefore poorly developed secondary sexual characteristics and small firm testes. T replacement will masculinize these men, but testicular growth and the initiation of spermatogenesis require gonadotropin replacement (16). Hypogonadotropic hypogonadism is usually due to a pituitary tumor, with the most common pituitary lesion being a benign prolactinoma. These are usually associated with a decreased libido, an elevated serum prolactin level, and decreased serum T and LH levels. Both macro- and microadenomas are often best treated with dopamine agonists such as bromocriptine or cabergoline (Dostinex). Serum estrogens, prolactin, and adrenal steroids are measured only if clinically indicated (low serum T, decreased libido, gynecomastia, or a history of precocious puberty). (For further information on this topic, please refer to Chapter 12.)

Genital Tract Imaging Studies

Transrectal ultrasonography is indicated in azoospermic patients with palpable vasa and low ejaculate volumes to determine if ejaculatory duct obstruction exists. Scrotal ultrasonography is indicated in those patients in whom physical examination of the scrotum is difficult or inadequate or in whom a testicular mass is suspected.

In the hands of an experienced sonographer, scrotal ultrasound with color flow Doppler is useful in the evaluation of questionable varicoceles, especially in obese men or men with a small, tight scrotum. The typical monographic criterion for the diagnosis of a varicocele is the presence of any internal spermatic veins greater than 3 mm in diameter associated with retrograde flow on Valsalva. Subclinical or questionable varicoceles are of limited clinical interest, as there is established data that have clearly shown that response to varicocelectomy is related to varicocele size (9). Men with large varicoceles sustain a greater improvement in semen quality following varicocele surgery than men with small or subclinical varicoceles.

Antisperm Antibody Testing

Antisperm antibodies can be produced either by the body of the male himself or by his female partner. Antisperm antibodies that are produced by the male and bound to sperm are associated with lower pregnancy rates. Risk factors for antibodies include torsion, epididymitis, orchitis, unilateral or partial obstruction, and large varicoceles. These are all conditions associated with impairment of the blood–testis barrier that usually prevents sperm antigens (which appear at puberty) from being exposed to the general circulation. An immunobead assay (Table 2) should be performed to detect antibodies on the sperm and in the serum. Antibodies adsorbed on the sperm surface can be detected by immunological assays using secondary, immunoglobulin (Ig) class-directed antibodies that are coupled to beads. The percentage of sperm adhering to the beads reflects in a semiquantitative manner the presence of antisperm antibodies. Mixed agglutination reaction (MAR)-test kits can detect antisperm-IgG in semen. Positive and dubious samples are subsequently tested for antisperm IgA (17). Some investigators have suggested that fertilization inhibition may be caused by a synergistic effect of IgG and IgA class antibodies in seminal plasma (18), as IgA antibodies rarely occur without associated IgG (19). Therefore, the test of

antisperm IgG antibodies in semen is sufficient for the first screening procedure. Antisperm IgG can be tested in serum, but this is of little benefit, as serum antisperm IgG does not correlate with antisperm Ig in semen and does not influence fertility prognosis.

High levels of antibodies are most often seen with obstruction, in particular before (in serum) and after (in serum and on sperm) vasectomy reversal. Low levels of antibodies on sperm and moderate levels in serum are usually seen in men with large varicoceles. A postcoital test is useful for evaluating sperm–cervical mucus interaction. A fair-to-good semen analysis associated with a poor postcoital test may suggest production of antisperm antibodies by the female partner and is usually considered an indication for intrauterine insemination (IUI). Although IUI can overcome cervical mucus antibodies or decreased counts, the success of IUI is dependent on the sperm's ability to fertilize an egg. Therefore prior to instituting IUI, a sperm penetration assay can be obtained that assesses the sperm's ability to bind and penetrate hamster oocytes, which have been rendered free of zona pellucida (20). Tests are interpreted as percent oocytes penetrated or sperm penetrations per oocyte. These tests are not perfect but do correlate about 80% with the ability to penetrate human eggs in vitro.

Other Special Investigations
Biochemical Analysis

Biochemical analysis (Table 2) of the secretory components from the prostate, seminal vesicles, and epididymis in semen give information about the functional state of these organs. These markers include fructose as a marker for the seminal vesicles, zinc, citric acid, or acid phosphatase as prostate markers, and α-glucosidase and carnitine as epididymal markers. Zinc can be measured by colorimetric assay, while fructose and carnitine are measured using enzymatic assays. (For further information on this topic, please refer to Chapter 24.) Seminal fructose is discussed below in further detail.

Seminal Fructose

Seminal fructose measurement is helpful in the evaluation of azoospermia (10). Fructose is normally produced by the seminal vesicles and transported into the vas deferens by the ejaculatory ducts; 13 mmol or more per ejaculate is considered normal (1). Absent seminal fructose usually indicates congenital absence of the seminal vesicles and vas deferens. Nonpalpable vas indicative of vasal agenesis is seen in 0.3% to 1.2% of infertile men and in up to 5% of azoospermic men (10). An examination of the scrotal contents of such patients may reveal the absence of the cauda epididymis and vas deferens. In most patients, an obstruction of the seminal excretory pathway occurs proximal to the excretory ducts of the seminal vesicles, with resultant normal semen fructose concentrations and normal testicular mass on examination. This may be the result of infectious damage or may be congenital in nature. Some patients may have both obstruction and germinal cell failure such as maturation arrest (the absence of mature spermatozoa) or Sertoli-cell-only syndrome, an idiopathic condition in which only Sertoli cells line the seminiferous tubules. These men will present with azoospermia and the absence of sperm in the ejaculate. In such cases, exploration, vasograms, and testicular biopsy studies may be needed to define the nature of the obstructive defect. Retrograde ejaculation is suggested by the presence of autonomic neuropathy and is most frequently seen in patients with diabetes mellitus. The presence of large numbers of sperm in the postejaculation urine specimen confirms the diagnosis.

Sperm Function Testing

As described above, abnormal sperm function may be evaluated further with sperm function tests. The evaluation of sperm interaction with cervical mucus (cervical mucus penetration test), the zona pellucida surrounding the oocyte (hemizona binding assay), or the oocyte itself (hamster-egg penetration assay) all require testing involving the female partner and are beyond the scope of this chapter (21,22). These specialized tests on semen are not required for the routine diagnosis of male infertility. They may be useful, however, in a small number of patients for identifying a male factor contributing to unexplained infertility, or for selecting therapy such as assisted reproductive technology.

Genetic Evaluation

Karyotyping and Y-chromosome analysis should be offered to the male who has nonobstructive azoospermia or severe oligospermia prior to performing ICSI. Genetic testing for the cystic fibrosis transmembrane conductance regulator (CFTR) mutations in the female partner should be offered before proceeding with treatments that utilize the sperm of men with congenital bilateral absence of the vas deferens (CBAVD). Normal serum FSH usually reflects normal spermatogenesis.

Testes biopsy and scrotal exploration are not necessary prior to therapy. (For further information on testicular biopsy, please refer to Chapters 25 and 33.) Because the vas deferens derives from the ureteral bud, CBAVD is associated with an 11% incidence of renal agenesis and abnormalities. A renal sonogram should be obtained in all men with CBAVD. Most men with CBAVD test positive for CFTR gene mutations, although they do not have any pulmonary manifestations of this disease. Typically, at this point, both the patient and the female partner are tested for cystic fibrosis CFTR gene mutations, and the couple must be referred for genetic counseling in order to have the opportunity to make a responsible and educated decision in choosing whether or not to pursue assisted reproductive technology (ART) (23).

Genetic counseling may be offered whenever a genetic abnormality is suspected in the male or female partner and should be provided whenever a genetic abnormality is detected (23). Men with nonobstructive azoospermia and severe oligospermia (less than 5–10 million sperm/mL) should be informed of the potential genetic abnormalities associated with azoospermia or severe oligospermia.

□ CONCLUSION

An initial screening evaluation of the male partner of an infertile couple should be done if pregnancy has not occurred within one year of unprotected intercourse. An earlier evaluation may be warranted if a known male or female infertility risk factor exists or if a man questions his fertility potential. The initial evaluation of male factor infertility should include comprehensive history taking, including a reproductive history, complete physical examination, and two properly performed semen analyses. Further, evaluation of the male partner should also be considered in couples with unexplained infertility and in couples in whom there is a treated female factor and persistent infertility.

☐ REFERENCES

1. World Health Organization. WHO Laboratory Manual for the Examination of Human Semen and Sperm-Cervical Mucous Interaction. 3rd ed. Cambridge, UK: Cambridge Press, 1992.

2. Crosignani PG, Rubin BL. Optimal use of infertility diagnostic tests and treatments. The ESHRE Capri Workshop Group. Hum Reprod 2000; 15(3): 723–732.

3. Honig SC, Lipshultz LI, Jarow J. Significant medical pathology uncovered by a comprehensive male infertility evaluation. Fertil Steril 1994; 62(5):1028–1034.

4. Kolettis PN, Sabanegh ES. Significant medical pathology discovered during a male infertility evaluation. J Urol 2001; 166(1):178–180.

5. Thonneau P, Marchand S, Tallec A, et al. Incidence and main causes of infertility in a resident population (1,850,000) of three French regions (1988–1989). Hum Reprod 1991; 6(6):811–816.

6. Jarow JP, Sharlip ID, Belker AM, et al. Best practice policies for male infertility. J Urol 2002; 167(5): 2138–2144.

7. Kim ED, Varicocele. http://www.emedicine.com/med/topic2757.htm, 2006.

8. Pasqualotto FF, Pasqualotto EB, Sobreiro BP, et al. Clinical diagnosis in men undergoing infertility investigation in a university hospital. Urol Int 2006; 76(2):122–125.

9. Cornell University, Weill Medical College. The Fertility Evaluation. Cornell Institute for Reproductive Medicine, Center for Male Reproductive Medicine and Microsurgery. http://www.maleinfertility.org/new-evaluation.html.

10. Swerdloff RS, Wang CW, Kandeel FR. Evaluation of the infertile couple. In: Young WF Jr, Klee GG, eds. Diagnostic Evaluation of Endocrine Disorders I. Endocrinology and Metabolism Clinics of North America. Vol. 17. 2nd ed. Philadelphia: WB Saunders Company, 1988.

11. Overstreet JW, Katz DF. Sperm transport, capacitations. In: Speroff L, Simpson JL, eds. Gynecology And Obstetrics Reproductive Endocrinology: Infertility And Genetics. Vol. 5. Philadelphia: JB Lippincott, 1981:1.

12. Eliasson R. Analysis of semen. In: Berrman SJ, Kistner RW, eds. Progress In Infertility. Boston: Little, Brown and Co, 1975:691.

13. Kruger TF, Acosta AA, Simmons KF, et al. Predictive value of abnormal sperm morphology in in vitro fertilization. Fertil Steril 1988; 49(1):112–117.

14. Chow V, Cheung AP. Male infertility. J Reprod Med 2006; 51(3):149–156.

15. Nallella KP, Sharma RK, Aziz N, et al. Significance of sperm characteristics in the evaluation of male infertility. Fertil Steril 2006; 85(3):629–634.

16. Liu PY, Handelsman DJ. The present and future state of hormonal treatment for male infertility. Hum Reprod Update 2003; 9(1):9–23.

17. Hjort T. Antisperm antibodies. Antisperm antibodies and infertility: an unsolvable question? Hum Reprod 1999; 14(10):2423–2426.

18. Culligan PJ, Crane MM, Boone WR, et al. Validity and cost-effectiveness of antisperm antibody testing before in vitro fertilization. Fertil Steril 1998; 69(5):894–898.

19. de Agostini A, Lucas H. Semen analysis. 9th Postgraduate Course for Training in Reproductive Medicine and Reproductive Biology. Department of Obstetrics and Gynecology, Geneva University Hospital. Geneva Foundation for Medical Education and Research. Online lecture, 2003. http://www.gfmer.ch/Endo/Lectures_09/semen_analysis.htm.

20. Schlegel PN, Girardi SK. Clinical review 87: in vitro fertilization for male factor infertility. J Clin Endocrinol Metab 1997; 82(3):709–716.

21. Liu DY, Baker HWG. Tests of human sperm function and fertilization in vitro. Fertil Steril 1992; 58(3):465–483.

22. Report on optimal evaluation of the infertile male. Baltimore, MD: American Urological Association, Inc.; 2001; 27.

23. Serebrovska ZA, Serebrovskaya TV, Pyle RL, et al. Transmission of male infertility and intracytoplasmic sperm injection (mini-review). Fiziol Zh 2006; 52(3): 110–118.

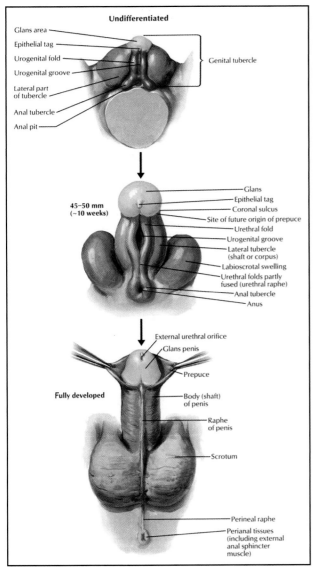

Figure 2.1 Differentiation of fetal penis and male gonads. *Source*: From Ref. 2.

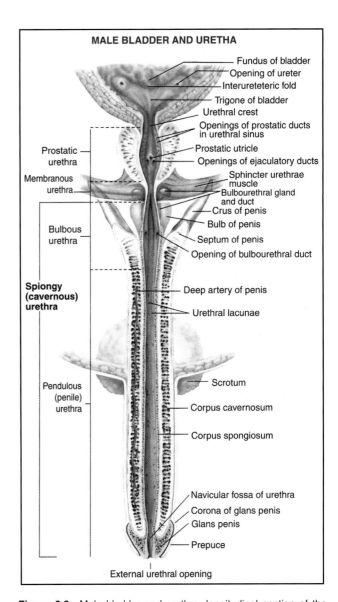

Figure 2.3 Male bladder and urethra: longitudinal section of the male penis, prostate, and bladder. The cross section through the penis also shows the urethra. *Source*: From Ref. 8.

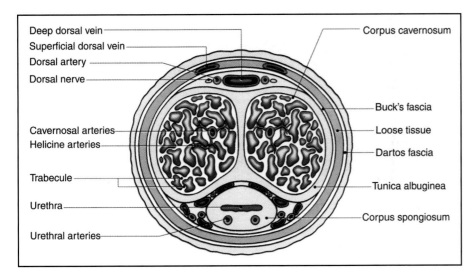

Figure 2.2 Cross section of the male penis showing the various structures. Note that the erectile tissue consists of two corpora cavernosa. Each corpus cavernosum is surrounded by a thick, fibrous sheath, the tunica albuginea. Each corpus has a centrally running cavernosal artery that supplies blood to the multiple lacunar spaces, which are interconnected and lined by vascular endothelium. *Source*: From Ref. 3.

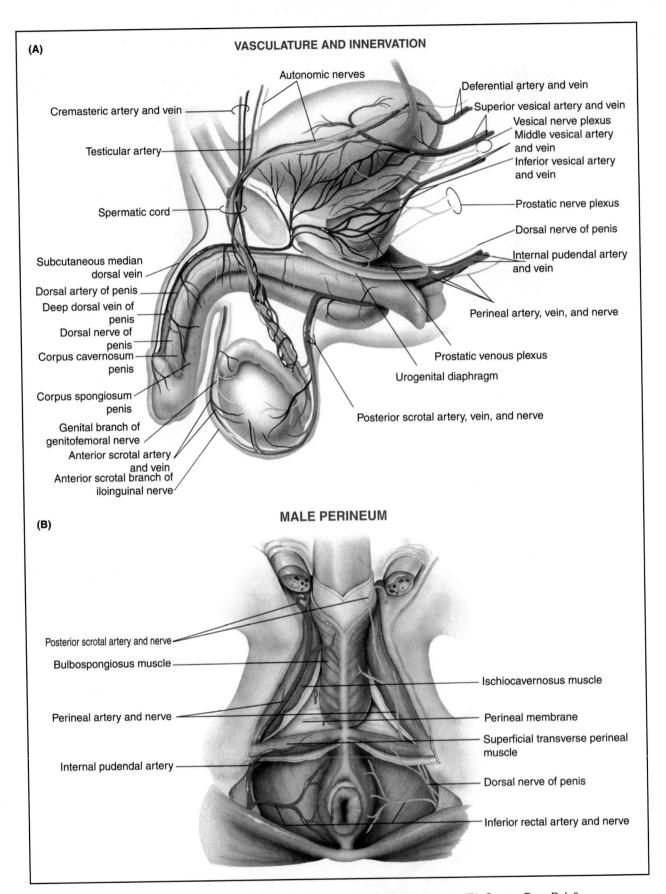

Figure 2.4 Vasculature and innervation of the male genitalia (**A**) and perineum (**B**). *Source*: From Ref. 8.

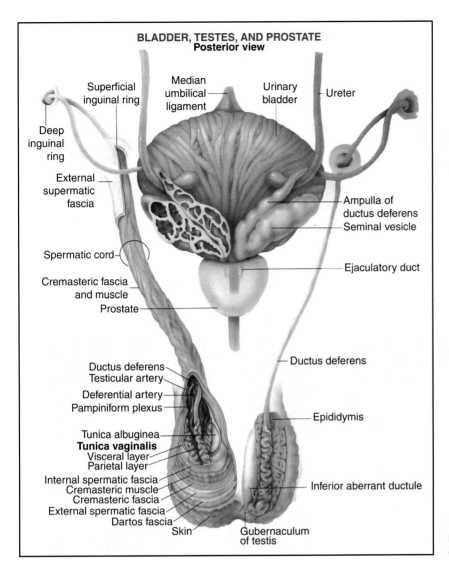

Figure 2.5 Bladder, testes, and prostate gland. *Source*: From Ref. 8.

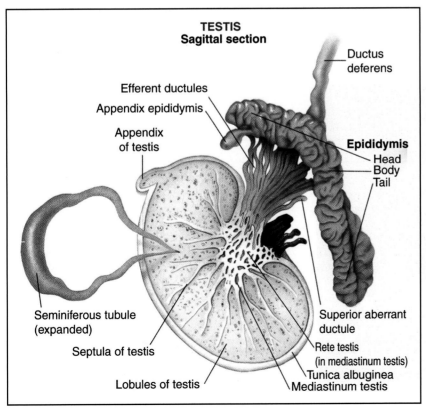

Figure 2.6 Testis and the epididymis, sagittal section. *Source*: From Ref. 8.

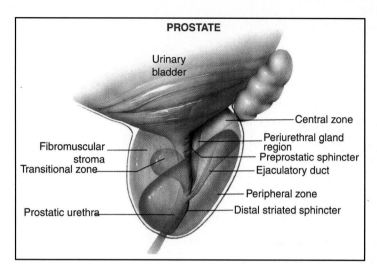

Figure 2.7 The prostate gland. *Source*: From Ref. 8.

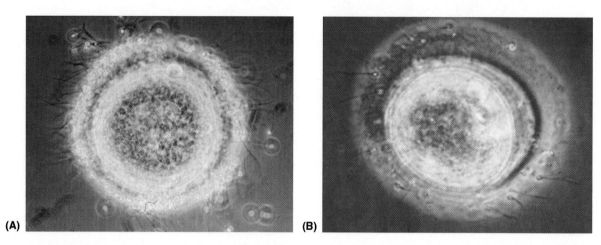

(A)   **(B)**

Figure 24.3 Oocyte after incubation with sperm and washing to remove loosely bound sperm (**A**), then after aspirating several times with a narrow bore glass pipette to shear off sperm bound to the surface of the zona pellucida leaving only those penetrating the zona pellucida or in the perivitelline space (**B**).

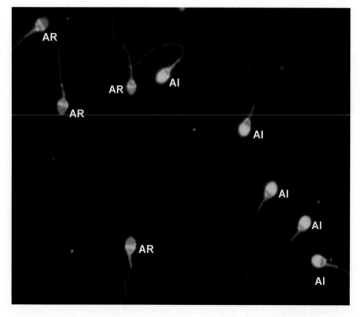

Figure 24.4 Sperm removed from the surface of the zona pellucida stained with pisum sativum agglutinin labelled with fluoresceine. Sperm with bright uniform fluorescence in the anterior part of the head are acrosome intact (AI). Those with bright fluorescence in the equatorial segment are acrosome reacted (AR).

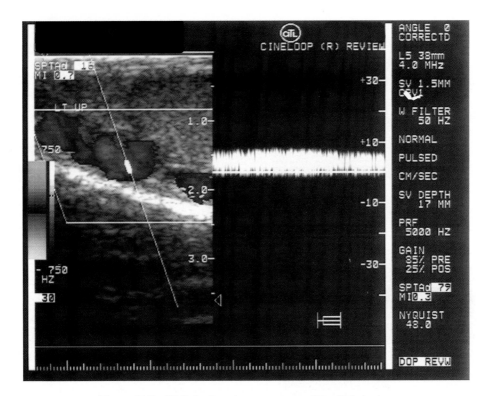

Figure 28.9 (**B**) Color Doppler appearance of the dilated veins.

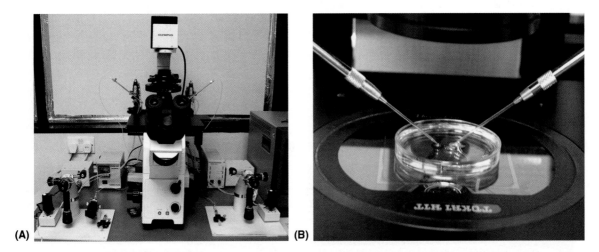

(A)   **(B)**

Figure 37.1 (**A**) Micromanipulation system that consists of: (1) a high-end inverted microscope, (2) pair of micromanipulators, (3) heating stage, (4) pair of micropipette holders, (5) a pair of injectors. (**B**) Micromanipulation set-up typically consists of a manipulation dish and two micopipettes.

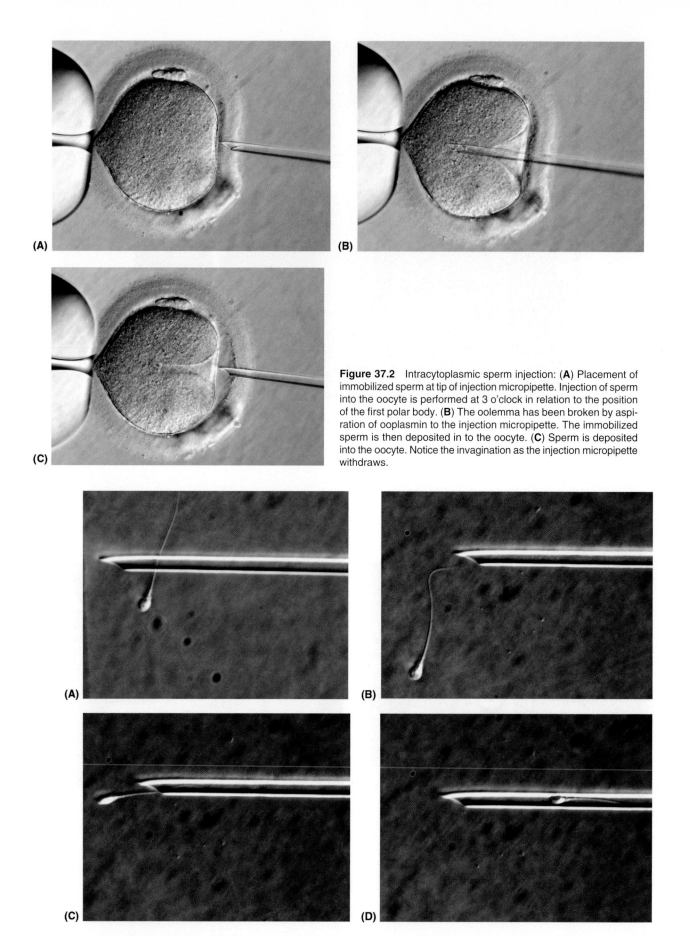

Figure 37.2 Intracytoplasmic sperm injection: (**A**) Placement of immobilized sperm at tip of injection micropipette. Injection of sperm into the oocyte is performed at 3 o'clock in relation to the position of the first polar body. (**B**) The oolemma has been broken by aspiration of ooplasmin to the injection micropipette. The immobilized sperm is then deposited in to the oocyte. (**C**) Sperm is deposited into the oocyte. Notice the invagination as the injection micropipette withdraws.

Figure 37.4 Immobilization of sperm: (**A**) A sperm is immobilized by crushing its tail by the injection micropipette. (**B–D**) Aspiration of immobilized sperm (tail-in) in to the injection.

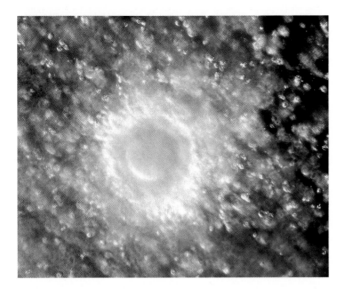

Figure 37.5 An oocyte retrieved by ovum pick-up (OPU). The oocyte is surrounded by hundreds of nurturing cumulus cells that are removed by hyaluronidase to assess its maturity stage (germinal vesicle, metaphase I or metaphase II) and for ICSI.

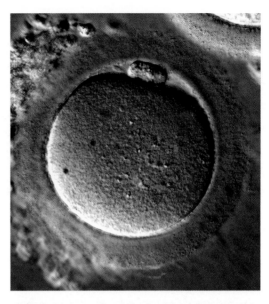

Figure 37.6 Human oocyte. A mature oocyte at metaphase II stage, partially denuded of its cumulus cells.

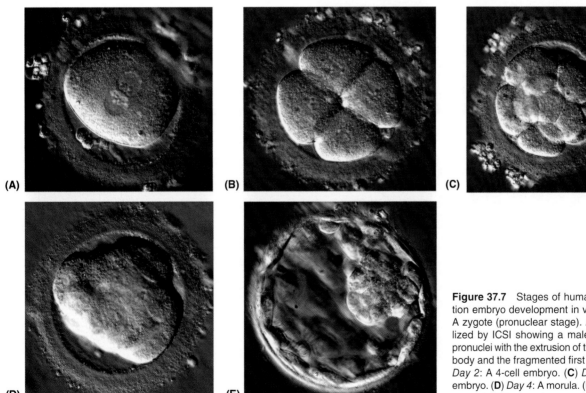

(A)

(B)

(C)

(D)

(E)

Figure 37.7 Stages of human preimplantation embryo development in vitro: (**A**) *Day 1*: A zygote (pronuclear stage). An oocyte fertilized by ICSI showing a male and a female pronuclei with the extrusion of the second polar body and the fragmented first polar body. (**B**) *Day 2*: A 4-cell embryo. (**C**) *Day 3*: An 8-cell embryo. (**D**) *Day 4*: A morula. (**E**) *Day 5*: A fully expanded blastocyst.

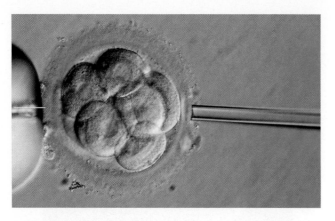

Figure 37.8 Assisted hatching of an 8-cell human embryo. Acidic Tyrode medium is used to thin the zona pellucida to assist hatching and implantation.

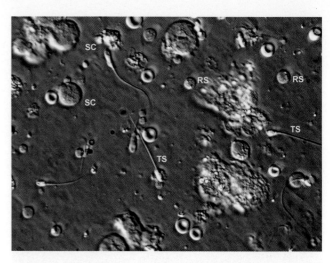

Figure 37.9 A testicular biopsy specimen showing immature sperm (TS), round spermatids (RS) and spermatocytes (SC).

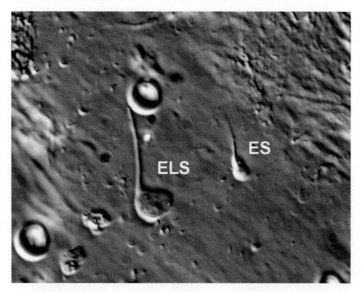

Figure 37.10 A testicular biopsy specimen showing an elongating spermatid (ELS) and an elongated spermatid (ES).

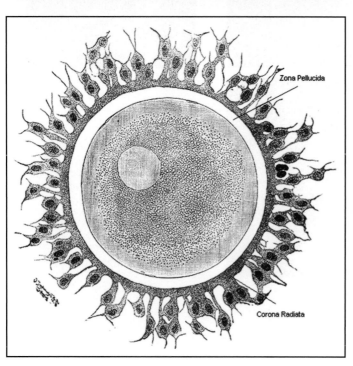

Figure 39.1 Human ovum. The zona pellucida is seen as a thick clear girdle surrounded by the cells of the corona radiata. The egg itself shows a central granular deutoplasmic area and a peripheral clear layer, and encloses the germinal vesicle, in which is seen the germinal spot. *Source*: From Ref. 96.

24

Semen Analysis and Sperm Function Testing

H. W. Gordon Baker

Department of Obstetrics and Gynaecology, University of Melbourne and The Royal Women's Hospital, Carlton, Victoria, Australia

Gary N. Clarke

Andrology Laboratory Division of Laboratory Services, The Royal Women's Hospital, Carlton, Victoria, Australia

De Yi Liu, Tanya M. Stewart, and Claire Garrett

Department of Obstetrics and Gynaecology, University of Melbourne, and The Royal Women's Hospital, Carlton, Victoria, Australia

☐ INTRODUCTION

In this chapter, we comment on standard semen analysis, computer-assisted semen analysis (CASA), sperm function tests (particularly of sperm–oocyte interaction), and some other assays currently used in clinical research. We also discuss evaluation of the clinical value of proposed new sperm tests. Details of methodology are omitted as these can be found in the literature. We concentrate on our own contributions.

☐ THE SCOPE OF MODERN SEMEN ANALYSIS

The process of semen analysis is critical in the management of patients with infertility. These techniques are also used to confirm that sperm have disappeared after vasectomy. Further, semen analyses are important research tools—for example in studies of factors affecting male reproductive health in the community (1). Although new methods of testing sperm, including CASA, have been developed over the last 30 years, the traditional semen analysis consisting of manual microscopy of sperm on slides and in counting chambers remains the standard method (2).

☐ STANDARD SEMEN ANALYSIS
World Health Organization Laboratory Manual

The World Health Organization (WHO) has made a significant contribution to improving techniques in semen analysis by producing successive revisions of the "WHO laboratory manual for the examination of human semen and sperm-cervical mucus interaction" (2). Although there are arguments about the tests included—for example, grades of motility, strict

assessment of morphology, and the need for duplicate assessments—the manual provides a useful reference that has gained wide acceptance as the standard for how semen analysis should be performed. It also has a substantial section in the fourth and later editions on quality control (QC) and the statistical aspects of counting and other errors involved in semen analysis.

Standard semen analysis requires macroscopic examination and measurement of the volume of the semen and microscopic measurement of sperm concentration and motility. The percentage of morphologically normal sperm is determined on a fixed and stained semen smear using oil immersion at a magnification of 1000×. All measurements involve counting at least 200 sperm in duplicate preparations. Each man is tested for sperm antibodies because none of the other aspects of the semen analysis is highly indicative of sperm autoimmunity and this condition would be missed without specific screening (see Chapters 26 and 36). We do not perform duplicate preparations as we consider that the mechanical mixing of semen samples and use of accurate automatic pipettes make sampling and dilution errors trivial when compared with counting error. We also use a simplified hematoxylin and eosin stain to expedite morphology assessment so that results can be available within the day of sample collection. Other tests are performed if indicated, such as sperm viability (determined by dye exclusion) for low sperm motility (<25% progressive) and seminal pH for azoospermia and low semen volume.

Errors of Semen Analysis: Measurement Uncertainty and QC

Semen analysis is subject to error. If the same semen sample is assessed in different laboratories, by different technicians within the same laboratory, or even by the same technician at different times, it is expected that the results will differ. There are a number of sources of error that result in measurement uncertainty (MU). The rigorous determination of MU is a complex process that requires careful calculation of the combined effect of all errors from each step in the testing process. Some laboratories report results that bear virtually no relationship to the true result as indicated by the results of large external quality assessment (EQA) schemes. For example, in the Australian External Quality Assurance Schemes for Reproductive Medicine, results for sperm concentration in 2006 for 144 laboratories had a wide range ($3.7–102 \times 10^6$/mL) for the same sample (3,4). For a laboratory that has each EQA result close to the All-Laboratory Trimmed Mean, a reasonable estimate of MU can be obtained by repeated analyses of pooled, well-mixed semen that has been cryopreserved. The ideal is to aim for a final sperm concentration around the normal range reference value of 20×10^6/mL after dilution with cryoprotectant and preferably a post-thaw motility in the mid-range of 30% to 50%. One of the frozen aliquots is analyzed daily (or, perhaps, weekly, but on different days each week) to take into account day-to-day changes in laboratory conditions including staff, reagents, ambient temperature, and so on. The results from approximately 30 analyses of the frozen pool can then be analyzed to estimate the MU for sperm concentration, motility, and morphology. For example, from the measurements, the mean, standard deviation, and coefficient of variation are calculated. The coefficient of variation is equivalent to the experimental standard deviation of the mean in MU terminology and is also known as the standard uncertainty (Uc). Next, calculate the expanded uncertainty (U) by multiplying the Uc by the coverage factor (2.04 for n=30), which is the t value for the appropriate degrees of freedom (n – 1). The laboratory then reports the MU at 20×10^6/mL + U with a confidence level of 95%. Further information on MU can be obtained at the ILAC website (3) or the APLAC website (4). The MU for different laboratories will vary depending on the procedures and the diligence of the laboratory manager and the staff in adhering to the procedure manual, care in the performance of the tests, equipment maintenance, and QC, including internal quality control (IQC) and EQA. There is unavoidable variability because only limited numbers of sperm can be assessed and there is additional variability due to preparation and assessment of samples (2). Good laboratory practice involves using procedures to minimize the latter variability from errors in sampling, dilution, chamber calibration and use, sperm counting, and calculation. Sampling errors can be a major source of variation because semen is not homogeneous on ejaculation and undergoes time-dependent coagulation and liquefaction. Sampling errors can be minimized by thorough mixing of specimens with a mechanical shaking stage or wheel, by carefully controlled syringing of specimens that have increased viscosity or aggregation and by correct pipetting techniques. Dilution errors can be minimized by using larger semen aliquots (e.g., 25–100 μL) and positive displacement pipettes that are

tested regularly for accuracy and precision. Using a standard technique and fixed volume minimizes errors of chamber filling. Regulating the workload of the scientists and QC can minimize counting and calculation errors.

QC involves monitoring ongoing performance. We have regular QC days when all laboratory staff perform "blind" readings on samples. This allows monitoring of intralaboratory precision and each scientist can gauge his performance against the laboratory mean. Weekly means QC charts are used to detect "drift" or unacceptable fluctuation in results (5). This type of QC is useful in our laboratory, which typically has a stable input of samples—mostly from patients being investigated for infertility—but may go out of control if the patient mix varies. EQA programs provide information on the overall agreement between laboratories (6–9). It is acknowledged, however, that no standards are available for semen analysis, that EQA is not performed under the same conditions as those used on fresh samples, and there can be significant differences between results of different EQA programs (7,10). We generally have our quarterly sperm concentration results within one standard deviation of the Australian laboratory EQA results. Thus, while technicians can be trained to produce results close to the theoretical counting error for sperm concentration, motility, and morphology, the wide variation in results between laboratories demonstrated by EQA indicates that standardization has not been achieved. In particular, sperm morphology is assessed very differently by different groups. Some prefer a strict assessment in which sperm with marginal defects of shape are considered abnormal, as this predicts low fertilization rates with standard in vitro fertilization (IVF) (2,11). Others find it ludicrous that fertile men could have 95% of their sperm classified as abnormal (12). Therefore, the clinician needs to be very familiar with his own laboratory in order to interpret patients' results, and researchers involved in multicenter studies need to establish centralized analyses of the semen or adjust results based on interlaboratory EQA.

☐ COMPUTER-ASSISTED SEMEN ANALYSIS

Image analysis and computer automation might have been expected to overcome the counting and interpretation errors associated with manual semen analysis; however, this has been difficult to achieve in practice. The human eye easily distinguishes sperm from similarly sized debris, but this is quite difficult with image analysis. This identification problem is compounded by the increase in the ratio of debris to sperm in poor semen samples. Early CASA equipment did not identify sperm accurately and gave inaccurate sperm concentrations and percentage motilities. In addition, collisions of motile sperm with other sperm or debris cause sperm concentration-dependent ambiguities for CASA assessment (2,13). Better image analysis and inclusion of sperm DNA staining with fluorescent dyes has improved the accuracy of CASA sperm counting. Assessment of sperm morphology remains a significant problem and full automation and standardization of sperm morphometry is not yet available commercially. Compared with manual methods of semen analysis, we believe that image analysis provides a major improvement in efficiency and reliability as well as new measures of sperm motion and morphology that are of prognostic value. Further exploration of other parameters of sperm motion and morphology will refine the clinical usefulness of CASA; however, CASA requires careful technical application and critical surveillance to achieve high levels of accuracy and reproducibility.

Kinematics

Even the earliest CASA systems allowed the trajectories of sperm to be analyzed in considerable detail, and the potential of newly derived "kinematic" measures of sperm motion, such as average straight-line velocity (VSL), were explored. Such measures may ultimately prove more clinically useful than classification assessments of percentage motility. We have found VSL is significantly related to fertilization rates in vitro and naturally conceived pregnancy rates in subfertile couples (see subsequently).

CASA for Routine Semen Analysis

For several years, our clinical laboratory has used the Hamilton–Thorne Motility Analyzer IVOS with Ident module and a specific protocol for routine measurement of sperm concentration, percentage progressive motility, and VSL for samples with sperm concentrations greater than 2×10^6/mL. The analyses are done at 37°C with bisbenzamide fluorescent DNA stain diluted 1:1 in Tyrode buffer with 5% bovine serum albumin to improve differentiation of sperm from debris. It is necessary to dilute samples with high sperm concentration with seminal plasma obtained by centrifuging the patient's semen at 16,000 G for five minutes in a mini centrifuge. Disposable 20 μ-deep MicroCell chambers are used, and it is essential to sample fields regularly across the counting chamber because of nonuniformity in the distribution of sperm caused by streaming while filling the chamber (14,15). Ideally, a minimum of 400 sperm is included in the analysis. As indicated above, IQC and EQA are good. Reproducibility for the IVOS system for repeated measurements on the same sample is better than that achieved by the technicians using the WHO manual methods: sperm concentration (~80× 10^6/mL) coefficient of variation 5.4%, progressive motility (~30%) 7.4%, and VSL (~35 μm/sec) 4.0%.

Morphometry

Early sperm morphometry was limited to quantification of sperm head dimensions, area, and regularity.

Some systems produce the conventional dichotomous classification of "normal" sperm based on some protocol such as strict morphology. Such classifications usually reflect the morphology of typical sperm in the semen of fertile men rather than characteristics of sperm capable of fertilization. It is recommended that selection of CASA variables should be based on a relevant functional end point (16). It is not possible to ascertain the fertilizing potential of the individual spermatozoon for direct comparison with its morphometry; however, it is possible to identify morphometric selectivity with some physiological end points such as sperm penetration of cervical mucus or sperm binding to the zona pellucida (ZP) of human oocytes (17). Image analysis enables identification of this selectivity for specific morphometric parameters. We have performed extensive studies comparing the sperm head morphometry of sperm in semen after swim-up and after binding to the ZP and found that a subset of 12 morphometry parameters exhibited significant selectivity. Selected sperm characteristics can be summarized as longitudinally symmetric heads, no neck anomalies, and a large acrosomal region. Interestingly, several parameters important to conventional classification of "normal" sperm, such as absolute head dimensions, elongation, and deviation from elliptical shape of the posterior region of the head, did not show significant selection (17). We defined a ZP-preferred morphometry (%Z) as the percentage of sperm in a sample conforming to within 1.5 SD of the optimal values of the 12 parameters. In a large follow-up study of natural pregnancies in subfertile couples, we found the most important factor was %Z (18). VSL and female age were also independently but less significantly related to pregnancy rate (see subsequently).

□ SPERM FUNCTION TESTS

During fertilization in vivo, sperm penetrate cervical mucus, traverse the female genital tract, penetrate the cumulus–corona complex of the oocyte, and then bind to the ZP, undergo the acrosome reaction (AR), penetrate the ZP, and finally fuse with the oolemma before entering the ooplasm. Tests of sperm functions involved in these events should provide useful information about fertility. Such tests should also give insights into sperm physiology and pathology. Several sperm function tests have been developed, covering the processes of capacitation (e.g., hyperactivated motility), sperm–mucus penetration, and sperm–oocyte interaction.

Sperm–Oocyte Interaction

Overstreet et al. first studied sperm–ZP binding and penetration using nonviable human oocytes (19,20). They also showed that human ZP could be stored in concentrated salt solution for use in sperm–ZP binding tests. In 1988, we developed the sperm–ZP binding ratio test using oocytes that had failed to fertilize during clinical IVF, and Burkman et al. developed a similar test, the hemizona assay (21,22). Extensions and modifications of the basic test have been developed for assessing other aspects of sperm–oocyte interaction, including sperm–ZP penetration, ZP-induced AR (ZPIAR), and sperm–oolemma binding (11,23).

Sources of Human Oocytes

Human oocytes are needed for tests of human sperm–ZP binding because human sperm usually do not bind to the ZP of other oocytes of other species (24,25). Oocytes that fail to fertilize in conventional clinical IVF provide an abundant source since 20% to 30% of oocytes are immature or fail to fertilize. Our patients sign consent forms permitting the use of their unfertilized gametes for research or test procedures. Most oocytes that show no evidence of two pronuclei or cleavage at 48 hours to 60 hours after insemination in the clinical IVF program are suitable for use. Although they have been exposed to sperm in IVF and their quality, age, and cortical granule reaction are unknown, the majority (>80%) are capable of binding sperm on reincubation with test sperm (21,26,27). Unfertilized oocytes with the ZP penetrated by a few (<10) sperm after IVF insemination have a similar capacity for subsequent sperm–ZP binding and ZPIAR compared with those with no sperm penetration (27). If the oocytes have sperm remaining bound to the ZP after the IVF insemination, these can be removed by repeated aspiration using a fine glass pipette with an inner diameter slightly smaller than the oocyte diameter (120 µm) (27,28). Immature (germinal vesicle or metaphase I) oocytes not suitable for intracytoplasmic sperm injection (ICSI) can also be used for the sperm–oocyte interaction tests; however, morphologically abnormal, degenerate or spontaneously activated oocytes are unsuitable. We find salt-stored oocytes are not useful for the tests of sperm penetration or ZPIAR (27).

Sperm–ZP Binding Tests

A test based on competitive binding of two differently labelled sperm populations incubated with the same group of oocytes allows variation in ZP to be controlled. A mixture of equal numbers of motile test and control sperm selected by swim-up or density gradient centrifugation and labeled with the fluorochromes fluorescein isothiocyanate (FITC) and tetramethylrhodamine isothiocyanate is incubated for two hours with a group of four oocytes. Loosely attached sperm are dislodged by aspiration with a large bore (250–300 µm) pipette and the number of sperm remaining tightly bound to the ZP are counted with a fluorescence microscope and the ratio of test to control sperm is calculated (21). For a simpler screening test not requiring control sperm, groups of four oocytes are incubated with 2×10^6 motile test sperm in 1 mL (Fig. 1). Under these experimental conditions of high insemination sperm concentration (20 times higher standard IVF

insemination), the number of sperm bound tightly to the ZP is greater than 100/ZP for fertile men. Samples with an average of less than 40 sperm per ZP are considered to have low binding (29,30).

ZPIAR Test

A simple method for assessment of the ZPIAR has been developed (27,31). Following the screening method (above) for sperm–ZP binding, the tightly bound sperm are sheared off the surface of the ZP by repeated aspiration using a glass pipette that is slightly smaller than the diameter of the oocyte (120 µm inner diameter). The ZP-bound sperm recovered from the four oocytes are collected and smeared on a glass slide and stained with Pisum sativum agglutinin labeled with FITC (Fig. 1). Sperm with more than half the head brightly and uniformly fluorescing under a fluorescence microscope have an intact acrosome and the percentage of ZPIAR is calculated after counting 200 sperm. As sperm must be alive and motile to bind to the ZP, there is no need to assess sperm viability.

Sperm–ZP Penetration Test

The technique developed to remove sperm bound to the surface of the ZP leaves sperm with their heads embedded in the ZP or perivitelline space (Fig. 1). These ZP-penetrating sperm are easy to count and histological examination of serial cross sections of some oocytes has confirmed the accuracy of this method (28). This test identifies defective sperm–ZP penetration. There is a strong correlation between the ZPIAR and sperm–ZP penetration. Men with ZPIAR above 20% have sperm penetrating the ZP of the majority of oocytes (27).

Sperm–Oolemma Binding Ratio Test

This test is similar to the sperm–ZP binding ratio test (32). The ZP is removed by brief exposure to acidified (pH 2.5–3.0) saline with repeated aspiration using a glass pipette under a dissecting microscope. Once the ZP dissolves, the oocyte is immediately transferred to culture medium supplemented with protein and washed with three to four changes of the medium over 30 to 60 minutes. Usually four ZP-free oocytes are incubated with a mixture of test and control sperm labeled with the different fluorochromes. We find that defective sperm–oolemma binding is an uncommon cause for failure of fertilization in clinical IVF (32). This test is useful, however, for studying the mechanism of sperm–oocyte interaction (33).

Alternative Tests

Since the source of test oocytes is limited, development of recombinant human ZP, particularly ZP3 (rhZP3) protein for tests of sperm–ZP binding and the ZPIAR, has been investigated. Although several groups have produced rhZP3, it is not consistently active (34–38). We expressed rhZP1, 2, and 3 alone or in combination

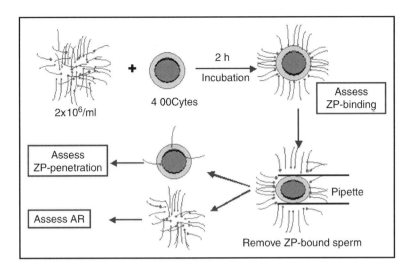

Figure 1 Combined test for sperm–ZP binding, sperm–ZP penetration and the ZP-induced AR. Four oocytes are incubated with 2×10^6/mL motile sperm (prepared by swim-up or colloidal silica gradient centrifugation) for two hours. The number of sperm tightly bound to the ZP is counted and then removed for assessment of AR (ZP-induced AR). The oocytes are then examined for sperm–ZP penetration. *Abbreviations*: AR, acrosome reaction; ZP, zona pellucida.

in a human kidney cell line to produce recombinant proteins glycosylated in a human pattern, but none bound sperm or induced the AR (39).

Most studies of the AR in the literature involve model systems (membrane preparations and permeabilized sperm) and other stimuli (progesterone and calcium ionophore), which may not provide useful information about the physiological human AR. For example, we have shown that there is no relationship between ZPIAR and either the calcium ionophore induced AR or the spontaneous AR occurring with incubation (27,40). In contrast, there is a close relationship between ZPIAR and the AR induced with solubilized ZP (27,41). There is currently no substitute for human ZP and therefore human oocytes that fail to fertilize in clinical IVF remain a valuable resource (23).

Sperm and Oocyte Characteristics Related to Sperm–Oocyte Interaction

Abnormalities in either sperm or oocyte could affect sperm–ZP interaction. In clinical IVF, there is no relationship between the number of sperm bound to the ZP and oocyte quality or maturity assessed morphologically and oocyte quality is not a common cause for low average sperm–ZP binding and penetration affecting all or most oocytes collected from the one patient (42,43). Complete failure of fertilization in standard IVF with low sperm–ZP binding or failure of sperm–ZP penetration is usually the result of sperm defects rather than oocyte defects (43).

Several sperm characteristics affect the sperm–ZP interaction. Before the advent of ICSI, low sperm binding to oocytes in clinical IVF was usually due to obvious sperm defects of motility or morphology (11,44,45). Sperm bind to the ZP by the plasma membrane overlying the flat surface of the acrosome; this probably explains why normal sperm morphology had such a highly significant relationship with IVF fertilization rates (Fig. 2) and also why %Z morphometry is

related to natural pregnancy rate in subfertile couples (18). Both the ZP and oolemma are selective for binding sperm with normal morphology (26,28). Sperm with gross head abnormalities such as amorphous or small heads with a small acrosome area do not bind well to the ZP (28). Also, a normal intact acrosome is required for sperm–ZP binding (26,33,46). Round-headed sperm without an acrosome do not bind to or penetrate the ZP (47). Sperm motility, concentration, and the proportion of sperm with a normal intact acrosome in the insemination medium are all correlated with sperm–ZP binding (21,42,48–50). The sperm–ZP binding test reflects multiple sperm functions, which is reflected in a highly significant correlation with fertilization rate in standard IVF (11,23).

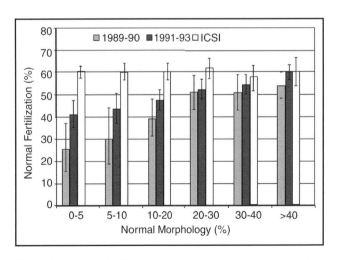

Figure 2 Average fertilization rates related to strict sperm morphology assessed by manual semen analysis before IVF treatment in different eras: 1989 to 1990 oocytes incubated with 2×10^5/mL motile sperm, 1991 to 1993 oocytes incubated with up to 2×10^6/mL motile sperm if normal sperm morphology <10%, ICSI introduced in 1993 and used for patients with oligospermia and teratospermia. Error bars show 95% confidence limits. *Abbreviations*: ICSI, intracytoplasmic sperm injection; IVF, in vitro fertilization.

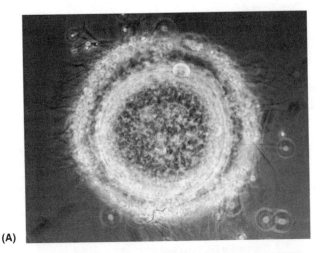

(A)

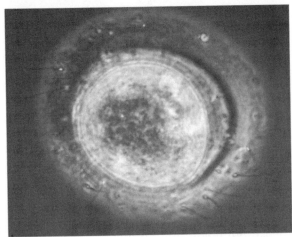

(B)

Figure 3 (*See color insert.*) Oocyte after incubation with sperm and washing to remove loosely bound sperm (**A**), then after aspirating several times with a narrow bore glass pipette to shear off sperm bound to the surface of the zona pellucida leaving only those penetrating the zona pellucida or in the perivitelline space (**B**).

Insights into Sperm Physiology and Pathology Resulting from Research on Human Sperm–Oocyte Interaction

Our work in developing human sperm–oocyte interaction tests has lead to a number of interesting findings that exemplify the value of the human sperm–oocyte interaction tests for clinical research.

Only a Limited Proportion of Motile Sperm Are Capable of Sperm–Oocyte Interaction

The sperm–ZP binding test was modified to provide excess ZP-binding sites by repeated exposure of the same sperm in a small droplet to successive groups of 10 oocytes. This enabled estimation of the proportion of motile sperm that are capable of binding to the ZP (30). We found that less than 25% (average 14%, range 8–25%) of motile sperm from normal fertile men were able to bind to the ZP (30). Also, only an average of 48% of ZP-bound sperm undergo the AR (51). Thus, we estimate that only an average of less than 7% of motile sperm in fertile men can bind to the ZP and

subsequently undergo an acrosome reaction. This low proportion of human sperm capable of oocyte penetration has important implications for clinical tests of sperm-fertilizing ability, particularly for developing improved sperm morphology assessments (see "Morphometry" above). It also underlines the need to assess the subpopulation of sperm capable of interacting with the ZP, rather than the whole sperm population in semen or those that are free-swimming in the culture medium.

Defects of Sperm–Oocyte Interaction

Two major defects of sperm–ZP interaction have been identified from application of the combined sperm–ZP binding and ZPIAR tests (Fig. 1). Defective sperm–ZP binding (DSZPB) is defined as an average of less than 40 sperm bound/ZP when four oocytes are incubated with 2×10^6/mL motile sperm and disordered ZP-induced AR (DZPIAR) is defined as less than 16% ZPIAR.

There are two types of DSZPB. Type I DSZPB patients have obvious sperm abnormalities including oligospermia, asthenospermia, or teratospermia, often in combination. Morphological defects of sperm head shape are common to this group who make up about 70% of patients with DSZPB (11,23). Type II DSZPB patients have no obvious abnormalities in routine semen analysis and diagnosis can only be made by sperm–ZP binding tests or failure of sperm–ZP binding in standard IVF. Type II DSZPB might have defective or absent ZP-binding sites in the sperm plasma membrane. Further investigations of patients with type II DSZPB may reveal the human sperm receptors for the ZP. Our studies show that about 13% of men with unexplained infertility have DSZPB II (23,43).

In 1994, we first reported the sperm defect called DZPIAR. This defect was the cause of failure of

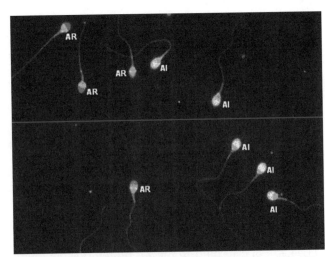

Figure 4 (*See color insert.*) Sperm removed from the surface of the zona pellucida stained with pisum sativum agglutinin labeled with fluoresceine. Sperm with bright uniform fluorescence in the anterior part of the head are acrosome intact (AI). Those with bright fluorescence in the equatorial segment are acrosome reacted (AR).

sperm–ZP penetration in a group of patients with a long duration of infertility and persistent zero or low (<30%) fertilization rates with standard IVF (31). They had complete failure of sperm–ZP penetration despite normal sperm–ZP binding. When sperm were tested with other patients' oocytes, ZPIAR was low (mean 6.5%, range 1–16%, normal: mean 53%, range 27–98%). These patients were previously classified as having idiopathic infertility since they had normal sperm analysis, no sperm autoimmunity, normal nuclear maturity, acridine orange (AO) staining of DNA, and normal acrosomes assessed by fluorescent lectin staining and electron microscopy. ICSI is very effective for these patients (52,53).

We had suspected the existence of this condition from observations that the ZPIAR for a sample is highly correlated with the proportion of oocytes showing ZP penetration by sperm from that sample (27,29,46,53). Also, incubation with a trypsin inhibitor prevented sperm penetration of the ZP while not affecting sperm motility or ZP-binding ability (54). Subsequently, in a prospective study of 65 patients undergoing standard IVF, we found those with ZPIAR below 16% had a low (average, 23%) fertilization rate (53). The frequency of low ZPIAR is high in patients with idiopathic infertility (normal semen): 25%, pre-IVF patients with normal semen: 29%, teratozoospermia (strict normal sperm morphology < 5% with normal sperm concentration) 48%, and oligozoospermia (sperm concentration $<20\times10^6$/mL): 69% (23,29, 43,51,53,55,56). We also found that ZPIAR was related to sperm concentration, low ZPIAR being more frequent in patients with sperm concentrations below 60×10^6/mL (23).

The existence of DZPIAR proves the critical importance of the ZPIAR for human fertility; however, the causes of DZPIAR are currently unknown. The biochemical mechanisms including the signal transduction and effector pathways of the human ZPIAR are poorly understood (57). Lengthening the time of preincubation of sperm did not increase the ZPIAR in the patients, suggesting it is not due to inadequate capacitation. Transmission EM shows the sperm bound to the ZP of fresh oocytes had intact outer acrosomal and overlying plasma membrane (PM); indicating that defective dispersal of the acrosome was not the cause of DZPIAR (31). Deficient or defective acrosin is not likely to cause DZPIAR because the patients had normal acrosin by gelatine slide test (31). Also, although they have delayed fertilization, acrosin knockout mice are not infertile (58,59). A similar phenotype with infertility due to reduced ZPIAR and sperm–ZP penetration has been reported in transgenic mice with disruption of two forms of phospholipase C (PLC), PLCδ4, or PLCδ1 (60,61); however, collaborative studies showed no difference in total PLC activity or expression of PLCδ4 in the sperm of DZPIAR and fertile men. This suggests that human DZPIAR is unlikely to be commonly caused by defects of PLCδ4 (60).

Studies of the Biochemical Pathways Involved in Human Sperm–Oocyte Interaction

Immunofluorescence with the monoclonal antibody PY20 labeled with FITC localizes tyrosine phosphorylated proteins mainly in the principal piece in capacitated human sperm. The proportion of tyrosine phosphorylated human sperm is related to sperm–ZP binding (62,63). This can be differentially modulated by osmolality of the culture medium (64).

Using different fluorescent markers for actin and acrosome contents on the same human sperm, we showed that actin was present in the acrosomal region but was lost following the AR (65). Blocking actin polymerization with cytochalasin B or D strongly inhibited the ZPIAR and an anti-actin monoclonal antibody had a similar effect (65,66). During in vitro culture, about 10% of motile sperm expose actin on the plasma membrane over the equatorial segment and acrosome. This actin on the outer surface of the PM can be detected with a monoclonal antibody and second antibody-coated beads or immunofluorescence (66,67). About 50% of the sperm removed from the ZP after binding display actin on the surface and this is correlated with the proportion of sperm in the insemination medium exposing actin (67). We suspect this phenomenon is related to sperm capacitation or preparation of sperm for ZP binding and the ZPIAR.

Immunohistological studies show protein kinase C-α (PKCα) in the acrosomal region (68). PKC stimulation with phorbol myristate acetate (PMA) and inhibition with staurosporine, calphostin C, sangivamycin, and bisindolylmeleimide have major effects on the ZPIAR (68,69).

We also reported that PMA induces a marked change in acrosomal shape. Many acrosomes had an irregular wavy appearance similar to ruffling of the plasma membrane of migrating cells in culture (69). Although PMA was unable to stimulate the AR in the absence of ZP, the percentage of sperm with ruffling was correlated with the PMA-enhanced ZPIAR. We also showed that actin polymerization is involved as cytochalasin B and C significantly reduced PMA-induced acrosomal ruffling. At this stage, the role of this ruffling in normal sperm–oocyte interaction is uncertain.

Clinical Application of Sperm–Oocyte Interaction Tests

In the clinical management of male infertility, if the prognosis for natural conception is low and there are no treatable conditions (such as genital tract obstruction, gonadotrophin deficiency, coital disorders, and reversible toxin exposure or illness), a decision must be made between offering standard IVF or ICSI (70). Standard IVF is preferred where fertilization is likely to occur since it has a lower cost and may produce more usable embryos. The choice is generally based on the results of semen analysis; however, standard semen analysis provides only limited information about sperm-fertilizing ability since many patients with sperm defects cannot be identified. In most clinics, unexplained infertility is usually treated by standard IVF. If this fails in the initial cycle, then ICSI would be used subsequently. Choice of first treatment in patients with idiopathic infertility and isolated teratozoospermia may be aided by results of sperm–oocyte interaction tests. Patients with normal results should do well with IVF, whereas those with low ZP binding or ZPIAR below 16% require ICSI.

□ SPERM CHROMATIN, DNA, AND OTHER TESTS

The mechanisms involved in the cause of common forms of male infertility associated with oligospermia, asthenospermia, and teratospermia are not understood. Abnormal sperm produce reactive oxygen species that could damage sperm DNA and result in defects of implantation or pregnancy loss (71); however, the results of ICSI to date do not reveal such problems (72). It is possible that abnormal sperm with redundant cytoplasm are excluded in natural or assisted fertilization by poor or zero motility and sperm aggregation caused by heavy coating with clusterin (73). There is a correlation between sperm with abnormal morphology and motility, and abnormal sperm DNA measured by a variety of techniques, including AO fluorescence and the sperm chromatin structure assay (74,75). There are similar correlations with other techniques that measure DNA strand breaks, including chromomycin staining and the terminal transferase dUTP nick end labeling (TUNEL) and comet assays (76).

AO Fluorescence

In a large study performed before the introduction of ICSI, we found a highly significant positive relationship between fertilization rate in IVF and the percentage of normal sperm assessed by the microscopic AO test, independent of other sperm characteristics (44). A flow cytometry acridine orange test (FCM-AOT) of sperm chromatin integrity involving DNA denaturation by exposure to acid was developed by Evenson (74). Red and green fluorescence intensities are measured for individual sperm and the resulting red–green cytograms are generally summarized in terms of the percentage of sperm with an abnormally high proportion of red to total fluorescence (DFI) (76). We found that FCM-AOT is efficient and the results are highly reproducible due to the rapid multiparametric analysis of large numbers of cells by FCM (75). FCM-AOT variables display significant correlations with motility (r=−0.557), vitality (r=−0.469), and morphology (r=−0.464, n=201), which are similar in magnitude to correlations between the standard semen variables. In a large group of IVF/ICSI patients, we showed DFI had additional predictive value for fertilization rates in standard IVF but could not confirm relationships with of implantation rate or pregnancy loss (75).

There are some problems with the FCM-AOT methodology and interpretation of the results. The DFI changes with acid concentration, and the acid denaturation medium is not appropriately buffered. There is no relationship between DFI and the percentage of normal sperm assessed in the microscopic AOT (75). The mechanism of some patterns of AO fluorescence from sperm is unclear. FCM-AOT performed on motile sperm in swim-up samples shows a major reduction in red fluorescence over that seen in semen, consistent with DFI being related to the proportion of dead sperm in the ejaculate. Also, a high number of FCM events from swim-up samples fall within the red and green fluorescence background gates set for semen samples. Cell sorting might help identify the nature of the different populations. It is possible that cellular debris may contribute to the abnormal DNA signal, particularly in samples with low sperm concentration that limit testing of oligospermic samples.

□ ASSESSMENT OF THE VALUE OF SPERM TESTS

Despite the advances in methodology, semen analysis and other sperm tests remain subject to misinterpretation. In addition, some methods of testing sperm have reached clinical usage stage but have been found to be of limited value. For example, the zona-free hamster oocyte penetration test was expected to improve semen testing, but in practice, it did not prove useful for predicting fertilization rates with standard IVF (2). It is important that innovations in semen analysis be investigated in detail by prospective studies to establish their value before they are introduced into the clinic.

Interpretation of Semen Analysis

Subject and collection factors may affect the results of semen analysis to the extent that these always need to be considered in the interpretation of results. For example, classical patterns of semen abnormality can be caused by incomplete collection, spillage, exposure of sperm to high or low temperatures, contamination with sperm toxins, or coincidental illness in the man (Table 1). Semen analysis results can also be extremely variable from day to day (77). Some of this variation may be attributable to illness, variations in the length of abstinence before the semen analysis, or a patient's exposure to heat. Often, however, there is no clear explanation. It is important that unless the clinical diagnosis dictates otherwise, patients have at least two semen analyses performed several weeks apart to guide discussions about prognosis for natural conception.

Relationships of Sperm Tests with Standard IVF

Investigation of the causes of failure of fertilization in standard IVF and the relationship between results of

Table 1 Pathological and Extraneous Causes of Semen Abnormalities

Volume (mL) 1–6[a]	Concentration (10^6/mL)>20[a]	Motility (%)>50	Normal morphology (%)>15	Comment	Pathological cause	Extraneous cause
0.4	0	–	–	Fructose 1 nmol/L (low) pH 6.5 (low)	Congenital absence of vasa Ejaculatory duct obstruction Partial retrograde ejaculation Testicular failure with androgen deficiency	Spill, incomplete collection
4.0	0	–	–	Fructose 15 nmol/L	Genital tract obstruction Primary seminiferous tubal failure Drugs: opiates, androgens	Transient impairment of spermatogenesis: illness Secondary seminiferous tubule failure with androgen treatment
3.0	100	0	35	Live 70%	Immotile cilia	Contamination condom collection
3.0	100	5	35	Live 20%	Necrospermia contamination Temperature effect: low or high	Delayed examination Sperm autoimmunity

[a]Normal range.

sperm tests and fertilization rates should provide useful information about the sperm tests relevant to fertility (21). There are a large number of publications on the relationships of various tests of sperm function, including sperm–oocyte interaction tests and fertilization rate in IVF (11). Some of the studies have also included oocyte characteristics such as maturity (presence of germinal vesicle and number of polar bodies) and morphological quality (good, fair, and poor) (21). Most of the studies involve sperm function tests performed on sperm from the same ejaculate as that used for insemination of oocytes in IVF. The results are analyzed using multiple logistic regression to determine which groups of sperm function results or oocyte factors are independently significantly related to fertilization rate. In general, the sperm–oocyte interaction tests, including sperm–ZP penetration and sperm–ZP binding assessed by either the ZP-binding ratio or the hemizona assay, were found to be most significantly related to fertilization rate (11,23). Sperm morphology assessed by strict criteria was also highly significant in the regression models (Fig. 2) (21). Other semen variables such as mean VSL and microscopic AOT were related to fertilization rates in some studies (44,78). The spontaneous AR of sperm in the insemination medium was inversely related to fertilization rate (49). Although some studies showed that the calcium ionophore A23187-induced AR may be useful for prediction of IVF, we found a significant correlation between the ionophore-induced AR and fertilization rate only in patients with teratozoospermia (79). The ionophore-induced AR was not correlated with either the ZPIAR or sperm–ZP penetration and so does not reflect the capacity of sperm to undergo the physiological AR (27,40). Many other sperm characteristics, including total sperm count, motility, hypo-osmotic swelling, nuclear maturity (acidic aniline blue stain), total acrosin activity, and oocyte morphological characteristics were not significant (11,48–50). Because the sperm concentration, motility, and morphology are all significantly related to sperm–ZP binding, sperm–ZP interaction tests reflect multiple sperm functions. This is likely why results of sperm–ZP interaction tests were so significantly related to standard IVF (11).

The use of fertilization rate in standard IVF as a surrogate for human fertility for evaluating sperm tests is no longer available because ICSI is used when the semen is not normal to minimize the risk of low or zero fertilization rates with standard IVF (72,80). Thus, the relationships between semen analysis results and IVF are not as strong since the introduction of ICSI (11,23). Tests of sperm function, particularly of sperm–oocyte interaction, can also be used as indicators of fertility but these tests are not widely available and have low precision (23).

Relationships of Sperm Tests with Natural Conception Rates

Normal reference ranges for semen tests can be determined by assessing semen in groups of men presumed to be fertile (because their partners are pregnant or have children) or infertile (because they present to infertility clinics) and then applying statistical techniques developed for screening tests, such as receiver operator curves, to determine cut-off values for each semen parameter; however, this is generally an unsatisfactory way of advancing the clinical evaluation of male fertility. Not only is the critical female component not considered in such evaluations, but also most patients seen for infertility are subfertile and may conceive if a sufficient number of attempts are made. Therefore, the time element needs to be included in the analysis. An additional issue is the interrelatedness of semen variables in groups of subjects: generally, sperm concentration, motility, and normal morphology are correlated. Regression modeling to select groups of variables that significantly affect the pregnancy rate independently is useful to select the important semen variables and to determine if a new test adds to the model or replaces previously significant factors. The nature of the relationship between a semen variable and pregnancy rate can also be investigated to determine if it is continuous or discontinuous and if there is evidence of the latter where the discontinuity occurs. This has been called a threshold effect, meaning there is a level below which fertility decreases with decreasing values of the variable and above which there is no effect. A slope–threshold logistic regression model has been used to identify the threshold for sperm concentration (81,82). A remaining problem is that semen variables usually explain only a small part of the variance of pregnancy rate if absolute problems are excluded, such as azoospermia.

Although studies to determine which groups of prognostic factors are related to pregnancy rates are important for the management of infertility and for understanding the nature of human fertility, these are not simple to perform. Such studies require extensive follow-up of large numbers of subjects to achieve sufficient statistical power (18,83). There are only a limited number of studies relating semen quality to fertility via pregnancy rate, determined either retrospectively or prospectively (18,81–86). Reported threshold levels vary for example for concentration: 20×10^6/mL (84), 40×10^6/mL (81), 55×10^6/mL (82), and for strict morphology 8% (86) and 18% (82), while others find no threshold effect (18,83,86). Other semen test results and subject characteristics are also variably reported to affect pregnancy rates such as sperm motility and coital frequency (84). Some find no effect of semen volume or sperm motility (81,82).

We performed a follow-up study (70) of 1367 subfertile couples initially investigated for male infertility between 1970 and 1984 who were not known to have an absolute barrier to fertility such as persistent azoospermia or bilateral tubal obstruction in the female partner. On follow up over six years, 448 couples conceived without receiving any effective treatment. Life table analysis showed about 30% conceived by one year and 45% by two years. Cox proportional hazards regression analysis was used to explore factors affecting pregnancy rates, which included in order of significance and direction: duration of infertility (negative), mean sperm concentration at initial testing (positive), previous fertility for the male (positive), size of left varicocele (positive), female age (negative), and sperm autoimmunity (negative) (70). Treatments such as varicocelectomy had no significant effect on pregnancy rate (83); however, these prognostic factors although statistically significant only explained 17% of the variance in pregnancy rates. Interestingly, sperm concentration and sperm autoimmunity (defined as positive sperm antibodies and failure of sperm-cervical mucus penetration) (see Chapters 26 and 36) were the only semen factors significant in the regression model. In a subsequent study of subfertile patients who conceived and were matched with similar patients who remained infertile, however, we found that sperm motility was higher in the oligospermic subjects who conceived (87). It is possible the relationship between sperm motility and fertility in such groups of subfertile couples may also be obscured by the inclusion of patients with necrospermia, who appear to have a better-than-expected prognosis for natural conception (88,89).

We conducted another follow-up study in the late 1990s of natural conceptions in 1191 subfertile couples to test the predictive value of the morphometry assessment %Z based on the "ZP-preferred" characteristics. We found %Z, VSL, and female age were independently significantly related to the pregnancy rate. (18). Intriguingly, the pregnancy rates in this study at one (30%) and two (45%) years were similar to those of the earlier study (83).

□ CONCLUSIONS AND FUTURE DIRECTIONS

Semen analysis and sperm function tests are complex procedures that require considerable care in performance and interpretation. CASA can be used routinely for sperm concentration and motility and reliable morphology by computer image analysis should be possible in the near future; however, clinically important severe abnormalities such as azoospermia and severe oligospermia cannot be assessed by CASA. Sperm–oocyte interaction tests remain difficult to perform routinely because of the requirement for human oocytes from an IVF program. Development of tests based on recombinant human zona proteins has not been successful. Although the sperm–ZP binding and ZPIAR tests may be useful for directing patients with idiopathic and mild male infertility to standard IVF or ICSI, a prospective trial to test this is unlikely to be performed because of the ethical limitations. These tests will therefore continue to be used mainly for research. FCM may be useful but it is an expensive technology and not possible on low numbers of sperm. In the future, identification of specific protein abnormalities by proteomic analysis of sperm pathologies, defects of ZP binding sites, or other indicators of functional competence such as actin exposure may provide new tests that will improve semen analysis. Most importantly, any new tests will require thorough preclinical evaluation in large prospective studies to prove their value for predicting fertility.

□ REFERENCES

1. McLachlan RI, Baker HWG, Clarke GN, et al. Semen analysis: its place in modern reproductive medical practice. Pathology 2003; 35(1):25–33.
2. World Health Organization Laboratory Manual For The Examination Of Human Semen And Sperm-Cervical Mucus Interaction. Cambridge: Cambridge University Press, 1999.
3. http://www.ilac.org.
4. http://www.ianz.govt.nz/aplac.
5. Clarke GN. A simple monthly means chart system for monitoring sperm concentration. Hum Reprod 1997; 12(12):2710–2712.
6. Neuwinger J, Behre HM, Nieschlag E. External quality control in the andrology laboratory: an experimental multicenter trial. Fertil Steril 1990; 54(2):308–314.
7. Cooper TG, Bjorndahl L, Vreeburg J, et al. Semen analysis and external quality control schemes for semen analysis need global standardization. Int J Androl 2002; 25(5):306–311.
8. Matson PL. External quality assessment for semen analysis and sperm antibody detection: results of a pilot scheme. Hum Reprod 1995; 10(3):620–625.
9. Brazil C, Swan SH, Tollner CR, et al. Quality control of laboratory methods for semen evaluation in a multicenter research study. J Androl 2004; 25(4):645–656.
10. Auger J, Eustache F, Ducot B, et al. Intra- and inter-individual variability in human sperm concentration, motility and vitality assessment during a workshop involving ten laboratories. Hum Reprod 2000; 15(11):2360–2368.
11. Liu DY, Baker HWG. Tests of human sperm function and fertilization in vitro. Fertil Steril 1992; 58:465–483.
12. Eliasson R. Basic semen analysis. In: Matson P, ed. Current Topics in Andrology. Perth: Ladybook Publishing, 2003:35–89.
13. Ismail MTM, Howard EJ, Baker HWG. Comparative study of standard methods of semen analysis and correlation of their results to cellsoft's tm. Malaysian J Reprod Health 1988; 6: 59–63.
14. Douglas-Hamilton DH, Smith NG, Kuster CE, et al. Capillary-loaded particle fluid dynamics: effect on estimation of sperm concentration. J Androl 2005; 26(1): 115–122.
15. Douglas-Hamilton DH, Smith NG, Kuster CE, et al. Particle distribution in low-volume capillary-loaded chambers. J Androl 2005; 26(1):107–114.
16. ESHRE. Consensus workshop on advanced diagnostic andrology techniques. ESHRE (european society of human reproduction and embryology) andrology special interest group. Hum Reprod 1996; 11(7):1463–1479.
17. Garrett C, Liu DY, Baker HWG. Selectivity of the human sperm-zona pellucida binding process to sperm head morphometry. Fertil Steril 1997; 67(2):362–371.
18. Garrett C, Liu DY, Clarke GN, et al. Automated semen analysis: 'zona pellucida preferred' sperm morphometry and straight-line velocity are related to pregnancy rate in subfertile couples. Hum Reprod 2003; 18(8): 1643–1649.
19. Overstreet JW, Hembree WC. Penetration of the zona pellucida of nonliving human oocytes by human spermatozoa in vitro. Fertil Steril 1976; 27(7):815–831.
20. Overstreet JW, Yanagimachi R, Katz DF, et al. Penetration of human spermatozoa into the human zona pellucida and the zona-free hamster egg: a study of fertile donors and infertile patients. Fertil Steril 1980; 33(5):534–542.
21. Liu DY, Lopata A, Johnston WI, et al. A human sperm-zona pellucida binding test using oocytes that failed to fertilize in vitro. Fertil Steril 1988; 50(5):782–788.
22. Burkman LJ, Coddington CC, Franken DR, et al. The hemizona assay (hza): development of a diagnostic test for the binding of human spermatozoa to the human hemizona pellucida to predict fertilization potential. Fertil Steril 1988; 49(4):688–697.
23. Liu DY, Garrett C, Baker HW. Clinical application of sperm-oocyte interaction tests in in vitro fertilization—embryo transfer and intracytoplasmic sperm injection programs. Fertil Steril 2004; 82(5):1251–1263.
24. Bedford JM. Sperm/egg interaction: the specificity of human spermatozoa. Anat Rec 1977; 188(4):477–487.
25. Liu DY, Lopata A, Pantke P, et al. Horse and marmoset monkey sperm bind to the zona pellucida of salt-stored human oocytes. Fertil Steril 1991; 56(4):764–767.
26. Liu DY, Baker HWG. Morphology of spermatozoa bound to the zona pellucida of human oocytes that failed to fertilize in vitro. J Reprod Fertil 1992; 94(1):71–84.
27. Liu DY, Baker HWG. A simple method for assessment of the human acrosome reaction of spermatozoa bound to the zona pellucida: lack of relationship with ionophore a23187-induced acrosome reaction. Hum Reprod 1996; 11(3):551–557.
28. Liu DY, Baker HWG. A new test for the assessment of sperm zona pellucida penetration—relationship with results of other sperm tests and fertilization in vitro. Hum Reprod 1994; 9(3):489–496.
29. Liu DY, Clarke GN, Martic M, et al. Frequency of disordered zona pellucida (zp)-induced acrosome reaction in infertile men with normal semen analysis and normal spermatozoa-zp binding. Hum Reprod 2001; 16(6): 1185–1190.
30. Liu DY, Garrett C, Baker HWG. Low proportions of sperm can bind to the zona pellucida of human oocytes. Hum Reprod 2003; 18(11):2382–2389.
31. Liu DY, Baker HWG. Disordered acrosome reaction of sperm bound to the zona pellucida: a newly discovered sperm defect with reduced sperm-zona pellucida penetration and reduced fertilization in vitro. Hum Reprod 1994; 9:1694–1700.

32. Liu DY, Lopata A, Baker HWG. Use of oocytes that failed to be fertilized in vitro to study human sperm-oocyte interactions: comparison of sperm-oolemma and sperm-zona pellucida binding, and relationship with results of IVF. Reprod Fertil Dev 1990; 2(6):641–650.

33. Liu DY, Baker HWG. Inducing the human acrosome reaction with a calcium ionophore a23187 decreases sperm-zona pellucida binding with oocytes that failed to fertilize in vitro. J Reprod Fertil 1990; 89(1):127–134.

34. van Duin M, Polman JE, De Breet IT, et al. Recombinant human zona pellucida protein zp3 produced by Chinese hamster ovary cells induces the human sperm acrosome reaction and promotes sperm-egg fusion. Biol Reprod 1994; 51(4):607–617.

35. Brewis IA, Clayton R, Barratt CL, et al. Recombinant human zona pellucida glycoprotein 3 induces calcium influx and acrosome reaction in human spermatozoa. Mol Hum Reprod 1996; 2(8):583–589.

36. Whitmarsh AJ, Woolnough MJ, Moore HD, et al. Biological activity of recombinant human zp3 produced in vitro: potential for a sperm function test. Mol Hum Reprod 1996; 2(12):911–919.

37. Dong KW, Chi TF, Juan YW, et al. Characterization of the biologic activities of a recombinant human zona pellucida protein 3 expressed in human ovarian teratocarcinoma (pa-1) cells. Am J Obstet Gynecol 2001; 184(5):835–843; discussion 843–834.

38. Tanphaichitr N, Haebe J, Leader A, et al. Towards a more precise assay of sperm function in egg binding. J Obstet Gynaecol Can 2003; 25(6):461–470.

39. Martic M, Moses EK, Adams TE, et al. Recombinant human zona pellucida proteins zp1, zp2, and zp3 co-expressed in a human cell line. Asian J Androl 2004; 6(1):3–13.

40. Liu DY, Baker HWG. Relationship between the zona pellucida (zp) and ionophore a23187-induced acrosome reaction and the ability of sperm to penetrate the zp in men with normal sperm-zp binding. Fertil Steril 1996; 66(2):312–315.

41. Baker HW, Liu DY, Garrett C, et al. The human acrosome reaction. Asian J Androl 2000; 2(3):172–178.

42. Liu DY, Lopata A, Johnston WI, et al. Human sperm-zona pellucida binding, sperm characteristics and in-vitro fertilization. Hum Reprod 1989; 4(6):696–701.

43. Liu DY, Baker HWG. Defective sperm-zona pellucida interaction: a major cause of failure of fertilization in clinical in-vitro fertilization. Hum Reprod 2000; 15(3):702–708.

44. Liu DY, Baker HWG. Sperm nuclear chromatin normality: relationship with sperm morphology, sperm-zona pellucida binding, and fertilization rates in vitro. Fertil Steril 1992; 58(6):1178–1184.

45. Liu DY, Clarke GN, Lopata A, et al. A sperm-zona pellucida binding test and in vitro fertilization. Fertil Steril 1989; 52(2):281–287.

46. Liu DY, Baker HWG. Acrosome status and morphology of human spermatozoa bound to the zona pellucida and oolemma determined using oocytes that failed to fertilize in vitro. Hum Reprod 1994; 9(4):673–679.

47. Bourne H, Liu DY, Clarke GN, et al. Normal fertilization and embryo development by intracytoplasmic sperm injection of round-headed acrosomeless sperm. Fertil Steril 1995; 63(6):1329–1332.

48. Liu DY, Elton RA, Johnston WI, et al. Spermatozoal nuclear chromatin decondensation in vitro: a test for sperm immaturity. Comparison with results of human in vitro fertilisation. Clin Reprod Fertil 1987; 5(4):191–201.

49. Liu DY, Baker HWG. The proportion of human sperm with poor morphology but normal intact acrosomes detected with pisum sativum agglutinin correlates with fertilization in vitro. Fertil Steril 1988; 50(2):288–293.

50. Liu DY, Baker HWG. Relationships between human sperm acrosin, acrosomes, morphology and fertilization in vitro. Hum Reprod 1990; 5(3):298–303.

51. Liu DY, Stewart T, Baker HWG. Normal range and variation of the zona pellucida-induced acrosome reaction in fertile men. Fertil Steril 2003; 80(2):384–389.

52. Liu DY, Bourne H, Baker HWG. High fertilization and pregnancy rates after intracytoplasmic sperm injection in patients with disordered zona pellucida-induced acrosome reaction. Fertil Steril 1997; 67(5):955–958.

53. Liu DY, Baker HWG. Disordered zona pellucida-induced acrosome reaction and failure of in vitro fertilization in patients with unexplained infertility. Fertil Steril 2003; 79(1):74–80.

54. Liu DY, Baker HWG. Inhibition of acrosin activity with a trypsin inhibitor blocks human sperm penetration of the zona pellucida. Biol Reprod 1993; 48(2):340–348.

55. Liu DY, Baker HWG. Frequency of defective sperm-zona pellucida interaction in severely teratozoospermic infertile men. Hum Reprod 2003; 18(4):802–807.

56. Liu DY, Baker HWG. High frequency of defective sperm-zona pellucida interaction in oligozoospermic infertile men. Hum Reprod 2004; 19(2):228–233.

57. Barratt CL, Publicover SJ. Interaction between sperm and zona pellucida in male fertility. Lancet 2001; 358(9294):1660–1662.

58. Baba T, Azuma S, Kashiwabara S, et al. Sperm from mice carrying a targeted mutation of the acrosin gene can penetrate the oocyte zona pellucida and effect fertilization. J Biol Chem 1994; 269(50):31845–31849.

59. Adham IM, Nayernia K, Engel W. Spermatozoa lacking acrosin protein show delayed fertilization. Mol Reprod Dev 1997; 46(3):370–376.

60. Fukami K, Nakao K, Inoue T, et al. Requirement of phospholipase Cdelta4 for the zona pellucida-induced acrosome reaction. Science 2001; 292(5518):920–923.

61. Choi D, Lee E, Hwang S, et al. The biological significance of phospholipase C beta 1 gene mutation in mouse sperm in the acrosome reaction, fertilization, and embryo development. J Assist Reprod Genet 2001; 18(5):305–310.

62. Visconti PE, Bailey JL, Moore GD, et al. Capacitation of mouse spermatozoa. I. Correlation between the capaci-

tation state and protein tyrosine phosphorylation. Development 1995; 121(4):1129–1137.

63. Liu DY, Clarke GN, Baker HW. Tyrosine phosphorylation on capacitated human sperm tail detected by immunofluorescence correlates strongly with sperm-zona pellucida (zp) binding but not with the zp-induced acrosome reaction. Hum Reprod 2006; 21(4):1002–1008.

64. Liu DY, Clarke GN, Baker HW. Hyper-osmotic condition enhances protein tyrosine phosphorylation and zona pellucida binding capacity of human sperm. Hum Reprod 2006; 21(3):745–752.

65. Liu DY, Martic M, Clarke GN, et al. An important role of actin polymerization in the human zona pellucida-induced acrosome reaction. Mol Hum Reprod 1999; 5(10):941–949.

66. Liu DY, Martic M, Clarke GN, et al. An anti-actin monoclonal antibody inhibits the zona pellucida-induced acrosome reaction and hyperactivated motility of human sperm. Mol Hum Reprod 2002; 8(1):37–47.

67. Liu DY, Clarke GN, Baker HW. Exposure of actin on the surface of the human sperm head during in vitro culture relates to sperm morphology, capacitation and zona binding. Hum Reprod 2005; 20(4):999–1005.

68. Liu DY, Baker HWG. Protein kinase c plays an important role in the human zona pellucida-induced acrosome reaction. Mol Hum Reprod 1997; 3(12):1037–1043.

69. Liu DY, Martic M, Grkovic I, et al. Phorbol myristate acetate induces ruffling of the acrosome of human sperm. Fertil Steril 2002; 78(1):128–136.

70. Baker HWG. Male infertility. In: DeGroot LJ, Jameson JL, eds. Endocrinology. Philadelphia: Elsevier Saunders, 2006:3199–3225.

71. Aitken RJ. Koopman P, Lewis SE. Seeds of concern. Nature 2004; 432(7013):48–52.

72. Baker HWG. Marvellous ICSI: the viewpoint of a clinician. Int J Androl 1998; 21(5):249–252.

73. O'Bryan MK, Murphy BF, Liu DY, et al. The use of anti-clusterin monoclonal antibodies for the combined assessment of human sperm morphology and acrosome integrity. Hum Reprod 1994; 9(8):1490–1496.

74. Evenson D, Jost L. Sperm chromatin structure assay: DNA denaturability. Meth Cell Biol 1994; (42 Pt B):159–176.

75. Apedaile AE, Garrett C, Liu DY, et al. Flow cytometry and microscopic acridine orange test: relationship with standard semen analysis. Reprod Biomed Online 2004; 8(4):398–407.

76. Evenson DP, Larson KL, Jost LK. Sperm chromatin structure assay: its clinical use for detecting sperm DNA fragmentation in male infertility and comparisons with other techniques. J Androl 2002; 23(1):25–43.

77. Mallidis C, Howard EJ, Baker HWG. Variation of semen quality in normal men. Int J Androl 1991; 14(2):99–107.

78. Liu DY, Clarke GN, Baker HWG. Relationship between sperm motility assessed with the hamilton-thorn motility analyzer and fertilization rates in vitro. J Androl 1991; 12(4):231–239.

79. Liu DY, Baker HWG. Calcium ionophore-induced acrosome reaction correlates with fertilization rates in vitro in patients with teratozoospermic semen. Hum Reprod 1998; 13(4):905–910.

80. Harari O, Bourne H, McDonald M, et al. Intracytoplasmic sperm injection—a major advance in the management of severe male subfertility. Fertil Steril 1995; 64(2):360–368.

81. Bonde JP, Ernst E, Jensen TK, et al. Relation between semen quality and fertility: a population-based study of 430 first-pregnancy planners. Lancet 1998; 352(9135): 1172–1177.

82. Slama R, Eustache F, Ducot B, et al. Time to pregnancy and semen parameters: a cross-sectional study among fertile couples from four european cities. Hum Reprod 2002; 17(2):503–515.

83. Baker HWG, Burger HG, de Kretser DM, et al. Testicular vein ligation and fertility in men with varicoceles. Br Med J (Clin Res Ed) 1985; 291(6510):1678–1680.

84. MacLeod J, Gold R. The male factor in fertility and infertility. VI. Semen quality and certain other factors in relation to ease of conception. Fertil Steril 1953; 4:10–33.

85. Sherins RJ. Are semen quality and male fertility changing? N Engl J Med 1995; 332(5):327–328.

86. Zinaman MJ. Brown CC, Selevan SG, et al. Semen quality and human fertility: a prospective study with healthy couples. J Androl 2000; 21(1):145–153.

87. Zaini A, Jennings MG, Baker HWG. Are conventional sperm morphology and motility assessments of predictive value in subfertile men? Int J Androl 1985; 8(6): 427–435.

88. Wilton LJ, Temple-Smith PD, Baker HWG, et al. Human male infertility caused by degeneration and death of sperm in the epididymis. Fertil Steril 1988; 49(6): 1052–1058.

89. Fang S, Baker HWG. Male infertility and adult polycystic kidney disease are associated with necrospermia. Fertil Steril 2003; 79(3):643–644.

25

Testicular Biopsy of the Infertile Male

Brett C. Mellinger

Department of Clinical Urology, SUNY Stony Brook, Stony Brook, New York, U.S.A.

☐ INTRODUCTION

Testicular biopsy is utilized to assess testicular spermatogenesis qualitatively in the infertile male. The value of this procedure was demonstrated in the 1940s by early reports from Charny (1) and Hotchkiss (2). The primary role of testis biopsy is to distinguish patients with ductal obstruction who are candidates for reconstructive surgery from patients with ablative testicular pathology that is not amenable to conventional therapies. Very little has changed over the last 60 years regarding the surgical technique, methods of processing tissue, and interpretation of the histopathology; however, with the advent of intracytoplasmic sperm injection (ICSI) and published results of live births achieved with testicular sperm (3), the indications for performing testis biopsy have expanded.

There are two main types of testicular biopsy: fine needle aspiration (FNA) and percutaneous testicular biopsy. FNA of the testis has been described as a minimally invasive method of obtaining testis tissue for cytological evaluation.

FNA cytology has been shown to demonstrate high correlation with histological studies (4). Few clinicians have access to flow cytometry and cytological analysis, however, limiting the routine use of this technique in clinical practice. Additionally, most male reproductive specialists have the knowledge and experience to accurately evaluate testicular histology.

Percutaneous testicular biopsy has been described and has been shown to correlate well with the standard open biopsy technique (5). This technique has the advantages of an office-based, minimally invasive procedure: less patient anxiety, quick return to normal activity, and reduced costs.

This chapter will review the absolute and relative indications for performing testicular biopsy in the evaluation of the infertile male. The different methods of performing testicular biopsy will be described, as well as the methods for processing the tissue. The more common histopathological findings will be presented and described. These techniques for performing testicular biopsy for diagnostic purposes can be utilized when performing therapeutic testicular biopsy for sperm retrieval/ICSI. This chapter, however, will primarily focus on the diagnostic aspects.

☐ INDICATIONS
Azoospermia

Patients with azoospermia due to anatomical obstruction or ejaculatory disorders often present with historical or physical findings suggestive of obstruction. Infertile men who are candidates for testicular biopsy are selected after the performance of a thorough history, physical examination, and specific laboratory studies.

The most common absolute indication is in the male with normal size and consistency of the testes, with follicle-stimulating hormone (FSH) levels less than two to three times the upper limit of normal. The primary role of the biopsy is to determine if spermatogenesis is normal; if so, this implies the presence of ductal obstruction anywhere from the efferent ducts to the ejaculatory ducts. The history may reveal prior surgical procedures associated with the potential of ductal injury or resultant neurological injury with associated ejaculatory disorders. Physical examination may reveal an indurated epididymis consistent with obstruction. Laboratory evaluation may reveal low-volume azoospermia or severe oligospermia suggestive of ejaculatory disorder or obstruction of the ejaculatory ducts. Ultrasound examination of the prostrate and ejaculatory ducts may reveal dilated ducts and seminal vesicles or a midline cyst, findings consistent with ejaculatory duct obstruction.

When the FSH is greater than three times the upper limit of normal, severe impairment of testicular spermatogenesis is the most likely cause for the azoospermia. Any degree of FSH elevation above the normal range associated with testicular atrophy is invariably associated with some degree of impaired spermatogenesis. In this scenario, ductal obstruction is highly unlikely, but biopsy will provide a definitive diagnosis. This information may be important for some patients who may wish to choose either donor sperm insemination or adoption instead of proceeding with sperm retrieval/ICSI.

With the advent of ICSI, almost any man has the potential of fathering offspring with his own sperm, regardless of the azoospermia being associated with FSH elevation or testicular atrophy. In this scenario, if focal spermatogenesis is determined by biopsy, testicular sperm extraction (TESE) combined with ICSI and in vitro fertilization offers a reasonable chance of conception (3).

The value of testicular biopsy for azoospermia associated with varicocele has recently been demonstrated. Biopsy would be indicated in patients with absolute azoospermia associated with varicocele. Patients with biopsies demonstrating hypospermatogenesis or maturation arrest–spermatid stage will often respond to varicocelectomy with a return of sperm to the ejaculate. Patients with biopsies demonstrating germ-cell aplasia (i.e., Sertoli-cell-only) are unlikely to respond to varicocelectomy (6).

□ TECHNIQUE

A unilateral biopsy is all that is necessary in most patients. The healthiest testis, as determined by size and consistency, should be biopsied. When an asymmetric lesion is suspected, then bilateral biopsy is indicated. Differences in testicular volume, unilateral absence of the vas deferens, or indurated epididymis is a finding that suggests an asymmetric lesion and requires affirmation that spermatogenesis is normal bilaterally. Unilateral biopsy is adequate in the absence of any signs of a unilateral problem (7).

Window Technique

Open biopsy using the window technique may be performed in the office or outpatient setting, utilizing local anesthesia with spermatic cord block, regional anesthesia, or general anesthesia. Because of the minimally invasive nature of the procedure, local anesthesia with intravenous sedation would be suitable for most patients. Lidocaine (1% or 2%) with 0.5% bupivacaine in a 1:1 mix provides immediate and long-acting anesthesia. The spermatic cord block is performed with a 27-gauge, 1.5-inch needle. The needle is advanced along the vasal sheath while injecting the anesthetic. If bilateral biopsies are being performed, then both spermatic cords are blocked at the same time. After delivering the cord block, the testis is firmly grasped and the scrotal skin is stretched over the testis, keeping the epididymis positioned posteriorly to prevent accidental injury (Fig. 1). The skin at the site of incision is then infiltrated with the anesthetic and a 0.5- to 1-cm horizontal incision is made in the scrotal skin with the scalpel. While continuing to incise, the dartos layer and then the parietal layer of the tunica vaginalis are encountered and the tunica albuginea of the testis is identified. At this point, an eyelid retractor may be placed to separate the incision to provide more exposure. The site of the biopsy is crucial to prevent significant injury to the intratesticular arterial supply. The best location to avoid significant arterial injury is the medial or lateral aspect of the upper pole (8). Additionally, the subsurface vasculature is often readily visualized, especially when some form of magnification is used, such as loupes or the operating

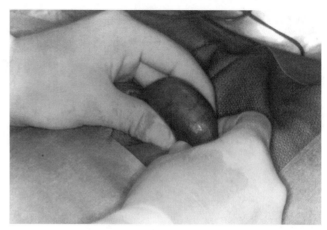

Figure 1 Proper positioning of the testis with epididymis positioned posteriorly.

microscope. After identifying the appropriate location for performing the biopsy, a 3-0 or 4-0 absorbable suture, such as polyglycolic acid, is placed as a stay suture with the needle left on (Fig. 2). With the scalpel, a 0.5 cm incision is made in the tunica albuginea of the testis. Pressure on the testis causes extrusion of parenchyma, which is then sharply excised with clean scissors. The tissue is first processed for cytological analysis and the remaining tissue is immediately placed in appropriate fixative for formal histopathologic analysis. The incision in the tunica albuginea is then closed in a running fashion using the same absorbable stay suture. The dartos and scrotal skin is then closed in the usual manner.

The window technique is the preferred method of performing an open biopsy to prevent formation of adhesions, which often makes subsequent reconstructive surgery more difficult. Biopsy can be performed after delivering the testis from the scrotal compartment during scrotal exploration if the surgeon intends to attempt microsurgical ductal repair. In this scenario, clinical findings may strongly suggest obstruction, and

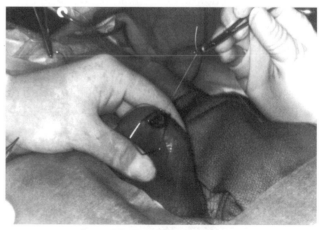

Figure 2 Window technique using an eyelid retractor and stay suture to secure position of the testis in the window.

the experienced microsurgeon may anticipate immediate repair. Frozen section analysis of testicular tissue is unreliable, but the surgeon can obtain immediate results by wet-prep analysis.

Older textbooks indicate that vasotomy and vasogram may be performed in conjunction with testicular biopsy. Current thinking, however, strongly argues against performing the vasogram at the time of the biopsy. Since many of the biopsies will reveal testicular pathology as the etiology of the azoospermia, simultaneous vasogram would be an unnecessary procedure in these patients. Vasotomy and vasogram are not without potential risks, such as vasal arterial injury and ductal obstruction, especially when performed by a surgeon with limited microsurgery experience. The vasotomy and vasogram should be performed at the time of definitive repair, unless it is the intent of the experienced reproductive surgeon to attempt immediate ductal reconstruction. Therefore, vasotomy and vasogram, in conjunction with testis biopsy, should be performed only by experienced microsurgeons if the plan is to attempt immediate and definitive repair. Typically, many clinicians will obtain tissue that is then sent to the andrology lab for analysis and freezing of the sperm at the same time. This often results in not having to do a later testicular sperm aspiration (TESA) or TESE as a separate procedure.

Percutaneous Needle Biopsy

The advantages of needle biopsy over open biopsy techniques are less cost, less tissue removed, less testicular bleeding, and less postprocedure fibrosis (9). All needle biopsy techniques, however, involve the limitation of providing relatively few tubular cross-sections for examination, with the resultant loss of some histological information. Needle biopsy techniques have been described as being best suited for the azoospermic patient as a simple means of documenting spermatogenesis in the office setting, so that subsequent operative exploration with microsurgical capability can be planned. Although further studies comparing needle biopsies with concurrent standard surgical biopsies are needed to determine the accuracy of needle biopsy techniques in quantifying spermatogenesis, Kessaris et al. have described a 95% correlation between percutaneous needle and open biopsy techniques in 24 testes (19 patients) in whom both techniques were applied, both for histologic assessment and touch imprint interpretation (5).

Percutaneous needle biopsy is performed in the office with local anesthesia. The type of anesthesia and technique for performing the spermatic cord block are as described previously for open biopsy techniques. The skin is stretched tightly over the testis with the epididymis positioned posteriorly. After infiltrating the skin with the anesthetic mixture, a small skin incision is made to facilitate placement of the needle. Several different needles have been described for use in performing needle biopsy, such as the Tru-cut needle

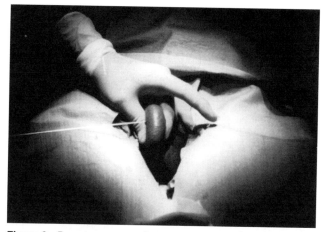

Figure 3 Percutaneous needle biopsy with the grasping hand positioned to avoid injury from the needle should it exit the scrotum.

or automated systems such as the Microvasive ASAP18 core biopsy system, which is 18-gauge with a 17-mm notch (5,10). The automated systems allow for rapid and repeat tissue sampling. As noted previously, the best location to obtain tissue and avoiding intratesticular arterial injury is the medial or lateral aspect of the upper pole. The surgeon must take notice of the location of his hand when grasping the testis to avoid accidental needle injury, as the needle may pass through the testis and exit the scrotum opposite the site of entry (Fig. 3). Two passes with the needle are usually all that are necessary to obtain an adequate amount of tissue for cytological and histopathologic analysis (Fig. 4). More than two passes are required for TESE in healthy, normal testes. The tissue is handled and processed in the same manner as in open biopsy.

Fine Needle Aspiration

FNA of the testis provides tissue for cytological examination and DNA flow cytometry. DNA flow cytometry is a quick and reproducible method previously

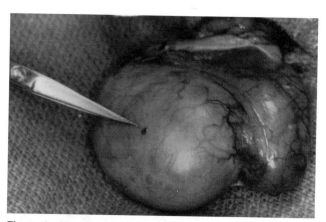

Figure 4 Site of needle biopsy at subsequent reconstructive surgery. Note that intratesticular blood vessels can be visualized just beneath the tunica albuginea.

described in the evaluation of male infertility (4,11). Abnormal testicular DNA distributions in infertile men could provide a prognosis and guide appropriate therapy. Normal testicular DNA flow cytometry associated with clinical findings suggestive of obstruction would indicate the need for microsurgical ductal reconstruction. Many clinicians, however, do not have access to DNA flow cytometry equipment nor are most clinicians familiar with or experienced in interpreting the results. These drawbacks have limited the routine use of this technique.

FNA for cytological evaluation, however, is ideal for immediate assessment of the presence and location of mature sperm. The technique for FNA is similar to the method used for percutaneous needle biopsy. The testis is positioned posteriorly after delivery of local anesthesia. A fine needle, 23-gauge, with a sharp, beveled tip is connected to a 10-mL syringe that is then placed in a syringe holder. A small amount of buffer solution such as human tubal fluid or Ham's F-10 is aspirated into the needle and syringe. The buffer solution facilitates expelling the aspirated testis tissue. The technique consists of advancing the needle into the testis while maintaining constant suction. The suction must be released just prior to withdrawing the needle. After withdrawal, the specimen is immediately transferred to a glass slide for cytological preparation or placed in a small test tube with buffer if therapeutic use is intended.

A recent study reported the use of systematic FNA of the testis to guide TESE by constructing a map detailing diagnostic biopsies (12). Although helpful in defining extratesticular obstruction, the testis biopsy offers limited information on nonobstructive azoospermic testes. Guided by diagnostic biopsies, testis sperm extraction procedures fail in 25% to 50% of patients with nonobstructive azoospermia, largely because it is clinically difficult to know where sperm are located. FNA mapping, however, uses systematic and multiple FNA of the testis to localize sperm for subsequent TESE. This novel report also demonstrates the heterogeneity of spermatogenesis in men with nonobstructive azoospermia. This technique requires the collaboration of an experienced cytopathologist. Multiple needle biopsies put the testis at risk for significant intratesticular arterial injury with resultant testicular atrophy. Although this study reported no evidence of testicular atrophy, adequate follow-up was available in only 20% of the patients studied. Additionally, other studies have compared sperm retrieval rates for FNA with open biopsy and have demonstrated that open biopsy is more likely to identify sperm than FNA in men with nonobstructive azoospermia (13). A recent study demonstrated that testicular microdissection permits the direct observation of tubules likely to contain sperm, thus increasing the yield with less tissue extracted (14). For the above reasons, the role of FNA with mapping appears limited and should be attempted by only the most experienced reproductive surgeons.

Cytology

Cytological examination of testicular tissue complements the histological evaluation and should be routinely performed with diagnostic biopsy. The histological pattern appears normal in late maturation arrest but the absence of mature sperm in cytological examination reveals the diagnosis. Immediately after obtaining the biopsy tissue, the tissue is gently touched and slid across a glass slide for the touch imprint (Fig. 5). The slide is immediately sprayed with a cytofixative or immersed in 95% ethyl alcohol before air drying. The slide can be stained with hematoxylin and eosin or Papanicolaou stain. A testicular wet prep is prepared by placing a small amount of tissue on a glass slide followed by several drops of normal saline before placing the cover slip. The slide is immediately examined for the presence of sperm. Motile sperm on the wet prep suggests ductal obstruction (15).

Tissue Handling

After obtaining the biopsy, the tissue requires immediate processing so as to preserve the delicate testicular histological architecture. Using the "no-touch" technique, the tissue is first processed for cytological analysis as described above. For diagnostic biopsy, the tissue is immediately placed in Bouin's or Zenker's solution. For therapeutic biopsy, several different media can be used, such as human tubal fluid, Ham's F-10, or Biggers, Whitten, and Whittingham solution.

Cryopreservation of sperm should be considered during a diagnostic biopsy. The ability to offer this to patients is limited to those centers with cryopreservation equipment and experienced personal. Testicular biopsy is often performed in the office or ambulatory surgery centers where cryopreservation facilities are often not available. With open biopsy techniques, enough sperm may be retrieved for freezing for subsequent ICSI, should this be necessary. Needle biopsy methods in nonobstructive azoospermic patients,

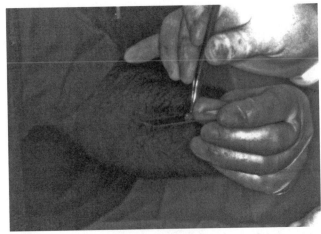

Figure 5 Testicular tissue is gently touched and slid across the slide for the touch imprint.

however, may not yield enough sperm to survive the freezing and thawing process. The specimen should be placed in buffer as outlined above prior to transportation to the cryopreservation facility.

Complications

Complications associated with testicular biopsy are few and infrequent. Scrotal hematoma is probably the most common complication associated with testicular biopsy. The bleeding is generally from the scrotal layers and not the testis. Treatment may consist of observation for small hematomas or drainage either with needle aspiration or open drainage for large hematomas. Injury to the epididymis and vas deferens are uncommon but may occur in situations in which significant adhesions from previous scrotal surgery prevent adequate exposure. Testicular atrophy following a single biopsy is rare, but multiple biopsies for sperm extraction increase the risk of significant intratesticular arterial injury. Direct observation of the tunica albuginea with magnification prevents accidental injury to the vessels visualized just beneath the surface of the tunica.

☐ HISTOPATHOLOGY

Evaluation of testicular biopsy utilizes light microscopy. Testicular biopsy does not provide information regarding the underlying etiology of the testicular lesion but only a descriptive evaluation. Testicular biopsy provides qualitative and not quantitative information about the status of the testicular parenchyma. Electron microscopy has been used but provides very little useful additional information and has not been used extensively in clinical practice.

Multiple cross sections of the seminiferous tubules are required for complete and accurate interpretation of the histopathology. Most reports indicate that approximately 100 cross-sections of seminiferous tubules are necessary (16). A more recent report, however, suggests that 20 to 30 cross-sectioned tubules are adequate in evaluating the biopsy specimen (17).

Normal

The testicular parenchyma consists of seminiferous tubules, which contribute to most of the testicular volume; blood vessels, lymphatics, and Leydig cells are found in the interstitial compartment. The seminiferous tubules consist of a basement membrane surrounded by a layer of myoid cells. Immature germ cells, spermatogonia, and Sertoli cells lie on the basement membrane. The Sertoli cells serve to support germ-cell maturation and are in intimate contact with the germ cells as they proceed through the stages of maturation. The germ cells go through an orderly process of maturation from spermatogonia, to primary spermatocytes, to secondary spermatocytes, to spermatids, and to mature spermatozoa. The

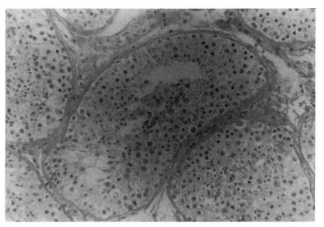

Figure 6 Normal testis biopsy demonstrating all stages of spermatogenesis.

sequence of germ-cell maturation is not present in each cross-sectioned tubule examined because spermatogenesis proceeds in a wave-like pattern along the seminiferous tubule. In humans, several different stages of spermatogenesis may be present in different areas of the cross-sectioned tubule. This explains the need to examine large numbers of cross-sectioned tubules when attempting to quantify the biopsy specimen (Figs. 6 and 7) (16).

Measuring the diameter of the seminiferous tubules is important when evaluating the biopsy specimen. Normal tubules have a mean diameter of almost 200 Mm (17). Smaller tubules contain diminished or absent germ cells. This observation provides important clinical information when performing therapeutic testicular biopsy (14). (For further information on the anatomy of the testes, see Chapter 2.)

Hypospermatogenesis

Hypospermatogenesis represents a generalized diminution of the number of germ cells with a thinning of the seminiferous epithelium. The tubular diameters

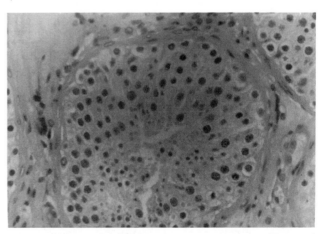

Figure 7 Higher magnification of normal testis biopsy. Elongated spermatids are identified near the lumen of the seminiferous tubule. Leydig cells are seen in the interstitium.

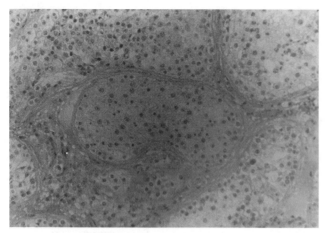

Figure 8 Maturation arrest with the absence of the elongated spermatids seen in Figures 6 and 7.

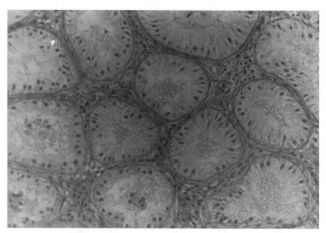

Figure 10 Sertoli-cell-only pattern with normal interstitium.

are smaller than normal, but spermatogenesis is present in all stages. It can be subjectively quantified as mild, moderate, or severe. This histological pattern is often associated with maturation arrest. It has been suggested that these two conditions often overlap, and when combined, represent up to 55% of ablative testicular lesions (16).

Maturation Arrest

Maturation arrest is a failure of the germ cells to progress beyond a particular stage of development. There usually are a normal number of germ cells in the proceeding stage of maturation. Both early and late maturation arrests occur and are usually clearly recognized. Late arrest at the spermatid stage is uncommon. This condition demonstrates a normal appearing pattern but mature sperm are not seen on the touch prep (Figs. 8 and 9).

Sertoli-Cell-Only Syndrome (Germ-Cell Aplasia)

Sertoli-cell-only syndrome is a condition in which there is a complete lack of germ cells within the seminiferous

tubules, which contain only Sertoli cells. This pattern is present in up to 13% of patients presenting with azoospermia (18). The basement membrane appears normal and tubule diameter may be normal or decreased in diameter. The interstitium contains a normal number of Leydig cells (Figs. 10 and 11). Sertoli-cell-only pattern may rarely be associated with areas of focal spermatogenesis (19). This condition may be acquired by exposure to gonadotoxins, chemotherapy, or radiation therapy. Most cases are of unknown etiology although genetic mutations involving the Y chromosome are increasingly identified.

Basement Membrane Hyalinization, Tubular Sclerosis, and Peritubular Fibrosis

This condition is represented by a thickening of the inner basement membrane due to hyaline, an eosinophilic fibrous substance. The severity may be mild to severe in which the germ and Sertoli cells are completely replaced with hyaline. Diffuse-and-severe hyalinization is termed "tubular sclerosis" and represents end-stage testicular failure. Tubular sclerosis with areas

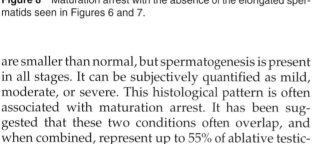

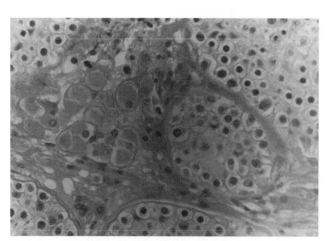

Figure 9 Maturation arrest with Leydig-cell hyperplasia.

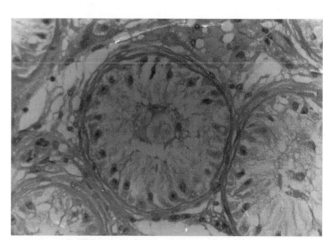

Figure 11 Higher magnification demonstrating Sertoli-cell-only pattern. Sertoli cells rest on the basement membrane and have prominent nucleoli.

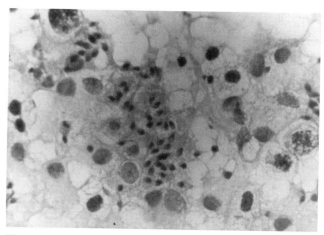

Figure 12 Touch prep demonstrating germ cells at different stages of maturation with mature spermatozoa.

of hyperplastic Leydig-cell nodules is often seen in Klinefelter's syndrome. The most common causes are ischemia, androgen deprivation, postinflammation, or exposure to gonadotoxic agents (17). Peritubular sclerosis is thickening of the myoid layer of the tunica propria. Causes include gonadotoxins and inflammatory conditions involving the interstitium (16).

Cytology

Testicular cytology can be assessed with the touch or wet-prep technique as previously described. Cytology is invaluable in distinguishing normal histology from later maturation arrest, sparing the patient from

unnecessary scrotal exploratory surgery. Immediate assessment with the wet-prep method allows the experienced reconstructive microsurgeon to proceed with definitive repair. Normal cytological specimens demonstrate germ cells at different stages, including the presence of mature sperm (Fig. 12). This is a good prognostic finding when subsequent TESE is planned.

□ CONCLUSION

Testicular biopsy qualitatively assesses spermatogenesis. The primary role of testicular biopsy is to distinguish patients with normal spermatogenesis and ductal obstruction from patients with ablative testicular pathology. With the introduction of ICSI and its successful application in cases of severe male factor infertility, the indications for testicular biopsy have expanded. The techniques developed for diagnostic biopsy have been applied to therapeutic biopsy—e.g., TESE. Despite technological advances in the field of reproductive medicine, little has changed over the last six decades in the technique and interpretation of testicular biopsy. Recent efforts have focused on methods to limit the amount of tissue extracted and increase the success and yield for therapeutic biopsy. Techniques to identify sperm-rich regions of the testis have been hampered by the invasive nature of these procedures and the heterogeneous nature of testicular histology and spermatogenesis. It is apparent that for the foreseeable future, clinicians will continue to perform and interpret testicular biopsy as has been done over the last half a century.

□ REFERENCES

1. Charny CW. Testicular biopsy. J Am Med Assoc 1940; 115: 1429–1433.

2. Hotchkiss RS. Testicular biopsy in the diagnosis and treatment of sterility in the male. Bull N Y Acad Med 1942; 18:600–605.

3. Silber SJ, Van Steirteghem AC, Liu J, et al. High fertilization and pregnancy rate after intracytoplasmic sperm injection with spermatozoa obtained from testicle biopsy. Hum Reprod 1995; 10(1):148–152.

4. Hellstrom WJ, Tesluk H, Deitch AD, et al. Comparison of flow cytometry to routine testicular biopsy in male infertility. Urology 1990; 35(4):321–326.

5. Kessaris DN, Wasserman P, Mellinger BC. Histopathological and cytopathological correlation of percutaneous testis biopsy and open testis biopsy in infertile men. J Urol 1995; 153(4):1151–1155.

6. Kim ED, Leibman BB, Grinblat DM, et al. Varicocele repair improves semen parameters in azoospermic men with testicular failure. J Urol 1999; 162(3 Pt 1):737–740.

7. Posinovec J. The necessity for bilateral biopsy in oligo- and azoospermia. Int J Fertil 1976; 21:189–191.

8. Jarow J. Intratesticular arterial anatomy. J Androl 1990; 11(3):255–259.

9. Harrington TG, Scheuer D, Gilbert BR. Percutaneous testis biopsy: an alternative to open testicular biopsy in the evaluation of the subfertile man. J Urol 1996; 156(5): 1647–1651.

10. Cohen MS, Frye S, Warner RS, et al. Testicular needle biopsy in diagnosis of infertility. Urol 1984; 24(5): 439–442.

11. Hellstrom WJG, Kaack B. Optimum testicular aspiration technique for deoxyribonucleic acid flow cytometric analysis of spermatogenesis in primates. Fertil Steril 1990; 54(3):517–521.

12. Turek PJ, Ljung B, Cha I, et al. Diagnostic findings from testis fine needle aspiration mapping in obstructed and nonobstructed azoospermic men. J Urol 2000; 163(6):1709–1716.

13. Friedler S, Raziel A, Strassburger D, et al. Testicular sperm retrieval by percutaneous fine needle sperm aspiration compared with testicular extraction by open

biopsy in men with non-obstructive azoospermia. Hum Reprod 1997; 12(7): 1488–1493.

14. Schlegel PN. Testicular sperm extraction: microdissection improves sperm yield with minimal tissue excision. Hum Reprod 1999; 14(1):131–135.

15. Jow WW, Steckel J, Schlegel PN, et al. Motile sperm in human testis biopsy specimens. J Androl 1993; 14(3): 194–198.

16. Coburn M, Wheeler T, Lipshultz LI. Testicular biopsy: its use and limitations. Urol Clin North Am 1987; 14(3): 551–561.

17. Nistal M, Paniagua R. Testicular biopsy: contemporary interpretation. Urol Clin North Am 1999; 26(3): 555–593.

18. Turek PJ, Kim M, Gilbaugh JH, et al. The clinical characteristics of 82 patients with Sertoli-cell-only testis histology. Fertil Steril 1995; 64(6): 1197–1200.

19. Levin HS. Testicular biopsy in the study of male infertility: its current usefulness, histologic techniques and prospects for the future. Hum Pathol 1979; 10(5); 569–584.

26

Immunological Evaluation of Male Infertility

Gary N. Clarke

Andrology Laboratory Division of Laboratory Services, The Royal Women's Hospital, Carlton, Victoria, Australia

H. W. Gordon Baker

Department of Obstetrics and Gynaecology, University of Melbourne and The Royal Women's Hospital, Carlton, Victoria, Australia

☐ INTRODUCTION

There is considerable support from clinical studies that sperm antibodies impair fertility (1–5) and are detectable in either the male or female partner in a significant proportion of couples presenting with infertility problems (6,7). Sperm antibodies may impair human fertility principally by blocking spermatozoan cervical mucus (CM) penetration, although inhibition of fertilization may also occur. The extent to which these effects are differentially expressed is related to the antibody level, immunoglobulin (Ig) class, and regional specificity of the antibodies concerned. For example, tail-tip antibodies do not significantly affect CM penetration (8) or fertilization (9) and often occur in fertile individuals (10–12). In addition, there is evidence that sperm-bound antibodies of the IgA class are more effective at blocking CM penetration than those of the IgG class (9). Other research has indicated that antibody titer is correlated directly with the severity of sperm functional impairment (13) and inversely with fecundability (1).

Historically, sperm immunity was assessed by observing the sperm agglutinating or immobilizing properties of the patient's serum. With the expansion of immunological knowledge in the 1970s, however, it became apparent that circulating antibodies are not necessarily indicative of local antibodies in either titer or Ig class. Work on the Immunobead Test (IBT) was initiated by the authors' laboratory in 1979 and first published in 1982 (14). The IBT has since proven to be an excellent test for sperm antibody screening. A slightly different version of the IBT was developed independently by Bronson et al. (15).

The preliminary investigation of the male partner of an infertile couple should include an IBT or mixed antiglobulin reaction screen for sperm-bound antibodies. A positive result should be followed up with a repeat test and mucus penetration testing to make a preliminary assessment of the functional significance of the antibodies. Selected men can be treated with corticosteroids to reduce their sperm antibody levels as well as to improve sperm function concomitantly

(16). The female partner should also be tested for circulating sperm antibodies. High levels of circulating antibodies may severely reduce the chances of successful treatment by in vitro fertilization (IVF) or donor insemination. Assessment of in vitro sperm–mucus interaction by means of the capillary (Kremer) test and/or the semen CM contact test (SCMCT) may suggest the likely presence of sperm antibodies in CM, even though circulating antibodies may have been weak or undetectable. The presence of antibodies in CM should be confirmed by testing liquefied CM using the indirect IBT. The presence of high CM antibody levels and associated negative or weak circulating antibodies suggests a good prognosis for treatment of the couple by intrauterine artificial insemination. On the other hand, the presence of high antibody levels both locally and systemically gives a poor prognosis. Couples with intractable immunoinfertility can be effectively treated using intracytoplasmic sperm injection (ICSI) (17).

In this chapter, the development of the IBT for sperm antibodies is described together with results of studies to validate the method and determine reference values. Some instances of the clinical importance of the IBT are given. Then methodology and interpretation of results of the IBT and the indirect IBT are detailed.

☐ BASIC PRINCIPLES OF THE IMMUNOBEAD TEST

The IBT is, in essence, a rosetting assay that relies on microscopic observation to determine the extent of interaction between the marker beads (immunobeads) and the target cells (motile spermatozoa). Immunobeads (Irvine Scientific, Santa Ana, California, U.S.A.) consist of spherical polyacrylamide beads of 2- to 10-μ diameter, with covalently attached rabbit antibodies directed against one class of human Ig (IgG-Cat# 15375, IgA-Cat# 15376). The interactions involved in generating a positive reaction are shown diagrammatically in Figure 1. The IBT is scored by determining the percentage of motile sperm with two or more immunobeads bound

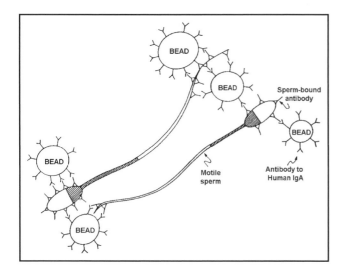

Figure 1 Diagram showing the interactions between immunobeads and motile sperm in a positive immunobead test. *Abbreviation*: Ig, immunoglobulin.

to their surface and by recording the regional pattern of bead binding (i.e., head, tail, main piece, or both). It is important to note that tail-tip bead binding should be ignored when scoring the IBT because tail-tip immunobead binding is not relevant clinically (see above, "Introduction"). The IBT result is classed as positive when greater than 50% of motile sperm have attached beads. These results are obtained for each Ig class separately. It is important that the spermatozoa be washed prior to performing the test because free Igs will inhibit interaction between immunobeads and sperm-bound antibodies. It is also necessary to wash the immunobeads to remove the preservative, which can have a deleterious effect on the spermatozoa. The IBT can be used either as a "direct" test for detecting antibodies bound to a patient's spermatozoa or as an "indirect" test for detecting sperm antibodies in serum or various reproductive tract fluids (18,19). In the indirect IBT, donor spermatozoa known to be negative by direct IBT are incubated for one hour at 37°C in the appropriately prepared fluid. If sperm antibodies are present in the fluid, they will attach to the spermatozoa and subsequently be detected by interaction with immunobeads. Positive and negative controls (prepared by preincubating the spermatozoa in appropriate pooled sera) are included in each test run. The amount of antispermatozoal antibody in a fluid can also be quantitated using a titration procedure (19).

□ SPECIFICITY AND REPRODUCIBILITY

The specificity of the direct IBT was originally investigated in several ways. Initially, a cross-inhibition test was used with purified human Igs representative of each Ig class (18). Thus, of 10 samples that were strongly positive (i.e., 90–100% of sperm-bound beads) for IgG-class antibodies, all were inhibited by purified IgG but none were inhibited by identical concentrations of

purified IgA or IgM. Similarly, strongly positive IgA–IBT reactions were inhibited by purified IgA but not by purified IgG or IgM. The second approach involved the comparison of direct IBT results in semen with sperm immobilization test (SIT) results in serum (Table 1). The SIT is an immunologically specific test because of the requirement for both antibody binding and complement fixation on the sperm surface to cause immobilization (20). The high degree of concordance between the IBT and SIT, therefore, provided further evidence of the specificity of the IBT (18,21). Finally, direct IBT results were compared with results of the SCMCT. Strongly positive "shaking" reactions in SCMCT have previously been found to be associated with the presence of sperm antibodies of IgA class in semen or CM (22). As described below in "Cervical Mucus Penetration," the authors of this chapter have found a strong correlation between IBT (particularly IgA) results and the proportion of shaking sperm in the SCMCT.

The reproducibility of the direct IBT was determined from results on 123 patients who had repeat tests. In 120 patients (97.5%), the subsequent tests agreed with the initial test, while in three patients, the result changed from negative to weak-positive or vice versa (18).

□ NORMAL GROUP STUDIES

The authors have recently performed an analysis of data obtained from direct IBT testing on the semen of a group of "normal" men. The subjects were either prospective semen donors being screened for the Royal Women's Hospital donor insemination program, or men participating in a normal fertility study whose partners were pregnant at the time of testing. Only one man out of 252 subjects was found to be positive for IgG-class antibodies (0.4%), and none were positive for IgA-class antibodies. Thus, only 0.4% of "normal" men were positive for IgG- and/or IgA-class antibodies as against 3.4% of a group of 1364 men presenting for infertility investigations during the same time period (Chi-squared, $p < 0.001$).

□ CM PENETRATION

The IBT was used by the authors of this chapter to study the Ig class of antibodies on sperm before and

Table 1 Relationship Between SIT and Direct IgG-IBT in Semen

		IgG–IBT <20	(% coated) ≥20
SIT (immobility index)	<2.0	136	5
	≥2.0	1	17

Note: Concordance = 96.2%.
Abbreviations: IBT, immunobead test; IgG, immunoglobulin G; SIT, sperm immobilization test.
Source: From Ref. 18.

after penetration through a microcolumn of CM. Of the men, 16 with positive sperm antibodies (positive SIT) and sperm that penetrated CM in prior tests were selected for study. At the time of study, however, sperm from seven subjects could not be recovered from the microcolumn. The nine subjects from whom motile sperm were obtained after passage through the column had better sperm mucus penetration tests, lower proportions of sperm binding to anti-IgA immunobeads, and a higher proportion of sperm with tail-tip-only binding. Sperm recovered after penetration through the mucus microcolumn displayed a greatly reduced binding to anti-IgA immunobeads in all nine subjects, whereas similar reductions in anti-IgG binding occurred in only four. These results confirm that IgA and sperm-head-directed antibodies are more important than IgG and sperm tail-tip-directed antibodies in impairing sperm penetration of CM (8).

In a second study, the authors analyzed the relationship between direct IgA–IBT results in semen and SCMCT results. A couple's results were included if they had in vitro capillary (Kremer) mucus penetration testing (showing normal penetration or semen factor), an SCMCT, and a direct IBT result on the husband's spermatozoa. Because of the findings in the first study, tail-tip-only antibody specificities were excluded for this analysis. The observed relationship between these two tests is apparent from this data and a Spearman's correlation of 0.85 ($p<0.001$). These results agree with earlier work that suggested antibodies of IgA class are responsible for generation of positive shaking reactions in the SCMCT (22,23).

☐ IN VITRO FERTILIZATION

A significant amount of evidence in favor of antibody-induced inhibition of fertilization has been obtained from studies of animal fertilization and of the fertilization of zona-free hamster ova by human spermatozoa (24,25). It should be noted, however, that the latter system does not measure the ability of the spermatozoa to penetrate the cumulus oophorus or the zona pellucida and hence may have little relevance to IVF or to natural fertilization in humans. To obtain more relevant information, the authors originally studied the effect of sperm isoantibodies and autoantibodies on the human fertilization process by analyzing the Royal Women's Hospital IVF data.

The effect of sperm autoantibodies on fertilization was investigated in a group of 17 IVF couples in which the male partners had sperm-bound antibodies determined by positive IBT results (9). In the subgroup ($n=8$) of couples in which the IBT showed that 80% or more of the motile spermatozoa were coated with IgG- and IgA-class antibodies, an overall fertilization rate of only 27% (18/55 ova) was obtained. In contrast, in a second subgroup ($n=9$) with less than 80% of motile spermatozoa coated with IgG- and IgA-class antibodies, a normal fertilization rate of 72% (47/75 ova) was obtained. Subsequently, using an experimental approach

with spare oocytes from consenting IVF patients, it was confirmed that sperm antibodies from human serum could inhibit human fertilization (26).

☐ LABORATORY PROCEDURES FOR PERFORMING THE IMMUNOBEAD TEST
Reagents
Buffer

Tyrode solution or Dulbecco's phosphate buffered saline (PBS) can be used as the buffer medium for the IBT. Both are available commercially from JRH Biosciences, Inc. (Lenexa, Kansas, U.S.A., www.jrhbio.com) or from Gibco (Grand Island, New York, U.S.A.). Alternatively, the buffers can be prepared in the laboratory. The JRH Biosciences catalog numbers are 55026 for Tyrode solution and 59300 for Dulbecco's PBS.

Bovine Serum Albumin

The source or purity of the bovine serum albumin (BSA) is unlikely to affect the performance of the IBT. It is important to obtain the BSA, however, in dried or powder form without preservatives and to filter the dissolved BSA before use, as explained below. Preservatives such as sodium azide can affect sperm viability and some bacterial contaminants of crude BSA products can cause false positive interactions between immunobeads and spermatozoa. BSA can be obtained from many companies. The authors use Bovostar (Cat# BSAS 0.1) from Bovogen (Melbourne, Australia, www.bovogen.com).

Tyrode Solution Containing 0.3% BSA

Tyrode solution containing 0.3% BSA (TBSA) is prepared on the day of use. For example, to prepare 300 mL of TBSA, weigh out 0.9 g of BSA, dissolve this in approximately 20 mL of Tyrode solution, then filter (0.45 μm Millipore) the solution into a conical flask, and make up to 300 mL with Tyrode solution. Warm the mixture to 30°C to 37°C before use.

Tyrode Solution Containing 5% BSA

Tyrode solution containing 5% BSA (TBSA-5) is prepared occasionally, aliquoted in 2 to 5 mL volumes, and stored frozen (below −30°C). The BSA (5 g/100 mL) is weighed out, dissolved in Tyrode solution, filtered through a 0.45-μm filter, and then aliquoted. A vial is removed from the freezer when required, thawed, and warmed to a temperature between 30°C and 37°C before use.

Immunobeads

Immunobeads are obtained from Irvine Scientific and consist of polyacrylamide beads of 2- to 10-μm diameter with covalently bound rabbit antibodies directed against human Ig classes (IgG Cat. No. 15375; IgA Cat. No. 15376). The beads are initially in dry form and are reconstituted by adding 10 mL of plain Tyrode solution (prefiltered, 0.45 µm) to a bottle containing 50 mg of beads (i.e., 5 mg/mL working solution). After reconstitution, the beads can be used for up to two months if kept at 4°C. Because the beads contain preservative, they must be washed once in TBSA immediately prior to use. This can usually be done at the same time as the second sperm wash.

Bromelain

Bromelain (Sigma Cat# B4882) is prepared occasionally and stored frozen at –70°C in the freezer. Bromelain powder is weighed out and dissolved in Tyrode solution at a concentration of 2 mg/mL, then aliquoted in 2-mL volumes before freezing. Bromelain is used to dissolve CM prior to testing.

Direct Immunobead Test
Application

The direct IBT (Fig. 2) is used to detect sperm-bound Igs of IgG or IgA Ig classes in a patient's semen sample. The direct IBT should be applicable to most semen samples with greater than 2.0×10^6 sperm/mL and motile sperm present, assuming that the sample is of normal volume.

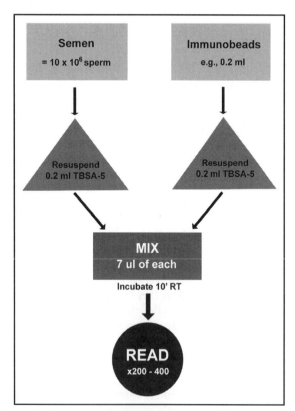

Figure 2 Direct Immunobead Test protocol. *Abbreviations*: IBT, immunobead test; RT, room temperature; TBSA-5, tyrode solution containing 5% bovine serum albumin.

Positive Control

The positive control for the direct IBT should consist of sera that are strongly positive (greater than or equal to 90%) for IBT–IgG and IBT–IgA in the indirect IBT (see section "Indirect Immunobead Test"). The appropriate sera are occasionally pooled, aliquoted (100 µL) into 10-mL centrifuge tubes, and stored frozen until used. On the day of use, a tube is thawed, 50 µL of semen (best available on the day) is added, and the mixture is preincubated at 37°C for 15 to 30 minutes.

Negative Control

Transfer 50 µL of the positive control mixture to a separate tube and do not wash this tube. The free serum-derived Igs will inhibit any specific sperm-bead binding.

Procedure

1. Dispense an aliquot of the semen to be tested into a 10-ml plastic conical centrifuge tube. The volume of semen dispensed is determined by the sperm count and motility. The aliquot should preferably contain 5×106 to 10×106 motile spermatozoa.
2. The volume is then made up to 10 mL with TBSA. The TBSA should be prewarmed to 30°C to 37°C and checked using a thermometer.
3. The tube is centrifuged at 500 g (2000 rpm) for five minutes. The supernatant is then aspirated down to approximately 0.2 mL and the pellet is resuspended and made up to 10 mL again with TBSA. Aliquots (e.g., 0.2 mL) of the appropriate immunobead reagents can be washed at the same time as the second sperm wash.
4. Repeat centrifugation and finally resuspend the sperm and immunobead pellets in 0.2 mL TBSA-5. If the density of motile sperm is too low to obtain an accurate reading, then centrifuge again (without adding washing buffer), remove 150 µL of the supernatant, and set up the slide preparations again. If this fails, then request a second semen sample or perform an indirect IBT on seminal plasma. The test is performed by mixing 7 µL of washed sperm with 7 µL of the appropriate immunobead reagent on a slide and covering with a standard (22 × 22 mm) cover slip. The slide is incubated at room temperature in a moist chamber for 10 minutes before grading under phase-contrast optics (200× to 400× magnification). Set up slides for both IgG and IgA.
5. A test is positive if at least 50% of the motile sperm have two or more attached beads. The percentage of motile sperm bound to beads is recorded and also the pattern of binding, that is, the head (H), tail mainpiece (M), tail endpiece (E), or all (A).

Indirect Immunobead Test
Application

The indirect test (Fig. 3) is used to detect sperm antibodies in seminal plasma (6), serum (27), follicular fluid (19), or CM (7). In the past, the authors of this chapter have recommended preliminary screening of sera using immunobeads directed against whole human Ig (IBT–GAM), followed by secondary testing of positives by IBT–IgG, IBT–IgA, and IBT–IgM (28). It is the authors' experience over the last few years, however, that has led to the conclusion that it is much more cost effective to screen for IgG- and IgA-class antibodies only. This is because sera are rarely positive for IgM-class antibodies alone, and it is not believed that IgM-class antibodies are of clinical significance.

Positive Control

The positive control for the indirect IBT is sera that are strongly positive for IBT–IgG and/or IBT–IgA. In the indirect IBT, this is occasionally pooled, passing through a 0.45 μm disposable Millipore filter, diluted 1/10 in Tyrode solution, aliquoted (500 μL), and frozen (–70°C) until used. On the day of use, a tube is thawed and processed with the batch of sera to be tested.

Negative Control

Sera that are negative for IBT–IgG and IBT–IbA are pooled and processed as above.

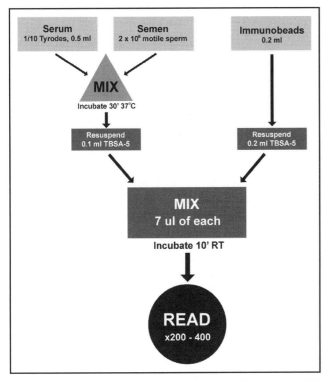

Figure 3 Indirect immunobead test protocol. *Abbreviations*: RT, room temperature; TBSA-5, tyrode solution containing 5% bovine serum albumin.

Sample Preparation
Seminal Plasma

An indirect IBT is performed on seminal plasma if there are not enough motile sperm to perform a direct test. Seminal plasma is prepared by filtering the semen through a 0.45 or 0.8 μm Millipore filter (disposable). Semen with increased viscosity must be syringed before filtering. Seminal plasma can be tested without inactivation of complement. Dilute 0.25 mL seminal plasma with an equal volume of Tyrode solution to test. Store at –70°C until tested.

Cervical Mucus

CM is prepared by adding an equal volume of Tyrode solution containing 2 mg/mL of Bromelain and incubating the mixture at room temperature for 10 to 15 minutes with frequent shaking. Check the viscosity by dropping the solution from a Pasteur pipette: if the drop hangs on at all, then syringe the mixture several times. The mixture is then centrifuged at 600 g (2000 rpm) for five minutes to remove debris and inactivated at 5°C for 30 minutes prior to testing. If not tested on the same day, freeze at –70°C.

Serum or Follicular Fluid

Inactivate at 56°C for 30 minutes. Store at –70°C until tested. The initial screening test is performed on sera diluted 1/10 in TBSA:

> 1/10 = 50 μL serum + 450 μL TBSA

Samples that are strongly positive (i.e., at least 80% of sperm with attached beads for IgG or IgA classes) at 1/10 dilution can then be titrated in tenfold steps and retested immediately:

> 1/100 = 50 μL of 1/10 dilution + 450 μl TBSA
> 1/1000 = 50 μL of 1/100 dilution + 450 μL TBSA

Procedure

Add 20 to 50 μL (approximately 2×10^6 motile sperm) of semen, previously found negative (less than 5% of sperm coated) by direct IBT, to 0.5 mL of the fluid to be tested. Mix and then incubate the mixture at 37°C for 30 minutes. At the completion of incubation, perform steps two to four as described for the "direct test" except that final sperm resuspension is in 80 μL of TBSA-5. The "indirect test" can be semiquantitated as a titer by preparing tenfold dilutions of the fluid to be tested, then processing, as described above.

Quality Control Procedures
Positive and Negative Controls

The procedures for generating positive and negative controls have been described above. Pooled serum containing sperm antibodies is used to produce a positive control for the direct IBT. This is necessary because of the logistic problem of obtaining natural positive semen on a day-to-day basis. The negative control is generated by inhibiting specific immunobead binding with serum-derived Igs. Alternatively, it might be feasible for some laboratories to use fresh or cryopreserved semen from an individual previously found to be negative by direct IBT. This would provide a "true" negative control that would be preferable to the artificially generated control. In any case, it is important to include a negative control with each test batch in order to determine if significant nonspecific bead–sperm binding may be occurring. The positive control demonstrates that the immunobead preparation is functionally intact; this controls against deterioration during storage or the possible introduction of extraneous factors—for example, if the technician accidentally used a buffer containing human serum, the positive control would give a weak or negative result.

In the event of a weak positive control result, the following should be checked:

1. The date of reconstitution of the immunobead preparation. If the immunobeads have been reconstituted and stored at 4°C for more than eight weeks, it would be advisable to discard them and open a new bottle. If the laboratory were only testing small numbers of samples, it would prove more economical to weigh out perhaps 10 mg of the lyophilized immunobeads instead of reconstituting the full 50 mg.
2. The immunobead stock for fungal or bacterial contamination. Discard immunobead stock if contaminated.
3. Whether the negative rather than a positive control tube was mistakenly used.
4. Whether the BTSA could have been contaminated with human serum.
5. If the incorrect buffer was used by mistake.

In the event of positive results occurring in the negative control, the following should be checked for:

1. Bacterial contamination of immunobeads: discard stock if contaminated.
2. Bacterial contamination of TBSA: was the BSA filtered? Is the TBSA more than 24 hours old or has it been maintained at 37°C for many hours? Prepare from fresh TBSA if indicated.
3. Mix-up of control tubes?
4. Mix-up of slide preparations?
5. If the semen sample was heavily contaminated with bacteria? If so, repeat the IBT on a fresh semen sample.

Crossed Inhibition Test

This procedure may be useful for troubleshooting or as an extra proof that a positive IBT result is due to immunologically specific binding between immunobeads and sperm-bound antibodies. The inhibition test is performed as follows:

1. Add an equal volume of pure IgG or IgA (Sigma Cat# I 4506 or I 1010, respectively, 2 mg/mL) to an aliquot of the appropriate immunobead preparation (e.g., anti-IgG immunobeads).
2. Incubate the Ig/bead mixture for 30 minutes at 37°C to allow binding between the rabbit anti-human IgG antibodies attached to the beads and the pure Igs added.
3. Retest the sperm preparation that was positive for sperm-bound antibodies of IgG class, but using the beads preincubated with pure Ig. A specific positive result for IgG should be inhibited by purified IgG but not by IgA. Similarly, a specific positive for IgA-class antibodies should be inhibited by pure IgA but not by IgG.

Cross Referencing

It is important for the scientist or technician performing the IBT to note if there are other indications of the presence of sperm antibodies, rather than relying entirely on a single test result. Did the patient have pronounced sperm agglutination in his semen? Has he had a vasectomy reversal (vasovasostomy) operation performed? Did his sperm penetrate normal CM? Did they show the shaking phenomenon in the SCMCT? Have any tests for circulating sperm antibodies been performed? Has the couple had negative postcoital tests (PCT)? Have they had unexplained poor fertilization results in IVF? Similar points need to be noted for a positive IBT for sperm antibodies in CM. It is important to note that there is not an exact relationship between these variables and IBT results. Cross-referencing is a useful exercise, however, particularly when first establishing the IBT protocol in a laboratory, because it will give confidence that the test is detecting sperm antibodies of clinical relevance—especially when strong IBT results are obtained.

Interpretation of Results

The authors of this chapter consider 50% sperm coating at 1/10 serum dilution to be the minimum indirect IBT result likely to have any clinical significance. This is a conservative criterion, considering the sensitivity of the IBT. It is possible that 1/100 may be a more appropriate serum dilution to use. This may also vary with the Ig class of the antibody for which the test is being used.

With respect to the direct IBT, the authors believe that a minimum of 50% of motile spermatozoa must be coated with antibodies for the IBT result to have any likely clinical significance because of several considerations. Firstly, from a statistical point of view, it is unlikely that sperm function will be significantly impaired if less than 50% of the motile sperm are coated with antibodies. This opinion was confirmed by comparison of IBT results with IVF, CM penetration, PCT, and conception rates. Therefore, the criterion of more than two beads bound to at least 50% of sperm is used as the criterion of positivity that is likely to have clinical significance. This criterion alone, however, is not sufficient to conclude that a patient has "immunoinfertility" or "sperm autoimmunity." The use of these terms is restricted to cases in which both sperm antibodies have been unequivocally detected *and* there is evidence of poor CM penetration by spermatozoa and/or repeated negative PCT, suggesting functional impairment consistent with infertility or subfertility.

What Is the Appropriate Course of Action after Sperm Antibodies Have Been Detected in Either Husband or Wife, or Both?

If the antibody test was initially performed on the patient's serum, then the following steps should be performed:

1. Repeat the indirect IBT on serum, including 1/100 and 1/1000 serum dilutions.
2. Perform an IBT on semen or CM.
3. If not already done, test for sperm/CM penetration.

If, as is preferable, tests for local antibodies have been performed first, then proceed as follows:

1. Test for sperm/CM penetration.
2. Repeat IBT tests on semen and/or CM.
3. Test sera by indirect IBT.

How Should the Various Results Be Interpreted in Order to Advise and Treat the Couple for Their Infertility Problem?

If a man has a positive direct IBT associated with a poor capillary (Kremer) test result (less than 2 cm in two hours), then the patient can be treated with ICSI or corticosteroids such as prednisolone (16). Before proceeding with corticosteroid treatment, it is imperative that the female partner is thoroughly evaluated to ascertain whether she is ovulating, has patent fallopian tubes, and does not have endometriosis. If any of these findings are indicated, she may require prior or concomitant treatment to ensure optimal chances for a successful outcome. The man must be thoroughly screened and counseled regarding the possible side effects of corticosteroid treatment. Any evidence of a peptic ulcer, high blood pressure, tuberculosis, diabetes, or any serious illness is a contraindication for corticosteroid treatment.

What Course Should Be Followed if the Female Partner Has Sperm Antibodies?

If the patient has a positive indirect IBT for IgA-class antibodies in CM associated with poor CM penetration results but a relatively low titer (less than 1/100) of circulating antibodies, then the patient has a reasonable chance of conceiving by intrauterine insemination of husband's semen or washed spermatozoa (assuming essentially normal semen quality). High-titer antibodies (>1/1000) give a generally poor prognosis.

☐ TREATMENT

The traditional treatment for sperm autoimmunity has involved the use of immunosuppressive doses of corticosteroids such as prednisolone taken continuously (16) or intermittently (29). This therapy is successful in helping approximately 25% of men with definite immunoinfertility to impregnate their partners. This treatment, however, is only suitable for men who are in good health. Unpleasant side effects lead some men to discontinue treatment, and it is not advisable to continue treatment for extended periods. Although corticosteroid treatment remains an option, immunoinfertility can now be circumvented using ICSI procedures (17).

☐ CONCLUSION

The IBT is an excellent test for assisting the clinical management of human infertility. All patients should be screened for sperm antibodies, and if the IBT is positive, tests of sperm function, such as sperm CM penetration, should be performed to assess the significance of the positive antibody test. Patients with positive IBT and severely impaired sperm function are unlikely to conceive naturally, by artificial insemination, or by standard IVF, but can be treated by ICSI. In the future, refinements of the IBT, such as using mixtures of beads with different Ig antibodies bound to different colored beads, may be used. New approaches to the quantitation of sperm antibodies may be developed, but tests that are specific for epitopes involved in the fertilization process are still only theoretical.

☐ REFERENCES

1. Menge AC, Medley NE, Mangione CM, et al. The incidence and influence of antisperm antibodies in infertile human couples on sperm-cervical mucus interactions and subsequent fertility. Fertil Steril 1982; 38(4):439–446.

2. Rumke P, Amstel NV, Messer EN, et al. Prognosis of fertility of men with sperm agglutinins in the serum. Fertil Steril 1974; 25(5):393–393.

3. Rumke P, Renckens CN, Bezemer PD, et al. Prognosis of fertility in women with unexplained infertility and sperm agglutinins in the serum. Fertil Steril 1984; 42(4): 561–567.

4. Ayvaliotis B, Bronson R, Rosenfeld D, et al. Conception rates in couples where autoimmunity to sperm is detected. Fertil Steril 1985; 43(5):739–742.

5. Witkin SS, David SS. Effect of sperm antibodies on pregnancy outcome in a subfertile population. Am J Obstet Gynecol 1988; 158(1):59–62.

6. Clarke GN. Sperm antibodies and human fertilization. Am J Reprod Immunol Microbiol 1988; 17(2):65–71.

7. Clarke GN, Stojanoff A, Cauchi MN, et al. Detection of antispermatozoal antibodies of IgA class in cervical mucus. Am J Reprod Immunol 1984; 5(2):61–65.

8. Wang C, Baker HW, Jennings MG, et al. Interaction between human cervical mucus and sperm surface antibodies. Fertil Steril 1985; 44(4):484–488.

9. Clarke GN, Lopata A, McBain JC, et al. Effect of sperm antibodies in males on human in vitro fertilization (IVF). Am J Reprod Immunol Microbiol 1985; 8(2): 62–66.

10. Hammitt DG, Muench MM, Williamson RA. Antibody binding to greater than 50% of sperm at the tail tip does not impair male fertility. Fertil Steril 1988; 49(1):174.

11. Jager S, Rumke P, Kremer J. A fertile man with a high sperm agglutination titer in the seminal plasma: a case report. Am J Reprod Immunol Microbiol 1987; 15: 29–32.

12. Clarke GN. Sperm antibodies in normal men: association with a history of nongonococcal urethritis (NGU). Am J Reprod Immunol Microbiol 1986; 12:31–32.

13. Fjallbrant B. Interrelation between high levels of sperm antibodies, reduced penetration of cervical mucus by spermatozoa and sterility in men. Acta Obstet Gynecol Scand 1968; 47:102–118.

14. Clarke GN, Stojanoff A, Cauchi MN. Immunoglobulin class of sperm-bound antibodies in semen. In: Bratanov K, ed. Proc Int Symp Immunology of Reproduction. Bulgaria: Bulgarian Academy of Sciences Press, 1982:482.

15. Bronson RA, Cooper GW, Rosenfeld DL. Correlation between regional specificity of antisperm antibodies to the spermatozoan surface and complement-mediated sperm immobilization. Am J Reprod Immunol Microbiol 1982; 2(4):222–224.

16. Baker HW, Clarke GN, Hudson B, et al. Treatment of sperm autoimmunity in men. Clin Reprod Fertil 1983; 2(1):55–71.

17. Clarke GN, Bourne H, Baker, HW. Intracytoplasmic sperm injection for treating infertility associated with sperm autoimmunity. Fertil Steril 1997; 68(1):112–117.

18. Clarke GN, Elliott PJ, Smaila C. Detection of sperm antibodies in semen using the immunobead test: a survey of 813 consecutive patients. Am J Reprod Immunol Microbiol 1985; 7(3):118–123.

19. Clarke GN, Hsieh C, Koh SH, et al. Sperm antibodies, immunoglobulins, and complement in human follicular fluid. Am J Reprod Immunol 1984; 5(4):179–181.

20. Isojima S, Li TS, Ashitaka Y. Immunologic analysis of sperm-immobilizing factor found in sera of women with unexplained sterility. Am J Obstet Gynecol 1968; 101:677–683.

21. Jennings MG, McGowan MP, Baker HW. Immunoglobulins on human sperm: validation of a screening test for sperm autoimmunity. Clin Reprod Fertil 1985; 3(4):335–342.

22. Kremer J, Jager S. Characteristics of anti-spermatozoal antibodies responsible for the shaking phenomenon with special regard to immunoglobulin class and antigen-reactive sites. Int J Androl 1980; 3(2):143–152.

23. Clarke GN. Induction of the shaking phenomenon by IgA class antispermatozoal antibodies from serum. Am J Reprod Immunol 1985; 9(1):12–14.

24. Alexander NJ. Antibodies to human spermatozoa impede sperm penetration of cervical mucus or hamster eggs. Fertil Steril 1984; 41(3):433–439.

25. Dor J, Rudak E, Aitken RJ. Antisperm antibodies: their effect on the process of fertilization studied in vitro. Fertil Steril 1981; 35(5):535–541.

26. Clarke GN, Hyne RV, du Plessis Y, et al. Sperm antibodies and human in vitro fertilization. Fertil Steril 1988; 49(6):1018–1025.

27. Clarke GN, Stojanoff A, Cauchi MN, et al. The immunoglobulin class of antispermatozoal antibodies in serum. Am J Reprod Microbiol 1985; 7(4):143–147.

28. Clarke GN. An improved immunobead test procedure for detecting sperm antibodies in serum. Am J Reprod Immunol Microbiol 1987; 13(1):1–3.

29. Hendry WF, Treehuba K, Hughes L, et al. Cyclic prednisolone therapy for male infertility associated with autoantibodies to spermatozoa. Fertil Steril 1986; 45(2): 249–254.

27

Genetic Evaluation of the Infertile Male

Edward D. Kim

Department of Surgery, Division of Urology, University of Tennessee Medical Center, Knoxville, Tennessee, U.S.A.

□ INTRODUCTION

The treatment of severe male-factor infertility has seen remarkable advances since 1992, with the introduction and widespread use of intracytoplasmic sperm injection (ICSI), a micromanipulation technique in which a single mature sperm is injected into the oocyte to initiate fertilization (1). This procedure now provides men who were previously thought to be irreversibly infertile the chance to initiate their own biologic pregnancy. When examining the offspring, the physician should keep in mind that abnormalities may be transmitted from either parent or may arise de novo, depending on the specific defect. While transmission of these genes may cause problems with male infertility in the offspring (2), unknown consequences may also be attendant.

The present genetic screening of subfertile men is directed toward azoospermic and severely oligozoospermic men (Table 1). It is estimated that 11% to 30% of these men may have an identifiable genetic abnormality (3,4). Men with spermatogenic failure are offered Y-chromosome microdeletion testing and karyotype analysis. Those men with congenital absence of the vas deferens require cystic fibrosis (CF) transmembrane-conductance regulator (CFTR) gene-mutation testing. At a minimum, the couple should be made aware of the availability and significance of this testing.

□ CF GENE MUTATIONS

Azoospermic men with vasal or epididymal abnormalities should be screened for CFTR gene mutations. The most common clinical presentation is that of azoospermia, low-volume ejaculate, and congenital bilateral absence of the vas deferens (CBAVD) (Fig. 1), which occurs in 1% to 2% of men presenting with infertility (5,6). The carrier status for this autosomal recessive condition is quite common, being present in 1/25 to 1/30 persons of Northern European descent. Over 800 CFTR gene mutations have been reported (4,7). Because of the potentially fatal nature of this autosomal recessive disorder for the offspring, screening should now be considered routine when vasal or epididymal abnormalities are suspected.

CF is a fatal disorder most prominently characterized by pulmonary and pancreatic disease.

Approximately 97% to 98% of men with CF also have CBAVD, although it is possible that 2% to 3% of men with CF are fertile (8). This lifelong illness, typically diagnosed in childhood, is progressive and inherited. Common symptoms include chronic cough, wheezing, sinus infections, nasal polyps, excessive mucus production, recurrent pneumonia, poor growth, frequent foul-smelling stools, enlarged fingertips, and skin that is salty to the taste. Because there is no cure, treatment is directed toward symptomatically improving the length and quality of life. Aerosols are used to ease breathing, and postural drainage or chest physical therapy helps to remove mucus from the lungs. Pancreatic enzymes are taken with meals to help digest food. Currently, 50% of CF patients are expected to live until their thirties.

The CFTR gene, also called ABCC7, is located on chromosome 7 at 7q31 and was identified in 1989 (9–11). The CFTR gene is 250 kb in length and contains 27 exons. ΔF508 is a three-base-pair deletion in exon 10 and is the most common mutation responsible for CF, accounting for approximately 70% of CF alleles (9). Other less common deletions include G542X (2.9%), N1303K (2.1%), and 1717-1G > A (1.3%) (12). Only 11 mutations have relative frequencies of over 0.4%. Ethnic and geographic variations exist. Testing should also be performed for the 5 thymidine (5T) allele on intron 8 because of the high frequency of abnormal findings. Since the 5T allele causes reduced levels of normal CFTR mRNA, this variant would appear to be likely involved in the pathogenesis of CBAVD. Chillon et al. concluded that the combination of the 5T allele in one copy of the CFTR gene with a CF mutation in the other copy is the most common cause of CBAVD (13). The 5T allele mutation has a wide range of clinical presentations, occurring in patients with CBAVD or moderate forms of CF and in fertile men.

Between 50% and 82% of men with CBAVD and approximately 43% with unilateral absence of the vas deferens will have at least one detectable CFTR gene mutation (14–16). Jarvi et al. reported that at least 47% of otherwise healthy men with idiopathic epididymal obstruction had a CFTR gene mutation (17). CFTR gene mutation analysis may reveal a variable mutation pattern (18). For example, ΔF508 mutations result in true CF, not just CBAVD. In contrast, milder mutations such as the R117H or 5T variant of intron 9 result in CBAVD, not CF. The determining factor for disease

Table 1 Common Genetic Testing for Male Infertility

Testing	Indications
Cystic fibrosis gene mutation	Congenital absence of the vas deferens Vasal or epididymal abnormalities
Y chromosome microdeletion	Spermatogenic failure characterized by sperm density <5 million sperm/mL
Simple karyotyping	Spermatogenic failure characterized by sperm density <5 million sperm/mL

severity is the total amount of normal CFTR protein produced. Up to 20% of CBAVD men may be carriers of two different mutations, also known as being compound heterozygotes.

These *CFTR* gene mutations may result in Wolffian duct abnormalities as the only somatic manifestations (including defects of the epididymis, vas, or secondary involvement as absence of a kidney), as sperm production is typically normal. The semen profile is characterized by azoospermia, reduced semen volume, and absent or decreased fructose levels. A defect in the Wolffian duct at or before the formation of the ureteral bud at seven weeks of age results in malformation of the entire Wolffian duct and subsequent vasal agenesis. Other clinical manifestations include unilateral renal agenesis and seminal vesicle aplasia or hypoplasia. Because renal agenesis is present in about 11% of men with bilateral congenital absence and 26% of infertile men with unilateral congenital absence of the vas deferens (14), a renal ultrasound should be recommended for men in whom a vas is not palpable.

Ideally, both the male and female should be tested. If resources are limited, then it is reasonable to test the female alone. If she is negative, the risk of the offspring having CF or CBAVD is 1:960 (19,20). If both partners are carriers for the same mutation, the rules of autosomal recessive inheritance are followed. The offspring will have a quarter chance of having full-blown CF, a half chance of being a carrier, and a quarter chance of having no gene mutations. If both are

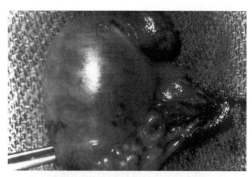

Figure 1 Congenital absence of the vas deferens. This patient's epididymis contains only a small portion of the caput. Variable amounts of the epididymis may be present.

carriers for the mutation, preimplantation blastomere biopsy analysis may be performed by several specialty research centers under investigational protocol (21).

In men with CBAVD, pregnancy rates of approximately 50% per cycle have been obtained with ICSI in contrast to 10% with standard in vitro fertilization (IVF), after sperm harvesting from the epididymis (22–24). (For further information on the techniques of sperm harvesting including microsurgical epididymal sperm aspiration and percutaneous epididymal sperm aspiration, see Chapter 33.) Cryopreservation of sperm does not appear to adversely affect outcome (24). Unless testicular atrophy is present, testicular biopsy prior to ICSI is unnecessary because spermatogenesis is preserved in the vast majority of men. It is generally believed that the presence of *CF* mutations in the male partner does not compromise in-vitro fertilization treatment outcomes or the opportunity for healthy live births (24).

CFTR gene mutation testing, obtained from a peripheral blood specimen or buccal mucosal smear, is available at most major medical centers and commercially (25,26). Testing is based on the polymerase chain reaction (PCR). The physician should be aware that not all possible mutations are detected because of limited allele testing—typically for only 30 of the most common loci.

☐ Y-CHROMOSOME MICRODELETIONS

Men who are azoospermic and severely oligozoospermic (<1–5 million sperm/mL) should be offered Y-chromosome microdeletion testing and karyotype analysis. Structural chromosomal abnormalities of the Y chromosome were suspected to have a role in male infertility by Tiepolo and Zuffardi in as early as 1976, but their findings and significance did not produce much clinical impact until the introduction and widespread use of ICSI (27). Deletions in the Deleted in Azoospermia gene (*DAZ*), which is a novel transcription unit that is usually present in the azoospermia factor locus (AZF) region in men of normal fertility gene, are present in 10% to 15% of otherwise normal 46,XY men with nonobstructive azoospermia (28–30). This defect is clearly phenotypically diverse, as approximately 6% to 10% of men with severe oligozoospermia (sperm density less than 5 million sperm/mL) have this deletion (31,32). In contrast, *DAZ* deletions are found in only approximately 2% of normal men.

It is well established that the long (q) arm of the Y chromosome is required for spermatogenesis (27) and that microdeletions on the Y chromosome are associated with infertility (33,34). The specific region of the Y chromosome implicated in male infertility based on mapping studies is called the AZF, containing approximately 5×10^6 base pairs and present in band q11.23 (Fig. 2) (35). Four distinct interstitial deletions causing azoospermia or severe oligozoospermia occurring in nonoverlapping subregions of Yq11 are called AZFa,

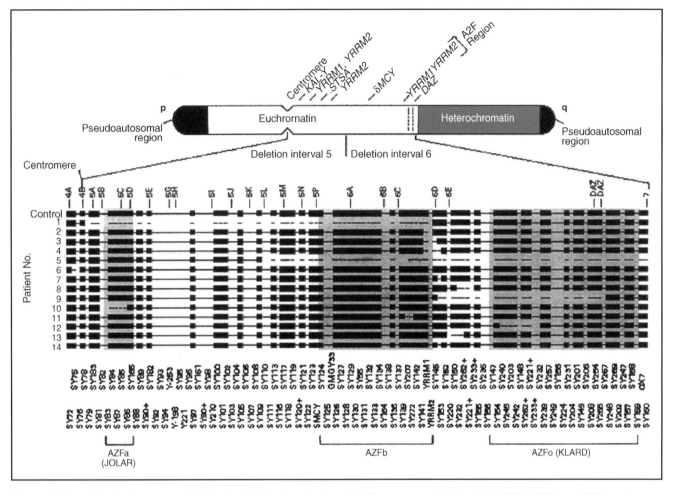

Figure 2 Map of the Y chromosome. STS in the deletion intervals 5 and 6 of the q arm are indicated. The AZFa, AZFb, and AZFc regions are highlighted. The patient numbers correspond to specific analysis from Pryor's study on Y-chromosome microdletions. The dashes represent deleted areas. *Abbreviations*: AZF, azoospermia factor locus; STS, sequence-tagged sites. *Source*: From Ref. 31.

b, c, and d (36,37). AZFa, AZFb, and AZFc correspond to the proximal, central, and distal segments of Yq11, respectively. These subregions appear to regulate different stages of spermatogenesis. Testicular biopsies in these men have demonstrated a range of spermatogenic defects from Sertoli-cell-only syndrome (SCO) (no sperm-forming elements) to maturation arrests (sperm-forming cells present, but not mature sperm) at the spermatid stage (28). Ferlin et al. suggest that 35% of men with SCO and 25% of men with severe hypospermatogenesis have microdeletions (38). In contrast, no deletions were found in testiculopathies of known etiology, obstructive azoospermia, and normal fertile men (38). Deletions in the AZFc region involving the *DAZ* gene were the most frequent finding and were more often observed in severe hypospermatogenesis than in SCO, suggesting that deletions of this region are not sufficient to cause complete loss of the spermatogenic line.

AZFa deletions are quite rare and have been associated with SCO. The Drosophila fat facets related Y (*DFFRY*) gene is a candidate gene for fertility that has been mapped to the AZFa subregion. Deletions of the AZFb region especially have been correlated with

the absence of mature spermatozoa and presence of round spermatids in testis biopsy specimen (39). It is likely that different AZFb subtypes result in specific spermatogenic abnormalities. Vogt first described that complete AZFb deletions (sY113-sY143) result in a maturation arrest at the spermatocyte or spermatid stage (36). The RNA-binding motif (*RBMY*) gene family is located in AZFb. Whole AZFb deletions with AZFa and/or AZFc are associated with SCO (40). Partial AZFb deletions are associated with a heterogenous phenotype, including oligozoospermia (40).

Isolated AZFc deletions are the most common type and coincide with the *DAZ* gene. Deletions including and extending beyond the AZFc region (AZFb + c, AZFa + b + c) are associated with a total absence of testicular spermatozoa (41). AZFc deletions alone, however, are associated with the presence of mature sperm in about 50% of azoospermic men (42). Foci of spermatogenesis within a predominant SCO pattern may be identified with AZFc deletions. AZFd associated with mild oligozoospermia or even normal sperm counts associated with abnormal sperm morphology has also been recently described (43). Deletions of the *DAZ* gene result in severe impairments of spermatogenesis, but not always. Microdeletions may also be responsible for severe bilateral testicular damage that could be phenotypically expressed by unilateral cryptorchidism as well as by idiopathic infertility (44).

As can be inferred from the preceding discussion, the type of AZF deletion may have implications on patient management (40). If a patient has a partial AZFb or a complete AZFc deletion, there is a higher likelihood of finding sperm than a complete AZFb deletion. These results are preliminary, and larger series may confirm that a complete AZFb deletion is associated with complete absence of mature sperm, thereby contraindicating testicular sperm extraction (TESE) attempts for such a patient. The specific type of deletion can guide the aggressiveness of TESE for finding mature sperm; however, data interpretation is still preliminary and caution should be used (45).

The immediate concern of these Y-chromosome microdeletions is that transmission to the offspring may occur (46–48). Page et al. demonstrated transmission in four sons fathered by three men with AZFc deletion through ICSI (47). All four sons were found to have inherited the Y-chromosome microdeletions. While the male offspring may be infertile, the answer may not be apparent for at least another decade, when these children reach reproductive age. Early indications from familial case reports, however, clearly demonstrate the inheritability of Y-chromosome microdeletions and impaired spermatogenesis, including a family in which four sons were either severely oligozoospermic or azoospermic and shared a DAZ deletion (49). The father was azoospermic at the time of analysis but demonstrated previous fertility. Interestingly, fathers of infertile men with microdeletions have been found to have the same deletions as their sons, while other microdeletions appear to arise de novo (31,32).

Y-chromosome microdeletion testing is performed using PCR. The three key steps to PCR are (i) denaturation, which results in separation of the double-stranded DNA, (ii) annealing of primers (short sequences of DNA specific to the boundaries of the region to be analyzed) to the target DNA, and (iii) extension with a Taq polymerase to synthesize sequences complementary to the original DNA. The PCR products are separated by electrophoresis and visualized with gel electrophoresis. Modifications including nested PCR, multiplex PCR, fluorescent PCR, and quantitative PCR can further enhance the accuracy and yield of PCR. This testing is available at many major universities as well as commercially (e.g., Promega's Y detection kit; Promega, Madison, Wisconsin, U.S.A.).

The number of sequence-tagged sites (STSs) examined is variable. Pryor et al. have suggested that 20 to 30 STSs are sufficient to provide adequate sensitivity and specificity (31). According to the European Academy of Andrology's recommendations, multiplex PCR should be used in two steps (50). First, two STS loci in each AZF subregion are tested, allowing for

above 90% detection of an AZF deletion. Second, if a deletion is detected, specific primer sets that can determine the extent of the deletion are used.

☐ CHROMOSOMAL ABNORMALITIES

Karyotype analysis can uncover numerical or structural chromosomal disorders such as Klinefelter's syndrome (classic 47,XXY; 1 in 500 live male births), mixed gonadal dysgenesis, and XYY (1 in 1000 live births) syndromes. Breakage and rearrangement of chromosomes can lead to abnormalities such as translocations (reciprocal, balanced, and Robertsonian), ring chromosome formation, and pericentric inversions. Identification is important because with the advent of ICSI, patients with mosaic (51,52) or nonmosaic patterns (53,54) may be able to have sperm harvested from testis biopsies and be able to initiate a pregnancy with resultant genetically normal embryos (55). However, failure to identify these chromosomal disorders prior to fertilization may have potential genetic consequences on the offspring.

The incidence of these abnormalities in infertile men ranges between 2.2% and 14.3%, and is markedly increased above baseline population levels (Table 2) (56,57). Therefore, it is recommended that all men with severe male-factor infertility have this cytogenetic analysis performed. In a study of 261 couples with male-factor infertility, abnormal karyotypes were found in 4.2% of the men and 1.2% of the women (58). Meschede et al. found a 2.1% chromosomal abnormality rate in men in a large, prospective series from Germany (57). Similarly, Pandiyan reported that 3.6% of 1201 men with abnormal semen analyses had either autosomal or sex chromosomal aberrations (59). Gekas et al. identified an abnormal karyotype in 6.1% of 2196 men participating in their French ICSI program (60). The most common abnormality was a numerical sex chromosome aberration (3.3%), followed by reciprocal translocations (1.2%), Robertsonian translocations (0.8%), and inversions (0.1%). The specific numerical chromosomal errors were 47,XXY (2.2%), 47,XYY

Table 2 Abnormal Karyotype Rates in Men with Spermatogenic Failure Undergoing ICSI

Series	Men screened	Abnormal karyotype rate (%)
Baschat (1996)	32	6.2
Peschka (1996)	200	3.0
Testart (1996)	261	4.2
Pandiyan (1996)	1,201	3.6
Yoshida (1997)	1,007	6.2
van der Ven (1997)	158	3.8
Mau (1997)	150	12.0
Meschede (1998)	432	2.1
Scholtes (1998)	1,140	4.5
Tuerlings (1998)	1,792	4.0
Le Bourhis (2000)	181	10.0
Gekas (2001)	2,196	6.1

Abbreviation: ICSI, intracytoplasmic sperm injection.

(0.3%), and mosaicism for numerical sex chromosome anomalies (0.8%). Men with spermatogenic failure and azoospermia had a much higher incidence of chromosomal abnormalities (6.3%) compared to men with oligozoospermia (2.8%) and normal sperm density (2.2%).

Klinefelter's syndrome (47, XXY) is relatively common, with an incidence of 1 in 500 live male births (Fig. 3). The mosaic form (46, XY/47, XXY) is present in 10% of Klinefelter's men. The extra X chromosome may be of maternal or paternal origin. Although men with Klinefelter's syndrome are classically described as having tall stature, gynecomastia, feminine hair distribution, and small testes, many of these somatic manifestations are absent. In a Japanese series of 148 Klinefelter's patients with sterility, small testes were observed in 95% of the patients and gynecomastia was seen in 12.4% (62). Half of the patients showed hypergonadotropic hypogonadism, while others showed normogonadism. There is a wide phenotypic appearance of men with Klinefelter's syndrome. Men with mosaic and nonmosaic Klinefelter's syndrome may have sperm within the seminiferous tubules. The characteristic finding on testis biopsy is seminiferous tubule hyalinization with Leydig cell hyperplasia. Preimplantation genetic diagnostic testing, chorionic villus sampling (CVS), or amniocentesis should be offered to couples prior to ICSI, although many couples may decline testing.

The XYY male syndrome occurs in about 1 in 1000 live births (63,64). Most men are phenotypically normal with a predisposition to greater than normal height, decreased intelligence, and increased incidence of leukemia. Numerous mosaic patterns may be present. Other less common, whole chromosomal abnormalities include the 46, XX male, which occurs in 1 in 20,000 live male births, and mixed gonadal dysgenesis. Mixed gonadal dysgenesis (46, XY or 45, X/46, XY) results in a phenotypic male or female with a unilateral testis and contralateral streak gonad. Both conditions result in azoospermia.

Translocations involve the exchange of segments of two different chromosomes without loss of genetic material. This exchange usually occurs during meiosis I and has been associated with male infertility by interrupting genes involved in spermatogenesis or various processes associated with gonadal differentiation, sperm structure, and androgen biosynthesis or action. The presence of Robertsonian translocations appears to cause fewer abnormal embryos and a higher rate of implantation than reciprocal translocations (65). A high percentage (87%) of embryos may be chromosomally abnormal, however, when parental Robertsonian translocations are present (66). Preimplantation genetic diagnosis substantially increases the couple's chances of sustaining a pregnancy to full term with chromosomally normal children when translocations are present (67,68).

Chromosomal abnormalities detected in the offspring of male-factor couples undergoing ICSI may be inherited or may arise de novo in a nonfamilial fashion. In't Veld et al. raised concerns when they reported four (27%) cytogenetic abnormalities in 15 pregnancies initiated by ICSI (69); however, these results may have been biased because of the advanced maternal age and the series being quite small. Wisanto et al., in contrast, studied a younger population and identified only six (1%) chromosomal abnormalities using CVS or amniocentesis from 585 prenatal diagnoses (70). Karyotype abnormalities may be inherited maternally or paternally. Bonduelle et al. determined fetal karyotypes in 1082 cases using prenatal diagnosis and identified 28 (2.6%) abnormalities (71). Testing of the parents indicated that 10 cases were inherited; nine (including eight balanced structural aberrations and one unbalanced trisomy 21) were transmitted from the father.

Karyotyping is indicative of gross chromosomal rearrangements and is easily assessed from a peripheral blood smear. Cells are cultured and arrested at the metaphase stage of meiosis to reveal the characteristic banding associated with each chromosome.

□ SYNDROMES AND UNCOMMON CONDITIONS

Numerous syndromes of uncommon occurrence may result in abnormal spermatogenesis. These conditions should be considered in terms of their principal level of action on sperm production and function: (i) hypothalamic–pituitary–gonadal axis (HPG), (ii) androgen biosynthesis/action, and (iii) sperm function. Kallmann's syndrome is an example of an HPG disorder resulting in an isolated defect of gonadotropin-releasing hormone (GnRH) from the hypothalamus. This syndrome is due to a deletion of the *KALIG-1* gene, located on Xp22.3, which is responsible for encoding a protein necessary for olfactory and GnRH axonal migration from the olfactory placode to the septal–preoptic nuclei (72). Clinical features include

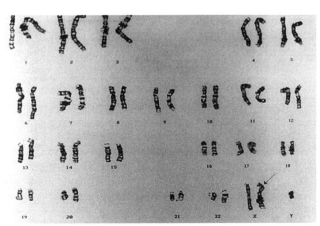

Figure 3 47, XXY karyotype analysis in an azoospermic male with Klinefelter's syndrome. The arrow indicates an extra X chromosome.

delayed onset of puberty, prepubertal size testes, and anosmia. HCG therapy combined with FSH may be used to stimulate sperm production. Other uncommon syndromes with a genetic basis affecting the HPG axis include abnormalities of the LH and FSH receptors, Prader–Willi syndrome (mutation/deletion in the paternal 15q11–q13), and cerebellar ataxia.

Syndromes that affect androgen production or action include defects in androgen biosynthesis, 5α-reductase deficiency, androgen-insensitivity syndrome, and Kennedy's disease. Milder forms of congenital adrenal hyperplasia can result in impaired testosterone production in otherwise healthy men but are extremely uncommon causes of male infertility. These errors of testosterone biosynthesis are presumed to be inherited in autosomal recessive or X-linked recessive fashion. 5α-reductase deficiency is inherited in autosomal recessive fashion and presents with incompletely virilized external genitalia. The intracellular conversion of testosterone to dihydrotestosterone is impaired by mutations in the gene for isoenzyme 2 (*SRD5A2*), mapped to 2p23, of 5α-reductase. The testes are typically cryptorchid or found in the labia. Although spermatogenesis is reduced, the major cause of reduced fertility is the inability to achieve vaginal penetration because of the markedly abnormal external genitalia.

Androgen-insensitivity syndromes include testicular feminization, Lub's syndrome, Reifenstein's syndrome, and Rosewater's syndrome. These syndromes all involve defects in the androgen receptor (AR), likely secondary to an *AR* gene defect. The *AR* gene is 90 kb in length, maps to Xq11-12, and consists of eight exons. An area of active research is the CAG repeat length in exon 1 in phenotypically normal men with idiopathic azoospermia (73,74). The CAG repeat length is shorter in normal men (21–24) than in men with spermatogenic failure (23,24,27–29), suggesting that this CAG trinucleotide expansion may be etiologic in some of these men (75–77). Other investigators, however, believe that differences in CAG repeat length are ethnically based and not causative of impaired spermatogenesis (78,79). Kennedy's disease, also known as spinal and bulbar muscular atrophy, is characterized by an amplification of CAG repeats in exon 1 of the transcriptional activation domain of the *AR* gene. This X-linked recessive disorder results in subtle androgen insensitivity manifest by gynecomastia and testicular atrophy. Although these men may be fertile early in life, oligozoospermia and azoospermia often result with age and disease progression, characterized by muscle weakness in the proximal spinal and bulbar muscles. Reifenstein's syndrome represents a form of partial androgen insensitivity. These men have impaired spermatogenesis, inadequate ductal morphogenesis, and incomplete external virilization.

Primary ciliary dyskinesia describes a number of syndromes that directly affect sperm function. The best known of these disorders is Kartagener's syndrome, characterized by immotile sperm as a result of a defect in the ultrastructure of the axoneme. Inherited in a predominantly autosomal recessive fashion, Kartagener's syndrome also is marked by chronic sinusitis, bronchiectasis, and situs inversus. Usher's syndrome is similar, but additionally features retinitis pigmentosa and deafness.

Finally, a number of syndromes with a probable genetic cause may cause male infertility as a result of variable effects on the reproductive tracts. These syndromes include prune belly syndrome, Noonan's syndrome, bladder exstrophy/epispadias, myotonic dystrophy, myelodysplasia, and β-thalassemia (80).

□ CONCERNS AND FUTURE DIRECTIONS
Consequences of Abnormal Testing
A Couple's Decision

Although genetic testing for men with azoospermia or severe oligozoospermia is advisable prior to ICSI, a couple may choose to decline evaluation, but it should be ensured that adequate genetic counseling has been provided. The effect of abnormal testing is influenced by the specific genetic abnormality and the attendant consequences. Further availability and refinement of technique of preimplantation genetic diagnostic testing in the future may influence a couple's decision to proceed with ICSI if a genetic abnormality is present.

The decision to proceed with ICSI when an AZFc microdeletion was present was unchanged in 79% of couples in a European series (81). In a Taiwanese series of 11 couples with Y-chromosome microdeletions, three (27%) thought microdeletion was a serious defect and opted against ICSI, while five (45%) chose ICSI as their treatment choice (82). The couples who proceeded with ICSI were likely influenced by the fact that the only known consequence of an AZFc microdeletion to date is spermatogenic failure, rather than a life-threatening or chronic illness. In contrast, when both parents are carriers of a *CFTR* gene mutation, cystic fibrosis may be the result in one in four offspring. With this significantly more serious known consequence, couples may be inclined to pursue preimplantation genetic diagnostic testing or the use of donor sperm. Even when chromosomal abnormalities are present and genetic counseling is provided, many couples choose to proceed with ICSI as evidenced in a Dutch series in which 42/75 couples (56%) proceeded with the ICSI (83).

Unknown Consequences of Abnormal Genetic Testing

Although ICSI represents one of the most significant advances in the treatment of the subfertile male, significant concerns exist regarding the potential for transmission of abnormal genes to the offspring because many of the natural barriers to conception have been bypassed. Although these abnormal genes may result in similar types of infertility problems in the offspring (as in the father), an unanswered question is whether these genes may result in other disease states or systemic problems (84). Thus far, no untoward effects have been observed (85). The true effect of ICSI on the offspring, however, cannot be determined without long-term follow-up (86).

Ethical Concerns

From a practical standpoint, it is possible that lack of confidentiality or release of the results of testing may cause genetic discrimination, whether subtle or overt (87–90). For example, if the male offspring of an ICSI pregnancy is known to have a Y-chromosome microdeletion or worse, his chances at establishing a marriage-type relationship with a significant other may be affected. Whether legally justified or not, patients with potential disease states may not wish for testing to be performed regardless of the genetic consequences for themselves or their offspring, fearing that obtaining health or life insurance would be jeopardized. Advances in computerized DNA chip technology for the rapid identification of DNA mutations will undoubtedly test these issues in the near future.

Promising Candidate Genes for Future Testing

All human cells contain 22 pairs of autosomes and one pair of sex chromosomes (XX-female, or XY-male) for a total of 23 pairs of chromosomes. Although most causes of poor sperm production are unknown, undoubtedly many genetic abnormalities will be identified on autosomal chromosomes. Animal studies are identifying numerous potential candidate genes (91). An example of a possible candidate male infertility gene is *DAZLA*, a new member of the *DAZ* family of genes and located at 3p25 (92). Other candidate genes such as *RBM* (*RBMY*), *DBY* (dead box on the Y), and *DFFRY* (*Drosophila* fat-facet-related Y) have been proposed in addition to *DAZ* (93).

The presence of human leukocyte antigen (HLA) class 1 may predispose men to idiopathic azoospermia (94,95). Miura et al. reported that the frequency of HLA-A33, B13, and B44 was significantly increased in Japanese men with idiopathic azoospermia compared to controls (94). Errors in genes responsible for DNA mismatch enzymes may also cause mutations in infertile men with meiotic arrest (96). For example, defects in the homologs of the DNA repair genes involved in hereditary nonpolyposis colon cancer lead to meiotic arrest in the testes of the offspring (97). Although many of the conceptions with defective DNA repair will likely result in a spontaneous abortion (98) with ICSI, it is possible that viable offspring may be born. Defects in chromatin packaging (99) and mitochondrial DNA (mtDNA) deletions (100) also have been correlated with either low fertilization rates or failure to achieve a pregnancy.

Preimplantation Genetic Diagnosis

Preimplantation genetic diagnosis (PGD) may be performed on IVF- or ICSI-derived embryos as a form of prenatal diagnosis aimed at eliminating embryos carrying serious genetic diseases before implantation (101–104). In PGD, a single cell is removed from an early eight-cell embryo (Fig. 4) and tested for various genetic disorders typically using fluorescence in-situ hybridization (FISH) or PCR. The most common technique used to biopsy the embryo involves the use of acidic Tyrode's drilling. FISH techniques allow the direct visualization of single genes and can be applied to single cells. The first clinical application of PGD was described in 1990 by Handyside, who amplified Y-chromosome-specific sequences using PCR to determine the sex of embryos from couples at risk of X-linked diseases (105). PGD may be used clinically for the detection of disease states associated with male infertility, such as cystic fibrosis and numerical chromosomal abnormalities. PGD has also been used for detection of numerous other disease states including Duchenne's muscular dystrophy, thalassemia, Huntington's disease, Tay-Sachs disease, fragile X, and Marfan syndrome.

The use of PGD in cases of severe male-factor infertility with additional adverse contributors such as advanced maternal age, repeated IVF failures, and altered peripheral blood karyotype was addressed by Gianaroli (106). In this series of 40 men and 28 normal controls, no increase in chromosomally abnormal embryos was detected. With regard to translocations, Pierce et al. demonstrated the beneficial use of PGD for the diagnosis of reciprocal translocations within the chromosomes 5 and 8 (107) for couples with Robertsonian translocations (66).

In a recent report from the European Society for Human Reproduction and Embryology (ESHRE) PGD Consortium, successful embryo biopsy was achieved in 96% to 99% of cases (101). An interpretable diagnosis was possible in 63% to 86% of embryos, and 36% to 43% of the embryos were diagnosed as suitable for transfer. Although diagnostic accuracy is excellent, a 4/116 (3.4%) fetal sac misdiagnosis rate was confirmed with the use of CVS and amniocentesis. Technical advances such as multiplex PCR may help to decrease this misdiagnosis rate. Altogether, the ESRHE PGD Consortium has reported on 241 births.

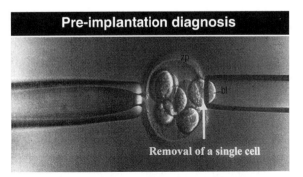

Figure 4 Removal of a single cell from an 8-cell embryo for preimplantation genetic diagnostic testing. *Source*: From Ref. 61.

FISH

Most FISH studies on sperm aneuploidy in infertile men have shown an increased rate of aneuploidy and disjunctional errors. Especially when the sperm density is below 5×10^6 sperm/mL, sperm disomy and diploidy rates may nearly double (108–112). Regarding sex chromosomes, reported frequencies of abnormalities range from 0.018% to 0.7% for XXY disomy, 0.009% to 0.6% for YY disomy, and 0.062% to 0.42% for CY disomy. The diploidy rates range from 0.06% to 0.97% (113,114). The variation in results is due to differences in selection criteria, differing FISH protocols, and variable scoring criteria. The use of multicolor FISH suggests that infertility patients had an increased risk of disomy for chromosome 1, 13, 21, and XY (115). These findings suggest that the offspring may have an increased risk of aneuploidy as a result.

To date, the application of FISH in clinical male infertility for evaluation of sperm aneuploidy has been research focused rather than as a widely used clinical assay for decision making. FISH is used to detect aneuploidies and chromosomal rearrangements (116). This technique uses a fluorescently labeled probe that binds or hybridizes to a chromosomal target (117). The two critical steps are: (i) denaturation of the DNA probe and the metaphase chromosomes on a slide, enabling separation of the double-stranded DNA, and (ii) hybridization of the probe to the chromosomal target. The fluorescent signal is observed by fluorescent microscopy.

Aneuploidy rates are also increased in spermatogenic cells in men with testicular failure. Using three-color FISH on testis biopsy tissue, Huang et al. found direct evidence of an increased aneuploidy rate in both mitotic and meiotic spermatogenic cells (118). The conclusion was that chromosomal instability may be the result of altered genetic control occurring during meiosis, mitosis, and spermatogonial proliferation.

Genetic Evaluation of the Offspring

The first large-scale study of genetic abnormalities in offspring conceived through ICSI was by Palermo et al. (119). A total of 751 couples undergoing 987 ICSI cycles for male-factor infertility were studied and had an overall clinical pregnancy (fetal heartbeat) rate of 44.3% and a resultant delivery rate per ICSI cycle of 38.7% (n = 382). In 8 of 11 miscarriages for which cytogenetic data were available, one autosomal trisomy was found, and seven additional pregnancies were terminated because of a chromosomal abnormality after prenatal diagnosis. Of the 578 neonates resulting from treatment by ICSI, 15 (2.6%) presented with congenital abnormalities (nine major and six minor abnormalities). This frequency of malformations, however, was lower than that observed in offspring born after standard IVF at the same institution. This study concluded that the chromosomal abnormality rate was not higher in ICSI compared to IVF. The true effect of ICSI on the offspring, however, cannot be determined without long-term follow-up. Similarly, several reviews and subsequent reports have concluded that ICSI does not appear to cause any significant increase in known genetics-based diseases or infertile males (120–122).

☐ CONCLUSION

Although ICSI represents one of the most significant advances in the treatment of the subfertile male, concerns exist regarding the potential for transmission of abnormal genes to the offspring because many of the natural barriers to conception have been bypassed. Genetic abnormalities related to male infertility should be considered in terms of being (i) causative for male infertility and (ii) potentially transmissible to the offspring. This chapter reviews genetic alterations such as Y-chromosome microdeletion, Klinefelter's syndrome, and *CF* gene mutations.

☐ REFERENCES

1. Palermo G, Joris H, Devroey P, et al. Pregnancies after intracytoplasmic injection of single spermatozoon into an oocyte. Lancet 1992; 340(8810):17–18.
2. Meschede D, Lemcke B, Behre HM, et al. Clustering of male infertility in the families of couples treated with intracytoplasmic sperm injection. Hum Reprod 2000; 15(7):1604–1608.
3. Rucker GB, Mielnik A, King P, et al. Preoperative screening for genetic abnormalities in men with non-obstructive azoospermia before testicular sperm extraction. J Urol 1998; 160:2068–2071.
4. Kupker W, Schwinger E, Hiort O, et al. Genetics of male subfertility: consequences for the clinical workup. Hum Reprod 1999; 14(suppl 1):24–37.
5. Greenberg SH, Lipshultz LI, Wein AJ. Experience with 425 subfertile male patients. J Urol 1978; 119: 507–510.
6. Jequier AM, Ansell ID, Bullimore NJ. Congenital absence of the vasa deferentia presenting with infertility. J Androl 1985; 6:15–19.
7. Cystic Fibrosis Genetic Analysis Consortium. Population variation of common cystic fibrosis mutations. Hum Mutation 1994; 4:167–177.
8. Welsh MJ, Smith AE. Cystic fibrosis. Sci Am 1995; 273: 52–59.

9. Kerem B, Rommens JM, Buchanan JA, et al. Identification of the cystic fibrosis gene: genetic analysis. Science 1989; 245:1073–1080.

10. Riordan JR, Rommens JM, Kerem B, et al. Identification of the cystic fibrosis gene: cloning and characterization of complementary DNA. Science 1989; 8:245(4922): 1066–1073.

11. Rommens JM, Iannuzzi MC, Kerem B, et al. Identification of the cystic fibrosis gene: chromosome walking and jumping. Science 1989; 245(4922): 1059–1065.

12. Claustres M, Guittard C, Bozon D, et al. Spectrum of CFTR mutations in cystic fibrosis and in congenital absence of the vas deferens in France. Hum Mutat 2000; 16(2):143–156.

13. Chillon M, Casals T, Mercier B, et al. Mutations in the cystic fibrosis gene in patients with congenital absence of the vas deferens. N Engl J Med 1995; 332: 1475–1480.

14. Schlegel P, Shin D, Goldstein M. Congenital absence of the vas deferens. J Urol 1996; 155:1644–1648.

15. Donat R, McNeill AS, Fitzpatrick DR, et al. The incidence of cystic fibrosis gene mutations in patients with congenital bilateral absence of the vas deferens in Scotland. Br J Urol 1997; 79(1):74–77.

16. Anguiano A, Oates RD, Amos JA, et al. Congenital bilateral absence of the vas deferens: a primarily genital form of cystic fibrosis. JAMA 1992; 267:1794–1797.

17. Jarvi K, Zielenski J, Wilschanski M, et al. Cystic fibrosis transmembrane conductance regulator and obstructive azoospermia. Lancet 1995; 345:1578.

18. Mickle JE, Cutting GR. Genotype-phenotype relationships in cystic fibrosis. Med Clin North Am 2000; 84(3): 597–607.

19. Lewis-Jones DI, Gazvani MR, Mountford R. Cystic fibrosis in infertility: screening before assisted reproduction. Hum Reprod 2000; 15:2415–2417.

20. Shin D, Gilbert F, Goldstein M, et al. Congenital absence of the vas deferens: incomplete penetrance of cystic fibrosisgene mutations. J Urol 1997; 158(5):1794–1798.

21. Goossens V, Sermon K, Lissens W, et al. Clinical application of preimplantation genetic diagnosis for cystic fibrosis. Prenat Diagn 2000; 20(7):571–581.

22. Schlegel PN, Palermo GD, Alikani M, et al. Micropuncture retrieval of epididymal sperm with in vitro fertilization: importance of in vitro micromanipulation techniques. Urology 1995; 46:238–241.

23. Silber SJ, Nagy ZP, Liu J, et al. Van Steirteghem AC. Conventional in-vitro fertilization versus intracytoplasmic sperm injection for patients requiring microsurgical sperm aspiration. Hum Reprod 1994; 9(9): 1705–1709.

24. Phillipson GT, Petrucco OM, Matthews CD. Congenital bilateral absence of the vas deferens, cystic fibrosis mutation analysis and intracytoplasmic sperm injection. Hum Reprod 2000; 15(2):431–435.

25. Genzyme Genetics at http://www.genzyme.com.

26. Genetics & IVF Institute at http://www.givf.com.

27. Tiepolo L, Zuffardi O. Localization of factors controlling spermatogenesis in the non-fluorescent portion of the human Y chromosome long arm. Hum Genet 1976; 89:292–300.

28. Reijo R, Lee T-Y, Salo P, et al. Diverse spermatogenic defects in humans caused by Y chromosome deletions encompassing a novel RNA-binding protein gene. Nature Genet 1995; 10:383–393.

29. Najmabadi H, Huang V, Yen P, et al. Substantial prevalence of microdeletions of the Y-chromosome in infertile men with idiopathic azoospermia and oligozoospermia detected using a sequence-tagged site-based mapping strategy. J Clin Endocrinol Metab 1996; 81:1346–1352.

30. Vogt P, Chandley AC, Hargreave TB, et al. Microdeletions in interval 6 of the Y chromosome of males with idiopathic sterility point to disruption of AZF, a human spermatogenesis gene. Hum Genet 1992; 89:491–496.

31. Pryor JL, Kent-First M, Muallem A. Microdeletions in the Y chromosome of infertile men. N Engl J Med 1997; 336:534–539.

32. Stuppia L, Mastroprimiano G, Calabrese G, et al. Microdeletions in interval 6 of the Y chromosome detected by STS-PCR in 6 of 33 patients with idiopathic oligo- or azoospermia. Cytogenet Cell Genet 1996; 72:155–158.

33. Chandley AC, Cooke HJ. Human male fertility—Y-linked genes and spermatogenesis. Hum Mol Genet 1994; 3:1449–1452.

34. Ma K, Inglis JD, Sharkey A, et al. A Y chromosome gene family with RNA-binding protein homology: candidates for the azoospermia factor AZF controlling spermatogenesis. Cell 1993; 75:1287–1295.

35. Bardoni B, Zuffardi O, Guioli S, et al. A deletion map of the human Yq11 region: implications for the evolution of the Y chromosome and tentative mapping of a locus involved in spermatogenesis. Genomics 1991; 11: 443–451.

36. Vogt PH, Edelmann A, Kirsch S, et al. Human Y chromosome azoospermia factors (AZF) mapped to different subregions in Yq11. Hum Mol Genet 1996; 5:933–943.

37. Krausz C, Quintana-Murci L, Barbaux S, et al. A high frequency of Y chromosome deletions in males with nonidiopathic infertility. J Clin Endocrinol Metab 1999; 84:3606–3612.

38. Ferlin A, Moro E, Garolla A, et al. Human male infertility and Y chromosome deletions: role of the AZF-candidate genes DAZ, RBM and DFFRY. Hum Reprod 1999; 14(7):1710–1716.

39. Brandell RA, Mielnik A, Liotta D, et al. AZFb deletions predict the absence of spermatozoa with testicular sperm extraction: preliminary report of a prognostic genetic test. Hum Reprod 1998; 13:2812–2815.

40. Krausz C, Quintana-Murci L, McElreavey K. Prognostic value of Y deletion analysis: what is the clinical prognostic value of Y chromosome microdeletion analysis? Hum Reprod 2000; 15(7):1431–1434.

41. Silber S, Alagappan R, Brown LG, et al. Y chromosome deletions in azoospermic and severely oligozoospermic men undergoing intracytoplasmic sperm injection after testicular sperm extraction. Hum Reprod 1998; 13:3332–3337.

42. Mulhall JP, Reijo R, Alagappan R, et al. Azoospermic men with deletion of the DAZ gene cluster are capable of completing spermatogenesis: fertilization, normal embryonic development and pregnancy occur when retrieved testicular spermatozoa are used for intracytoplasmic sperm injection. Hum Reprod 1997; 12: 503–509.

43. Kent-First M, Muallem A, Shultz J, et al. Defining regions of the Y-chromosome responsible for male infertility and identification of a fourth AZF region (AZFd) by Y-chromosome microdeletion detection. Mol Reprod Dev 1999; 53(1):27–41.

44. Foresta C, Moro E, Garolla A, et al. Y chromosome microdeletions in cryptorchidism and idiopathic infertility. J Clin Endocrinol Metab 1999; 84(10): 3660–3665.

45. Liow SL, Yong EL, Ng SC. Prognostic value of Y deletion analysis. Hum Reprod 2001; 16:9–12.

46. Kleiman SE, Yogev L, Gamzu R, et al. Three-generation evaluation of Y-chromosome microdeletion. J Androl 1999; 20(3):394–398.

47. Page DC, Silber S, Brown LG. Men with infertility caused by AZFc deletion can produce sons by intracytoplasmic sperm injection, but are likely to transmit the deletion and infertility. Hum Reprod 1999; 14(7): 1722–1726.

48. Kent-First MG, Kol S, Muallem A, et al. The incidence and possible relevance of Y-linked microdeletions in babies born after intracytoplasmic sperm injection and their infertile fathers. Mol Hum Reprod 1996; 2: 943–950.

49. Chang PL, Sauer MV, Brown S. Y chromosome microdeletion in a father and his four infertile sons. Hum Reprod 1999; 14:2689–2694.

50. Simoni M, Bakker MC, Eurlings MCM, et al. Laboratory guidelines for molecular diagnosis of Y chromosomal microdeletions. Int J Androl 1999; 22:292–299.

51. Estop AM, Munne S, Cieply KM, et al. Meiotic products of a Klinefelter 47,XXY male as determined by sperm fluorescence in-situ hybridization analysis. Hum Reprod 1998; 13(1):124–127.

52. Kruse R, Guttenbach M, Schartmann B, et al. Genetic counseling in a patient with XXY/XXXY/XY mosaic Klinefelter's syndrome: estimate of sex chromosome aberrations in sperm before intracytoplasmic sperm injection. Fertil Steril 1998; 69(3):482–485.

53. Nodar F, De Vincentiis S, Olmedo SB, et al. Birth of twin males with normal karyotype after intracytoplasmic sperm injection with use of testicular spermatozoa from a nonmosaic patient with Klinefelter's syndrome. Fertil Steril 1999; 71(6):1149–1152.

54. Ron-El R, Strassburger D, Gelman-Kohan S, et al. A 47,XXY fetus conceived after ICSI of spermatozoa from a patient with non-mosaic Klinefelter's syndrome: case report. Hum Reprod 2000; 15:1804–1806.

55. Palermo GD, Schlegel PN, Sills ES, et al. Births after intracytoplasmic injection of sperm obtained by testicular extraction from men with nonmosaic Klinefelter's syndrome. N Engl J Med 1998; 338(9):588–590.

56. Mau UA, Bäckert IT, Kaiser P, et al. Chromosomal findings in 150 couples referred for genetic counseling prior to intracytoplasmic sperm injection. Hum Reprod 1997; 12:930–937.

57. Meschede D, Lemcke B, Exeler JR, et al. Chromosome abnormalities in 447 couples undergoing intracytoplasmic sperm injection—Prevalence, types, sex distribution and reproductive relevance. Hum Reprod 1998; 13:576–582.

58. Testart J, Gautier E, Brami C, et al. Intracytoplasmic sperm injection in infertile patients with structural chromosome abnormalities. Hum Reprod 1996; 11: 2609–2612.

59. Pandiyan N, Jequier AM. Mitotic chromosomal anomalies among 1210 infertile men. Hum Reprod 1996; 11:2604–2608.

60. Gekas J, Thepot F, Turleau C, et al. Chromosomal factors of infertility in candidate couples for ICSI: an equal risk of constitutional aberrations in women and men. Hum Reprod 2001; 16:82–90.

61. Schimmel TW, Crumm KF. Images in medicine. Microsurgical fertilization and blastomere removal for genetic analysis. N Engl J Med 1994; 331(18):1200.

62. Okada H, Fujioka H, Tatsumi N, et al. Klinefelter's syndrome in the male infertility clinic. Hum Reprod Apr 1999; 14(4):946–952.

63. Smyth CM, Bremner WJ. Klinefelter syndrome. Arch Intern Med 1998; 158(12):1309–1314.

64. Diemer T, Desjardins C. Developmental and genetic disorders in spermatogenesis. Hum Reprod Update 1999; 5(2):120–140.

65. Munne S, Sandalinas M, Escudero T, et al. Outcome of preimplantation genetic diagnosis of translocations. Fertil Steril 2000; 73(6):1209–1218.

66. Conn CM, Harper JC, Winston RM, et al. Infertile couples with Robertsonian translocations: preimplantation genetic analysis of embryos reveals chaotic cleavage divisions. Hum Genet 1998; 102(1): 117–123.

67. Munne S, Morrison L, Fung J, et al. Spontaneous abortions are reduced after pre-conception diagnosis of translocations. J Assist Reprod Genet 1998; 15: 290–296.

68. Giltay JC, Tiemessen CH, van Inzen WG, et al. One normal child and a chromosomally balanced/normal twin after intracytoplasmicsperm injection in a male with a de-novo t(Y;16) translocation. Hum Reprod 1998; 13(1O):2745–2747.

69. In't Veld P, Brandenburg H, Verhoeff A, et al. Sex chromosomal abnormalities and intra-cytoplasmic sperm injection. Lancet 1995; 346:773.

70. Wisanto A, Bonduelle M, Camus M, et al. Obstetric outcome of 904 pregnancies after intracytoplasmic sperm injection. Hum Reprod 1996; 11(suppl 4):121–129.

71. Bonduelle M, Camus M, De Vos A, et al. Seven years of intracytoplasmic sperm injection and follow-up of 1987 subsequent children. Hum Reprod 1999; 14(suppl 1):243–264.

72. Bick D, Franco B, Sherins RJ, et al. Brief report: intragenic deletion of the KALIG-1 gene in Kallmann's syndrome. N Engl J Med 1992; 326(26):1752–1755.

73. Hiort O, Holterhus PM, Horter T, et al. Significance of mutations in the androgen receptor gene in males with idiopathic infertility. J Clin Endocrinol Metab 2000; 85(8):2810–2815.

74. Gottlieb B, Beitel LK, Lumbroso R, et al. Update of the androgen receptor gene mutations database. Hum Mutat 1999; 14(2):103–114.

75. Yoshida KI, Yano M, Chiba K, et al. CAG repeat length in the androgen receptor gene is enhanced in patients with idiopathic azoospermia. Urology 1999; 54(6): 1078–1081.

76. Dowsing AT, Yong EL, Clark M, et al. Linkage between male infertility and trinucleotide repeat expansion in the androgen-receptor gene. Lancet 1999; 354(9179): 640–643.

77. Komori S, Kasumi H, Kanazawa R, et al. CAG repeat length in the androgen receptor gene of infertile Japanese males with oligozoospermia. Mol Hum Reprod 1999; 5(1):14–16.

78. Dadze S, Wieland C, Jakubiczka S, et al. The size of the CAG repeat in exon 1 of the androgen receptor gene shows no significant relationship to impaired spermatogenesis in an infertile Caucasoid sample of German origin. Mol Hum Reprod 2000; 6(3):207–214.

79. Giwercman YL, Xu C, Arver S, et al. No association between the androgen receptor gene CAG repeat and impaired sperm production in Swedish men. Clin Genet 1998; 54(5):435–436.

80. Jaffe T, Oates RD. Genetic aspects of infertility. In: Lipshultz L, Howards S, eds. Infertility in the Male. 3rd ed. St. Louis: Mosby, 1997:280–304.

81. Nap AW, Van Golde RJ, Tuerlings JH, et al. Reproductive decisions of men with microdeletions of the Y chromosome: the role of genetic counseling. Hum Reprod 1999; 14(8): 2166–2169.

82. Lin WM, Chen CW, Sun S, et al. Y-chromosome microdeletion and its effect on reproductive decisions in Taiwanese patients presenting with nonobstructive azoospermia. Urology 2000; 56:1041–1046.

83. Giltay JC, Kastrop PM, Tuerlings JH, et al. Subfertile men with constitutive chromosome abnormalities do not necessarily refrain from intracytoplasmic sperm injection treatment: a follow-up study on 75 Dutch patients. Hum Reprod 1999; 14(2):318–320.

84. Lamb DJ. Debate: is ICSI a genetic time bomb? Yes. J Androl 1999; 20(1):23–33.

85. Schlegel PN. Debate: is ICSI a genetic time bomb? No: ICSI is safe and effective. J Androl 1999; 20(1):18–22.

86. Tripp BM, Kolon TF, Bishop C, et al. Intracytoplasmic sperm injection and potential transmission of genetic disease. JAMA 1997; 277(12):963–964.

87. Blanck PD, Marti MW. Genetic discrimination and the employment provisions of the Americans with Disabilities Act: emerging legal, empirical, and policy. Behav Sci Law 1996; 14:411–432.

88. Kegley JA. Using genetic information: a radical problematic for an individualistic framework. Med Law 1996; 15:715–720.

89. Miller K, Kohm LM. Designer babies: are test tubes and microbes replacing romance? relevant legal issues and DNA. Am J Forensic Med Pathol 1996; 17(4): 305–307.

90. Lapham EV, Kozma C, Weiss JO. Genetic discrimination: perspectives of consumers. Science 1996; 274(5287):621–624.

91. Kim ED, Lamb DJ, Bischoff FZ, et al. Genetic concerns of ICSI. Prenat Diag 1998; 18:1349–1365.

92. Seboun E, Barbaux S, Bourgeron T, et al. Gene sequence, localization, and evolutionary conservation of DAZLA, a candidate male sterility gene. Genomics 1997; 41(2):227–235.

93. Vogt PH, Edelmann A, Habermann B, et al. Y chromosome and male fertility genes. In: Kempers RD, Cohen J, Haney AF, Younger AF, eds. Fertility and Reproductive Medicine. Proceedings of the XVI World Congress on Fertility and Sterility, San Francisco, New York: Elsevier 1998:765–739.

94. Miura H, Tsujimura A, Nishimura K, et al. Susceptibility to idiopathic azoospermia in Japanese men is linked to HLA class I antigen. J Urol 1998; 159(6):1939–1941.

95. Van der ven K, Fimmers R, Engels G, van der Ven H, Krebs D. Evidence for major histocompatibility complex-mediated effects on spermatogenesis in humans. Hum Reprod 2000; 15:189–196.

96. Nudell D, Castillo M, Turek PJ, et al. Increased frequency of mutations in DNA from infertile men with meiotic arrest. Hum Reprod 2000; 15(6): 1289–1294.

97. Baker SM, Plug AW, Prolla TA, et al. Involvement of mouse Mlh1 in DNA mismatch repair and meiotic crossing over. Nat Genet 1996; 13(3):336–342.

98. Spandidos DA, Koumantakis E, Sifakis S, et al. Microsatellite mutations in spontaneously aborted embryos. Fertil Steril 1998; 70(5):892–895.

99. Evenson DP, Jost LK, Marshall D, et al. Utility of the sperm chromatin structure assay as a diagnostic and prognostic tool in the human fertility clinic. Hum Reprod 1999; 14(4):1039–1049.

100. St John JC, Cooke ID, Barratt CL. Mitochondrial mutations and male infertility. Nat Med 1997; 3(2): 124–125.

101. ESHRE Preimplantation genetic diagnosis (PGD) consortium: data collection II (May 2000). Hum Reprod 2000; 15:2673–2683.

102. Grifo JA, Tang YX, Krey L. Update in preimplantation genetic diagnosis. Age, genetics, and infertility. Ann N Y Acad Sci 1997; 828:162–165.

103. Harper JC, Handyside AH. The current status of preimplantation diagnosis. Curr Obstet Gynecol 1994; 4:143–149.

104. Harper JC. Preimplantation diagnosis of inherited disease by embryo biopsy: an update of the world figures. J Assist Reprod Genet 1996; 13:90–95.

105. Handyside AH, Kontogianni EH, Hardy K, et al. Pregnancies from biopsied human preimplantation embryos sexed by Y-specific DNA amplification. Nature 1990; 344:768–780.

106. Gianaroli L, Magli MC, Ferraretti AP, et al. Preimplantation genetic diagnosis increases the implantation rate in human in vitro fertilization by avoiding the transfer of chromosomally abnormal embryos. Fertil Steril 1997; 68(6):1128–1131.

107. Pierce KE, Fitzgerald LM, Seibel MM, et al. Preimplantation genetic diagnosis of chromosome balance in embryos from a patient with a balanced reciprocal translocation. Mol Hum Reprod 1998; 4(2): 167–172.

108. Bernardini L, Martini E, Geraedts JP, et al. Comparison of gonosomal aneuploidy in spermatozoa of normal fertile men and those with severe male factor detected by in-situ hybridization. Mol Hum Reprod 1997; 3: 431–438.

109. Bernardini L, Borini A, Preti S, et al. Study of aneuploidy in normal and abnormal germ cells from semen of fertile and infertile men. Hum Reprod 1998; 13: 3406–3413.

110. Ushijima C, Kumasako Y, Kihaile PE, et al. Analysis of chromosomal abnormalities in human spermatozoa using multi-colour fluorescence in-situ hybridization. Hum Reprod 2000; 15:1107–1111.

111. Martin RH, Spriggs E, Rademaker AW. Multicolor fluorescence in situ hybridization analysis of aneuploidy and diploidy frequencies in 225,846 sperm from 10 normal men. Biol Reprod 1996; 54(2):394–398.

112. Moosani N, Pattinson HA, Carter MD, et al. Chromosomal analysis of sperm from men with idiopathic infertility using sperm karyotyping and fluorescence in situ hybridization. Fertil Steril 1995; 64(4): 811–817.

113. Egozcue J, Blanco J, Vidal F. Chromosome studies in human sperm nuclei using fluorescence in-situhybridization (FISH). Hum Reprod Update 1997; 3(5): 441–452.

114. Vegetti W, Van Assche E, Frias A, et al. Correlation between semen parameters and sperm aneuploidy rates investigated by fluorescence in-situ hybridization in infertile men. Hum Reprod 2000; 15(2): 351–365.

115. Martin RH. Genetics of human sperm. J Assist Reprod Genet 1998; 15(5):240–245.

116. St John JC. Incorporating molecular screening techniques into the modern andrology laboratory. J Androl 1999; 20(6):692–701.

117. Downie SE, Flaherty SP, Matthews CD. Detection of chromosomes and estimation of aneuploidy in human spermatozoa using fluorescence in-situ hybridization. Mol Hum Reprod 1997; 3(7):585–598.

118. Huang WJ, Lamb DJ, Kim ED, et al. Germ-cell nondisjunction in testes biopsies of men with idiopathic infertility. Am J Hum Genet 1999; 64(6): 1638–1645.

119. Palermo GD, Colombero LT, Schattman GL, et al. Evolution of pregnancies and initial follow-up of newborns delivered after intracytoplasmic sperm injection. JAMA 1996; 276:1893–1897.

120. Engel W, Murphy D, Schmid M. Are there genetic risks associated with microassisted reproduction? Hum Reprod 1996; 11:2359–2370.

121. Loft A, Petersen K, Erb K, et al. A Danish national cohort of 730 infants born after intracytoplasmic sperm injection (ICSI) 1994–1997. Hum Reprod 1999; 14(8): 2143–2148.

122. Wennerholm UB, Bergh C, Hamberger L, et al. Incidence of congenital malformations in children born after ICSI. Hum Reprod 2000; 15:944–948.

28

Imaging of the Reproductive Tract in Male Infertility

Ewa Kuligowska
Department of Radiology, Boston Medical Center, Boston, Massachusetts, U.S.A.

Erik N. Nelson
Department of Radiology, Massachusetts General Hospital, Boston, Massachusetts, U.S.A.

Helen M. Fenlon
Department of Radiology, Mater Misericordiae Hospital, Dublin, Ireland

□ INTRODUCTION

Reproductive infertility, defined as the inability to conceive after one year of unprotected intercourse, affects 15% of couples in the United States (1). In up to 50% of these cases, a male factor is responsible. Scrotal abnormalities resulting in the disordered production of normal sperm count represent almost half of all male infertility cases (2); other conditions that produce male infertility include congenital and developmental anomalies such as cryptorchidism, Klinefelter's syndrome, and agenesis of the vas deferens, seminal vesicles, and ejaculatory ducts, as well as varicoceles, hypopituitarism, and other endocrinopathies. Distal duct obstruction (including cysts and stones of the vas deferens, seminal vesicles, and ejaculatory ducts), and inflammatory or infective conditions such as mumps orchitis, syphilis, and bacterial infections involving the testes, epididymis, vas deferens, seminal vesicles, ejaculatory ducts, and prostate are also possible causes for male infertility (3).

Since the causes of male reproductive dysfunction can be broadly categorized as being either correctable or noncorrectable, good clinical management depends on the accurate identification and diagnosis of the underlying disorder. Abnormalities that cause testicular failure and impaired spermatogenesis generally cannot be surgically corrected (with the notable exception of surgical varicocele repair), whereas obstructive processes involving the sperm transport system are more often curable (4,5). Therefore, a combination of thorough clinical evaluation and seminal analysis helps differentiate patients with irreversible defects from those with distal duct obstruction that may be amenable to surgical or radiologic intervention.

A complete physical examination of the patient should be performed after a thorough history and review of all prior laboratory testing, including semen analyses. Attention is then directed to the testes (size and consistency), vas deferens (palpability), epididymis (length and consistency), and the presence or absence of varicoceles. Repeated semen analyses, further endocrine testing, and postejaculatory urine analysis are performed when appropriate to exclude retrograde ejaculation (5). Patients with clinically irreparable testicular failure or impaired spermatogenesis usually present with either azoospermia or oligospermia and normal ejaculate volumes (greater than 2 mL), as most of the ejaculate volume is elaborated by the unobstructed seminal vesicles. Therefore, patients with azoospermia (the total absence of sperm cells in the ejaculate) or severe oligospermia (less than 2.0×10^6 spermatozoa/mL) who have low ejaculate volumes (less than 1 mL) in the absence of retrograde ejaculation should be investigated for distal duct abnormalities. These may include conditions such as agenesis or hypoplasia of the vas deferens, seminal vesicles, and ejaculatory ducts, distal ductal obliteration by fibrosis and calcification, and distal duct obstruction by calculi or cysts.

Traditional evaluation of the distal male reproductive tract was limited until recently by an inability to visualize the distal portions of the vas deferens, seminal vesicles, ejaculatory ducts, and prostate directly and noninvasively (4–11). Clinical examination provides little or no anatomic information regarding the distal ductal system. Vasography, although effective in delineating distal ductal structures, is invasive and may result in iatrogenic damage to the vas deferens (2–4). Technical improvement in equipment, such as the development of high-resolution small parts and endorectal transducers, as well as additional color Doppler and power Doppler capabilities, has enabled the radiologist to make a specific diagnosis and direct appropriate patient management. Noninvasive imaging modalities, including computerized tomography (CT), magnetic resonance imaging (MRI), and transrectal ultrasound (TRUS), are increasingly used to evaluate infertile male patients. TRUS is the most widely accepted of the cross-sectional imaging

Table 1 Imaging Recommendations for Male Infertility Conditions

Condition	Imaging modality
Congenital abnormalities of the vas deferens or seminal vesicles	TRUS, MRI[a]
Cryptorchidism	Pelvic ultrasound, CT, MRI[a]
Ejaculatory duct obstruction	TRUS (sagittal views), MRI[a]
Low-volume azoospermia	TRUS
Prostatic and periurethral cysts	TRUS, ultrasound-guided needle aspiration
Seminal vesicle and vas deferens cysts	TRUS
Testicular neoplasm	Ultrasound (Doppler), MRI[a]
Testicular pathology (epididymitis and orchitis, hydrocele, spermatocele, testicular atrophy, testicular microlithiasis, torsion ischemia, trauma, varicocele)	Ultrasound (Doppler)

[a]Recommended only for more complex, problematic cases due to cost and limited availability.
Abbreviations: CT, computed tomography; MRI, magnetic resonance imaging; TRUS, transrectal ultrasound.

techniques and has almost totally replaced vasography in many institutions (4–10).

This chapter outlines the pathologic variants that may be seen in infertile men and highlights the contribution of new imaging technologies such as MRI, scrotal ultrasound, and TRUS in dictating appropriate patient management. Please refer to Table 1 for a concise summary of imaging modality recommendations organized by clinical condition.

☐ RADIOGRAPHIC EVALUATION OF MALE INFERTILITY
Overview of Imaging Modalities
Ultrasound

Modern ultrasound equipment uses the pulsed-echo technique, converting electrical impulses into intermittent waves of sound that are transmitted into live tissue. These waves are then absorbed or reflected in varying degrees depending on the density of the tissues with which they interact. Reflected sound waves are received by the transducer and translated back into electrical impulses. The ultrasound machine analyzes the intervals between sound transmission and reception and subsequently displays the information as an image composed of different shades of gray. Very dense tissues produce more reflections of sound ("echoes") that are depicted as a bright, or "hyperechoic" pattern. Fluid- containing tissues reflect fewer sound waves, yielding a relatively dark, or "anechoic" pattern (12).

Most medical applications employ ultrasound transducers with frequencies between 2 and 15 MHz. At the expense of diminished depth of penetration, greater spatial resolution can be obtained with higher frequency transducers. This property makes high-resolution ultrasound equipment particularly well suited for imaging superficial structures such as joints, the thyroid gland, or the scrotum; the latter organ is usually scanned with a 7 to 10 MHz transducer (10).

Additional functional information can be obtained through the use of color Doppler and power Doppler imaging. These modalities detect the direction and relative velocity of flowing blood as the result of the apparent sound wave frequency shift that occurs when blood

flows past a stationary transducer. Blood predominantly moving away from the transducer shifts the transmitted sound wave to a lower frequency, while blood moving toward the transducer shifts the transmitted sound wave to a higher frequency. The magnitude of the frequency shift is determined by the velocity of blood flow. Color Doppler superimposes this information on the gray-scale image, typically illustrating blood moving either toward or away from the transducer in the colors red and blue, respectively, with lighter shades indicating higher velocities. Power Doppler imaging offers the additional advantage of greater slow-flow sensitivity, as well as being nondirectionally dependent (12,13).

Scrotal Ultrasound

For ultrasound examination of the testes, the patient is positioned supine on the examining table, with the penis retracted onto the abdomen and the scrotum supported on a towel. Adequate amounts of gel and avoidance of air bubbles are important to ensure minimization of artifacts. Selection of the correct transducer, gain, and Doppler scale settings are critical and is best established on the normal or asymptomatic testis first.

Transrectal Ultrasound

TRUS should be performed using a dedicated high-frequency endorectal transducer (5–9 MHz). Patients are examined in the left lateral decubitus position with the transducer placed in the rectum. The terminal vas deferens, seminal vesicles, ejaculatory ducts, and prostate are examined in a systematic manner in both axial and sagittal planes, with measurements recorded in two dimensions. Careful consideration of the dimensions of the distal ductal structures as well as the internal architecture and echotexture of the vas deferens and seminal vesicles is necessary. Additional attention should be given to the kidneys in order to detect potential associated renal anomalies (4,5,14,15).

Magnetic Resonance Imaging

The advantages of the lack of ionizing radiation and increased anatomic detail offered by MRI make this modality an attractive choice for imaging of the male reproductive tract. For example, visualization of unde-scended or ectopic testes is often possible in cases of cryptorchidism, and the vas deferens and seminal vesicles can be assessed easily for evidence of obstruction, structural abnormality, or inflammation, as well. The general recommendation is to use T1- and T2-weighted images for optimal tissue contrast, detection of hemorrhage, and differentiation of fluid collections. Recently, fast-spin echo techniques have been substituted for conventional scans due to the significant reduction in scanning time (16).

Within the scrotum, MRI is also useful in identifying both malignant and benign processes. Testicular tumors appear as well-defined areas of low signal on T2-weighted images, demarcated from the high-signal background of testicular parenchyma. Tumor invasion may be seen as disruption of the dark line of the tunica albuginea. Accurate demonstration of abdominal and pelvic lymphadenopathy allows for reliable staging. MRI may assist in distinguishing seminomas from nonseminomatous tumors, the latter of which are more heterogeneous on both T1- and T2-weighted images, due to the greater amount of hemorrhage and necrosis present in these tumors. This heterogeneity corresponds well with the mixed echogenicity similarly seen on ultrasound. Nonseminomatous tumors may also often demonstrate a well-defined, dark capsule. In contrast, seminomas are more homogeneous and nodular, hypodense relative to testicular parenchyma on T2-weighting, and lack a well-defined capsule (17). It should be noted, however, that the only definitive method of differentiating these tumors remains surgical pathology, and sometimes the presence of tumor markers.

Epididymal cysts appear on MRI as well-defined extratesticular fluid collections, low signal on T1-weighted images, and high signal on T2-weighted images. Conversely, spermatoceles contain more debris and sediment than epididymal cysts and thus provide more heterogeneous signal intensities (17).

Typical congenital and obstructive abnormalities of the seminal vesicles, vas deferens, ejaculatory ducts, and prostate are best approached with TRUS, and MRI should be reserved for more problematic cases. Cysts in the seminal vesicle, vas deferens, ejaculatory ducts, and prostate can be clearly depicted on T1- and T2-weighted images, except when hemorrhage coexists. MRI using dedicated endorectal coils is effective in demonstrating the distal male reproductive system but its use is unfortunately limited by cost and availability. CT provides only limited visualization of the distal ducts and is rarely indicated.

□ EMBRYOLOGIC CONSIDERATIONS

Because the Wolffian duct ultimately gives rise to the renal collecting system, ureter, bladder trigone, vas deferens, seminal vesicles, ejaculatory ducts, epididymis, paradidymis, and appendix epididymis, complex

associations of congenital anomalies of the distal male reproductive tract and urinary tract can often be explained by their common embryological origin. The nature and severity of such anomalies are related to the stage at which developmental arrest or insult occurs in utero (11,18,19). Similarly, irregular closure of the processus vaginalis may result in the formation of testicular or spermatic cord hydroceles (12,13,20).

□ ANATOMIC IMAGING OF THE NORMAL MALE REPRODUCTIVE TRACT

Testis

On ultrasound examination, the scrotal wall appears as a single layer with maximal thickness of 8 mm. There is a midline septum bisecting the scrotal cavity, and a thin layer of fluid (1–2 mL in volume) lines the serosal sac. The testes are symmetric in shape and size, with each adult testis measuring approximately 4 cm in length, 3 cm in width, and 2.5 cm in anterior–posterior diameter; all of these parameters decrease slightly with age. The testes are homogeneous in echotexture, with intermediate echogenicity. The mediastinum, however, appears as a thick, brightly echogenic line extending longitudinally through the testis (Fig. 1A and B). The epididymis demonstrates less homogeneity and slightly increased echogenicity compared to the testis and can be found parallel and posterior to the linear mediastinum. The head is located immediately posterior to the superior pole of the testis and measures approximately 7 mm in diameter, while the tapering body is 1 to 2 mm in width (12,21).

Doppler waveforms of the normal intratesticular arteries contain wide systolic peaks with relatively high diastolic flow, due to the low vascular resistance within the testis (22).

Vas Deferens

The vas deferens are paired tubular structures that pass from the scrotum into the pelvis through the inguinal canal. At the internal ring, they curve laterally and then pass medially and downward into the pelvis toward the base of the bladder. On axial TRUS imaging, the distal portion of each vas deferens is seen passing posteromedial to the ipsilateral seminal vesicle and has a mean diameter of 3 to 5 mm. The tortuous and dilated terminal of each vas is known as the ampulla, which has an external diameter of approximately 5 to 8 mm (Figs. 2A, 2B, and 3) (4–10).

Seminal Vesicles

The normal seminal vesicles are paired, saccular, elongated organs lying above the prostate and posterior to the bladder. Normal seminal vesicles are hypoechoic relative to the prostate, with multiple fine internal echoes corresponding to the folds of the excretory epithelium. Laterally, the seminal vesicles diverge in the perivesical fat while medially, they converge to

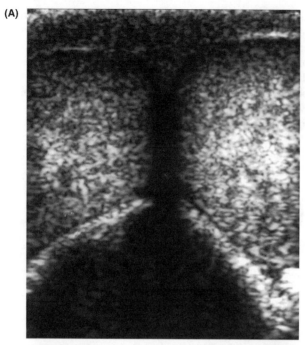

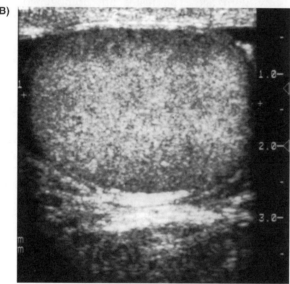

Figure 1 Normal testis. (**A**) Transverse view of the normal testis demonstrates homogeneous intermediate echogenicity with smooth margins. (**B**) Sagittal view of the normal testis.

join with the ampulla of the vas deferens to form the ejaculatory ducts, producing the typical "bow–tie" appearance on axial TRUS images (Figs. 2A and 2B).

Seminal vesicles may vary in size, shape, and degree of distension. They are, however, usually symmetric and measure no more than 5 to 10 cm in length and 2 to 5 cm in width with an estimated mean volume of approximately 15 mL. Caution is advised, however, in measuring seminal vesicle volume in only two dimensions as a seemingly small vesicle may extend a long way cephalad behind the bladder and thus have a normal volume (6).

Ejaculatory Ducts

The confluence of the vasal ampullae and seminal vesicles to form paired ejaculatory ducts is normally identified at the level of the prostatic capsule or just within the substance of the prostate. The intraprostatic course of each duct within a fibromuscular envelope is usually visible on TRUS and is identified as a fine, curvilinear, hypoechoic structure. The lumen of the ejaculatory duct should not exceed 2 mm in maximum width. On sagittal images, the course of each ejaculatory duct can normally be traced down to a focal area of hyperechogenicity corresponding to the verumontanum (Fig. 4). Small echogenic foci, representing concretions in the periurethral glands at the level of the verumontanum, provide a useful sonographic landmark for the junction of the ejaculatory ducts and the urethra (4–10).

It is important to note that on TRUS, careful attention should be given not only to the dimensions of the distal ductal structures but also to their echotexture and internal architecture. The normal vas deferens and seminal vesicles are hypoechoic relative to the normal prostate. If, however, the vas deferens or seminal vesicles should appear isoechoic or hyperechoic compared to the prostate, obliteration by fibrosis or calcification should be suspected. In the presence of diffuse fibrosis or calcification, the normal internal convolutions of the seminal vesicles and vas deferens corresponding to normal tubular epithelium are not identifiable on TRUS.

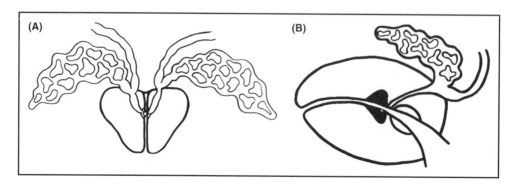

Figure 2 Normal transrectal ultrasound anatomy. (**A**) Diagrammatic representation of the distal male reproductive system, axial plane. (**B**) Diagrammatic representation of the distal male reproductive system, sagittal plane.

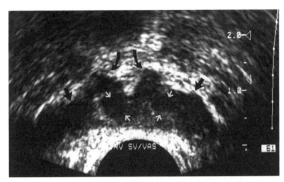

Figure 3   Normal transrectal ultrasound anatomy. Axial view demonstrates the distal vas deferens (*curved arrows*) joining the seminal vesicles (*straight black arrows*) to form the ampullary portion of the vas deferens bilaterally (*white arrows*).

□ RADIOLOGIC DETECTION OF MALE REPRODUCTIVE PATHOLOGY

Scrotal Abnormalities

Congenital Abnormalities

Cryptorchidism

Thirty percent of premature infants and 3.4% of term infants are born with an undescended testis. Many of these, however, undergo spontaneous descent in infancy, and the overall incidence of cryptorchidism is thus reduced to approximately 0.8% by one year of life (23). This condition is slightly more common on the right, while roughly 10% are bilateral. Although surgical correction with orchiopexy has been reportedly effective in preserving fertility if accomplished by age two, a history of cryptorchidism is generally associated with testicular atrophy and abnormal spermatogenesis in both testes, regardless of the timing of repair (24). Indeed, as many as 15% of instances of oligospermia may be secondary to failure of testicular descent. Although both endocrine and autoimmune mechanisms have been proposed, the likely etiology for cryptorchid-related infertility is the deleterious effect of the higher ambient body temperatures of nonscrotal locations on spermatogenesis within the seminiferous tubules (3).

In addition to infertility issues, cryptorchid patients also maintain a four- to fivefold risk increase

for germ cell tumors and other malignancies; increased incidence of tumor is seen in the contralateral, normally descended testis, as well. Therefore, surgical orchiopexy is done primarily to allow examination of the testis. Malignant degeneration is more common in abdominal and ectopic testes than in other types of cryptorchidism.

Uncorrected cryptorchid testes may be located anywhere along the path of descent and are often found in intra-abdominal, inguinal (also termed canalicular or emergent testes), or high scrotal locations. The most common location is within the inguinal canal, and this type is visible on ultrasound 70% to 80% of the time. Approximately one-fourth of these are retractile testes that slide back and forth between the scrotum and the external inguinal ring. An undescended testis will appear on ultrasound as an atrophic, homogeneously hypodense gonad with a relatively large epididymis (Fig. 5A). It should be noted that the presence of a linear, echogenic mediastinum is invaluable in distinguishing an undescended testis from an inguinal lymph node or other object (3,17,23,24).

When an undescended testis cannot be visualized in the inguinal canal by ultrasound, intra-abdominal cryptorchidism should be suspected. Intra-abdominal testes are typically located adjacent to the iliopsoas

(A)

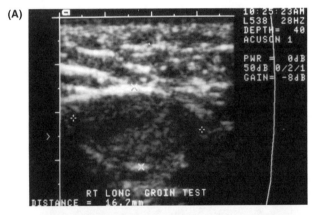

(B)

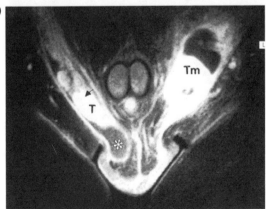

Figure 5   Cryptorchidism. (**A**) Small, atrophic testis with heterogenous echotexture, located in the right groin. (**B**) Coronal T2-weighted magnetic resonance imaging of bilateral cryptorchidism. Right inguinal testis (T) and left inguinal testis with germ cell tumor (Tm) are clearly shown outside the scrotal sac.

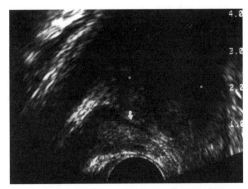

Figure 4   Normal transrectal ultrasound anatomy. The ejaculatory duct (*arrow*), sagittal view.

muscle above the internal inguinal ring, but they may be retroperitoneal or even ectopically placed in the perineum, anterior abdominal wall, thigh, or penis. Both CT and MRI are often quite sensitive in detecting this type of cryptorchidism, as gonadal tissue is typically intermediate signal on T1-weighted MR images and high signal on T2-weighted sequences (Fig. 5B) (17).

Cryptorchidism is sometimes associated with genetic disorders such as Prader–Willi, Klinefelter, and Noonan syndromes. Anorchia, or complete absence of a testis, is a very rare condition that is the result of either failed embryonic development or atresia following a gestational insult. Anorchia is frequently accompanied by decreased fertility. When bilateral, anorchia is usually part of a collection of phenotypic and endocrinologic abnormalities comprising a familial syndrome. Differentiation of anorchia from bilateral cryptorchidism can be made via the radiologic absence of identifiable gonadal tissue on ultrasound, CT, or MRI, and medical confirmation may be obtained by documenting high baseline gonadotropin levels and a lack of testosterone response to exogenous human chorionic gonadotropin (17,25).

Testicular Microlithiasis

An uncommon but potentially significant finding on scrotal sonography is testicular microlithiasis. This is seen as multiple hyperechoic foci within the testis ranging in size from 0.3 to 3 mm and does not cause the shadowing associated with larger calculi such as gallstones or nephrolithiasis. Microlithiasis is usually diffusely distributed, with five or more foci visible per field of view, and is almost always bilateral (Fig. 6). Prevalence varies from 0.05% in autopsy specimens to an estimated 0.7% in patients referred for scrotal ultrasound. On gross pathologic examination, the microliths correspond to calcified sediment and lamellated collagen fibers within atrophic seminiferous tubules. These are likely markers of a prior insult to the affected testis and not specific for an individual disease process, but strong associations with subfertility, cryptorchidism,

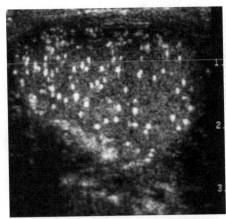

Figure 6 Testicular microlithiasis. Numerous nonshadowing, hyperechoic foci are diffusely distributed throughout the testicular parenchyma.

Klinefelter's syndrome, pseudohermaphroditism, Down's syndrome, and pulmonary alveolar microlithiasis have been documented. Most importantly, a link has been established between testicular microlithiasis and testicular malignancies, particularly among pediatric and young adult patients. Follow-up surveillance with annual sonography and testicular self-examination is therefore recommended for men in whom testicular microlithiasis is identified (3,26).

Acquired Abnormalities
Torsion and Ischemia

Testicular ischemia may be caused by severe epididymitis, embolic endocarditis, trauma, or vasculitis, but in the absence of epididymo-orchitis, the acute onset of scrotal pain is most frequently the result of testicular torsion (12). Since the chances of salvaging a torsed testis are greatly increased by performing surgery within four hours of the onset of pain, prompt and accurate diagnosis is essential. Recent improvements in color Doppler imaging have made reliable ultrasonographic identification of torsion possible, supplanting scintigraphy as the diagnostic modality of choice.

There is an increased risk of torsion with the "bell-clapper" deformity of the tunica vaginalis, in which a narrowed attachment of the tunica to the posterior testis results in a mobile stalk, allowing the testis to rotate. This condition is most commonly observed during adolescence, but it may also occur in children and adults. The bell-clapper deformity is often bilateral, so that patients with torsion of one testis are at higher risk for future torsion of the contralateral testis (21). Occult torsion or inability to salvage an infarcted testis leads to testicular atrophy, decreased sperm production, and subfertility, while bilateral testicular infarction results in sterility. Some reports indicate that testicular volume and sperm counts remain reduced even if surgical detorsion is accomplished within a few hours (13).

Ultrasound demonstrates decreased or completely absent blood flow within the affected testis, which must be compared with the presumably normal, opposite side to ensure proper gain settings. A heterogeneous mass may be visible superior or lateral to the testis, corresponding to the twisted vascular pedicle. With time, the ischemic testis becomes hypoechoic and enlarged with edema and then progressively more heterogeneous as coalescent cystic fluid collections and atrophy develop. These findings are easily distinguished from the hyperemia associated with acute inflammatory conditions, allowing reliable triage of those patients requiring urgent surgical exploration. (For further information on this topic, please refer to Chapter 13.)

Epididymitis and Orchitis

Epididymitis is responsible for more than half of all cases of scrotal inflammation. *Neisseria gonorrhea* and *Chlamydia trachomatis* are the primary causative agents among sexually active males, while gram-negative organisms from the urinary tract are more common among male children and the elderly. On ultrasound, the affected epididymis will be enlarged with diffusely decreased echogenicity, and Doppler images will confirm an increase in the number and size of epididymal blood vessels, as well as the increase in blood flow within them (Fig. 7A and B). Scrotal wall thickening and a reactive hydrocele are common associated findings in the acute setting, while calcifications may be present with chronic epididymitis (12).

Isolated inflammation of the testis is far less common than epididymitis or epididymo-orchitis and is usually secondary to viral infection such as mumps or influenza. Other causes include infection by fungal, parasitic, or bacterial agents (including tuberculosis), as well as inflammation as the result of direct trauma to the testis. Most patients with orchitis experience significant discomfort, but occasionally, asymptomatic individuals may be encountered. Ultrasound shows dramatically increased blood flow and diffuse hypoechogenicity. Diffuse enlargement of the testis is also often seen with mumps and tuberculosis. Involvement may be focally limited, however, especially if it is the result of contiguous spread from epididymitis or a urinary tract infection (Fig. 8A–D) (13,21,23).

Untreated infection within the epididymis or testis can progress to an intrascrotal abscess that appears sonographically as a relatively avascular mass with increased blood flow at the periphery. Although such abscesses are typically located within the epididymis or testis, it is not uncommon for rupture to occur into the surrounding tissues, possibly even involving the scrotal wall itself (13). Prolonged inflammation may result in scarring, with resultant deleterious effects upon testicular function and ductal obstruction, as well as the accompanying impairment of fertility.

Neoplasm

Testicular tumors are common among men in the same age group as those that present with infertility. They may cause alterations in endocrine function and decreased spermatogenesis, and they may also be discovered incidentally during the evaluation for infertility. Most appear on ultrasound as well-defined intratesticular masses that are often hypoechoic with increased blood flow on color Doppler. The radiologic detection of a primary testicular neoplasm should also provoke suspicion for the presence of a small attendant hydrocele, as the two lesions frequently accompany one another. (For further information on hydroceles, see "Hydrocele" below.)

The most common primary testicular neoplasms—accounting for 95%—are of germ cell origin such as seminoma (50%), embryonal cell carcinoma, teratoma, choriocarcinomas, and mixed types. Seminomas exhibit less-aggressive behavior and are radiosensitive; they appear as homogenous, hypoechoic masses that tend to displace adjacent normal testicular parenchyma without invasion. Nonseminomatous germ cell tumors tend to be more heterogeneous, with areas of calcification, cysts, and irregular margins corresponding to areas of necrosis and hemorrhage (12,21).

Nongerm cell tumors are much less frequent in young males and include Leydig cell and Sertoli cell tumors, epidermoids, dermoids, leukemias, lymphomas, and metastases. Both lymphoma and metastases (especially renal cell and prostate carcinoma) are more common than germ cell tumors in men over age 50; they will appear as diffusely enlarged testes with decreased echogenicity, without the well-defined margins of other neoplasms. Benign stromal tumors of Leydig and Sertoli cell origin are indistinguishable in

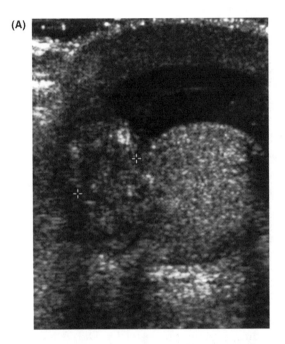

(A)

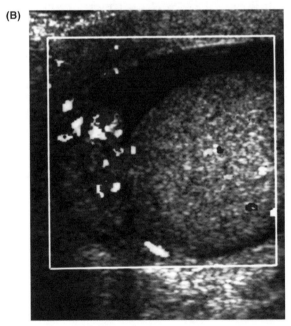

(B)

Figure 7   Epididymitis. (**A**) Sagittal view of the epididymis shows diffuse enlargement and heterogeneity. (**B**) Sagittal view of the epididymis with dramatically increased blood flow on Doppler analysis.

320   Kuligowska et al.

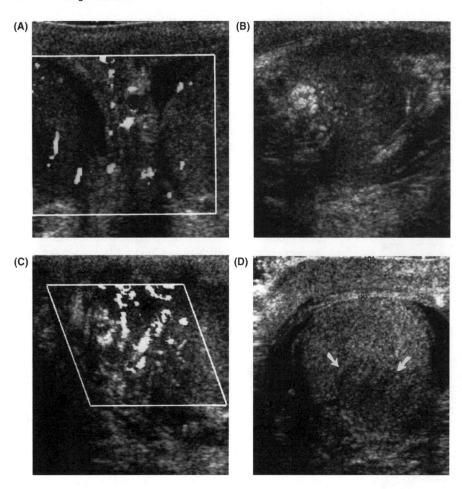

Figure 8 Epididymo-orchitis: 95-year-old diabetic man with painful enlargement of the scrotum. (**A**) Transverse view showing edema of the scrotal wall and increased blood flow within both testes. (**B**) Sagittal section of the epididymal head showing enlargement and increased echogenicity. (**C**) Significantly increased vascularity within the epididymal head. (**D**) Transverse view of the right testis demonstrating abnormal hypoechoic area within posterior portion of testis, compatible with orchitis (*arrows*).

sonographic appearance from other testicular tumors but are more likely to cause hormonal derangements and consequent altered spermatogenesis (3,12).

Unfortunately, currently available therapies for testicular neoplasm with surgery, radiation, and chemotherapeutics have all been linked to abnormal sperm counts, motility, morphology, and transport. Disruption of sympathetic nerves and ganglia during lymph node dissection may lead to impaired or retrograde ejaculation. Although generally dose-dependent, azoospermia from radiation and chemotherapy can be permanent (23).

Varicocele

Of the surgically reversible scrotal abnormalities associated with infertility, the most prevalent is the varicocele. Although clinically present in 10% to 15% of all adult males, it is seen in 35% to 40% of men with infertility. If nonpalpable, "subclinical" varicoceles are included in this estimate, the prevalence rate among infertile men increases to 60% compared with 35% among the general male population (8).

A varicocele is a dilatation of the pampiniform plexus of veins draining the testes, usually the result of incompetent venous valves that produce stasis or even retrograde flow. It is thought that venous stasis within the varicocele raises the temperature within the scrotum to a level above that optimal for spermatogenesis

(8,10). On physical examination, the engorged pampiniform plexus may be palpable as a "bag of worms." A grading system proposed by Dubin and Amelar classifies clinical varicoceles as Grade 1 if palpable only during Valsalva, Grade 2 if palpable at rest, and Grade 3 if visible to the naked eye. Varicoceles are usually left-sided but are bilateral in approximately 25%. A unilateral varicocele can impair both testes, causing bilateral atrophy, histologic changes, hormonal dysfunction, and an abnormal semen analysis (23,24).

Ultrasound clearly demonstrates palpable varicoceles and is also able to detect nonpalpable, subclinical varicoceles with reliable sensitivity. Criteria for ultrasound diagnosis of varicoceles include either the detection of multiple grouped dilated veins in the wall of the scrotum with diameters greater than 2 mm or the demonstration of a single dilated vein with a diameter greater than 3 mm, with augmentation of size during Valsalva (10). Color Doppler may facilitate more confident identification of smaller varicoceles by improving the distinction of dilated veins from other cystic structures within the scrotum (Fig. 9A and B) (13,24).

Surgical ligation and varicocelectomy have been shown to improve seminal quality parameters in approximately half of all patients, regardless of the size of the varicocele (27). (For further information on varicoceles, please refer to Chapter 15.)

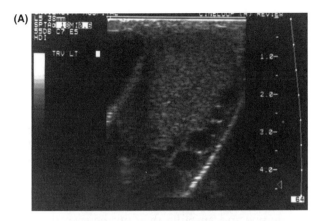

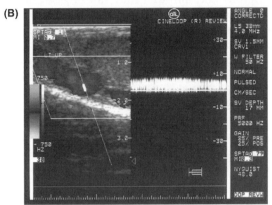

Figure 9 Varicocele: 32-year-old infertile male. (**A**) Transverse view of left hemiscrotum demonstrates dilated pampiniform plexus surrounding the left testis, compatible with varicocele. (**B**) (*See color insert.*) Color Doppler appearance of the dilated veins (gray-scale image).

Testicular Atrophy

Testicular atrophy of any cause, particularly when bilateral, can lead to decreased spermatogenesis and hormonal production. Atrophic testes appear on ultrasound as small and homogeneously hypoechoic, with decreased flow on Doppler analysis. Intrinsic abnormalities associated with testicular atrophy include myotonic dystrophy, trauma, infarction, and torsion, or genetic disorders such as Klinefelter's or Kallmann's syndromes (21).

Hydrocele

A hydrocele is an abnormal collection of serous fluid between the visceral and parietal layers of the tunica vaginalis. It usually presents with painless swelling of the scrotum and is most frequently idiopathic in origin; alternative causes include torsion, inflammation, and malignancy. Ultrasound reveals an accumulation of anechoic fluid around the testis without internal architecture, often accompanied by concomitant scrotal wall calcification (Fig. 10A–C). The presence of septations or heterogeneity within the fluid collection is consistent with either hemorrhage (hematocele) or infection (pyocele).

It should be noted that since most primary testicular neoplasms are accompanied by a small hydrocele, the identification of peritesticular fluid in an infertile patient should prompt a diligent search for a possible underlying malignancy (12).

Spermatocele

A spermatocele is a collection of small cysts within the head of the epididymis. Smaller collections, described simply as epididymal cysts, are epithelial-lined and contain debris, immobile sperm, and lipids. Spermatoceles are exceedingly common (up to 40% of normal men) and are almost always asymptomatic. They may vary greatly in size, from as small as 2 mm to larger than 4 cm, and are usually of no clinical significance; very large spermatoceles, however, may cause obstruction of the efferent ductules, replacement of the epididymal head, and production of a mass effect upon the testis (12). The presence of a large spermatocele and epididymal head enlargement in an oligospermic or azoospermic male may warrant further investigation to exclude the possibility of epididymal obstruction (Fig. 11).

Trauma

Traumatic injury to the scrotum may result in hematoma, hematocele, or testicular fracture. A fractured testis may demonstrate disrupted borders with extracapsular protrusion of testicular parenchyma into the scrotal sac. Evacuation of this extruded parenchyma must be performed without delay to ensure future

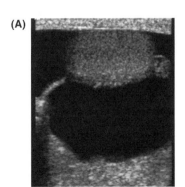
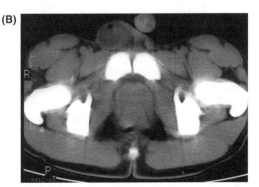
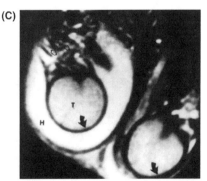

Figure 10 Hydrocele in right testis. (**A**) Ultrasound shows abnormal anechoic fluid collection surrounding right testis. (**B**) Computed tomography scan demonstrating abnormal fluid collection within right hemiscrotum. (**C**) T2-weighted magnetic resonance imaging showing fluid between the parietal and visceral layers of the tunica vaginalis.

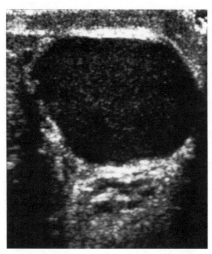

Figure 11 Spermatocele. Abnormal fluid collection with debris within the epididymal head.

fertility, as it is thought that the extracapsular parenchyma may incite an autoimmune response (13).

Pathology of the Distal Ducts
Vas Deferens

Congenital abnormalities of the vas deferens are the most common finding seen on TRUS in males with azoospermia and low ejaculate volumes (4–10). Congenital aplasia of the vas deferens is reported in 1% to 2.5% of most series of infertile men and accounts for 4.4% to 17% of cases of azoospermia. Agenesis of the vas deferens may be partial or complete, unilateral or bilateral, and associated with hypoplasia of the epididymis (Fig. 12A–C). The combination of low

ejaculate volume, azoospermia, normal testicular size and consistency, and a nonpalpable vas deferens on physical examination is diagnostic of agenesis.

True vasal agenesis is always associated with an ipsilateral seminal vesicle anomaly, as the two structures share a common embryological derivation from the Wolffian duct. Similarly, agenesis of the vas deferens is always associated with absence of the ipsilateral ejaculatory duct (4,5). A sonographically absent or atrophic seminal vesicle in a patient with no palpable ipsilateral vas deferens is conclusive evidence of vasal aplasia. In the extremely rare condition of vasal atrophy secondary to infection or obstruction, while the distal vas deferens and ampulla may not be seen on ultrasound, the proximal vas deferens may still be palpable; there may also be a normal ipsilateral seminal vesicle identifiable on TRUS.

The spectrum of TRUS findings in patients with vasal agenesis ranges from complete absence of the vas to persistence of a vestigial remnant, the latter of which may be identified as a diminutive, isoechoic or hyperechoic oval structure measuring less than 3 mm in diameter posterior to the bladder. On TRUS, vasal hypoplasia is recognized as a unilateral or bilateral reduction in size of the vas deferens (Fig. 13A and B). As clinical palpation of the vas deferens may be difficult, particularly when there is thickening of the spermatic cord, TRUS should be routinely performed when vasal agenesis is suspected (i.e., in all patients with low-volume azoospermia) to confirm or refute the clinical diagnosis as well as to detect other associated distal ductal anomalies. If a unilateral vasal agenesis or hypoplasia is indeed detected, a mandatory search for a contralateral ductal abnormality is in order to account for infertility in patients with azoospermia and low ejaculate volumes (4,5).

(A)

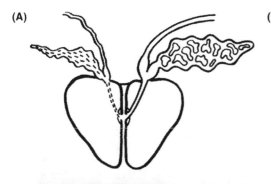

(B)

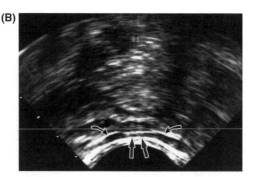

(C)

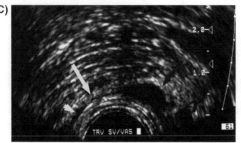

Figure 12 Absence and hypoplasia of the vas deferens. (**A**) Diagrammatic representation of the distal ducts demonstrating ipsilateral absence of vas deferens and seminal vesicle. (**B**) Axial view showing complete bilateral absence of vas deferens (*straight arrows*) associated with bilateral rudimentary seminal vesicles (*curved arrows*). (**C**) Unilateral absence of vas deferens. Axial view shows absence of right vas deferens (*straight white*) and rudimentary right seminal vesicle (*white arrow head*). Normal left vas deferens (*straight black arrow*) and normal left seminal vesicle (*curved black arrow*). *Source*: From Ref. 15.

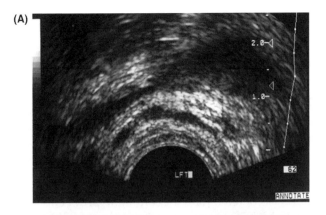

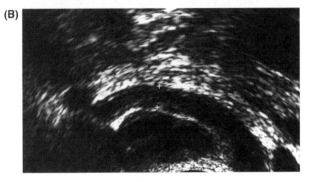

Figure 13   Hypoplasia of vas deferens. (**A**) Sagittal view demonstrates small, narrow, and echogenic vas deferens. (**B**) Compare to the diameter of the normal vas deferens (*cursors*) in Fig. 17A.

Other vasal abnormalities in infertile male patients that may be identified on TRUS include increased echogenicity representing occlusion of the vas deferens by fibrosis or calcification (Figs. 6, 14A, 14B, 15, and 16A–C), obstructing cysts of the vas deferens and vas deferens calculi. The TRUS findings in patients with vasal occlusion by fibrosis or calcification range from subtle alterations in echotexture to frank calcification. Similar textural changes are usually present in the seminal vesicles and ejaculatory ducts. The pathogenesis of such diffuse distal ductal fibrosis or calcification is unclear. A congenital etiology is likely in patients with diffuse, bilateral, and symmetrical textural abnormalities, but some cases may be secondary to chronic indolent infection. Cysts and calculi are most commonly seen in the terminal ampullary portion of the vas deferens (Figs. 14A, 14B, 15, and 16A–C). Ampullary cysts and calculi frequently produce dilatation of the proximal vas deferens as well as obstruction of the ipsilateral seminal vesicle. Occasionally, ampullary cysts may reach a size sufficient enough to cause both ipsilateral and contralateral ductal obstruction (4–10).

There are a number of interesting findings associated with vasal agenesis. For example, sonographic evaluation of the scrotum may also demonstrate hypoplasia of the distal two-thirds of the epididymis. In addition to seminal vesicle and ejaculatory abnormalities, however, 16% to 43% of patients with unilateral vasal agenesis will harbor renal anomalies including renal agenesis, crossed fused ectopia or an ectopic pelvic kidney (more commonly on the left side), whereas patients with congenital bilateral absence of the vas deferens (CBAVD) generally do not exhibit renal agenesis (4,6–11,14–16,19,20,28). Further, vasal aplasia syndromes may also occur as part of the clinical spectrum of cystic fibrosis (28–33). Males with cystic fibrosis will present with bilateral vasal aplasia and recognizable cystic fibrosis gene mutations. Conversely, up to 82% of patients with CBAVD have at least one detectable cystic fibrosis gene mutation. Of patients with unilateral absence of the vas deferens, cystic fibrosis gene mutations are found only in patients with partial occlusion of the single-formed vas deferens. Yet, despite the presence of gene mutations, most patients with unilateral or even bilateral vasal agenesis do not demonstrate significant clinical symptoms of cystic fibrosis, and 75% have normal sweat tests. Interestingly, patients with vasal agenesis who also possess concurrent renal anomalies will not typically demonstrate mutations on cystic fibrosis gene analysis (30).

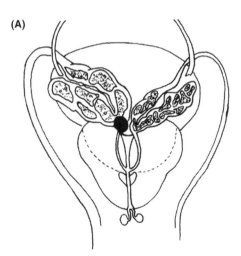

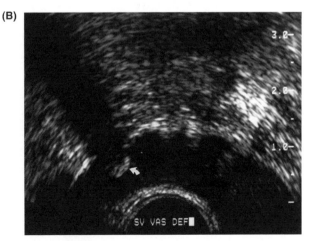

Figure 14   Vas deferens calculi. (**A**) Diagrammatic representation of ampullary stone. (**B**) Axial view demonstrates a 5-mm calculus in the right vasal ampulla (*arrow*).

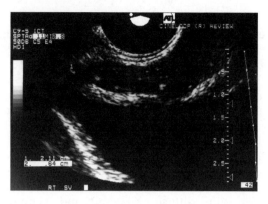

Figure 15 Vas deferens obstruction. Sagittal view shows abnormally dilated right vas deferens, obstructed by multiple stones. Compare to the normal vas deferens in Fig. 17B.

Seminal Vesicles

Embryologically, the seminal vesicles arise as saccular dilatations of the distal Wolffian duct (the future vas deferens) near its junction with the urogenital sinus. Because 80% to 90% of the ejaculate volume is elaborated by the seminal vesicles, congenital anomalies and obstructive pathology of the seminal vesicles will result in a diminished ejaculate volume, low pH and reduced fructose levels in the seminal fluid.

Abnormalities of the seminal vesicles associated with infertility include seminal vesicle agenesis, hypoplasia (Fig. 12), obliteration by calcification and fibrosis, and obstruction secondary to cysts (Fig. 17A–C) and calculi. As stated previously, seminal vesicle abnormalities occur in all patients with agenesis of the vas deferens (Fig. 13A and B), in which cases the seminal vesicle may be totally absent, atrophic, or hypoplastic (less than 30% of normal volume). Seminal vesicles are considered normal when greater than 25 mm in length, hypoplastic when greater than 16 mm but less than 25 mm in length, atrophic when less than 16 mm in length, and absent when no tissue is identified. It should be noted, however, that although there may be complete histological absence of the seminal vesicle, a diminutive, rudimentary, and fibrotic remnant may still be seen on TRUS posterior to the bladder (Fig. 12A–C).

Occlusion of the seminal vesicles by calcification or fibrosis is thought to be congenital in origin, although some cases may occur secondary to chronic infection (seminal vesiculitis). This is perhaps the most difficult diagnosis to make on TRUS in infertile male patients, as only subtle alterations in echotexture may be present. In addition to increased echogenicity and lack of normal internal convolutions, the seminal vesicle may be either diminished or increased in size. Frequently, similar textural abnormalities are identified in the ipsilateral vas deferens and the contralateral ductal system. Chronic seminal vesiculitis also predisposes the patient to seminal vesicle stone formation, likely due to chronic urinary reflux from the prostatic urethra. Calculi may also form as the result of concretions of static fluid and cellular debris in an obstructed seminal vesicle.

Seminal vesicle cysts are rare entities, more often congenital than acquired, that generally result from a discontinuity between the seminal vesicle and the ejaculatory duct (Fig. 17A–C). The congenital types of seminal vesicle cysts are commonly associated with anomalies of the ipsilateral Wolffian duct, such as the kidney, ureter, or bladder trigone. These anomalies include ipsilateral renal dysgenesis (present in 80% to 90% of cases), duplication of the renal collecting system, ectopic insertion of the ureter, and ectopic location of the kidney (4,6,34–37). The association of seminal vesicle cysts and ipsilateral renal and ureteric anomalies may be explained by an abnormally cephalic origin of the ureteric bud from the Wolffian duct that may cause the developing ureter to fail to meet and stimulate the differentiation of the nephrogenic blastema. Alternatively, the more cephalic ureter may, in fact, reach the nephrogenic blastema, but then terminate ectopically into a Wolffian duct derivative such as the bladder or seminal vesicle. The likelihood of renal anomalies increases as the origin of the ureteric bud becomes more cephalic.

Patients with adult polycystic kidney disease may also demonstrate seminal vesicle cysts, but these are typically bilateral. As only 60% of patients will report a relevant family history of polycystic kidney

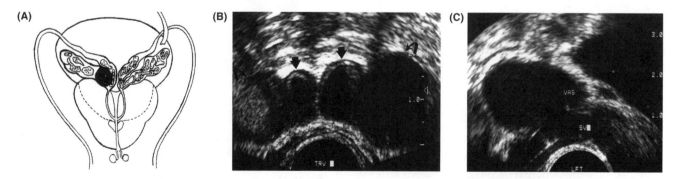

Figure 16 Vas deferens cyst. (**A**) Diagrammatic representation of a right vas deferens cyst. (**B**) Axial view demonstrates bilateral vas deferens cyst (*straight arrows*) causing obstruction of the seminal vesicles (*curved arrows*). (**C**) Sagittal view of the cyst in left vas deferens.

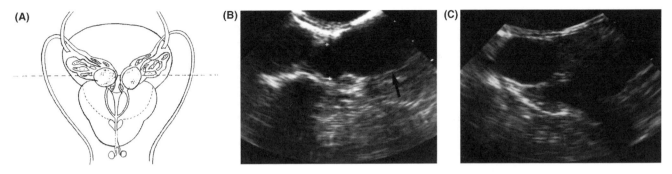

Figure 17   Seminal vesicle cysts. (**A**) Diagrammatic representation of the distal ducts demonstrating bilateral cysts of the seminal vesicle. (**B**) A cyst of the left seminal vesicle (*arrow*), axial view. (**C**) A cyst of the left seminal vesicle, sagittal view. *Source*: From Ref. 3.

disease, the presence of bilateral seminal vesicle cysts should suggest the presence of polycystic kidneys and thus prompt a full renal evaluation. Seminal vesicle cysts should also be differentiated from cystic dilatation secondary to obstruction of the ejaculatory ducts, as the latter is best treated by transurethral resection. Some infertility specialists believe that increased seminal vesicle width (greater than 2 cm) demonstrated on TRUS is actually diagnostic of ejaculatory duct obstruction.

Ejaculatory Ducts

Ejaculatory duct dysfunction may occur via several mechanisms, including obstruction secondary to extrinsic compression of the duct by periurethral and prostatic cysts (such as utricular and Mullerian duct cysts), obstruction as the result of the duct orifices entering blindly into a cyst (such as an ejaculatory duct cyst, an ejaculatory duct diverticulum, or a Wolffian duct cyst), obstruction secondary to occlusion by calcification, fibrosis, or calculi, or even as the result of agenesis or hypoplasia of the duct itself (Figs. 18A–C and 19A–C) (3–10,36). Most cases of ejaculatory duct obstruction are associated with proximal dilatation of the seminal vesicles and vas deferens; in those cases involving agenesis, hypoplasia, and atrophy, however, proximal atrophic changes or agenesis are more often seen.

Sagittal TRUS images demonstrate the intraprostatic course of the ejaculatory duct as a thin, curvilinear structure extending from the vasal ampulla to the verumontanum, which is identified as a focal area of hyperechogenicity (Fig. 4) (4–10). The lumen of the ejaculatory duct may be visible but should not exceed 2 mm in maximum dimension. Cysts, calcification, fibrosis, and stones are also best appreciated on sagittal images (37).

Prostatic and Periurethral Cysts

A variety of intraprostatic and periurethral cysts, clearly identifiable on TRUS, may result in proximal obstruction of the male reproductive tract (Figs. 20A–C) (6,8,11,38). These cysts may be classified according to their location and the presence or absence of spermatozoa within the cystic fluid (4–6). Midline cysts without spermatozoa are likely to be utricular cysts. Such cysts are considered embryologic remnants of an incompletely regressed Mullerian duct system (Mullerian duct cysts). The normal utricle is no more than a 6 mm depression on the surface of the verumontanum; in 10% of males, however, the utricle is larger and extends in a cephalad direction over a variable distance. A tense utricular cyst may cause ejaculatory duct obstruction via extrinsic compression. Large and persistent utricular cysts are also associated with various congenital anomalies including proximal hypospadias,

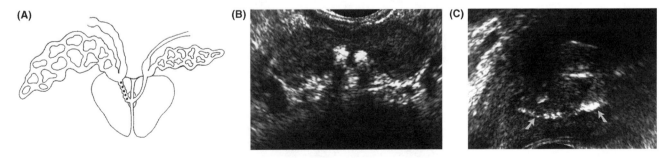

Figure 18   Ejaculatory duct calculi. (**A**) Diagrammatic representation of ejaculatory duct stones. (**B**) Axial view of the prostate, demonstrating ejaculatory ducts with bilateral calculi. (**C**) Sagittal view of the ejaculatory duct with diffuse calcification and fibrosis (*arrows*). *Source*: From Ref. 3.

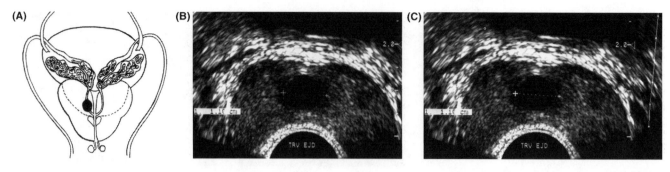

Figure 19 Ejaculatory duct cyst. (**A**) Diagrammatic representation of the distal male reproductive system, demonstrating right ejaculatory duct cyst. (**B**) Axial view demonstrating ejaculatory duct cyst (*cursors*). (**C**) Sagittal view of ejaculatory duct cyst (*cursors*). Note the typical elongated appearance of an ejaculatory duct seen on sagittal projection. *Source*: From Ref. 3.

posterior urethral valves, prune belly syndrome, imperforate anus, and Down's syndrome (6).

Midline intraprostatic cysts containing spermatozoa are known as ejaculatory duct cysts, and embryologically are of Wolffian duct origin (39). Although actually paramedian in location and not strictly "midline," these cysts nevertheless appear to have a midline location on TRUS. In contrast, prostatic retention cysts are more peripherally located, are degenerative, and do not contain spermatozoa. Although prostatic retention cysts are a frequent finding in normal fertile males, they are even more commonly observed in infertile patients, suggesting that such cysts are not simply incidental TRUS findings. In general, however, these degenerative prostatic cysts rarely reach sufficient size to compress the adjacent ejaculatory ducts.

The sonographic appearance of midline cysts is variable. Although cysts are clearly demonstrated on TRUS, it is not usually possible to classify them on the basis of sonographic findings alone. In general, a small midline cyst close to the verumontanum is most likely an enlarged utricle or utricular cyst (Mullerian duct cyst), while cysts located along the line of the ejaculatory duct are likely to be of Wolffian or ejaculatory duct origin. A useful distinguishing feature of ejaculatory duct cysts is an elongated, oval appearance on sagittal images (Fig. 19C). Definitive differentiation of the various types of prostatic cysts requires ultrasound-guided direct needle aspiration and subsequent analysis of the resulting aspirate for the presence or absence of sperm.

☐ THE ROLE OF IMAGING TECHNOLOGY IN THE MANAGEMENT OF MALE INFERTILITY

Although representing only a small proportion of all infertile male patients, patients with certain congenital and acquired ductal anomalies can be treated with surgical intervention (36,37,40–45). Determination of suitability for surgery and the optimum operative approach, however, demands precise delineation of the nature and level of the abnormality. Thus, radiographic imaging can be a very useful tool in the management and treatment of male infertility. In general, distal ductal anomalies can be classified as being either surgically correctable or nonsurgically correctable depending on the level and nature of obstruction. Surgically correctable causes of infertility are confined to lesions involving the distal two-thirds of the ejaculatory ducts, including ejaculatory duct cysts, calculi, fibrosis, and calcification. Agenesis or occlusion of the ductal system above this level is, by definition, nonsurgically correctable, and fertility can only be achieved via in vitro fertilization following epididymal aspiration (Fig. 21A–C).

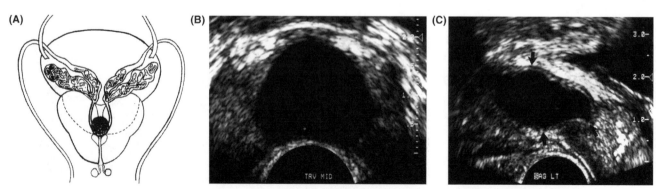

Figure 20 Midline cyst. (**A**) Diagrammatic representation of the distal male reproductive system demonstrating a midline cyst. (**B**) Axial view demonstrates a large midline cyst (*arrows*). (**C**) Sagittal view demonstrates a large midline cyst (*arrows*). *Source*: From Ref. 3.

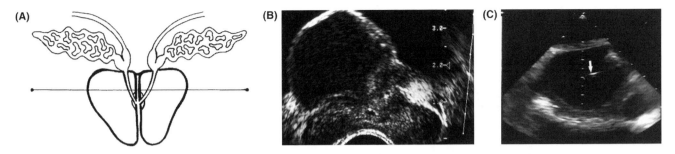

Figure 21 TRUS-guided cyst aspiration. (**A**) Diagrammatic representation of the distal male reproductive system. The horizontal line demarcates surgically correctable from nonsurgically correctable lesions based on their location. Lesions below the line causing ejaculatory duct obstruction are amenable to surgical correction by transurethral resection of the verumontanum or ejaculatory ducts. Ductal obstruction or occlusion above this level is not amenable to surgical correction. (**B**) Axial view demonstrates a large cyst, extending above the prostate and protruding into the urinary bladder. Note multiple internal echoes indicating the presence of spermatozoa. (**C**) TRUS-guided cyst aspiration was performed. According to previous convention, the transducer is displayed at the top of this image. Tip of the needle is visualized (*arrow*). Aspiration yielded spermatozoa for in vitro fertilization. *Abbreviation*: TRUS, transrectal ultrasound.

Congenital Abnormalities

Infertility as the result of congenital bilateral agenesis of the vas deferens is, by definition, nonsurgically correctable; these patients may instead be successfully treated with microscopic epididymal sperm aspiration and in vitro fertilization. Because up to one-third of bilateral vasal agenesis cases will be missed on the basis of physical examination alone, TRUS is indicated in all patients with low-volume azoospermia in order to detect vasal agenesis as well as to identify potential associated anomalies similarly missed on physical exam. Scrotal ultrasound is recommended prior to epididymal sperm aspiration as 30% of patients with vasal agenesis will have hypoplasia of the distal two-thirds of the epididymis; the side with the longest epididymal remnant should be selected for surgery. Alternatively, testicular sperm extraction (TESE) may be performed.

If a midline cyst or ejaculatory duct calculus is identified, the optimum surgical approach is simple transurethral resection of the distal portion of the ejaculatory ducts (Fig. 4). If TRUS fails to define a midline obstructing cyst or stone but instead demonstrates diffuse ejaculatory duct obliteration by calcification or fibrosis with proximal dilatation, more extensive surgery is required, typically involving incisions in the prostatic floor from just distal to the bladder neck to the verumontanum, lateral to the midline, and sufficiently deep to enter the ejaculatory ducts from their origin posterolaterally to their termination in the prostatic urethra (40–45).

Distal Ductal Anomalies

Seminal vesicle and vas deferens cysts may be treated with TRUS-guided needle aspiration, although it should be noted that this therapeutic benefit is not permanent, as the cysts will recur (Fig. 19). Cyst aspiration may be therapeutic in two ways: first, decompression of the cyst may help relieve proximal ductal obstruction and second, such cysts may contain spermatozoa, which may be harvested for the purposes of in vitro fertilization.

Treatment of testicular causes of male infertility is somewhat controversial. Surgical correction of undescended testes is generally recommended in boys and young men in order to enable examination of the affected testis for possible malignancy as well as to improve future fertility. Varicoceles are amenable to treatment either by surgical ligation or by angiographic sclerotherapy, a relatively noninvasive and effective technique (26). The effectiveness of the surgery or sclerotherapy may be confirmed by postinterventional color Doppler sonography to demonstrate involution of the varicocele. Approximately half of treated patients will have improved fertility following either type of treatment (3,8,23,25). There is also anecdotal evidence to support the treatment of hydrocele and spermatocele, but caution is advised if attempting surgical correction as postoperative scarring may cause duct obstruction and actual worsening of infertility.

□ CONCLUSION

There are many possible etiologies for male infertility. A systematic, logical, and thorough evaluation of infertile male patients is mandatory to distinguish patients with correctable defects from those with noncorrectable abnormalities. Scrotal ultrasound and TRUS are safe and effective methods of visualizing the distal male reproductive system that can help identify patients appropriate for either surgical or radiologic intervention, thereby eliminating unnecessary further investigations and interventions in patients unlikely to reap treatment benefits.

□ REFERENCES

1. Templeton A. Infertility-epidemiology, aetiology, and effective management. Health Bull (Edinb) 1995; 53(5): 294–298.
2. Benson CB. Scrotal abnormalities associated with infertility. In: Goldstein SR, Benson CB, eds. Imaging of the Infertile Couple. London: Martin Dunitz Ltd., 2001:111–120.
3. de Kretser DM. Male infertility. Lancet 1997; 349: 787–790.
4. Kuligowska E, Baker CE, Oates RD. Male infertility: role of transrectal US in diagnosis and management. Radiology 1992; 185(2):353–360.
5. Kuligowska E. Transrectal ultrasonography in diagnosis and management of male infertility. In: Jaffe R, Pierson RA, Abramowicz JS, eds. Imaging in Infertility and Reproductive Endocrinology. Philadelphia: JB Lippincott Co, 1994:217–229.
6. Carter V, Shinohara K, Lipshultz LI. Transrectal ultrasonography in disorders of the seminal vesicles and ejaculatory ducts. Urol Clin North Am 1989; 16(4):773–790.
7. Abbitt PL, Watson L, Howards S. Abnormalities of the seminal tract causing infertility: diagnosis with endorectal sonography. AJR Am J Roentgenol 1991; 157(2):337–339.
8. Jarow JP. Role of ultrasonography in the evaluation of the infertile male. Semin Urol 1994; 12(4):274–282.
9. Jarow JP. Transrectal ultrasonography of infertile men. Fertil Steril 1993; 60(6):1035–1039.
10. Honig SC. Use of ultrasonography in the evaluation of the infertile man. World J Urol 1993; 11(2):102–110.
11. Parsons RB, Fisher AM, Bar-Chama N, et al. MR imaging in male infertility. Radiographics 1997; 17(3):627–637.
12. Brant WE. Genital tract and bladder ultrasound. In: Brant WE, Helms CA, eds. Fundamentals of Diagnostic Radiology. 2nd ed. Baltimore: Lippincott, Williams & Wilkins, 1999:859–880.
13. Horstman WG, Middleton WD, Melson GL, et al. Color Doppler US of the scrotum. Radiographics 1991; 11(6): 941–957.
14. Kuligowska E, Pomeroy OH. Prostate. In: McGahan J, Goldberg B, eds. Diagnostic Ultrasound, a Logical Approach. Philadelphia: Lipincott-Raven, 1997: 863–884.
15. Kuligowska E, Fenlon HM. Role of transrectal ultrasound in male infertility. In: Goldstein SR, Benson CB, eds. Imaging of the Infertile Couple. London: Martin Dunitz, 2001:121–135.
16. Foran, Popovich MJ. Magnetic resonance imaging of the testes and seminal vesicles. In: Papanicaolaou N, ed. Lippincott's Review of Radiology. Philadelphia: J.B. Lippincott Co, 1992:586–603.
17. Fritzsche PJ, Stark DD. MRI of the Body, The Raven MRI Teaching File. New York: Raven Press, 1993: 164–179.
18. Tanagho EA. Embryologic basis for lower ureteral anomalies: a hypothesis. Urology 1976; 7(5):451–464.
19. Moore KL. The Developing Human: Clinically Oriented Embryology. 3rd ed. Philadelphia: 1991; 29: 365–382.
20. Sadler TW. Langman's Medical Embryology. 7th ed. Baltimore: Williams & Wilkins, 1995:286–309.
21. Gooding GA. Scrotal ultrasonography. Radiologist 1994; 1:297–307.
22. Hattery RR, King BF Jr, Lewis RW, et al. Vasculogenic impotence. Duplex and color Doppler sonography. Radiol Clin North Am 1991; 29(3):629–645.
23. Papanicolaou NP, Kuligowska E, Lee MJ, et al. Scrotal and lower genitourinary tract sonography in male infertility. In: Papanicaolaou N, ed. Lippincott's Review of Radiology. Philadelphia: J.B. Lippincott Co, 1992:552–585.
24. Min Hoan M, Seung Hyup K, Jeong Yeon C, et al. Scrotal US for evaluation of infertile men with azoospermia. Radiology 2006; 239(1):168–173.
25. Hargreave TB, Ghosh C. Male infertility disorders, Endocrinol Metab Clin North Am 1998; 27(4):765–782.
26. Cast JE, Nelson WM, Early AS, et al. Testicular microlithiasis: prevalence and tumor risk in a population referred for scrotal sonography. AM J Roentgenol 2000; 175(6):1703–1706.
27. Chuang AT, Howards SS. Male infertility: evaluation and nonsurgical therapy. Urol Clin North Am 1998; 25(4):703–713.
28. Trigaux JP, Van Beers B, Delchambre F. Male genital tract malformations associated with ipsilateral renal agenesis: sonographic findings. J Clin Ultrasound 1991; 19(1):3–10.
29. Patel PJ, Pareek SS. Scrotal ultrasound in male infertility. Eur Urol 1989; 16(6):423–425.
30. Mulhall JP, Oates RD. Cystic fibrosis-associated vasal aplasia. Current Opin Urol 1995; 5:316–319.
31. Augarten A, Yahav Y, Kerem BS, et al. Congenital bilateral absence of the vas deferens in the absence of cystic fibrosis. Lancet 1994; 344(8935):1473–1474.
32. Mickle J, Milunsky A, Amos JA, et al. Congenital unilateral absence of the vas deferens: a heterogeneous disorder with two distinct subpopulations based upon aetiology and mutational status of the cystic fibrosis gene. Hum Reprod 1995; 10(7):1728–1735.
33. Oates RD, Amos JA. The genetic basis of congenital bilateral absence of the vas deferens and cystic fibrosis. J Androl 1994; 15(1):1–8.
34. Chillon M, Casals T, Mercier B, et al. Mutations in the cystic fibrosis gene in patients with congenital absence

of the vas deferens. N Engl J Med 1995; 332(22): 1475–1480.

35. Asch MR, Toi A. Seminal vesicles. Imaging and intervention using transrectal ultrasound. J Ultrasound Med 1991; 10(1):19–23.

36. Gevenois PA, Van Sinoy ML, Sintzoff SA Jr, et al. Cysts of the prostate and seminal vesicles: MR imaging findings in 11 cases. AJR Am J Roentgenol 1990; 155(5):1021–1024.

37. Meacham RB, Hellerstein DK, Lipshultz LI. Evaluation and treatment of ejaculatory duct obstruction in the infertile male. Fertil Steril 1993; 59(2):393–397.

38. Poore RE, Jarow JP. Distribution of intraprostatic hyperechoic lesions in infertile men. Urology 1995; 45(3):467–469.

39. Hamilton S, Fitzpatrick JM. Ultrasound diagnosis of a prostatic cyst causing acute urinary retention. J Ultrasound Med 1987; 6(7):385–387.

40. Namiki M. Recent concepts in the management of male infertility. Int J Urol 1996; 3:249–255.

41. Costabile RA. Infertility–is there anything we can do about it? J Urol 1997; 157(1):158–159.

42. Sokol RZ. The diagnosis and treatment of male infertility. Curr Opin Obstet Gynecol 1995; 7(3):177–181.

43. Madgar I, Seidman DS, Levran D, et al. Micromanipulation improves in-vitro fertilization results after epididymal or testicular sperm aspiration in patients with congenital absence of the vas deferens. Hum Reprod 1996; 11(10):2151–2154.

44. Schlegel PN, Girardi SK. Clinical review 87: in vitro fertilization for male factor infertility. J Clin Endocrinol Metab 1997; 82(3):709–716.

45. Kuligowska E, Fenlon HM. Transrectal US in male infertility:spectrum of findings and role in patient care. Radiology 1998; 207:173–181.

Part IV

Treatment of Male Reproductive Dysfunction

The treatment of the many causes of male reproductive dysfunction may be broadly classified as being either surgical or nonsurgical. Of the nonsurgical treatments, both pharmacologic and psychosocial therapies are available. The chapters in Part IV of this volume first describe the appropriate etiology-based management of each of the conditions that may threaten male fertility. Special consideration is given to the problems of sperm autoimmunity and the preservation of fertility in males with spinal cord injury, as well as those experiencing cancer and/or undergoing current cancer treatment.

One exciting area of development in the field of reproductive medicine involves the restoration of male fertility utilizing various new forms of assisted reproductive technology (ART), including in vitro fertilization (IVF) and intracytoplasmic sperm injection (ICSI). The successful implementation of these methods, however, requires the assumption that the traditional barriers to fertilization will be breached by directly placing an operator-selected sperm with the ovum; thus, there may be ethical considerations regarding the future genetic health of any offspring created using such techniques.

Although the overall goal of this volume is to describe and provide solutions for the problem of male factor infertility, one additional topic raised in this section is actually antithetical to the trend of the rest of the book, but represents another exciting area of current research in reproductive medicine: male hormonal contraception. While "the pill" has long been a female-initiated mainstay of preventing unwanted pregnancy, similar drugs for male-only use have recently been developed; thus, these treatments are also included in Part IV of this volume.

Androgen Replacement Therapy

Ronald S. Swerdloff

Division of Endocrinology and Metabolism, Harbor-UCLA Medical Center,
Torrance, California and Department of Medicine, David Geffen School of Medicine, University of California,
Los Angeles, California, U.S.A.

□ PRINCIPLES OF THE ANDROGEN TREATMENT OF HYPOGONADISM

The indications for androgen treatment are shown in Table 1 (1). Primary Leydig cell failure must be treated with androgens to relieve clinical symptoms and signs. Response to androgen replacement therapy is monitored by checking for improvement in the clinical features of hypogonadism. Typically, an improvement in sexual function, frequency of shaving, secondary sexual characteristics, and general well being occurs rapidly after the initiation of treatment. It is often useful to monitor minimum and peak testosterone levels during the start of therapy and in patients who do not show adequate clinical response.

Androgen treatment does not reverse infertility. Secondary Leydig cell dysfunction can be corrected by normalizing blood luteinizing-hormone (LH) levels. Until patients with hypothalamic–pituitary disorders associated with hypogonadotropic hypogonadism are desirous of a pregnancy, however, they are also treated with androgens because of the ease of administration and low cost. When a patient with hypogonadotropic hypogonadism desires fertility, the testes must be stimulated with LH- and follicle-stimulating hormone (FSH)-like hormones. This is usually done with human chorionic gonadotropin (hCG) or recombinant human LH, followed by combined hCG or LH and human menopausal gonadotropin or purified FSH. As an alternate method, pulsatile gonadotropin-releasing hormone (GnRH) injections may be given to induce spermatogenesis and fertility (2,3).

Pulsatile treatment requires the patient to continuously wear a micropump device for delivering small amounts of GnRH every two hours. Prior treatment with testosterone does not jeopardize the chances of fertility in patients with hypogonadotropic hypogonadism.

In young children with micropenis, a short course of low-dose androgen therapy is often tried. In adolescent boys with constitutional delay of puberty in whom the psychological effects of delayed puberty are significant, short-term treatment with testosterone for three to four months may be indicated.

As described in earlier sections, total and free testosterone levels decrease with age (please refer to Chapter 12). This decline in Leydig cell function occurs at a time when various androgen-responsive end organs show signs of abnormal function (i.e., penis, bone, and muscle). Although a decrease in sexual function is often observed in older men, many aged men have other causes for erectile dysfunction (ED), and thus do not experience a reversal of impotence when treated with testosterone alone. Combined PDE-5 inhibitors and testosterone may be beneficial on sexual function when decreased libido and ED are present in hypogonadal, older men. Although it has not been proved that androgen therapy in older men with borderline or normal range testosterone levels will improve sexual function, prevent bone and muscle loss, or improve the quality of life (4–7), clinical trials are underway to determine its efficacy in symptomatic men with definitely low serum testosterone levels. The possible beneficial effect of androgens must be balanced against the possible adverse effects on lipids, prostate, and sleep-related breathing disorders (7–9).

Testosterone has been given alone or in conjunction with other steroids and GnRH analogs as experimental male contraceptives (10–13). Recent data indicate that pharmacologic doses of testosterone will successfully suppress sperm counts to levels incompatible with fertility (13). These effects are reversible (14). In these regimens, androgens function both to suppress sperm production by inhibiting gonadotropins and to replace endogenous androgen levels. The dosage of testosterone used in successful male contraceptive trials is higher than replacement, and long-term data on possible adverse effects on the prostate and cardiovascular system are not yet available.

In hereditary angioneurotic edema, anabolic steroids have been used to prevent attacks. These anabolic steroids increase the synthesis of complement 1 inhibitor, which is deficient in these patients. Because of the known side effects of these agents, they are not recommended for use in pregnant women and in children.

Table 1 Indications for Androgen Therapy

Definite	Male hypogonadism
Probable or possible	Micropenis in children
	Constitutional delayed puberty
	Aging men (with evidence of androgen deficiency)
	Male contraception
	Hereditary angioneurotic edema
Dubious or controversial	Hematological disorders such as aplastic anemia, myelofibrosis with myeloid metaplasia hemolytic anemia, autoimmune thrombocytopenia, and leukopenia
	Improvement of nitrogen balance in non-androgen-deficient catabolic state
	Improvement of libido in hypogonadal women
Not indicated	Anemia associated with renal failure
	Improvement of muscle strength and endurance in athletes, body builders

The role of androgens in the treatment of hematological disorders remains controversial; and newer, more specifically targeted treatments are available. Treatment of refractory hypoplastic anemia with androgens may be tried for three to six months, but in responders, treatment must be continued for a much longer period. Because of the availability of recombinant human erythropoietin, with its more specific action and its lack of side effects, androgens are no longer the primary treatment for patients with anemia associated with chronic renal failure.

Androgens have been used in clinical situations such as severe trauma or chronic illness, in which the patient is in long-term negative nitrogen balance. The long-term results are generally disappointing, but trials in cancer and HIV-infected patients are underway.

There is an increasing trend toward the use of androgenic steroids by athletes and body builders. The pattern of androgen use by athletes involves the intermittent and cyclical administration of pharmacological doses of a combination of oral and parenteral agents. These unprescribed androgens may include huge doses of drugs, including veterinary agents that either are potentially toxic or have not been tested in humans (15). Androgens increase muscle mass and strength in women and prepubertal children. In normal adult men, it has been debated whether the administration of additional androgens enhances athletic performance. Most information is anecdotal; however, a number of studies including several well-controlled protocols have been performed. Results of double-blind studies are contradictory; there are reports indicating both positive and nonbeneficial effects on athletic performance in postpubertal males (9,15,16). A careful dose–response study was performed in which normal men were given a GnRH antagonist to markedly suppress serum LH levels. Groups of men were then given increasing doses of testosterone from subphysiological to markedly pharmacological amounts. The effect on muscle size and strength was progressive, indicating that the performance-enhancing effects of androgens are dose related (17). Even in those studies in which increased strength and performance was seen, the changes induced by these agents were small; thus, documentation of clinically significant improvement in muscle strength and endurance has not been obtained (15). Despite the controversy, some athletic trainers and physicians have argued that even small changes in performance justify the use of these agents by high-performance, competitive athletes. Nevertheless, the policies of all international and U.S. athletic regulatory agencies are unambiguously opposed to "doping" with androgens or other medicines to improve performance. Furthermore, physicians believe that the unsupervised use of androgens and high-dose androgen treatment impose some risk of undesired toxic effects. The long-term abuse of supraphysiological doses of androgens in men may lead to gynecomastia, hepatic toxicity (caused by 17-alkylated androgens), polycythemia, lipid changes (lowering of high-density cholesterol), and suppression of spermatogenesis (due to decreased LH and FSH secretion and decreased testosterone biosynthesis by the Leydig cells). These toxic side effects are suffcient to discourage the use of androgens for nonmedical reasons in people of all ages, even adult men.

☐ ADVERSE EFFECTS OF ANDROGEN TREATMENT

In general, testosterone and its esters have fewer side effects than the synthetic 17-alkylated androgens (8,9,13). Acne and increased oiliness of skin are frequently experienced by patients at the initiation of androgen supplementation. Because testosterone is metabolized to estradiol, gynecomastia may develop. The gynecomastia is often mild, and treatment is usually unnecessary. Most patients gain weight when administered androgens. The weight gain is due to water retention, increased blood volume, and increased lean body mass. With the exception of severely hypogonadal men with preexisting azoospermia and decreased testicular volume, patients given exogenous androgen therapy have suppression of spermatogenesis and a decrease in testicular size. The decreases in sperm production and seminiferous tubule volume are consequences of the suppression of GnRH, LH, and FSH.

Androgens cause virilization in women and prepubertal children. In addition, androgens promote premature epiphyseal closure of the long bones in children and will result in reduced ultimate height. There have been several studies on androgen effects on hypodesire states in women. The results indicate positive effects over placebo. Androgens are not approved in the United States for this condition, presumably because of the sparseness of safety data. For these reasons, androgens should not be used in women and in children of either sex except for the specific indications discussed previously.

Changes in liver function and hepatic disorders are dependent on the type of androgen given. Liver dysfunction is not observed with testosterone or its esters. In contrast, the 17-alkylated androgens can produce liver dysfunction, including cholestasis, elevation of plasma alkaline phosphatase, and conjugated bilirubin. Methyltestosterone causes cholestatic jaundice with minimal parenchymal liver damage. Recovery is usually rapid after drug discontinuation. Two more serious liver problems, peliosis hepatis and hepatic tumors, may occur rarely after androgen therapy, and only when high pharmacological doses of androgens are used to treat conditions such as refractory aplastic anemia. Because most of these reports involved patients with preexisting conditions that are associated with increased evidence of neoplasms, the implications of such reports in the treatment of hypogonadal men remain controversial. The majority of studies in which testosterone was given in physiologic doses for hypogonadism or pharmacologic doses for male contraception have not demonstrated evidence of hepatic toxicity.

Testosterone treatment influences cholesterol and apolipoprotein synthesis and metabolism. When a 17-alkylated androgen, stanozolol, is administered to normal men, high-density lipoprotein (HDL) cholesterol and apolipoprotein A-I and A-II levels are decreased, and low-density lipoprotein cholesterol and apolipoprotein B levels are increased. These changes in lipid profiles have been identified as risk factors for coronary atherosclerosis. Such changes in lipid profile occur to a much lower extent with testosterone esters such as testosterone enanthate, perhaps because some of the testosterone is converted to estrogens that have effects on lipid profile opposite those of androgens. Another explanation for the difference in lipid profiles may be that the orally active anabolic steroids (17-alkylated androgens) have a first-pass effect on the liver, leading to effects on lipids not apparent with the parenterally administered testosterone esters. More data are needed in larger groups of men to quantify the degree to which testosterone esters are associated with adverse effects on lipid profiles and to determine if these small effects are associated with an increased risk of atherosclerosis. The findings of decreased HDL cholesterol after high-dose testosterone and 17-alkylated androgens need to be balanced by the failure to document these changes in many replacement studies (6,17–19).

Androgens cause small increases in hemoglobin, hematocrit, and total red cell count when administered to normal or hypogonadal men (20). Androgens both stimulate erythropoietin production by the kidneys and have a direct effect on the bone-marrow stem cells. Clinically significant polycythemia is uncommon in hypogonadal men given androgen replacement except in patients who are likely to develop polycythemia—for example, those with chronic obstructive pulmonary disease or sleep apnea.

The 17-alkylated androgens have been given to men with coagulation disorders. Although small increases of clotting factors have been recorded, these anabolic steroids increase fibrinolysis and antithrombin III levels (a natural anticoagulant). The net effect is that increased bleeding episodes occur. The increase in fibrinolysis may counterbalance the negative effects of lipid profiles on the risk of coronary heart disease.

In hypogonadal men treated with androgen replacement, sleep-related breathing disorders (sleep apnea) have been reported. In obese patients and those with chronic obstructive airway disease, the physician should question the patient about sleep-related breathing disorders before the commencement of androgen replacement.

Although reports of androgen-induced mild resistance to insulin action exist, the usual doses of testosterone esters, when given to normal men, are not associated with changes in glucose or insulin levels. Although adverse effects on glucose control in diabetic patients given androgen replacement have been reported, many studies now suggest that testosterone may benefit the metabolic syndrome by reducing body and visceral fat.

Benign prostatic hypotrophy and prostate cancer rarely occur in men who developed androgen deficiency prior to puberty. Despite this fact, no clear evidence indicates that androgen replacement given to men who become hypogonadal after puberty increases the risk of prostatic disease. For all adult men, especially older men on long-term androgen therapy, regular digital rectal examination must be performed and prostate-specific antigen levels should be monitored. If there is a suspicion of prostatic enlargement, a transrectal prostatic ultrasound should be performed and/or final needle biopsy of a suspicious nodule.

The effects of androgen on behavior and cognitive function have been topics of broad public interest. Anecdotal reports of androgen rage or increased aggressive behavior after androgen therapy have not been substantiated by controlled studies. A recent report (9) has shown improved mood, lessened depression, and general well being when hypogonadal men are treated with testosterone.

☐ CONCLUSION

Disorders of Leydig cell function can be primary or secondary to abnormal secretion of LH and FSH. These disorders can be congenital or acquired. The clinical manifestations depend on the following: (*i*) location of the defect (hypothalamic, pituitary, and gonadal) or mimicking by abnormalities of androgen-responsive end organs; (*ii*) age at onset of the disorder; and (*iii*) the nature of associated nonreproductive problems. Because of the actual role of intratesticular testosterone in germ cell maturation, Leydig cell dysfunction usually leads to infertility. Testosterone replacement therapy is required for androgen-deficient males with primary Leydig cell underfunction. Males with hypogonadotropic hypogonadism may be treated with either LH (hCG) or testosterone to normalize serum testosterone levels, but reversal of infertility requires gonadotropic hormone treatment.

□ REFERENCES

1. Wang C, Swerdloff RS. Androgens. In: Smity CM, Revard AM, eds. Essentials of Pharmacology. Philadelphia, PA: WB Saunders Company, 1995:555–562.

2. Sherins RJ. Evaluation and management of men with hypogonadotropic hypogonadism. In: Garcia CR, Mastroianni I, Amelar RD, et al. eds. Current Therapy in Infertility. Philadelphia: BC Decker, 1984:147–151.

3. Wang C, Swerdloff RS. Male infertility—overview of current therapy. In: Boutaleb MB, ed. Proceedings of 13th World Congress on Fertility and Sterility. Casterton Hall, UK: Parthenon Publishing, 1990.

4. Allan CA, McLachlan RI. Age-related changes in testosterone and the role of replacement therapy in older men. Clin Endocrinol (Oxf) 2004; 60(6):653–670.

5. Gruenewald DA, Matsumoto AM. Testosterone supplementation therapy for older men: potential benefits and risks. J Am Geriatr Soc 2003; 51(1):101–115.

6. Liu PY, Swerdloff RS, Veldhuis JD. The rationale, efficacy and safety of androgen therapy in older men: future research and current practice recommendations. J Clin Endocrinol Metab 2004; 89(10):4789–4796.

7. Liverman CT, Blazer DG. Testosterone and Aging: Clinical Research Directions. Washington, DC: National Academies Press, 2004.

8. Bardin CW, Swerdloff RS, Santen RJ. Androgens: risks and benefits. J Clin Endocrinol Metab 1991; 73(1):4–7.

9. Wang C, Alexander G, Berman N, et al. Testosterone replacement therapy improves mood in hypogonadal men-a clinical research center study. J Clin Endocrinol Metab 1996; 81(10):3578–3583.

10. Cummings DE, Bremner WJ. Prospects for new hormonal male contraceptives. Endocrinol Metab Clin North Am 1994; 23(4):893–922.

11. Swerdloff RS, Steiner B, Callegari C, et al. GnRH analogues and male contraception. In: Bhasin S, Gabelnick H, Spieler J, Swerdloff RS, Wang C, eds. Biology, Pharmacology and Clinical Application of Androgens. New York: Wiley-Liss, 1995.

12. World Health Organization. Laboratory Manual for the Examination of Human Semen and Sperm Cervical Mucus Interaction. 4th ed. Cambridge University Press, 1999.

13. World Health Organization Task Force on methods for the regulation of male fertility. Contraceptive efficacy of testosterone-induced azoospermia and oligozoospermia in normal men. Fertil Steril 1996; 65(4): 821–829.

14. Liu PY, Swerdloff RS. Rate, extent, and modifiers of spermatogenic recovery after hormonal male contraception: an integrated analysis. Lancet 2006; 367(9520):1412–1420.

15. Wilson JD. Androgen abuse by athletes. Endocr Rev 1988; 9(2):181–199.

16. Casaburi R, Storer T, Bhasin S. Androgen effects on body composition and muscle performance. In: Bhasin S, Gabelnick H, Spieler J, et al., eds. Biology, Pharmacology, and Clinical Applications of Androgens. New York, New York: Wiley-Liss, 1995.

17. Bhasin S, Woodhouse L, Casaburi R, et al. Testosterone dose-response relationships in healthy young men. Am J Physiol Endocrinol Metab 2001; 281(6):E1172–E1181.

18. Cunningham G, Swerdloff RS. Endocrine Society Consensus Statement. 2001. Tertiary Endocrine Society Consensus Statement.

19. Wang C, Swedloff RS, Iranmanesh A, et al. Transdermal testosterone gel improves sexual function, mood, muscle strength, and body composition parameters in hypogonadal men. Testosterone Gel Study Group. J Clin Endocrinol Metab 2000; 85(8):2839–2853.

20. Palacios A, Campfield LA, McClure RD, et al. Swerdloff RS. Effect of testosterone enanthate on hematopoiesis in normal men. Fertil Steril 1983; 40(1):100–104.

30

Hormonal Induction of Spermatogenesis in Males with Hypogonadotropic Hypogonadism

Peter Y. Liu

Division of Endocrinology, Harbor-UCLA Medical Center, Torrance, California, U.S.A. and Department of Andrology, ANZAC Research Institute, University of Sydney, New South Wales, Australia

☐ INTRODUCTION

Approximately 10% of all couples will seek fertility assessment (1), and of these, a male factor will be found in up to two-thirds (2–5). Fertility assessment may be the first presentation of adult gonadotropin deficiency due to adult-onset or neglected pubertal delay (5,6). Missed diagnosis at this stage may have adverse long-term general health consequences (e.g., osteoporosis, sarcopenia, reduced quality of life), and may also immediately expose both the male and female partners, as well as any progeny, to the unnecessary risks of assisted reproduction (7).

Conventionally, gonadotropin deficiency is treated with androgen replacement therapy (see Chapter 29) to induce and maintain virilization since steroids are cheaper and more easily administered than gonadotropins; however, testis development, spermatogenesis, and fertility cannot be induced by exogenous testosterone alone (8), since the resulting intratesticular testosterone concentrations are two orders of magnitude lower than that achieved with luteinizing hormone (LH) stimulation. Hence, gonadotropin or pulsatile gonadotropin–releasing hormone (GnRH) therapy is required for gonadotropin-deficient men who seek fertility. Since pregnancy is the desired outcome, spermatogenic and testicular parameters are only surrogate markers of fertility. Nevertheless, sperm output is a critical, quantifiable (9), and prospectively quantitative (10) determinate of male fertility (see Chapter 24).

Although gonadotropin deficiency remains one of the few disorders of male fertility responsive to specific treatment, it accounts for less than 1% of all causes of infertility (2–4). Furthermore, affected men seek fertility on few occasions and successful pregnancy typically requires years (rather than months) of treatment. For these reasons, prospective randomized efficacy studies are not feasible, and even retrospective studies in specialized centers require decades to accumulate sparse and incomplete data (11–13). Among the larger studies of gonadotropin replacement (12–29), only six examined more than 20 men (12–17). These six include four multi-center studies (14–17) where consistency of therapy may not

have been maintained. Fertility outcome data following pulsatile GnRH therapy are even sparser (11,13,24, 25,30–33).

Important differences in the use and effect of gonadotropin therapy between men and women limit extrapolation. Gonadotropin therapy is typically used pharmacologically for ovarian hyperstimulation in women as part of a nonspecific infertility treatment (7). Furthermore, the effectiveness and risk of ovarian hyperstimulation syndrome with pharmacological gonadotropin therapy and the physiological variation in gonadotropin and steroid secretion during the menstrual cycle and with age (menopause) has no parallel in men. These important differences limit extrapolation, except when assessing pharmacokinetics, local tolerability, and antigenicity of specific gonadotropin preparations.

This chapter will therefore highlight studies performed specifically in gonadotropin-deficient men that examined pregnancy outcomes and predictors of fertility; however, since fertility data are so limited, with few studies including it as an important endpoint (12,13,26,28,34,35), other studies will also be included if quantitative spermatogenic data are provided, even if few participants actually sought fertility (11,14–17,19,22–24,25,27). The clinical application of this information will be emphasized.

☐ INDUCTION OF SPERMATOGENESIS IN GONADOTROPIN DEFICIENCY

Gonadotropin deficiency is caused by structural or functional disorders of the pituitary and/or hypothalamus. Genetic defects in the synthesis, secretion, and action of GnRH, LH, or follicle-stimulating hormone (FSH) ligands and receptors are increasingly being recognized as important causes of gonadotropin deficits (36–40). However, other acquired causes of gonadotropin deficiency should be considered, as specific treatments may be effectively applied. Iron chelation in hemochromatosis (41), dopamine agonist treatment of macroprolactinoma (42,43), and surgery and/or radiotherapy for pituitary tumors each may occasionally restore fertility. Concurrent evaluation of tubal patency and ovulation in the female partner is also required, since male and female factors may coexist in up to one-third of all cases of infertility (2–4).

Androgen replacement therapy (if used) must be stopped prior to commencement of gonadotropin or GnRH therapy. Both treatments are effective, but GnRH therapy is not approved by regulatory authorities in some countries (including the United States). In addition, GnRH therapy is ineffective in men lacking pituitary gonadotroph function (44), and can only be considered in gonadotropin-deficient men without pituitary disease; however, such therapy requires continuous use of a portable pump to deliver pulsatile therapy, which is inconvenient, costly to maintain, and is now rarely used outside of highly specialized centers (11,13,30). For this reason, gonadotropin therapy has become standard therapy and data regarding the outcome of GnRH therapy remains limited.

Clinical features (androgenic effects, Tanner pubertal stage, and testis size), blood (plasma testosterone), and semen (semen analysis) should be assessed at baseline and monitored throughout therapy. Assessment of testis volume by ultrasound (otherwise by Prader orchidometer), and monthly examination of blood and semen is ideal (see Chapter 12). If initiation of spermatogenesis is slow or sperm output remains poor, assisted reproductive technologies may be introduced cautiously (45). Gonadotropin-deficient men with smaller initial testicular volumes or incomplete puberty are more likely to require such additional treatment (11,12,46).

After pregnancy is confirmed, continuation of therapy until completion of the first trimester is prudent. During this time, GnRH or human chorionic gonadotropin (hCG)/FSH can be converted to hCG treatment alone (31,47), since such therapy is less costly and more convenient, and the potential reduction in sperm output is less important once pregnancy has been confirmed. This is consistent with the classical view that FSH is necessary for quantitatively normal spermatogenesis (8,48). Cryostorage of sperm for future pregnancies is also advisable (49), but may be of poor quality post-thaw.

□ GONADOTROPIN THERAPY
Preparations

Successful initiation of spermatogenesis in primates requires FSH and LH secretion by the pituitary gland, although the relative importance of FSH to initiate or maintain spermatogenesis remains controversial (50,51). In gonadotropin-deficient men, hCG therapy alone may be sufficient to induce (21,52), maintain (29,53), or reinitiate (48,53) qualitatively normal spermatogenesis, but FSH is required for quantitatively normal spermatogenesis (47,52). Gonadotropins have been clinically available for almost four decades (54,55) and are highly effective. Successful regimens have been reported using hCG purified from urine of

pregnant women alone (21), or combined with FSH purified from human pituitaries (29), urine of menopausal women (13), or recombinant FSH (56). However, gonadotropin therapy is ineffective in the absence of gonadotropin deficiency (7).

Recombinant FSH

Recombinant human FSH is manufactured from genetically engineered Chinese Hamster Ovary (CHO) cells in which the genes encoding the α and β chains of human FSH are introduced through recombinant DNA technology (57,58). Two recombinant FSH preparations are commercially available: follitropin α (Gonal F®, Ares-Serono, Geneva, Switzerland) and follitropin β (Follistim®, Organon, West Orange, New Jersey, or Puregon®, NV Organon, Oss, The Netherlands). Follitropin α is purified from the cell culture supernatant by ultrafiltration followed by five chromatographic stages, which include reversed-phase, high-performance liquid chromatography and immunoaffinity. The chromatographic stages in the purification of follitropin β include anion and cation exchange, hydrophobic interaction, and size exclusion. Both compounds are structurally very similar, and possess similar immunopotency, in vitro potency, and internal carbohydrate complexity (59). Hence, they are likely to be equally effective for induction of spermatogenesis, although direct comparisons are not available.

In women, both forms of FSH are equally effective and safe for in vitro fertilization (IVF) treatment (60–62). The use of a pen delivery device improves effectiveness in women, which is most likely explained by reduced waste, increased convenience, and better compliance (63). Similar studies in the context of male infertility have not yet been published.

Recombinant human FSH has advantages in formulation over urinary FSH preparations due to its greater purity, higher specific activity, and more consistent composition (59,64), and it is also theoretically available in an unlimited supply; however, the manufacture of urinary compounds has correspondingly become more sophisticated to compensate for these perceived limitations. Whereas the first available preparations [human menopausal gonadotropin (hMG) or menotropin] contained protein impurities and possessed both FSH and LH activity, modern purification procedures have resulted in preparations that contain trace quantities of other proteins and have greater batch-to-batch consistency (through bioactivity testing) (65). Other purification methods have also been developed to reduce intrinsic LH activity (producing urofollitropin compounds); however, these compounds have no specific clinical advantages for the induction of spermatogenesis. Critically, urinary and recombinant FSH appear to be equally effective in inducing spermatogenesis and causing pregnancy (12,56), although formal comparisons are not available. This is consistent with the comparable pregnancy rates determined by meta-analysis in various groups of women undergoing assisted reproduction (66–69). Local tolerability of either highly or regularly purified compounds is also equivalent to recombinant FSH (65,70).

Nevertheless, urinary FSH preparations are increasingly supplanted by recombinant FSH, despite being approximately half the cost in some countries (71). This trend is not due to rigorous cost-effectiveness analysis since formal cost-effectiveness studies are not available in men, and cannot be derived from analyses in the context of assisted reproduction (72–74). The decreased availability of urinary FSH may be partly due to reduced donor pool availability after more stringent screening to limit the risk of transmissible prion disease was instituted. Although pituitary extracts have a known risk of prion disease transmission (75–79), and are no longer available, no cases of transmission have been documented for either urinary or recombinant preparations (68,80). Such transmission remains a theoretical possibility since both compounds require either potentially infectious human urine or bovine serum as part of the manufacturing process.

Recombinant hCG

Recombinant hCG, which is commercially available as chorionic gonadotropin α (Ovidrel®, Ares-Serono, Geneva, Switzerland), has recently received regulatory approval in the United States for assisted reproduction. Based on the impact of recombinant FSH on the availability of urinary FSH, it is likely that urinary hCG will also be progressively replaced. Recombinant hCG is otherwise pharmacokinetically bioequivalent to urinary hCG (81), but has fewer local side effects (82–84). Whether local tolerability of urinary hCG could be improved with more stringent purification procedures is not known. Although recombinant hCG has been used in men (85), studies of its use in the context of male infertility are awaited. Recombinant LH (86) is also available, but its potential role in spermatogenesis induction has not yet been defined.

New Preparations

Other novel FSH agonists are being developed using recombinant technology in CHO cell lines. Some have already been tested in clinical trials and their commercial availability is anticipated. The development of these compounds has followed two general approaches. One approach was to develop proteins of reduced size and complexity but with full bioavailability in the hope of producing compounds, that could be administered nasally rather than by injection (87). Although less painful to administer, these compounds would probably be less convenient if more frequent dosing was required. The other approach was to develop larger, more heavily glycosylated and acidic proteins with increased duration of action due to reduced renal clearance and/or increased intrinsic activity (59,88). Such compounds would be more convenient if less frequent administration was required and are ideally suited for induction

of spermatogenesis rather than ovarian hyperstimulation, since careful dose titration is not necessary in men. FSH–CTP manufactured by fusion of the C terminal sequence of the chorionic gonadotropin β subunit to the follitropin β subunit (89) is one such compound. Prolonged duration of action has been observed in men due to the resultant introduction of four O-linked glycosylation sites as well as the induction of the Sertoli cell and fertility marker, inhibin B, and minimal antigenicity (90); however, the effect of FSH–CTP on spermatogenesis has not yet been reported. Administration in women has resulted in similar results as well as clinical pregnancies (91,92).

More recent innovations include techniques to insert N-linked glycosylation sites and to produce fusion proteins. Fusion proteins (including an FSH–CTP-like protein) contain both α and β subunits on a single chain (93,94). The covalent linkage reduces subunit dissociation and results in prolonged duration of action and increased efficiency of subunit assembly. The introduction of N-linked glycosylation sites into the α subunit (95) or β subunit (94) has also been reported. A novel protein combining these extra sites within a fusion protein has been created (94), although further increase in duration of action has not been formally demonstrated. The construction of a modified hCG protein containing extra N-linked glycosylation sites is also anticipated, since the α subunit is common to all gonadotropins. However, the bioactivity of this protein, particularly with multiple dosing, would still need to be formally established since desensitization may be limiting (96–98).

Regimens

Conventionally, hCG is commenced at a dose of 1000 to 2000 IU administered two to three times each week. Patients are reassessed after the first month. If the trough plasma testosterone (measured immediately before the next injection) is subnormal (below the eugonadal range) and/or if there is inadequate testicular or androgenic response, the same dosage is increased to three times or, rarely, four times weekly. A trial of hCG treatment alone is warranted since spermatogenesis can be effectively induced in some men (21,53), particularly those with larger testicular volume (26) or those who have completed puberty (28); however, if no sperm has appeared by 6 to 12 months of adequate hCG treatment, FSH is added. The usual dose of FSH required is 75 to 150 IU three times weekly. Provided total dose is the same, frequency of administration does not appear important (14). If testis growth and sperm output are inadequate, the dose is can be increased, rarely, to 150 IU daily.

All commercially available gonadotropins (urinary or recombinant FSH or hCG) can be administered intramuscularly or subcutaneously (22,81,99–102) even in the presence of obesity (103). Nevertheless, the subcutaneous route is preferable since it is more amenable to self-administration, is more convenient, and less painful. When administering hCG with FSH, both can be mixed and injected in the same syringe.

Rarely, antibodies can develop against urinary gonadotropins (104). Since the antibodies may be directed against other protein impurities, a trial of recombinant (105,106) or highly purified preparations is indicated. As a last resort, pulsatile GnRH therapy may be attempted, but may not necessarily be successful (104).

☐ GnRH THERAPY

GnRH is secreted by specific neuroendocrine cells located in the arcuate region of the mediobasal hypothalamus into a closed portal system through which it reaches the anterior pituitary gonadotropes, which secrete LH and FSH (107). Endogenous GnRH is secreted in a pulsatile fashion, typically every 90 to 120 minutes (108), and this pulsatility is essential to its action (109). Since small quantities are secreted into a closed system, systemically administered synthetic GnRH (gonadorelin) must be given at much higher doses. Furthermore, long-acting analogues downregulate GnRH action and are not useful in for the treatment of gonadotropin deficiency.

Regimens

Therapeutic studies in men with GnRH deficiency (110–112) confirm that 5 to 20 µg (25 to 600 ng/kg) per bolus administered every 90 to 120 minutes subcutaneously by portable pump through an indwelling butterfly needle results in physiological LH and FSH response. The needle is usually placed in the abdominal wall and changed every two days. Therapy is monitored by serum LH, FSH, and testosterone usually every two weeks initially, and then every two months. Although intravenous administration produces the most physiologic pulse characteristics (113,114) and can successfully induce spermatogenesis and pregnancy (115), subcutaneous administration is more practical for long-term treatment. Intranasal GnRH can maintain already induced spermatogenesis (116), but the need for frequent dosing every two hours also renders this clinically impractical.

Failure of GnRH therapy may result from anti-GnRH antibody formation (117–119), which requires conversion to or supplementation with gonadotropin therapy. Although supplementary hCG/hMG treatment may further increase spermatogenesis in men with poor testosterone response to GnRH therapy (30), it is not possible to determine if modification of GnRH therapy alone would have been sufficient.

☐ EXPECTED RESPONSE TO THERAPY

Response to therapy can be quantified using pregnancy, induction of spermatogenesis or testicular growth as endpoints. Ideally, time to endpoint variables should be summarized using median rather than mean estimates, since mean estimates are biased by ignoring the contribution of men who never achieve the endpoint (120); however, any of these estimates can be highly skewed by sample heterogeneity. Many factors, including testicular volume, cryptorchidism, completion of puberty, and prior androgen or gonadotropin therapy, are known to predict response and may be present to varying degrees in different populations. A further complication is that these predictors are interrelated and correlated—for example, smaller testis volumes occur in the presence of cryptorchidism and incomplete puberty.

To determine the relative contribution of each predictor of response, all variables must be simultaneously assessed in a multivariate analysis (12). Using this analysis, revealed that higher testicular volume and prior completion of puberty were the two most important predictors of faster induction of sperm output and pregnancy. This is consistent both with other major reports (46) and with anatomical function, since testis volume is predominantly physically determined by the amount of spermatogenic tissue present. For this reason, estimates of response times can be most usefully expressed according to testis volume.

The three major endpoints used to determine response to hormone therapy (induction of spermatogenesis, pregnancy, and testisticular growth) are reviewed individually below.

Induction of Spermatogenesis

The most extensive response data exists for spermatogenic endpoints. This is summarized in the bivariate plot of initial testicular volume versus duration of therapy required to induce spermatogenesis (Fig. 1). We found 13 studies that reported baseline testis volume and estimates (mean or median) of time to appearance of sperm in at least seven men receiving gonadotropin treatment (12–18,20,24,25,34,35,121). One study (121) was subsequently incorporated into a larger analysis (13) and was excluded. All these studies used gonadotropin dose regimens similar to that described in this chapter except one study, which appeared to use much lower doses and was excluded (20). The total number of subjects represented is almost 330. An additional seven studies of GnRH therapy were found using the same criteria (13,24,25,30–32,122). Pulsatile dose-titrated subcutaneous GnRH was administered in all studies but one, as described before, which used less frequent, eight-hour administration and was excluded (122). The total number of subjects represented is almost 80.

As illustrated, initial testis volume (calculated as the average of the left and right testis volume) consistently predicts spermatogenic response, with sperm first appearing within six months in men with larger (>4 mL) testis volumes and after nine months in men with smaller (≤4 mL) testis volumes. In some cases, spermatogenesis may be delayed by as long as 20

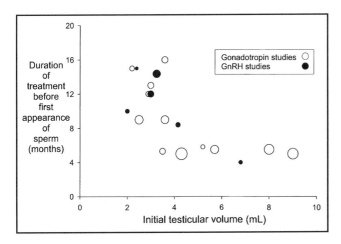

Figure 1 Bivariate bubble plot of larger published studies relating testicular volume with first appearance of sperm. Bivariate bubble plot of central estimates (mean or median) of initial testicular volume (mL) against duration of treatment required before first appearance of sperm (months). Each point represents a single published study of gonadotropin (*open symbols*) or pulsatile GnRH (*closed symbols*) therapy. The area of each point is, proportional to the sample size of that study. *Abbreviation*: GnRH, gonadotropin-releasing hormone.

months (20,24,123), particularly if dosage is low (20,123). These estimates are consistent with other studies of gonadotropin (23,52,124) and GnRH (11,32,122) therapy.

Pregnancy

Less extensive data regarding pregnancy outcomes after gonadotropin therapy is available. The largest studies (reporting altogether 34 successful pregnancies) suggest that half of all pregnancies will occur by approximately 20 months of treatment (12,18). Another large study has reported a shorter estimate of approximately 10 months (13) but was biased by use of assisted reproduction and statistical censoring. Smaller studies (seven pregnancies each) of long-term hCG treatment report that half of all pregnancies will occur by approximately 20 (26) or 45 (21) months of treatment. However, these are likely to be overestimates of combined gonadotropin treatment, which should result in more rapid response. Altogether, these studies have reported almost 75 pregnancies. Individual studies consistently report that approximately one- to two-thirds of all couples seeking fertility will eventually be successful (12,13,15–19,21,24,26,34,35).

The data regarding pregnancy outcomes after pulsatile GnRH therapy is so limited that conclusions cannot be drawn. Altogether, only approximately 20 pregnancies have been reported in five (13,24,25,30,31) of the eight larger studies identified (11,13,24,25,30–32,122). These pregnancies typically occur at low (3–8 million/mL) sperm concentrations (12,13,18,21,26,29). This cutoff is not specific to gonadotropin-treated men since a similar sperm output threshold demarcating subnormal from normal pregnancy rates was reported in normal men treated with spermatogenesis-suppressing contraceptive regimens (125). Similar relationships are likely to exist for pulsatile GnRH

therapy, but extensive quantitative data is not available.

Testicular Growth

Other response variables include testicular growth and hormonal response, but these are less useful if fertility is the desired outcome. Combined gonadotropin therapy typically results in testicular growth of approximately 7 mL (3–10 mL) (13–18,23,24,26,27,34, 35,52,56,124). This is consistent with studies of GnRH therapy (11,13,24,25,30–32,122), and may be useful in the rare patient whose goal is testicular growth rather than fertility. Normalization of hormonal parameters typically occurs by two to three months.

☐ PREDICTORS OF RESPONSE
Testicular Factors

As discussed above, testis volume is an important predictor of sperm output, which is interrelated with other known predictors. The testis volume level of 4 mL suggested empirically from Figure 1 has ancillary theoretical support since this same cutoff demarcates partial from complete gonadotropin deficiency, and the likelihood of completion of puberty (11). Indeed, below this level, induction of spermatogenesis often requires protracted therapy, although conception can rarely occur (21). Furthermore, within individual studies, most large studies (12–14,18,21,26,30) have reported a significant relationship between initial testicular volume and spermatogenic response. Studies that did not report such a relationship (17,22,34,35,52) often had a restricted range of testis volume or selected subjects specifically on the basis of another confounding variable.

Cryptorchid testes are less responsive to gonadotropin or GnRH therapy, and this effect is additional to that explained by testis volume. In a study of 13 cryptorchid men, matched for testicular volume (<4 mL) with 13 noncrypt-orchid men, gonadotropin therapy resulted in statistically lower testicular volume and sperm output (19). The remainder of the studies have largely confirmed this relationship (11,12,14,28,34), although fewer cryptorchid men were examined, testis volume was not matched, and some studies have reported equivocal (13,22) or no (35) association.

Previous Gonadotropin or Androgen Exposure

Testicular exposure to endogenous gonadotropin secretion during puberty is associated with improved testicular response to subsequent gonadotropin or GnRH therapy. Spermatogenesis, pregnancy, and/or normal serum testosterone are more rapidly attained with appropriate treatment in adult gonadotropin-deficient men who have previously completed puberty spontaneously (11,12,17,23,28,126). These beneficial effects are not mediated solely by testis volume (12).

Furthermore, degree of pubertal development seems to define specific phenotypes (46). Although these data suggest that endogenous gonadotropin exposure primes the testis, the current studies do not exclude the possibility that pubertal completion is simply a marker of disease severity.

Previous testicular exposure to exogenous gonadotropin therapy at any age also results in more rapid attainment of sperm production (12) or pregnancy (13,121) with subsequent therapy, although improved response rates have not been observed in all studies (17). Indeed, this seems to be due, in part, to persistently increased testicular volume (12), providing additional evidence for a true testis priming effect. Another study reported that previous age-specific use of hCG for the induction of puberty reduced the dose subsequently required for testicular growth and testosterone normalization (18). These data strengthen the hypothesis that previous gonadotropin exposure, whether due to natural puberty or prior gonadotropin treatment, actually primes the testis and results in enhanced spermatogenic response to subsequent gonadotropin therapy. Long-term gonadotropin therapy in adolescent males to induce spermatogenesis and androgenization has been attempted to mimic natural gonadotropin exposure at puberty (127,128). Recently, early postnatal treatment with recombinant human LH and FSH, has been used to mimic the early postnatal gonadotropin surge (129). These studies show that age-appropriate gonadotropin treatment is feasible, and suggest that chronologically appropriate testis growth and spermatogenesis may improve the prospect of future fertility (127,129). This concept is further supported by the greater delay in inducing spermatogenesis reported when treatment of acquired gonadotropin deficiency is delayed by more than two years (123). These approaches may become more widespread with the increased availability of recombinant FSH, although the greater cost and inconvenience of gonadotropins persists. A formal clinical trial examining this hypothesis would be highly desirable, but would be a formidable undertaking.

Prior androgen therapy does not preclude subsequent response to gonadotropin therapy (130) and has no relationship with subsequent induction of spermatogenesis, attainment of pregnancy, or testicular response (12,20,121); however, if age-appropriate gonadotropin exposure is beneficial, then androgen exposure may be detrimental insofar as it is an indicator of neglected gonadotropin use.

☐ NONPREDICTORS OF RESPONSE
Choice of Gonadotropin or Pulsatile GNRH Therapy

As indicated by the above discussion, optimal gonadotropin or GnRH therapy results in equivalent pregnancy rates, and spermatogenic and testicular response. As illustrated in Figure 1, the same relationship between initial testicular volume and treatment duration to induce spermatogenesis exists regardless of whether gonadotropin or pulsatile GnRH therapy is used. Direct comparisons between therapies have been performed in three studies (13,25,31), but none were randomized and one was retrospective (13). Differences in pregnancy outcome have never been reported and only one (24) of these three studies, recruiting only 18 men who self-selected therapy, found that GnRH therapy was superior to gonadotropin therapy due to significantly faster onset of spermatogenesis and larger final testicular volume. Two separate single- case reports have also reported that pulsatile GnRH can successfully induce spermatogenesis and cause pregnancy after failed gonadotropin therapy (131,132). Although there is insufficient data to conclude that GnRH is more effective than gonadotropin therapy, a clinical trial of GnRH after failed gonadotropin therapy may be warranted if feasible.

Cause of Gonadotropin Deficiency

Larger studies have consistently reported that the cause of gonadotropin deficiency is not a significant predictor of spermatogenic endpoints (12,13,17,18). Smaller studies (fewer than five men) have variably reported hypopituitarism as being advantageous (27) or detrimental (34). Since hypopituitarism generally occurs postpubertally and is also associated with larger testicular volume (121), these other confounders must be adjusted for. Similar confounding variables may explain why various hypothalamic causes of gonadotropin deficiency may differ in response to GnRH therapy (31). It therefore appears unlikely that the cause of gonadotropin deficiency is an important predictor of response if the effect of testicular volume and puberty are first accounted for.

☐ CONCLUSION

The induction of spermatogenesis with gonadotropin replacement in gonadotropin-deficient men has long been the prototype for successful management of male infertility. Indeed, the effectiveness of urinary gonadotropins (12,13,16–20,22–28,34,35,133–135) in these men has long rendered placebo-controlled studies unethical. Throughout this time, various gonadotropin regimens (subcutaneous vs. intramuscular and urinary vs. recombinant) have been available, differing in cost and convenience, but not in effectiveness.

Methods to improve the effectiveness of treatment have been unsuccessful so far. The superiority of pulsatile GnRH therapy has not been definitively demonstrated, and hence the greater inconvenience is difficult to justify. Furthermore, gonadotropin or GnRH dose escalation eventually becomes ineffective due to a ceiling in response. This fact combined with the unsuccessful attempts to apply these therapies more broadly to other causes of male infertility (7) suggest that, in contrast to ovarian hyperstimulation, hormonal overdrive of spermatogenesis is not feasible. For these reasons, although the commercial availability of longer-acting, more conveniently administered, recombinant gonadotropin analogues are anticipated, effectiveness is unlikely to be improved. Protein- or gene-based treatments to enhance the effect of gonadotropin therapy may eventually be developed. Such research is highly desirable, and resultant therapies may have broad application to other causes of male infertility.

In the meantime, vigilance is required to limit exposure to transmissible prion disease, since decades may elapse between infection and symptoms. The application of quantitative multivariate statistical methods in larger datasets should be encouraged to better quantify clinically useful time-dependent variables and key predictors. Standard therapy needs to be continually reassessed to adjust for more accurate response estimates and advances in assisted reproduction: currently, judicial use of IVF or ICSI may be worthwhile if sperm density remains consistently less than 3 million/mL and spermatogenesis or pregnancy has been slow (more than 10 or 20 months, respectively). The role of recombinant LH, in relation to hCG, needs appraisal, particularly in the context of pubertal, and eventually postnatal, testicular priming. The accumulating evidence supporting the importance of age-appropriate gonadotropin exposure requires formal evaluation.

□ ACKNOWLEDGMENTS

The author acknowledges the mentorship and intellectual stimulation in the area of male fertility by Professor David J. Handelsman, and the National Health and Medical Council of Australia (Grant 262025).

□ REFERENCES

1. Snick HK, Snick TS, Evers JL, et al. The spontaneous pregnancy prognosis in untreated subfertile couples: the Walcheren primary care study. Hum Reprod 1997; 12(7):1582–1588.

2. Comhaire FH, de Kretser DM, Farley TM, et al. Towards more objectivity in diagnosis and management of male fertility. Int J Androl 1987; 7(suppl):1–53.

3. Nieschlag E. Classification of andrological disorders. In: Nieschlag E, Behre HM, eds. Andrology: Male Reproductive Health and Dysfunction. 2nd ed. New York: Springer, 2000:83–87.

4. Hurst T, Lancaster P. Assisted conception Australia and New Zealand 1999 and 2000. Sydney, Australian Institute of Health and Welfare National Perinatal Statistics Unit, 2001.

5. Baker HWG. Male infertility. In: DeGroot LJ, Jameson JL, eds. Endocrinology. 4th ed. Philadelphia: Saunders, 2001:2308–2328.

6. Nachtigall LB, Boepple BA, Pralong FP, et al. Adult-onset idiopathic hypogonadotropic hypogonadism—a treatable form of male infertility. N Engl J Med 1997; 336(6):410–415.

7. Liu PY, Handelsman DJ. The present and future state of hormonal treatment for male infertility. Hum Reprod Update 2003; 9(1):9–23.

8. Schaison G, Young J, Pholsena M, et al. Failure of combined follicle-stimulating hormone—testosterone administration to initiate and/or maintain spermatogenesis in men with hypogonadotropic hypogonadism. J Clin Endocrinol Metab 1993; 77(6):1545–1549.

9. World Health Organization. WHO Laboratory Manual For The Examination of Human Semen and Sperm-Cervical Mucus Interaction. 4th ed. Cambridge: Cambridge University Press, 1999:1–107.

10. WHO. Annual Technical Report 1994. Geneva, World Health Organization, 1994.

11. Pitteloud N, Hayes FJ, Dwyer A, et al. Predictors of outcome of long-term GnRH therapy in men with idiopathic hypogonadotropic hypogonadism. J Clin Endocrinol Metab 2002; 87(9):4128–4136.

12. Liu PY, Gebski VJ, Turner L, et al. Predicting pregnancy and spermatogenesis by survival analysis during gonadotrophin treatment of gonadotrophin-deficient infertile men. Hum Reprod 2002; 17(3): 625–633.

13. Buchter D, Behre HM, Kliesch S, et al. Pulsatile GnRH or human chorionic gonadotropin/human menopausal gonadotropin as effective treatment for men with hypogonadotropic hypogonadism: a review of 42 cases. Eur J Endocrinol 1998; 139(3):298–303.

14. Bouloux PM, Nieschlag E, Burger HG, et al. Induction of spermatogenesis by recombinant follicle-stimulating hormone (puregon) in hypogonadotropic azoospermic men who failed to respond to human chorionic gonadotropin alone. J Androl 2003; 24(4):604–611.

15. Bouloux P, Warne DW, Loumaye E. Efficacy and safety of recombinant human follicle-stimulating hormone in men with isolated hypogonadotropic hypogonadism. Fertil Steril 2002; 77(2):270–273.

16. European Metrodin HP Study Group. Efficacy and safety of highly purified urinary follicle-stimulating hormone with human chorionic gonadotropin for treating men with isolated hypogonadotropic hypogonadism. Fertil Steril 1998; 70(2):256–262.

17. Burgues S, Calderon MD. Subcutaneous self-administration of highly purified follicle stimulating

hormone and human chorionic gonadotrophin for the treatment of male hypogonadotrophic hypogonadism. Spanish Collaborative Group on Male Hypogonadotropic Hypogonadism. Hum Reprod 1997; 12(5):980–986.

18. Kung AW, Zhong YY, Lam KS, et al. Induction of spermatogenesis with gonadotrophins in Chinese men with hypogonadotrophic hypogonadism. Int J Androl 1994; 17(5):241–247.

19. Kirk JM, Savage MO, Grant DB, et al. Gonadal function and response to human chorionic and menopausal gonadotrophin therapy in male patients with idiopathic hypogonadotrophic hypogonadism. Clin Endocrinol (Oxf) 1994; 41(1):57–63.

20. Okada Y, Kondo T, Okamoto S, et al. Induction of ovulation and spermatogenesis by hMG/hCG in hypogonadotropic GH-deficient patients. Endocrinol Jpn 1992; 39(1):31–43.

21. Vicari E, Mongioi A, Calogero AE, et al. Therapy with human chorionic gonadotrophin alone induces spermatogenesis in men with isolated hypogonadotrophic hypogonadism—long-term follow-up. Int J Androl 1992; 15(4):320–329.

22. Saal W, Happ J, Cordes U, et al. Subcutaneous gonadotropin therapy in male patients with hypogonadotropic hypogonadism. Fertil Steril 1991; 56:319–324.

23. Mastrogiacomo I, Motta RG, Botteon S, et al. Achievement of spermatogenesis and genital tract maturation in hypogonadotropic hypogonadic subjects during long term treatment with gonadotropins or LHRH. Andrologia 1991; 23(4):285–289.

24. Schopohl J, Mehltretter G, von Zumbusch R, et al. Comparison of gonadotropin-releasing hormone and gonadotropin therapy in male patients with idiopathic hypothalamic hypogonadism. Fertil Steril 1991; 56(6):1143–1150.

25. Liu L, Banks SM, Barnes KM, et al. Two-year comparison of testicular responses to pulsatile gonadotropin-releasing hormone and exogenous gonadotropins from the inception of therapy in men with isolated hypogonadotropic hypogonadism. J Clin Endocrinol Metab 1988; 67(6):1140–1145.

26. Burris AS, Rodbard HW, Winters SJ, et al. Gonadotropin therapy in men with isolated hypogonadotropic hypogonadism: the response to human chorionic gonadotropin is predicted by initial testicular size. J Clin Endocrinol Metab 1988; 66(6):1144–1151.

27. Nakamura M, Namiki M, Okuyama A, et al. Testicular responsiveness to long-term administration of hCG and hMG in patients with hypogonadotrophic hypogonadism. Horm Res 1986; 23(1):21–30.

28. Finkel DM, Phillips JL, Snyder PJ. Stimulation of spermatogenesis by gonadotropins in men with hypogonadotropic hypogonadism. N Engl J Med 1985; 313(11):651–665.

29. Burger HG, Baker HW. Therapeutic considerations and results of gonadotropin treatment in male hypogonadotropic hypogonadism. Ann NY Acad Sci 1984; 438:447–453.

30. Christiansen P, Skakkebaek NE. Pulsatile gonadotropin-releasing hormone treatment of men with idiopathic hypogonadotropic hypogonadism. Horm Res 2002; 57(1–2):32–36.

31. Delemarre-Van de Waal HA. Induction of testicular growth and spermatogenesis by pulsatile, intravenous administration of gonadotrophin-releasing hormone in patients with hypogonadotrophic hypogonadism. Clin Endocrinol (Oxf) 1993; 38(5):473–480.

32. Aulitzky W, Frick J, Galvan G. Pulsatile luteinizing hormone-releasing hormone treatment of male hypogonadotropic hypogonadism. Fertil Steril 1988; 50(3):480–486.

33. Spratt DI, Finkelstein JS, O'Dea LS, et al. Long-term administration of gonadotropin-releasing hormone in men with idiopathic hypogonadotropic hypogonadism. A model for studies of the hormone's physiological effects. Ann Intern Med 1986; 105(6):848–855.

34. Ley SB, Leonard JM. Male hypogonadotropic hypogonadism: factors influencing response to human chorionic gonadotropin and human menopausal gonadotropin, including prior exogenous androgens. J Clin Endocrinol Metab 1985; 61(4):746–752.

35. Jones TH, Darne JF. Self-administered subcutaneous human menopausal gonadotrophin for stimulation of testicular growth and the initiation of spermatogenesis in hypogonadotrophic hypogonadism. Clin Endocrinol (Oxf) 1993; 38(2):203–208.

36. Seminara SB, Hayes FJ, Crowley WF Jr. Gonadotropin-releasing hormone deficiency in the human (idiopathic hypogonadotropic hypogonadism and Kallmann's syndrome): pathophysiological and genetic considerations. Endocr Rev 1998; 19(5):521–539.

37. Layman LC. Genetics of human hypogonadotropic hypogonadism. Am J Med Genet 1999; 89(4):240–248.

38. de Roux N, Young J, Brailly-Tabard S, et al. The same molecular defects of the gonadotropin-releasing hormone receptor determine a variable degree of hypogonadism in affected kindred. J Clin Endocrinol Metab 1999; 84(2):567–572.

39. Seminara SB, Messager S, Chatzidaki EE, et al. The GPR54 gene as a regulator of puberty. N Engl J Med 2003; 349(17):1614–1627.

40. Dode C, Levilliers J, Dupont JM, et al. Loss-of-function mutations in FGFR1 cause autosomal dominant Kallmann syndrome. Nat Genet 2003; 33:463–465.

41. Siemons LJ, Mahler CH. Hypogonadotropic hypogonadism in hemochromatosis: recovery of reproductive function after iron depletion. J Clin Metab 1987; 65(3):585–587.

42. De Rosa M, Colao A, Di Sarno A, et al. Cabergoline treatment rapidly improves gonadal function in hyperprolactinemic males: a comparison with bromocriptine. Eur J Endocrinol 1998; 138(3):286–293.

43. Laufer N, Yaffe H, Margalioth EJ, et al. Effect of bromocriptine treatment on male infertility associated with hyperprolactinemia. Arch Androl 1981; 6(4):343–346.

44. Wang C, Tso SC, Todd D. Hypogonadotropic hypogonadism in severe beta-thalassemia: effect of chelation and pulsatile gonadotropin-releasing hormone therapy. J Clin Endocrinol Metab 1989; 68(3):511–516.

45. Yong EL, Lee KO, Ng SC, et al. Induction of spermatogenesis in isolated hypogonadotrophic hypogonadism with gonadotrophins and early intervention with intracytoplasmic sperm injection. Hum Reprod 1997; 12(6):1230–1232.

46. Pitteloud N, Hayes FJ, Boepple PA, et al. The role of prior pubertal development, biochemical markers of testicular maturation, and genetics in elucidating the phenotypic heterogeneity of idiopathic hypogonadotropic hypogonadism. J Clin Endocrinol Metab 2002; 87:152–160.

47. Depenbusch M, von Eckardstein S, Simoni M, et al. Maintenance of spermatogenesis in hypogonadotropic hypogonadal men with human chorionic gonadotropin alone. Eur J Endocrinol 2002; 147(5):617–624.

48. Matsumoto AM, Karpas AE, Bremner WJ. Chronic human chorionic gonadotropin administration in normal men: evidence that follicle stimulating hormone is necessary for the maintenance of quantitatively normal spermatogenesis in man. J Clin Endocrinol Metab 1986; 62(6):1184–1192.

49. Kelleher S, Wishart SM, Liu PY, et al. Long–term outcomes of elective human sperm cryostorage. Hum Reprod 2001; 16(12):2632–2639.

50. Moudgal NR, Sairam MR. Is there a true requirement for follicle stimulating hormone in promoting spermatogenesis and fertility in primates? Hum Reprod 1998; 13(4):916–919.

51. Plant TM, Marshall GR. The functional significance of FSH in spermatogenesis and the control of its secretion in male primates. Endocr Rev 2001; 22(6):764–786.

52. De Sanctis V, Vullo C, Katz M, et al. Induction of spermatogenesis in thalassaemia. Fertil Steril 1998; 50(6):969–975.

53. Johnsen SG. Maintenance of spermatogenesis induced by HMG treatment by means of continuous HCG treatment in hypogonadotrophic men. Acta Endocrinol (Copenh) 1978; 89(4):763–769.

54. Gemzell C, Kjessler B. Treatment of infertility after partial hypophysectomy with human pituitary gonadotrophins. Lancet 1964; 15:644.

55. MacLeod J, Pazianos A, Ray BS. Restoration of human spermatogenesis by menopausal gonadotrophins. Lancet 1964; 13:1196–1197.

56. Liu PY, Turner L, Rushford D, et al. Efficacy and safety of recombinant human follicle stimulating hormone (Gonal-F) with urinary human chorionic gonadotrophin for induction of spermatogenesis and fertility in gonadotrophin-deficient men. Hum Reprod 1999; 14(6):1540–1545.

57. Olijve W, de Boer W, Mulders JW, van Wezenbeek PM. Molecular biology and biochemistry of human recombinant follicle stimulating hormone (Puregon). Mol Hum Reprod 1996; 2(5):371–382.

58. Recombinant Human FSH Product Development Group. Recombinant follicle stimulating hormone: development of the first biotechnology product for the treatment of infertility. Hum Reprod Update 1998; 4(6):862–881.

59. Horsman G, Talbot JA, McLoughlin JD, et al. A biological, immunological and physico-chemical comparison of the current clinical batches of the recombinant FSH preparations Gonal-F and Puregon. Hum Reprod 2000; 15(9):1898–1902.

60. Tulppala M, Aho M, Tuuri T, et al. Comparison of two recombinant follicle-stimulating hormone preparations in in-vitro fertilization: a randomized clinical study. Hum Reprod 1999; 14(11):2709–2715.

61. Brinsden P, Akagbosu F, Gibbons LM, et al. A comparison of the efficacy and tolerability of two recombinant human follicle-stimulating hormone preparations in patients undergoing in vitro fertilization-embryo transfer. Fertil Steril 2000; 73(1):114–116.

62. Harlin J, Aanesen A, Csemiczky G, et al. Delivery rates following IVF treatment, using two recombinant FSH preparations for ovarian stimulation. Hum Reprod 2002; 17(2):304–309.

63. Platteau P, Laurent E, Albano C, et al. An open, randomized single-centre study to compare the efficacy and convenience of follitropin beta administered by a pen device with follitropin alpha administered by a conventional syringe in women undergoing ovarian stimulation for IVF/ICSI. Hum Reprod 2003; 18(6):1200–1204.

64. Gervais A, Hammel YA, Pelloux S, et al. Glycosylation of human recombinant gonadotrophins: characterization and batch-to-batch consistency. Glycobiology 2003; 13(3):179–189.

65. The European and Israeli study group on highly purified menotropin versus recombinant FSH. Efficacy and safety of highly purified menotropin versus recombinant follicle-stimulating hormone in in vitro fertilization/intracytoplasmic sperm injection cycles: a randomized, comparative trial. Fertil Steril 2002; 78(3):520–528.

66. Van Wely M, Bayram N, Van der Veen F. Recombinant FSH in alternative doses or versus urinary gonadotrophins for ovulation induction in subfertility associated with polycystic ovary syndrome: a systematic review based on a Cochrane review. Hum Reprod 2003; 18(6):1143–1149.

67. Van Wely M, Westergaard LG, Bossuyt PMM, et al. Human menopausal gonadotropin versus recombinant follicle stimulation hormone for ovarian stimulation in assisted reproductive cycles. Cochrane Database Syst Rev 2003; 1:1.

68. Jansen C. Bye-bye urinary gonadotrophins? Reply to Debate. Hum Reprod 2003; 18(4):895–896.

69. Al-Inany H, Aboulghar M, Mansour R, et al. Meta-analysis of recombinant versus urinary-derived FSH: an update. Hum Reprod 2003; 18(2):305–313.

70. Recombinant Human FSH Study Group. Clinical assessment of recombinant human follicle-stimulating

hormone in stimulating ovarian follicular development before in vitro fertilization. Fertil Steril 1995; 63(1):77–86.

71. Dyer SJ. The conflict between effective and affordable health care--a perspective from the developing world. Hum Reprod 2002; 17(7):1680–1683.

72. Daya S, Ledger W, Auray JP, et al. Cost-effectiveness modelling of recombinant FSH versus urinary FSH in assisted reproduction techniques in the UK. Hum Reprod 2001; 16(12):2563–2569.

73. Sykes D, Out HJ, Palmer SJ, et al. The cost-effectiveness of IVF in the UK: a comparison of three gonadotrophin treatments. Hum Reprod 2001; 16(12):2557–2562.

74. Silverberg K, Daya S, Auray JP, et al. Analysis of the cost effectiveness of recombinant versus urinary follicle-stimulating hormone in in vitro fertilization/intracytoplasmic sperm injection programs in the United States. Fertil Steril 2002; 77(1):107–113.

75. Cochius JI, Burns RJ, Blumbergs PC, et al. Creutzfeldt-Jakob disease in a recipient of human pituitary-derived gonadotrophin. Aust N Z J Med 1990; 20(4): 592–593.

76. Cochius JI, Hyman N, Esiri MM. Creutzfeldt-Jakob disease in a recipient of human pituitary-derived gonadotrophin: a second case. J Neurol Neurosurg Psychiatry 1992; 55:1094–1095.

77. Dumble LJ, Klein RD. Creutzfeldt-Jakob legacy for Australian women treated with human pituitary gonadotropins. Lancet 1992; 340(8823):847–848.

78. Healy DL, Evans J. Creutzfeldt-Jakob disease after pituitary gonadotrophins. BMJ 1993; 307:517–518.

79. Collins S, Masters CL. Iatrogenic and zoonotic Creutzfeldt-Jakob disease: the Australian perspective. Med J Aust 1996; 164(10):598–602.

80. Reichl H, Balen A, Jansen CA. Prion transmission in blood and urine: what are the implications for recombinant and urinary-derived gonadotrophins? Hum Reprod 2002; 17(10):2501–2508.

81. Trinchard-Lugan I, Khan A, Porchet HC, et al. Pharmacokinetics and pharmacodynamics of recombinant human chorionic gonadotrophin in healthy male and female volunteers. Reprod Biomed Online 2002; 4(2):106–115.

82. The European Recombinant Human Chorionic Gonadotrophin Study Group. Induction of final follicular maturation and early luteinization in women undergoing ovulation induction for assisted reproduction treatment--recombinant HCG versus urinary HCG. Hum Reprod 2000; 15(7): 1446–1451.

83. The International Recombinant Human Chorionic Gonadotropin Study Group. Induction of ovulation in World Health Organization group II anovulatory women undergoing follicular stimulation with recombinant human follicle-stimulating hormone: a comparison of recombinant human chorionic gonadotropin (rhCG) and urinary hCG. Fertil Steril 2001; 75(6):1111–1118.

84. Ludwig M, Doody KJ, Doody KM. Use of recombinant human chorionic gonadotropin in ovulation induction. Fertil Steril 2003; 79(5):1051–1059.

85. Liu PY, Wishart SM, Handelsman DJ. A double-blind, placebo-controlled, randomized clinical trial of recombinant human chorionic gonadotropin on muscle strength and physical function and activity in older men with partial age-related androgen deficiency. J Clin Endocrinol Metab 2002; 87(7): 3125–3135.

86. The European Recombinant Human LH Study Group. Recombinant human luteinizing hormone (LH) to support recombinant human follicle-stimulating hormone (FSH)-induced follicular development in LH- and FSH-deficient anovulatory women: a dose-finding study. J Clin Endocrinol Metab 1998; 83(5):1507–1514.

87. Heikoop JC, Huisman-de Winkel B, Grootenhuis PD. Towards minimized gonadotropins with full bioactivity. Eur J Biochem 1999; 261(1):81–84.

88. Vitt UA, Kloosterboer HJ, Rose UM, et al. Isoforms of human recombinant follicle-stimulating hormone: comparison of effects on murine follicle development in vitro. Biol Reprod 1998; 59(4):854–861.

89. Fares FA, Suganuma N, Nishimori K, et al. Design of a long-acting follitropin agonist by fusing the C-terminal sequence of the chorionic gonadotropin beta subunit to the follitropin beta subunit. Proc Natl Acad Sci USA 1992; 89(10): 4304–4308.

90. Bouloux PM, Handelsman DJ, Jockenhovel F, et al; FSH-CTP study group. First human exposure to FSH-CTP in hypogonadotrophic hypogonadal males. Hum Reprod 2001; 16(8): 1592–1597.

91. Duijkers IJ, Klipping C, Boerrigter PJ, et al. Single dose pharmacokinetics and effects on follicular growth and serum hormones of a long-acting recombinant FSH preparation (FSH-CTP) in healthy pituitary-suppressed females. Hum Reprod 2002; 17(8): 1987–1993.

92. Beckers NG, Macklon NS, Devroey P, et al. First live birth after ovarian stimulation using a chimeric long-acting human recombinant follicle-stimulating hormone (FSH) agonist (recFSH-CTP) for in vitro fertilization. Fertil Steril 2003; 79(3):621–623.

93. Klein J, Lobel L, Pollak S, et al. Pharmacokinetics and pharmacodynamics of single-chain recombinant human follicle-stimulating hormone containing the human chorionic gonadotropin carboxyterminal peptide in the rhesus monkey. Fertil Steril 2002; 77(6): 1248–1255.

94. Klein J, Lobel L, Pollak S, et al. Development and characterization of a long-acting recombinant hFSH agonist. Hum Reprod 2003; 18(1):50–56.

95. Perlman S, Van Den Hazel B, Christiansen J, et al. Glycosylation of an N-terminal extension prolongs the half-life and increases the in vivo activity of follicle stimulating hormone. J Clin Endocrinol Metab 2003; 88(7):3227–3235.

96. Smals AG, Pieters GF, Drayer JI, et al. Leydig cell responsiveness to single and repeated human chorionic gonadotropin administration. J Clin Endocrinol Metab 1979; 49(1):12–14.

97. Glass AR, Vigersky RA. Resensitization of testosterone production in men after human chorionic gonadotropin-induced desensitization. J Clin Endocrinol Metab 1980; 51(6):1395–1400.

98. Smals AG, Pieters GF, Boers GH, et al. Differential effect of single high dose and divided small dose administration of human chorionic gonadotropin on Leydig cell steroidogenic desensitization. J Clin Endocrinol Metab 1984; 58(2):327–331.

99. Saal W, Glowania HJ, Hengst W, et al. Pharmacodynamics and pharmacokinetics after subcutaneous and intramuscular injection of human chorionic gonadotropin. Fertil Steril 1991; 56(2):225–229.

100. le Cotonnec JY, Porchet HC, Beltrami V, et al. Clinical pharmacology of recombinant human follicle-stimulating hormone (FSH). I. Comparative pharmacokinetics with urinary human FSH. Fertil Steril 1994; 61(4): 669–678.

101. Porchet HC, le Cotonnec JY, Loumaye E. Clinical pharmacology of recombinant human follicle-stimulating hormone. III. Pharmacokinetic-pharmacodynamic modeling after repeated subcutaneous administration. Fertil Steril 1994; 61(4):687–695.

102. Handelsman DJ, Turner L, Boylan LM, et al. Pharmacokinetics of human follicle-stimulating hormone in gonadotropin-deficient men. J Clin Endocrinol Metab 1995; 80(5):1657–1663.

103. Steinkampf MP, Hammond KR, Nichols JE, et al. Effect of obesity on recombinant follicle-stimulating hormone absorption: subcutaneous versus intramuscular administration. Fertil Steril 2003; 80(1): 99–102.

104. Thau RB, Goldstein M, Yamamoto Y, et al. Failure of gonadotropin therapy secondary to chorionic gonadotropin-induced antibodies. J Clin Endocrinol Metab 1988; 66(4):862–867.

105. Albano C, Smitz J, Camus M, et al. Pregnancy and birth in an in-vitro fertilization cycle after controlled ovarian stimulation in a woman with a history of allergic reaction to human menopausal gonadotrophin. Hum Reprod 1996; 11(8):1632–1634.

106. Whitman-Elia GF, Banks K, O'Dea LS. Recombinant follicle-stimulating hormone in a patient hypersensitive to urinary-derived gonadotropins. Gynecol Endocrinol 1998; 12(3): 209–212.

107. Schally AV, Arimura A, Kastin AJ, et al. Gonadotropin-releasing hormone: one polypeptide regulates secretion of luteinizing and follicle-stimulating hormones. Science 1971; 173(4001):1036–1038.

108. Crowley WF Jr, Filicori M, Spratt DI, et al. The physiology of gonadotropin-releasing hormone (GnRH) secretion in men and women. Recent Prog Horm Res 1985; 41:473–531.

109. Belchetz PE, Plant TM, Nakai Y, et al. Hypophysial responses to continuous and intermittent delivery of hypopthalamic gonadotropin-releasing hormone. Science 1978; 202(4368): 631–633.

110. Shargil AA. Treatment of idiopathic hypogonadotropic hypogonadism in men with luteinizing hormone-releasing hormone: a comparison of treatment with daily injections and with the pulsatile infusion pump. Fertil Steril 1987; 47(3):492–501.

111. Spratt DI, Finkelstein JS, Butler JP, et al. Effects of increasing the frequency of low doses of gonadotropin-releasing hormone (GnRH) on gonadotropin secretion in GnRH–deficient men. J Clin Endocrinol Metab 1987; 64(6):1179–1186.

112. Finkelstein JS, Badger TM, O'Dea LS, et al. Effects of decreasing the frequency of gonadotropin-releasing hormone stimulation on gonadotropin secretion in gonadotropin-releasing hormone-deficient men and perifused rat pituitary cells. J Clin Invest 1988; 81(6): 1725–1733.

113. Handelsman DJ, Jansen RPS, Boylan LM, et al. Pharmacokinetics of gonadotropin-releasing hormone: comparison of subcutaneous and intravenous routes. J Clin Endocrinol Metab 1984; 59(4):739–746.

114. Spratt DI, Crowley WF Jr, Butler JP, et al. Pituitary luteinizing hormone responses to intravenous and subcutaneous administration of gonadotropin-releasing hormone in men. J Clin Endocrinol Metab 1985; 61(5):890–895.

115. Blumenfeld Z, Makler A, Frisch L, et al. Induction of spermatogenesis and fertility in hypogonadotropic azoospermic men by intravenous pulsatile gonadotropin-releasing hormone (GnRH). Gynecol Endocrinol 1988; 2(2):151–164.

116. Klingmuller D, Schweikert HU. Maintenance of spermatogenesis by intranasal administration of gonadotropin-releasing hormone in patients with hypothalamic hypogonadism. J Clin Endocrinol Metab 1985; 61(5): 868–872.

117. Blumenfeld Z, Frisch L, Conn PM. Gonadotropin-releasing hormone (GnRH) antibodies formation in hypogonadotropic azoospermic men treated with pulsatile GnRH—diagnosis and possible alternative treatment. Fertil Steril 1988; 50(4):622–629.

118. Meakin JL, Keogh EJ, Martin CE. Human anti-luteinizing hormone-releasing hormone antibodies in patients treated with synthetic luteinizing hormone-releasing hormone. Fertil Steril 1985; 43(5):811–813.

119. Lindner J, McNeil LW, Marney S, et al. Characterization of human anti-luteinizing hormone-releasing hormone (LRH) antibodies in the serum of a patient with isolated gonadotropin deficiency treated with synthetic LRH. J Clin Endocrinol Metab 1981; 52(2):267–270.

120. Peto R, Pike MC, Armitage P, et al. Design and analysis of randomised clinical trials requiring prolonged observation of each patient: I. Introduction and design. Br J Cancer 1976; 34(6):585–612.

121. Kliesch S, Behre HM, Nieschlag E. High efficacy of gonadotrophin or pulsatile gonadotrophin-releasing hormone treatment in hypogonadotrophic hypogonadal men. Eur J Endocrinol 1994; 131(4):347–354.

122. Mortimer CH, McNeilly AS, Fisher RA, et al. Gonadotrophin-releasing hormone therapy in hypogonadal males with hypothalamic or pituitary dysfunction. Br Med J 1974; 4(5945):617–621.

123. Tachiki H, Ito N, Maruta H, et al. Testicular findings, endocrine features and therapeutic responses of men with acquired hypogonadotropic hypogonadism. Int J Urol 1998; 5(1):80–85.

124. Tachiki H, Kumamoto Y, Itoh N, et al. Testicular findings, endocrine features and therapeutic responses of men with idiopathic hypogonadotropic hypogonadism. Nippon Naibunpi Gakkai Zasshi 1995; 71(4): 605–622.

125. WHO Task Force on Methods for the Regulation of Male Fertility. Contraceptive efficacy of testosterone-induced azoospermia and oligozoospermia in normal men. Fertil Steril 1996; 65(4):821–829.

126. Spratt DI, Crowley WF Jr. Pituitary and gonadal responsiveness is enhanced during GnRH-induced puberty. Am J Physiol 1988; 254(5 Pt 1):E652–E657.

127. Bouvattier C, Tauber M, Jouret B, et al. Gonadotropin treatment of hypogonadotropic hypogonadal adolescents. J Pediatr Endocrinol Metab 1999; 12(suppl 1):339–344.

128. Barrio R, de Luis D, Alonso M, et al. Induction of puberty with human chorionic gonadotropin and follicle-stimulating hormone in adolescent males with hypogonadotropic hypogonadism. Fertil Steril 1999; 71(2):244–248.

129. Main KM, Schmidt IM, Toppari J, et al. Early postnatal treatment of hypogonadotropic hypogonadism with recombinant human FSH and LH. Eur J Endocrinol 2002; 146(1):75–79.

130. Burger HG, de Kretser DM, Hudson B, et al. Effects of preceding androgen therapy on testicular response to human pituitary gonadotropin in hypogonadotropic hypogonadism. Fertil Steril 1981; 35(1):64–68.

131. Donald RA, Wheeler M, Sonksen PH, et al. Hypogonadotrophic hypogonadism resistant to hCG and responsive to LHRH: report of a case. Clin Endocrinol (Oxf) 1983; 18(4):385–389.

132. Berezin M, Weissenberg R, Rabinovitch O, et al. Successful GnRH treatment in a patient with Kallmann's syndrome, who previously failed HMG/HCG treatment. Andrologia 1988; 20(4):285–288.

133. Gayral MN, Millet D, Mandelbaum J, et al. Male hypogonadotrophic hypogonadism: successful treatment of infertility with HMG + HCG (author's transl). [Article in French]. Ann Endocrinol (Paris) 1975; 36(5):227–241.

134. Mattei A, Roulier R. Neopergonal treatment in male hypogonadotropic hypogonadism (author's transl). [Article in French]. Sem Hop 1978; 54(25–28): 875–877.

135. Gattuccio F, D'Alia O, Lo Bartolo G, et al. Gonadotropic therapy in men with hypogonadotropic hypogonadism. J Androl 1984; 5:106–110.

31

Progress in Male Contraception

Christina Wang
General Clinical Research Center, Harbor-UCLA Medical Center, Torrance, California and Department of Medicine,
David Geffen School of Medicine, University of California, Los Angeles, California, U.S.A.

Ronald S. Swerdloff
Division of Endocrinology and Metabolism, Harbor-UCLA Medical Center, Torrance, California and
Department of Medicine, David Geffen School of Medicine, University of California, Los Angeles, California, U.S.A.

□ INTRODUCTION

Family planning remains an important challenge for sexually active men and women. For women, a wide array of options has been made available to prevent pregnancies, including oral contraceptive pills, transdermal patches, subcutaneous implants, injectables that may be administered every month or as infrequently as every three months, intrauterine systems, vaginal rings, intravaginal spermicides, and female condoms. Recent surveys, however, have indicated that men would be willing to share family planning responsibilities, including the use of newly developed methods (1–3). Yet, the only approved and available methods of male contraception are using condoms and surgical vasectomy. It is clear to many interested parties that the development of new contraceptives should include a male focus (4). In fact, real progress has occurred in the past few years, with the most advanced and promising methods currently in development relying on the suppression of spermatogenesis via the exogenous administration of hormones. This chapter will describe the recent state-of-the-art progress in male hormonal contraception.

□ CURRENT METHODS

Condoms offer dual protection against pregnancy and sexually transmitted infections. The failure rate of condom users is about 12% (5). Although condoms are recommended for use in casual sexual encounters and in environments where sexually transmitted infections are prevalent, they may not be acceptable to all couples in stable relationships. Further, while nonlatex condoms are preferred by subjects in comparison studies of the efficacy of latex and nonlatex condoms, the breakage rate is higher with nonlatex condoms, although the contraceptive efficacy appears to be similar (6). (For further information on sexually transmitted diseases, see Chapter 16.)

The morbidity of surgical vas occlusion has decreased with the introduction of the no-scalpel vasectomy technique (7). Theoretically, vas occlusion is very effective, with a low failure rate of less than 1%. Recent prospective studies, however, have showed that the failure rate may be much higher, indicating that couples should receive appropriate counseling (8,9). The success of vas occlusion depends on the competence of the operator as well as on the method (10). Fascial interposition appears to result in lower failure rate (11). Cauterizing one of the vasal ends has also ensured effectiveness (12). Although percutaneous intravasal injection of occlusive substances and the placement of stents have both been tried, these methods have not shown advantages over standard methods and often have high failure rates. It is important to note that after vasectomy, the spermatozoa are not emptied instantaneously from the male accessory glands and the ejaculatory systems. Men are advised to use another method of contraception until 20 ejaculations or 12 weeks have elapsed since the vasectomy date. A recent prospective study, however, has indicated that a greater number of ejaculations or more time is required for the spermatozoa to be fully cleared from the accessory glands and the ejaculatory system (13).

Vasectomy is offered as an irreversible method. Although reanastomosis of the two cut ends is possible and is associated with high rates of spermatozoa reappearance, pregnancy rates remain much lower—presumably because of the development of antisperm antibodies associated with vas occlusion. (For further information on vasectomy and vasectomy reversal, see Chapter 34.)

□ HORMONAL CONTRACEPTION
Basis of Hormonal Contraception

Like the female hormonal methods that attempt to suppress ovulation, male hormonal methods are based on the suppression of hypothalamic gonadotropin-releasing hormone (GnRH) that in turn inhibits the secretion and production of luteinizing hormone (LH) and follicle-stimulating hormone (FSH). LH normally stimulates the Leydig cells to secrete testosterone (T), resulting in a sufficiently high intratesticular T concentration to maintain spermatogenesis. FSH, through its receptors on the Sertoli cells within the seminiferous tubules, stimulates and maintains spermatogenesis. In all currently tested male hormonal methods, total or near-total suppression of both LH and FSH is required to produce the marked suppression of spermatogenesis required for azoospermia or near azoospermia (Fig. 1). Selective suppression of FSH by FSH immunization has not resulted in the severe decrease in sperm production. Similarly, experiments involving FSH receptor mutations in both mice and men did not produce a severe and uniform suppression of spermatogenesis (14).

Because LH suppression and the consequent marked reduction in endogenous T production are necessary components of male hormonal contraceptive methods, androgen supplementation is thus required to prevent hypogonadism. Androgen activity is necessary for patients to maintain normal sexual function, mood, muscle, and bone mass. The regimens of hormonal male contraception that have been tested include androgens alone (T alone) or androgens plus another gonadotropin suppressive agent such as progestin or a GnRH antagonist (T plus progestins). The details of the recent studies on various T alone or T plus progestins regimens have been reviewed (15–18). (For more information on the hormones of the male reproductive system, see Chapters 3 and 4.)

Mechanisms of Action of Male Hormonal Contraception

Studies indicate that hormonal male contraception relies on the marked suppression of FSH, LH, and intratesticular T. In the mature rat, intratesticular T deprivation, achieved by treatment with a GnRH antagonist (19,20) or exogenous T implants (21), caused stage- and cell-specific activation of germ-cell apoptosis, predominantly at stages VII and VIII of the rat spermatogenic cycle (19,20). The involvement of the intrinsic pathway signaling in male germ-cell apoptosis in rats after hormone deprivation has been demonstrated (22). The initiation of apoptosis is associated with a cell-type specific increase in the expression of the proapoptotic protein, Bax, involving only those germ cells undergoing apoptosis; this is accompanied by a marked decrease in levels of the antiapoptotic protein, Bcl-2. Other investigators have reported that failure of sperm release from the germinal epithelium may also contribute to decreased sperm output after FSH inhibition or T suppression (23). The use of a GnRH antagonist or T implants in monkeys resulted in inhibition of spermiation with a rapid and marked decrease in germ-cell development from type A pale spermatogonia and type B spermatogonia onward (24–26), demonstrating that suppression of FSH is essential to attain consistent azoospermia (27). Testicular samples obtained from human subjects participating in clinical trials of male contraceptive agents (T alone or T plus progestin) similarly showed a marked decrease in type B spermatogonia. Impairment of spermatogenesis from that stage onward and

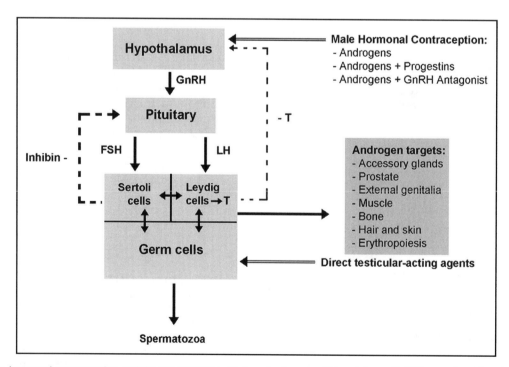

Figure 1   Male hormonal contraception and the hypothalamic–pituitary–testis axis. *Abbreviations*: GnRH, gonadotropin-releasing hormone; FSH, follicle-stimulating hormone; LH, luteinizing hormone; T, testosterone.

inhibition of spermiation were important determinants of sperm output (25,28,29). (For further information on spermatogenesis, see Chapter 5.)

Efficacy of Male Hormonal Contraception

To study whether hormonally induced azoospermia or severe oligospermia (arbitrarily defined as less than 3 million sperm cells/mL of ejaculate) has contraceptive efficacy, the World Health Organization conducted two pivotal studies in the 1990s. In the first study, when azoospermia was induced by exogenous administration of weekly testosterone enanthate (TE) injections, the contraceptive efficacy was 0.8 per 100 person-years (30). In the second study, when suppression of spermatogenesis reached severe oligospermia with exogenous TE injections in 357 couples, the contraceptive efficacy was 1.4 per 100 person-years. Four pregnancies occurred in the second study, with the pregnancy rate being proportional to the residual sperm concentration (31). This contraceptive efficacy rate is similar to those of currently available female methods of contraception such as injectables, pills, and patches. More recently, two studies demonstrated similar contraceptive efficacy utilizing undecanoate alone (32) and T pellets with depot medroxyprogesterone acetate (DMPA) injections (33).

Androgens-Alone Regimens
Testosterone

Various androgen preparations have been used alone for the suppression of spermatogenesis, including early studies performed with weekly or bi-weekly injections of TE and implantable T pellets, both of which demonstrated suppression of spermatogenesis to severe oligospermia in most men (Table 1) (30,31,34). Weekly intramuscular injections and the insertion of implants every four months, however, were not considered acceptable and practical methods. T patches did not deliver adequate androgens to allow for adequate suppression of spermatogenesis (35).

The most promising androgen preparation currently being tested is T undecanoate (TU). Oral TU has been available for the treatment of hypogonadal men for many years in Europe, Asia, and Canada, as well as in many other regions. TU administered intramuscularly in oil was first used by Chinese investigators for T replacement in hypogonadal men (36).

Subsequently, the intramuscular administration of TU at a dose of 1000 mg every 12 weeks has been shown to provide adequate androgen replacement for hypogonadal men (37,38). When TU was administered to normal Chinese men at a dose of 500 mg or 1000 mg every four weeks, azoospermia was induced in most of the subjects (39). Subsequently, Gu et al. administered 1000 mg of TU as a loading dose followed by 500 mg every four weeks intramuscularly to over 300 couples (32). Azoospermia or severe oligospermia was achieved in 95% of the men. When the couples used only this method for contraception, no pregnancy occurred. Currently, there is an ongoing Phase III study that aims to test the same TU regimen for two years on a large scale of 1000 male recruits in China. Studies in non-Asian men showed that TU administered at 1000 mg every six to eight weeks resulted in azoospermia in about 50% to 60% of subjects, and severe oligospermia in 80% to 90% of subjects (40).

Potential Adverse Effect of Androgens

In these short-term androgen-alone regimens, the adverse events are few and related to the dose of androgen administered. Acne and weight gain were present in the early studies of TE. With long-acting T esters, the side effects are related to androgen actions, including an increase in hematocrit/hemoglobin and a decrease in high-density lipoprotein (HDL) cholesterol. These side effects are usually mild and rarely lead to discontinuation from the clinical trials. If any, the long-term adverse effects of androgens in younger men on the prostate or the cardiovascular system are not known. Long-term epidemiological studies will be able to address these questions only when a male hormonal contraceptive becomes available to the public. Based on current knowledge, however, a lower androgen dose is presumed to be associated with fewer short-term side effects.

Androgens with Selective Actions

Androgens with more selective actions have been studied for male contraceptive development. For example, the selective androgen 7-α-methyl-19-nortestosterone (MENT) is not converted by 5-α-reductase to dihydrotestosterone (DHT). In rodents and monkeys, MENT is about 10 times more potent than T in suppressing gonadotropins, and only four times more efficacious than T in supporting unwanted prostate growth in castrated animals (41,42). Subcutaneous implants of MENT can maintain sexual function but are unable to maintain bone mass in comparison to TE (43,44). With four subcutaneous implants of MENT, sperm concentration was suppressed after six months of treatment to azoospermia and severe oligospermia in 64% and 82% of men, respectively, without any change in serum prostatic–specific antigen levels or prostate volume (45). When the subjects were followed for longer periods, all became oligospermic, and five out of six men remained azoospermic. The efficacy of

Table 1 Androgens in Male Contraception

Oral T	T undecanoate (not efficacious)
Buccal T	Not yet tested
Injectables	TE
	TU
Implants	T
	MENT
Transdermal	Patches—not efficacious
	Gels—not yet tested

Abbreviations: T, testosterone; TE, testosterone enanthate; TU, testosterone undecanoate; MENT, 7-α-methyl-19 nor-testosterone.

MENT alone or in combination with progestogens in male contraceptive studies must still be confirmed with larger, multicenter studies.

To date, many pharmaceutical companies are developing tissue-selective androgen-receptor modulators (SARMs) that may be steroidal or nonsteroidal compounds. The steroidal compounds are designed to have less stimulatory effects on prostate growth while still being aromatizable, thus conferring the beneficial effects of estrogens on bone and lipid profiles. The nonsteroidal SARMs are neither aromatizable nor 5-α-reduced, but may have selective action on tissues. If it possible to develop selective gonadotropin-suppressing SARMs that can maintain androgenic effects on sexual function, bone, muscle, and mood without stimulating the prostate, these SARMs would be the ideal androgens for male hormonal contraception and the treatment of male hypogonadism.

Variation in Responsiveness to Exogenous Androgens

In the multicenter androgen-alone studies, it was noted that azoospermia was achieved in over 90% of Asian men as against approximately 60% of non-Asian men (30,31). These observations have been confirmed in studies utilizing androgens plus progestins (46). The reason for the differences in the suppression of spermatogenesis in response to exogenous hormones is not known. When exogenous T was administered to both Asian and non-Asian men, serum LH pulse amplitude suppressed at a lower dose of T in Asian men, suggesting that their GnRH-LH axis may be more sensitive to exogenous T (47). The clearance of T is not different between Asian and white men but T production rates may be slightly lower in Asian men (48,49). It has been shown that Asian men have a smaller average testis volume and seminiferous tubular volume, and fewer number of Sertoli cells, all of which are associated with an increased basal apoptotic rate of germ cells (50). Other researchers have shown that 5-α-reductase activity may be higher in those who failed to achieve near-complete suppression of sperm concentrations in semen, allowing DHT to maintain residual spermatogenesis (51). It has also been demonstrated that longer CAG repeats in exon 1 of the androgen receptor are more common in nonresponders, indicating lower androgen receptor activity in men who failed to demonstrate severe suppression of spermatogenesis to hormones administered exogenously (52).

Because of the smaller inhibitory response of non-Asians to androgen-alone male contraceptive regimens, it is generally thought that the addition of another gonadotropin-suppressive agent would be necessary to achieve more significant suppression of spermatogenesis in most men.

Androgens and Progestins

Table 2 lists the combination of androgens and progestins that have undergone testing in more recent

Table 2 Androgen and Progestin Combinations

Progestins	Androgens
Injectables	
DMPA	+TE
	+TU[a]
	+pellets
	+19 nortestosterone
NET-EN	+TU[a]
Oral	
LNG	+TE
	+TU[a]
	+T patch
	+DHT gel
	+T pellets
DSG	+TE
	+T pellets
	+MENT
Implants	
ENG	+T pellets
	+TU[a]
LNG	+TE injections
	+T pellets
	+TU[a]
Agents with antiandrogen activity	
CPA	+TE
	+TU oral

[a]Intramuscular injection.
Abbreviations: CPA, cyproterone acetate; DHT, dihydrotestosterone; DMPA, depot medroxyprogesterone acetate; DSG, desogestrel; ENG, etonogestrel; LNG, levonorgestrel; MENT, 7-α-methyl-19 nortestosterone; NET-EN, norethisterone enanthate; T, testosterone; TE, testosterone enanthate; TU, testosterone undecanoate.

clinical trials. Reviews of these androgen- and plus-progestin studies have been published (16–18). These include oral levonorgestrel (LNG) and desogestrel (DSG), injectables such as DMPA and norethisterone enanthate (NET-EN), and implants of LNG and DSG [etonogestrel (ENG)]. These studies, conducted in both Asian and non-Asian men, indicate that the addition of a progestin to an androgen induces more rapid suppression of spermatogenesis, with greater than 90% of non-Asian men becoming azoospermic with some combinations (e.g., NET-EN plus TU, DMPA plus T pellets, and oral DSG with TE). The addition of progestins primarily acts to suppress GnRH and the gonadotropins, although recent studies suggest that progestins may also have direct actions on the testis. Addition of androgenic oral progestins such as LNG and DSG results in weight gain and greater suppression of HDL cholesterol and serum sex hormone–binding globulin than androgen-alone regimens.

One of the most promising combinations may be that of TU plus NET-EN, given as an injection every six to eight weeks. In studies involving a small number of men, this combination of steroids resulted in over 90% of men achieving azoospermia, with severe oligospermia in the remainder (53,54). TU is also being studied in combination with ENG implants as an injectable preparation given every 10 to 12 weeks, designed to release adequate ENG for suppression of gonadotropins in men. Single or double ENG implants are also being tested in combination with T pellets and with

MENT implants. LNG implants have also been tested with T and MENT implants.

All of these studies have the objective of developing either a practical bimonthly injectable or a yearly implant system for men. Although the oral progestins are very potent and active, at present, there is no oral T preparation that can be used with these oral progestins. An orally active, potent androgen without significant adverse effects is yet to be developed for achieving the goal of having a male equivalent of the female "pill." Combinations of androgen plus progestin in a transdermal application have not yet been tested.

Progestins with Antiandrogenic Activity

The progestin cyproterone acetate (CPA) has antiandrogenic effects. A study with a small number of men showed that when CPA was used in combination with TE, the resulting suppression was sufficient to induce azoospermia in all subjects. When TE injections were substituted with oral TU, however, the suppression of spermatogenesis was incomplete (55,56).

Role of Androgens in Progestin–Androgen Combinations

When LNG implants were used in combination with transdermal T patches, azoospermia occurred in about 25% of the men. This percentage was markedly increased when TE injections were administered with LNG implants (35). These studies indicate that the androgen component in the androgen–progestin combination plays an important role in the inhibition of gonadotropins and enhances the contraceptive efficacy of progestins in addition to providing androgen supplementation.

GnRH Antagonists and Androgens

Although GnRH agonists are very safe, they fail to suppress LH and FSH levels consistently enough to induce complete inhibition of spermatogenesis even with high doses or continuous infusions (57–59). In contrast, GnRH antagonists are extremely effective in suppressing the secretion of both LH and FSH as they completely block GnRH action. In combination with androgens, GnRH antagonists suppress sperm production to achieve azoospermia in most men (60–62). The earlier GnRH antagonists, however, produced the unwelcome side effects of local skin reaction when administered subcutaneously. The recently synthesized GnRH antagonist acyline, however, does not appear to have this problem, and when administered at a relatively high dose, it can maintain suppression of the gonadotropins for about 14 days (63). Currently, acyline is being developed for male contraception by the National Institutes of Health. Because GnRH antagonists are expensive to synthesize, a more user-friendly, long-acting delivery system is also under development. Several pharmaceutical companies are also developing nonpeptide antagonists via receptor drug modeling methods.

The potential for the oral activity of these agents may be a great contribution to the development of male contraceptive methods.

Maintenance of Spermatic Suppression with Androgens Alone

Another theoretical approach examines whether the GnRH antagonist plus androgen-induced suppression of spermatogenesis can be maintained by androgens alone. If maintenance of suppression can indeed be achieved with androgens alone, this approach may offer considerable advantages in terms of less long-term steroid exposure for men and the overall economy of a treatment that only employs a single agent. Swerdloff et al. showed that when severe oligospermia is induced by a potent GnRH antagonist (Nal-Glu GnRH) and TE injections, the suppression can be maintained for four months with TE injections alone (64). Other studies using 19 nor-T alone, however, failed to maintain the suppression of spermatogenesis to azoospermia induced by the same regimen (65).

Reversibility of Hormonal Male Contraception

A recent integrated multivariate time-to-event analysis of data from individual participants in 30 studies published between 1990 and 2005 demonstrated full reversibility of male hormonal contraception within a predictable time course. The typical probability of recovery of 20,000,000 sperm/mL of semen was 67% within 6 months, 90% within 12 months, and 100% within 24 months (66).

□ NONHORMONAL MALE CONTRACEPTION

Gossypol, a derivative from cottonseed oil, has been found to be a very effective oral contraceptive in China. Because of its direct action on germ cells, however, men treated with gossypol may sustain irreversible infertility (67). In some men, gossypol also led to hypokalemic paralysis. A second compound derived from the root of Tripterygium wilfordii and aptly named "triptolide" was initially thought to reduce sperm motility via direct actions on the epididymis; however, long-term studies in rodents have showed that triptolide has toxic effects on the germinal epithelium with the potential to cause irreversible infertility as well (68).

Lonidamine is a nonsteroidal antispermatogenic agent with direct effects on the germinal epithelium. An analog of lonidamine has been studied that also works on the germinal epithelium, but without the toxic effects of lonidamine on the kidney and liver (69,70). These agents are currently being tested in animal models.

Most recently, alkylated imino sugars were reported to have contraceptive activity in mice (71). When these imino sugars were administered orally in mice, epididymal sperm were discovered to have abnormal heads, acrosome reaction was blocked, and sperm motility was reduced. These mice became infertile three weeks after dosing was initiated, implicating an effect on mature sperm via interference with the biosynthesis of glucosylceramide-based sphingolipids.

There has also been research to identify possible novel targets in spermiogenesis and sperm maturation in the epididymis. These protein targets, including receptors, ligands, enzymes, and ion channels, are excellent targets for drug development (4). The functional roles of these targets can be tested in knockout or knock-in mouse models. Although many laboratory discoveries have since been made, these potential targets will not be available for clinical testing for the next 10 to 20 years.

□ CONCLUSION

The currently available male-controlled methods of contraception consisting of condoms and vasectomies are not acceptable to many couples. Male hormonal contraceptive methods may be the most promising for men and women in stable relationships who desire

family planning or spacing. For Asian men, androgen-alone methods may be adequate for suppression of spermatogenesis. In non-Asian men, androgens in combination with a progestin or GnRH antagonist appear to be more effective. It is anticipated that within the next 7 to 10 years, an injectable male contraceptive and possibly implants may become available. Improvements in delivery systems and the availability of SARMs and nonpeptide GnRH antagonists may result in male contraceptives that are affordable, safe, generally available, reversible, and user-friendly. Research efforts are directed toward identifying targets that regulate spermatogenesis, spermiogenesis, or sperm maturation and motility that can be developed into drugs for male contraception.

□ ACKNOWLEDGMENTS

Supported by grants: M01 RR00425 to the General Clinical Research Center at Harbor-UCLA Medical Center Contraceptive Research and Development Program and The Population Council. The authors would also like to acknowledge Sally Avancena, M.A., for her assistance in the preparation of this manuscript.

□ REFERENCES

1. Martin CW, Anderson RA, Cheng L, et al. Potential impact of hormonal male contraception: cross-cultural implications for development of novel preparations. Hum Reprod 2000; 15(3):637–645.
2. Weston GC, Schlipalius ML, Bhuinneain MN, et al. Will Australian men use male hormonal contraception? A survey of a postpartum population. Med J Aust 2002; 176(5):208–210.
3. Saad F, White S, Heinemann K. Attitudes toward hormonal male fertility control: USA results of a multinational survey. Proceedings of the 86th Annual Meeting of the Endocrine Society, New Orleans, LA, June 16–19, 2004.
4. Nass SJ, Strauss JF III, eds. New Frontiers in Contraceptive Research: A Blueprint for Action. Washington, D.C.: The National Academies Press, 2004:1–217.
5. Trussell J, Kost K. Contraceptive failure in the United States: a critical review of the literature. Stud Fam Plann 1987; 18(5):237–283.
6. Gallo MF, Grimes DA, Schulz KF. Nonlatex vs. latex male condoms for contraception: a systematic review of randomized controlled trials. Contraception 2003; 68(5):319–326.
7. Liu X, Li S. Vasal sterilization in China. Contraception 1993; 48(3):255–265.
8. Nazerali H, Thapa S, Hays M, et al. Vasectomy effectiveness in Nepal: a retrospective study. Contraception 2003; 67(5):397–401.
9. Jamieson DJ, Costello C, Trussell J, et al. The risk of pregnancy after vasectomy. Obstet Gynecol 2004; 103(1):848–850.
10. Labrecque M, Dufresne C, Barone MA, et al. Vasectomy surgical techniques: a systematic review. BMC Med 2004; 2:21.
11. Sokal D, Irsula B, Hays M, et al. Vasectomy by ligation and excision, with or without fascial interposition: a randomized controlled trial. BMC Med 2004; 2:6.
12. Barone MA, Irsula B, Chen-Mok M, et al. Effectiveness of vasectomy using cautery. BMC Urol 2004; 4:10.
13. Barone MA, Nazerali H, Cortes M, et al. A prospective study of time and number of ejaculations to azoospermia after vasectomy by ligation and excision. J Urol 2003; 170(3):892–896.
14. Themmen APN, Huhtaniemi IT. Mutations of gonadotropins and gonadotropin receptors: elucidating the physiology and pathophysiology of pituitary-gonadal function. Endocr Rev 2000; 21(5):551–583.
15. Anderson RA, Baird DT. Male contraception. Endocr Rev 2002; 23(6):735–762.
16. Meriggiola MC, Farley TM, Mbizvo MT. A review of androgen-progestin regimens for male contraception. J Androl 2003; 24(4):466–483.

17. Kamischke A, Nieschlag E. Progress towards hormonal male contraception. Trends Pharmacol Sci 2004; 25(1): 49–57.
18. Wang C, Swerdloff RS. Male hormonal contraception. Am J Obstet Gynecol 2004; 190(suppl 4):S60–S68.
19. Hikim AP, Wang C, Leung A, et al. Involvement of apoptosis in the induction of germ cell degeneration in adult rats after gonadotropin-releasing hormone antagonist treatment. Endocrinology 1995; 136(6): 2770–2775.
20. Sinha Hikim AP, Rajavashisth TB, Sinha Hikim I, et al. Significance of apoptosis in the temporal and stage-specific loss of germ cells in the adult rat after gonadotropin deprivation. Biol Reprod 1997; 57(5): 1193–1201.
21. Lue Y, Hikim AP, Wang C, et al. Testicular heat exposure enhances the suppression of spermatogenesis by testosterone in rats: the "two-hit" approach to male contraceptive development. Endocrinology 2000; 141(4):1414–1424.
22. Sinha Hikim AP, Lue Y, Diaz-Romero M, et al. Deciphering the pathways of germ cell apoptosis in the testis. J Steroid Biochem Mol Biol 2003; 85(2–5): 175–182.
23. Saito K, O'Donnell L, McLachlan RI, et al. Spermiation failure is a major contributor to early spermatogenic suppression caused by hormone withdrawal in adult rats. Endocrinology 2000; 141(8):2779–2785.
24. Zhengwei Y, Wreford NG, Royce P, et al. Stereological evaluation of human spermatogenesis after suppression by testosterone treatment: heterogeneous pattern of spermatogenic impairment. J Clin Endocrinol Metab 1998; 83(4):1284–1291.
25. Zhengwei Y, Wreford NG, Schlatt S, et al. Acute and specific impairment of spermatogonial development by GnRH antagonist-induced gonadotrophin withdrawal in the adult macaque (Macaca fascicularis). J Reprod Fertil 1998; 112(1):139–147.
26. O'Donnell L, Narula A, Balourdos G, et al. Impairment of spermatogonial development and spermiation after testosterone-induced gonadotropin suppression in adult monkeys (Macaca fascicularis). J Clin Endocrinol Metab 2001; 86(4):1814–1822.
27. Narula A, Gu YQ, O'Donnell L, et al. Variability in sperm suppression during testosterone administration to adult monkeys is related to follicle stimulating hormone suppression and not to intratesticular androgens. J Clin Endocrinol Metab 2002; 87(7): 3399–3406.
28. McLachlan RI, O'Donnell L, Stanton PG, et al. Effects of testosterone plus medroxyprogesterone acetate on semen quality, reproductive hormones, and germ cell populations in normal young men. J Clin Endocrinol Metab 2002; 87(2):546–556.
29. McLachlan RI, O'Donnell L, Meachem SJ, et al. Identification of specific sites of hormonal regulation in spermatogenesis in rats, monkeys, and man. Recent Prog Horm Res 2002; 57:149–179.
30. World Health Organization Task Force on Methods for the Regulation of Male Fertility. Contraceptive efficacy of testosterone-induced azoospermia in normal men. Lancet 1990; 336(8721):955–959.
31. World Health Organization Task Force on Methods for the Regulation of Male Fertility. Contraceptive efficacy of testosterone-induced azoospermia and oligozoospermia in normal men. Fertil Steril 1996; 65(4):821–829.
32. Gu YQ, Wang XH, Xu D, et al. A multicenter contraceptive efficacy study of injectable testosterone undecanoate in healthy Chinese Men. J Clin Endocrinol Metab 2003; 88(2):562–568.
33. Turner L, Conway AJ, Jimenez M, et al. Contraceptive efficacy of a depot progestin and androgen combination in men. J Clin Endocrinol Metab 2003; 88(10): 4659–4667.
34. Handelsman DJ, Conway AJ, Boylan LM. Suppression of human spermatogenesis by testosterone implants. J Clin Endocrinol Metab 1992; 75(5):1326–1332.
35. Gonzalo IT, Swerdloff RS, Nelson AL, et al. Levonorgestrel implants (Norplant II) for male contraception clinical trials: combination with transdermal and injectable testosterone. J Clin Endocrinol Metab 2002; 87(8):3562–3572.
36. Zhang GY, Gu YQ, Wang XH, et al. A pharmacokinetic study of injectable testosterone undecanoate in hypogonadal men. J Androl 1998; 19(6):761–768.
37. Behre HM, Abshagen K, Oettel M, et al. Intramuscular injection of testosterone undecanoate for the treatment of male hypogonadism: phase I studies. Eur J Endocrinol 1999; 140(5):414–419.
38. Nieschlag E, Buchter D, von Eckardstein S, et al. Repeated intramuscular injections of testosterone undecanoate for substitution therapy in hypogonadal men. Clin Endocrinol (Oxf) 1999; 51(6):757–763.
39. Zhang GY, Gu YQ, Wang XH, et al. A clinical trial of injectable testosterone undecanoate as a potential male contraceptive in normal Chinese men. J Clin Endocrinol Metab 1999; 84(10):3642–3647.
40. Kamischke A, Ploger D, Venherm S, et al. Intramuscular testosterone undecanoate with or without oral levonorgestrel: a randomized placebo-controlled feasibility study for male contraception. Clin Endocrinol (Oxf) 2000; 53(1):43–52.
41. Kumar N, Didolkar AK, Monder C, et al. The biological activity of 7 alpha-methyl-19-nortestosterone is not amplified in male reproductive tract as is that of testosterone. Endocrinology 1992; 130(6):3677–3683.
42. Cummings DE, Kumar N, Bardin CW, et al. Prostate-sparing effects in primates of the potent androgen 7alpha-methyl-19-nortestosterone: a potential alternative to testosterone for androgen replacement and male contraception. J Clin Endocrinol Metab 1998; 83(12): 4212–4219.
43. Anderson RA, Martin CW, Kung AW, et al. 7Alpha-methyl-19-nortestosterone maintains sexual behavior and mood in hypogonadal men. J Clin Endocrinol Metab 1999; 84(10):3556–3562.

44. Anderson RA, Wallace AM, Sattar N, et al. Evidence for tissue selectivity of the synthetic androgen 7 alpha-methyl-19-nortestosterone in hypogonadal men. J Clin Endocrinol Metab 2003; 88(6):2784–2793.

45. von Eckardstein S, Noe G, Brache V, et al. A clinical trial of 7 alpha-methyl-19-nortestosterone implants for possible use as a long-acting contraceptive for men. J Clin Endocrinol Metab 2003; 88(11):5232–5239.

46. World Health Organization Task Force on Methods for the Regulation of Male Fertility. Comparison of two androgens plus depot-medroxyprogesterone acetate for suppression to azoospermia in Indonesian men. Fertil Steril 1993; 60(6):1062–1068.

47. Wang C, Berman NG, Veldhuis JD, et al. Graded testosterone infusions distinguish gonadotropin negative-feedback responsiveness in Asian and white men—clinical Research Center study. J Clin Endocrinol Metab 1998; 83(3):870–876.

48. Santner SJ, Albertson B, Zhang GY, et al. Comparative rates of androgen production and metabolism in Caucasian and Chinese subjects. J Clin Endocrinol Metab 1998; 83(6):2104–2109.

49. Wang C, Catlin DH, Starcevic B, et al. Testosterone metabolic clearance and production rates determined by stable isotope dilution/tandem mass spectrometry in normal men: influence of ethnicity and age. J Clin Endocrinol Metab 2004; 89(6):2936–2941.

50. Hikim AP, Wang C, Lue Y, et al. Spontaneous germ cell apoptosis in humans: evidence for ethnic differences in the susceptibility of germ cells to programmed cell death. J Clin Endocrinol Metab 1998; 83(1):152–156.

51. Anderson RA, Wallace AM, Wu FC. Comparison between testosterone enanthate-induced azoospermia and oligozoospermia in a male contraceptive study. III. Higher 5 alpha-reductase activity in oligozoospermic men administered supraphysiological doses of testosterone. J Clin Endocrinol Metab 1996; 81(3): 902–908.

52. Eckardstein SV, Schmidt A, Kamischke A, et al. CAG repeat length in the androgen receptor gene and gonadotrophin suppression influence the effectiveness of hormonal male contraception. Clin Endocrinol (Oxf) 2002; 57(5):647–655.

53. Kamischke A, Venherm S, Ploger D, et al. Intramuscular testosterone undecanoate and norethisterone enanthate in a clinical trial for male contraception. J Clin Endocrinol Metab 2001; 86(1):303–309.

54. Kamischke A, Heuermann T, Kruger K, et al. An effective hormonal male contraceptive using testosterone undecanoate with oral or injectable norethisterone preparations. J Clin Endocrinol Metab 2002; 87(2):530–539.

55. Meriggiola MC, Bremner WJ, Paulsen CA, et al. A combined regimen of cyproterone acetate and testosterone enanthate as a potentially highly effective male contraceptive. J Clin Endocrinol Metab 1996; 81(8):3018–3023.

56. Meriggiola MC, Bremner WJ, Costantino A, et al. An oral regimen of cyproterone acetate and testosterone undecanoate for spermatogenic suppression in men. Fertil Steril 1997; 68(5):844–850.

57. Bhasin S, Heber D, Steiner B, et al. Hormonal effects of GnRH agonist in the human male: II. Testosterone enhances gonadotrophin suppression induced by GnRH agonist. Clin Endocrinol (Oxf) 1984; 20(2): 119–128.

58. Bhasin S, Heber D, Steiner BS, et al. Hormonal effects of gonadotropin-releasing hormone (GnRH) agonist in the human male. III. Effects of long term combined treatment with GnRH agonist and androgen. J Clin Endocrinol Metab 1985; 60(5):998–1003.

59. Bhasin S, Steiner B, Swerdloff R. Does constant infusion of gonadotropin-releasing hormone agonist lead to greater suppression of gonadal function in man than its intermittent administration? Fertil Steril 1985; 44(1): 96–101.

60. Tom L, Bhasin S, Salameh W, et al. Induction of azoospermia in normal men with combined Nal-Glu gonadotropin-releasing hormone antagonist and testosterone enanthate. J Clin Endocrinol Metab 1992; 75(2):476–483.

61. Bagatell CJ, Matsumoto AM, Christensen RB, et al. Comparison of a gonadotropin releasing-hormone antagonist plus testosterone (T) versus T alone as potential male contraceptive regimens. J Clin Endocrinol Metab 1993; 77(2):427–432.

62. Behre HM, Kliesch S, Puhse G, et al. High loading and low maintenance doses of a gonadotropin-releasing hormone antagonist effectively suppress serum luteinizing hormone, follicle-stimulating hormone, and testosterone in normal men. J Clin Endocrinol Metab 1997; 82(5):1403–1408.

63. Herbst KL, Anawalt BD, Amory JK, et al. Acyline: the first study in humans of a potent, new gonadotropin-releasing hormone antagonist. J Clin Endocrinol Metab 2002; 87(7):3215–3220.

64. Swerdloff RS, Bagatell CJ, Wang C, et al. Suppression of spermatogenesis in man induced by Nal-Glu gonadotropin releasing hormone antagonist and testosterone enanthate (TE) is maintained by TE alone. J Clin Endocrinol Metab 1998; 83(10):3527–3533.

65. Behre HM, Kliesch S, Lemcke B, et al. Suppression of spermatogenesis to azoospermia by combined administration of GnRH antagonist and 19-nortestosterone cannot be maintained by this non-aromatizable androgen alone. Human Reprod 2001; 16(12): 2570–2577.

66. Liu PY, Swerdloff RS. Rate, extent, and modifiers of spermatogenic recovery after hormonal male contraception: an integrated analysis. Lancet 2006; 367(9520): 1412–1420.

67. Waites GM, Wang C, Griffin PD. Gossypol: reasons for its failure to be accepted as a safe, reversible male antifertility drug. Int J Androl 1998; 21(1):8–12.

68. Huynh PN, Hikim AP, Wang C, et al. Long-term effects of triptolide on spermatogenesis, epididymal sperm

function, and fertility in male rats. J Androl 2000; 21(5): 689–699.

69.   Cheng CY, Mo M, Grima J, et al. Indazole carboxylic acids in male contraception. Contraception 2002 65(4):265–268.

70.   Cheng CY, Silvestrini B, Grima J, et al. Two new male contraceptives exert their effects by depleting germ cells prematurely from the testis. Biol Reprod 2001; 65(2):449–461.

71.   van der Spoel AC, Jeyakumar M, Butters TD, et al. Reversible infertility in male mice after oral administration of alkylated imino sugars: a nonhormonal approach to male contraception. Proc Natl Acad Sci USA 2002; 9(26): 17173–17178.

Retrograde Ejaculation

Avner Hershlag

Department of Obstetrics and Gynecology, North Shore University Hospital, New York University School of Medicine, Manhasset, New York, U.S.A.

Sarah K. Girardi

Department of Urology, Weill Medical College of Cornell University, North Shore University Hospital, Manhasset, New York, U.S.A.

□ INTRODUCTION

The term "retrograde ejaculation" (RE) refers to a condition in which failure of bladder neck closure results in the retrograde flow of semen into the bladder. This is an uncommon cause of infertility, accounting for only 1% of male-factor cases. RE can result from a variety of causes. The purpose of this chapter will be to review the anatomy and physiology of ejaculation, examine the different etiologies of RE, and discuss current treatment options in light of the recent advances in assisted reproductive technologies (ART).

□ ANATOMY AND PHYSIOLOGY

There are two phases of ejaculation. During the initial phase coined "emission," semen is deposited into the posterior urethra. Emission is under the control of the sympathetic nervous system: afferent stimuli from the genitalia travel via the pudendal nerve to the cerebral cortex. Efferent impulses travel by way of the anterolateral columns to the sympathetic nerves, T12 to L3. Through the hypogastric nerve, impulses cause the contraction of the vas deferens, seminal vesicles, and prostate gland, as well as bladder neck closure. These two simultaneous events governed by the sympathetic nervous system result in emission of the ejaculate into the posterior urethra.

During the second phase, propulsion, semen is propelled out of the posterior urethra. Normal propulsion occurs in an antegrade direction and results from (*i*) bladder neck closure and (*ii*) a strong contraction of the bulbospongiosus and perineal muscles. The latter is under the control of the parasympathetic nervous system: impulses travel via the parasympathetic outflow of S2 to S4 to the internal pudendal nerve. Stimulation of the internal pudendal nerve results in contraction of the bulbocavernosus and the deep and superficial perineal muscles, resulting in expulsion of the ejaculate. If there is failure of the sympathetic nerves to effect bladder neck closure, the contraction of perineal and bulbospongiosus muscles will result in retrograde flow of the ejaculate into the urinary bladder, thereby causing RE. (For further details on the anatomy and physiology of ejaculation, please refer to the chapters in Part I.)

□ ETIOLOGY

A careful history will often reveal the etiology of RE and will help guide the treatment plan. Table 1 summarizes the different conditions that can result in RE. This discussion will be limited to the five most common causes of RE.

Transurethral prostatectomy (TURP) remains the most common surgical cause of RE. In this procedure, the hyperplastic tissue in the center of the prostate gland is removed by endoscopic resection. This results in a large opening at the bladder neck, which may temporarily or permanently alter effective coaptation. It has been reported that between 40% and 95% of patients who undergo TURP will have RE (1,2). For this reason, in young men with bladder outlet obstruction due to an enlarged prostate gland, transurethral incision of the prostate (TUIP) is the recommended procedure-of-choice. In TUIP, two incisions are made in the bladder neck extending from the ureteral orifices toward the verumontanum (posterior urethra). Because there is no removal of prostatic tissue, the procedure is associated with RE in less than 5% of men (3). (For further details on prostate cancer, see Chapter 41.)

In the past, retroperitoneal lymph node dissection (RPLND) for testis cancer was a common reason for RE and other ejaculatory disturbances (4), as RPLND involves the dissection of lymphatic tissue along the sympathetic chains bilaterally. Since most men undergoing lymphadenectomy for testis cancer are in the reproductive age group, ejaculatory dysfunction presented a major problem. Modifications to RPLND were first proposed in the early 1980s by Narayan et al. (5). By preserving the sympathetic chain on one side below the level of the inferior mesenteric artery, ejaculation continued to be antegrade in approximately half of the patients. Richie (6) reported 94% antegrade ejaculation postoperatively in a prospective study of 85 men with clinical stage I nonseminomatous

Table 1   Etiologies of Retrograde Ejaculation

Anatomical
   Congenital
      Posterior urethral valves
      Utricular cyst
      Extrophy or hemitrigone
   Acquired
      Transurethral resection of the prostate
      Retropubic prostatectomy
      Y-V plasty
      Pelvic trauma
Neurogenic
   Spinal cord lesions
   Surgical injury
      Lumbar sympathectomy
      Retroperitoneal lymphadenectomy
      Aortoiliac surgery
      Abdominoperineal resection
   Neuropathies
      Diabetes mellitus
      Multiple sclerosis
Pharmacological
   α-adrenergic blockade
      Phenoxybenzamine
      Prazosin
      Terazosin
   Peripheral sympatholytics
      Guanethidine
   Ganglion blockers
      Hexamethonium
   Antipsychotics
      Chlorpromazine
      Haloperidol
Mechanical obstruction
   Urethral stricture
   Meatal stenosis
   Urethral valves
   Urethrocele
Idiopathic

germ cell tumors who had undergone the modified RPLND.

Lumbar sympathectomy is performed in patients who are symptomatic from excessive sympathetic output. The consequences of sympathectomy may range from RE in less-extensive cases to total ejaculatory failure when bilateral sympathetic chains are destroyed from T8 to L3 (7).

Presacral nerve damage caused by aortoiliac surgery or abdominoperineal resection can also result in RE. When care is taken to preserve the presacral nerves in aneurysmectomy, antegrade ejaculation is retained in 90% of patients (8).

Diabetes mellitus has been associated with RE, probably due to a peripheral neuropathy involving the bladder neck. Diabetic neuropathy may also be associated with erectile dysfunction and ejaculatory failure.

Pharmacological agents may also lead to RE. Any medication that disturbs α-adrenergic receptors at the bladder neck may be a culprit. The most common of these is the class of antihypertensive medications known as α-blockers, which are currently prescribed

for the treatment of obstructive urinary symptoms due to benign prostatic hyperplasia. Certain antipsychotic agents have also been associated with RE. A partial list of medications associated with RE is provided in Table 1.

$\square$ DIAGNOSIS

RE should be suspected in men with low-volume ejaculates and any of the aforementioned underlying conditions. It should be noted, however, that the most common reason for a low-volume ejaculate in the absence of the medical conditions listed above is a sampling error. Men who consistently make a low-volume specimen through masturbation should be encouraged to collect via condom during sexual intercourse.

Because the seminal vesicles contribute most of the ejaculate volume, ejaculatory duct obstruction and absent or atretic seminal vesicles are also common explanations for low-volume ejaculate. To differentiate these conditions from RE, a postejaculate urine sample is obtained. The patient is asked to empty his bladder into a container immediately after intercourse or masturbation. The urine is centrifuged at 300 g for 10 minutes and the pellet is examined under 40× power magnification. If the patient has absent sperm in his antegrade ejaculate, the presence of 6 to 10 sperm per high power field confirms the diagnosis of RE. If the patient has a low-volume ejaculate and low sperm concentration, the presence of a higher concentration of sperm in the postejaculatory urine than the ejaculated specimen confirms a significant component of RE. If the patient has low-volume azoospermia and no sperm are recovered from the urine, a transrectal ultrasound should be performed to evaluate for ejaculatory duct obstruction. A low-volume ejaculate with oligospermia and no sperm in the postejaculatory urine suggests absent or atretic seminal vesicles, and, again, a transrectal ultrasound is indicated.

$\square$ TREATMENT

Several different treatment options have been proposed for RE. These are summarized in Table 2. The primary treatment is sympathomimetics to restore bladder neck closure. Several α-adrenergic medications have been used. Until recently, the most common was phenylpropanolamine hydrochloride (Omade), 25 mg twice daily (9–12). Reports of hemorrhagic stroke associated with the first-time use of phenylpropanolamine hydrochloride may make this a less-attractive alternative, however (13). Oxedrine (Synephrine, Boehringer Ingleheim, Ridgefield, Connecticut) has been effective in a single dose of 15 to 60 mg (14,15).

Anticholinergics have also been used successfully, the most common being brompheniramine maleate (Dimetane), 8 mg twice daily (16).

Table 2 Methods for Restoring Antegrade Ejaculation

Medications
  α adrenergics
    Imipramine 25 mg by mouth 2–4 times daily
    Phenylpropanolamine HCl by mouth twice daily
    Ephedrine 25 mg by mouth 4 times daily
    Pseudoephedrine 60 mg by mouth 4 times daily
    Pseudoephedrine (sustained release) 120 mg daily × 4 days
  Anticholinergics
    Brompheniramine maleate
  Other
    Imipramine
Surgical treatment
    Abrahams vesical neck reconstruction
    Young–Dees procedure

Imipramine (chlorpropamide hydrochloride) 25 to 50 mg daily has also been used successfully (17–20). Although the precise mechanism by which imipramine works is unknown, it appears to have both anticholinergic and α-adrenergic properties.

When RE is the result of bladder neck surgery, bladder neck reconstruction has been suggested. Two procedures have been proposed to correct bladder neck dysfunction. The first is the Young–Dees procedure, which involves fashioning a 1.5 cm strip of posterior urethral mucosa over a catheter to create a new bladder neck. The prostatic mucosal remnant is stripped and the denuded prostatic and posterior urethral muscles are imbricated over the urethral reconstruction (21).

A second procedure, proposed by Abrahams et al., involves a transvesical approach to the bladder neck. A U-shaped incision is made at the bladder neck through the mucosa beginning at 8 o'clock and ending at 4 o'clock. The mucosa is elevated for 1 cm into the prostatic urethra and incised. The scar tissue is removed and four zero-chromic catgut sutures are used to close the defect. The vesical sphincter is reconstructed to the diameter of a 16-Foley catheter. In their small series, Abrahams et al. reported that antegrade ejaculation was restored in two patients who had previously undergone Y-V plasty of the bladder neck (22).

Improved sperm recovery techniques combined with the success of ART today have rendered surgical treatment for RE of historic significance only.

□ SPERM RECOVERY AND USE IN ASSISTED REPRODUCTION

When antegrade ejaculation cannot be restored medically, it may be necessary to use spermatozoa from the bladder. The obvious limitation is the deleterious effect of acidic urine on sperm quality. Due to the contribution of an alkaline secretion from the seminal vesicles, the fresh ejaculate maintains a pH ranging from 7.2 to 8.2, and an osmolarity ranging from 300 mOsm/kg to 380 mOsm/kg. Acidification causes immobilization of

spermatozoa, while exposure to hypertonic urine can lead to disruption of the cell membrane. These effects are duration dependent. Makler et al. observed that neutralization of the pH is therefore not sufficient to restore motility and should be accompanied by adjustments in osmolarity as well (10). The pH of the medium can be adjusted with NaOH to be alkaline, while serum albumin may be used to buffer pH fluctuations.

Different protocols have been proposed to obtain the optimal sample from the patient with RE. One of the earliest, proposed by Hotchkiss in 1955, involves passing a catheter into the patient's bladder after he has urinated to wash the bladder with a buffer solution. Two milliliters of buffer are left in the bladder and the patient masturbates. The bladder is catheterized again to retrieve the specimen, which is prepared as above (23).

To avoid catheterization, Urry et al. (24) suggested giving patients two tablets of sodium bicarbonate in a glass of water every two hours, beginning 8 to 12 hours before sperm recovery. Thirty minutes to one hour before insemination, the husband is asked to empty his bladder, ejaculate via masturbation or intercourse, and then urinate. The latter urine sample is collected and diluted with modified Ham's F-10 medium (Gibco, Grand Island, New York, U.S.) at a ratio of one to two parts medium per one part urine. Samples are gently mixed and centrifuged at 250 g for 10 minutes. Extra care is taken since spermatozoa from retrograde ejaculates are more fragile. The supernatant is removed, and the pellet is resuspended in 0.5 to 1 mL of Ham's F-10 medium. Urry et al. reported pregnancies in six of seven patients treated with this technique.

Brassesco et al. (25) used a different protocol that involved adjusting the pH and osmolarity of the urine the day of insemination only. They instructed the patient to drink a solution containing sodium bicarbonate 4 gm in 250 mL of water on the day of insemination. The patient would void every 15 minutes thereafter, and the urine pH and osmolarity were determined. When a pH between 6.5 and 8.0 and an osmolarity between 300 and 500 mOsm/kg were reached, the patient was instructed to masturbate and then urinate. This protocol has the advantage of no catheterization for sperm recovery, and no preparation prior to the insemination day. With this technique and using three intracervical inseminations per cycle, the authors reported pregnancies in seven couples.

An even more simplified approach is suggested by a case report, in which a couple achieved a pregnancy through self-inseminations with semen collected through urination (26). In this case, the husband had RE secondary to bladder neck surgery as a child. Just prior to insemination, the patient was asked to masturbate and then urinate. In the urine–semen mixture, the unliquefied semen was identifiable as a gelatinous mass measuring 2 mL in volume. This mass was easily aspirated into a syringe, and the couple used the specimen for intravaginal insemination at home. Of note, because the semen was retrieved from the urine immediately, no adjustments in bladder pH or osmolarity were necessary. Using this technique, the couple achieved a pregnancy after their fifth cycle of inseminations.

Based on reports such as these, the authors no longer require alkalinization in RE patients prior to sperm procurement, provided the exposure to urine is limited. In patients for whom bladder catheterization is necessary, alkalinization is not advised. Similarly, in patients who "urinate" their ejaculate, alkalinization is not advised provided the specimen can be processed within 30 minutes of production. Only in rare instances, when a specimen is expected to remain exposed to urine for greater than 30 minutes, is alkalinization recommended with one of the regimens described above. This approach has simplified considerably the management of patients with RE.

□ RESULTS

Few centers report separate pregnancy success rates in couples with RE. One of the few reports in the literature is by Okada et al. and describes seven men with RE treated with a variety of methods (27). In their small series, three men achieved antegrade ejaculation with imipramine, while three additional patients required retrieval of sperm from the bladder after alkalinization. Further, two patients achieved pregnancies with intercourse after imipramine, one patient achieved a pregnancy with artificial insemination, and two required in vitro fertilization (IVF) to achieve a pregnancy. Of the remaining two patients, one was unmarried and the other failed IVF with intracytoplasmic sperm injection (ICSI). Since the wife of this latter patient was 42 years of age, additional treatment was not pursued. Although this series is small, it illustrates the importance of making available a variety of assisted reproductive techniques depending on the quality of the sperm retrieved.

□ A RATIONAL APPROACH TO ACHIEVE PREGNANCIES IN RE

Patients with RE have presented a challenge to fertility specialists for years. Procuring optimal quality semen

Table 3 Rational Approach to Treating the Infertile Couple with Retrograde Ejaculation

- Restore antegrade ejaculation pharmacologically when possible.
- Obtain voided postejaculate urine when antegrade ejaculation cannot be restored.
- Catheterize bladder after alkalinizing, if voided specimen unsatisfactory.
- If 5 million or greater total motile sperm, proceed to intrauterine insemination.
- Less than 5 million total motile sperm, consider in vitro fertilization/intracytoplasmic sperm injection.

with the least inconvenience to the patient requires a thorough understanding of the physiology of ejaculation and the available armamentarium for treatment. A rational approach combines effective sperm retrieval with the appropriate assisted reproductive technique.

ICSI has not changed the basic approach to sperm procurement in men with RE. The specimen can be retrieved from voided urine or through catheterization. The development of ICSI as a highly successful reproductive technique has allowed for the use of extremely poor-quality semen specimens for fertilization in vitro.

A rational approach to the patient with RE is summarized in Table 3. One should start with efforts to restore antegrade ejaculation by pharmacological means. When such measures fail, or if drugs cannot be tolerated (such as the patient with hypertension in whom α-adrenergic medications are contraindicated), retrieval of sperm from postejaculatory urine is the next step. Depending on the quality of the sperm obtained, that specimen can be used for artificial insemination or IVF. Most practitioners feel that 5 million total motile sperm are adequate for intrauterine insemination. A lower number constitutes a relative indication for IVF in most centers. Other factors relating to the female partner should be elucidated prior to such decisions. This is one of several conditions where a team approach, consisting of a reproductive urologist, a reproductive endocrinologist, and a quality andrology laboratory, allows for optimal management. Patients with RE should be counseled that in the absence of additional major infertility factors, the prognosis for a pregnancy is excellent.

☐ REFERENCES

1. Reiser C. The etiology of retrograde ejaculation and a method of insemination. Fertil Steril 1961; 12: 488–492.

2. Turner-Warwick R. A urodynamic review of bladder outlet obstruction in the male and its clinical implications. Urol Clin North Am 1979; 6:171–192.

3. Dorflinger T, Jensen FS, Kraup T, et al. Transurethral prostatectomy compared with incision of the prostate in the treatment of prostatism caused by small benign prostate glands. Scand J Urol Nephrol 1992; 26(4): 333–338.

4. Kedia K, Markland C, Fraley E. Sexual function following high retroperitoneal lymphadenectomy. J Urol 1975; 114(2):237–239.

5. Narayan P, Lange PH, Fraley EE. Ejaculation and fertility after extended retroperitoneal lymph node dissection for testicular cancer. J Urol 1982; 127(4): 685–688.

6. Richie JP. Clinical Stage I testicular cancer: the role of modified retroperitoneal lymphadenectomy. J Urol 1990; 144(5):1160–1163.

7. Rose S. An investigation into sterility after lumbar ganglionectomy. Br Med J 1953; 1(4804):247–250.

8. Sabri S, Cotton L. Sexual function following aortoiliac reconstruction. Lancet 1971; 2(7736):1218–1219.

9. Sandler B. Idiopathic retrograde ejaculation. Fertil Steril 1979; 32(4):474–475.

10. Makler A, David R, Blumenfeld Z, et al. Factors affecting sperm motility. VII. Sperm viability as affected by change of pH and osmolarity of semen and urine specimens. Fertil Steril 1981; 36(4):507–511.

11. Thiagarajah S, Vaughan ED, Kitchin JD. Retrograde ejaculation: successful pregnancy following combined sympathomimetic medication and insemination. Fertil Steril 1978; 30(1):96–97.

12. Stewart BH, Bergant JA. Correction of retrograde ejaculation by sympathomimetic medication: preliminary report. Fertil Steril 1974; 25(12):1073–1074.

13. Kernan WN, Viscoli CM, Brass LM, et al. Phenyl-propanolamine and the risk of hemorrhagic stroke. N Engl J Med 2000; 343(25):1826–1832.

14. Stockamp K, Schreiter F, Altwein J. Alpha-adrenergic drugs in retrograde ejaculation. Fertil Steril 1974; 25(9): 817–820.

15. Jonas D, Linzbach P, Weber W. The use of midodrin in the treatment of ejaculation disorders following retroperitoneal lymphadenectomy. Eur Urol 1979; 5(3): 184–187.

16. Androloro VA Jr, Dube A. Treatment of retrograde ejaculation with brompheniramine, Urology 1975; 5(4): 520–522.

17. Wein AJ, Van Arsdalen KN. Drug-induced male sexual dysfunction. Urol Clin N Am 1988; 15(1):23–31.

18. Brooks ME, Sidi A. Treatment of retrograde ejaculation using imipramine. Urology 1981; 18(6):633.

19. Nijman JM, Jager S, Boer PW, et al. The treatment of retrograde ejaculation disorder after retroperitoneal lymph node dissection. Cancer 1982; 50(12): 2967–2971.

20. Eppel SM, Berzin M. Pregnancy following treatment of retrograde ejaculation with clomipramine hydrochloride. A report of 3 cases. S Afr Med J 1984; 66(23): 889–891.

21. Middleton RG, Urry RL. The Young-Dees operation for the correction of retrograde ejaculation. J Urol 1986; 136:1208–1209.

22. Abrahams JI, Solish GI, Boorjian P, et al. The surgical correction of retrograde ejaculation. J Urol 1975; 114(6): 888–890.

23. Hotchkiss R, Pinto A, Kleegman S. Artificial insemination with semen recovered from the bladder. Fertil Steril 1954; 6(1):37–42.

24. Urry RL, Middleton RG, McGavin S. A simple and effective technique for increasing pregnancy rates in couples with retrograde ejaculation. Fertil Steril 1986; 46(6):1124–1127.

25. Brassesco M, Viscasillas P, Burrel L, et al. Sperm recuperation and cervical insemination in retrograde ejaculation. Fertil Steril 1988; 49(5):923–925.

26. Cleine JH. Retrograde ejaculation: can sperm be retrieval be simpler and non-invasive? Fertil and Steril 2000; 74(2):416–417.

27. Okada H, Fujioka H, Hitoshi F, et al. Treatment of patients with retrograde ejaculation in the era of modern assisted reproduction technology. J Urol 1998; 159(3):848–850.

33

Surgical Treatment of Male Infertility

Peter N. Schlegel

Departments of Urology and Reproductive Medicine, Weill Medical College of Cornell University, New York, New York, U.S.A.

Jeremy Kaufman

Department of Urology, The New York-Presbyterian Hospital, New York Center for Biomedical Research, and The Rockefeller University Hospital, New York, New York, U.S.A.

□ INTRODUCTION

The treatment of male infertility will often involve surgical therapy. Additionally, surgery allows diagnostic information to be gathered regarding the cause and prognosis for treatment success. For azoospermic men, surgical sperm retrieval may be required to allow successful treatment with assisted reproduction. Surgical treatment of male infertility can be very successful at providing high rates of pregnancy and is typically more cost-effective than alternative forms of treatment such as assisted reproduction procedures alone.

□ TESTIS BIOPSY

A testis biopsy is performed to determine whether obstruction is present for an azoospermic man with palpable vasa deferentia. Testis biopsy can also provide some, but not absolute, diagnostic information for men with nonobstructive azoospermia (NOA). Only men with a serum follicle-stimulating hormone (FSH) level that is less than three times the upper limit of normal levels will have normal sperm production. Azoospermic men with small or soft testes are highly unlikely to have sperm production, but some of these men have limited foci of spermatogenesis that can provide sperm for assisted reproduction. In the authors' experience, all men with congenital absence of the vas deferens, normal serum FSH levels, and normal volume testes (greater than 15 cc) had sperm production, obviating the need for diagnostic biopsy. Biopsy should be performed on both testes, since substantial differences in sperm production may be present without a palpable difference in the testes.

A second relative indication for testis biopsy is for the evaluation of azoospermic men with presumed abnormal production. These men with NOA will have soft or small testes and an elevated FSH level in most cases. Although these patients are not expected to have reproductive tract obstruction, in selected cases, sperm may be retrieved from the testis and used with assisted reproduction techniques such as intracytoplasmic sperm injection (ICSI). A biopsy may be of value in providing some prognostic information on which patients are candidates for ICSI. Unfortunately, a diagnostic biopsy is performed randomly and evaluates only 5 to 10 of the highly coiled seminiferous tubules within the testis. Subsequent attempts at sperm retrieval are dependent on finding the most advanced spermatogenic pattern of production in the 600 to 1000 tubules present within each testis. An initial, random diagnostic biopsy that demonstrates at least one spermatozoon predicts the subsequent finding of sperm on attempted testicular sperm extraction (TESE) in over 80% of patients (1). The observation of at least germ cells (spermatogonia or spermatocytes) on diagnostic biopsy predicts subsequent sperm retrieval with TESE for about 50% of patients (1). In all cases, the chance of sperm retrieval is determined by the most advanced pattern of sperm production on diagnostic biopsy, not the predominant pattern. For men who have only tubules with Sertoli cells in their lumen, the chance of sperm retrieval from another area of the testis is at least 25% (1). Therefore, the prognostic value of a diagnostic biopsy in NOA is limited.

Diagnostic information on the status of spermatogenesis is most reliably determined on evaluation of a thin-sectioned, stained, fixed tissue specimen. Adequate specimens for tissue evaluation can be obtained by open biopsy, needle biopsy, or, occasionally, fine needle aspiration (FNA). Given the potential inadequacy of needle biopsy or FNA, with the attendant risks to the vasculature of the testis, the open biopsy technique is preferable. The biopsy should be performed prior to reconstruction (rather than simultaneous to vasoepididymostomy), so that a definitive analysis of sperm production is possible on fixed sections prior to further exploration. In addition, vasography is superfluous at the time of biopsy and should be avoided because of the risk of vasal injury or stricture. Techniques of biopsy are described briefly below. (For further information on testicular biopsy, please refer to Chapter 25.)

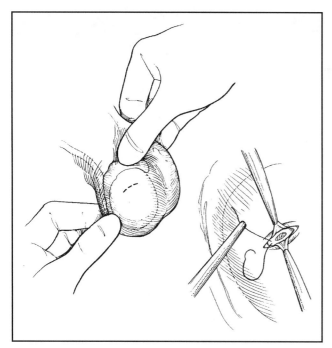

Figure 1 Location of incision and "window" technique for diagnostic testicular biopsy.

Testicular Biopsy Technique

For open biopsy, the testis must be accurately positioned with the scrotal skin tightly stretched over the testis, and the epididymis must be secured in a posterior position. A 1 cm incision is made transversely over the midportion of the testis (Fig. 1). The incision is carried out down to the tunica vaginalis. Cutting through this tunic is confirmed intraoperatively by the release of a small amount of clear fluid, expressed from within the space of the tunica vaginalis. A stay suture is placed through a nonvascularized region of the testis, preferably in a superior, medial, or lateral position. Optical loupes or an operating microscope may help identify vessels under the tunica albuginea, avoiding the risk of injury to the testicular blood supply. Nonreactive suture such as nylon or polypropylene is preferred. A 0.5 cm incision is made through the tunica albuginea with a sharp #15 blade or a fine ophthalmic knife. A small sample of seminiferous tubules should extrude easily through this incision. If a sample is not easily delivered, the incision may not be long or deep enough. Excessive pressure to extrude tubules may adversely affect the architecture of the specimen. The sample should be cut off sharply and placed directly into Bouin's solution or buffered glutaraldehyde. The use of formalin is avoided because of the deleterious effects that it has on tubular architecture. A wet prep of the cut seminiferous tubular surface or a "squash prep" of a separate piece of tubule on a glass slide, bathed with lactated Ringer's and compressed with a cover slip, can be immediately examined under the microscope. The presence of sperm alone does not guarantee obstruction; however, distal obstruction is highly likely in men with motile sperm.

The tunical levels and the skin should both be closed to encourage hemostasis. Generous injection of 0.25% bupivacaine into the tunica vaginalis space and the subcutaneous areas provides excellent local anesthesia postoperatively.

"Quick-Prep" Cytologic Evaluations for Men with Presumed Obstruction

Since Hotchkiss (2) and Charney's (3) introduction of the testis biopsy as a diagnostic tool, a variety of refinements in the technique have been proposed to improve its usefulness. The role of a testis biopsy is to evaluate spermatozoal production—and, indirectly, the presence or absence of reproductive tract obstruction. Since formal testis biopsy requires fixation and the embedding and staining of specimens for interpretation, biopsy and reproductive tract reconstruction must occur at different times. Quantitative analysis of testicular sperm production is possible by counting the number of mature spermatids per round tubule, as described by Silber and Rodriguez-Rigau (4). Several techniques have attempted to provide additional "quick analysis" information from testis biopsy specimens.

Technique: Touch Prep

The touch prep, or testicular touch imprint, is a cytological smear of fluid from the cut surface of testicular parenchyma. The touch prep is performed during testis biopsy by taking a clean glass slide and placing it on the cut surface of seminiferous tubules after obtaining a specimen for permanent section. The slide is applied to the cut surface in several areas and immediately cytofixed with a commercial spray or 95% ethyl alcohol. The smear is subsequently stained via the Papanicolaou technique (5,6). Identification of individual spermatogenic cells as well as mature spermatozoa is possible. The most important role of the touch prep is to differentiate between late maturation arrest and complete spermatogenesis. Late maturation arrest may be difficult to assess on biopsy, since mature sperm with tails are not commonly seen on the thin slice of a histologic slide, and quantitation of spermatozoal production is usually inferred from the number of mature spermatids present on fixed testis biopsy specimens. Quantitation of spermatozoa on touch prep allows direct evaluation of whether late maturation arrest is present. Detection of fully formed testicular sperm morphology is also possible. A diagnosis of late maturation arrest spares the patient unnecessary scrotal exploration and even possible partial epididymectomy in a futile attempt at reconstruction.

Little published data exist regarding the frequency of late maturation arrest, or the sensitivity (or specificity) of the touch prep technique. If late maturation arrest is very uncommon, and false positive results occur with the touch prep, then it is possible that more patients may be denied reconstructive microsurgery than are benefited by the diagnosis of late maturation arrest. Certainly, the touch prep can be of great value when late maturation arrest is suspected.

Technique: Wet Prep

A wet prep is performed after the standard biopsy specimen has been atraumatically transferred into Bouin's solution (5). For the wet prep, a small additional piece of testis is placed on a clean glass slide with Ringer's lactate, and the tissue is compressed under a glass cover slip. Analysis of this specimen can be performed immediately in the operating room. The presence or absence of sperm is documented, and the motility of sperm can also be evaluated.

The presence or absence of sperm is not very predictive of the findings on fixed permanent sections, but the presence of sperm motility may be of importance. A review of 100 consecutive testis biopsy and wet prep evaluations at Cornell (6) indicated that histology (complete spermatogenesis) and cytology (presence of sperm on wet prep) were concordant in only 81% of biopsies; however, the presence of motile sperm had a 100% positive predictive value for the presence of reproductive tract obstruction. For the 18 cases in which motile sperm were present, it would have been safe to proceed with microsurgical reconstruction of the reproductive tract. The converse, however, is not applicable: the absence of motile sperm did not predict the absence of obstruction. In fact, 47 out of 65 (72%) men with obstruction did not have motile sperm present on wet prep.

Further data collection will be helpful for fully evaluating the relevance of sperm motility on wet prep examination during testis biopsy. Based on the data available, the presence of motile testicular sperm is highly suggestive of the presence of distal obstruction.

Technique: Cytospin

Coburn et al. (7) described the technique of cytospin evaluation of testis tissue obtained during testis biopsy. Cytospin evaluation involves placement of a small segment of testicular tissue into cold tissue culture solution, with subsequent agitation of that specimen for one minute. The specimen is removed and placed into Bouin's solution prior to paraffin sectioning. The supernatant is centrifuged in a cytospin processor, stained, and examined for the presence or absence of spermatozoa.

Studies at Baylor have demonstrated mature sperm in all specimens from testes affected by obstructive lesions (8). The remaining patients showed no sperm cytologically and were found to have germinal cell aplasia or complete maturation arrest on formal histological evaluation. One patient had maturation arrest found only because of the addition of cytological evaluation to routine histology. This finding supports the value of cytospin or touch prep for the detection of late maturation arrest during routine testis biopsy.

Summary

Testis biopsy is a diagnostic technique to assess spermatogenesis. It is most useful to determine whether obstruction is the cause of azoospermia. It is also possible to take additional tissue during this diagnostic procedure that can be frozen for subsequent therapeutic trials of assisted reproduction. Cytologic evaluation, when performed concurrently with standard testicular biopsy, may provide important adjunctive information. Cytospin and touch prep techniques allow for the detection of late maturation arrest—not evaluable on fixed permanent sections. Additionally, cytospin and touch prep techniques allow the evaluation of the presence of sperm within the seminiferous tubule without the removal of an additional piece of testicular parenchyma. The wet prep technique allows the evaluation of sperm motility. The presence of sperm motility appears to be highly indicative of the presence of obstruction. Further information regarding the frequency of late maturation arrest and the endurance of the predictive value of wet prep sperm motility is needed. At present, cytological techniques should best be considered adjuncts to, but not replacements of, careful evaluation of fixed permanent testicular biopsy specimens. (For additional information on semen analysis, please refer to Chapters 23 and 24.)

☐ VASOGRAPHY

Vasography should not be performed as a separate procedure since it can injure the vas deferens or cause leakage of sperm at the cannulation site with subsequent formation of a sperm granuloma, and thus should also be avoided at the time of biopsy. It can, however, be performed most easily by simply injecting 4 to 5 cc of saline or Ringer's lactate into the lumen of the vas deferens. Absence of back pressure confirms the absence of obstruction. If back pressure is detected, methylene blue is injected and the patient catheterized to confirm that the dye passes into the posterior urethra and bladder. Vasography may be of value during transurethral resection or dilation. An assistant can perform the injection of dilute methylene blue through a soft, nonreactive 2Fr umbilical artery catheter placed in the vas deferens during transurethral management of partial or complete ejaculatory duct obstruction. Alternatively, the seminal vesicle can be injected with dye using transrectal ultrasound (TRUS) guidance.

Technique

To perform a vasotomy, the vas is isolated just distal to the convoluted vas deferens under the skin of the lateral scrotum. The vas is delivered into a small scrotal incision and dissected free of associated perivasal vessels (Fig. 2). Under the operating microscope, a longitudinal incision is made over the vas in its straight portion, just beyond the convoluted region of the vas. The incision is carried out with a 15° ultrasharp knife

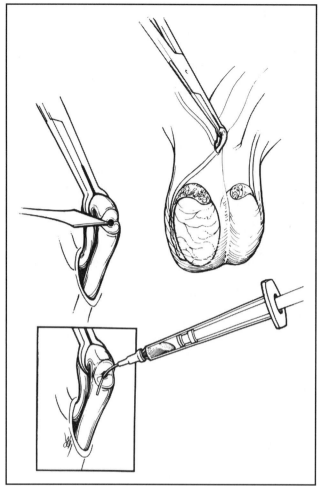

Figure 2 Delivery of the vas deferens for hemivasotomy and sampling of intravasal fluid for vasography.

down to the muscular layers of the vas. The vas is mobilized and isolated with a small straight clamp or thin piece of Penrose drain. A hemivasotomy is performed so that the posterior half of the vas is preserved. Vasal fluid must be tested for the presence of sperm. A 22- or 24-gauge angiocatheter can be used to perform a noncontrast vasogram with methylene blue dye. Catheterization of the bladder with return of blue urine will demonstrate patency of the reproductive tract. Inability to inject fluid, or high pressure with injection, should lead to a contrast vasogram with 50% or higher concentration of Renografin. During contrast vasography, a Foley catheter should be placed into the bladder. Filling the Foley balloon with air will provide double contrast to allow localization of the bladder neck. The hemivasotomy is subsequently closed with 9-0 and 10-0 monofilament sutures, as described below for microsurgical vasovasostomy.

□ VARICOCELECTOMY

Varicocelectomy is indicated for men with symptomatic varicoceles, for men with confirmed infertility

and persistently abnormal sperm quality, and for adolescents with large varicoceles and associated testicular hypotrophy. An International WHO study on varicoceles has also supported the finding that varicoceles are clearly related to infertility (9,10). (For further information on varicoceles, please refer to Chapter 15.)

Approaches to varicocele correction include inguinal, retroperitoneal, and laparoscopic techniques (Fig. 3). Transvenous balloon embolization is also highly successful, with minimal morbidity, but its application is limited to those with significant experience in this technique. Correction of right-sided varicoceles is frequently not possible by retrograde balloon embolization because of the acute angle of the right internal spermatic vein at its junction with the vena cava. Laparoscopic approaches appear to be fairly successful (Fig. 4). Laparoscopy, however, takes the subcutaneous procedure of inguinal varicocelectomy and converts it into an intra-abdominal approach, which is of higher risk. There are currently few indications for laparoscopic varicocelectomy.

Varicocelectomy involves ligation of all internal spermatic veins to prevent the retrograde flow of blood in this system that is pathognomonic of a varicocele. In order to effectively and safely correct a varicocele, one should (*i*) leave the vas deferens and its associated vessels intact, (*ii*) divide all internal spermatic veins (and external spermatic veins if the inguinal approach is used), and (*iii*) leave the lymphatic vessels and

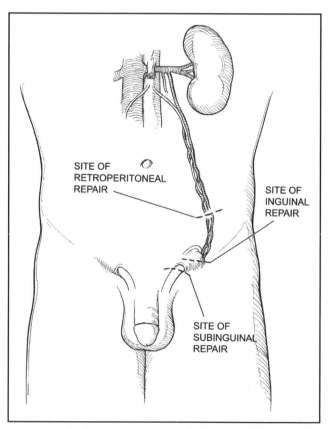

Figure 3 Incisional approaches for repair of varicocele.

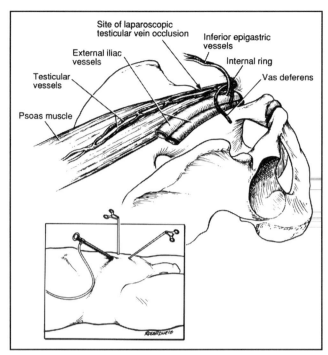

Figure 4 Schematic view of laparoscopic approach to varicocele repair.

testicular arteries intact. Difficulty in visualizing any small internal spermatic vessels in the retroperitoneum explains the 10% clinical recurrence/persistence rate after a "Palomo varicocelectomy" (older, retroperitoneal approach) (11). Even with a muscle-splitting approach, more morbidity occurs with this approach than an inguinal approach.

The optimal surgical approach to varicocelectomy is an inguinal or a subinguinal one, with at least 6 to 8× optical magnification (12). If it is readily available, an operating microscope provides the ability to use variable magnification during the procedure. In the authors' experience with both approaches, the use of an operating microscope clearly provides better visualization of the lymphatics and the testicular arteries during varicocelectomy. Although it is tedious to perform a microsurgical dissection, the advantages are significant: testicular arteries can be identified and preserved in over 99.5% of cases, the varicocele recurrence/persistence rate is less than 0.5%, and hydroceles occur postoperatively in less than 0.5% of cases (13–15). It is highly upsetting to both patient and physician when painful testicular atrophy occurs because of inadvertent injury to the testicular artery, or when a massive, symptomatic hydrocele is present postoperatively. Considering the gravity of these postoperative complications, it certainly seems worth extending the intraoperative case time by 15 or 20 minutes in order to decrease the postoperative complication rate from 10% to approximately 1%. Therefore, there is little rationale for performing varicocele repair without optical magnification.

Delivery of the testis probably contributes very little to decreasing recurrence rates. Although some

dilated veins are present in the gubernaculum in many men with varicoceles, these are usually "vents" for the return of refluxing blood down the internal spermatic veins. There is little evidence that the gubernacular veins actually can form collaterals to the internal spermatic system, thereby causing persistence of a varicocele.

Technique

The procedure can be performed under local or general anesthesia. A 1- to 1.5-in. incision is made over the external inguinal ring. Blunt dissection is carried out down to the external ring with Kelly clamps. The subcutaneous tissues are separated. If the external ring is reasonably capacious, then the entire spermatic cord is grasped with a Babcock clamp as it passes over the pubis. If the external ring is very small, then the external spermatic fascia is opened with careful identification of the ilioinguinal nerve. The spermatic cord is delivered, leaving the ilioinguinal nerve on the floor of the canal. The canal must be carefully examined to preclude the presence of any perforating veins. The spermatic cord is draped over a Penrose drain or Penrose-covered tongue blade, and the operating microscope is brought into position. The position of the vas is determined by palpation, and the external and internal fascias are incised longitudinally. Usually, the artery is identified readily by sprinkling a mixture of papaverine and lidocaine on the cord. If no pulsations are detected, a Doppler probe is helpful for identification of the artery. In 50% of cases, more than one artery is present in the spermatic cord. All veins are either doubly ligated (note that the use of undyed and black sutures is helpful in keeping the ties separate) or clipped with small or medium hemoclips. The external spermatic veins are also ligated and divided, with preservation of all perivasal vessels (Fig. 5).

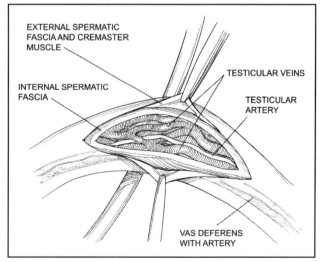

Figure 5 Schematic view of the spermatic cord during dissection for microsurgical varicocele repair. Vasal vessels, the vas deferens, testicular arteries, and lymphatics are the only structures preserved after repair.

The lymphatic vessels must be irrigated to confirm the absence of blood in their lumina. Typically, six to eight lymphatics can be identified and preserved in the spermatic cord. This procedure—many components of which were popularized by Goldstein (13)—is also very similar to that described by Marmar (16) in the early 1980s.

Complications

Complications of open surgical varicocele repair include those generally associated with surgery (bleeding, infection, and risks of anesthesia) as well as those specific to the varicocele procedure (hydrocele, testicular atrophy, and varicocele recurrence/persistence). Significant complications of varicocelectomy are rare; reoperation for a major hematoma or infection occurs in approximately 1 in 500 cases (in the authors' experience) (17,18). Hydrocele formation rates are related to the ability of the surgeon to identify and preserve lymphatics during dissection of the internal spermatic vessels. For microsurgical approaches, hydroceles form in less than 1% of cases and are usually transient. Testicular atrophy can occur if the testicular artery is compromised during varicocele repair; this may happen from division of the artery or compromise of the spermatic cord by excessive tightening of the external inguinal ring. With microsurgical approaches, atrophy is essentially never seen. With macrosurgical approaches, atrophy occurs in less than 1% of cases, although these statistics are rarely published. Persistence of the varicocele occurs if a large internal spermatic vein is missed and the varicocele is easily detected in the early postoperative period. Varicocele recurrence is caused by the persistence of microscopic veins that subsequently enlarge as the result of communication with the remainder of the pampiniform plexus. The rate of varicocele recurrence has been reported to be between 0.4% and 1% with microsurgical techniques, and up to 15% with high-ligation techniques. Varicocele persistence after balloon embolization is dependent on the skill of the radiologist and ranges from 3% to 25% (19,20).

Results

Several reviews of varicocelectomy have almost uniformly suggested that 60% to 70% of patients who undergo varicocele repair will have demonstrable improvement in semen parameters, with 35% to 40% of the patients contributing to a pregnancy within a year (14,15,21). Two-year follow-up data have suggested that pregnancy rates may increase up to 70% in the second year, at least for couples with no female factor infertility. Semen parameters are known to be highly variable in normal and infertile men, however, and some of these reported pregnancies may have occurred without any intervention. Therefore, it is important to consider controlled series of varicocele repair, in which men who have varicocelectomy are compared to those who have no treatment, counseling,

or medical therapy, or other comparable patient groups. A review of these studies demonstrated a statistically significant benefit of varicocele repair in improving pregnancy rates (22). It is clear from these results that subfertile men with a varicocele are likely to have a real—albeit moderate—benefit from varicocele treatment. Results of varicocelectomy are definitively related to the varicocele size as well as the patient's age (Table 1). The larger the varicocele, the greater the expected postoperative change in semen parameters. This finding, coupled with controversial results after repair of subclinical (smaller, nonpalpable) varicoceles, supports the importance of repair of the clinical varicocele alone. Some studies (23) have suggested that men with clinical varicoceles will typically have internal spermatic veins that are 2.7 mm or larger in diameter on scrotal ultrasonography. The chance of improvement in semen parameters is related to varicocele size on scrotal ultrasonography. In men who have varicoceles less than 2.7 mm in diameter, equal proportions of men have improved semen parameters after varicocelectomy and decreased semen parameters.

Summary

Varicoceles are sometimes "red herrings" that do not cause infertility. For many couples in whom varicocele-associated male infertility factor is present, however, initial treatment with varicocelectomy is strongly recommended. Controlled studies of varicocelectomy support the effectiveness of this treatment for male factor infertility. Varicocele repair is a cost-effective treatment for male infertility, especially when compared to treatment using ICSI.

□ VASECTOMY REVERSAL

Reversal of vasectomy is now technically possible and highly successful for a majority of men. The duration of time after vasectomy is important. Secondary obstruction of the epididymis becomes increasingly more common when more than 10 years have passed after vasectomy. The modern techniques for vasovasostomy are modifications of the microsurgical approaches described in the mid-1970s by Drs. Owen (24) and Silber (25). Microsurgical techniques generally have approximately 85% to 90% postoperative patency rates in experienced hands (26). Yet, only 60%

Table 1 Percent Change in Semen Parameters after Varicocelectomy

Varicocele grade	Motile sperm concentration (%)	Sperm concentration (%)	Motility (%)
I	27	21	15
II	21	24	3
III	128	94	37

of couples actually achieve a pregnancy after vasovasostomy. Antisperm antibodies, female infertility, secondary obstruction in the epididymis, or recurrent obstruction at the anastomotic site may all contribute to the inability of nearly half of all men with established patency after vasovasostomy to contribute to pregnancies (27).

The technique for vasectomy reversal (i.e., vasovasostomy vs. vasoepididymostomy) depends on the intravasal findings at the time of surgical exploration. In addition, obstructive lesions may occur in the vas deferens at the inguinal level after hernia repair. Testis biopsy is not routinely indicated prior to vasectomy reversal. Optimal results with vasovasostomy (or vasoepididymostomy) are achieved when these principles are followed: (*i*) accurate mucosa-to-mucosa anastomosis to allow a leak-proof anastomosis, (*ii*) tension-free anastomosis, (*iii*) adequate blood supply to the ends of the vas with healthy mucosa and muscularis, and (*iv*) atraumatic technique. Adherence to these fundamental principles is far more important than the number of layers performed or the exact suture material used. The two approaches are described briefly below. (For further information on vasectomy reversal, please refer to Chapter 34.)

Vasovasostomy

High vertical scrotal incisions are performed bilaterally over the testis, directed toward the external inguinal ring (Fig. 6). The testis is delivered; the site of vasectomy is then isolated and dissected free. The testicular side of the vas is isolated and cleanly divided at a 90° angle with the aid of a slotted nerve clamp. Vasal fluid is carefully collected after bipolar control of bleeding. The epididymis is milked, and the presence or absence of sperm is evaluated. If sperm are present and the abdominal side of the vas is patent, then an anastomosis is performed. If no sperm are present, the vasal fluid should be sequentially sampled during evaluation of the contralateral vasectomy site. The abdominal side of the vas is similarly divided with the slotted nerve clamp, and saline vasography is performed. Formal vasography is only necessary if saline vasography is not possible or is abnormal. The two ends of the vas are carefully examined under the operating microscope to confirm that the cut ends of the vasa are healthy (Fig. 7). The vasa are stabilized in a vasal approximator and the anastomosis performed over a Penrose-covered tongue blade at 25× magnification. Double-armed fish-hook 70 μm needles with 10-0 monofilament nylon sutures are used on the top half of the anastomosis. The fish-hook configuration with double arming essentially prevents back walling. Accurate mucosal apposition is possible with mucosally based sutures and an ample width of muscle. Additional sutures are placed from the outer wall of the vas, without penetrating the mucosa, using a cutting 9-0 nylon suture. A couple of sutures in the adventitial layer of the vas can help to minimize tension on the anastomosis.

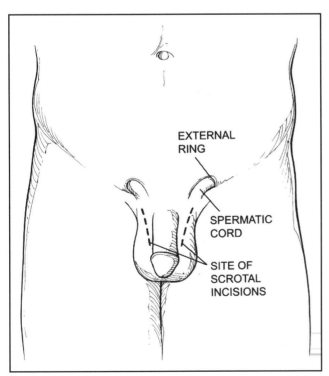

Figure 6   Position of high vertical incisions in the scrotum for vasovasostomy or vasoepididymostomy. The incisions are placed high in the scrotum and directed toward the external ring to avoid tension on the anastomosis and facilitate dissection of the vas deferens.

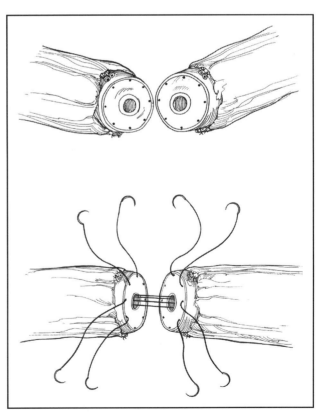

Figure 7   Preparation of the cut ends of the vas deferens for vasovasostomy with preservation of adequate perivasal tissue to allow maintenance of good blood supply to the vas.

If multiple tears of the mucosa or other technical misadventures occur, the vasa should be cut back and the anastomosis performed again. If excessive bleeding is seen, then Penrose drains should be placed through dependent puncture sites in the scrotum.

Microsurgical Vasoepididymostomy

Patency results with microsurgical vasoepidymostomy in experienced hands are only about 70%. Of all patients who undergo the operation, only 30% actually contribute to a pregnancy (28). It must be noted, however, that the single-tubule anastomotic results are far better than those previously obtained with "slash and fistula" techniques. Anastomosis can be performed in either an end-end or an end-side approach to the epididymis. The choice of technique is dependent on operator experience and vasal length. Sometimes, it is not possible to perform a low end-side anastomosis with a short vas deferens. Some surgeons find it very difficult to sort out which epididymal tubules should be used to perform the anastomosis during an end-end vasoepididymostomy because of the multiple divided tubules present on the bloody cut surface of the epididymis. An end-side anastomosis is easiest to perform when a clear level of obstruction is easily seen on visual inspection of the epididymis, allowing set-up of the anastomosis prior to performing an incision in the epididymal tunics. When tubular dilation is not as clear, an end-end technique is preferred. Serial sectioning of the epididymis is performed until a gush of cloudy fluid is obtained from a single dominant epididymal tubule.

Technique

High vertical scrotal incisions are performed, as with the approach for vasovasostomy. The testis is delivered and vasography performed at the junction of the straight and convoluted vas deferens. The absence of

sperm is confirmed. Saline vasograms are performed. The vas is completely divided and hemostasis obtained with a slotted nerve clamp. The tunica vaginalis is opened. For end-side anastomoses, the vas can be brought through a puncture site in the tunics with later closure of the tunica.

End–End Approach

The epididymis is sharply dissected free of the testis and swung up toward the inguinal ring. The epididymis is sequentially divided with a slotted nerve clamp and examined for the presence of a single dominantly effluxing epididymal tubule. The presence of sperm is confirmed by performing a wet prep of the cut edge of the epididymis. Intact sperm (not sperm heads or other fragments) should be detected. The anastomosis is performed with both the vas and the epididymis stabilized by a vas–epididymis approximating clamp. Methylene blue or a fresh marking pen can be used to help outline the cut edge of the mucosa of the epididymal tubules. A minimum of four (and preferably six) 10-0 nylon mucosal sutures are placed between the effluxing epididymal tubule and the mucosa of the vas. A second row of 9-0 sutures is placed between the muscularis layer of the vas and epididymal tunics. It is important to avoid including any dilated epididymal tubules in either of these sets of sutures, as that may obstruct the epididymis more proximally.

End–Side Approach

When the level of obstruction is obvious, the planned anastomotic site can be set up prior to opening the epididymal tunic. In this case, a row of 9-0 nylon sutures is used to stabilize the back wall of the muscular layer of the vas to the epididymal tunic (Fig. 8A). Anastomosis is performed to the incised epididymal tubule with subsequent closure of the vasal adventitia and muscle

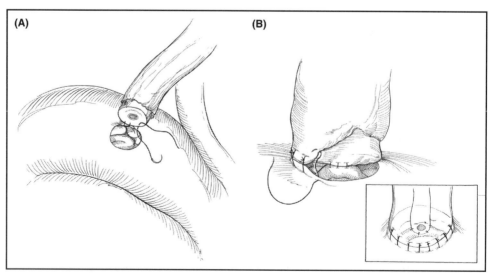

Figure 8 Vasoepididymostomy: end-side approach. (**A**) The vas deferens is attached to the edge of the epididymal tunic with interrupted 9-0 sutures in preparation for an end-side anastomosis during vasoepididymostomy. (**B**) Suture of epididymal tunics to vasal adventitia during vasoepididymostomy.

to the epididymal tunic (Fig. 8B). An improved technique for vasoepididymostomy involves invagination of an epididymal tubule into the vas deferens with triangulating sutures (Fig. 9A). After these three sutures are placed in the epididymis, a single tubule is dissected free, and a linear incision is made in the isolated epididymal tubule. The sutures that were previously placed into the epididymis are then placed into the lumen of the vas deferens (Fig. 9B). The muscular layer of the vas is then anastomosed circumferentially to the epididymal tunic with interrupted 9-0 sutures (Fig. 8B). If the vas has been brought through a puncture site in the tunica vaginalis, then the adventitia of the vas can be sutured to the outer layer of the parietal tunica with one or two 6-0 polypropylene sutures to avoid any direct tension of the anastomosis. If possible, the tunica vaginalis is closed.

□ SPERM RETRIEVAL FOR ASSISTED REPRODUCTION
Background

To understand clinical approaches to sperm retrieval in men with obstructive and NOA, it is necessary to consider how the male reproductive system is affected by these conditions. (For further information on the anatomy and physiology of the male reproductive tract, please refer to Chapters 2, 5, and 6.)

Obstructive Azoospermia: Inverted Motility

It had long been thought that sperm exiting the testis lack maturity, motility, and fertilizing capability, and that transit through the epididymis is essential for the acquisition of these features. In the unobstructed setting, sperm quality improves as the spermatozoa travel

from caput to cauda; this is not true, however, in the obstructed setting. In reproductive tract obstruction, improved motility is seen in sperm retrieved from the caput epididymis compared to the cauda, as sperm extracted from the tail of an obstructed epididymis are in advanced stages of degeneration and necrosis. Here, normal sperm are absent or rare, and macrophages filled with phagocytized sperm remnants are seen in abundance (Fig. 10). This finding is often referred to as "inverted motility."

Thus, in the case of obstruction, better-quality sperm can be found proximally in the rete testis, vasa efferentia, or caput epididymis; the more distal cauda epididymis is the site of sperm degeneration. These factors should be taken into account during any attempt at sperm removal.

NOA: Heterogeneity of Sperm Production

It has previously been shown that human testicular histology is heterogeneous; there can be small foci of abnormal spermatogenesis adjacent to normal seminiferous tubules. This formerly casual observation is now the cornerstone of treatment for men with NOA. Successful sperm-retrieval is possible in most testicular sperm-retrieval attempts in men with NOA, despite diagnostic testis-biopsy specimens showing predominantly maturation arrest. The ability to retrieve sperm from the testes of men with NOA is independent of testicular size and FSH level, but dependent on the most advanced level of spermatogenesis identified. All standard parameters of testicular evaluation (testicular volume, FSH, and inhibin B levels) are used to evaluate overall function of the testis. Since sperm retrieval and pregnancy are dependent on finding sperm in just one small focus of the testis, the only predictor of successful treatment is the most developed region of the

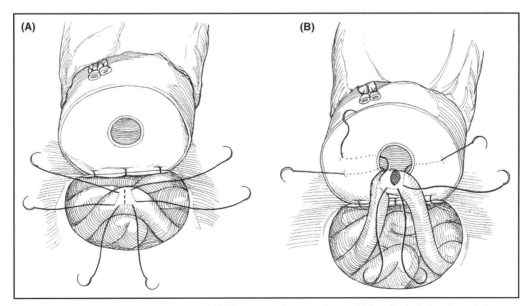

Figure 9 Vasoepididymostomy: triangulation technique. (**A**) Placement of sutures into epididymal tubule for triangulation anastomosis during vasoepididymostomy (line of incision in tubule is shown as interrupted line). (**B**) Mucosal suture placement into vas deferens for triangulation technique of vasoepididymostomy.

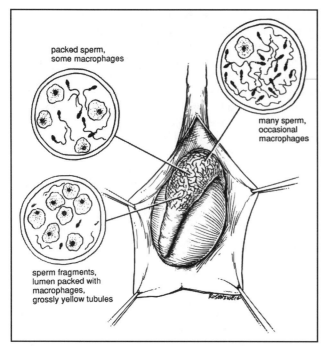

packed sperm,
some macrophages

many sperm,
occasional
macrophages

sperm fragments,
lumen packed with
macrophages,
grossly yellow tubules

Figure 10 The content of epididymal fluid from different levels of the epididymis in men with obstructive azoospermia is shown.

testis, not the predominant pattern of testicular histology, overall testicular volume, or FSH level. These observations suggest that nearly all cases of male factor infertility can potentially be treated.

Intracytoplasmic Sperm Injection

Without question, the most significant advance in the treatment of male infertility has been the technique of ICSI. The procedure involves the deposition of a single sperm directly into the oocyte cytoplasm with a micropipette. The advantage of this technique is that it bypasses all oocyte barriers so that even severely abnormal spermatozoa can successfully fertilize, as long as the spermatozoon is viable. To date, ICSI has been applied successfully to both obstructive and NOA with fresh and thawed spermatozoa obtained from the epididymis and testis.

Background: Etiology of Azoospermia

Evaluation of the type of azoospermia (obstructive vs. nonobstructive) may superficially seem irrelevant, since sperm can usually be retrieved for ICSI. The definition of etiology, however, is critical for the direction of genetic testing of male and female partners, as well as for the consideration of medical conditions associated with azoospermia. In men with severely impaired sperm production, the presence of osteoporosis or osteopenia should be considered, with testis tumors occasionally detected; on the other hand, many men with obstructive azoospermia due to congenital unilateral absence of the vas deferens present with renal agenesis. Genetic anomalies that have been defined

presently include partial deletions of the Y-chromosome and other karyotypic abnormalities for men with NOA, whereas men with obstructive azoospermia may be carriers of cystic fibrosis gene defects. The presence of some of these abnormalities may be of life-threatening importance to the azoospermic man, for whom infertility may well be the only initial symptom. Genetic anomalies may provide indications for preimplantation genetic diagnoses in order to avoid affecting offspring produced via infertility treatment. (For further information on this topic, please refer to Chapter 27.)

Techniques for Sperm Retrieval

The following is a summary of the various sperm retrieval techniques best suited for obstructive azoospermia versus NOA.

Obstructive Azoospermia
Microsurgical Epididymal Sperm Aspiration
In cases of unreconstructable reproductive tract obstruction, including cases of congenital bilateral absence of the vas deferens or when the patient chooses not to have surgical reconstruction, epididymal sperm can be aspirated as an isolated surgical procedure. When performed as an operative microsurgical procedure, these techniques are referred to as microsurgical epididymal sperm aspiration (MESA).

To avoid contamination of sperm with blood cells during aspiration, the technique of micropuncture of the epididymal tubule was developed (29). Briefly, single epididymal tubules can be identified under the operating microscope and individually aspirated with an atraumatic technique (Fig. 11). Sequential micropunctures can be performed until optimal sperm quality has been obtained. Puncture sites are closed or cauterized. Typically, over 100×10^6 sperm with good motility are retrieved using this approach. An alternative approach is to incise tubules and gather fluid after it flows out of the tubules. Because sperm in the epididymal fluid are so highly concentrated (roughly 1×10^6 sperm/μL), only microliters of fluid need to be retrieved. Thus, MESA provides for more than adequate numbers of sperm for immediate use with ICSI, as well as for cryopreservation. MESA can be performed with local or general anesthesia.

Percutaneous Epididymal Sperm Aspiration
In addition to microsurgical techniques, percutaneous procedures are part of the armamentarium currently available for sperm retrieval. These procedures have many advantages: they can be performed without surgical scrotal exploration, can be repeated easily and at low cost, and do not require an operating microscope or expertise in microsurgery. Percutaneous epididymal sperm aspiration can be performed under local or general anesthesia. After induction of anesthesia, the testis is stabilized and the epididymis is held between the surgeon's thumb and forefinger. A butterfly needle

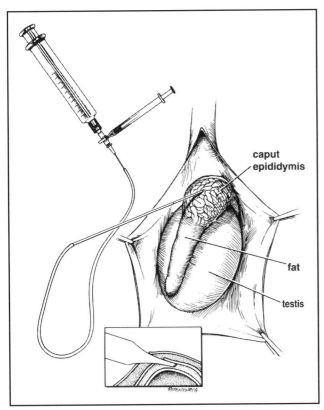

Figure 11 Micropuncture apparatus for epididymal sperm retrieval is shown. The sharpened tip of a micropuncture pipet is shown entering an epididymal tubule through the epididymal tunic.

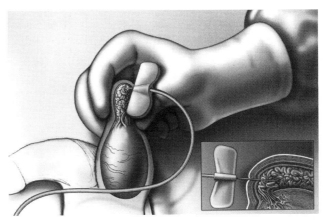

Figure 12 Technique for percutaneous epididymal sperm aspiration.

attached to a 20-mL syringe is inserted into the caput epididymis and withdrawn gently until fluid can be seen entering the tubing of the aspiration set (Fig. 12). The procedure is repeated until adequate amounts of epididymal fluid are retrieved. If no sperm are retrieved, as occurs in at least 20% of sperm retrieval attempts, then it is necessary to proceed with MESA, testis biopsy, or testicular aspiration.

Percutaneous Testicular Sperm Aspiration

As mentioned above, it was previously thought that sperm retrieved from the testis were incapable of fertilization. It is now well established, however, that testicular sperm can be used effectively with ICSI, although the cytogenetic abnormality rate is higher with testicular sperm than with epididymal or ejaculated sperm. Although testicular sperm retrieval has been reported in cases of obstructive azoospermia after failure of epididymal aspiration attempts, the primary indication for open testicular sperm retrieval today should be for sperm acquisition in NOA.

Testicular sperm can be recovered using an FNA, a percutaneous biopsy, or an open technique. The technique of percutaneous FNA of the testis was initially described as a diagnostic procedure in azoospermic men (29). In this procedure, the testis is stabilized between the surgeon's thumb and forefinger and a needle is inserted along the long axis of the testis (Fig. 13). The needle is then slightly withdrawn and

redirected in order to disrupt the testicular architecture. The procedure is repeated until adequate testicular material has been aspirated. A Franzen needle holder can be used to provide negative pressure for needle aspiration.

Percutaneous Testicular Biopsy

The technique of percutaneous biopsy of the testis has also been described (29). A 14-gauge biopsy gun with a short (1 cm) excursion is used to retrieve testicular tissue (Fig. 14). Anesthesia is achieved with a spermatic cord block, and multiple biopsies can be obtained through a single entry site. The patient may be prepared for this procedure by the topical application of local anesthetic such as EMLA cream (lidocaine 2.5% and prilocaine 2.5%, manufactured by Astra-Zeneca Pharmaceuticals, Worcester, Massachusetts, U.S.A.). The core needle provides better sperm yield than the FNA technique, and is relatively simple to use.

Testicular Sperm Extraction

Testicular sperm retrieval using an open biopsy technique (TESE) is rarely, if ever, indicated for men with obstructive azoospermia. The procedure is more

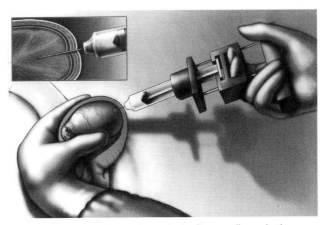

Figure 13 Technique for testicular fine needle aspiration.

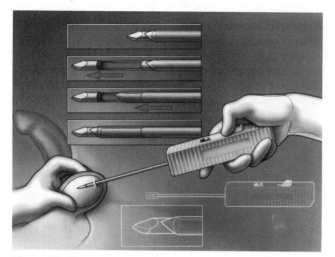

Figure 14 Percutaneous testis biopsy with a 14-gauge automatic biopsy gun.

invasive, is not needed in obstructive azoospermia to allow sperm retrieval, and carries higher risks than alternative open or percutaneous procedures. If an open procedure is performed, in the authors' experience, over 99% (184/185) of men with obstructive azoospermia will have approximately 100×10^6 sperm retrieved from the epididymis with MESA (30). Sperm retrieval from the epididymis is far more efficient than testicular biopsy extraction in that it provides better sperm yield and motility when compared to that obtained with TESE in obstructive azoospermia. MESA provides sperm quantities sufficient for a virtually unlimited number of ICSI attempts. If testicular sperm retrieval is planned because of patient preference or if microsurgical expertise is not available, then PercBiopsy is the recommended approach.

Nonobstructive Azoospermia

Testicular access is required for sperm retrieval in NOA since pockets of sperm production are limited and evaluation of large areas of the testis or multiple biopsies are usually needed to retrieve sperm. Although testicular FNA has been used to retrieve spermatozoa in azoospermic men, documentation of its effectiveness is lacking for men with NOA. Two controlled studies (31,32) have shown that open biopsy produces a substantially higher yield of sperm in men with NOA. An alternative approach is to perform testis biopsies with intentional cryopreservation. This approach may lead to unnecessary biopsies, however, since up to 35% of "azoospermic" men will have sperm found with careful examination of the ejaculate on the day of planned simultaneous TESE–ICSI. Additionally, sperm "retrieved" from the testis and frozen may not survive the freeze–thaw process in NOA. Further, multiple biopsies may be needed to retrieve sperm in men with NOA, thus requiring a careful, simultaneous biopsy-by-biopsy analysis by an experienced embryologist.

Microsurgical TESE

Microsurgical TESE offers the advantages of improved yield of spermatozoa per biopsy, less tissue removal (and thus less risk of testicle loss), and improved identification of blood vessels within the testicle, resulting in the minimization of the risk of vascular injury and loss of remaining functional areas of the testis.

On the day of oocyte retrieval, scrotal exploration is performed through a median raphe incision under local or general anesthesia. Sperm are retrieved using an open testicular biopsy technique. In order to avoid undue injury to the testis, all testicular vessels are first identified; delivery of the testis is routinely performed to prevent injury to the epididymis.

Testicular blood vessels under the tunica albuginea are identified with 6 to 8× optical magnification. An avascular region near the midportion of the medial, lateral, or anterior surface of the testis is chosen, and a generous incision in the tunica albuginea is created with a 15° ultrasharp knife, avoiding any capsular testicular vessels. With this approach, direct visualization of large areas of the testis can be achieved, which allows for either large sample biopsies or microdissection (Fig. 15). Because the incision is directed at an avascular region, the sperm retrieval procedure is less traumatic than multiple "blind" biopsies. The testis is opened widely to allow direct examination of all areas of testicular parenchyma. Dissection between the

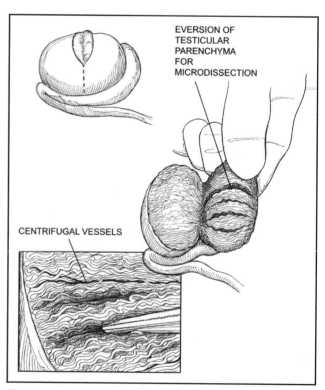

Figure 15 Incision in the tunica albuginea for wide exposure of seminiferous tubules in preparation for microdissection testicular sperm extraction with exposure of the parenchyma and dissection between septae of the testis.

tubules is also needed to view tubules that are not exposed with the initial approach. The recent microdissection technique applied by the authors allows the removal of tiny (2–3 mm; 3–5 mg) testicular tissue with improved sperm yield. The tubules containing sperm can often be identified visually under an operating microscope after opening the testis, when approximately 20× magnification is used to assist the biopsies. The tubules containing sperm production are directly identified based on their large size and white color. If all tubules appear uniform at high-power magnification, then dissection is performed to allow access to other regions of the testis. Finally, if no sperm are seen in microdissected samples, a limited number of larger random biopsies are performed, avoiding testicular vessels between the septae that separate seminiferous tubules.

The excised testicular biopsy specimen is placed in human tubal fluid (HTF) culture medium supplemented with 6% Plasmanate. Isolation of individual tubules from the mass of coiled testicular tissue is achieved by initial dispersal of the testis biopsy specimen with two sterile glass slides, stretching the testicular parenchyma to isolate individual seminiferous tubules. Subsequently, mechanical disruption of the tubules is accomplished by mincing the extended tubules with sterile scissors in HTF/Plasmanate medium. Additional dispersion of tubules is achieved by passing the suspension of testicular tissue through a 24-gauge angiocatheter. For minimal tissue specimens, little dissection is performed in the operating room, since the tissue sample is so small and opening of the individual tubules may need to be done in the embryology laboratory immediately prior to ICSI.

Intraoperatively, a "wet preparation" of the suspension is examined under phase contrast microscopy at 200× power. If no spermatozoa are seen, then (*i*) additional samples of tissue are obtained through the same tunical incision, (*ii*) the remainder of the testis is examined by evaluating the exposed regions of testicular tissue, (*iii*) exposure of deeper tubules is effected by dissecting between the septae and everting the testicular tissue, and (*iv*) examination of the contralateral testis is then performed, if no sperm have been found. After dispersal, a member of the in vitro fertilization (IVF) laboratory in the operating room performs immediate intraoperative evaluation of each specimen at 200× magnification using a phase contrast microscope. The sperm extraction process is complete when sperm are reliably identified in the wet preparation of a biopsy specimen. Otherwise, sperm extraction attempts cease when all areas of the testis have been examined. Care must be taken to preserve vessels between and within the septae of the testis that contain the tubules. At no time should additional incisions be made that could adversely affect the blood supply to the testis. Subsequent processing of the testicular tissue suspension, including mechanical disruption and/or additional enzymatic digestion of the specimens, is

performed in the IVF laboratory. Aliquots of tissue are also processed for cryopreservation.

Summary

Sperm retrieval for use with the advanced form of assisted reproduction, ICSI, is now possible for many men with NOA. Men with azoospermia may have unique genetic or associated urogenital defects that should be evaluated prior to an attempt at conception. In obstructive azoospermia, several options exist to allow for sperm retrieval rates approaching 100%. In NOA, TESE is required and sperm retrieval is less certain. At The New York Hospital-Cornell Medical Center, 59% of couples have had sperm retrieved from the testis with TESE, and 58% of couples achieved a clinical pregnancy using testicular sperm in NOA. Since some couples will not have sperm retrieved with TESE, the use of frozen donor spermatozoa as backup should be discussed with couples prior to simultaneous TESE–ICSI attempts.

☐ EJACULATORY DUCT OBSTRUCTION

Ejaculatory duct obstruction may contribute to male infertility. Men with bilateral complete ejaculatory duct obstruction will typically present with low-volume, fructose-negative, and acidic semen devoid of sperm. Men with partial ejaculatory duct obstruction may have a more variable presentation of semen parameters. In the authors' experience, up to 4.4% of infertile men will have ultrasonographic findings suggestive of ejaculatory duct obstruction.

Ejaculatory duct obstruction is a treatable abnormality that can affect semen parameters and cause male infertility. Unfortunately, safe treatment for partial ejaculatory duct obstruction is not always possible. Transurethral resection for partial obstruction may result in the reflux of urine into the vas deferens, causing subsequent epididymitis.

Indications for evaluation, treatment approaches, and the results of therapy for ejaculatory duct obstruction are presented here. Together, both partial and complete ejaculatory duct obstruction are treatable abnormalities that affect a significant proportion of patients with male factor infertility. (For further information on ejaculatory duct obstruction, please refer to Chapter 18.)

Indications for Evaluation

Ejaculatory duct obstruction may occur because of congenital maldevelopment, genitourinary infections, prostatic disease, or prior pelvic surgery. Obstructed patients may report hematospermia, pain on or after ejaculation in the prostatic region that may radiate to the testes, a sudden change in ejaculate volume, tenesmus and other difficulty with bowel movements, or even no symptoms at all. A prior history of prostatic surgery, urethral instrumentation, rectal surgery, or prostatic disease should be sought. Episodes of urinary tract infections or penile discharge may increase the risk of ejaculatory duct or epididymal obstruction. Congenital maldevelopment of variable lengths of the ejaculatory ducts can occur. Since ejaculatory duct obstruction is associated with congenital absence of the vas deferens, a condition that is nonsurgically correctable, it is essential to confirm that the vasa are palpable bilaterally before proceeding with further evaluation of possible ejaculatory duct obstruction.

Complete Ejaculatory Duct Obstruction

Bilateral complete ejaculatory duct obstruction results in only prostatic fluid contributing to the ejaculate. The prostatic contribution has 0.5 to 10.0 cc of volume with a watery appearance and a typical pH of 6.5. Both the fructose and the coagulum contained in the ejaculate are produced by the seminal vesicles. In the presence of bilateral ejaculatory duct obstruction, the ejaculate will lack sperm, coagulum, and fructose. Men with palpable vasa and low-volume azoospermia with an acidic semen specimen should be evaluated for the presence of complete bilateral ejaculatory duct obstruction.

Partial Ejaculatory Duct Obstruction

The clinical presentation of partial ejaculatory duct obstruction is highly variable. Therefore, the indications for evaluation of partial ejaculatory duct obstruction are controversial. Previously published indications for evaluation (33) include low ejaculate volume (less than 1.5 cc), very poor sperm motility (less than 30%), or oligospermia (less than 20×10^6 sperm/cc) in the presence of normal testicular volume (greater than 18 cc). Abnormal serum testosterone levels and a lack of response to known, effective treatments such as varicocelectomy are also factors that should prompt evaluation. Infertile men who fail to respond with an improvement in semen parameters after varicocelectomy, as well as those with low ejaculate volume, and impaired motility or oligospermia in the presence of normal testicular volume and serum testosterone level (greater than 350 ng/dL) should be evaluated for partial ejaculatory duct obstruction.

Evaluation for Ejaculatory Duct Obstruction

The level of ejaculatory duct obstruction can be evaluated with high-resolution TRUS, vasography, or transrectal injection of the seminal vesicles with contrast media. In most cases, TRUS may be considered a simple, minimally involved procedure to image the prostate, ejaculatory ducts, seminal vesicles, and vas deferens in an effort to detect the presence and site of ejaculatory duct obstruction. (For further information on TRUS and other imaging modalities, please refer to Chapter 28.)

The seminal vesicles are located lateral to the vasal ampullae. In typically symmetrical, paired organs, multiple attempts have been made to characterize the normal TRUS appearance of seminal vesicles. Carter et al. (34) recommended that only the greatest length on sagittal images and the anteroposterior diameter were useful in describing seminal vesicle size. Seminal vesicles have been arbitrarily defined as enlarged when the anteroposterior dimension exceeds 1.5 cm. Volumetric criteria have also been proposed, but Jarow (35) found that none of these criteria were useful in distinguishing a population of fertile from infertile men. Sufficient data do not currently exist to identify men with ejaculatory duct obstruction based on TRUS evaluation of the seminal vesicles alone. More recent studies by Jarow et al. (36) have suggested that evaluation of an aspirated specimen from the seminal vesicles provides greater insight into the presence or absence of obstruction: Men who have ejaculated within 24 hours should have less than 3 sperm/hpf in the seminal vesicle fluid in contrast to men with ejaculatory duct obstruction, who have many sperm in the seminal vesicle fluid. This diagnostic procedure may be combined with injection of radiographic or visual dye and transurethral resection or dilation of the ejaculatory ducts to effect successful treatment of obstruction.

Vasal segments can be visualized by TRUS behind the bladder to their junction with the seminal vesicles. Dilation of the vasa, defined by the presence of intraluminal anechoic fluid or hyperechoic material, strongly suggests dysfunction or obstruction of the vas. Vasal dilation may be present in neurogenic abnormalities of ejaculation such as in men with diabetes or spinal cord injury, as well as obstruction to the vas deferens. Vasal obstruction is typically untreatable because the obstruction is outside of the prostate and unresectable. Therefore, vasal dilation in the presence of ejaculatory duct dilation may support a diagnosis of ejaculatory duct obstruction and should be sought. The presence of vasal dilation without ejaculatory duct obstruction, however, does not support the diagnosis of a treatable obstruction.

Treatment of Ejaculatory Duct Obstruction

The standard treatment of ejaculatory duct obstruction involves transurethral resection of the ejaculatory ducts. Prior to transurethral resection of presumed ejaculatory duct obstruction in an azoospermic man, it is important to document sperm production. This may be provided with a formal testis biopsy and confirmatory wet prep evaluation; however, less-invasive approaches described below are equally effective when ejaculatory duct obstruction exists in the absence of a Mullerian duct cyst. Transurethral resection has been described with (*i*) no adjunctive guides for identification of the ejaculatory ducts, (*ii*) injection of dye into the seminal vesicles prior to resection, (*iii*) concomitant TRUS, (*iv*) simultaneous vasotomy and vasography (dilute methylene blue), or (*v*) after injection of the seminal vesicles with radiographic contrast and methylene blue or indigo carmine dye. Clearly, vasography is the most involved procedure, requiring microsurgical closure of the vasotomy sites.

Transurethral Resection

The candidate for treatment of presumed ejaculatory duct obstruction with transurethral resection is brought to the operating room and given broad-spectrum antibiotics. TRUS is performed and the seminal vesicles aspirated with a long 18-gauge needle. The aspirate is examined using a phase contrast microscope. If many sperm (greater than 3/hpf) are seen in the aspirate, then a mixture of radiographic contrast tinged with methylene blue is injected into the seminal vesicles under TRUS control. A radiograph may be taken, preferably with an air-filled Foley balloon in the bladder, to help identify the bladder neck and avoid spillage of contrast into the bladder. The patient is placed on the operating table either in the dorsal lithotomy position or in a position that enables the ability to adduct the patient's legs. As an alternative to this approach, vasotomies may be performed under the operating microscope. Vasal fluid is sampled by 2Fr catheters placed well into the vasa. Cystoscopy is performed and the lateral side of the verumontanum resected on the side(s) of the obstruction. If a Mullerian cyst is present in the midline, then further resection is performed in

the midline of the prostate proximal to the verumontanum to completely unroof the cyst. If no Mullerian cyst is present, then the standard treatment is to resect the obstructed ejaculatory duct(s) until a dilated region of the ejaculatory duct is seen, or free flow of dye into the urethra is seen with injection of dye through the vas (Fig. 16). Resection along the ejaculatory duct is a hazardous procedure if the obstruction is proximal, the ejaculatory duct cannot be visualized, or the surgeon is inexperienced with the procedure. Because the typical infertility patient is young and has a small prostate, therefore, resection is carried out very close to the rectum, sphincter, and bladder neck. Some surgeons may be more comfortable with an O'Connor sheath in the rectum to digitally assess the proximity of resection to the rectum as well as having dye injectable through the vas deferens to guide resection. Hemostasis is obtained with minimal cautery to avoid structuring the newly opened ejaculatory ducts.

Balloon Dilatation

An alternative approach is to perform a minimum of resection until direct access to the ducts is obtained. For occasional patients, no resection is necessary prior to transurethral dilation of the ejaculatory ducts. Most patients, however, will require at least partial resection of the verumontanum prior to dilation. The obstructed ejaculatory duct(s) are cannulated and dilated to 4 mm. A catheter that is 4 mm wide (dilated width) and 2 cm long is used for transurethral dilation. The presence of a narrow silicone or Teflon leader on the balloon dilation catheter facilitates intubation of the ejaculatory duct. Prior to dilation, the balloon catheter is less than 0.04 in. in diameter and is able to be passed through most ejaculatory duct strictures (Fig. 17). Long-term follow-up with dilation is necessary before this technique can be considered the standard approach to replace transurethral resection of obstructed ejaculatory ducts.

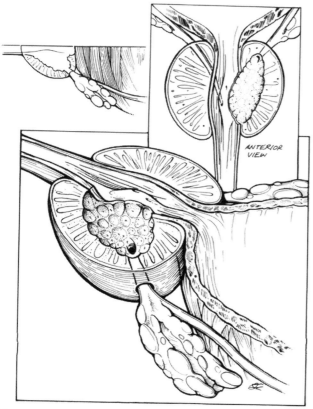

Figure 16   Results of standard technique for resection of obstructed ejaculatory ducts. Note the large defect in the prostatic fossa that may allow pooling of urine in the prostatic fossa and contamination of the ejaculate with urine.

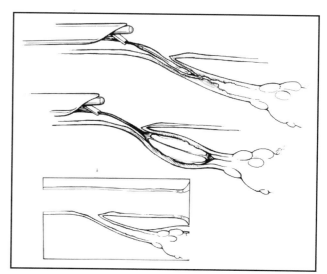

Figure 17   Schematic depiction of technique for balloon dilation of ejaculatory duct strictures.

When free flow of fluid through the vasotomy is obtained after resection or dilation, the procedure is terminated and a 22Fr urethral catheter with a 30 cc balloon is carefully placed in the bladder with a mandarin stylet. Blind passage of catheter should be avoided as it can easily enter a large Mullerian cyst, resulting in a large false passage and undermining of the bladder neck. The vasotomy sites are closed with 10-0 and 9-0 monofilament nylon as typically performed in a two-layer vasovasostomy. The catheter can be removed the next morning and the patient discharged from the hospital.

Results of Treatment of Ejaculatory Duct Obstruction

Most published series of treatment of ejaculatory duct obstruction are small. Several publications in the early 1990s suggested than an increased number of cases of ejaculatory duct obstruction can be found with application of TRUS to the infertile male (37–41). Overall, only about one half of all patients who undergo attempted surgical treatment for ejaculatory duct obstruction will have sperm appear in the ejaculate postoperatively; of these, only one half of those patients who have a patent reconstruction will contribute to a pregnancy, or a quarter of all men who undergo treatment. These results are far less successful than those achieved after reconstruction of other reproductive tract obstructions such as microsurgical vasovasostomy. For the 50% of men who have no sperm in the ejaculate postoperatively, the questions that need to be answered are: (i) is the treated site of obstruction patent and (ii) are sperm present in the vas proximal to the treated site of obstruction? The high rate of failure of patency achievement reinforces the importance of documenting the presence of sperm in the seminal vesicles by aspiration, or within the vas deferens with a vasotomy at the time of reconstruction. Given the overall low success rate of treatment, cryopreservation of sperm retrieved at the time of reconstructive surgery for ejaculatory duct obstruction is suggested.

Additional reasons for failure to achieve pregnancy after relief of ejaculatory duct obstruction may relate to the anatomical effects of transurethral resection of the ejaculatory ducts. Resection of the prostate to reach the ejaculatory ducts will necessarily result in an increased diameter of the prostatic urethra. The prostatic urethra will fill with urine between ejaculations. Emission of fluid from the seminal vesicles, prostate, and vas deferens will then mix with urine in the prostatic fossa, with urine contaminating the ejaculate. Many men will note a yellow color and urinary odor to the ejaculate after transurethral resection of the ejaculatory ducts. Men with these findings after surgery for ejaculatory duct obstruction should be instructed to alkalinize the urine with Poly-citra (potassium citrate, 5 cc orally, taken eight hours and two hours prior to producing a specimen; manufactured by Alza Pharmaceuticals, Mountain View, California, U.S.A.).

In addition, men should dilute the urine as much as possible to minimize any adverse effects of high osmolarity on sperm function. This is achieved by drinking one liter of water or other liquid during the hour prior to producing a semen specimen, and urinating just prior to producing the specimen.

Complications of ejaculatory duct resection may be severe and significant. Proper attention to resection of only the ejaculatory ducts can avoid the most significant side effects. Complications can occur because of the small prostate in younger infertility patients and the relatively deep resection necessary to reach some obstructions. Most complications, such as a rectourethral fistula and incontinence due to sphincteric injury, are avoided by careful delineation of the ejaculatory ducts during the resection. If the surgeon is able to follow the course of the ejaculatory ducts during resection, then inadvertent injury to the rectum and other normal organs is highly unlikely.

Unfortunately, deep resection may affect ejaculatory function, allowing retrograde ejaculation due to undermining of, or direct injury to, the bladder neck. Scarring at the bladder neck may cause urinary (bladder neck) obstruction from contractures. Impairment of sperm quality may occur because of excessive coagulation near the ejaculatory ducts, causing scarring and obstruction of these narrow structures. High (proximal) obstructions may also restrict when the prostatic fossa heals and the resected ejaculatory duct is sequestered above the prostatic fossa, if the site of resection was above and posterior to the bladder neck.

Normally, reflux of urine from the urethra into the ejaculatory ducts during voiding is prevented by the angle of entry of the ejaculatory ducts into the verumontanum and urethra. After resection of the ejaculatory ducts and prostate, this anatomical relationship is destroyed, and reflux of urine up the vasa is possible during micturition. Clinically, urinary reflux after transurethral resection of the ejaculatory ducts is detectable with voiding cystourethrography and may be associated with a deterioration in semen parameters. Balloon dilation appears to have a lower rate of urinary contamination of the ejaculate after treatment of ejaculatory duct obstruction. Similarly, an improvement in semen parameters occurs after balloon dilation when compared to transurethral resection alone.

The frequency of complete bilateral ejaculatory duct obstruction is low. The benefits of treatment for men with partial ejaculatory duct obstruction are not always certain and must be balanced against the potential complications of treatment such as urinary reflux. Although balloon dilation for ejaculatory duct obstruction apparently has lower complication rates, long-term follow-up of postprocedural success rates is needed.

☐ ORCHIOPEXY

The incidence of undescended testes (UDT) at birth is approximately 3%, and 15% of these are bilateral (42).

Spontaneous descent may occur up to one year of age, when the incidence of UDT falls to 0.8%. It is well known that cryptorchidism is associated with a high incidence of infertility, even when it is unilateral. This is presumably due to an elevation in scrotal temperature, as an adverse effect of higher temperature on spermatogenesis for infertile adult males with retractile or UDT has been suggested (43). It is thought that orchiopexy may restore spermatogenesis, and thus fertility potential may be restored by early intervention, preferably around one year of age. Therefore, orchiopexy may improve spermatogenic function and sperm counts for some infertile men with retractile or UDT, albeit not as adults. (For further information on cryptorchidism, please refer to Chapter 13.)

Surgery to correct retractile or UDT requires relocation of the testes to the scrotum without tension. This requires testis localization, mobilization, cord dissection, and isolation of the patent processus vaginalis. Both inguinal and scrotal approaches can be used to effect the correction of these conditions.

Inguinal Approach

An initial inguinal approach is needed for all testes that are on tension when they are brought into the scrotum on initial examination, as well as those testes that cannot be brought into the scrotum at all on physical examination. In cases where the testis cannot be secured in the scrotum by an inguinal approach alone, the testis must be secured in the scrotum with a combined inguinal and scrotal approach.

Retractile Testes

Retractile testes may be placed in the scrotum using an inguinal incision with release of all external spermatic vessels and muscles (specifically, the cremasteric musculature). To effect this release, a subinguinal incision is fashioned and the spermatic cord is isolated over the pubis. The spermatic cord is delivered and the external

spermatic fascia is opened. Identification and preservation of the vas deferens and its associated paired arteries and lymphatics are carried out, followed by division of all external spermatic structures. The cremaster muscles are further dissected off of the exposed internal spermatic fascia until a dependent position is secured for the testis (Fig. 18). In rare cases, it may be necessary to secure the testis in a subdartos scrotal pouch using a scrotal approach.

Undescended Testes

Approach to the UDT should be made using an inguinal incision. The spermatic cord should be isolated above the testis. To isolate the cord, the external spermatic attachments to the cord should be divided, starting at the lateral attachments to the cord. Care should be taken at all times to avoid entering the internal spermatic fascia that surrounds the testicular vessels, which will prevent inadvertent injury to the blood supply to the testis. The testis is progressively mobilized until it can be brought without tension into the scrotum. The testis is secured in the scrotum within a subdartos pouch.

Scrotal Approach

A scrotal approach is used for the unusual cases of testes that are pushed back up into the subcutaneous tissues of the low inguinal region by a hyperactive scrotum that can result from overactive dartos contractions. In addition, a scrotal approach may augment inguinal dissection of UDT and help to secure a dependent position of the testes within the scrotum.

The incision for the creation of a subdartos pouch is made transversely over a dependent portion of the scrotum. The dartos muscle is dissected off of the scrotal skin to create an area of adequate volume that will comfortably hold the testis and epididymis. Care must be taken to create this pouch in a dependent portion of the scrotum, remaining in the relatively avascular plane between skin and dartos muscle. The testis is then brought through a small opening in the dartos muscles and arranged comfortably in the subdartos pouch. If there is any tension whatsoever on the scrotal skin, a nylon suture may be placed through the inferior medial or lateral tunica albuginea that is brought out through the dependent scrotal skin and tied over a cotton pledget or Kitner dissector. The pledget is left in place for 10 days to two weeks, and then removed with the entire nylon suture. Closure is carried out in two layers, subcutaneous and skin level, using absorbable synthetic sutures to avoid the risk of the testis eviscerating through the incision.

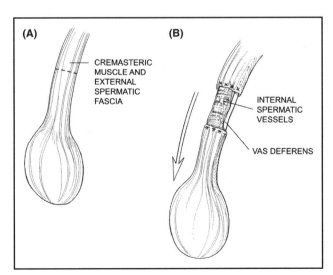

Figure 18 Release of external spermatic (cremasteric) musculature during inguinal approach to orchiopexy for retractile testes in the adult.

☐ TREATMENT CHOICE: COST-EFFECTIVENESS CONSIDERATIONS

With the introduction of advanced reproductive technologies, the options for the specific treatment of male infertility, or even bypassing the problem entirely using ICSI, now exist. For azoospermic men, sperm retrieval with ICSI is possible. Several studies (18,44,45) have attempted to compare these treatments using a cost-effectiveness analysis that examines cost per success rate (cost per infant delivery). For men with vasectomy-associated infertility, the chance of pregnancy and the cost-per-delivery were significantly higher for vasectomy reversal when compared with sperm retrieval-ICSI.

In order to evaluate the relative cost-effectiveness of varicocelectomy versus ICSI for varicocele-associated infertility, the authors have created a model for U.S. costs and expected results from controlled series of varicocelectomy, as well as ICSI studies published in the United States (18). In this study, the overall expected U.S. delivery rate at the best centers was 28% per attempt, whereas a 30% delivery rate was obtained after surgical varicocelectomy alone. The cost-per-delivery (taking into account all costs of treatment, including the costs of complications of varicocelectomy or ICSI) was over $89,000 for ICSI, but only $26,268 after varicocelectomy. The dramatic cost-effectiveness of varicocelectomy must be considered when selecting potential treatment options during the initial management of varicocele-associated infertility.

There are certain circumstances in which immediate treatment with assisted reproduction may be a better alternative than varicocelectomy. If significant female factors are present, including advanced maternal age that could adversely affect the chances of natural pregnancy occurring after varicocelectomy, then ICSI may be the best initial treatment. For younger couples, however, especially in the case of men who present with a large clinical varicocele, the benefits of varicocelectomy are compelling. Varicocele repair in this situation may allow a young couple a better chance to have several children at their own pace, with lower risks involved than with assisted reproduction.

□ CONCLUSION

Surgical treatment can be an effective approach for the diagnosis and treatment of the infertile male. Accurate identification of the cause of infertility and microsurgical approaches to its management will often provide more effective treatment with lower morbidity. Appropriate training in microsurgery and overall experience with surgical techniques will produce the most effective treatment of the infertile man.

□ REFERENCES

1. Glina S, Soares JB, Nelson A Jr, et al. Testicular histopathological diagnosis as a predictive factor for retrieving spermatozoa for ICSI in non-obstructive azoospermic patients. International Braz J Urol 2005; 131(4):338–341.

2. Hotchkiss RS. Testicular biopsy in the diagnosis and treatment of sterility in the male. Bull N Y Acad Med 1942; 18:600–605.

3. Charney CW. Testicular biopsy. Its value in male sterility. JAMA 1940; 115:1429.

4. Silber SJ, Rodriguez-Rigau LJ. Quantitative analysis of testicle biopsy: determination of partial obstruction and prediction of sperm count after surgery for obstruction. Fertil Steril 1981; 36(4):480–485.

5. Choyke PL, Bluth EI, Bush WH Jr, et al. (Expert Panel on Urologic Imaging. Staging of testicular malignancy). [online publication]. Reston (VA): American College of Radiology (ACR); 2005.

6. Jow WW, Steckel J, Schlegel PN, et al. Motile sperm in human testis biopsy specimens. J Androl 1993; 14(3): 194–198.

7. Coburn M, Wheeler T, Lipshultz LI. Testicular biopsy. Its use and limitations. Urol Clin North Am 1987; 14(3):551–561.

8. Moreira SG Jr, Lipshultz LI. Management of male infertility. Scientific World Journal 2004; 4:214–248.

9. World Health Organization. The influence of varicocele on parameters of fertility in a large group of men presenting to infertility clinics. Fertil Steril 1992; 57(6):1289.

10. Kass EJ, Freitas JE, Bour JB. Adolescent varicocele: objective indications for treatment. J Urol 1989; 142(2 Pt 2):579–582.

11. Palomo A. Radical cure of varicocele by a new technique: preliminary report. J Urol 1989; 61:604-607.

12. Cayan S, Acar D, Ulger S, et al. Adolescent varicocele repair: long-term results and comparison of surgical techniques according to optical magnification use in 100 cases at a single university hospital. J Urol 2005; 174(5):2003–2006; discussion 2006–2007.

13. Goldstein M, Gilbert BR, Dicker AP, et al. Microsurgical inguinal varicocelectomy with delivery of the testis: an artery and lymphatic sparing technique. J Urol 1992; 148(6):1808–1811.

14. Matthews GJ, Matthews ED, Goldstein M. Induction of spermatogenesis and achievement of pregnancy after microsurgical varicocelectomy in men with azoospermia and severe oligoasthenospermia. Fertil Steril 1998; 70(1):71–75.

15. Marmar Jl, Kim Y. Subinguinal microsurgical varicocelectomy: a technical critique and statistical analysis of semen and pregnancy data. J Urol 1994; 152(4): 1127–1132.

16. Marmar JL, De Benedictis TJ, Praiss D. The management of varicoceles by microdissection of the spermatic cord at the external inguinal ring. Fertil Steril 1985; 43(4):583–588.

17. Schlegel PN, Goldstein M. Anatomical approach to varicocelectomy. Semin Urol 1992; 10(4):242–247.

18. Schlegel PN. Is assisted reproduction the optimal treatment for varicocele-associated male infertility? A cost-effectiveness analysis. Urology 1997; 49(1):83–90.

19. Grober ED, Chan PT, Zini A, Goldstein M. Microsurgical treatment of persistent or recurrent varicocele. Fertil Steril 2004; 82(3):718–722.

20. Watanabe M, Nagai A, Kusumi N, et al. Minimal invasiveness and effectivity of subinguinal microscopic varicocelectomy: a comparative study with retroperitoneal high and laparoscopic approaches. Int J Urol 2005; 12(10):892–898.

21. Su LM, Goldstein M, Schlegel PN. The effect of varicocelectomy on serum testosterone levels in infertile men with varicoceles. J Urol 1995; 154(5):1752–1755.

22. Schlegel PN, Girardi SK. Clinical review 87: in vitro fertilization for male factor infertility. J Clin Endocrinol Metab 1997; 82(3):709–716.

23. Jarow JP, Ogle SR, Eskew LA. Seminal improvement following repair of ultrasound detected subclinical varicoceles. J Urol 1996; 155(4):1287–1290.

24. Owen ER. Microsurgical vasovasostomy: a reliable vasectomy reversal. Aust N Z J Surg 1977; 47(3): 305–309.

25. Silber SJ. Microscopic technique for reversal of vasectomy. Surg Gynecol Obstet 1976; 143(4):631.

26. Chan PT, Goldstein M. Superior outcomes of microsurgical vasectomy reversal in men with the same female partners. Fertil Steril 2004; 81(5):1371–1374.

27. Amarin ZO, Obeidat BR. Patency following vasectomy reversal. Temporal and immunological considerations. Saudi Med J 2005; 26(8):1208–1211.

28. Schiff J, Chan P, Li PS, et al. Outcome and late failures compared in 4 techniques of microsurgical vasoepididymostomy in 153 consecutive men. J Urol 2005; 174(2):651–655; quiz 801.

29. Van Peperstraten A, Proctor ML, Johnson NP, et al. Techniques for surgical retrieval of sperm prior to ICSI for azoospermia. Cochrane Database Syst Rev 2006; 3: CD002807.

30. Schlegel PN, Berkeley AS, Goldstein M, et al. Epididymal micropuncture with in vitro fertilization and oocyte micromanipulation for the treatment of unreconstructable obstructive azoospermia. Fertil Steril 1994; 61(5): 895–901.

31. Schlegel PN, Palermo GD, Goldstein M, et al. Testicular sperm extraction with ICSI for non-obstructive azoospermia. Urology 1997; 49:435–440.

32. Kahraman S, Ozgur S, Altas C, et al. Fertility with testicular sperm extraction and intracytoplasmic sperm injection in non-obstructive azoospermic men. Hum Reprod 1994; 756–760.

33. Coppens L. Diagnosis and treatment of obstructive seminal vesicle pathology. Acta Urol Belg 1997; 65(2): 11–19.

34. Carter SS, Shinohara K, Lipshultz LI. Transrectal ultrasonography in disorders of the seminal vesicles and ejaculatory ducts. Urol Clin North Am 1989; 16(4): 773–790.

35. Jarow JP. Transrectal ultrasonography in the diagnosis and management of ejaculatory duct obstruction. J Androl 1996; 17(5):467–472.

36. Jarow JP. Diagnosis and management of ejaculatory duct obstruction. Zhonghua Nan Ke Xue 2002; 8(1): 10–17.

37. Colpi GM, Negri L, Nappi RE, et al. Is transrectal ultrasonography a reliable diagnostic approach in ejaculatory duct sub-obstruction? Hum Reprod 1997; 12(10): 2186–2191.

38. Jones TR, Zagoria RJ, Jarow JP. Transrectal US-guided seminal vesiculography. Radiology 1997; 205(1):276–278.

39. Cornud F, Belin X, Delafontaine D, et al. Imaging of obstructive azoospermia. Eur Radiol 1997; 7(7):1079–1085.

40. Kim ED, Lipshultz LI. Role of ultrasound in the assessment of male infertility. J Clin Ultrasound 1996; 24(8):437–453.

41. Ruiz Rubio JL, Fernandez Gonzalez I, Quijano Barroso P, et al. The value of transrectal ultrasonography in the diagnosis and treatment of partial obstruction of the seminal duct system. J Urol 1995; 153(2):435–436.

42. Leung AK, Robson WL. Current status of cryptorchidism. Adv Pediatr 2004; 51:351–377.

43. Hjollund NH, Storgaard L, Ernst E, et al. Impact of diurnal scrotal temperature on semen quality. Reprod Toxicol 2002; 16(3):215–221.

44. Karpman E, Williams DH, Lipshultz LI. IVF and ICSI in male infertility: update on outcomes, risks, and costs. Scientific World J 2005; 5:922–932.

45. Garceau L, Henderson J, Davis LJ, et al. Economic implications of assisted reproductive techniques: a systematic review. Hum Reprod 2002; 17(12):3090–3109.

34

Vasectomy and Vasectomy Reversal

Peter T. K. Chan

Department of Urology, McGill University Health Centre, Montreal, Quebec, Canada

Marc Goldstein

Cornell Institute for Reproductive Medicine, Department of Urology, New York-Presbyterian Hospital and Weill Medical College of Cornell University, New York, New York, U.S.A.

□ VASECTOMY

Vasectomy is a safe and effective method of permanent contraception (1). In the United States, it is employed by nearly 7% of all married couples and performed on approximately one-half million men per year—more than any other urological surgical procedures. Impressive as these numbers may seem, far fewer vasectomies are performed, than female sterilizations by tubal ligation worldwide (2); this is in spite of the fact that vasectomy is less expensive and associated with much less morbidity and mortality than tubal ligation. Some men fear pain and complications, whereas others falsely equate vasectomy with castration or loss of masculinity. Although vasectomy is conceptually a very simple procedure, its technical difficulty is reflected in the markedly increased incidence of postoperative complications in the hands of surgeons who perform relatively few vasectomies per year (3). Efforts to enhance the popularity of vasectomy have led the Chinese to develop refined methods of vasectomy that minimize trauma, pain, and complications.

Local Anesthesia for Vasectomy

Vasectomy can be safely performed as an outpatient procedure using local anesthetics. Poor local anesthetic technique can result in pain and hematoma formation. Valium 10 mg, given orally one hour before the procedure, relaxes the patient and his scrotum.

The vas deferens is separated from the spermatic cord vessels, manipulated to a superficial position under the scrotal skin, and firmly trapped between the middle finger, the index finger, and thumb of the left hand (Fig. 1). A 1 cm-diameter superficial skin wheal is raised using a 1.5 in., 25-gauge needle, and 1% plain lidocaine (without epinephrine). The needle is then advanced within the perivasal sheath toward the external inguinal ring, and 2 to 5 mL of lidocaine is injected around the vas without moving the needle in and out (Fig. 2). This produces a vasal nerve block (4) and minimizes edema at the actual vasectomy site. The original

skin wheal is pinched to reduce local edema. The relatively large amount of anesthetic used assures a complete block and is well below the limits of toxicity. Injection away from the vasectomy site into the perivasal sheath prevents interference with exposure due to local edema. Avoidance of multiple punctures and excess needle movement minimizes the risk of hematoma. The site of the needle puncture hole is indicated with a marking pen so that the anesthetized area can be readily reidentified.

Conventional Incisional Techniques of Vasectomy

With the vas mobilized to a superficial position under the scrotal skin, two 1 cm bilateral transverse incisions or a single median raphe incision are carried down through the vas sheath until the bare vas is exposed (Fig. 3) and delivered. The deferential artery, veins, and accompanying nerves are dissected free of the vas and spared. A small segment is removed and the ends occluded using one of the techniques described later in this section. Suture closure of the scrotal wounds is optional. Leaving the small incisions open helps prevent hematoma formation. The wound seals itself in 24 hours. Fluff gauze dressings are held in place by a snug-fitting athletic supporter.

No-Scalpel Vasectomy

An elegant method for gaining access to the vas deferens though a single tiny puncture hole was developed in China in 1974 (5) and introduced to the United States in 1985 (4). This method eliminates the use of the scalpel, results in fewer hematomas and infections, and leaves a much smaller wound than conventional methods of accessing the vas deferens for vasectomy (6).

The vas deferens is fixed under the median raphe, and vasal nerve block is performed as described previously. After both vasa have been anesthetized, the right vas is again fixed under the previously marked needle puncture site, with the left hand, using the three-finger method. The ring-tipped fixation clamp (Fig. 4) is grasped with the right hand and opened

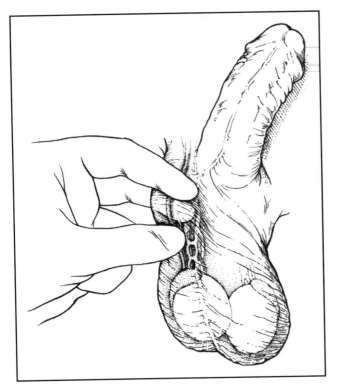

Figure 1   Three-finger technique of fixing the right vas deferens with the left hand. The surgeon is standing on the patient's right side.

while pressing downward, stretching the scrotal skin tightly over the vas and locking the vas within the clamp.

The ringed clamp is placed in the left hand and the trapped vas elevated with the left thumb, tightening the scrotal skin over the vas (Fig. 5). Using one blade, a sharp, pointed, curved mosquito hemostat

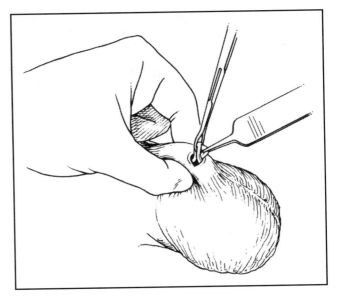

Figure 3   Incisional technique of accessing the vas.

(Fig. 6) is introduced through the same needle puncture hole used for anesthesia to puncture the scrotal skin, vas sheath, and vas wall (Fig. 7).

If the scrotum is thick or tight, the skin is first punctured with the sharp, curved hemostat and spread until the vertical slit-like opening in the median raphe is just large enough to introduce the ringed clamp. The ringed clamp is introduced into the opening, and the vas is grasped and brought up to the opening; the procedure then follows as described above.

The single blade of the hemostat is withdrawn, and the closed tip of the instrument is introduced through the same puncture hole. The blades of the clamp are gently opened, spreading all layers until the

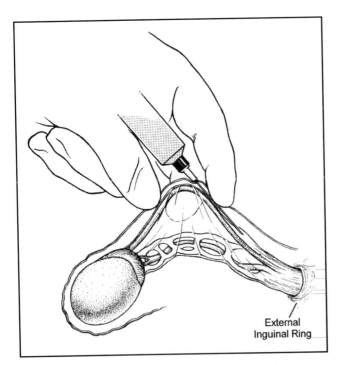

Figure 2   Vasal nerve block away from the vasectomy site.

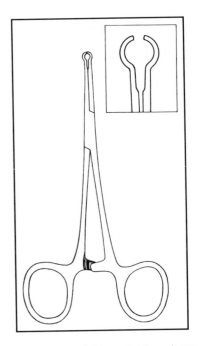

Figure 4   Ring-tipped vas deferens fixation clamp: cantilevered design prevents injury to the scrotal skin.

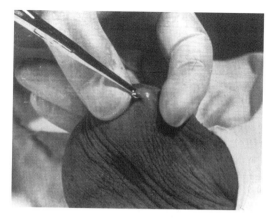

Figure 5 Vas fixed in the ring clamp. Scrotal skin is tightly stretched over the most prominent portion of the vas.

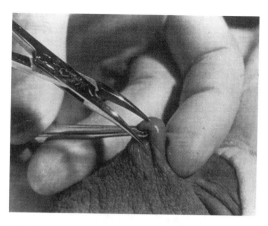

Figure 7 Puncture of the skin, vas sheath, and wall into the lumen.

bare vas can be visualized. Using the right blade of the hemostat, the vas wall is skewered from inside the lumen out at a 45° angle, and the hemostat is rotated laterally 180° (Fig. 8). The vas is delivered through the puncture hole, while the ringed fixation clamp is released (Fig. 9). The ring clamp is used to secure the delivered vas. The sharp hemostat is used to clean the vasal vessels away from the vas, yielding a clean segment at least 2 cm in length (Fig. 10).

At this point, the vas is divided and occlusion performed using one of the techniques described later in this section.

After checking for bleeding, the ends of the right vas are returned to the scrotum. The left vas is then fixed directly under the same puncture hole using the three-finger technique. Alternatively, the ring clamp can first be introduced through the puncture hole, encircling the vas without the overlying skin. The remainder of the procedure is identical to that described for the right side. After both vasa are returned to the scrotum, the puncture hole is pinched for a minute and inspected for bleeding. The puncture hole contracts and is virtually invisible. Antibiotic ointment is applied to the site and sterile fluff dressings held in place with a snug-fitting athletic supporter.

Studies in the United States and China (4), as well as a large controlled study carried out in Thailand, comparing no-scalpel to conventional vasectomy (7), have clearly shown that the no-scalpel technique results in a significantly reduced incidence of hematoma, infection, and pain. In addition, the no-scalpel vasectomy is performed in about 40% less time.

Although this method of vasectomy appears deceptively simple, it is more difficult to learn than conventional vasectomy and requires intensive hands-on training. Its use, however, may enhance the popularity of vasectomy and make it a more significant part of the urologist's practice.

Methods of Vasal Occlusion and Vasectomy Failure

The technique employed for occlusion of the vasal lumina, as well as the length of vas removed, determines the incidence of recanalization. Suture ligature, still the most common method employed worldwide, may result in necrosis and sloughing of the cut end distal to the ligature. If this occurs on the testicular end of the cut vas, a sperm granuloma will result. If both ends slough, recanalization is more likely to occur.

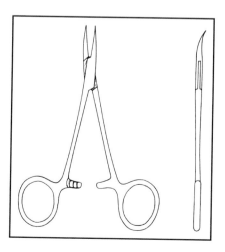

Figure 6 Sharp, curved mosquito hemostat.

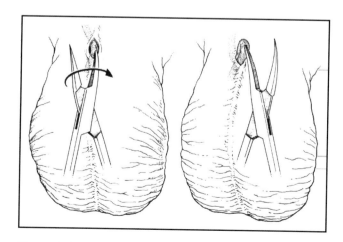

Figure 8 Vas wall is skewered from inside the lumen with one blade of the clamp and the vas delivered.

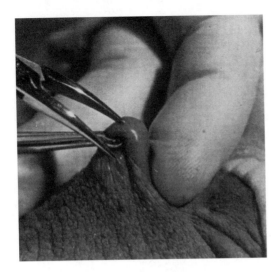

Figure 9 Delivery of clean vas.

The incidence of vasectomy failure ranges from 1% to 5% when ligatures alone are used for occlusion.

When the vasa are sealed with two medium hemoclips on each end, failure rates are reduced to less than 1% (8,9). The wider diameter of hemoclips compared to sutures more evenly distributes pressure on the vasal wall, resulting in less necrosis and sloughing.

Intraluminal occlusion with needle electrocautery or battery-driven thermal cautery, set at a power sufficient to destroy mucosa but not high enough to cause transmural destruction of the vas, reduces recanalization rates to less than 0.5% (10). At least 1 cm of lumen should be cauterized in each direction. Thermal wires should be rotated to cauterize the entire mucosal surface. The appearance of smoke is a good endpoint.

Interposing fascia between the cut ends, folding back of the vasal ends, and securing one end within the dartos muscle are all techniques that have been

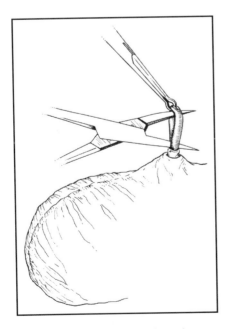

Figure 10 Segment cleaned.

advocated with the intent of reducing vasectomy failure rates (11). No controlled studies have been performed that document the efficacy of any of these methods in reducing failure rates. Moreover, these techniques complicate vasectomy and increase the time required to perform the procedure.

The length of vas removed undoubtedly influences the rate of vasectomy failure. Removing very long segments will reduce the possibility of recanalization. Such destructive procedures are more likely to be associated with postoperative hematomas and will lessen the possibility of future vasectomy reversal. Most urologists insist on removal of a segment of vas for pathologic verification, primarily for medicolegal reasons. Even from the legal point of view, a pathologist's report confirming the presence of vas in the vasectomy specimen offers little or no protection from litigation. Documented counseling, diligent follow-up to obtain at least one and preferably two azoospermic semen specimens postoperatively, and careful selection of appropriate candidates for vasectomy in the first place will provide the best protection from malpractice suits.

Preferred Methods of Occlusion

Occlusion techniques that result in very low rates of recanalization without destruction of excessively long segments of vas or complicated, time-consuming strategies include the following:

1. Removal of a 1 cm segment followed by intraluminal thermal cautery with a battery-driven device for a distance of 1 cm in each direction, plus application of a medium hemoclip on each end distal to the cauterized segment (this is the authors' preferred technique)
2. Intraluminal cautery as described above plus separation of the vasal ends into different tissue planes with or without removal of a segment
3. Sealing with double-medium hemoclips on each end, 1 cm apart, after removal of a 1 cm segment, with or without separation into different tissue planes

Postoperative Semen Analysis

No technique of vasal occlusion, short of removing the entire scrotal vas, is 100% effective (12). Follow-up semen analysis with the goal of obtaining at least one and preferably two absolutely azoospermic specimens four to six weeks apart is recommended. If any motile sperm are found in the ejaculate three months after vasectomy, the procedure should be repeated. If rare, nonmotile sperm are found, contraception may be cautiously discontinued and repeat semen analysis done every three months. Rare, motile, and nonmotile complete sperm in a spun semen analysis pellet are found in 10% of semen specimens at a mean of 10 years after vasectomy (13).

Complications of Vasectomy

Hematoma and Infection

Hematoma is the most common complication of vasectomy, with an average incidence of 2% ranging from 0.09% to 29% (3). Infection is surprisingly common, with an average rate of 3.4%, but several series report rates from 12% to 38% (14–16). The experience of the vasectomist is the single most important factor relating to the occurrence of complications (3). The hematoma rate was significantly higher among physicians performing 1 to 10 vasectomies per year (4.6%) than among those performing 11 to 50 vasectomies per year (2.4%), or greater than 50 vasectomies per year (1.6%). A similar relationship was seen for hospitalization rate.

Sperm Granuloma

Sperm granulomas form when sperm leak from the testicular end of the vas. Sperm are highly antigenic, and an intense inflammatory reaction occurs when sperm escape outside the reproductive epithelium. Sperm granulomas are rarely symptomatic. The presence or absence of a sperm granuloma at the vasectomy site seems to be of importance in modulating the local effects of chronic obstruction on the male reproductive tract. The sperm granuloma's complex network of epithelialized channels provides an additional absorptive surface that helps vent the high intraluminal pressure in the obstructed excurrent ducts. Numerous animal studies have correlated the presence or absence of sperm granuloma at the vasectomy site with the degree of epididymal and testicular damage. Species that always develop granulomas after vasectomy have minimal damage to the seminiferous tubules. Some studies of men undergoing vasectomy reversal have revealed somewhat higher success rates in men who have a sperm granuloma at the vasectomy site (17), whereas another large study has not (18).

Although sperm granulomas at the vasectomy site are present, microscopically, in 10% to 30% of men undergoing reversal, it is likely that, given enough time, virtually all men will develop sperm granulomas at the vasectomy site, the epididymis, or the rete testis.

When chronic postvasectomy pain is localized to the granuloma, excision, and occlusion of the vasa with intraluminal cautery usually relieves the pain and prevents recurrence (19). On the other hand, men with postvasectomy congestive epididymitis may be relieved of their pain by open-ended vasectomy designed to purposefully produce a pressure-relieving sperm granuloma; however, it should be pointed out that some investigators have raised concern of potential vasectomy failure with the open-ended technique (20).

Long-Term Effects of Vasectomy

Long-term effects of vasectomy in humans include vasitis nodosa, chronic testicular and/or epididymal pain, alterations in testicular function, chronic epididymal obstruction, postulated systemic effects of vasectomy, and, possibly, an increased incidence of prostate cancer (21). Vasitis nodosa is a benign disorder characterized macroscopically by nodularity of the vas. Microscopically, there is perivasal proliferation of tubules lined with epithelium and stromal inflammation with infiltration of histiocytes, polymorphonuclear leukocytes, and Langerhans giant cells. Although vasitis nodosa has been reported in up to 66% of vasectomy specimens in men undergoing vasectomy reversal (22), this entity does not appear to be associated with pain or significant medical sequelae.

In humans, micropuncture studies have revealed that the markedly increased pressures that occur on the testicular side of the vas as well as the epididymis after vasectomy are not transmitted to the seminiferous tubules (23). Therefore, little disruption of spermatogenesis is expected in humans. Biopsies up to 15 years after vasectomy show the testes to be essentially normal by light microscopy. Electron microscopic studies, however, have revealed thickening of the basal lamina and scattered areas of disrupted spermatogenesis in portions of the biopsy specimens (24). Chronic orchalgia and/or epididymal pain after vasectomy may occur in up to 15% of patients (25). In some cases, vasectomy reversal—or, alternatively, an open-ended vasectomy, as described previously—might be considered. The brunt of pressure-induced damage after vasectomy falls on the epididymis and efferent ductules. These structures become markedly distended, adapting to reabsorb large volumes of testicular fluid and sperm products. When pain and tenderness are localized in the epididymis, total epididymovasectomy, including removal of the testicular vasal remnant, relieves pain in 95% of men (26).

Systemic effects of vasectomy have been postulated. Vasectomy disrupts the blood–testis barrier, resulting in detectable levels of serum antisperm antibodies in 60% to 80% of men (27,28). Some studies suggest that the antibody titers diminish two or more years after vasectomy, while others suggest that these antibody titers persist; however, neither circulating immune complexes nor deposits are increased after vasectomy in man (29). Studies in animals and man have failed to find any association between antisperm antibodies and immune complex–mediated diseases such as lupus erythematosus, scleroderma, rheumatoid arthritis, or myasthenia gravis (30). Although one study in cynomolgus monkeys found more frequent and extensive atherosclerosis of the major vessels in previously vasectomized monkeys fed a high-cholesterol diet (31), no evidence of excess cardiovascular disease (32), illness requiring hospitalization (33,34), or biochemical alterations (35) have been found in more than 15 reports (with 12 of these employing matched controls) examining thousands of men (36).

Major among the controversies is the possible link between vasectomy and prostate cancer. Studies have found an increased risk of prostate cancer in men who had a vasectomy 20 years ago. Two large-scale cohort studies, however, evaluated men from a wide range of socioeconomic strata and did not find a link between vasectomy and prostate cancer. Another study of vasectomy sequelae found no increased incidence of cancer or other diseases (36).

The most likely explanation for the increased diagnosis of prostate cancer in vasectomized men is detection bias. Vasectomized men are more likely to visit a urologist and, therefore, are more likely to have cancer diagnosed earlier. Further, men who choose to undergo vasectomy may be more likely to seek health care, increasing their opportunity for prostate cancer detection. A multidisciplinary National Institutes of Health panel concluded that the epidemiologic associations between vasectomy and prostate cancer are weak. It recommended no change in clinical or public health practice and said that screening for prostate cancer should not be any different for vasectomized men (37).

Nevertheless, men seeking vasectomy should be informed of these and other related studies and should be counseled about the controversies. The American Urological Association now recommends annual digital rectal examination and serum prostate-specific antigen (PSA) assay for men who had had a vasectomy more than 20 years ago, or who had been older than 40 at the time of vasectomy.

□ VASOVASOSTOMY

The number of American men who undergo vasectomy has remained stable at about 500,000 per year, as has the divorce rate of 50%. Surveys suggest that 2% to 6% of vasectomized men will ultimately seek reversal. Furthermore, obstructive azoospermia can be the result of iatrogenic injuries to the vas deferens, usually from hernia repair (38), in 6% of azoospermic men (39). Recent cost-effectiveness analyses (40,41) have shown that microsurgical reconstruction, in cases that are feasible, is a more cost-effective initial approach and typically yields better pregnancy rates than sperm retrieval combined with in vitro fertilization (IVF) and intracytoplasmic sperm injection (ICSI).

Preoperative Evaluation

Prior to attempted surgical reconstruction of the reproductive tract, spermatogenesis in the patient should be evident. A prior history of natural fertility prevasectomy is usually adequate. In other cases, a testicular biopsy may be indicated to confirm the presence of spermatogenesis.

Physical Examination

1. *Testis*: a small or soft testes suggests impaired spermatogenesis and predicts a poor outcome.
2. *Epididymis*: an indurated, irregular epididymis often predicts secondary epididymal obstruction, necessitating vasoepididymostomy.

3. *Hydrocele*: the presence of a hydrocele in the face of excurrent ductal system obstruction is often associated with secondary epididymal obstruction. Surgeons attempting reconstruction should be aware of the possibility of requiring a vasoepididymostomy.
4. *Sperm granuloma*: a sperm granuloma at the testicular end of the vas suggests that sperm have been leaking at the vasectomy site. This vents the high pressures away from the epididymis and is associated with a better prognosis for restored fertility regardless of the time interval since vasectomy.
5. *Vasal gap*: when a very destructive vasectomy has been performed, most of the scrotal straight vas may be absent or fibrotic, and the patient should be advised that inguinal extension of the scrotal incision will be necessary to mobilize an adequate length of vas to enable a tension-free anastomosis.
6. *Scars from previous surgery*: operative scars in the inguinal or scrotal region should alert the surgeon to the possibility of iatrogenic vasal or epididymal obstruction.

Laboratory Tests

1. *Preoperative semen analysis*: preoperative semen analysis with centrifugation and examination of the pellet for sperm may provide helpful information. Complete sperm with tails are found in 10% of preoperative pellets at a mean of 10 years after vasectomy (13). Under these circumstances, sperm are certain to be found in the vas on at least one side, indicating a favorable prognosis for restored fertility. Men with a low semen volume should have a transrectal ultrasound to alert one to the possibility of an additional ejaculatory duct obstruction.
2. *Serum and antisperm antibody studies*: the presence of serum antisperm antibodies corroborates the diagnosis of obstruction and the presence of active spermatogenesis. At present, this test is of unknown prognostic value and is optional.
3. *Serum follicle-stimulating hormone (FSH)*: men with small, soft testes should have serum FSH measured. An elevated FSH predicts impaired spermatogenesis and a poorer prognosis.
4. *PSA*: all vasectomy reversal candidates over age 40 should have serum PSA measured.

Anesthesia

Light general anesthesia is preferred. Slight movements are greatly magnified by the operating microscope and will disturb performance of the anastomosis. In cooperative and motivated patients, regional, or even local, anesthesia with sedation can be employed if the vasal ends are easily palpable, a sperm granuloma is present, and/or the time interval since vasectomy is short, decreasing the likelihood of secondary epididymal obstruction. When large vasal gaps are present, extensions of the incisions high into the inguinal canal may be necessary. Furthermore, if vasoepididymostomy is necessary, the operating time could exceed four or five hours. Local anesthesia limits the options available to the surgeon. Hypobaric spinal anesthesia with long-acting agents such as Marcaine can provide four to five hours of anesthesia time; these have the additional advantage of eliminating lower body motion. Epidural anesthesia with an indwelling catheter can be equally effective.

Surgical Approaches
Scrotal Incisions

Bilateral high vertical scrotal incisions provide the most direct access to the obstructed site in cases of vasectomy reversal. Length is usually a problem on the abdominal end but not on the testicular end. The location of the external inguinal ring is marked (Fig. 11). If the vasal gap is large, or the vasectomy site is high, this incision can easily be extended inguinally toward the external ring. If the vasectomy site is low, it is easy to pull up the testicular end. This incision should be made at least 1 cm lateral to the base of the penis. The testis should be delivered with the tunica vaginalis left intact; this provides excellent exposure of the entire scrotal vas deferens and, if necessary, the epididymis.

Inguinal Incision

An inguinal incision is the preferred approach in men when obstruction of the inguinal vas deferens from prior herniorrhaphy or orchiopexy is strongly suspected. Incision through the previous scar usually leads directly to the site of obstruction. If the obstruction turns out to be scrotal or epididymal, it is a simple matter to deliver the testis through the inguinal incision or through a separate scrotal incision to perform the anastomosis.

Preparation of the Vasa

The vas should be mobilized enough to allow a tension-free anastomosis. To preserve good blood supply, the vas should not be stripped of its periadventitial sheath. Transillumination of the sheath, by properly adjusting the operating light, allows clear visualization of the blood vessels, which facilitates dissection of the periadventitial sheath and prevents damage to the vasal vessels. The obstructed segment—and, if present, the sperm granuloma at the vasectomy site—should be dissected and excised. By staying right on the vas and/or sperm granuloma during this dissection, the risk of injuring the testicular artery is reduced. Injury to adjacent cord structures, especially the testicular artery, is likely to result in testicular atrophy, since the vasal artery has usually been interrupted at the vasectomy site.

When the vasal gap is extremely large, additional length can be achieved by blunt dissection with a gauze-wrapped index finger to separate the cord structures from the vas. Blunt finger dissection through the external ring will free the vas to the internal inguinal ring if additional abdominal side length is necessary. These maneuvers will leave all the vasal vessels intact. In addition, the entire convoluted vas can be dissected free of its attachments to the epididymal tunica (Fig. 12), allowing the testis to drop upside-down. These maneuvers can provide an additional 4 to 6 cm of length. To maintain the integrity of the vasal vessels, this dissection is performed best using magnifying loupes or the operating microscope under low power. If the amount of vas removed is so large that even these

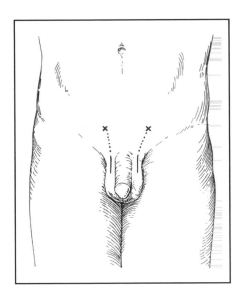

Figure 11 Preferred incisions (*solid lines*) for vasectomy reversal allow extension (*dotted lines*) to external inguinal ring (marked by "*X*") when abdominal vas is short.

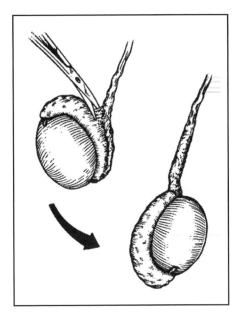

Figure 12 Convoluted vas dissected off of epididymal tunica provides additional length on testicular side.

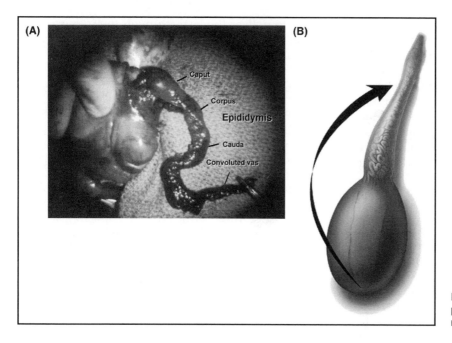

Figure 13 (**A,B**) Entire vasoepididymal complex dissected to caput epididymis to bridge massive vasal gaps.

measures fail to allow a tension-free anastomosis, the incision can be extended to the internal inguinal ring, the floor of the inguinal canal cut, and the vas rerouted under the floor, as in a difficult orchiopexy. An additional 4 to 6 cm of length can be obtained by dissecting the epididymis off of the testis from the vasoepididymal (VE) junction to the caput epididymis (Fig. 13A and B). The superior-epididymal vessels are left intact to provide adequate blood supply to the testicular end of the vas. With this combination of maneuvers, up to 10 cm gaps can be bridged.

After the vasa have been freed, the testicular end of the vas is cut transversely. An ultrasharp knife drawn through a slotted 2, 2.5, or 3 mm-diameter nerve-holding clamp (Accurate Surgical and Scientific Instrument Corp., Westbury, New York, U.S.A.) yields a perfect 90° cut (Fig. 14). The cut surface of the testicular end of the vas deferens is inspected using 15- to 25-power magnification. A healthy, white mucosal ring

should be seen that springs back immediately after gentle dilation. The muscularis should appear smooth and soft. A gritty-looking muscularis layer indicates the presence of scar/fibrotic tissues. The cut surface should look like a bull's eye, with the three vasal layers distinctly visible. Healthy bleeding should be noted from both the cut edge of the mucosa and the surface of the muscularis. If the blood supply is poor or the muscularis is gritty, the vas is recut until healthy tissue is found. The vasal artery and vein are then clamped and ligated with 6-0 nylon sutures. Small bleeders are controlled with a microbipolar forceps set at low power. Once a patent lumen has been established on the testicular end, the vas is milked and a clean glass slide is touched to its surface. The vasal fluid is immediately mixed with a drop or two of saline or Ringer's lactate and preserved under a cover slip for microscopic examination. The abdominal end of the vas deferens is prepared in a similar manner, and the lumen is gently dilated with a microvessel dilator and cannulated with a 24-gauge angiocatheter sheath. Injection of saline or Ringer's lactate confirms its patency. After Ringer's injection and test dilation, the vas is recut to obtain a fresh surface. Minimal instrumentation of the mucosa should be performed.

After preparation, the ends of the vasa are stabilized with a Microspike approximating clamp (42) to remove all tension prior to performing the anastomosis. Isolating the field through a slit in a rubber dam prevents microsutures from sticking to the surrounding tissue. A sterile tongue blade covered with a large Penrose drain is placed beneath the ends of the vasa to provide a platform on which to perform the anastomosis.

Examination of Vasal Fluid

The gross appearance of fluid expressed from the testicular end of the vas is usually predictive of findings

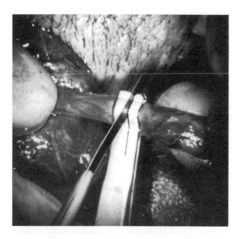

Figure 14 Ultrasharp knife drawn through a 2- to 3-mm slotted nerve-holding clamp (from Accurate Surgical and Scientific Instrument Corp., Westbury, New York, U.S.A.) produces a perfect 90° cut.

Table 1   Relationship Between Gross Appearance of Vasal Fluid and Microscopic Findings

Vasal fluid appearance	Most common findings on microscopic exam	Surgical procedure indicated
Copious, crystal clear, watery	No sperm in fluid	Vasovasostomy
Copious, cloudy thin, water soluble	Usually sperm with tails	Vasovasostomy
Copious, creamy yellow, water soluble	Usually many sperm heads, occasional sperm with short tails	Vasovasostomy
Scant fluid, granuloma present at vasectomy site	Barbitage fluid reveals sperm	Vasovasostomy
Copious, thick, white, toothpaste-like, water insoluble	No sperm	Vasoepididymostomy
Scant, white, thin fluid	No sperm	Vasoepididymostomy
Dry, spermless vas; no sperm at vasectomy site	No sperm	Vasoepididymostomy

on microscopic examination (Table 1). If microscopic examination of the vasal fluid reveals the presence of sperm with tails, vasovasostomy is performed. If no fluid is found, a 24-gauge angiocatheter sheath is inserted into the lumen of the testicular end of the vas and barbotage with 0.1 mL of saline while the convoluted vas is vigorously milked. The barbotage fluid is expressed onto a slide and examined. Men with large sperm granulomas often have virtually no dilation of the testicular end of the vas and little or no fluid initially; however, with barbotage and vigorous milking, invariably, sperm will be found in this scant fluid. If there is no sperm granuloma and the vas is absolutely dry and spermless after multiple samples are examined, vasoepididymostomy is indicated. If the fluid expressed from the vas is found to be thick, white, water insoluble, and toothpaste-like in quality, microscope examination rarely reveals sperm. Under these circumstances, the tunica vaginalis is opened and the epididymis inspected. If clear evidence of obstruction is found, i.e., an epididymal sperm granuloma with dilated tubules above and collapsed tubules below, vasoepididymostomy is performed. When in doubt, or if not very experienced with vasoepididymostomy, vasovasostomy should be performed. Only 15% of men with bilateral absence of sperm in the vasal fluid after barbotage and an intensive search, however, will have sperm return to the ejaculate after vasovasostomy (43).

When copious, crystal-clear, water-like fluid squirts out from the vas and no sperm are found in this fluid, a vasovasostomy is performed because there is a likelihood of sperm returning to the ejaculate after vasovasostomy is performed.

Multiple Vasal Obstructions

If saline injection reveals that the abdominal end of the vas deferens is not patent, a 2-0 nylon or polypropylene suture is gently threaded into the vas lumen to determine the site of obstruction. If the obstruction is within 5 cm of the original vasectomy site, the abdominal end of the vas deferens may be dissected to this site and excised. The incision should then be extended inguinally to free the vas extensively up toward the internal inguinal ring. To gain additional length, the testicular end should be freed up to the VE junction. If the site of the second obstruction is so far from the

vasectomy site that two vasovasostomies are necessary, alternative surgical approaches, such as a single crossed vasovasostomy, should be considered, e.g., if the contralateral testis is atrophic or absent, precluding a proper reconstruction. If this is not possible, the aspiration of vasal or epididymal sperm into micropipettes and cryopreservation for future IVF with ICSI (Fig. 15) should be considered. Simultaneous vasovasostomies at two separate sites may lead to devascularization of the intervening segment with fibrosis and necrosis.

Anastomotic Techniques: Keys to Success

All successful vasovasostomy techniques depend on adherence to surgical principles that are universally applicable to anastomoses of all tubular structures. These include

1. Accurate mucosa-to-mucosa approximation. In human vasovasostomy, the lumen on the testicular side is usually dilated, often to diameters two to five times that of the abdominal side. Techniques that work well with lumina of equal diameters may be less successful when applied to lumina of markedly discrepant diameters.
2. Leakproof anastomosis. Sperm are highly antigenic and provoke an inflammatory reaction when they escape from the normally intact lining of the excurrent ducts of the male reproductive tract. Extravasated sperm adversely influence the success of

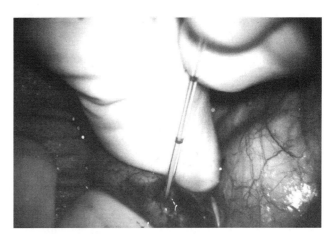

Figure 15   Sperm drawn into the micropipette by capillary action.

vasovasostomy (44). Unlike blood vessel anastomoses, where platelets and clotting factors seal the gaps between sutures, vasal and epididymal fluid contain no platelets or clotting factors; so the watertightness of the anastomosis is entirely dependent on the mucosal sutures.

3. Tension-free anastomosis. When an anastomosis is performed under tension, sperm may appear in the ejaculate for several months after surgery. Ultimately, sperm counts and motility will decrease and azoospermia may ensue. At re-exploration, only a thin, fibrotic band is found at the anastomotic site. This can be prevented by adequately freeing up the vasa and placing reinforcing sutures in the sheath of the vas.

3. Good blood supply. If the cut vas exhibits poor blood supply, it should be recut until healthy bleeding is encountered. If extensive resection is necessary, additional length should be obtained using the techniques previously described.

4. Healthy mucosa and muscularis. If the mucosa or cut surface of the vas exhibits poor distensibility after dilation, peels away from the underlying muscularis, or shreds easily, then the vas should be cut back until healthy mucosa is found. Surgeons should be aware that if a needle electrocautery was used in vasectomy, the area of damage to the mucosa and muscularis by the electric current may extend far beyond the tip of the needle cautery. If the muscularis is found to be fibrotic or gritty, the vas must be recut until healthy tissue is found.

5. Good atraumatic anastomotic technique. If multiple surgical errors occur during the procedure, such as inadvertent cutting of the mucosa with needles when placing sutures, tearing through of sutures, or backwalling of the mucosa, the anastomosis should be resected and redone immediately.

Set-Up

An operating microscope providing variable magnification from 6- to 32-power is employed. A diploscope providing identical fields for both surgeon and assistant is preferred. Foot pedal controls for a motorized zoom and focus leave the surgeon's hands free.

Both surgeon and assistant should be comfortably seated on microsurgical chairs that stabilize the chest and arms. This dramatically improves stability and accuracy (Fig. 16). An inexpensive alternative is a simple rolling stool with a round beanbag (meditation pillow) taped on top for padding. Two arm boards, placed on either side of the surgeon, and built up to the appropriate height with folded blankets taped to the board, provide excellent arm support. A right-handed surgeon should sit on the patient's right side, so that the forehand stitch is always thrown on the smaller, more difficult, abdominal side of the lumen.

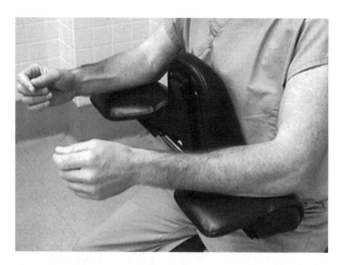

Figure 16 Microsurgery chair stabilizes lower body, chest, and arms, substantially enhancing stability and accuracy.

Microsurgical Multilayer Microdot Method

This method of vasovasostomy can handle lumina of markedly discrepant diameters in the straight or convoluted vas. The microdot technique ensures precise suture placement by exact mapping of each planned suture. The microdot method separates the planning from the placement (45). This allows focus on only one task at a time, and results in substantially improved accuracy.

A microtip marking pen (Devon Skin Marker Extra Fine #151; 1-800-DEVON PO) is used to map planned needle exit points. Exactly six mucosal sutures are used for every anastomosis because it is easy to map and always results in a leakproof closure even when the lumen diameters are markedly discrepant (Fig. 17). Monofilament 10-0 nylon sutures, double armed with 70 μm-diameter taper-point needles bent

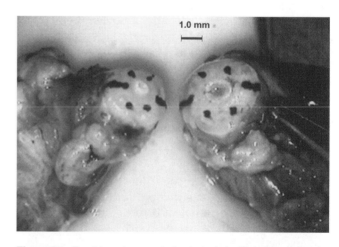

Figure 17 Precision placement of sutures is facilitated by drying the cut surface of the vas with a Weck cell and using a microtip marking pen to map out planned needle exit points. Lines are drawn at 3 o'clock and 9 o'clock to help match them up. This mapping prevents dog-ears and leaks when the lumen diameters are discrepant.

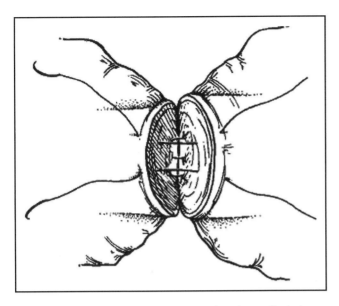

Figure 18 Deep muscularis sutures placed exactly between mucosal sutures.

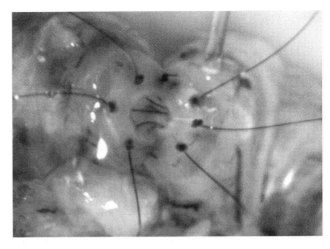

Figure 20 Placement of three additional 10-0 mucosal sutures. Note sutures exit through microdots.

into a fish-hook configuration (available from sharpoint, Reading PA, U.S.A. and Ethicon, Somerville, NJ, U.S.A.), are utilized. Double-armed sutures allow inside-out placement, eliminating the need for manipulation of the mucosa and the possibility of backwalling. If the mucosal rings are not sharply defined, the cut surfaces of the vasal ends are stained with indigo carmine to highlight the mucosa (46). The anastomosis is begun with the placement of three 10-0 mucosal sutures anteriorly. On the small abdominal side lumen, the lumen is gently and momentarily dilated with a microvessel dilator just prior to placement of the sutures. For accurate mucosal approximation, only a small amount of mucosa is included—one-third to one-half of the muscle wall thickness. Exactly the same amount of tissue is included in the bites on each side. The needle should exit through the center of each dot. After placement, the three mucosal sutures are tied.

Two 9-0 monofilament nylon deep muscularis sutures are placed exactly in between the three previously placed mucosal sutures, just above, but not through the mucosa (Fig. 18) and are then tied. These sutures seal the gaps between the mucosal sutures (Fig. 19) without trauma to the mucosa from the larger 100 μm-diameter cutting needle required to penetrate the tough vas muscularis and adventitia. The vas is rotated 180° and three additional 10-0 sutures are placed through each microdot and then tied to complete the mucosal portion of the anastomosis (Fig. 20). Just prior to tying the last mucosal suture, the lumen is irrigated with heparinized Ringer's solution to prevent the formation of clot in the lumen. After completion of the mucosal layer (Fig. 21), four more 9-0 deep muscularis sutures are placed exactly in between each mucosal suture—just above, but not penetrating the mucosa. Four to six 9-0 nylon interrupted sutures are placed between each muscular suture. This is a purely adventitial layer that covers the innermost mucosal sutures. The anastomosis is completed by approximating the

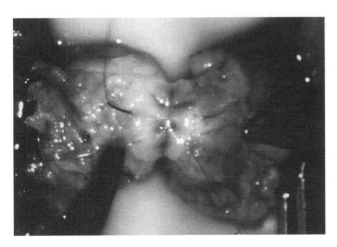

Figure 19 9-0 sutures placed just above but not through the mucosa to seal gaps between mucosal sutures. The single suture pictured is the third layer (adventitial).

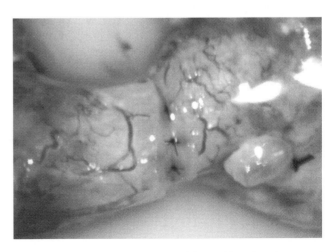

Figure 21 Completed 10-0 mucosal layer. Note the absence of dog-ears.

vasal sheath with six interrupted sutures of 7-0 PDS that completely cover the anastomosis and relieve it of all tension.

Anastomosis in the Convoluted Vas

Vasovasostomy performed in the convoluted portion of the vas deferens is technically more demanding than anastomoses in the straight portion. Fear of cutting back into the convoluted vas in order to obtain healthy tissue may lead surgeons to complete an anastomosis in the straight portion when the testicular end of the vas has poor blood supply, unhealthy or friable mucosa, or gritty fibrotic muscularis. Adherence to the following principles will enable anastomosis in the convoluted vas to succeed as often as those in the straight portion:

1. A perfect transverse cut yielding a round ring of mucosa and a lumen directed straight down is essential (Fig. 22). A very oblique lumen with a thin flap of muscle and mucosa on one side is not acceptable (Fig. 22). The vas should be recut at 0.5 mm intervals until a perfect cut with good blood supply and healthy tissue is obtained. A slotted nerve clamp, 2.5 or 3 mm in diameter, and an ultrasharp knife facilitate this part of the procedure (Fig. 14). Often, the vas must be recut two or three times until a satisfactory cut is obtained.
2. The convoluted vas should not be unraveled. This disturbs the blood supply at the anastomotic line.
3. The sheath of the convoluted vas may be carefully dissected free of its attachments to the epididymal tunica (Fig. 12). This will minimize disturbance of its blood supply and provide the necessary length to perform a tension-free anastomosis.
4. Care must be taken to avoid taking large bites of the muscularis and adventitial layers on the convoluted side to prevent inadvertent perforation of adjacent convolutions.
5. The anastomosis is reinforced by approximating the vasal sheath of the straight portion to the sheath of the convoluted portion with six interrupted sutures of 7-0 PDS. This will remove all tension from the anastomosis.

Crossed Vasovasostomy

This is a useful procedure that often provides an easy solution for otherwise difficult problems (38,47,48). Crossover is indicated in the following circumstances:

1. Unilateral inguinal obstruction of the vas deferens associated with an atrophic testis on the contralateral side. A crossover vasovasostomy should be performed to connect a healthy testicle to the contralateral unobstructed vas.
2. Obstruction or aplasia of the inguinal vas or ejaculatory duct on one side and epididymal obstruction on the contralateral side.

It is preferable to perform one anastomosis with a high probability of success (vasovasostomy) than two operations with a much lower chance of success, that is, unilateral vasoepididymostomy and contralateral transurethral resection of the ejaculatory ducts.

Technique

The vas attached to the atrophic testis at the junction of its straight and convoluted portion is transected, and its patency is confirmed with a Ringer's or indigo carmine vasogram (Fig. 23). The contralateral vas is dissected with the normal testis toward the inguinal obstruction and is clamped and transected as high up as possible with a right angle clamp. The testicular end of the vas is crossed through a capacious opening made in the scrotal septum, and vasovasostomy should proceed as described above. This procedure is much easier than an inguinal vasovasostomy, which requires finding both ends of the vas within the dense scar of a previous inguinal operation.

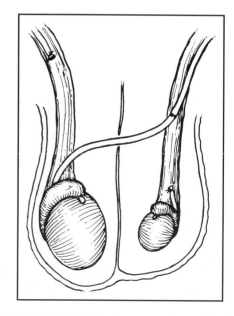

Figure 23 Transeptal crossed vasovasostomy. The right testis with normal sperm production is connected to a patent vas on the contralateral side.

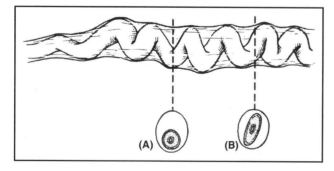

Figure 22 (**A**) Round lumen essential for success in convoluted anastomoses. (**B**) Oblique cut not acceptable.

Transposition of the Testis

Occasionally, when the vasal length is critically short, a tension-free crossed anastomosis can best be accomplished by testicular transposition. The spermatic cord is always longer than the vas. The testes will comfortably cross through a generous opening in the septum and sit nicely in the contralateral scrotal compartment.

Wound Closure

If the vasal dissection is extensive, Penrose drains are brought out of the dependent portion of the right and left hemiscrota and fixed in place with sutures and safety pins, preferably prior to beginning the anastomosis. Placement of drains at the end of the procedure may potentially disturb the anastomosis. The dartos layer is approximated with interrupted 4-0 absorbable sutures and the skin with subcuticular sutures of 5-0 Monocryl. The wound heals with a fine scar. The use of through-and-through skin closures, which give an unacceptable "railroad-track"-looking scar, should be avoided. Virtually all of the authors' procedures are performed on an ambulatory basis. If drains are placed, the patients are given detailed instructions (with explicit drawings) on how to remove the drains the next morning.

Postoperative Management

Sterile fluff gauze dressings are held in place with a snug-fitting scrotal supporter. Only perioperative antibiotics are used. Patients are discharged with a prescription for acetaminophen with codeine. They shower 48 hours after surgery. They wear a scrotal supporter at all times (except in the shower), even when sleeping, for six weeks postoperatively. Thereafter, a scrotal supporter is worn during athletic activity until pregnancy is achieved. Desk-type work may be resumed in three days. No heavy work or sports are allowed for three weeks. No intercourse or ejaculation is allowed for four weeks postoperatively. Semen analyses are obtained at one, three, and six months postoperatively and every six months thereafter. In the authors' experience, persistent azoospermia beyond six months has rarely resulted in subsequent return of sperm in the ejaculate. In these cases, a redo vasovasostomy or vasoepididymostomy will be necessary.

Postoperative Complications

The most common complication is hematoma. In 2100 operations, seven small hematomas occurred. None required surgical drainage. Most were walnut-sized and perivasal. These take 6 to 12 weeks to resolve. Wound infection has not occurred. Late complications include sperm granuloma at the anastomotic site (approximately 5%); this usually is a harbinger of eventual obstruction. Late stricture and obstruction are disappointingly common (see below). Progressive loss of motility followed by decreasing sperm counts indicates stricture. The authors' recent switch back to nylon sutures (49), use of the microdot system to prevent leaks, extensive dissection of the vas until healthy mucosa and muscularis and a good blood supply is obtained, and generous use of scrotal support until pregnancy is established may reduce this incidence. Because of the significant rate of late stricture and obstruction, the authors strongly encourage cryopreservation of semen specimens as soon as motile sperm appear in the ejaculate.

Long-Term Follow-Up Evaluation after Vasovasostomy

When sperm are found in the vasal fluid on at least one side at the time of surgery, the anastomotic technique described results in the appearance of sperm in the ejaculate in 99.5% of men (45). Late obstruction, after initial patency, may occur in up to 12% of men by 14 months postoperatively (50). Pregnancy has occurred in 52% of couples followed for at least two years, and 63% when female factors are excluded.

□ VASOEPIDIDYMOSTOMY

Detailed knowledge of epididymal anatomy and physiology is essential prior to undertaking surgery of this delicate but important structure. Sperm motility and fertilizing capacity progressively increase during passage through the 200 μm-diameter, 12- to 15-foot long, tightly coiled single tubule. When the epididymis is obstructed and functionally shortened after vasoepididymostomy, even very short lengths of epididymis are able to adapt and allow some sperm to acquire motility and fertilizing capacity (51,52). Adaptation may gradually continue up to two years after surgical reconstruction, with progressive improvement in the fertility and motility of sperm. Nevertheless, preservation of the greatest possible length of functional epididymis is most likely to result in the best sperm quality after vasoepididymostomy (53,54). Furthermore, because the wall of the epididymis is thinnest in the caput region and gradually thickens, due to the increasing numbers of smooth muscle cells in its more distal (inferior) end, anastomoses are technically easier to perform and more likely to succeed in its distal regions. Since the corpus and cauda epididymis comprise a single tubule with a very small diameter, injury or occlusion of a tubule anywhere along its length will lead to total obstruction of outflow at that level. For these reasons, magnification, with loupes for macrodissection and the operating microscope for anastomosis, is essential for performing all epididymal surgery.

Fortunately, the epididymis is blessed with a rich blood supply derived from the testicular vessels superiorly and the deferential vessels inferiorly. Because of the extensive interconnections between these branches, either the testicular or the deferential branches (but not both) to the epididymis may be divided without compromising on epididymal viability.

Conversely, since the epididymal branches of the testicular artery are medial to and separate from the main testicular artery and veins, surgical procedures may be performed on the epididymis without compromise to testicular blood supply.

Prior to the development of microsurgical techniques, accurate approximation of the vasal lumen to that of a specific epididymal tubule was not possible. Vasoepididymostomy was performed by aligning the vas deferens adjacent to a slash made in multiple epididymal tubules with the hope that a fistula would form. Results with this primitive technique were poor. Microsurgical approaches allow the accurate approximation of the vasal mucosa to that of a single epididymal tubule (55), resulting in the marked improvement of patency and pregnancy rates (54,56). Microsurgical vasoepididymostomy, however, is the most technically demanding procedure in all of microsurgery. In virtually no other operation are results so dependent upon technical perfection. Microsurgical vasoepididymostomy should only be attempted by experienced microsurgeons who perform the procedure frequently.

Indications

The indications for vasoepididymostomy at the time of vasectomy reversal are reviewed below. For obstructive azoospermia not due to vasectomy, vasoepididymostomy is indicated when the testis biopsy reveals complete spermatogenesis and scrotal exploration reveals the absence of sperm in the vasal lumen with no vasal or ejaculatory duct obstruction. The preoperative evaluation is identical to that described for vasovasostomy.

Microsurgical End-to-Side Vasoepididymostomy

End-to-side techniques of vasoepididymostomy have the advantage of being minimally traumatic to the epididymis and relatively bloodless (57–60). The end-to-side technique does not disturb the epididymal blood supply. When the level of epididymal obstruction is clearly demarcated by the presence of markedly dilated tubules proximally and collapsed tubules distally, the site at which the anastomosis should be performed is readily apparent. The end-to-side approach has the advantage of allowing accurate approximation of the muscularis and adventitia of the vas deferens to a precisely tailored opening in the tunica of the epididymis. This is the preferred technique when vasoepididymostomy is performed simultaneously with inguinal vasovasostomy, because it is possible to preserve the vasal blood supply deriving from the epididymal branches of the testicular artery. This provides blood supply to the segment of vas intervening between the two anastomoses. Maintenance of the deferential artery's contribution to the testicular blood supply is also important in situations in which the integrity of the testicular artery is in doubt due to prior surgery such as orchiopexy, nonmicroscopic varicocelectomy, or hernia repair.

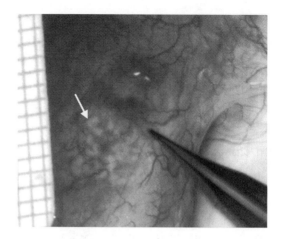

Figure 24 Inspection of the epididymis for dilated tubules (*arrow*) seen beneath the epididymal tunica.

After opening the tunica vaginalis, the epididymis is inspected under the operating microscope. An anastomotic site is selected above the area of suspected obstruction, proximal to any visible sperm granulomas, where dilated epididymal tubules are clearly seen beneath the epididymal tunica (Fig. 24). A relatively avascular area is grasped with sharp jeweler's forceps and the epididymal tunica tented upward. A 3 to 4 mm buttonhole is made in the tunica with microscissors to create a round opening that matches the outer diameter of the previously prepared vas deferens. The epididymal tubules are then gently dissected with a combination of sharp and blunt dissection until dilated loops of tubule are clearly exposed (Fig. 25). If the level of obstruction is not clearly delineated, after the buttonhole opening is made in the tunic, a 70 μm-diameter tapered needle from the 10-0 nylon microsuture is used to puncture the epididymal tubule, beginning as distally as possible, and fluid is sampled from the puncture site. When sperm are found, the puncture sites are sealed with microbipolar forceps, a new buttonhole is made in the epididymal tunic just proximally, and the tubule is prepared as described previously.

The vas deferens is drawn up through an opening in the tunica vaginalis and secured in proximity to

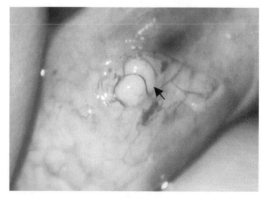

Figure 25 Dissection exposing dilated loops of epididymal tubule (*arrow*).

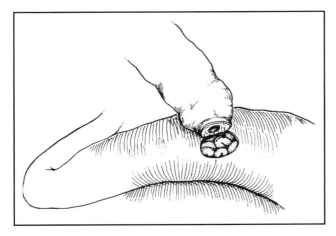

Figure 26 Preparation for end-to-side vasoepididymostomy. 9-0 sutures approximate the posterior lip of vasal adventitia to lower edge of the opening tailored in the epididymal tunica.

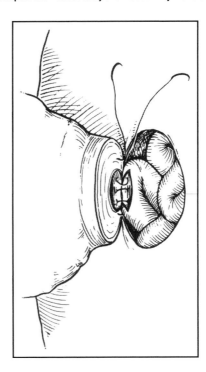

Figure 28 Posterior row of 10-0 mucosal sutures placed inside out.

the anastomotic site with two to four interrupted sutures of 6-0 polypropylene placed through the vasal adventitia and the tunica vaginalis. The vasal lumen should reach the opening in the epididymal tunica easily with length to spare. The posterior edge of the epididymal tunica is then approximated to the posterior edge of the vas muscularis and adventitia with two to three interrupted sutures of double-armed 9-0 nylon (Figs. 26 and 27). This is done in such a way as to bring the vasal lumen in close approximation to the epididymal tubule selected for anastomosis.

Classic End-to-Side Technique

Under 25- to 32-power magnification, using a small curved microscissors or a 15° microknife, an opening about 0.3 to 0.5 mm in diameter is made in the selected tubule. Epididymal fluid is touched to a slide, diluted with saline or Ringer's, and inspected under the microscope for sperm. If no sperm are found, the opening in the tubule is closed with 10-0 sutures, the vas detached, and the tunica incision closed with 9-0 nylon sutures. The procedure is then repeated more proximally in the epididymis.

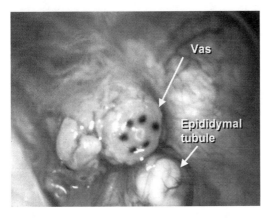

Figure 27 As in vasovasostomy, the use of microdots on the cut surface of the vas can enhance precision in suture placement.

Once sperm are identified, they are aspirated into glass capillary tubes and flushed into media for cryopreservation (Fig. 15) (50). Indigo carmine solution is dripped on the cut tubule to outline the mucosa (46). The posterior mucosal edge of the epididymal tubule is approximated to the posterior edge of the vasal mucosa with two interrupted sutures of 10-0 monofilament nylon sutures double armed with fish-hook 70 μm-diameter tapered needles (Fig. 28). The lumen is irrigated with Ringer's solution just prior to placement of each suture to keep the epididymal lumen open. After these mucosal sutures are tied, the anterior mucosal anastomosis is completed with two to four additional 10-0 sutures. The outer muscularis and adventitia of the vas is then approximated to the cut edge of the epididymal tunica with 6 to 10 additional interrupted sutures of 9-0 nylon double-armed with 100 μm-diameter needles (Fig. 29). The vasal sheath is secured to the epididymal tunica with three to five sutures of 9-0 nylon. The testis and epididymis are gently returned to the tunica vaginalis, which is closed with 5-0 Vicryl. The scrotum is closed as previously described for vasovasostomy.

End-to-Side Intussusception Technique

This method is also known as the triangulation technique and was introduced by Berger (56). There are several advantages of this method over previous techniques, and it is now the authors' preferred method for all vasoepididymostomies (61). The set-up is identical to that for the classical end-to-side vasoepididymostomy. After the vas is fixed to the opening in the epididymal tunica, six microdots are placed on the cut

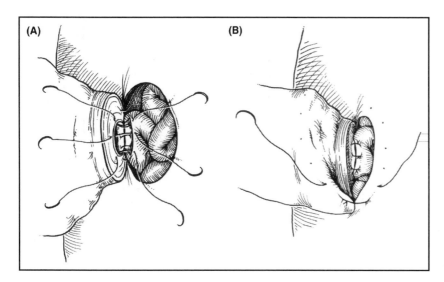

Figure 29 (A,B) After completion of anterior mucosal portion of the anastomosis, the second layer of 9-0 nylon sutures are placed to provide a water-tight seal.

surface of the vas in a fashion identical to that described for vasovasostomy. The selected epididymal tubule is dissected with blunt microscissors and the microneedle holder until it is free of surrounding tissue and prominent. The tubule is then stained with indigo carmine. Using 10-0 monofilament nylon sutures approximately two inches in length, double-armed with 70 cm-diameter fish-hook-shaped, tapered needles, three sutures are placed in the epididymal tubule in a triangulation fashion. The apex of the triangle faces the inferior edge of the vasal mucosa (Fig. 30). The needles are not pulled through but left in situ, creating a triangle of needles (Fig. 31). Using a 15° microknife with the blade pointing upward, a generous opening is made in the epididymal tubule in the center of the triangle created by the three needles (Fig. 32). The three needles are then pulled through. The six needles are now laid out so as to avoid a spaghetti-like tangle. A glass slide is touched to the fluid exuding from the opening in the epididymal tubule and mixed with human tubal fluid media, covered with a cover slip, and examined by the surgeon using the separate

bench microscope under 400-power magnification. If whole sperm (whether motile or not) or abundant sperm heads/fragments are present, the decision is made to proceed with the anastomosis. Sperm are aspirated into micropipettes first (Fig. 33), expressed into human tubal fluid media, and sent for cryopreservation if motility is observed. Sperm that initially appear immotile, when mixed with human tubule fluid, often regain motility adequate for successful cryopreservation. Even immotile sperm should be placed in the media and evaluated for potential cryopreservation. If the needles are pulled through prior to placing all three sutures or before making an opening in the epididymal tubule, epididymal fluid and sperm will immediately leak through the suture hole, causing the tubules to collapse. This makes the placement of subsequent sutures and the creation of the opening in the center of the triangle considerably more difficult. Leaving the needles in the epididymal tubule prior to making the opening also prevents accidental cutting of the sutures when making the opening in the center of the triangle. After abundant sperm have been

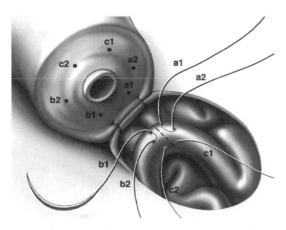

Figure 30 Intussusception end–side vasoepididymostomy. The first two sutures (a1-2 and b1-2) are placed in a V-shaped configuration with the point of the "V" aimed at the 6 o'clock position on the vas deferens.

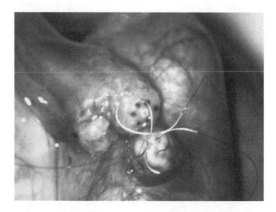

Figure 31 The 70 μm needle is larger than the 17 μm diameter of the suture. To avoid leaking of fluid, which will lead to collapse of the tubule and difficult placement of subsequent sutures, the needles are left in place. In addition, accidental cutting of the sutures is avoided when opening the tubule with a sharp microknife.

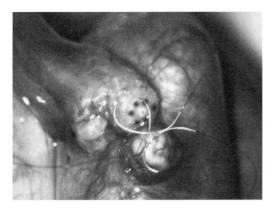

Figure 32 Position of sutures in the epididymal tubule once the tubule is opened.

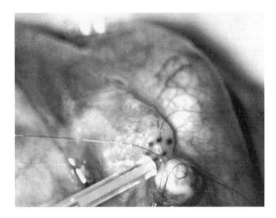

Figure 33 Once the presence of sperm in the epididymal tubule has been confirmed, epididymal fluid is aspirated by capillary action into the micropipette for cryopreservation.

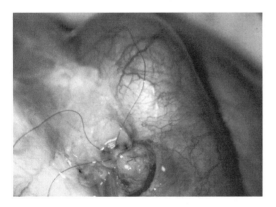

Figure 34 The six needles are passed inside-out the vas deferens, exiting through the six microdots.

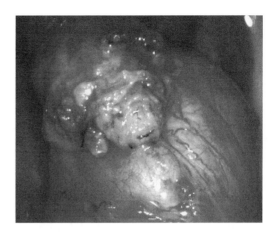

Figure 35 Tying the sutures intussuscepts the epididymal tubule into the vas lumen.

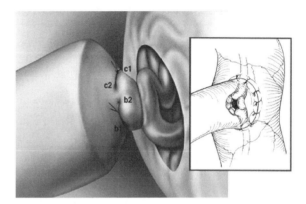

Figure 36 Schematic illustration of the intussusception of the epididymal tubule into the vas lumen.

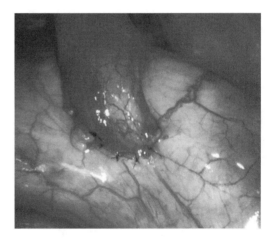

Figure 37 Completion of closure of the second layer.

aspirated into micropipettes and cryopreserved, the six needles are passed inside-out the vas deferens, exiting through the six previously placed microdots in the order indicated (Fig. 34). Each pair of sutures is then sequentially tied, beginning with suture a1 and a2, then b1 and b2, and finally c1 and c2. Tying of these sutures intussuscepts the epididymal tubule into the vas lumen (Figs. 35 and 36). This creates a water-tight

closure. Additionally, the flow of epididymal fluid from the epididymal tubule into the vas deferens tends to plaster the edges of the epididymal tubule against the mucosal walls of the vas deferens, further helping create a leakproof closure. The second layer of the anastomosis is completed in a fashion identical to that described for the classical end-to-side operation above (Fig. 37).

Two-Stitch Variation of the Intussusception Technique

For anastomoses to very small epididymal tubules such as those found in the caput or to the efferent ductules (62), the three-stitch triangulation technique may be impossible. For these anastomoses, a two-stitch intussusception technique is much easier to perform and may be almost as successful (63). With this method, four microdots are marked on the cut surface of the vas deferens and two parallel sutures are placed in the distended epididymal tubule but not pulled through (Fig. 38). Marmar (63) suggests mounting two needles in the needle holder and placing them simultaneously; however, if the needles are not pulled through to avoid leakage of fluid and tubular collapse, they can be placed one at a time with greater control and accuracy. Using a 15° microknife, an opening is made exactly between and parallel to the two previously placed sutures. After the fluid is tested for sperm and aspirated into micropipettes for cryopreservation, the four needles are passed inside-out the vas deferens and tied. The anastomosis is completed as described previously.

Microsurgical Vasoepididymostomy: End-to-End Anastomosis

End-to-end anastomosis was introduced by Silber (55), representing the first specific tubule VE anastomosis. When this method was first described, it was far superior to any of the nonmicroscopic techniques previously employed. With this method, the epididymis is dissected completely to the VE junction, and then serially and transversely transected until a gush of fluid is seen exuding from the cut surface, indicating the correct level of the anastomosis (Fig. 39). The single tubule from which fluid is effluxing is identified and anastomosed directly to the vas mucosa with three to

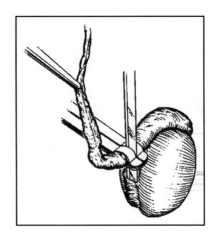

Figure 39   Preparation for end-to-end vasoepididymostomy.

five interrupted sutures of 10-0 monofilament nylon (Fig. 40). The advantage of this technique is that the correct level in the epididymis at which the anastomosis should be performed can be rapidly and accurately assessed. In addition, if vasal length is compromised, the epididymis can be dissected to the caput by ligating the inferior and medial epididymal vessels and flipping the epididymis up, providing additional length (Fig. 39). A major disadvantage of this technique is that the diameter of the transversely sectioned epididymal tunica is far larger than the outer diameter of the vas deferens, making a water-tight closure of the outer layer difficult to achieve (Fig. 41). Finally, because of the difficulty in obtaining good hemostasis, it is far more difficult to aspirate clean, blood-free sperm for cryopreservation than it is with the end-to-side techniques.

Technique when Vasal Length Is Severely Compromised

When there is inadequate length of the vas deferens to reach the dilated epididymal tubule without tension, the epididymis can be dissected down to the VE junction and then dissected off the testes as in the older end-to-end operation.

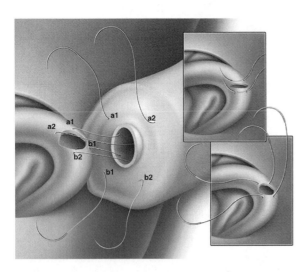

Figure 38   Two-needle intussusception vasoepididymostomy. This is particularly useful for anastomoses to very small epididymal tubules as in the caput epididymis or efferent ductules.

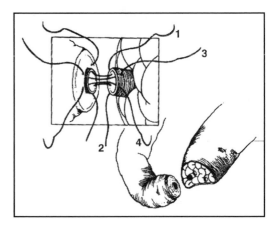

Figure 40   The scheme for the placement of 10-0 mucosal sutures for end-to-end vasoepididymostomy.

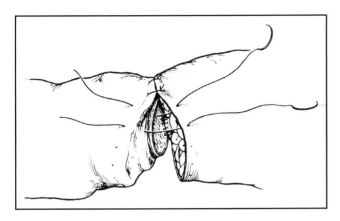

Figure 41 Second layer of 9-0 nylon sutures approximating vasal adventitia and perivasal sheath to cut edge of the epididymal tunica.

After the vas has been prepared, the tunica vaginalis is opened and the testis delivered. Inspection of the epididymis under the operating microscope may reveal a clearly delineated site of obstruction. Often, a discrete yellow sperm granuloma is noted, above which there is indurated epididymis and dilated tubules, and below which the epididymis is soft and the tubules collapsed. If the level of obstruction is not clearly delineated, a 70 μm tapered needle from the 10-0 nylon microsuture is used to puncture the epididymal tubule beginning as distally as possible and fluid is sampled from the puncture site until sperm are found. At that level, the puncture is sealed with microbipolar forceps and the epididymis is ligated just proximal to the puncture site with a 6-0 nylon suture. The epididymis is then dissected off the testis and flipped up to obtain additional length. To do this, the epididymis is encircled with a small Penrose drain at the level of obstruction and, using 2.5 power loupe magnification, dissected off of the testis for 3 to 5 cm, yielding sufficient length to perform the anastomosis. Usually, a nice plane can be found between the epididymis and testis, and injury to the epididymal blood supply can be avoided by staying right on the tunica albuginea of the testis. The inferior, and, if necessary, middle epididymal branches of the testicular artery are doubly ligated and divided to free an adequate length of epididymis. The superior-epididymal branches entering the epididymis at the caput are always preserved and can provide adequate blood supply to the entire epididymis. The tunica vaginalis in then closed over the testis with 5-0 Vicryl, which prevents drying of the testis and thrombosis of the surface testicular vessels during the anastomosis. The dissected epididymis remains outside the tunica vaginalis.

If the epididymis is indurated and dilated throughout its length, the epididymis is dissected to the VE junction. This dissection is often facilitated by first dissecting the convoluted vas to the VE junction from below, and then, after encircling the epididymis with a Penrose drain, dissecting the epididymis to the VE junction from above. In this way, the entire VE junction can be freed up. This will allow preservation of maximal epididymal length in cases of distal obstruction near the VE junction. After the epididymis is dissected off of the testis and flipped upward, a three-stitch end-to-side intussusception anastomosis is performed as described above.

Long-Term Follow-Up Evaluation and Results

Microsurgical vasoepididymostomy in the hands of experienced and skilled microsurgeons will result in the appearance of sperm in the ejaculate in 50% to 85% of men. Patency rates with the intussusception technique can exceed 80% (56,63,64). With the classic end-to-side or older end-to-end method, the patency rate is about 70%, and 43% of men with sperm will impregnate their wives after a minimum follow-up of two years (54,65). Pregnancy rates are higher the more distal the anastomosis is performed. With the older end-to-end or end-to-side method, at 14 months after surgery, 25% of initially patent anastomoses are found to be shut down (50). For this reason, the authors recommend banking sperm both intraoperatively (66) and as soon as they appear in the ejaculate postoperatively. In men with very low counts or poor sperm quality postoperatively and men who remain azoospermic, the sperm intraoperatively cryopreserved can be used for IVF with intracytoplasmic sperm injection. Persistently azoospermic men without cryopreserved sperm can opt for either a redo vasoepidymostomy and/or a microscopic epididymal sperm aspiration combined with IVF and intracytoplasmic sperm injection.

☐ CONCLUSION

With the increasing awareness of the safety and efficacy of vasectomy, as well as the introduction of the less invasive no-scalpel vasectomy, the role of men in family planning has increased tremendously worldwide. In recent years, advancements in the surgical management of male fertility have further extended to microsurgical reconstruction procedures—namely, vasovasostomy and vasoepididymostomy—allowing many infertile and subfertile men with excurrent ductal obstruction to father children through natural conception. In the era of IVF/ICSI, surgical treatment for obstructive male infertility still remains the safest and most cost-effective management option for couples. Clinicians specialized in treating male infertility should therefore be familiar with the indications and techniques of microsurgical reconstruction procedures.

☐ REFERENCES

1. Schwingl PJ, Guess HS. Safety and effectiveness of vasectomy. Fertil Steril 2000; 73(5):923–936.
2. Wilson EW. Sterilization. Bailliees Clin Obstet Gynaecol 1996; 10(1):103–119.
3. Kendrick J, Gonzales B, Huber D, et al. Complications of vasectomies in the United States. J Fam Prac 1987; 25(3):245–248.
4. Li S, Goldstein M, Zhu J, et al. The no-scalpel vasectomy. J Urol 1991; 145:341–344.
5. Li S. Ligation of vas deferens by clamping method under direct vision. Chin Med J 1976; 4:213–214.
6. Sokal D, McMullen S, Gates D, et al. A comparative study of the no scalpel and standard incision approaches to vasectomy in 5 countries. The Male Sterilization Investigator Team. J Urol 1999; 162(5):1621–1625.
7. Nirapathopongporn A, Huber DH, Krieger JN. No-scalpel vasectomy at the King's birthday vasectomy festival. Lancet 1990; 335(8694):894–895.
8. Moss WM. Sutureless vasectomy, an improved technique; 1300 cases performed without failure. Fertil Steril 1974; 27(9):1040–1045.
9. Bennett AH. Vasectomy without complication. Urology 1976; 7(2):184–185.
10. Schmidt SS. Vasectomy. Urol Clin North Am 1987; 14(1):149–154.
11. Esho JO, Cass AS. Recanalization rate following methods of vasectomy using interposition of fascial sheath of vas deferens. J Urol 1978; 120(2):178–179.
12. Maatman TJ, Aldrin L, Carothers GG. Patient noncompliance after vasectomy. Fertil Steril 1997; 68(3):552–555.
13. Lemack GE, Goldstein M. Presence of sperm in the pre-vasectomy reversal semen analysis: incidence and implications. J Urol 1996; 155(1):167–169.
14. Appell R, Evans P. Vasectomy: etiology of infectious complications. Fertil Steril 1980; 33(1):52–53.
15. Randall PE, Ganguli L, Marcuson RW. Wound infection following vasectomy. Br J Urol 1983; 55(5):564–567.
16. Randall PE, Ganguli LA, Keaney MGL, et al. Prevention of wound infection following vasectomy. Br J Urol 1985; 57(2):227–229.
17. Silber SJ. Sperm granulomas and reversibility of vasectomy. Lancet 1977; 2(8038):588–589.
18. Belker AM, Thomas AV, Fuchs EEF. Results of 1469 microsurgical vasectomy reversals by vasovasostomy study group. J Urol 1991; 145(3):505–511.
19. Schmidt SS. Spermatic granuloma: an often painful lesion. Fertil Steril 1979; 31(2):178–181.
20. Sokal D, Irsula B, Chen-Mok M, et al. A comparison of vas occlusion techniques: cautery more effective than ligation and excision with fascial interposition. BMC Urol 2004; 4(1):12.

21. Choe JM, Kirkemo AK. Questionnaire-based outcomes study of nononcological post-vasectomy complications. J Urol 1996; 155(4):1284–1286.
22. Freund MJ, Weidmann JE, Goldstein M, et al. Microrecanalization after vasectomy in man. J Androl 1989; 10(2):120–132.
23. Johnson AL, Howards SS. Intratubular hydrostatic pressure in testis and epidydimis before and after vasectomy. Am J Physiol 1975; 228(2):556–564.
24. Jarow JP, Budin RE, Dym M, et al. Quantitative pathological changes in the human testis after vasectomy. N Engl J Med 1985; 313(20):1252–1256.
25. Awsare NS, Krishnan J, Boustead GB, et al. Complications of vasectomy. Ann R Coll Surg Engl 2005; 87(6):406–410.
26. Selikowitz AM, Schned AR. A late post-vasectomy syndrome. J Urol 1985; 134(3):494–497.
27. Lepow IH, Crozier R. Vasectomy: Immunologic and Pathophysiologic Effects in Animal and Man. New York: Academic Press, 1979.
28. Fuchs EF, Alexander N. Immunologic considerations before and after vasovasostomy. Fertil Steril 1983; 40(4):497–499.
29. Witkin SS, Zelikovsky G, Bongiovanni AM. Sperm-related antigens, antibodies, and circulating immune complexes in sera of recently vasectomized men. J Clin Invest 1982; 70(1):33–40.
30. Massey FJ Jr, Bernstein GS, O'Fallon WM, et al. Vasectomy and health. Results from a large cohort study. JAMA 1984; 252(8):1023–1029.
31. Alexander NJ, Clarkson TB. Vasectomy increases the severity of diet-induced atherosclerosis in Macaca fascicularis. Science 1978; 201(4355):538–541.
32. Walker AM, Hunter JR, Watkins RN, et al. Vasectomy and non-fatal myocardial infarction. Lancet 1981; 1(8210):13–15.
33. Walker AM, Jick H, Hunter JR, et al. Hospitalization rates in vasectomized men. JAMA 1981; 245(22):2315–2317.
34. Petitti DB, Klein R, Kipp H, et al. Vasectomy and the incidence of hospitalized illness. J Urol 1982; 129(4):760–762.
35. Smith MS, Paulson DF. The physiologic consequences of vas ligation. Urological Survey 1980; 30(2):31–33.
36. Schuman LM, Coulson AH, Mandel JS, et al. Health status of American Men—a study of post-vasectomy sequalae. J Clin Epidemiol 1993; 46(8):697–958.
37. Healy B. Does vasectomy cause prostate cancer? From the National Institutes of Health. JAMA 1993; 269(20):2620.
38. Sheynkin YR, Hendin BN, Schlegel PN, et al. Microsurgical repair of iatrogenic injury to the vas deferens. J Urol 1998; 159(1):139–141.
39. Hendin BN, Schlegel PN, Goldstein M. Microsurgical reconstruction of iatrogenic injury to the vas deferens.

Proceedings of the 48th Annual meeting of the American Fertility Society, New Orleans, LA, Nov 2–5, 1992 (abstr), 1992; 140:1545–1548.

40. Kolettis PN, Thomas AJ Jr. Vasoepididymostomy for vasectomy reversal: a critical assessment in the era of intracytoplasmic sperm injection. J Urol 1997; 158(2): 467–470.

41. Pavlovich CP, Schlegel PN. Fertility options after vasectomy: a cost-effectiveness analysis. Fertil Steril 1997; 67(1):133–141.

42. Goldstein M. Microspike approximator for vaso-vasostomy. J Urol 1985; 134(1):74.

43. Sheynkin YR, Chen ME, Goldstein M. Intravasal azoospermia: a surgical dilemma. B J U Int 2000; 85(9): 1089–1092.

44. Hagan KF, Coffey DS. The adverse effects of sperm during vasovasostomy. J Urol 1977; 118(2):269–273.

45. Goldstein M, Li PS, Matthews GJ. Microsurgical vasovasostomy: the microdot technique of precision suture placement. J Urol 1998; 159(1):188–190.

46. Sheynkin YR, Starr C, Li PS, et al. Effect of methylene blue, indigo carmine, and renografin on human sperm motility. Urology 1999; 53(1):214–217.

47. Lizza EF, Marmar JL, Schmidt SS, et al. Transseptal crossed vasovasostomy. J Urol 1985; 134(6):1131–1132.

48. Hamidinia A. Transvasovasostomy--an alternative operation for obstructive azoospermia. J Urol 1988; 140(6):1545–1548.

49. Sheynkin YR, Li PS, Magid ML, et al. Comparison of absorbable and nonabsorbable sutures for microsurgical vasovasostomy in rats. Urology 1999; 53(6): 1235–1238.

50. Matthews GJ, Schlegel PN, Goldstein M. Patency following microsurgical vasoepididymostomy and vasovasostomy: temporal considerations. J Urol 1995; 154(6):2070–2073.

51. Silber SJ. Role of epididymis in sperm maturation. Fertil Steril 1989; 33(1):47–51.

52. Jow WW, Steckel J, Schlegel PN, et al. Motile sperm in human testis biopsy specimens. J Androl 1993; 14(3): 194–198.

53. Schoysman RJ, Bedford JM. The role of the human epididymis in sperm maturation and sperm storage as reflected in the consequences of epididymovasostomy. Fertil Steril 1986; 46(2):292–299.

54. Schlegel PN, Goldstein M. Microsurgical vasoepididymostomy: refinements and results. J Urol 1993; 150(4):1165–1168.

55. Silber SJ. Microscopic vasoepididymostomy: specific microanastomosis to the epididymal tubule. Fertil Steril 1978; 30(5):565–571.

56. Berger R. Triangulation end-to-side vasoepididymostomy. J Urol 1998; 159(6):1951–1953.

57. Wagenknecht LV, Klosterhalfen H, Schirren C. Microsurgery in andrologic urology. I. Refertilization. J Microsurg 1980; 1(5):370–376.

58. Krylov VS, Borovikov AM. Microsurgical method of reuniting ductus epididymis (sic). Fertil Steril 1984; 41(3):418–423.

59. Fogdestam I, Fall M, Nilsson S. Microsurgical epididymovasostomy in the treatment of occlusive azoospermia. Fertil Steril 1986; 46(5):925–929.

60. Thomas AJ Jr. Vasoepididymostomy. Urol Clin North Am 1987; 14(3):527–538.

61. Goldstein M, McCallum S, Li PS. Microsurgical vasoepididymostomy: end-to-side triangulation technique. American Urologic Association Meeting, Dallas, TX, May 2, 1999, (abstr #V 17). J Urol 1999; 161(suppl 4):93.

62. Chan PTK, Goldstein M. Microsurgical reconstruction of pre-epididymal obstructive azoospermia. American Urological Annual Meeting, Atlanta, GA, May 2, 2000, (abstr). J Urol 2000; 163(suppl 4):258.

63. Marmar JL. Modified vasoepididymostomy with simultaneous double needle placement, tubulotomy and tubular invagination. J Urol 2000; 163(2):483–486.

64. Brandell RA, Goldstein M. Reconstruction of the male reproductive tract using the microsurgical triangulation technique for vasoepididymostomy. American Urologic Association Meeting, Dallas, TX, May 5, 1999, (abstr #1355). J Urol 1999; 161(suppl 4):350.

65. Pasqualotto FF, Agarwal A, Srivastava M, et al. Fertility outcome after repeat vasoepididymostomy. J Urol 1999; 162(5):1626–1628.

66. Matthews GJ, Goldstein M. A simplified technique of epididymal sperm aspiration. Urology 1996; 47(1): 123–125.

Psychological Effects of Infertility and Its Treatment in Males

Kenneth Gannon
School of Psychology, University of East London, Stratford, London, U.K.

Lesly Glover
Department of Clinical Psychology, The University of Hull, Hull, U.K.

Paul David Abel
Division of Surgery, Oncology, Reproduction and Anaesthesia, Imperial College School of Medicine, London, U.K.

☐ INTRODUCTION

Approximately 20% of cases of infertility are due solely to male factor problems and 20% to a female factor; 30% involve both male and female factors, and 30% have no identifiable cause (1). Although it is widely recognized that infertility can present psychological as well as medical challenges and difficulties, literature dealing with the psychological aspects has tended to focus on women's reactions to the situation. Men have either been neglected, or it has been assumed that their reactions will be similar to those of their partner. There is a growing body of research that suggests that infertility has a specific impact on men, especially in the case of male-factor problems. The purpose of this chapter is to review this research and to provide some guidelines for applying this information in clinical practice.

☐ SOCIAL PERSPECTIVES ON REPRODUCTION AND INFERTILITY

Although reproduction is a biological imperative in humans, it occurs within an intensely social context. In order to better understand how infertility affects the individual, it is necessary to consider both the value attached to conceiving and bearing children and the meanings ascribed to motherhood and fatherhood. It is also important to recognize the way in which sex roles and gender are viewed within a particular society in order to understand the impact on the individual of alterations in gender-normative life events.

Importance of Reproduction

Individual views and attitudes about fertility are inevitably influenced by prevailing societal and cultural standpoints. Fertility and parenthood are highly valued in almost all societies. Anthropologists have documented the extremes to which infertile women across cultures are willing to go to have children (2). These range from poor urban women bathing with miscarried fetuses and stillborn infants to Western women repeatedly undergoing risky medical procedures with unknown long-term effects; however, comparable information on the lengths to which men will go to father a child is lacking. In a small-scale study based in the United Kingdom, Dalton and Lilford (3) examined the trade-off values in infertility. They found that individuals (presumably women although the authors did not specify gender) drawn from the general population (N=32) and from an infertile population (N=16) in England would be willing to shorten their life span by 12 years in order to become pregnant once. In addition, the infertile population would accept a 35% risk of death to have one child. In another study of 108 infertile couples, over 20% of the women and 7% of the men said that they were willing to give up everything to have children, with 30% of women and 28% of men willing to give up a great deal to have a child (4).

Infertility, Impotence, and Masculinity

There is a perception that "being a man" is synonymous with fathering a child. Work by Mason (5) asserted that manliness is traditionally viewed as relating more to the ability to make a woman pregnant as opposed to undertaking the role of father. Another study interviewing infertile men suggested that fertility is central to men's gender identity (6). There is an apparent underlying societal assumption that infertility is a threat to male sexuality or at least to masculinity (5,7). Whatever its origin, this confounding of impotence and infertility has consequences for infertile men. Fathering a child is seen as proof of masculinity (8) and it follows therefore that not fathering one is seen as a failure to achieve this level of manhood. Nachtigall et al. (6) found that approximately two-thirds of infertile men were preoccupied with the loss of their "physical potency." On the other hand, few men raised this concern when infertility had an identified female cause.

Not all studies, however, have found an association between masculinity and infertility. Edelmann et al. (7), asked 205 couples with male-factor subfertility if they agreed with the following statement: "a man can never be sure about his masculinity until he is a father." Although they found few couples agreeing with the statement, it was suggested that this atypical finding was because their sample was drawn from a self-help organization and may not have been typical of infertile couples. Men who did agree with the statement, however, reported greater distress than those who did not, suggesting that, for some men at least, infertility may compromise masculine identity.

Goffman (9) used the term "stigma" to describe the way in which a person's identity can become compromised or "spoiled." Nachtigall et al. (6) specifically addressed the issue of stigma in infertile men. They found that two-thirds of the infertile men in their sample felt stigmatized and identified infertility as relating to their perceived loss of masculinity. Miall (10) interviewed 71 men and 79 women with no fertility problems about their views of infertile men and women. Male infertility was associated with higher levels of stigma than female infertility; half the sample felt that society views male and female infertility differently. Miall (10) identified three themes that emerged from the interviews: infertile men were more likely to be ridiculed than infertile women; infertile women were more likely to be offered sympathy than their male counterparts; and the inability to have children was more likely to be attributed to the woman. When the cause of infertility was attributed to the man, it was seen as the result of sexual dysfunction. The majority of men (83%) and half the women in the sample felt that infertile men would experience more difficulty with their self-perception than infertile women. Almost all who responded linked infertile men's difficulties to their "tarnished" male ego or to worries about male sexual prowess. At an individual level, it seems that for men, the experience of infertility may relate not only to the fact of not having a child but also to the effect this has on individual self-perceptions.

Social theorists have developed the concept of hegemonic masculinity to describe the idealized form of masculinity at a given place and time (11). Beliefs and behaviors associated with contemporary Western hegemonic masculinity are the denial of weakness or vulnerability, emotional and physical control, the appearance of being strong and robust, dismissal of any need for help, a ceaseless interest in sex, the display of aggressive behavior, and physical dominance. Given this prevailing generalized set of powerful cultural values and expectations, and the particular issues encountered in confronting male-fertility problems, we might expect that men presenting with subfertility or infertility will experience psychological distress and that this may well differ from that being experienced by their partners. How they cope with this may have implications for their response to investigation and treatment.

The prevailing concepts of masculinity may have hindered research into male-factor subfertility and infertility, particularly in the psychological dimension. For example, Bents (12) suggested that male infertility has not been researched because the confusion between potency and fertility led to it being a taboo subject. The perception that infertility is less significant for men than for women may also have contributed to the lack of research in this area.

Motherhood and Fatherhood

It is a fundamental view of society that motherhood is the ultimate expression of being a woman and that a woman cannot achieve her full potential without becoming a mother (13,14). Motherhood is idealized and highly valued but such strong constructions do not apply to fatherhood. While motherhood is central to the ways in which women are defined both by themselves and by others (14), fatherhood remains simply one aspect of many in men's lives and yet another way in which they define themselves. In a study exploring attitudes to parenthood, Humphrey (15) found that men, especially childless men, were likely to associate fatherhood with masculinity, while women associated motherhood with contentment. Men were less likely to associate fatherhood with contentment. The study of roles and meanings of fatherhood is relatively new. Although it is argued that children benefit from the presence of a father, scant research is available on the importance to men of raising children (16). At least in Western societies, it seems that the primary role of men in reproduction is viewed as enabling women to become mothers (17).

Newton et al. (18) investigated the motives for parenthood in couples undergoing in vitro fertilization (IVF). They found that the primary reason given by the majority of men was a desire for marital completion while in women the emphasis was on the need to fulfill gender requirements. They suggested that men are less likely to see infertility as a threat to self-worth than as a threat to their marital relationship. Van Balen and Trimbos-Kemper (4) found both men and women cite happiness as their primary motive for having a child, with well-being and fatherhood being second and third motives for men, respectively.

□ PSYCHOLOGICAL SEQUELAE OF INFERTILITY

The understanding of men's psychological experience of infertility and its investigation has been made difficult by limited data. In addition, treatment procedures have changed rapidly over the past few years. The introduction of intracytoplasmic sperm injection (ICSI) in the early 1990s opened up the possibility that many men who had previously had little or no hope of enabling their partners to conceive could now do so. Such advances in treatment have influenced men's experiences of infertility and make it more difficult to have a clear, up-to-date picture of how men respond psychologically to being infertile. The studies reviewed in this section document the individual experience, but because so few have focused on men alone, it will be necessary to include studies that describe the experiences and reactions of both men and women. This approach also allows men's responses to be compared with those of women.

Impact of Infertility
Studies of Men

Although very few studies have focused on men alone, those that did identified a range of negative effects of infertility on psychological well-being. Higher levels of generalized distress have been identified in men with fertility problems than in men from the general population. For example, Kedem et al. (19) compared 107 men attending a specialist infertility clinic for semen analysis with a control group of 30 men without known fertility problems. They found that the infertile men had significantly lower self-esteem and were more anxious than the controls. Wright et al. (20) studied 449 couples who were assessed for infertility on their first clinic attendance and found that the men were significantly more distressed than average. In another study by Morrow et al. (21), 65% of the male partners of infertile couples scored above the normative mean on the Global Severity Index subscale of the Symptom Checklist 90-Revised, indicating that they suffered greater psychological distress than men in the general population.

Other studies have even identified clinically significant levels of distress. McEwan et al. (22) reported clinically significant scores on the General Health Questionnaire (a screening measure for psychological distress) in 13% of their sample of 45 men from couples with different types of infertility. Glover et al. (23) carried out a longitudinal study of subfertile men attending a specialist clinic. At the initial consultation, they were found to be highly anxious, with 51% scoring in either a borderline or a clinical range on the Hospital Anxiety and Depression Scale. They blamed themselves for their fertility problems and felt less of a man because of them. They considered their life satisfaction to be less than it would be if they were able to father a child. Measures of mood, life-satisfaction, and self-blame were unchanged at 6-week and 18-month follow-up.

Not all studies have found elevated levels of distress, however. Raval et al. (24) conducted individual interviews to evaluate distress in 47 couples attending an infertility clinic with various diagnoses. They found that, compared with control groups, the male scores were "unremarkable." Nevertheless, most studies agree that infertility has a range of negative psychological consequences for men including anxiety, psychological distress, dissatisfaction, and self-blame.

Comparison of Men and Women

Most studies have indicated that psychological consequences of infertility are worse for women than men, irrespective of whether it is due to male or female factor(s). Women had greater overall intensity of emotional response to subfertility (25). They were also both more depressed (26) and distressed (20) than subfertile men. In addition, women perceived their relationship with their partner as more adversely affected (24).

In interviews with 174 primary infertile couples versus 74 presumed-to-be-fertile couples, it was found that infertile wives perceived having children as more important and being subfertile as more stressful than their husbands (27). Furthermore, men in the infertile group reported greater home-life stress than men in the control group. They also found that both infertile and presumed-to-be-fertile women experienced more depression and lower self-esteem than their husbands. Collins et al. (28) examined perceptions of infertility and treatment stress in a consecutive series of 200 couples entering an IVF treatment program. Using an unpublished measure called the Infertility Reaction Scale, they found that women had significantly higher scores than men, suggesting that they experienced greater emotional and social effects of infertility than did men.

Not all studies, however, have found women to be more distressed. Stanton et al. (29) developed a scale to measure infertility specific distress in a study of 54 subfertile couples. They found that although women acknowledged more distress specific to infertility than their partners, there was no difference between men and women in their general emotional distress.

Berg et al. (30) found no difference in the level of emotional strain, marital adjustment, or sexual satisfaction between men and women in their study of 104 infertile couples, but they did identify differences in the context of distress for men and women. Women were more likely than men to report having a child as being important to them, to locate the cause of their infertility as being within them, and to feel that their infertility was a punishment for something they had done. Women experienced more discomfort than men in the presence of fertility-related stimuli. Also, men were less likely than women to reveal their fertility problem to relatives or individuals outside the family.

Sexual Functioning and Marital Relationship

Andrews et al. (31) conducted separate interviews with 157 infertile couples and found that fertility-related stress was associated with decreases in sexual self-esteem, satisfaction with own sexual performance, and frequency of intercourse. The negative association between this stress and frequency of intercourse was greater for husbands than for wives.

Kedem et al. (19) found that men with partners with an identified fertility problem had a higher incidence of sexual dysfunction than did those men whose partners had no problems. Elstein (32) reported a decrease in libido when sexual function became primarily a reproductive process and intercourse was reduced to a goal-oriented exercise in semen delivery. In a study of 51 couples attending a fertility clinic for postcoital testing, Drake and Grunert (33) found that 10% of the men reported sexual dysfunction (inability to maintain an erection or ejaculatory failure) during their partner's ovulation but at no other time during the menstrual cycle. It may be that for these couples, the influence of "this-is-the-night syndrome" is even greater, with the goal-oriented nature of intercourse being emphasized.

Raval et al. (24) reported changes in sexual functioning over time, with a peak in problems following recognition of infertility but prior to treatment. Overall, however, there was no significant difference between the incidence of sexual dysfunction in the sample and rates in the general population. This supports the hypothesis of Drake and Grunert (33) that the mild and acute nature of mid-cycle sexual dysfunction is not detectable by standard assessment techniques. Berger (34) found that 10 out of 16 couples interviewed after the husband was discovered to be azoospermic reported a period of impotence lasting between one and three months following the discovery, suggesting that sexual dysfunction in men with fertility problems is not solely the result of pressure to achieve a pregnancy.

A number of authors have looked at the impact of infertility on relationships, particularly on marital and sexual satisfaction. Several studies and reviews (35,36) have concluded that satisfaction with the relationship remains high, even in the presence of sexual dysfunction. Greater satisfaction has been found to be associated with longer periods of trying to conceive (37) and with men's acceptance of a childless lifestyle (38); however, greater marital difficulties have been found to be associated with male-factor infertility (39), and some (31) have reported that fertility-related stress increased marital conflict.

Change Over Time

The following sections examine the impact of continuing subfertility and psychological outcomes of pregnancy following fertility problems.

Continuing Subfertility

There have been few long-term follow-up studies of those undergoing fertility investigation and treatment. Slade et al. (40) interviewed couples attending a subfertility clinic four months after their initial appointment and again three years later. Of the original 47 couples, 25 took part in the follow-up, and, of these, 14 had continuing subfertility. The majority of couples with continuing subfertility had a male-factor problem. The authors found that psychological functioning did not improve over time if there was continuing infertility. They also reported deterioration in both the marital relationship and the sexual relationship and

found evidence of a decline in the men's self-esteem, suggesting a more negative emotional outcome in men where a male-factor problem has been identified. This is supported by Connolly et al. (41) who compared attendees at an infertility clinic at first visit and after seven months. Based on the General Health Questionnaire, they found increased distress in men ($N=39$) with a male-factor problem.

Pregnancy as an Outcome

In the aforementioned Slade et al. (40) study, 11 couples had produced their own biological child at three-year follow up. No change was found in mood or self-esteem for women regardless of whether or not they had continuing fertility problems. Men who subsequently became fathers, however, showed an improvement in self-esteem. From their cohort of infertile couples, Abbey et al. (42) found that the women experienced greater benefits of parenthood than did the men. Both partners had reduced marital well-being on becoming parents; men also reported decreased home-life stress (but not the women). Abbey et al. (42) suggested that after years of trying to have a child, previously infertile men may be more sensitive to their changed household responsibilities and their wives' expectations of their performance in the home. In an 18-month longitudinal study of 165 couples, of whom 48 became pregnant, Benazon et al. (43) found that marital functioning decreased as treatment progressed. Marital distress was greater in those who did not conceive than those who did. Glover et al. (44) reported follow-up data on 50 male subfertility clinic attendees, comparing outcomes in those men whose partners became pregnant and those who remained childless. At initial clinic visits, there was no difference between the groups. At 18-month follow-up visits, there was a significantly greater positive change in life-satisfaction scores in the pregnant as against the nonpregnant group.

Although there are some inconsistencies among these studies, some general conclusions may be drawn. Continuing infertility is stressful (partly as a consequence of ongoing treatment), but many couples adapt well to their childless state and enjoy a good relationship and average levels of satisfaction with life. Having a child satisfies some needs, such as that of men to demonstrate their fertility, but brings its own stresses. Such stresses are, of course, a natural concomitant to parenting, but an important (and as yet unanswered) question is the extent to which they may be increased by an overly idealized view of parenthood developed over many years of unsuccessful attempts.

☐ INVESTIGATION AND TREATMENT

The process of investigation for subfertile women is less performance oriented than that experienced by subfertile men. Infertility requires men to perform sexually, both for tests (semen analysis and postcoital testing) and in attempts to conceive (natural and assisted). This means that men are provided with opportunities for both immediate and future success or failure (i.e., test results or pregnancy). Carmeli and Birenbaum-Carmeli (45) interviewed infertile men in Israel and Canada about their experiences of infertility treatment and suggested that men often felt marginalized because treatment tended to focus on women, even when there was a male-factor problem. Male partners were also sometimes excluded from attending procedures that their partner underwent, such as egg retrieval and insemination. They concluded that these experiences could undermine men's position in conjugal decision-making with respect to infertility.

One study compared 18 men undergoing ICSI and 22 men undergoing IVF for one complete treatment cycle (46). The men completed a daily chart, which assessed emotional, physical, and social reactions to infertility treatment. They found that distress changed across the cycle, with the active stages of oocyte retrieval and embryo transfer and the pregnancy test day being most distressing. Another study comparing the distress of men in couples undergoing ICSI versus those undergoing IVF found that distress levels were similar in each group, apart from a marginal difference just prior to retrieval of sperm when men undergoing ICSI were found to be slightly more distressed (47).

Daniluk (26) performed psychological tests on 63 couples attending an infertility clinic over four sessions: immediately following initial consultation with the doctor, four weeks after initial consultation, one week after diagnosis, and six weeks after diagnosis. Psychological distress was highest for both men and women at the time of the initial medical interview. In another study, Takefman et al. (48) assessed couples at the beginning and end of their investigation for fertility problems over a minimum period of three months; they reported that men whose psychological distress levels increased over the sessions had higher neuroticism scores and higher intercourse frequency than those whose levels remained unchanged.

A study on the immediate impact of medical consultation on anxiety, depression, self-blame, information appraisal, and perceptions of future fertility in subfertile men found that anxiety levels were high before the consultation, but afterwards, anxiety and self-blame had reduced while depression had increased (49). Even when a poor prognosis was given during the consultation, participants remained overly optimistic about their chances of achieving a pregnancy. Similarly, a study of 103 men attending a specialized fertility clinic looked at how they rated their partner's chances of achieving a pregnancy (23). Before consultation, patients expected that their chance of pregnancy would be increased following the clinic visit. Post consultation, their perceptions of their chances of pregnancy were often inaccurate and were more influenced by their preconsultation expectations than the consultant's view.

A subsequent study had 29 subfertile men complete questionnaires before and after consultation to assess expectations (50). Subfertile men rated increasing the chances of their partner conceiving as most important, with gaining information also receiving high ratings. Following the consultation, patients felt that they had gained understanding and their expectations of receiving help with decision-making had been fulfilled. They rated their satisfaction with the consultation as high and distress during the consultation as low despite the fact that many of their initial expectations had not been fulfilled.

In summary, the evidence seems to suggest that investigation and treatment of infertility is experienced as a process punctuated by events (e.g., clinic visits, giving semen samples, and receiving test results) and that these events may provide more or less stress. In addition to these particular events, it seems likely that the process has a cumulative effect, with stress increasing over time. Consultations appear to be perceived as a valuable experience even in the absence of a "cure"; however, understanding and recall of information may often be poor and influenced more by expectations than by the information actually given.

☐ FACTORS AFFECTING RESPONSES TO INFERTILITY

A variety of factors, including demography, diagnosis, and individual differences, have been shown to influence responses to infertility.

Demographic Factors

The most significant demographic factors are briefly reviewed here. Other factors have also been investigated but there are few or inconclusive data relating to them.

Age does seem to relate to distress in men with fertility difficulties. A study of 86 men (mean age: 34 years) and 120 women (mean age: 32 years) found that increased age added to the prediction of psychological distress in men but not in women (21). Although men do not have time constraints on their ability to reproduce, their partners do; as a result, men may still have a feeling that time is running out. Alternatively, it may be that men's desire for children and family life develops as time goes on and so the inability to have children becomes more distressing with age.

Duration of infertility has also been investigated. The majority of studies report no relationship between length of time trying to conceive and level of distress (19,22,24,26,39); however, Berg et al. (30) found that couples where the male partner was more distressed than the female partner (male-distressed group) had been undergoing investigation for a significantly shorter time than other groups. They suggested that men in the male-distressed group might be responding to problems of scheduling sex. Also, most of these studies have focused on couples with primary infertility, although some have included those with secondary problems. Again results are inconclusive, although Morrow et al. (21) found that not having biological children added to the prediction of psychological distress in men but not in women.

Diagnosis and Location of Cause

A factor often overlooked in these studies is the cause of the fertility problem. Edelmann and Connolly (51) suggested that resolution of uncertainty, whether it be by pregnancy or knowledge of azoospermia, is associated with less distress than not knowing. Another study found no difference in scores of distress and marital problems between diagnosed and undiagnosed couples (39). It may be that even with a diagnosis, uncertainty remains and that knowledge about the cause of the fertility problem may only be useful if it leads to definite statements about outcome. When the cause of infertility was found to be with the man, it was judged by both partners to create more marital difficulties than when the cause was found to be with the woman or with both partners (39). Infertility in men increased men's feelings of guilt, isolation, and depression; in the wives of infertile men, it led to increased feelings of guilt and lack of success. McEwan et al. (22) found that women who felt personally more responsible for their infertility were more distressed than those who did not; however, they also found that 44% of women without a diagnosis and 30% of women with a partner with a clear diagnosis still felt responsible for the problem. In a study by Daniluk (26), participants identified as having an organic fertility problem reported higher levels of depression than their partners did at the time of diagnosis.

Additional support for the presence of greater distress in men with male-factor infertility comes from the longitudinal literature. One study followed-up couples for seven to nine months after an initial visit to an infertility clinic. Using the General Health Questionnaire, they found that infertile men scored lower than men in couples with female factors only, male and female factors, or unexplained infertility (41). In another study, Slade et al. (40) followed patients three years after consultation; they again found infertile men were the least adjusted. Nachtigall et al. (6) interviewed couples undergoing infertility treatment and found that men with a male-factor problem experienced a more negative emotional response to infertility (in terms of feelings of stigma, loss, and self-esteem) than men without a male factor. Van Balen and Trimbos-Kemper (4), in a study of 108 couples with long-term infertility (mean 8.6 years), found more feelings of guilt and blame in infertile men than in involuntarily childless men with no identified fertility problem; however, no similar relationship existed between cause and negative feelings in women. Mikulincer et al. (52) found that for both men and women, a diagnosis of male-factor infertility was significantly more distressing and participants reported less well-being than for a diagnosis of female infertility.

Placing emphasis solely on who has the identified problem, however, may be unhelpful, as it does not take into account the fact that feelings of responsibility for infertility are not solely related to the location of the problem (22,27). An additional complicating factor is that patients' views of the source of the problem may differ from the medical diagnosis. Buttler et al. (53) examined the concordance between the perceptions of men attending a subfertility clinic and the medical diagnosis. Interestingly, they found that 17% of men with a male-factor diagnosis disagreed with the medical opinion, while 42.5% of men whose partner was diagnosed as infertile agreed with the diagnosis. Men in couples with a female factor who disagreed with the medical opinion reported a joint or unexplained diagnosis.

Individual Differences

The experience of infertility has multiple factors and thus has been examined using a variety of models. The complex and unique nature of infertility, however, makes it difficult to find a single model that adequately takes into account all aspects of this experience. Infertility has been seen to be a process (54), a life crisis (55), and a developmental crisis (56).

Drawing on the work of Lazarus and Folkman, recent infertility research has focused on the stress-coping aspect (57). At its core is the idea that an event is not stressful per se; rather, for an individual, it is the meaning of the event and the ability to find and use effective coping strategies that determine how the event is experienced. A situation is stressful if the individual perceives that environmental demands exceed his or her resources and endanger his or her well-being. This theory of psychological stress identifies cognitive appraisal and coping as critical mediators of person–environment relationships. This framework has three key processes: (i) primary appraisal (the perception of a potential threat), (ii) secondary appraisal (the perception of the ability to cope with a threat and consideration of a response), and (iii) coping (the process of executing a response to the threat). Situations likely to be appraised as stressful are characterized by unpredictability, negativity, uncontrollability, and ambiguity. Coping comprises two major functions: addressing the problem that is causing the distress (problem focus) and regulating emotion (emotion focus). The framework of Lazarus and Folkman has yielded important results, summarized below.

Cognitive Appraisal

Cognitive appraisal describes the process by which individuals ascribe causes to and explain events. Stanton et al. (29) assessed cognitive appraisal of infertility in a group of 76 women and 54 men with mixed infertility diagnoses. They developed a measure of appraisal to distinguish between perceptions of infertility as a threat or as a challenge. They found no relationship between cognitive appraisal and distress (infertility specific or general) in men, although men whose wives appraised infertility as more challenging were less distressed than other men.

Perceived Control

The inability to conceive may represent a loss of control for infertile individuals. Although Mahlstedt (58) referred to the loss of control observed in couples experiencing fertility problems, there has been relatively little research into how loss of control is perceived. Stanton et al. (29) examined control perceptions in their study of cognitive appraisal and found that couples appraised infertility as relatively uncontrollable but that control perceptions did not relate to general distress or infertility-specific distress in men. In an early study of perceived control in infertility, Platt et al. (59) examined locus of control in 25 couples seeking infertility treatment. They found that infertile men and women had higher scores on the external control scale (indicating that they felt that their situation was determined by forces outside of their control) than a control group of individuals with either no knowledge of their fertility status or with children.

Abbey et al. (27) reported that perceived control was the strongest predictor of fertility-related stress for both sexes. The more control over their infertility individuals perceived, the less distress was reported. Glover (60) investigated perceived control and coping in 83 subfertile men and found that high levels of perceived control were associated with lower anxiety. Infertility distress was lower in those who coped by interpreting their experiences in a positive fashion and by accepting their status and higher in those who focused on their emotions. Additionally, it was found that only infertility control significantly predicted anxiety.

Coping Strategies

Coping is the process by which individuals attempt to manage stress. Although findings from studies about coping with infertility are mixed, it appears there is a relationship between distress and using avoidance as a coping mechanism. Morrow et al. (21) used the 55-item Ways of Coping—Revised Questionnaire to examine coping strategies in 86 men from infertile couples with mixed location of diagnosis. They derived three factors from the questionnaire scores: self-blame and avoidance, informational and emotional support seeking, and cognitive restructuring. Self-blame and avoidance coping were identified as the best predictors of psychological distress in these men.

Stanton et al. (62) used the Ways of Coping Questionnaire to examine the relationship between coping strategies and general distress in 96 women and 72 men (including 72 couples) with fertility problems. For both men and women, there was a significant correlation between the use of avoidance coping strategies and general distress. Compared with their partners, men were more likely to cope through distancing, self-control, and problem solving, and they were less likely to cope through mobilizing support and avoidance. The partner's coping style was also an important factor. Wives who used more self-controlling coping had more distressed husbands. Use of this strategy may reflect more limited communication about the infertility problem. Notably, women (but not men) who coped by accepting responsibility for their infertility were found to be more distressed.

Stanton (62,63) also reported on the way in which infertile individuals compared their coping efforts with those of other infertile individuals. In a sample of 52 couples with mixed diagnosis (13% male factor only), the majority of men thought they coped better than same-sex others. They most often reported being in a better position because of a personal or motivational characteristic, such as their degree of motivation to have a child. Those men who felt they were coping worse than same-sex others attributed it to a personal characteristic such as being too emotional. Men who felt they were coping better than same-sex others were less threatened by infertility. Half of the men saw no difference between their own and their partner's coping although the tendency was for men to see themselves as coping better than their partner. Overall, the partners did not differ in their appraisals of infertility and, in general, felt relatively little control over their fertility problems. When infertility was perceived as a greater threat, men reported lower well-being, while those men who felt greater control reported a greater sense of well-being. Confrontational coping was the most powerful predictor of distress in men. Participants evidenced more global distress than would be expected in the general population, although general well-being was comparable. There was no difference between the men and women in their general emotional distress.

Edelmann et al. (37) examined coping and mood in their study of 152 couples entering an IVF program. Their results indicated that the strategies of acceptance, redefinition of the situation, and direct action were adaptive for the men in their sample.

The results of Morrow et al. (21) revealed that self-blame and avoidance coping were the strongest predictors of psychological distress among infertile men and women. This is consistent with the finding of Stanton et al. (61) that infertile individuals who engage in self-blame and avoidance are at risk for psychological distress. Cook et al. (63) found that infertile individuals who were anxious and/or depressed were more likely to use avoidance-coping strategies than those who did not have emotional problems. The evidence implies that avoidance coping, denying the existence of the problem, and self-blame are risk factors for adverse psychological strain during infertility.

Social support is often viewed as a mediating or buffering factor in the coping process. It has been well documented that seeking social support can have benefits for psychological well-being, particularly for infertile women (40,61). Satisfaction with social support has been found to correlate with lower levels of distress in women in infertile couples but not in men (27). This supports the assertion by Sarason et al. (64) that women receive and value social support to a greater extent than men do. Thus, access to support may be more important for women experiencing stress than for men; however, seeking social support may present infertile men with a particular difficulty since individuals are less likely to pursue social support in situations that threaten self-esteem (65). These potential sources of support cannot ameliorate anxiety for these men since revealing their fertility problem will further lower their self-esteem (66). Slade et al. also found that less effective coping reflects increased levels of distress in infertile men compared with fertile men (40). In their sample of fertile and infertile couples, infertile men used fewer coping strategies, and men with continuing infertility showed the lowest use of social support strategies. Self-blame and detachment were particularly associated with poor marital adjustment.

☐ APPRAISAL, COPING, AND LOCATION OF CAUSE

In the light of the evidence suggesting that men with male-factor infertility experience greater distress than those with a joint, unexplained, or female-factor diagnosis, some studies have sought to examine differences in appraisal and coping between these groups. Hurst et al. (67) looked specifically at stress and coping mechanisms employed by fertile and subfertile men. They found similar levels of perceived stress in 24 fertile and 25 subfertile men as categorized by their semen samples. Subfertile men, however, had to use more coping resources to maintain the same emotional level as the men in the fertile group.

In order to evaluate the effects of a gender-specific diagnosis of infertility on men, Gannon et al. (68) conducted a study that included men with a male-factor fertility problem (MMF) and men whose partner had a fertility problem (MFF). They focused on the way these men appraised their infertility (for example, whether they saw it as a threat or as a challenge) and the way they coped with it (for example, whether they sought support from others or tried to ignore it). There was no overall difference between the groups in their appraisals of infertility or in their level of adjustment. In both groups, those who appraised infertility in terms of threat and loss showed higher levels of distress, and those who saw themselves as having some control showed greater well-being. The MMF group was significantly more likely to cope through seeking instrumental social support and through mental disengagement than the MFF group. Appraising infertility as a threat and focusing on and venting of emotions were associated with more distress for MMF. For men in the MFF group, a wider range of appraisals and coping styles were associated with distress.

☐ DONOR INSEMINATION

Although much of the literature on the impact of infertility and individual responses applies to all those experiencing fertility difficulties, some specific issues arise for couples who use donor insemination (DI). For many years, DI was the only treatment strategy for couples with male-factor infertility. It was first used in the late 1930s and has become common since the 1950s. Initially, DI was received with outrage, although views have changed over the years due to a changing social and moral climate. It challenges societal ideas about paternity and biological versus social fatherhood. In the 1940s, men who donated sperm and men who allowed their wife to have another man's biological child were regarded with great suspicion. At one time, registering a DI child as that of the social father was in fact a crime (69).

Although DI is less researched than male infertility in general, there have been some important findings. It has been suggested that DI still carries a stigma and is often shrouded in secrecy (70). Donors are anonymous and remain untraceable by their offspring. Parents of DI children frequently decide not to tell the child about his or her origins and thus create a secret that may be known only by the parents, but which, in many cases, is known also by other family members and friends. Research suggests that the majority of couples undergoing DI treatment do not intend to tell their child about his or her origins (71,72). Parents who do not intend to tell their child have higher distress levels than those who do (73). Although achieving a pregnancy was the main concern of couples undergoing DI treatment, they also expressed concern about the donor, telling the child (and the impact that might have on the child's well-being), and the father's relationship with the child (73).

☐ COUNSELING

The process of infertility is often conceptualized in terms of a bereavement process, with couples needing to mourn the losses associated with childlessness (e.g., control of fertility, hopes of parenting, and self-esteem). Menning (56) suggested that bereavement provides a useful model for counseling infertile couples and argued that the need to grieve is often unmet because of the lack of a concrete object. Grieving may be more difficult if there is no finality in the situation; that is, a hope of conceiving continues. In contrast, couples for whom conception is impossible may more easily accept their infertility, process their emotions, and plan for the future. Viewing the knowledge of infertility as a process has implications for applying a bereavement model. Rather than thinking of infertility as a single bereavement, it may be more useful to see it as consisting of multiple monthly losses, with each monthly occurrence reawakening the wide range of emotions associated with being unable to have a child. Such ongoing losses may have a compounding effect, and rather than becoming immune to the experience, each monthly disappointment may draw on decreasing reserves and make coping more difficult.

Although the bereavement model is widely used in counseling infertile couples, it is derived largely from clinical observation and there is little empirical support for it. Certainly, there is evidence that couples describe feelings of loss (56). Nachtigall et al. (6) found that approximately half their sample of subfertile men reported the discovery of their infertility as a loss, of which two kinds were identified: the loss of potency and the loss of biological children. A much higher proportion of women, however, identified loss and the authors concluded that this reflected the different expectations of parenthood held by men and women. Furthermore, while there are undoubtedly losses associated with infertility, individuals may not necessarily respond to these in ways similar to other losses.

Although many women may find the bereavement model of infertility useful, such a model may be less appropriate for men where feelings of threat and anxiety appear to be more salient and should be considered in counseling (19,74). In addition, cultural issues related to models of masculinity should be borne in mind as they form an important context for the male experience. Lee (75) acknowledges that the changing role of men in society is an important contributor to male distress in relation to fertility problems (although he fails to integrate this insight into his approach to therapy in a systematic way). An additional challenge in counseling for infertility is that men and women are usually seen as a couple; thus, counseling must simultaneously address the different issues confronting both partners. One potentially useful approach would be to assist the couple to explore and acknowledge their different reactions to the situation and to draw on these insights to improve communication and understanding as well as to assist in making decisions concerning their course of action.

☐ SUMMARY
Reactions to Infertility

There can be little doubt that men are distressed by infertility. This tends to be greater when a male factor is implicated, and for a sizeable proportion of men, the distress will reach clinically significant levels. The presentation of distress appears to differ for men and women, with anxiety being a more prominent feature in men. This suggests that clinical interventions to address anxiety rather than depression are likely to be useful in male-factor infertility. Levels of distress are mediated by a number of variables: greater age, the absence of children, and male-factor problems are all associated with greater distress in men. A successful pregnancy will generally result in improvements in self-esteem and life satisfaction for men but will

inevitably bring its own stresses and challenges, many of which may have been unanticipated. It may be helpful to encourage couples to look beyond the immediate context of diagnosis and treatment to consider these unanticipated events.

The Consultation—Investigation and Treatment

The whole process of investigation and treatment is stressful, with peaks at particular stages, such as egg and sperm collection. The consultation is perceived as being valuable, even when it is not possible to give a firm diagnosis or to offer specific treatment options. The main benefits appear to be derived from the opportunity to discuss concerns and to receive information. Nevertheless, recall of this information may be poor, and the beliefs of patients concerning their diagnosis may differ from those of the clinician. The consultation should, therefore, be viewed as an important opportunity to provide accurate information, to address concerns, and to be therapeutic in its own right. Care should be taken to assess patient understanding and to address any misapprehensions. This could be done, for example, by asking the patient to summarize the information provided.

Dealing with Infertility

Individuals vary widely in the way in which they attempt to manage their reactions to their infertile status. Those who view matters as being beyond their control are likely to be more distressed than those who see themselves as being able to exert some control over the situation. How individuals cope with these stresses is also important. There are some gender differences in coping responses. In general, however, coping through self-blame and avoidance of the issues is associated with heightened distress. Conversely, responses such as redefining the situation (e.g., seeing a challenge rather than a threat), taking positive action, and acceptance can be beneficial. Social support can also be valuable, although men generally find it more difficult than women to access this type of support.

Even men who appear to be coping effectively may be doing so at the expense of deploying a great many coping responses. As coping imposes its own costs (76), this may have implications for longer-term psychological well-being. It is probably useful to enhance the individual's sense of control, for example, by involving them as much as possible in decision-making. Coping responses that involve taking positive action, redefining the situation in more positive ways, and moving toward acceptance should be identified and promoted. Men in particular should be encouraged to seek support and to identify other individuals with whom they can discuss their feelings. Having said this, it is important to note that the overriding issue to remember when working with infertile couples is that they are all different. Listening to and understanding individual responses are of paramount importance in providing useful and appropriate support.

□ REFERENCES

1. Hargreave TB. Human infertility. In: Hargreave TB, ed. Male Infertility. 2nd ed. New York: Springer-Verlag, 1994:1–16.

2. Inhorn MC. Interpreting infertility: medical anthropological perspectives. Introduction. Soc Sci Med 1994; 39(4):459–461.

3. Dalton M, Lilford R. Benefits of in-vitro fertilisation. (Letter). Lancet 1989; 2(8675):1327–1329.

4. van Balen F, Trimbos-Kemper TC. Involuntarily childless couples: their desire to have children and their motives. J Psychosomat Obstet Gynecol 1995; 16(3):137–144.

5. Mason MC. Male Infertility—Men Talking. London: Routledge, 1993.

6. Nachtigall RD, Becker G, Wozny M. The effects of gender-specific diagnosis on men's and women's response to infertility. Fertil Steril 1992; 57(1):113–121.

7. Edelmann RJ, Humphrey M, Owens DJ. The meaning of parenthood and couples' reactions to male infertility. Br J Med Psychol 1994; 67(Pt 3):291–299.

8. Owens DJ. The desire to father: reproductive ideologies and involuntary childless men. In: McKee L, O'Brien M, eds. The Father Figure. London: Tavistock Publications, 1982.

9. Goffman E. Stigma: Notes on the Management of Spoiled Identity. Englewood Cliffs, NJ: Prentice-Hall, 1963.

10. Miall C. Community constructs of involuntary childlessness: sympathy, stigma, and social support. Can Rev Sociol Anthropol 1994; 31(4):392–421.

11. Courtenay WH. Constructions of masculinity and their influence on men's well-being: a theory of gender and health. Social Sci Med 2000; 50(10):1385–1401.

12. Bents H. Psychology of male infertility—a literature survey. International J Androl 1985; 8(4):325–336.

13. Ussher J. The Psychology of the Female Body. London: Routledge, 1989.

14. Phoenix A, Woolett A. Motherhood: social construction, politics & psychology. In: Phoenix A, Woolett A, Lloyd E, eds. Motherhood: Meanings, Practices, and Ideologies. London: Sage Publications, 1991:13–27.

15. Humphrey M. Sex differences in attitude to parenthood. Hum Relat 1977; 30(8):737–749.

16. Lamb M. The changing roles of fathers. In: Lamb M, ed. The Father's Role: Applied Perspectives. London: John Wiley & Sons, 1986:3–27.

17. Marsiglio W. Procreative Man. New York: New York University Press, 1998.

18. Newton CR, Hearn MT, Yuzpe AA, et al. Motives for parenthood and response to failed in vitro fertilization: implications for counseling. J Assist Reprod Genet 1992; 9(1):24–31.

19. Kedem P, Mikulincer M, Nathanson YE, et al. Psychological aspects of male infertility. Br J Med Psychol 1990; 63(Pt 1):73–80.

20. Wright J, Duchesne C, Sabourin S, et al. Psychosocial distress and infertility: men and women respond differently. Fertil Steril 1991; 55(1):100–108.

21. Morrow KA, Thoreson RW, Penney LL. Predictors of psychological distress among infertility clinic patients. J Consult Clin Psychol 1995; 63(1):163–167.

22. McEwan KL, Costello CG, Taylor PJ. Adjustment to infertility. J Abnorm Psychol 1987; 96(2):108–116.

23. Glover L, Gannon K, Sherr L, et al. Differences between doctor and patient estimates of outcome in male subfertility clinic attenders. Br J Clin Psychol 1996; 35(Pt 4):531–542.

24. Raval H, Slade P, Buck P, et al. The impact of infertility on emotions and the marital and sexual relationship. J Reprod Infant Psychol 1987; 5(4):221–234.

25. Brand H. The influence of sex differences on the acceptance of infertility. J Reprod Infant Psychol 1989; 7(2):129–131.

26. Daniluk JC. Infertility: intrapersonal and interpersonal impact. Fertil Steril 1988; 49(6):982–990.

27. Abbey A, Andrews F, Halrnan L. Gender's role in responses to infertility. Psychol Women Q 1991; 15(2):295–316.

28. Collins A, Freeman EW, Boxer AS, et al. Perceptions of infertility and treatment stress in females as compared with males entering in vitro fertilization treatment. Fertil Steril 1992; 57(2):350–356.

29. Stanton A, Tennen H, Affleck G, et al. Cognitive appraisal and adjustment to infertility. Women Health 1991; 17(3):1–15.

30. Berg BJ, Wilson JF, Weingartner PJ. Psychological sequelae of infertility treatment: the role of gender and sex-role identification. Soc Sci Med 1991; 33(9):1071–1080.

31. Andrews FM, Abbey A, Halman LJ. Stress from infertility, marriage factors, and subjective well-being of wives and husbands. J Health Soc Behav 1991; 32(3):238–253.

32. Elstein M. Effect of infertility on psychosexual function. Br Med J 1975; 3(5978):296–299.

33. Drake TS, Grunert GM. A cyclic pattern of sexual dysfunction in the infertility investigation. Fertil Steril 1979; 32(5):542–545.

34. Berger DM. Couples' reactions to male infertility and donor insemination. Am J Psychiatry 1980; 137(9):1047–1049.

35. Berg BJ, Wilson JF. Patterns of psychological distress in infertile couples. J Psychosom Obstet Gynaecol 1995; 16(2):65–78.

36. Leiblum SR. The impact of infertility on sexual and marital satisfaction. In: Bancroft J, Davis CM, Ruppel HJ Jr, eds. Annual Review of Sex Research. Vol. 4, 1993: 99–120.

37. Edelmann RJ, Connolly KJ, Bartlett H. Coping strategies and psychological adjustment of couples presenting for IVF. J Psychosom Res 1994; 38(4):355–364.

38. Ulbrich PM, Coyle AT, Llabre MM. Involuntary childlessness and marital adjustment: his and hers. J Sex Marital Ther 1990; 16(3):147–158.

39. Connolly K, Edelmann R, Cooke I. Distress and marital problems associated with infertility. J Reproduct Infant Psychol 1987; 5(1):49–57.

40. Slade P, Raval H, Buck P, et al. A 3-year follow-up of emotional, marital and sexual functioning in couples who were infertile. J Reprod Infant Psychol 1992; 10(4): 233–243.

41. Connolly KJ, Edelmann RJ, Cooke ID, et al. The impact of infertility on psychological functioning. J Psychosom Res 1992; 36(5):459–468.

42. Abbey A, Andrews F, Halman L. Infertility and parenthood: does becoming a parent increase well-being? J Consult Clin Psychol 1994; 62(2):398–403.

43. Benazon N, Wright J, Sabourin S. Stress, sexual satisfaction, and marital adjustment in infertile couples. J Sex Marital Ther 1992; 18(4):273–284.

44. Glover L, Gannon K, Abel P. Eighteen-month follow-up of male subfertility clinic attenders: a comparison between men whose partner subsequently became pregnant and those with continuing subfertility. J Reprod Infant Psychol 1999; 17(1):83–87.

45. Carmeli Y, Birenbaum-Carmeli D. The predicament of masculinity: towards understanding the male's experience of infertility treatments. Sex Roles 1994; 30(9–10): 663–667.

46. Boivin J, Andersson L, Skoog-Svanberg A, et al. Psychological reactions during in-vitro fertilization: similar response pattern in husbands and wives. Hum Reprod 1998; 13(11):3262–3267.

47. Boivin J, Shoog-Svanberg A, Andersson L, et al. Distress level in men undergoing intracytoplasmic sperm injection versus in-vitro fertilization. Hum Reprod 1998; 13(5):1403–1406.

48. Takefman J, Brender W, Boivin J, et al. Sexual and emotional adjustment of couples undergoing infertility investigation and the effectiveness of preparatory information. J Psychosomat Obstet Gynecol 1990; 11(4): 275–290.

49. Glover L, Gannon K, Sherr L, et al. Psychological distress before and immediately after attendance at a male sub-fertility clinic. J R Soc Med 1994; 87(8): 448–449.

50. Glover L, Gannon K, Platt Z, et al. Male subfertility clinic attenders' expectations of medical consultation. Br J Health Psychol 1999; 4(1):53–61.

51. Edelmann RJ, Connolly KJ. Psychological aspects of infertility. Br J Med Psychol 1986; 59(Pt 3):209–219.

52. Mikulincer M, Horesh N, Levy-Shiff R, et al. The contribution of adult attachment style to the adjustment to infertility. Br J Med Psychol 1998; 71(Pt 3): 65–280.

53. Buttler S, Glover L, Gannon K, et al. Location of cause of subfertility--discrepancies between perceptions of men in subfertile couples and those of their doctors. J Reprod Infant Psychol 1999; 17(3):218–219.

54. Dunkel-Schetter C, Lobel M. Psychological reactions to infertility. In: Stanton AL, Dunkel-Schetter C, eds. Infertility: Perspectives from Stress and Coping Research. London: Plenum Press, 1991:29–57.

55. Menning BE. The emotional needs of infertile couples. Fertil Steril 1980; 34(4):313–319.

56. Menning B. Infertility: A Guide for the Childless Couple. Englewood Cliffs, NJ: Prentice-Hall, 1977.

57. Lazarus R, Folkman S. Stress, Appraisal and Coping. New York: Springer, 1984.

58. Mahlstedt PP. The psychological component of infertility. Fertil Steril 1985; 43(3):335–346.

59. Platt JJ, Ficher I, Silver MJ. Infertile couples: personality traits and self-ideal concept discrepancies. Fertil Steril 1973; 24(12):972–976.

60. Glover L. Psychological Aspects of Male Sub-Fertility and its Investigation. Ph.D. dissertation. University College, London, 1996.

61. Stanton AL, Tennen H, Affleck G, et al. Coping and adjustment to infertility. J Soc Clin Psychol 1992; 11(1): 1–13.

62. Stanton A. Downward comparison in infertile couples. Basic Appl Social Psychol 1992; 13(4):389–403.

63. Cook R, Parsons J, Mason B, et al. Emotional, marital and sexual functioning in patients embarking upon IVF and AID treatment for infertility. J Reprod Infant Psychol 1989; 7(2):7–93.

64. Sarason B, Sarason I, Hacker T, et al. Concomitants of social support: social skills, physical attractiveness, and gender. J Pers Soc Psychol 1985; 49(2): 469–480.

65. Folkman S, Lazarus R, Dunkel-Schetter C, et al. Dynamics of a stressful encounter: cognitive appraisal, coping, and encounter outcomes. J Pers Soc Psychol 1986; 50(5):992–1003.

66. Band D, Edelmann R, Avery S, et al. Correlates of psychological distress in relation to male infertility. Br J Health Psychol 1998; 3(3):245–256.

67. Hurst K, Dye L, Rutherford A, et al. Differential coping in fertile and sub-fertile males attending an assisted conception unit: a pilot study. J Reprod Infant Psychol 1999; 17(3):189–198.

68. Gannon K, Buttler S, Glover L, et al. The effect of location of cause on men's cognitive appraisal, coping and adjustment to infertility. Society of Reproductive and Infant Psychology Annual Conference, University of Birmingham, UK, 2000.

69. Pfeffer N. The Stork and the Syringe: A Political History of Reproductive Medicine. Cambridge: Polity Press, 1993.

70. Daniels K, Taylor K. Secrecy and openness in donor insemination. Politics Life Sci 1993; 12(2): 155–170.

71. Golombok S, Cook R, Bish A, et al. Families created by the new reproductive technologies: quality of parenting and social and emotional development of the children. Child Dev 1995; 66(2):285–298.

72. McWhinnie A. A study of parenting of IVF and DI children. Med Law 1995; 14(7–8):501–508.

73. Salter-Ling N, Hunter M, Glover L. Donor insemination: exploring the experience of treatment and intention to tell. J Reprod Infant Psychol 2001; 19(3): 175–186.

74. Glover L, Gannon K, Sherr L, et al. Distress in sub-fertile men: a longitudinal study. J Reprod Infant Psychol 1996; 4(1):23–36.

75. Lee S. Counseling in Male Infertility. London: Blackwell Science, 1996.

76. Cohen S, Evans G, Stokols D, et al. Behavior, Health and Environmental Stress. New York: Plenum Press, 1986.

Management of Immunological Factors in Male Infertility

H. W. Gordon Baker

Department of Obstetrics and Gynaecology, University of Melbourne and The Royal Women's Hospital, Carlton, Victoria, Australia

Gary N. Clarke

Andrology Laboratory Division of Laboratory Services, The Royal Women's Hospital, Carlton, Victoria, Australia

□ INTRODUCTION

Sperm autoimmunity is an important cause of male infertility. It is present in 4% to 10% of men seen for the treatment of infertility (1–3). In some surveys of infertile men, very high proportions of positive results have been reported (4). The condition is important to recognize as a cause of asthenozoospermia, idiopathic infertility, or the unexpected failure of standard in vitro fertilization (IVF). Yet, the significance of sperm autoimmunity is disputed because early tests for the detection of sperm antibodies were not very accurate, and even recent tests, such as those based on immuno-fluorescence, can still be misleading (see Chapter 26) (5, 6). It has also been suggested that screening for anti-sperm antibodies before IVF is not cost-effective, as a positive test has a low predictive value for the failure of fertilization and the need for intracytoplasmic sperm injection (ICSI) (7,8). This is an unfortunate attitude that, if extended, would result in minimal evaluation of patients and a consequent inability to counsel patients regarding their prognosis for conception without treatment, the evaluation of ART results for different conditions, or the prompt consideration of alternative approaches to couples management.

Despite considerable research effort, the pathogenesis of sperm autoimmunity remains unclear. In particular, the antigens involved in sperm autoimmunity are poorly understood (see Chapter 26). Experimental models such as autoimmune orchitis and immunization with testis- or sperm-specific proteins has yet to expose the causes and mechanisms of human sperm autoimmunity. More is known about the effects of sperm antibodies, however. In the male, these antibodies can impair sperm output and function, reducing penetration of the cervical mucus and oocyte vestments and causing severe infertility. Sperm isoimmunity is an equivalent condition in females that can also produce severe infertility, although this is difficult to predict from the currently used antibody tests

(9–11). The severity of the infertility associated with sperm autoimmunity and isoimmunity combined with the lack of other resultant effects elsewhere in the body both suggest that, if these conditions could be induced in a controlled manner, it is possible that they could be used to develop a method of long-term contraception (10,12,13). As with other organ-specific autoimmune conditions in which the autoantibody tests are positive in a considerable number of healthy people, however, sperm antibodies may also be present without an impairment of fertility (1). Therefore, the clinician must be careful not to over-interpret test results.

While acquired immune deficiency syndrome (AIDS) and other autoimmune diseases such as systemic lupus erythematosus, polyarteritis nodosa, and immunological hypopituitarism may also affect testicular function, these diseases will not be discussed in this chapter. For further information on these conditions, please refer Chapters 12, 14, 17, and 19. Similarly, immunological mechanisms that may contribute to testicular damage following orchitis are not covered. For further information on orchitis, please refer to Chapter 16.

□ DEFINITION

Sperm autoimmunity is an organ-specific autoimmune disease in which antibodies bind to sperm and impair their function, causing severe infertility. Therefore it is necessary for clinical diagnosis that there is both a positive antibody test and a test result demonstrating a detrimental effect on sperm function, typically that of impaired sperm-cervical mucus penetration. Historically, a positive Isojima sperm immobilization test (SIT) in blood serum combined with impaired sperm mucus penetration tests provided a useful algorithm for the provisional diagnosis (Chapter 26). The results were confirmed by a second set of tests before making a conclusive diagnosis of sperm autoimmunity.

The criteria for impaired mucus penetration consisted of either the absence of progressively motile sperm in a mid-cycle, post-coital test (PCT), or an in vitro sperm cervical mucus contact test (SCMCT), or alternatively, no sperm penetration beyond 2 cm in the Kremer capillary tube cervical mucus penetration test. Since the introduction of the immunobead test (IBT) in the 1980s, a positive IBT is used (greater than 50% of motile sperm with anti-IgA and/or anti-IgG beads bound), and a blocked Kremer test on two separate occasions. The indirect IBT on blood serum is used if there are no motile sperm in the semen. Positive sperm antibody tests without evidence of severe impairment of sperm function are termed "low-level sperm antibodies," and patients with such results should not be regarded as having sperm autoimmunity. In these patients, other causes for infertility should be sought. Failure to appreciate this important distinction between clinically insignificant positive sperm antibody tests and sperm autoimmunity is probably a major cause of the confusion in the literature about the significance of the condition (5).

☐ TYPES OF SPERM AUTOIMMUNITY

There are three types of sperm autoimmunity: that associated with genital tract obstruction, that accompanied by testicular inflammation, and a spontaneously occurring type that does not present with either of the preceding associated features.

Sperm Autoimmunity Associated with Genital Tract Obstruction

About 50% of men seen with positive sperm antibody tests also have genital tract obstruction—most commonly the result of vasectomies, post-inflammatory epididymal obstructions, or reconstructive surgery. More than 70% of men develop sperm antibodies in their serum within twelve months of vasectomy (14,15). The antibodies are more frequent in men who also have sperm granulomas associated with the vasectomy (16). The presence of these antibodies is an adverse factor for the future success of vasovasostomy, as well as surgery for other genital tract obstructions (17–19). Sperm autoimmunity is common in men with persisting infertility after vasectomy reversal (20).

The other types of genital tract obstruction associated with sperm autoimmunity appears to be that which occurs after puberty, such as post-gonococcal epididymitis or obstruction due to trauma, including iatrogenic vasal damage inflicted at the time of inguinal hernia surgery (21). Unilateral genital tract obstruction may also cause sperm antibody production (22). Sperm antibodies are less common with congenital epididymal obstructions, Young syndrome, and congenital absence of the vasa (19,23,24). The presence of antibodies in this group may be related to the length of unobstructed epididymis (25).

Sperm Autoimmunity Associated with Orchitis

Occasionally, inflammatory cell infiltrates are found in testicular biopsies of men with sperm antibodies. This "autoimmune orchitis" may follow an episode of epididymo-orchitis or it may occur spontaneously (1,26). Whether the infiltrates are related to the sperm antibodies is unknown, as they may exist in the absence of sperm antibodies. Sympathetic orchitis following testicular injury may occur, but it is very rare (27,28).

Spontaneous Sperm Autoimmunity

About half the men with sperm antibodies have no obvious genital tract obstruction or orchitis. Some may have a genetic or familial predisposition to autoimmunity. Wall et al. found thyroid antibodies to be more common in infertile men, some of whom had sperm antibodies (29). The authors of this chapter have previously reported 101 non-azoospermic men with positive sperm antibody tests who were found to have a higher frequency of family histories of other autoimmune diseases such as pernicious anemia and thyroid disorders (32% compared with 11% in 725 control infertile men) (1). In a study of 102 men with spontaneously occurring sperm autoimmunity and 277 control infertile men without azoospermia and negative SIT, a significantly higher frequency of positive thyroid microsomal antibodies was also found: 11.8% compared with 4.3% in controls. Positivity for any thyroid or gastric antibody was also higher than in controls (18.6% compared with 8.7%). The results for another 57 patients with sperm autoimmunity associated with genital tract obstruction were similar to the SIT negative control patients (30). Previously, several researchers had shown that vasectomy itself does not predispose to the development of any autoantibodies other than antisperm antibodies (31,32). The existence of patients with sperm autoimmunity and other concomitant autoimmune diseases, such as Hashimoto thyroiditis, however, has since been demonstrated. It is possible that there are HLA subtypes that predispose a patient to the development of sperm antibodies (33,34). Notably, the frequency of positive sperm antibody positive results tends to increase with age in men (35). These features suggest that this form of sperm autoimmunity has a similar pathogenesis to other organ-specific autoimmune diseases. It is interesting that neonatal thymectomy in some strains of mice and rats produces autoimmune endocrine gland disorders, orchitis, and infertility associated with sperm antibodies (36).

Other Associations of Sperm Antibodies

Associations between sperm antibodies and other conditions such as mumps orchitis, varicocele, sexually transmissible and non-specific male accessory gland inflammation, leprosy, chronic alcoholism, hyperprolactinemia, immotile cilia and failure of ejaculation of various causes including chronic spinal cord injury have been suggested but not confirmed (37–42). Testicular biopsy, orchiopexy for undescended testes, other scrotal surgery, testicular torsion and other injuries do not appear to cause or aggravate sperm autoimmunity (43–45). During the evaluation of a method for fine needle tissue aspiration biopsy of the testis, the authors attempted to observe a change in titre of sperm antibodies in men previously known to be positive. Serum was collected two weeks after the biopsy, when an anamnestic response would be expected to peak. There was, however, no change detected by the indirect IBT in any IgG, IgA, or IgM antibody class (44). Apart from the association with genital tract obstruction of post-pubertal onset, minor damage to the scrotal contents is unlikely to be relevant to the production of sperm antibodies. Histories of testicular trauma, inflammation and surgery appear to be no more frequent in men with sperm antibodies than in other infertile men (1).

□ PATHOPHYSIOLOGY
Sperm Autoantigens

The mechanisms of development of sperm antibodies in men are unclear. Multiple antigens appear to be involved in the pathogenesis of sperm autoimmunity, but most of the epitopes reacting with the autoantibodies are unknown (46–49). Some of the antigens identified are intracellular proteins, and it is difficult to understand how antibodies to these could cause an abnormality of sperm function (50). The antibodies may be naturally occurring to sperm-coating proteins from the epididymis. It is certain that non-peptide antigens are involved (51–54). Oligosaccharide or glycolipid epitopes may have cross-reactions with bacteria or other cells (55,56).

The different patterns of immunobead binding to the sperm surface: head, neck, tail, tail tip may result either from antibodies binding to different antigens in these locations, or from variations in the total amount of antibodies on the sperm (57).

Mechanism of Immunization

The mechanism of immunization is poorly understood. Alterations in immunomodulatory factors in the seminal plasma of men with sperm autoimmunity suggests that a loss of immune tolerance is involved in the pathogenesis (58–60). The autoantibodies could appear in the genital tract due to defects in the blood-testis barrier or possibly because of impairment of the immunomodulatory mechanisms that allow the testis to be an immunologically privileged organ. These antibodies may also be produced by lymphocytes resident in the epithelium of the epididymis (61,62).

Effect of Autoantibodies on Sperm

Sperm antibodies of different immunoglobulin classes can be found in the serum and seminal plasma as well as on the sperm itself. IgG and IgA sperm antibodies (particularly secretory IgA) locally produced in the male genital tract may cause the greatest interference with sperm function (57,63).

Sperm antibodies may impair fertility at several levels, potentially resulting in defective spermatogenesis, sperm agglutination in the male genital tract, reduced sperm motility, impaired cervical mucus penetration, impeded transit of the female genital tract, or ultimately, interference with the process of binding to the zona pellucida, the acrosome reaction (including premature acrosome loss), and penetration of the zona (64–66). Diverse immunologic effects of the antibodies are also possible, such as complement-dependent cytotoxicity and opsonization with macrophage removal of antibody-coated sperm (67). The importance of such mechanisms in vivo, however, is uncertain. Direct effects in the testis are not clear as inflammatory cell infiltration and immune deposits are not common (68). The main pathogenetic effects of sperm antibodies appear to include the direct effects of the antibodies bound to the surface of the sperm that cause sperm agglutination, impaired motility, blockage of sperm mucus penetration and impaired sperm–oocyte interaction.

Reduced sperm penetration of cervical mucus and the shaking phenomenon (active but nonprogressive motility typical of sperm heavily coated with antibodies in cervical mucus) is particularly caused by an interaction between the Fc parts of the sperm antibodies on the sperm and components of the mucus (69). Both IgA and IgG antibodies may be involved, but IgA antibodies appear to be particularly important in impairing sperm–cervical mucus penetration (57,63,70,71,72).

Early studies showed that sperm antibodies produced variable results with impaired or enhanced human sperm-zona free hamster oocyte penetration tests (73,74). It was apparent early on, however, that high levels of antibodies impaired human fertilization in vitro (75–77). Clarke et al. (78) conducted experiments on human fertilization in vitro indicating that human sera containing antisperm antibodies blocked fertilization and that IgA antibodies were particularly significant in interfering with fertilization. Reducing the antibody levels with glucocorticoid therapy resulted in reasonable results with standard IVF (75). Although there are some reports that do not demonstrate a relationship between antisperm antibody levels and low fertilization rates with standard IVF, most studies have confirmed these findings (79–81). Studies with human oocytes suggest that sperm antibodies interfere particularly with sperm zona pellucida binding, the zona pellucida-induced acrosome reaction, and sperm penetration of the zona pellucida (82–85). Impaired oolemma binding may also occur with high levels of sperm antibodies (86). There is a strong correlation between impaired IVF fertilization rates and impaired sperm mucus penetration.

Additional adverse effects of sperm antibodies have been suggested, such as the increased production of reactive oxygen species (87). DNA damage and its deleterious effects on stages subsequent to fertilization have been raised, but these do not appear to be important in humans as there is no evidence of reduced embryo utilization, implantation rates, or increased pregnancy wastage with immunological infertility of male origin (88–90). Immunological infertility of female origin may be associated with some embryonic losses (91,92).

□ PROGNOSIS FOR NATURAL FERTILITY AND STANDARD IVF

Poor prognosis for fertility in men with high levels of sperm antibody activity in serum was found in early follow-up studies (Table 1) (1, 93–95). It must be emphasized that these data were obtained with high-titer antibody positivity only (particularly SIT), or when blocked sperm mucus penetration was also present (1,94,95). Under these conditions, sperm auto-immunity causes persistent severe infertility. The authors studied 101 men with positive SIT who were not azoospermic. Of the 14 men not tested for sperm mucus penetration, four individuals achieved pregnancies within six months without medical treatment. Eight of 15 men who had sperm mucus penetration tests showing progressively motile sperm produced pregnancies within seven months. As summarized in Table 1, six pregnancies occurred during follow-up review of the 72 men with positive SIT and blocked sperm mucus penetration, and three of these pregnancies occurred with the use of glucocorticoid therapy. The pregnancy rate for these men with sperm autoimmunity (positive sperm antibody test and blocked sperm mucus penetration) was 0.67/100 months, compared with 2.6/100 months in 753 control infertile men not known to have sperm autoimmunity (1).

Table 1 Pregnancy Rates in Subfertile Couples with and without Sperm Autoimmunity

Group	Number of couples	Pregnant (%)	Pregnancy rate (pregnancies/ 100 cycles)
Control (sperm antibody test negative or not done)	753	30	2.6
Sperm autoimmunity (sperm antibody test positive and blocked sperm-mucus penetration)	72	8.3	0.67
Treated by AIH (1-6 cycles)	17	5.9	1.3
Treated with testosterone esters (250 mg 2 weekly for 3 months)	15	13	2.6
Treated with prednisolone (0.5–0.75mg/kg/day, 4–6 months)	14	21	4.6
No treatment	35	2.8	0.3

Source: From Ref. 1.

Similarly low pregnancy rates with sperm autoimmunity are apparent in the literature (93–95). If the definition of sperm autoimmunity is loosened to include all sperm antibody positive patients, the spontaneous pregnancy rates are higher, approaching 1.7% per cycle (96).

Occasionally, sperm autoimmunity may fluctuate in severity. The rare patients who produce pregnancies without treatment appear to have spontaneous improvements in semen quality, with a fall in antibody levels and increased sperm-mucus penetration (1). Sperm antibodies may also decrease after relief of genital tract obstruction, but this may take many months or years to occur (97). As explained in the following, glucocorticoid treatment typically produces only a transient benefit.

□ CLINICAL FEATURES
Diagnosis

Surveys comparing infertile men with and without sperm antibodies indicate that the former have longer durations of infertility and fewer previous pregnancies despite higher average sperm concentrations and less ovulatory disorders in the female partners (1). Sperm motility tends to be low, and sperm agglutination is common (98). Interestingly, however, there is no characteristic semen pattern with sperm autoimmunity. Sperm agglutination and low motility are not invariable; the semen analysis may vary from normal to azoospermic. Thus, all infertile men must be screened. The WHO laboratory manual for the examination of human semen and semen-cervical mucus interaction includes testing for sperm antibodies as a standard procedure (99). Either the IBT or the mixed antiglobulin reaction (MAR) test is recommended, although the IBT may be preferable, as it is a more robust test. It should be noted that the various agglutination tests and SIT are now obsolete for clinical purposes. A positive result must be evaluated further by a sperm mucus penetration test. An alternative to screening for antibodies would be to perform a sperm mucus penetration test. If there are no motile sperm in the semen, an indirect IBT may be performed on blood or seminal plasma.

□ DIFFERENTIAL DIAGNOSIS

Men with sperm autoimmunity must be distinguished from those with low-level sperm autoantibodies that are not relevant to the infertility. Previous suggestions that 20% IBT binding should be regarded as positive were misleading. Patients with positive bead binding to less than 50% of motile sperm do not have additional impairment of fertility (100,101). Such patients have mucus penetration tests that are normal or only marginally impaired. Treatment for the antibodies is not warranted, and other causes of the couple's infertility should be sought. Many patients with low-level sperm antibodies have immunobead binding only to the tail tips, or IBT results with less than 70% binding to the sperm heads (57).

If there are few or no sperm present in the semen, the main problem to be determined is whether the sperm antibodies are the only source of the pathology or whether there is also an obstruction or a spermatogenic disorder. Clinical features such as previous genital tract trauma, surgery, or palpable abnormalities in the epididymides or vasa may suggest obstruction, while testicular atrophy and elevated serum follicle-stimulatiing hormone (FSH) levels typically indicate a spermatogenic defect. Because the presence of sperm antibodies indicates that sperm are being produced; thus, a positive IBT in an azoospermic man suggests an obstructive element. A trial of glucocorticoid therapy may be useful to differentiate those patients with combined mechanical obstruction and sperm antibodies from those with azoospermia or very severe oligospermia as the result of sperm autoimmunity alone. In the latter case, there may be a dramatic increase in sperm output (1).

☐ TREATMENT

There is confusion about the value of treatment of sperm autoimmunity in the literature. This is partly related to the lack of understanding about the need to separate patients with sperm autoimmunity from those with low levels of sperm antibodies that do not contribute significantly to the infertility. The latter type of patient may achieve pregnancies by a variety of methods, including artificial insemination and standard IVF, both of which techniques produce very poor results in patients with sperm autoimmunity. Some studies, however, do not differentiate these patient groups, and thus produce controversial results (102). Because of the poor prognosis for natural conception, artificial insemination, or standard IVF in cases with sperm autoimmunity, donor insemination is also an option for these couples. If donor insemination is used, it is necessary to tell the couple to avoid coitus within 48 hours of insemination, as the antibodies in the man's semen could affect the donor sperm (103, 104).

ICSI

ICSI is now the primary method of treatment for sperm autoimmunity (105). Provided the sperm are alive, outcomes tend to be good. Sperm antibodies do not appear to have an adverse effect on the outcome of ICSI. In fact, reports indicate that ICSI generally produces good results when compared to historical controls that utilized standard IVF without glucocorticoid treatment of the men (106–108). There also have been comparative studies that clearly demonstrate higher fertilization rates with ICSI than standard IVF using a random selection of oocytes from each patient for ICSI or IVF (107).

Before the introduction of ICSI, standard IVF produced poor results with patients with severe sperm autoimmunity (109,110). If sperm antibody levels were reduced with prednisolone treatment the results were reasonable (75). A controlled trial by Lahteenmaki et al. (111) with prednisolone showed no improvement with fertilization rate over that with placebo, but the dosing regimen was very modest at only 20 mg daily for 10 days. As can be expected, there was no effect on antibody levels. It should be noted, however, that this group later found that a low dose of prednisolone was, in fact, able to reduce antibody levels in some patients if the treatment course were prolonged to a total of 21 days (112).

Methods

Standard methods are used for preparation and injection of sperm ICSI (113). Some protocols require the man to ejaculate into approximately 50 ml of culture medium in order to reduce the amount of antibodies bound to the sperm. If no motile sperm are present in the fresh or cryopreserved semen, pentoxifylline or hypoosmotic swelling may be used to select live sperm; testicular biopsy may also be used to obtain elongated spermatids for ICSI (113).

Results

Fertilization rates are low if immotile sperm are injected. Otherwise, the results appear to be the same as for other types of male infertility that can be treated successfully with ICSI. Not to be discounted are the influences of female factors, particularly age. In women under 35 years of age, about 35% to 40% will be able to conceive with embryo transfers obtained from each multiple oocyte collection.

Complications

The complications of ICSI in women include ovarian hyperstimulation syndrome, bleeding, infection from the oocyte collection procedure, and multiple pregnancies when more than one embryo is transferred. These complications are not specific to sperm autoimmunity, and occur with ICSI performed for other reasons.

☐ GLUCOCORTICOID TREATMENT

Although there is a range of differing opinions, the effectiveness of glucocorticoid treatment for sperm autoimmunity does have an evidence base in controlled clinical trials (3,97,114). This method of treatment is a reasonable choice when sperm autoimmunity is the only obvious cause for infertility in a healthy couple that wishes to do everything possible to achieve a natural pregnancy. Long-term glucocorticoid treatment is contraindicated if the woman is infertile or if the man has other illnesses that increase the risks of serious adverse effects, particularly peptic ulcer disease, hypertension, obesity, or diabetes mellitus. ICSI is an alternative treatment that has replaced the need for short-term glucocorticoid treatment before performing standard IVF (75,105). The couple may choose either ICSI or glucocorticoid treatment initially, and if the first treatment is unsuccessful, may simply try the other. The couple may also pursue donor insemination.

Clinical Trials

Initial reports of glucocorticoid treatment of sperm autoimmunity were unfortunately not controlled (1, 115–119). Some studies included combinations of treatments, such as testosterone suppression and glucocorticoids (120). Typical results included the reduction of antibody levels and increased sperm motility and mucus penetration. Large increases in sperm concentration were also reported in some men (1,121). Although the results were limited, pregnancy rates seemed higher than in historical controls (1,122).

Some comparative trials were performed that also suggested the potential benefits of glucocorticoid therapy, but of these, some included both men and women with sperm antibodies (123). It is likely that trials that produced results suggesting the ineffectiveness of glucocorticoid therapy involved insufficient doses of glucocorticoid drug or durations of therapy (124). A small randomized trial with 10 men who were given low-dose intermittent therapy only demonstrated reduced antibody levels (125). Keane et al. also showed a decrease in antibody levels in 10 men treated with intermittent high-dose prednisolone; four pregnancies occurred as a result (126). In a larger study of 48 patients, both a fall in antibody levels and an improvement in sperm motility were demonstrated with long-term moderate-dose intermittent therapy, resulting in 12 pregnancies (127). A crossover trial of intermittent moderate-dose prednisolone or placebo for three cycles produced neither a change in antibody levels nor pregnancy (128). In this trial, the dose and time of treatment was probably inadequate, as a number of the same patients later produced pregnancies with artificial insemination or IVF, subsequently suggesting that the trial subjects included patients with low-level sperm antibodies and that not all had severe sperm autoimmunity. The most encouraging trial reported to date involved 43 men with sperm antibodies and impaired cervical mucus penetration treated with 20 mg of prednisolone twice daily for the first 10 days of the partner's menstrual cycle for nine months or placebo tablets. The results of this study demonstrated nine pregnancies occurring in the prednisolone group, and two pregnancies occurring in the placebo group (114).

Regimen

Various regimens of prednisolone or other glucocorticoid therapy have been used. Because a number of cases of aseptic necrosis of the femoral head have been associated with high-dose (i.e., 96 mg) methylprednisolone, this regimen is no longer in use (119). Both continuous and intermittent prednisolone therapy regimens have been shown to be effective in placebo-controlled trials. Continuous therapy is considered to be 0.75 mg/kg or 50 mg/day given as a single dose each morning with breakfast until a pregnancy occurs, or for a maximum of four to six months. A typical intermittent regimen will use 20 mg to 25 mg of prednisolone each day from day 1 through day 10, or, alternatively, day 4 through 14 of the woman's menstrual cycle. If the semen quality and mucus penetration have not improved within three months, then the dosage is doubled at that time and again after six months. Treatment is usually stopped after a total of nine months.

A therapeutic trial of prednisolone 50 mg daily for four to eight weeks may be used to distinguish genital tract obstruction associated with sperm antibodies from sperm autoimmunity alone causing azoospermia or severe oligozoospermia.

Monitoring and General Management

Patients must be carefully monitored for improvement in semen quality and for adverse effects. Semen tests, IBT, and sperm mucus penetration tests are performed monthly about the time of the woman's menses. Findings of increased sperm concentration, motility, mucus penetration accompanied by a decreased IBT, particularly an IgA IBT of less than 70%, are indicative of a beneficial effect (Fig. 1).

The couple should have sexual intercourse frequently at the most fertile time of the cycle, preferably daily. If semen quality improves, sperm may be cryopreserved during the non-fertile times of the woman's cycle and stored for future use in subsequent artificial insemination or ICSI. Artificial insemination may be successful with stored semen from a previous course of prednisolone therapy (1).

Results

About 50% of men treated with glucocorticoids for sperm autoimmunity demonstrate a reduction in sperm antibody levels and an increase in sperm concentration, motility, and mucus penetration. Pregnancies occur in about 25% of couples during a four- to six-month course of continuous daily prednisolone or after a longer period of intermittent prednisolone therapy. Ovulatory disorders, endometriosis, and tubal abnormalities reduce the chances of a pregnancy occurring during treatment.

Complications

Adverse effects of prednisolone treatment are common. Insomnia and dyspepsia are frequent early problems. Cushingoid appearance, muscle weakness, and joint aches are frequent after more than two or three months of treatment. Transient decreases in

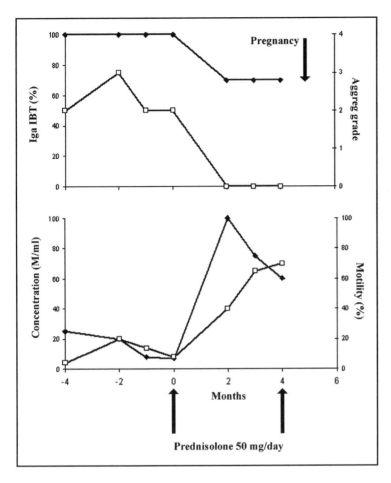

Figure 1 Glucocorticoid treatment of a patient with sperm autoimmunity. After two months treatment with prednisolone (50 mg/day), the antibody levels on the sperm were less (IgA IBT fell from 100% to 70%) (*upper panel, left axis, closed symbols*), sperm aggregation decreased (Aggreg grade) (*upper panel, right axis, open symbols*) and sperm concentration (*lower panel, left axis, closed symbols*), motility (*lower panel, right axis, open symbols*) and mucus penetration (not shown) increased. A natural conception occurred in the month after the 50 mg dose of prednisolone was stopped.

testosterone and SHBG levels, muscle and bone mass occur with a concurrent increase in fat mass (129). Occasional adverse effects resulting from depressed immunity include herpes zoster and severe folliculitis. More serious adverse effects, such as depression, cataracts, Addisonian crisis after cessation of treatment, and aggravation of peptic ulcer disease are rare. The most serious adverse effect of prednisolone treatment is aseptic bone necrosis, most commonly of the femoral head (130).

Unfortunately, this major side effect has been described in a number of men being treated for sperm autoimmunity. It is thought that heavy alcohol drinking may predispose patients to this complication, and thus patients need to be carefully advised due to the large number of litigation actions that have occurred as a result. Appropriate patient counselling should include a telephone number for emergency contact purposes if severe hip pain occurs, thus enabling early cessation of prednisolone and the immediate intervention of a rheumatologist or orthopaedic surgeon which may avoid serious bone necrosis and the need for hip replacement in up to 50% of patients. While other concomitant illnesses such as asthma and psoriasis are often improved during glucocorticoid treatment, they may flare up after stopping the treatment. Only rarely does semen quality deteriorate

during glucocorticoid treatment. There may also be loss of libido possibly related to the suppression of testosterone levels.

□ OTHER POSSIBLE TREATMENTS

Testosterone suppression of spermatogenesis, artificial insemination (AI), washing sperm to remove sperm antibodies, antibiotic therapy, and IVF or gamete intrafallopian transfer (GIFT) without prior prednisolone therapy are ineffective for sperm autoimmunity (1,116,131). Reports in the literature claiming success for these procedures do not separate patients with low-level sperm antibodies (132,133). Lahteenmaki et al. (133) performed a trial in 31 men with positive anti-sperm antibodies in order to compare intrauterine insemination (IUI) with low-dose prednisolone and timed intercourse. The latter course of treatment had a poorer outcome than the IUI without glucocorticoid therapy. Similarly, IUI was compared with IVF for patients with a positive MAR of greater than 50%, with no difference in results (134).

Also worthy of consideration are surgeries to relieve obstructions, such as repeat vasovasostomy and vasoepididymostomy, or the removal of an orchitic testis (113). Some experts suggest that partial obstruction is a more important cause of the development of sperm antibodies (135). In one open study, sperm antibody titers were reportedly decreased after the treatment of prostatitis (136). For further information on obstruction, please refer to Chapter 18.

Separation of sperm with less antibodies on the surface from those that are more heavily coated is possible in patients with low-level antibodies (57,137). This fact is not helpful for treatment, however, since the antibodies in such patients are not present in sufficient quantity to cause severe infertility. Removal of sperm-bound antibodies by washing cannot be successful due to the seven-day half-life of antibody-antigen dissociation interactions. It is possible that enzyme methods may be more successful, such as in the example of IgA protease (138,139). The use of pure antigen to block binding has also been considered (140). In the future, immunomodulatory approaches

may be available. Preliminary results with Levamisol and Cyclosporin have been reported (141,142). Other approaches using Fab fragments and anti-idiotypic antibodies have been postulated (143).

□ CONCLUSION

Sperm autoimmunity is an important cause of male infertility and it should be screened for routinely. Diagnosis should be made only after repeated tests demonstrate positive IBT and failure of sperm cervical mucus penetration. Patients with these characteristics are severely infertile and are unlikely to produce pregnancies without treatment with ICSI or glucocorticoids. These treatments have limited success rates and severe side effects are possible. Donor insemination or adoption may be a suitable alternative for some couples.

□ REFERENCES

1. Baker HW, Clarke GN, Hudson B, et al. Treatment of sperm autoimmunity in men. Clin Reprod Fertil 1983; 2(1):55–71.

2. Clarke GN, Elliott PJ, Smaila C. Detection of sperm antibodies in semen using the immunobead test: a survey of 813 consecutive patients. Am J Reprod Immunol Microbiol 1985; 7(3):118–123.

3. Mazumdar S, Levine AS. Antisperm antibodies: etiology, pathogenesis, diagnosis, and treatment. Fertil Steril 1998; 70(5):799–810.

4. Luckas MJ, Buckett WM, Aird IA, et al. Seminal plasma immunoglobulin concentrations in autoimmune male subfertility. J Reprod Immunol 1998; 37(2): 171–180.

5. Haas GG Jr. Immunologic infertility. Obstet Gynecol Clin North Am 1987; 14(4):1069–1085.

6. Clarke GN. Lack of correlation between the immunobead test and the enzyme-linked immunosorbent assay for sperm antibody detection. Am J Reprod Immunol Microbiol 1988; 18(2):44–46.

7. Culligan PJ, Crane MM, Boone WR, et al. Validity and cost-effectiveness of antisperm antibody testing before in vitro fertilization. Fertility and Sterility 1998; 69(5):894–898.

8. Montoya JM, Bernal A, Borrero C. Diagnostics in assisted human reproduction. Reprod Biomed Online 2002; 5(2): 198–210.

9. Check JH, Katsoff D, Bollendorf A, et al. The effect of sera antisperm antibodies in the female partner on in vivo and in vitro pregnancy and spontaneous abortion rates. Am J Reprod Immunol 1995; 33(1):131–133.

10. Clarke GN, Liu DY, Baker HW. Immunoinfertility: a case study with implications for immunocontraception. Arch Androl 1995; 35(1):21–27.

11. Eggert-Kruse W, Rohr G, Bockem-Hellwig S, et al. Immunological aspects of subfertility. Int J Androl 1995; 18(suppl 2): 43–52.

12. Diekman AB, Herr JC. Sperm antigens and their use in the development of an immunocontraceptive. Am J Reprod Immunol 1997; 37(1):111–117.

13. Kamada M, Maegawa M, Yan YC, et al. Antisperm antibody: a monkey wrench in conception/magic bullet of contraception? J Med Invest 1999; 46(1-2):19–28.

14. Tung KS. Human sperm antigens and antisperm antibodies I. Studies on vasectomy patients. Clin Exp Immunol 1975; 20(1):93–104.

15. Parslow JM, Royle MG, Kingscott MM, et al. The effects of sperm antibodies on fertility after vasectomy reversal. Am J Reprod Immunol 1983; 3(1):28–31.

16. Alexander NJ, Schmidt SS. Incidence of antisperm antibody levels and granulomas in men. Fertil Steril 1977; 28(6): 655–657.

17. Linnet L, Hjort H, Fogh-Andersen P. Association between failure to impregnate after vasovasostomy and sperm agglutinins in semen. Lancet 1981; 1(8212):117–119.

18. Fuchs EF, Alexander NJ. Immunologic considerations before and after vasovasostomy. Fertil Steril 1983; 40(4):497–499.

19. Hendry WF, Parslow JM, Stedronska J. Exploratory scrototomy in 168 azoospermic males. Br J Urol 1983; 55(6):785–791.

20. Gupta I, Dhawan S, Goel GD, et al. Low fertility rate in vasovasostomized males and its possible immunologic mechanism. Int J Fertil 1975; 20(3):183–191.

21. Friberg J, Fritjofsson A. Inguinal herniorrhaphy and sperm-agglutinating antibodies in infertile men. Arch Androl 1979; 2(4):317–322.

22. Hendry WF. Clinical significance of unilateral testicular obstruction in subfertile males. Br J Urol 1986; 58(6):709–714.

23. Amelar RD, Dubin L, Schoenfeld C. Circulating sperm-agglutinating antibodies in azoospermic men with congenital bilateral absence of the vasa deferentia. Fertil Steril 1975; 26(3):228–231.

24. Yamamoto M, Hibi H, Miyake K. The incidence of antisperm antibodies in patients with seminal tract obstructions. Nagoya J Med Sci 1996; 59(1-2):25–29.

25. de Kretser DM, Huidobro C, Southwick GJ, et al. The role of the epididymis in human infertility. J Reprod Fertil Suppl 1998; 53:271–275.

26. Tung KS. Autoimmunity to sperm. Andrologia 1978; 10(3):247–249.

27. Wyburn-Mason R. Sympathetic orchiopathia. Letter. Lancet 1981; 2(8260-8261):1417–1418.

28. Suominen JJ. Sympathetic auto-immune orchitis. Andrologia 1995; 27(4):213–216.

29. Wall JR, Stedronska J, David RD, et al. Immunologic studies of male infertility. Fertil Steril 1975; 26(10):1035–1041.

30. Baker HW, Clarke GN, McGowan MP, et al. Increased frequency of autoantibodies in men with sperm antibodies. Fertil Steril 1985; 43(3):438–441.

31. Mathews JD, Skegg DC, Vessey MP, et al. Weak autoantibody reactions to antigens other than sperm after vasectomy. Br Med J 1976; 2(6048):1359–1360.

32. Crewe P, Dawson L, Barnes RD, et al. Lack of association of the development of anti-sperm antibodies and other autoantibodies as a consequence of vasectomy. Int J Fertil 1977; 22(2):104–109.

33. Law HY, Bodmer WF, Mathews JD, et al. The immune response to vasectomy and its relation to the HLA system. Tissue Antigens 1979; 14(2):115–139.

34. Tsuji Y, Mitsuo M, Yasunami R, et al. HLA-DR and HLA-DQ gene typing of infertile women possessing sperm-immobilizing antibody. J Reprod Immunol 2000 46(1):31–38.

35. Fjallbrant B. Autoimmune human sperm antibodies and age in males. J Reprod Fertil 1975; 43(1):145–148.

36. Kojima A, Spencer CA. Genetic susceptibility to testicular autoimmunity: comparison between postthymectomy and postvasectomy models in mice. Biol Reprod 1983; 29(1): 195–205.

37. Van Thiel DH, Gavaler JS, Smith WI, et al. Testicular and spermatozoal autoantibody in chronic alcoholic males with gonadal failure. Clin Immunol Immunopathol 1977; 8(2):311–317.

38. Hargreave TB, Harvey J, Elton RA, et al. Serum agglutinating and immobilising sperm antibodies in men attending a sexually transmitted diseases clinic. Andrologia 1984; 16(2): 111–115.

39. Clarke GN. Sperm antibodies in normal men: Association with a history of nongonococcal urethritis (ngu). Am J Reprod Immunol Microbiol 1986; 12(2):31–32.

40. Comhaire FH, de Kretser DM, Farley TM. Towards more objectivity in diagnosis and management of male infertility. Int J Androl 1987; 7(suppl):1–53.

41. Eggert-Kruse W, Probst S, Rohr G, et al. Induction of immunoresponse by subclinical male genital tract infection? Fertil Steril 1996; 65(6):1202–1209.

42. Wolff H. The biologic significance of white blood cells in semen. Fertil Steril 1995; 63(6):1143–1157.

43. Hargreave TB, Elton RA, Webb JA, et al. Maldescended testes and fertility: a review of 68 cases. Br J Urol 1984; 56(6): 734–739.

44. Mallidis C, Baker HW. Fine needle tissue aspiration biopsy of the testis. Fertil Steril 1994; 61(2):367–375.

45. Steele EK, Ellis PK, Lewis SE, et al. Ultrasound, antisperm antibody, and hormone profiles after testicular Trucut biopsy. Fertil Steril 2001; 75(2):423–428.

46. Shetty J, Naaby-Hansen S, Shibahara H, et al. Human sperm proteome: Immunodominant sperm surface antigens identified with sera from infertile men and women. Biol Reprod 1999; 61(1):61–69.

47. Koide SS, Wang L, Kamada M. Antisperm antibodies associated with infertility: properties and encoding genes of target antigens. Proc Soc Exp Biol Med 2000; 224(3):123–132.

48. Chiu WW, Chamley LW. Use of antisperm antibodies in differential display Western blotting to identify sperm proteins important in fertility. Hum Reprod 2002; 17(4):984–989.

49. Bohring C, Krause W. Immune infertility: towards a better understanding of sperm (auto)-immunity: The value of proteomic analysis. Hum Reprod 2003; 18(5):915–924.

50. Neilson LI, Schneider PA, Van Deerlin PG, et al. cDNA cloning and characterization of a human sperm antigen (spag6) with homology to the product of the Chlamydomonas PF16 locus. Genomics 1999; 60(3):272–280.

51. Isojima S, Kameda K, Tsuji Y, et al. Establishment and characterization of a human hybridoma secreting monoclonal antibody with high titers of sperm immobilizing and agglutinating activities against human seminal plasma. J Reprod Immunol 1987; 10(1):67–78.

52. Diekman AB, Norton EJ, Westbrook VA, et al. Antisperm antibodies from infertile patients and their cognate sperm antigens: a review. Identity between SAGA-1, the H6-3C4 antigen, and CD52. Am J Reprod Immunol 2000; 43(3): 134–143.

53. Poulton TA, Everard D, Baxby B, et al. Characterisation of a sperm coating auto-antigen reacting with antisperm antibodies of infertile males using monoclonal antibodies. Br J Obstet Gynaecol 1996; 103(5): 463–467.

54. Norton EJ, Diekman AB, Westbrook VA, et al. A male genital tract-specific carbohydrate epitope on human CD52: implications for immunocontraception. Tissue Antigens 2002; 60(5):354–364.

55. Sarkar S. Carbohydrate antigens of human sperm and autoimmune induction of infertility. J Reprod Med 1974; 13(3):93–99.

56. Kurpisz M, Alexander NJ. Carbohydrate moieties on sperm surface: physiological relevance. Fertil Steril 1995; 63(1): 158–165.

57. Wang C, Baker HW, Jennings MG, et al. Interaction between human cervical mucus and sperm surface antibodies. Fertil Steril 1985; 44(4):484–488.

58. Imade GE, Baker HW, de Kretser DM, et al. Immunosuppressive activities in the seminal plasma of infertile men: relationship to sperm antibodies and autoimmunity. Hum Reprod 1997; 12(2):256–262.

59. Munoz MG, Jeremias J, Witkin SS. The 60 kDa heat shock protein in human semen: relationship with antibodies to spermatozoa and Chlamydia trachomatis. Hum Reprod 1996; 11(12):2600–2603.

60. Sakin-Kaindl F, Wagenknecht DR, Strowitzki T, et al. Decreased suppression of antibody-dependent cellular cytotoxicity by seminal plasma in unexplained infertility. Fertil Steril 2001; 75(3):581–587.

61. Ritchie AW, Hargreave TB, James K, et al. Intra-epithelial lymphocytes in the normal epididymis. A mechanism for tolerance to sperm auto-antigens? Br J Urol 1984; 56(1):79–83.

62. el-Demiry MI, Hargreave TB, Busuttil A, et al. Immunocompetent cells in human testis in health and disease. Fertil Steril 1987; 48(3):470–479.

63. Jager S, Kremer J, Kuiken J, et al. Immunoglobulin class of antispermatozoal antibodies from infertile men and inhibition of in vitro sperm penetration into cervical mucus. Int J Androl 1980; 3(1):1–14.

64. Francavilla F, Romano R, Santucci R, et al. Interference of antisperm antibodies with the induction of the acrosome reaction by zona pellucida (ZP) and its relationship with the inhibition of ZP binding. Fertil Steril 1997; 67(6):1128–1133.

65. Harrison S, Hull G, Pillai S. Sperm acrosome status and sperm antibodies in infertility. J Urol 1998; 159(5): 1554–1558.

66. Shibahara H, Shigeta M, Toji H, et al. Sperm immobilizing antibodies interfere with sperm migration from the uterine cavity through the fallopian tubes. Am J Reprod Immunol 1995; 34(2):120–124.

67. London SN, Haney AF, Weinberg JB. Macrophages and infertility: enhancement of human macrophage-mediated sperm killing by antisperm antibodies. Fertil Steril 1985; 43(2): 274–278.

68. Salomon F, Saremaslani P, Jakob M, et al. Immune complex orchitis in infertile men. Immunoelectron microscopy of abnormal basement membrane structures. Lab Invest 1982; 47(6):555–567.

69. Jager S, Kremer J, Kuiken J, et al. The significance of the Fc part of antispermatozoal antibodies for the shaking phenomenon in the sperm-cervical mucus contact test. Fertil Steril 1981; 36(6):792–797.

70. Jager S, Kremer J, Kuiken J, et al. Induction of the shaking phenomenon by pretreatment of spermatozoa with sera containing antispermatozoal antibodies. Fertil Steril 1981; 36(6):784–791.

71. Clarke GN. Induction of the shaking phenomenon by IgA class antispermatozoal antibodies from serum. Am J Reprod Immunol Microbiol 1985; 9(1):12–14.

72. Parslow JM, Poulton TA, Besser GM, et al. The clinical relevance of classes of immunoglobulins on spermatozoa from infertile and vasovasostomized males. Fertil Steril 1985; 43(4):621–627.

73. Haas GG Jr, Ausmanus M, Culp L, et al. The effect of immunoglobulin occurring on human sperm in vivo on the human sperm/hamster ova penetration assay. Am J Reprod Immunol Microbiol 1985; 7(3):109–112.

74. Bronson R, Cooper G, Rosenfeld D. Ability of antibody-bound human sperm to penetrate zona-free hamster ova in vitro. Fertil Steril 1981; 36(6):778–783.

75. Clarke GN, Lopata A, McBain JC, et al. Effect of sperm antibodies in males on human in vitro fertilization (IVF). Am J Reprod Immunol Microbiol 1985; 8(2):62–66.

76. Johnston WI, Oke K, Speirs A, et al. Patient selection for in vitro fertilization: physical and psychological aspects. Ann N Y Acad Sci 1985; 442:490–503.

77. Kamada M, Daitoh T, Hasebe H, et al. Blocking of human fertilization in vitro by sera with sperm- immobilizing antibodies. Am J Obstet Gynecol 1985; 153(3):328–331.

78. Clarke GN, Lopata A, Johnston WI. Effect of sperm antibodies in females on human in vitro fertilization. Fertil Steril 1986; 46(3):435–441.

79. Yeh WR, Acosta AA, Seltman HJ, et al. Impact of immunoglobulin isotype and sperm surface location of antisperm antibodies on fertilization in vitro in the human. Fertil Steril 1995; 63(6):1287–1292.

80. Ford WC, Williams KM, McLaughlin EA, et al. The indirect immunobead test for seminal antisperm antibodies and fertilization rates at in-vitro fertilization. Hum Reprod 1996; 11(7):1418–1422.

81. Taneichi A, Shibahara H, Hirano Y, et al. Sperm immobilizing antibodies in the sera of infertile women cause low fertilization rates and poor embryo quality in vitro. Am J Reprod Immunol 2002; 47(1):46–51.

82. Bronson RA, Cooper GW, Rosenfeld DL. Sperm-specific isoantibodies and autoantibodies inhibit the binding of human sperm to the human zona pellucida. Fertil Steril 1982; 38(6):724–729.

83. Tsukui S, Noda Y, Yano J, et al. Inhibition of sperm penetration through human zona pellucida by antisperm antibodies. Fertil Steril 1986; 46(1):92–96.

84. Liu DY, Clarke GN, Baker HW. Inhibition of human sperm-zona pellucida and sperm-oolemma binding by antisperm antibodies. Fertil Steril 1991; 55(2): 440–442.

85. Shibahara H, Shigeta M, Inoue M, et al. Diversity of the blocking effects of antisperm antibodies on fertilization in human and mouse. Hum Reprod 1996; 11(12):2595–2599.

86. Wolf JP, De Almeida M, Ducot B, et al. High levels of sperm-associated antibodies impair human spermoolemma interaction after subzonal insemination. Fertil Steril 1995; 63(3): 584–590.

87. Zalata A, Hafez T, Comhaire F. Evaluation of the role of reactive oxygen species in male infertility. Hum Reprod 1995; 10(6):1444–1451.

88. Clarke GN, Baker HW. Lack of association between sperm antibodies and recurrent spontaneous abortion. Fertil Steril 1993; 59(2):463–464.

89. Daitoh T, Kamada M, Yamano S, et al. High implantation rate and consequently high pregnancy rate by in vitro fertilization-embryo transfer treatment in infertile women with antisperm antibody. Fertil Steril 1995; 63(1):87–91.

90. Evans ML, Chan PJ, Patton WC, et al. Sperm artificially exposed to antisperm antibodies show altered deoxyribonucleic acid. J Assist Reprod Genet 1999; 16(8):443–449.

91. Daya S, Clark D. In vitro fertilisation in immunological infertility. Ann Acad Med Singapore 1992; 21(4):525–532.

92. Shibahara H, Mitsuo M, Ikeda Y, et al. Effects of sperm immobilizing antibodies on pregnancy outcome in infertile women treated with IVF-ET. Am J Reprod Immunol 1996; 36(2):96–100.

93. Rumke P, Van Amstel N, Messer EN, et al. Prognosis of fertility of men with sperm agglutinins in the serum. Fertil Steril 1974; 25(5):393–398.

94. Hargreave TB, Haxton M, Whitelaw J, et al. The significance of serum sperm-agglutinating antibodies in men with infertile marriages. Br J Urol 1980; 52(6):566–570.

95. Menge AC, Medley NE, Mangione CM, et al. The incidence and influence of antisperm antibodies in infertile human couples on sperm-cervical mucus interactions and subsequent fertility. Fertil Steril 1982; 38(4):439–446.

96. Mahmoud AM, Tuyttens CL, Comhaire FH. Clinical and biological aspects of male immune infertility: a case-controlled study of 86 cases. Andrologia 1996; 28(4):191–196.

97. Hendry WF. Detection and treatment of antispermatozoal antibodies in men. Reprod Fertil Dev 1989; 1(3):205–220; discussion 220-222.

98. Cookson MS, Witt MA, Kimball KT, et al. Can semen analysis predict the presence of antisperm antibodies in patients with primary infertility? World J Urol 1995; 13(5):318–322.

99. WHO. World Health Organization laboratory manual for the examination of human semen and sperm-cervical mucus interaction. Cambridge: Cambridge University Press, 1999:23–26.

100. Bronson RA, Cooper GW, Rosenfeld DW. Autoimmunity to spermatozoa: effect on sperm penetration of cervical mucus as reflected by postcoital testing. Fertil Steril 1984; 41(4): 609–614.

101. Barratt CL, Dunphy BC, McLeod I, et al. The poor prognostic value of low to moderate levels of sperm surface-bound antibodies. Hum Reprod 1992; 7(1):95–98.

102. Francavilla F, Romano R, Santucci R, et al. Naturally-occurring antisperm antibodies in men: interference with fertility and implications for treatment. Front Biosci 1999; 4:E9-E25.

103. Quinlivan WL, Sullivan H. Spermatozoal antibodies in human seminal plasma as a cause of failed artificial donor insemination. Fertil Steril 1977; 28(10): 1082–1085.

104. Quinlivan WL, Sullivan H. The immunologic effects of husband's semen on donor spermatozoa during mixed insemination. Fertil Steril 1977; 28(4): 448–450.

105. Clarke GN, Bourne H, Baker HW. Intracytoplasmic sperm injection for treating infertility associated with sperm autoimmunity. Fertil Steril 1997; 68(1): 112–117.

106. Nagy ZP, Verheyen G, Liu J, et al. Results of 55 intracytoplasmic sperm injection cycles in the treatment of male-immunological infertility. Hum Reprod 1995; 10(7):1775–1780.

107. Jun JH, Lim CK, Park YS, et al. Efficacy of intracytoplasmic sperm injection (ICSI) treatment in the immunological infertile patients. Am J Reprod Immunol 37(4):310–314.

108. Lahteenmaki A, Reima I, Hovatta O. Treatment of severe male immunological infertility by intracytoplasmic sperm injection. Hum Reprod 1995; 10(11):2824–2828.

109. Vazquez-Levin MH, Notrica JA, Polak de Fried F. Male immunologic infertility: sperm performance on in vitro fertilization. Fertil Steril 1997; 68(4):675–681.

110. Junk SM, Matson PL, Yovich JM, et al. The fertilization of human oocytes by spermatozoa from men with antispermatozoal antibodies in semen. J In Vitro Fert Embryo Transf 1986; 3(6):350–352.

111. Lahteenmaki A, Rasanen M, Hovatta O. Low-dose prednisolone does not improve the outcome of in-vitro fertilization in male immunological infertility. Hum Reprod 1995; 10(12): 3124–3129.

112. Rasanen M, Lahteenmaki A, Agrawal YP, et al. A placebo-controlled flow cytometric study of the effect of low-dose prednisolone treatment on sperm-bound antibody levels. Int J Androl 1996; 19(3): 150–154.

113. Baker G, Bourne H, Edgar D. Sperm preparation techniques. In: Gardner D, Weissman A, Howles C, Shoham Z, eds. Textbook of Assisted Reproductive Techniques: Laboratory and Clinical Perspectives. London: Martin Dunitz, 2001: 77–87.

114. Hendry WF, Hughes L, Scammell G, et al. Comparison of prednisolone and placebo in subfertile men with antibodies to spermatozoa. Lancet 1990; 335(8681):85–88.

115. De Almeida M, Soufir JC. Corticosteroid therapy for male autoimmune infertility. Lancet 1977; 2(8042): 815–816.

116. Kremer J, Jager S, Kuiken J. Treatment of infertility caused by antisperm antibodies. Int J Fertil 1978; 23(4):270–276.

117. Shulman S, Harlin B, Davis P, et al. Immune infertility and new approaches to treatment. Fertil Steril 1978; 29(3): 309–313.

118. Hendry WF, Stedronska J, Parslow J, et al. The results of intermittent high dose steroid therapy for male infertility due to antisperm antibodies. Fertil Steril 1981; 36(3):351–355.

119. Shulman JF, Shulman S. Methylprednisolone treatment of immunologic infertility in male. Fertil Steril 1982; 38(5): 591–599.

120. Dondero F, Isidori A, Lenzi A, et al. Treatment and follow-up of patients with infertility due to spermagglutinins. Fertil Steril 1979; 31(1):48–51.

121. De Almeida M, Jouannet P. Dexamethasone therapy of infertile men with sperm autoantibodies: immunological and sperm follow-up. Clin Exp Immunol 1981; 44(3):567–575.

122. Hargreave TB, Elton RA. Treatment with intermittent high dose methylprednisolone or intermittent betamethasone for antisperm antibodies: preliminary communication. Fertil Steril 1982; 38(5):586–590.

123. Alexander NJ, Sampson JH, Fulgham DL. Pregnancy rates in patients treated for antisperm antibodies with prednisone. Int J Fertil 1983; 28(2):63–67.

124. Haas GG Jr, Manganiello P. A double-blind, placebo-controlled study of the use of methylprednisolone in infertile men with sperm-associated immunoglobulins. Fertil Steril 1987; 47(2):295–301.

125. De Almeida M, Feneux D, Rigaud C, et al. Steroid therapy for male infertility associated with antisperm antibodies. Results of a small randomized clinical trial. Int J Androl 1985; 8(2):111–117.

126. Keane D, Jenkins DM, Higgins T, et al. The effect of intermittent steroid therapy on anti-sperm antibody levels. Eur J Obstet Gynecol Reprod Biol 1995; 63(1):75–79.

127. Sharma KK, Barratt CL, Pearson MJ, et al. Oral steroid therapy for subfertile males with antisperm antibodies in the semen: prediction of the responders. Hum Reprod 1995; 10(1): 103–109.

128. Bals-Pratsch M, Doren M, Karbowski B, et al. Cyclic corticosteroid immunosuppression is unsuccessful in the treatment of sperm antibody-related male infertility: a controlled study. Hum Reprod 1992; 7(1):99–104.

129. Pearce G, Tabensky DA, Delmas PD, et al. Corticosteroid-induced bone loss in men. J Clin Endocrinol Metab 1998; 83(3):801–806.

130. Pavelka K. Osteonecrosis. Baillieres Best Pract Res Clin Rheumatol 2000; 14(2):399–414.

131. Confino E, Friberg J, Dudkiewicz AB, et al. Intrauterine inseminations with washed human spermatozoa. Fertil Steril 1986; 46(1):55–60.

132. Grigoriou O, Konidaris S, Antonaki V, et al. Corticosteroid treatment does not improve the results of intrauterine insemination in male subfertility caused by antisperm antibodies. Eur J Obstetrics and Gynecology Reprod Biol 1996; 65(2): 227–230.

133. Lahteenmaki A, Veilahti J, Hovatta O. Intra-uterine insemination versus cyclic, low-dose prednisolone in couples with male antisperm antibodies. Hum Reprod 1995; 10(1):142–147.

134. Ombelet W, Vandeput H, Janssen M, et al. Treatment of male infertility due to sperm surface antibodies: IUI or IVF? Hum Reprod 1997; 12(6):1165–1170.

135. Carbone DJ Jr, Shah A, Thomas AJ Jr, et al. Partial obstruction, not antisperm antibodies, causing infertility after vasovasostomy. J Urol 1998; 159(3):827–830.

136. Fjallbrant B, Nilsson S. Decrease of sperm antibody titer in males, and conception after treatment of chronic prostatitis. Int J Fertil 1977; 22(4):255–256.

137. Zavos PM, Correa JR, Zarmakoupis-Zavos PN. Antisperm antibody treatment mode: levels of antisperm antibodies after incubation with TEST-yolk buffer and filtration using the SpermPrep II method. Fertil Steril 1998; 69(3):517–521.

138. Bronson RA, Cooper GW, Rosenfeld DL, et al. The effect of an IgA1 protease on immunoglobulins bound to the sperm surface and sperm cervical mucus penetrating ability. Fertil Steril 1987; 47(6): 985–991.

139. Kutteh WH, Kilian M, Ermel LD, et al. Antisperm antibodies in infertile women: subclass distribution of immunoglobulin (Ig) A antibodies and removal of IgA sperm-bound antibodies with a specific IgA1 protease. Fertil Steril 1995; 63(1):63–70.

140. Menge AC, Christman GM, Ohl DA, et al. Fertilization antigen-1 removes antisperm autoantibodies from spermatozoa of infertile men and results in increased rates of acrosome reaction. Fertil Steril 1999; 71(2): 256–260.

141. Luisi M, Gasperi M, Franchi F, et al. Levamisole treatment in male infertility due to spermagglutinins. Lancet 1982; 2(8288):47.

142. Bouloux PM, Wass JA, Parslow JM, et al. Effect of cyclosporin A in male autoimmune infertility. Fertil Steril 1986; 46(1): 81–85.

143. D'Cruz OJ, Haas GG Jr. Protection of sperm from isoimmune attack in vivo by pretreatment with antisperm Fab: fertility trials in the immune rabbit model. Res Commun Mol Pathol Pharmacol 1995; 88(3):243–270.

37

Micromanipulation of Male Gametes in the Treatment of the Subfertile Male

Soon-Chye Ng

O & G Partners Fertility, Gleneagles Hospital, Singapore

Swee-Lian Liow

Embryonics International, Gleneagles Hospital, Singapore

☐ INTRODUCTION

Male-factor infertility can be associated with a wide range of semen anomalies involving sperm count, motility, and morphology. In the inherently complex fertilization process, male-factor infertility, along with defects in sperm function, is the single most common cause of failure to achieve pregnancy. The etiology of impaired sperm production and function could be due to congenital or acquired obstruction to sperm passage from the testis or epididymes, genetic mutations, chromosomal abnormalities, endocrine factors and idiopathic factors.

In the last one-and-a-half decades of the twentieth century, many micromanipulation techniques, such as partial zona dissection (PZD) (1), subzonal sperm injection (SUZI) (2), and intracytoplasmic sperm injection (ICSI) (3) were developed and refined to overcome some of the problems of human infertility; when Palermo et al. (3) reported the first human pregnancies following ICSI, the direct injection of a single sperm into an oocyte, it was a major breakthrough in the field of assisted fertilization in humans. Since then, ICSI has evolved as the most effective treatment for severe oligoasthenoteratozoospermia (poor sperm count, poor motility, and high numbers of abnormal sperm), with many in vitro fertilization (IVF) centers reporting a significant improvement in pregnancy rate and live birth rates. It is also now possible to inject testicular spermatozoa and spermatids directly into the oocyte to enable conception. The direct injection of a spermatozoa (mature ejaculated or immature aspirated) into the oocyte bypasses critical physiological steps in sperm selection in a normal fertilization such as acrosome reaction, sperm binding to the zona pellucida, and sperm fusion with the oolemma (see Figure 1 in Chapter 39). There is a concern that ICSI may have opened a channel for the transmission of genetic defects to the next generation, as genetic mutations and chromosomal abnormalities have been linked to male infertility.

This review presents a brief history of the development of micromanipulation techniques and the application of these techniques in assisting conception in humans. The outcome and implications of these micromanipulation techniques in the treatment of male infertility are discussed.

A Brief History of Micromanipulation

Micromanipulation is defined as the art of performing microscopic procedures or microsurgery on individual cells with the aid of a microscope and apparatus in which very fine instruments are held and displaced in microdistances. The first microsurgical apparatus was developed by Schmidt (4). Schmidt's apparatus consisted of a special microscope stage that held a specimen of tissue. Surrounding the stage were three screw-controlled positioners that were used for operating a variety of microscopic dissection instruments such as metal needles, scissors, and scalpels. A fine motion of the microsurgical tool could be obtained by turning the screws. Chabry (5) further developed the micromanipulation apparatus and methodology that led to the first true embryological micromanipulation of embryos of ascidians. The embryos were manipulated by glass capillary tubing and very fine glass needles. Chabry (5) also described the technique for the fabrication of ultrafine glass needles by using a hot platinum wire to pull minute, sharp points from the tips of glass microneedles. Microforge techniques are adapted from this method. Since then, the micromanipulation apparatus and microtool fabrication techniques developed by Schmidt (4) and Chabry (5), respectively, have been further refined by other researchers, particularly those involved in the study of cell biology and mammalian embryology.

The first few decades of the twentieth century were devoted to the application of micromanipulation techniques in experimental cytology, bacteriology, cellular physiology, and embryology in invertebrates and amphibians. From 1940 onward, micromanipulation

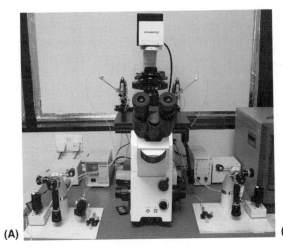 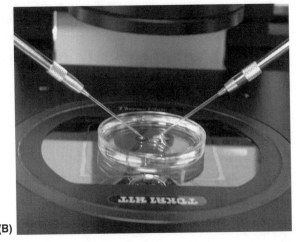

(A)   (B)

Figure 1 (*See color insert.*) (**A**) Micromanipulation system that consists of: (1) a high-end inverted microscope, (2) pair of micromanipulators, (3) heating stage, (4) pair of micropipette holders, (5) a pair of injectors. (**B**) Micromanipulation set-up typically consists of a manipulation dish and two micopipettes.

techniques were used to study oocytes in mammals: the rat (6), the human (7), the mouse (8), and the rabbit (9). The impetus for experimental mammalian embryology was provided by Lin (10), who conducted a series of experiments on the technical and experimental nature of micromanipulation of mouse oocytes. In 1966, Lin reported the first successful microinjection of mouse oocytes. He demonstrated that during the microinjection of bovine gamma globulin-citrate Locke's solution into these oocytes, penetration through the elastic zona pellucida requires a thrust of the microinjection pipette. On the other hand, injecting into the watery ooplasm requires the smooth and slow penetration of the microinjection pipette, because sudden penetration would cause the disruption of the oolemma and death of the oocyte. Lin concluded that microinjection was easier at the pronuclear stage than at the unfertilized stage. He (11) also demonstrated that the mouse oocyte remained intact after the removal of its ooplasm with a micropipette up to almost half its volume.

The early investigations regarding the injection of sperm into oocytes were primarily to elucidate the early events of fertilization, such as membrane fusion between homologous and heterologous gametes, oocyte activation, and pronuclear formation. With the advent of human IVF, it is possible to subject human oocytes and preimplantation embryos to micromanipulation. Micromanipulation in the human is presently limited to diagnosing and correcting genetic and chromosomal disorders and assisting embryo hatching and fertilization in severe male-factor infertility.

☐ MICROMANIPULATION TECHNIQUES IN ASSISTED REPRODUCTION

Since the birth of Louise Brown, the first test-tube baby in 1978, IVF has been used, with varying degrees of success to treat male infertility. The limitations to IVF

are azoospermia, severe oligoasthenoteratospermia, and thickening of the zona pellucida. Sperm with severe morphological defects are unable to penetrate the zona pellucida. Micromanipulation procedures were developed to assist fertilization via a bypass of the zona pellucida—the main barrier to sperm penetration. The different approaches of these micromanipulation procedures include (*i*) the creation of an opening in the zona pellucida to facilitate sperm passage, (*ii*) direct placement of a few sperm under the zona pellucida, and (*iii*) the microinjection of a single sperm directly into the ooplasm. The first two approaches rely solely on the ability of the sperm to bind to and fuse with the oolemma. On the other hand, microinjection of a single sperm directly into the ooplasm obviates the need for sperm–oocyte fusion. These procedures are performed by a clinical embryologist using the micromanipulation system (Fig. 1 and B).

Zona Pellucida Dissection

The thickness of the zona pellucida appears to affect sperm penetration and thus fertilization rate (FR) (12); however, micromanipulation of the zona pellucida alone is not efficient in enhancing assisted reproduction. Nevertheless, it marks the beginning of an evolution and development of more clinically efficient assisted reproductive techniques.

Zona Drilling

Zona drilling involves the use of an acidic solution to dissolve the zona pellucida so that a gap can be created within the zona. This allows sperm to swim into the perivitelline space (PVS) of an oocyte so that normal sperm–oocyte interaction can occur. Gordon and Talansky (13) successfully developed this technique in the mouse in the hopes that similar results could be obtained when applied to clinical IVF for patients with reduced sperm count. Although fertilization was frequently achieved, embryonic development was generally abnormal. Replacement of zona-drilled embryos did not result in pregnancies (14–16) except for only one early miscarriage (17). The failure of this technique appears to be related to the exposure of the oocyte to acidic conditions, which, possibly, could disrupt the capacity of the oocyte to complete the meiotic division (15) and also alter the morphology of the microvilli present on the oolemma (18), which are important for sperm–oocyte interaction. Furthermore, zona drilling also causes a significant drop in intracellular pH, which could disrupt the integrity of the oocyte, leading to cytoplasmic degeneration and death (19).

Partial Zona Dissection

PZD was developed to overcome the shortcomings of zona drilling. A gap is mechanically created in the zona pellucida by using a glass microneedle to pierce through one side of the zona pellucida at the one o'clock position and out through the zona at the 11 o'clock position (20). The oocyte is then released from the holding pipette that is used to abrade the zona until the oocyte drops off the microneedle, and a slit is made in the zona. Sucrose solution is used to shrink the oocyte so that the microneedle can be introduced into the PVS without damaging the oocyte. The morphology of the oocyte is restored by exposure to a medium with normal osmolarity, and then the oocyte is inseminated. This procedure was responsible for achieving the first human pregnancy via assisted fertilization by a micromanipulation technique (1).

Although PZD enhances fertilization of oligozoospermic men, there is no significant improvement in fertilization with normal sperm parameters. Polyspermic FRs of 5% to 15% for patients with abnormal sperm parameters (21–23) and 36% to 57% for normozoospermic patients (20,23,24) have been reported; however, severely reduced sperm concentrations and the presence of sperm defects (20,21,24,25) can result in the failure of sperm to traverse the slit in the zona pellucida and thus limit the success of PZD (22). Undesirable consequences of PZD include monozygotic twinning (26) and problems with variable gap size created by the piercing needle. The latter can cause strangulation of embryos during hatching when the opening is too narrow; an overlarge gap could cause polyspermy and the partial or complete loss of embryos during intrauterine replacement (27). Loss of trophoblastic tissue (28) can also occur.

Laser Zona Cutting

Laser has been considered as a superior alternative because of its ability to create precisely sized gaps. A variety of lasers have been proposed, including contact (optic fiber) and noncontact (objective lens). The zona is photoablated to create a 20 μm hole, and the oocyte is inseminated. Few pregnancies have been achieved with this technology (29,30); however, the application of this technique in assisted fertilization has been superceded by the successful application of ICSI.

Limitations of Zona-Opening Procedures

The major limitation of conventional (non-laser) zona-opening procedures is their inability to produce standardized and uniform gaps. In acid zona drilling, the size of the hole is determined by the size of the dispensing micropipette, the spread of the acidic medium upon dispensing, and the distance between the zona pellucida and the micropipette. In PZD, the size of the piercing micropipette and the degree of shearing forces induced by the operator through the micropipette determine the dimension of the slit in the zona pellucida. Simon et al. (31) have demonstrated that the average slit after PZD is rectangular, 10 to 20 μm in length, and 2 to 5 μm in width. Therefore, the likelihood of increasing polyspermic fertilization or extrusion of the oocyte from the zona pellucida remains with these zona-opening procedures.

Subzonal Injection of Sperm

Although fertilization of human oocytes was achieved by microinjecting sperm under the zona pellucida (32), the first success of this technique in a mammalian model was achieved by Mann (33) when a few capacitated mouse sperm were inserted under the zona pellucida of mouse oocytes, resulting in live birth. Subsequently, Ng et al. (2) reported the first human pregnancy using a modified technique. The successful fertilization of the ovum by placement of a few motile sperm within the PVS demonstrated for the first time that (i) the zona pellucida of the human oocyte can be penetrated with a microinjection pipette without damaging the oocyte, (ii) although a few motile sperm are placed within the PVS, monospermic fertilization can occur, and (iii) the rate of polyspermic fertilization is similar to both PZD and IVF. Many acronyms have been given to this technique, such as microinjection sperm transfer, sub-zonal insertion, and SUZI (subzonal insemination); however, SUZI is the most commonly used acronym. SUZI was initially applied in cases of severe oligozoospermia and previous failed IVF cycles, but was later found to be beneficial in those cases with defective sperm penetration of the zona pellucida.

Only acrosome-reacted sperm can fuse with the oolemma. FR was shown to increase linearly between one and three injected sperm, but above that, the FR plateaued around 25%. Polyspermic fertilization was also found to correlate with the number of sperm injected and usually did not exceed 5%. The capacity of the sperm to fuse with the oolemma was found to be dependent upon semen characteristics and sperm morphology (34). Differences in patient selection sperm preparation, and the skill of the technician are some of the factors that influence the success of SUZI. Compared with ICSI, SUZI is associated with lower monospermic FRs of 49.4% and 17.7%, respectively; however, more embryos were typically available for transfer using ICSI than SUZI (83.3% and 39.3%, respectively) and consequently, the pregnancy rate per oocyte retrieval was higher with ICSI than with SUZI (25% and 10.3%, respectively). Artificially induced acrosome reactions did not significantly increase the FR for SUZI (22% and 11% for monospermic and polyspermic fertilization, respectively) when compared with non-stimulated sperm (18% and 8%, respectively) (35). Thus, the above-mentioned results suggest that SUZI is not as efficient as ICSI in treating cases with severe male infertility.

Intracytoplasmic Sperm Injection

Early work in the direct injection of a single sperm into an oocyte was performed in both heterospecific and homospecific mammalian systems. During this early work, sperm nuclear decondensation and male pronuclear formation have been achieved, but the procedure often resulted in severe damage to the oocytes. In 1992, Palermo et al. (3) reported the first human pregnancy by direct injection of a single spermatozoon into the ooplasm. Although there was initial skepticism, ICSI has now evolved as the most effective treatment for severe oligoasthenoteratozoospermia, with many IVF centers reporting significant improvements in pregnancy and live birth rates. Generally, embryos obtained with ICSI have a lower potential to develop into blastocysts as compared with IVF

embryos; however, recent studies have indicated that there are no differences in the embryo development and blastocyst formation, irrespective of either ICSI or IVF (36–38). The timing of sperm injection does not significantly affect the survival and FRs of the oocytes and embryo quality (39), but higher numbers of good quality embryos can be obtained when ICSI is performed between one hour and nine hours after oocyte recovery (40).

Membrane Breakage

The ICSI technique (Fig. 2A–C) performed by most centers requires that the oolemma be broken at the point of injection before the sperm is delivered into the ooplasm (41–46). Palermo et al. (43) described three types of membrane breakage: normal, intermediate, and difficult. Normal membrane breakage refers to the rupture of an invagination that is created by passage of the injection needle into the oocyte. Intermediate and difficult breakage of the oolemma without creating a funnel and/or oolemma that breaks after several penetration attempts can affect subsequent embryonic development to the blastocyst stage (37,38). Joris et al. (45) described different patterns of membrane breakage to overcome this problem.

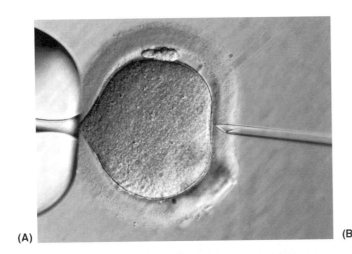

(A)

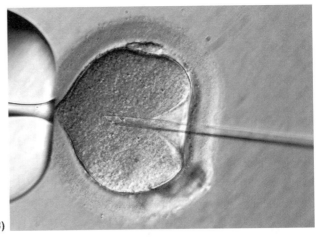

(B)

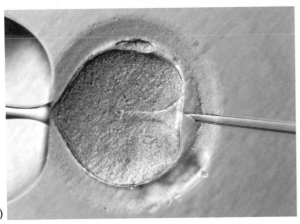

(C)

Figure 2 (*See color insert.*) Intracytoplasmic sperm injection: (**A**) Placement of immobilized sperm at tip of injection micropipette. Injection of sperm into the oocyte is performed at 3 o'clock in relation to the position of the first polar body. (**B**) The oolemma has been broken by aspiration of ooplasm into the injection micropipette. The immobilized sperm is then deposited into the oocyte. (**C**) Sperm is deposited into the oocyte. Notice the invagination as the injection micropipette withdraws.

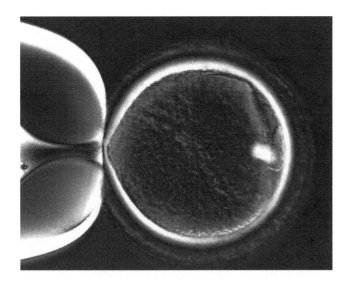

Figure 3 A mature oocyte as viewed by polarized microscopy (PolScope). A reflective meiotic spindle is clearly visible.

Aspiration of Ooplasm

Intimate contact of injected sperm with the ooplasm within the ovum is necessary for the formation of the male pronucleus (47,48). Ooplasmic aspiration is an integral part of the ICSI technique as it ensures that the sperm is in the oocyte and in intimate contact with the ooplasm. Ooplasmic aspiration is also thought to

trigger the initial steps in inducing activation of the oocyte via an artificial calcium influx generated by ICSI (49,50). The actual aspiration of the ooplasm into the needle to induce breakage is a delicate technical matter. Gentle handling of the ooplasmic aspiration within the needle results in higher survival rates of the oocytes and better embryo quality (38,44,46).

Recently, polarized microscopy has been used to identify the location of the meiotic spindle so as to avoid it being damaged by ICSI (Fig. 3).

Immobilization of Sperm

Immobilization of motile sperm prior to ICSI by crushing the tail (Fig. 4A–D) and avoiding damage to the mid-piece with the needle is a mandatory part of the ICSI technique, even with totally nonmotile spermatozoa (44,51,52). The method of sperm immobilization is important for the rapid release of sperm factors that initiate oocyte activation. Differences in sperm immobilization methods may affect the timing of initial Ca^{2+} oscillations and FR, but rates of cleavage and pregnancy were not significantly different (53). Immobilization of a spermatozoon induces permeabilization of the sperm membrane, which may result in the release of a cytosolic factor(s) that diffuses into the ooplasm with subsequent intracellular Ca^{2+} oscillations and hyperpolarization of the oocyte (54,55). Ca^{2+} oscillations due to sperm–oocyte interaction

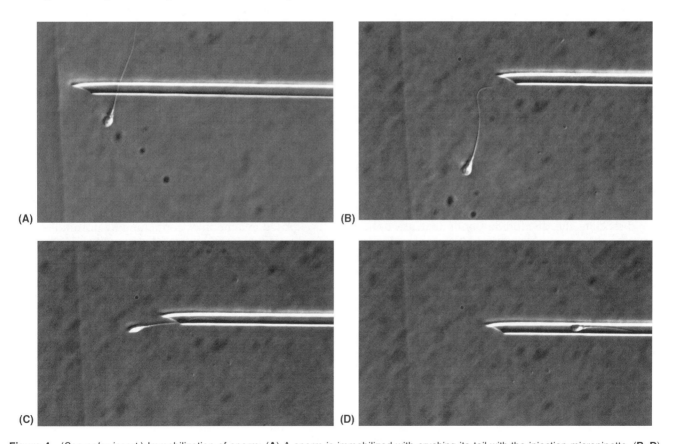

(A)
(B)
(C)
(D)

Figure 4 (*See color insert.*) Immobilization of sperm: (**A**) A sperm is immobilized with crushing its tail with the injection micropipette. (**B–D**) Aspiration of immobilized sperm (tail-in) into the injection micropipette.

were observed at about five minutes after ICSI (53). The activation of the oocyte triggers a series of biochemical processes in the ooplasm that eventually lead to sperm nuclear decondensation (47,48), second polar body extrusion, pronuclear formation, and exocytosis (56,57). Injection of this sperm cytosolic factor was shown to cause embryonic development up to at least the blastocyst stage in a mouse experimental model (58). The components of the sperm cytosolic factor have been shown to be heat-sensitive proteins, and are only effective when injected into the ooplasm (42,50,56,57,59,60). Full mammalian oocyte activation is initiated by the coordinated action of one or more heat-sensitive protein constituents of the peri-nuclear matrix and at least one heat-stable sub-membrane component of sperm-borne oocyte-activating factors (60,61).

Features of ICSI that Are Different from IVF and Fertilization In Vitro

The technique of ICSI bypasses many physiological barriers and/or processes that occur in IVF and natural insemination, for which sperm selection is an important process in fertilization. Only spermatozoa with progressive motility and generally normal morphology can penetrate a thick layer of cumulus cells and the zona pellucida. During this process, two major events—capacitation and the acrosome reaction—occur (62). Capacitation induces hyperactivity of the spermatozoon and, along with the release of an enzyme acrosin (acrosome reaction), that enables the spermatozoon to burrow through the zona pellucida to reach the oolemma (63,64). The spermatozoon aligns the equatorial region of its head with the oolemma so that both are in intimate contact with each other and fusion of their membranes follows (65). During sperm–oocyte fusion, an exchange of factors occurs: (*i*) the release of sperm cytosolic factors into the oocyte, which triggers a cascade of biochemical reactions characterized by Ca^{2+} oscillations and resulting in oocyte activation (54) and (*ii*) gradual entry of histones present in the ooplasm into the sperm head to replace protamines that eventually dissociate the disulphide bonds that are tightly bound to the sperm chromatin (48). Additionally, the spermatozoon introduces the centriole attached to its neck (66–69) that contributes to the first mitotic spindle of the fertilized zygote. Spermatozoon entry into the oocyte is completed by phagocytosis. Fertilization then culminates in the formation of a male and a female pronuclei within the oocyte with the extrusion of the second polar body.

In IVF and natural insemination, only spermatozoa that have undergone the acrosome reaction are capable of penetrating the zona pellucida and fusing with the oolemma (70,71). The events leading to fertilization differ in ICSI, from the IVF and natural insemination in that sperm capacitation and acrosome reaction are not essential. In ICSI, spermatozoa are exposed to a viscous medium containing 10% (v/v)

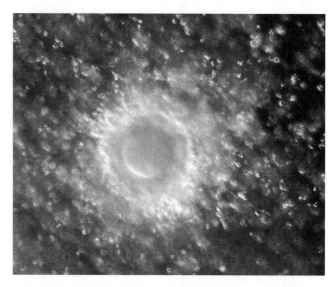

Figure 5 (*See color insert.*) An oocyte retrieved by ovum pick-up (OPU). The oocyte is surrounded by hundreds of nurturing cumulus cells that are removed by hyaluronidase to assess its maturity stage (germinal vesicle, metaphase I, or metaphase II) and for ICSI.

polyvinylpyrrolidone (PVP) to slow down their motility. A spermatozoon is selected by an embryologist on the basis of its motility and morphology. Then, immobilized by the crushing of its flagellum with a glass microinjection needle, aspirated into the needle and then finally injected into the ooplasm. Once the spermatozoon is deposited in the ooplasm, there is passive diffusion of sperm cytosolic factors from the site of the injured flagellum during the sperm nucleus swelling phase (72). These factors trigger a cascade of biochemical reactions that release intracellular Ca^{2+} from internal stores within the oocyte; these reactions are characterized by a series of Ca^{2+} oscillations (73). During this process, the oocyte is activated, pronuclear formation of the male and female gametes begins, and the extrusion of the second polar body follows (74,75).

Prior to the actual sperm injection, the oocyte is also handled in several steps. The freshly recovered oocyte surrounded by numerous cumulus cells (Fig. 5) is exposed in a medium containing hyaluronidase that facilitates the detachment of the cumulus cells from the zona pellucida. The oocyte is also manually handled with glass pipettes of variable sizes to hasten the process of denudation until an almost naked oocyte is obtained (Fig. 6).

During ICSI, the oocyte undergoes a series of unnatural events: the oocyte is penetrated by the microinjection needle, which causes a significant deformation resulting in a shape change from a sphere to a biconcave disk, and some of the ooplasm is aspirated into the microinjection needle to facilitate breakage of the oolemma. There is also regional homogenization of the ooplasm with the medium and PVP within the needle. The mixture, including the spermatozoon, is then deposited into the oocyte. The introduction of extracellular chemicals into the oocyte may alter the

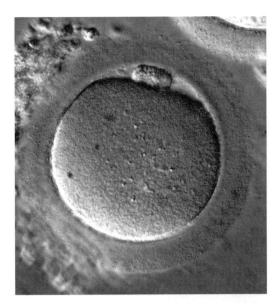

Figure 6 (*See color insert.*) Human oocyte. A mature oocyte at metaphase II stage, partially denuded of its cumulus cells.

intracellular pH and affect some physiological processes within the oocyte. The introduction of a spermatozoon that usually has not undergone an acrosome reaction further poses an additional burden to the oocyte. Nonetheless, the oocyte is able to neutralize the acrosomal enzymes, but their ultimate fates are still not established (76). The damage to the oolemma due to penetration by the microinjection needle also requires a period of healing for the membrane (75). These events do not happen in IVF or natural insemination where the entry of the spermatozoon into the oocyte is by sperm–oocyte fusion. Furthermore, only spermatozoa that have undergone acrosome reaction are capable of penetrating the zona pellucida and fusing with the oolemma (70,71). The stages of in vitro development of the human preimplantation embryos are shown in Figure 7. Assisted hatching of embryos is sometimes performed to improve implantation (Fig. 8).

Outcome of ICSI

Since the birth of the first ICSI baby in 1992, ICSI has become established as the most effective treatment for severe male-factor infertility. The use of ICSI has been extended to epididymal and testicular sperm and spermatids. The results from IVF centers vary with the level of competency of the embryologists. Nevertheless, the European Society of Human Reproduction and Embryology has established an ICSI Task Force to collect, annually, the clinical results obtained from participating IVF centers around the world, the outcome of pregnancy, and the follow-up of children conceived by ICSI. Tarlatzis and Bili (77) have reported results of one such survey collected from various IVF centers worldwide over a period of three years (1993–1995). During this period, the number of IVF centers performing ICSI increased from 35 to 101, and the total number of ICSI cycles performed per year increased from 3157

to 23,932. The incidence of damaged oocytes was low (<10%) and FRs obtained from ICSI with ejaculated, epididymal, and testicular sperm were 64%, 62.5%, and 52%, respectively. Consequently, about 90% of the couples had an embryo transfer resulting in viable pregnancy rates of 21% for ejaculated, 22% for epididymal, and 19% for testicular spermatozoa. Over 25% of these pregnancies, however, were mostly twin pregnancies. The etiology of azoospermia either obstructive (congenital or acquired) or nonobstrutive did not significantly influence the results of ICSI. In another survey, Nygren and Andersen (78) reviewed the results of IVF and ICSI from data collected from treatments initiated during 1997 in 18 European countries. ICSI and IVF shared similar clinical pregnancy rates per transfer and delivery rates per embryo transfer of 26% and 21%, respectively. Total multiple delivery rates for IVF and ICSI were 29.6% and 28.2%, respectively, with twin deliveries being the majority. It is noteworthy that the results thus far have indicated that both IVF and ICSI are effective in treating male-factor infertility, but IVF is limited by severe sperm parameters that can mostly be overcome by ICSI. As in other assisted reproductive techniques, the female age has an influential effect on the success rates of ICSI (79–86).

Loft et al. (87) reported a Danish national cohort study that included all clinical pregnancies with ICSI between January 1994 and July 1997 at five public and eight private fertility clinics. Laboratory and clinical data were obtained from the fertility clinics. Male-factor infertility was the main reason for performing ICSI in the majority of the couples who responded to a questionnaire on the pregnancy and health of the child. In this study, six cases with major chromosomal abnormalities (2.9%) were found in all interrupted or intra-uterine deaths with a gestational age <24 weeks, including triploidy, unbalanced t(17;22), trisomies 13, 18, and 21, and one case (0.5%) of inherited structural aberrations, t(9;22)pat. Minor birth defects such as congenital hip luxation, ranula, pilonidal cyst, short tongue frenulum, and syndactyly were found in nine children (1.2%). Unlike the results reported by Bonduelle et al. (88), there were no sex chromosome aberrations reported in this study.

In another report on children born after ICSI, Wennerholm et al. (89) reported the incidence of congenital malformations in a complete cohort of Swedish children. In this study, medical records were retrieved for 736 singletons, 200 sets of twins, and one set of triplets. A total of 87 infants (7.6%) had an identified congenital anomaly, including 40 infants with minor malformations. Based on the odds ratio (OR) analysis, the study found that for children born through ICSI, the increased rate of congenital malformations was mainly due to a high rate of multiple births. When delivery hospital, year of birth, and maternal age were matched, the OR for having a major or minor malformation was 1.75 [95% confidence interval (CI) 1.19–2.58]; the OR was reduced to

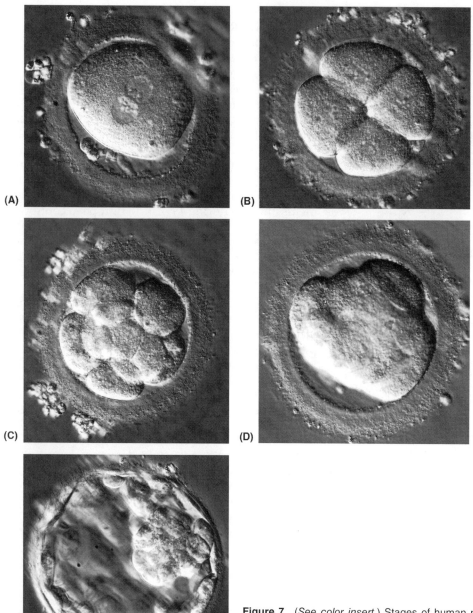

Figure 7 (*See color insert.*) Stages of human preimplantaton embryo development in vitro: (**A**) *Day 1*: A zygote (pronuclear stage). An oocyte fertilized by ICSI showing a male and a female pronuclei with the extrusion of the second polar body and the fragmented first polar body. (**B**) *Day 2*: A 4-cell embryo. (**C**) *Day 3*: An 8-cell embryo. (**D**) *Day 4*: A morula. (**E**) *Day 5*: A fully expanded blastocyst.

1.19 (95% CI 0.79–1.81) when adjustment was also done for singletons and twins. Interestingly, however, the study found that male children conceived by ICSI have a relative risk of acquiring hypospadia, which may be related to paternal subfertility (OR=3.0; 95% CI 1.09–6.50).

Aytoz et al. (90) investigated the obstetric outcome of pregnancies achieved after the transfer of cryopreserved or fresh embryos, in which the initial procedure was standard IVF and ICSI. The authors concluded that the cryopreservation process had no negative impact on the outcome of pregnancies over 20 weeks of gestation when the frequencies of preterm deliveries, infants with very low birthweight, intrauterine deaths, and major malformation rates were

compared between pregnancies resulting from transfer of fresh IVF and ICSI embryos and pregnancies resulting from the transfer of frozen IVF and ICSI embryos. The authors cautioned, however, that long-term follow-up studies are needed in order to prove the safety of the freezing–thawing process.

Should ICSI Be Done for All Cases?

ICSI has resulted in a dramatic improvement of FRs, especially in cases of severe oligoteratoasthenozoospermia; however, there have been contrasting reports on the implantation potential of ICSI-derived and IVF-derived embryos. Oehninger et al. (91) compared the implantation potential of embryos in patients with

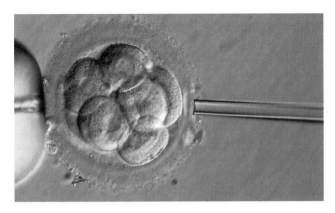

Figure 8 (*See color insert.*) Assisted hatching of an 8-cell human embryo. Acidic Tyrode medium is used to thin the zona pellucida to assist hatching and implantation.

severe teratozoospermia who were treated by either IVF with high insemination concentration (HIC) or ICSI. The authors found that IVF–HIC resulted in higher FRs than did ICSI, but a significantly higher proportion of good quality ICSI-derived embryos with a tendency toward a higher implantation potential were available for replacement. On the other hand, Hsu et al. (92) found that IVF-derived embryos had better cleavage rates and were morphologically superior to ICSI-derived embryos. Yet, the implantation potential of both IVF-derived and ICSI-derived embryos was similar when pregnancy and abortion rates were adjusted by age and number of embryos replaced. Recently, a few other studies have indicated that male factors can significantly influence embryo quality and implantation. Lundin et al. (93) found that abortion rates in ICSI from teratozoospermic patients were 31%, increasing to 67% when additional sperm factors were present. Furthermore, the development of embryos to blastocysts is compromised by unfavorable sperm morphology and motility (94). Defects in the sperm centrosome that result in numerical chromosomal abnormalities in embryos, loose packaging of sperm chromatin, and DNA strand breaks can also cause implantation failure (95–98) due to developmental arrest of the embryos.

A debate that still has no clear answer is whether ICSI should be performed for all cases of male-factor infertility. The success of conventional IVF is limited mainly by the quality of the spermatozoa (99,100), whereas sperm viability seems to be the limiting factor for ICSI (44). Fishel et al. (101) reported on different clinical scenarios of in vitro conception i.e., fertilization with conventional IVF, IVF–HIC, and ICSI among sibling oocytes. In their study, poor sperm factors and unexplained infertility did not have a negative impact on the outcome of ICSI with the partner's spermatozoa. In fact, the FR was found to be significantly higher in ICSI with partner's spermatozoa as compared with IVF or IVF with HIC with donor spermatozoa. Moreover, the study also found that ICSI improved the overall results of IVF in cases of oocytes that failed to

fertilize with conventional IVF in previous cycles. The overall conclusion reached by the authors was that ICSI as a first option offers a higher incidence of fertilization, maximizes the number of embryos, and minimizes the risk of complete failure of fertilization for all cases requiring in vitro conception. Concerns regarding the possible risks of transmission of genetic mutations (102–104) and the safety of the ICSI procedure (37,94), however, do not warrant the use of this procedure in the treatment of all cases of infertility.

Intracytoplasmic Injection of Immature Sperm Cells
Epididymal Sperm Injection

A great majority of mammalian spermatozoa attain their full fertilizing potential during their transit through the epididymis (105,106). Capacitation and acrosome reaction can only occur, however, when the spermatozoa leave the epididymis and reside in the female genital tract for some period of time (106,107). Successful pregnancies have been achieved when epididymal spermatozoa were artificially inseminated in a few mammalian species (108–114) including man (115). Epididymal spermatozoa were also capable of fertilizing oocytes (115–117), but pregnancy rates were significantly lower, particularly in human IVF (118) because of senescence and/or immaturity of the sperm (119) and the presence of sperm antibodies in men with obstructive azoospermia (120). In these cases, ICSI is the only effective treatment available at present for men with severe male-factor infertility.

There are two approaches to the surgical retrieval of epididymal sperm. These include microsurgical epididymal sperm aspiration (MESA) and percutaneous epididymal sperm aspiration (PESA). MESA is invasive and requires general anesthesia. The number of sperm retrieved is high so that cryopreservation is possible. PESA only requires local anesthesia, and cryopreservation is possible even though the yield of sperm may be lower (121). Although first pregnancies achieved through MESA–IVF have been described, initial attempts to perform IVF with epididymal sperm retrieved from men with obstructive azoospermia showed limited results owing to poor sperm quality after retrieval (115,117,122,123). Combining ICSI with epididymal sperm has improved fertilization and pregnancy rates to be equivalent to those achieved with ejaculated sperm (124–127). The ICSI procedure does not have stringent requirements for sperm quality in terms of sperm number, motility and morphology to achieve pregnancies. As long as the sperm is viable, fertilization and pregnancy can occur. Various studies have shown that there were no differences in the ICSI outcome when either fresh or frozen-thawed epididymal sperm were used (121,127–135). Sperm aspiration can be carried out at any given time to minimize the inconvenience associated with sperm retrieval performed concurrently with ovulation induction (129,136). Also, epididymal samples can be collected and frozen during a diagnostic procedure or during a vasectomy reversal operation (121).

Testicular Sperm Injection

Testicular sperm extraction (TESE) in combination with ICSI is a therapeutic technique for men with non-obstructive azoospermia since mature testicular spermatozoa could be found in these men (137–139), and successful pregnancies can be achieved (140). Surgical sperm recovery from men with nonobstructive azoospermia has become a routine part of clinical infertility treatment and as with the epididymis, cryopreservation of testicular spermatozoa has also become routine (141). Although global spermatogenic function is severely impaired, most of these azoospermic men have focal areas of spermatogenesis within the testes (142). TESE involves biopsy of the testis and allows isolation of spermatozoa from the focal areas of spermatogenesis for use with ICSI (143). Azoospermic men who have only minute foci of active spermatogenesis from which a very few number of spermatozoa can be extracted would require more testicular biopsies. Open biopsies, or biopsy gun samples, are preferred to fine needle aspiration in order to maximize the chances of finding these rare foci of active spermatogenesis. Multiple testicular biopsies, however, increase the risk of blood supply interruption (144), postsampling fibrosis or autoimmune response (145), and testicular atrophy (142).

Round Spermatid Injection and Elongating Spermatid Injection

In approximately 40% of azoospermic men with germinal failure, spermatozoa cannot be recovered, even if a few foci of complete spermatogenesis exist (146). Therefore, spermatids are the only germ cells that can be retrieved from a testicular biopsy or the ejaculate (147,148). The injection of round spermatid nuclei was first attempted in hamster and mouse oocytes (149,150), and subsequently resulted in the live birth in mice from round spermatid injection (ROSI) (151). Only four spermatid-derived live and apparently normal mice, however, were born after injections of 475 oocytes (<1% live birth rate). These preliminary results led other investigators to attempt spermatid injection in human oocytes; a late-stage spermatid was injected into an oocyte, which resulted in normal fertilization (152). Subsequently, the first human pregnancies from spermatid injection using round spermatids (Fig. 9) found in the spermatozoa-deficient ejaculate (153) and elongated spermatids (Fig. 10) from seminiferous tubules (154) were reported. Since then, successes with spermatid injections have been reported by a few Assisted Reproductive Technology (ART) clinics. The outcome of ROSI and elongating spermatid injection (ELSI) have been comprehensively reviewed by Aslam et al. (148). In 80 cycles performed by ROSI, 648 oocytes were injected, resulting in 203 fertilized oocytes (31.3%). Of these, 155 embryos were transferred

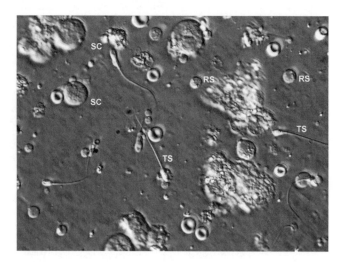

Figure 9 (*See color insert.*) A testicular biopsy specimen showing immature sperm (TS), round spermatids (RS) and spermatocytes (SC).

(76.3%), resulting in 10 clinical pregnancies and nine deliveries. Pregnancy rate per cycle and per embryo transfer were 12.5% and 13.3%, respectively, with an implantation rate of 6.5%. In ELSI, 55 cycles have been performed, from which 426 oocytes were injected, resulting in 245 fertilized oocytes (57.5%), 198 transferred embryos (80.8%), 12 clinical pregnancies, and 11 deliveries. Pregnancy rate per cycle and per embryo transfer were 21.8% each, with an implantation rate of 6.1%. Despite a high pregnancy rate with ELSI, ROSI and ELSI have low implantation rates per embryo as compared with IVF or ICSI (148). This could be attributed to poor embryo quality and slower cleavage rate, particularly in ROSI-derived embryos (155). In one study, blastocysts resulting from ROSI were of poor quality and spontaneous hatching was absent (156).

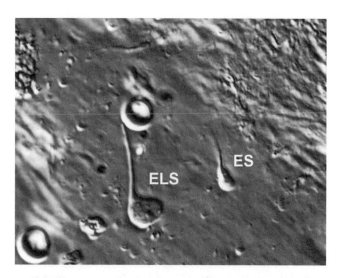

Figure 10 (*See color insert.*) A testicular biopsy specimen showing an elongating spermatid (ELS) and an elongated spermatid (ES).

The poor performance of ROSI could be improved when round spermatids were matured in vitro to elongated forms for microinjection (157).

In another recent study, Ghazzawi et al. (158) reported the injection of testicular round spermatids from patients with complete failure of spermiogenesis compared with that of mature epididymal and testicular spermatozoa. In this study, 180 azoospermic patients who had undergone a previous testicular biopsy were recruited into the ICSI program; 38 patients had pure obstructive azoospermia, while 142 patients had nonobstructive azoospermia. Mature spermatozoa were found in 93 patients, whereas spermatozoa were entirely absent, with a predominance of round spermatids, in 87 patients. In about 60% of the oocytes that were injected with round spermatids, the presence of two pronuclei stage was observed at 10 to 12 hours post-ICSI. By comparison, in oocytes that were injected with mature spermatozoa, the two pronuclei stage appeared at 16 hours post-ICSI. The authors also found that ROSI produced fewer zygotes that subsequently resulted in fewer embryos available for replacement. Owing to the less than desirable quality of the ROSI-derived embryos, no pregnancy could be achieved; however, 18 pregnancies were achieved from the injection of mature spermatozoa (pregnancy rate/cycle=20%). The authors concluded that ROSI from patients with complete failure of spermiogenesis resulted in a significantly lower FR and a higher developmental arrest compared with injection of mature spermatozoa. With no pregnancies achieved, the authors questioned the unusual variability of reported success rates and stressed the need for further research in order to improve the outcome of this novel technique.

Clinical pregnancies obtained from ROSI and ELSI, have been reported. These pregnancies resulted in the births of 8 and 12 healthy babies, respectively, after ROSI and ELSI (153,154,159–168). Subsequently, Zech et al. (169) reported that from four pregnancies obtained after injection of elongated spermatids, two cases of major malformation resulted. These were a male fetus with trisomy 9 (47,XY,+9) with hydrocephalus, spina bifida, and diaphragmatocele and a boy with open lumbosacral myelomeningocele (Arnold–Chiari Syndrome type II) that had not been detected during the pregnancy. Although the relationship between these anomalies and ICSI with spermatids could not be established, serious concerns regarding the safety of this procedure remain.

□ GENETIC MUTATIONS IN MALE-FACTOR INFERTILITY

The rapid advancement of molecular biology has provided evidence that many diseases have a genetic basis. Likewise, many causes of infertility have been linked to genetic defects. The risk of transmitting a genetic defect to an offspring would depend on the incidence and frequency of the mutation in a population.

Therefore, genetic abnormalities related to male infertility need to be considered in terms of being causative for male infertility and potentially transmissible to the offspring. A genetic evaluation on a male infertile patient is necessary so that information on the natural history, variation, and expression of a potential genetic defect can be obtained with the possibility of clarifying the pattern of inheritance.

Detections of chromosome aberrations or genetic mutations have been reported in a small proportion of infertile couples treated with ICSI (170–176). Not all of the genetic defects, however, can be detected with currently available techniques. Analysis of the recurrence pattern of infertility in infertile couples' families could define the importance of heritable factors in the pathogenesis of human infertility. Meschede et al. (177) subjected 621 consecutive infertile couples treated with ICSI to a comprehensive genetic workup, including documentation of the family history, karyotyping, and various DNA tests; 1302 fertile couples served as controls. In this study, 6.4% of the infertile couples were shown to have a fertility problem with a definite genetic basis. Further, male fertility problems displayed a distinct pattern of familial aggregation, and these, too, should be considered a potentially heritable condition. The authors conclude that the recurrence risk for infertility in the offspring of couples treated with ICSI could be substantial.

Cytogenetic investigations review that in oligozoospermic men with sperm counts below 10×10^6 spermatozoa/mL, the rate of chromosome aberrations is estimated to be 5% to 7%, with the percentage of cytogenically abnormal cases increasing up to 10% to 15% in azoospermic men (178). Sex chromosome aneuploidies are also frequently found. In a recent study to determine the type and frequency of chromosome aberrations in infertile couples undergoing ICSI because of severe male infertility or fertilization failures in previous IVF attempts, Peschka et al. (178) found that approximately 35% of the patients, including male and female partners, had chromosome abnormalities. Abnormal karyotypes were found in 13% of the patients, including chromosome aberrations in combinations of different types of abnormalities: constitutional aberrations (4.4%), fragile sites of autosomes (3.0%), low-level mosaicism of sex chromosomes (4.0%), and secondary structural chromosome aberrations (4.2%). Single cell aberrations were detected in another 22% of these patients, but the significance of these is not known. Interestingly, sex chromosomal abnormalities in the female partner were found to be exceptionally high, ranging from 6% to over 50% (172,174,178). This implies that in some cases of male-factor infertility, a hidden female chromosome factor may be present that cannot be identified by standard clinical evaluation. Therefore, chromosomal analysis and genetic counseling should be recommended to both partners prior to ICSI.

There are at least three nuclear DNA mutations that have an effect on spermatogenesis: mutations in the *androgen receptor* (*AR*) gene on the X chromosome, mutations in the *Azoospermia factor* (*AZF*) gene on the Y chromosome, and mutations in the *cystic fibrosis* (*CF*) gene on chromosome 7 in the presence of congenital bilateral absence of the vas deferens (CBAVD)—all have a significant effect on sperm production and fertility.

Androgen Receptor Gene Mutation

Androgens are essential for normal sperm production, and decreasing intratesticular androgens results in defective spermatogenesis (179). All androgens act through the AR that is encoded by a single copy gene located on the X chromosome and contains, in exon 1, a polymorphic glutamine (CAG) tract (180) that varies in length between individuals, with a normal range of 11 to 31 repeat units (181,182). Mutations in the *AR* gene are known to lead to androgen resistance or insensitivity that would compromise the process of spermatogenesis, resulting in azoospermia or severe oligospermia in men. Tut et al. (183) have shown that long polymorphic CAG tracts can increase the risk of defective spermatogenesis due to decreased transactivation capacity of the AR protein. In other words, infertile men with a CAG expansion of more than 28 in their AR would have a four-fold increased risk of defective spermatogenesis when compared to fertile controls. Approximately 25% of azoospermic men in fact have long CAG expansions of the *AR* gene, indicating a reduction in androgen sensitivity (184). Yet, most of the affected men have spermatozoa in their testes and many are able to have their genetic offspring with ICSI. Based on the Mendelian pattern of inheritance, the male offspring in the first generation would not be affected, but the AR mutation would be vertically transmitted to the female offspring. As carriers of the mutation, 50% of their sons would be expected to suffer from X-chromosomally determined infertility. Therefore, one could expect, over generations, a very slight increase in the frequency of male infertility.

Y Chromosome Microdeletions

There are a large number of genes on the Y chromosome that are known to play a role in male germ cell development. These genes are found within the *AZF* gene locus, which is located on the Yq11 region along the long arm (q) of the Y chromosome (185–192). Major deletions on the Yq can be detected in some azoospermic men in routine cytogenetic screening (193). About 10% of azoospermic men with unknown causes for their infertility will have microdeletions in the Y chromosome. These microdeletions can be detected by sequence-tagged sites (STSs) using the technique of polymerase chain reaction (PCR). Deletions of genes along Yq11 could result in complete lack of sperm cells or Sertoli-cell-only syndrome (SCOS), or oligospermia (189). In the case of the complete absence of sperm cells, ICSI is not possible. On the other hand, when sperm cells are available either in the ejaculate or in the testes, it is possible to perform ICSI. In this case, all the sons of these patients would be expected to have defective spermatogenesis. Therefore, the importance of microdeletions on Yq11 for male infertility, with respect to ICSI, depends on how often such microdeletions are found in patients with either severe oligospermia or azoospermia. The incidence of microdeletions is two times higher in azoospermic than severely oligospermic men (194). It is possible, with the availability of the STS–PCR technique, to analyze for the presence of microdeletions, and thus inform potential ICSI couples about possible infertility in a future male child. It is important to note that men with *AZF* microdeletions in Yq11 are perfectly healthy, despite having fertility disorders. Therefore, these couples should not be denied the conception of a child by ICSI. Their healthy sons can themselves fulfill a possible desire for children through the use of ICSI. Any daughters, and their children, would be expected to be fertile. Although there is a cause-and-effect relationship between microdeletions and male infertility, the precise role of these microdeletions in male infertility is still not absolutely clear (195).

Cystic Fibrosis

CF is a fatal autosomal recessive disorder that mainly manifests as a dysfunction of the pancreas and results in an increased propensity to respiratory tract infections. From a molecular point of view, the disease is caused by mutations in the structure of the *cystic fibrosis transmembrane conductance regulator* (*CFTR*) gene (196–198) and is mapped to the long arm of chromosome 7 (7q31.2) (196,197). As the name implies, the *CFTR* gene codes for a protein that functions as a transmembrane channel for chloride ions (199). This protein is present at high levels in the apical membranes of various epithelial cells within the organs commonly affected by CF. Typical CF is one of the most common diseases of Caucasians, affecting approximately 1 in 2500 newborns (200); 1 in 25 are carriers of gene mutations involving the *CFTR* gene (201). Atypical CF is often expressed as monosymptomatic forms of the disease and has underlying molecular pathology. There are at least 800 different mutations and 70 DNA sequence variants have been identified in the *CFTR* gene (202).

Perhaps the most frequent atypical form of CF is CBAVD, affecting about 25% of male patients with obstructive azoospermia (203) and 2% of all male patients (204). There is a very strong association between CF and CBAVD since CBAVD is found in a large cohort of men with mutations in the *CFTR* gene (205–214). It is estimated that the frequency of mutated *CFTR* genes in men with infertility due to CBAVD is twenty times higher than the carrier frequency detected in the general population (203). The malformation of the vas deferens is caused by a complex interplay between different mutations and/or intronic polymorphisms in the *CFTR* gene. The most common mutations found among the CBAVD patients are: ΔF508, R117H, R1070W, and

IVS8-5T. Mutations in the *CFTR* gene result in absent or severe reduction in the activity of CFTR protein in these men, causing an imbalance in ionic exchange and fluid content within the lumen of the epididymis. Consequently, the unfavorable environment can cause further reduction in CFTR activity, leading to a progressive sloughing of the epithelial lining of the lumen of the epididymis and vas deferens. This, in turn, leads to impediment of sperm passage from the testis or epididymis to the outer genital tract (215). *CFTR* gene mutations are the molecular cause for a variety of different forms of male infertility due to obstructive azoospermia, ranging from CBVAD to isolated abnormalities of epididymides or ejaculatory ducts (210,211). CBAVD is mostly but not always, caused by *CFTR* gene mutations (207); however, it has been found that *CFTR* gene mutations do not play a significant role in primary spermatogenic failure (207,210,216–218). Testicular biopsies of men with CF have shown hypospermatogenesis and highly abnormal spermatozoa (219–223). On the other hand, testicular histological findings in men with CBAVD showed completely normal spermatogenesis (224,225). Instead, the spermatogenic failure in men with CF may be the result of malnutrition (219), but a minor pathological effect on spermatogenesis or sperm maturation is still possible (205,226). Clinically, azoospermia, reduced sperm volume with abnormal sperm forms, increased acidity in semen, and absent or low concentrations of fructose in the ejaculate are some of the abnormal semen parameters identified in men with CF (219,220,222,226,227). In addition to these parameters, aplasia, hypoplasia or cystic dilatation, and the absence of the ejaculatory ducts are commonly found in the CF men (228).

Male infertility due to CBAVD can be treated with microsurgical epididymal sperm aspiration (MESA), testicular sperm aspiration (TESA), or testicular sperm extraction (TESE) and subsequent ICSI (124). Men who are affected by CBAVD, but not by CF, have a high penetrance (60%) of heterozygous mutations in the *CFTR* gene (206). Therefore, every couple in which the man suffers from CF-related infertility should undergo genetic counseling and both partners should be tested for the presence of mutations in the *CFTR* gene prior to ICSI. The couples should be made aware of the specific risk of CF in their offspring and the possibility of prenatal diagnosis and informed of the clinical symptoms and the risks of the different forms of CF due to *CFTR* gene mutations. Women with CF have a reduced fertility due to a retarded menarche.

Training for ICSI

The mastery of micromanipulation techniques requires a long learning curve. One of the significant challenges in ART is the achievement of technical proficiency in micromanipulation without an initial phase of low success rates. Usually, fertilization rates for "beginners" range from 30% to 40%, and oocyte damage rates can be as high as 20% to 30%. Gvakharia et al. (229) have established a standardized protocol for an experimental ICSI model using hamster oocytes and human sperm on the basis of the authors' experience with the optimized sperm penetration assay (SPA) and micro-SPA (230).

☐ CONCLUSION

The last two decades have brought rapid advancement in the understanding of mammalian embryology and the development of assisted reproductive techniques to alleviate the problems of human infertility. During this period, there has been much improvement in the set-up of the IVF laboratory to include the cryopreservation of oocytes and embryos, ICSI, and preimplantation genetic diagnostic capabilities. The skill of the laboratory personnel has been constantly upgraded through workshops and access to almost instant knowledge via the Internet. The introduction of ICSI into the IVF program has revolutionized the treatment of male-factor–related infertility. Since pregnancies can be achieved even with round and elongated spermatids, the approach to the treatment of male infertility should bear further improvement in the future. A male patient who seeks treatment for his predicament should not be viewed as infertile unless he suffers from severe hypospermatogenesis, such as SCOS.

The direct injection of sperm into the oocyte to treat severe male infertility bypasses critical physiological events of sperm selection leading to fertilization such as acrosome reaction, sperm binding to the zona pellucida, and sperm–egg membrane fusion. Moreover, immature spermatozoa are frequently used to achieve fertilization and pregnancy. ICSI was introduced for clinical therapy in ARTs without going through a carefully controlled series of experiments in animal models. Since ICSI has become the treatment of choice in most IVF laboratories and human infertility is often related to chromosome abnormalities or genetic mutations, many investigators have raised their concern about the potential risk of transmitting these defects to future generations. Several retrospective studies on ICSI in ART have reported no increase in the risk of major or minor congenital malformations, but a slight increase in sex chromosomal aberrations (77,231,232). Minor and major congenital malformations have been found in children conceived by ICSI with epididymal and testicular sperm and spermatids (233,234). Recently, there is direct evidence of a higher incidence of numerical chromosome abnormalities in sperm-fertilized human oocytes after ICSI (235). Moreover, transmission of genetic mutations to the offspring by ICSI has been reported (102–104). These studies were unable to conclude decisively, however, that there are no long-lasting and unanticipated consequences of ART using ICSI. There is therefore an urgent need to undertake clinically relevant research to resolve several questions on the cellular and molecular aspects of fertilization effected by ICSI. The mouse has been used extensively as a mammalian model system to investigate fertilization processes and embryonic development and implantation; however, the fertilization process in the mouse is fundamentally different from that in the human, in that maternal centrosome in the mouse oocyte has a significant role in fertilization (236–238); in humans and other primates, the sperm centrosome plays a major role in the fertilization process (66–69,239). Although the mouse model has contributed extensively to the understanding of basic mammalian fertilization processes, nonhuman primates would provide a more ideal research model (240).

□ REFERENCES

1. Cohen J, Malter H, Fehilly C, et al. Implantation of embryos after partial opening of oocyte zona pellucida to facilitate sperm penetration. Lancet 1988; 2(8603):162.

2. Ng SC, Bongso A, Ratnam SS, et al. Pregnancy after transfer of sperm under zona. Lancet 1988; 2(8614):790.

3. Palermo G, Joris H, Devroey P, et al. Pregnancies after intracytoplasmic injection of single spermatozoon into an oocyte. Lancet 1992; 340(8810):17–18.

4. Schmidt HD. On the minute structure of the hepatic lobules, particularly with reference to the relationship between the capillary blood vessels, the hepatic cells and the canals which carry off the secretions of the latter. Am J Med Sci 1859; 37:13–40.

5. Chabry L. Contribution a l'embryologie normal et teratologique des ascidies simples. J Anat Physiol (Paris) 1887; 23:167.

6. Nicholas JS, Hall BV. Experiments on developing rats. II. The development of isolated blastomeres and fused eggs. J Exp Zool 1942; 90:441–458.

7. Duryee WR. Microdissection studies on human ovarian eggs. Trans NY Acad Sci 1954; 17(2):103–108.

8. Tarkowski AK. Experimental studies on regulation in the development of isolated blastomeres of mouse eggs. Acta Theriologica 1959; 3:191–267.

9. Seidel F. Die Entwicklungsfahigkeiten isolierter Furchungszellen aus den Ei des kaninchens oryctolagus ciniculus. Arch Entwicklungsmech 1960; 152:33–37.

10. Lin TP. Microinjection of mouse eggs. Science 1966; 151(3708):333–337.

11. Lin TP. Micropipetting cytoplasm from the mouse egg. Nature 1967; 216(111):162–163.

12. Bertrand E, Van den Bergh M, Englert Y. Does zona pellucida thickness influence the fertilization rate? Hum Reprod 1995; 10(5):1189–1193.

13. Gordon JW, Talansky BE. Assisted fertilization by zona drilling: a mouse model for correction of oligospermia. J Exp Zool 1986; 239(3):347–354.

14. Gordon JW, Grunfeld L, Garrisi GJ, et al. Fertilization of human oocytes by sperm from infertile males after zona pellucida drilling. Fertil Steril 1988; 50(1):68–73.

15. Ng SC, Bongso A, Chang SI, et al. Transfer of human sperm into the perivitelline space of human oocytes after zona-drilling or zona-puncture. Fertil Steril 1989; 52(1):73–78.

16. Payne D, McLaughlin KJ, Depypere HT, et al. Experience with zona drilling and zona cutting to improve fertilization rates of human oocytes in vitro. Hum Reprod 1991; 6(3):423–431.

17. Jean M, Barriere P, Sagot P, et al. Utility of zona pellucida in cases of severe semen alterations in man. Fertil Steril 1992; 57(3):591–596.

18. Santella L, Alikani M, Talansky BE, et al. Is the human oocyte plasma membrane polarized? Hum Reprod 1992; 7(7):999–1003.

19. Depypere HT, Leybaert L. Intracellular pH changes during zona drilling. Fertil Steril 1994; 61(2):319–323.

20. Cohen J, Malter H, Wright G, et al. Partial zona dissection of human oocytes when failure of zona pellucida penetration is anticipated. Hum Reprod 1989; 4(4):435–442.

21. Calderon G, Veiga A, Penella J, et al. Two years of assisted fertilization by partial zona dissection in male factor infertility patients. Fertil Steril 1993; 60(1):105–109.

22. Levron J, Stein DW, Brandes JM, et al. Presence of sperm in the perivitelline space predicts fertilization rate after partial zona dissection. Fertil Steril 1993; 59(4):820–825.

23. Vanderzwalmen P, Barlow P, Nijs M, et al. Usefulness of partial dissection of the zona pellucida in a human in-vitro fertilization programme. Hum Reprod 1992; 7(4):537–544.

24. Tucker MJ, Bishop FM, Cohen J, et al. Routine application of partial zona dissection for male factor infertility. Hum Reprod 1991; 6(5):676–681.

25. Strehler E, Sterzik K, De Santo M, et al. Submicroscopic mathematical evaluation of spermatozoa in assisted reproduction. 3. Partial zona dissection (PZD) (Notulae seminologicae 12). J Submicrosc Cytol Pathol 1997; 29(3):387–391.

26. Alikani M, Noyes N, Cohen J, et al. Monozygotic twinning in the human is associated with the zona pellucida architecture. Hum Reprod 1994; 9(7):1318–1321.

27. Cohen J, Feldberg D. Effects of the size and number of zona pellucida openings on hatching and trophoblast outgrowth in the mouse embryo. Mol Reprod Dev 1991; 30(1):70–78.

28. Malter HE, Cohen J, Alikani M, et al. Microsurgical fertilization and zona pellucida micro-manipulation. In: Fishel S, Symonds M, eds. Gamete and Embryo

Micromanipulation in Human Reproduction. London: Edward Arnold, 1993:101.

29. Feichtinger W, Strohmer H, Fuhrberg P, et al. Photoablation of oocyte zona pellucida by erbium-YAG laser for in vitro fertilization in severe male infertility. Lancet 1992; 339(8796):811.

30. Antinori S, Versaci C, Fuhrberg P, et al. Seventeen live births after the use of an erbium-yytrium aluminum garnet laser in the treatment of male factor infertility. Hum Reprod 1994; 9(10):1891–1896.

31. Simon A, Palanker D, Harpaz-Eisenberg V, et al. Interaction between human sperm cells and hamster oocytes after argon fluoride excimer laser drilling of the zona pellucida. Fertil Steril 1993; 60(1):159–164.

32. Metka M, Haromy T, Huber J. Micromanipulatory sperm injection – a new method in the treatment of infertile males. Wien Med Wochenschr 1985; 135(3):55–59.

33. Mann J. Full term development of mouse eggs fertilized by a spermatozoon microinjected under the zona pellucida. Biol Reprod 1988; 38(5):1077–1083.

34. Wolf JP, Ducot B, Aymar C, et al. Absence of block to polyspermy at the human oolemma. Fertil Steril 1997; 67(6):1095–1102.

35. Tarin JJ. Subzonal insemination, partial zona dissection or intracytoplasmic sperm injection? An easy decision? Hum Reprod 1995; 10(1):165–170.

36. Griffiths TA, Murdoch AP, Herbert M. Embryonic development in vitro is compromised by the ICSI procedure. Hum Reprod 2000; 15(7):1592–1596.

37. Westphal LM, Hinckley MD, Pehr B, et al. Effect of ICSI on subsequent blastocyst development and pregnancy rates. J Assist Reprod Genet 2003; 20(3):113–116.

38. Van Landuyt L, De Vos A, Joris H, et al. Blastocyst formation in in vitro fertilization versus intracytoplasmic sperm injection cycles: influence of the fertilization procedure. Fertil Steril 2005; 83(5):1397–1403.

39. Van de Velde H, De Vos A, Joris H, et al. Effect of timing of oocyte denudation and micro-injection on survival, fertilization and embryo quality after intracytoplasmic sperm injection. Hum Reprod 1998; 13(11):3160–3164.

40. Yanagida K, Yazawa H, Katayose H, et al. Influence of oocyte preincubation time on fertilization after intracytoplasmic sperm injection. Hum Reprod 1998; 13(8):2223–2226.

41. Nagy Z, Liu J, Joris H, et al. The influence of the site of sperm deposition and mode of oolemma breakage at intracytoplasmic sperm injection on fertilization and embryo development rates. Hum Reprod 1995; 10(12):3171–3177.

42. Dozortsev D, Rybouchkin A, de Sutter P, et al. Sperm plasma membrane damage prior to intracytoplasmic sperm injection: a necessary condition for sperm nucleus decondensation. Hum Reprod 1995; 10(11):2960–2964.

43. Palermo GD, Alikani M, Bertoli M, et al. Oolemma characteristics in relation to survival and fertilization patterns of oocytes treated by intracytoplasmic sperm injection. Hum Reprod 1996; 11(1):172–176.

44. Vanderzwalmen P, Bertin G, Lejeune B, et al. Two essential steps for a successful intracytoplasmic sperm injection: injection of immobilized spermatozoa after rupture of the oolema. Hum Reprod 1996; 11(3): 540–547.

45. Joris H, Nagy Z, Van de Velde H, et al. Intracytoplasmic sperm injection: laboratory set-up and injection procedure. Hum Reprod 1998; 13(suppl 1):76–86.

46. Carrillo AJ, Atiee SH, Lane B, et al. Oolemma rupture inside the intracytoplasmic sperm injection needle significantly improves the fertilization rate and reduces oocyte damage. Fertil Steril 1998; 70(4): 676–679.

47. Tesarik J, Kopecny V. Developmental control of the human male pronucleus by ooplasmic factors. Hum Reprod 1989; 4(8):962–968.

48. Montag M, Tok V, Liow SL, et al. In vitro decondensation of mammalian sperm and subsequent formation of pronuclei-like structures for micromanipulation. Mol Reprod Dev 1992; 33(3):338–346.

49. Tesarik J, Sousa M, Testart J. Human oocyte activation after intracytoplasmic sperm injection. Hum Reprod 1994; 9(5):511–518.

50. Tesarik J. Oocyte activation after intracytoplasmic injection of mature and immature sperm cells. Hum Reprod 1998; 13(suppl 1):117–127.

51. Fishel S, Lisi F, Rinaldi L, et al. Systematic examination of immobilizing spermatozoa before intracytoplasmic sperm injection in the human. Hum Reprod 1995; 10(3): 497–500.

52. Van den Bergh A, Bertrand E, Biramane J, et al. Importance of breaking a spermatozoon's tail before intracytoplasmic injection: a prospective randomized trial. Hum Reprod 1995; 10:2819–2820.

53. Yanagida K, Katayose H, Hirata S, et al. Influence of sperm immobilization on onset of Ca2+ oscillations after ICSI. Hum Reprod 2001; 16(1):148–152.

54. Homa ST, Swann K. A cytosolic sperm factor triggers calcium oscillations and membrane hyperpolarizations in human oocytes. Hum Reprod 1994; 9(12): 2356–2361.

55. Dale B, Marino M, Wilding M. Sperm–induced calcium oscillations. Soluble factor, factors or receptors? Mol Hum Reprod 1999; 5(1):1–4.

56. Stice SL, Robl JM. Activation of mammalian oocytes by a factor obtained from rabbit sperm. Mol Reprod Dev 1990; 25(3):272–280.

57. Swann K. A cytosolic sperm factor stimulates repetitive calcium increases and mimics fertilization in hamster oocytes. Development 1990; 110(4):1295–1302.

58. Swann K, Lawrence Y. How and why spermatozoa cause calcium oscillations in mammalian oocytes. Mol Hum Reprod 1996; 2(6):388–390.

59. Palermo GD, Avrech OM, Colombero LT, et al. Human sperm cytosolic factor triggers Ca2+ oscillations and overcomes activation failure of mammalian oocytes. Mol Hum Reprod 1997; 3(4):367–374.

60. Perry AC, Wakayama T, Yanagimachi R. A novel trans-complementation assay suggests full mammalian oocyte activation is coordinately initiated by multiple, submembrane sperm components. Biol Reprod 1999; 60(3):747–755.

61. Perry AC, Wakayama T, Cooke IM, et al. Mammalian oocyte activation by the synergistic action of discrete sperm head components: induction of calcium transients and involvement of proteolysis. Dev Biol 2000; 217(2):386–393.

62. Fraser LR. Sperm capacitation and the acrosome reaction. Hum Reprod 1998; 13(suppl 1):9–19.

63. Chen C, Sathananthan AH. Early penetration of human sperm through the vestments of human eggs in vitro. Arch Androl 1986; 16(3):183–197.

64. Zaneveld LJ, De Jonge CJ, Anderson RA, et al. Human sperm capacitation and the acrosome reaction. Hum Reprod 1991; 6(9):1265–1274.

65. Tsuiki A, Hoshiai H, Takahashi K, et al. Sperm-egg interactions observed by scanning electron microscopy. Arch Androl 1986; 16(1):35–47.

66. Sathananthan AH, Kola I, Osborne J, et al. Centrioles in the beginning of human development. Proc Natl Acad Sci USA 1991; 88(11):4806–4810.

67. Palermo G, Munne S, Cohen J. The human zygote inherits its mitotic potential from the gamete. Hum Reprod 1994; 9(7):1220–1225.

68. Simerly C, Wu GJ, Zoran S, et al. The paternal inheritance of the centrosome, the cell's microtubule-organizing center, in humans, and the implications for infertility. Nature Med 1995; 1(1):47–52.

69. Sathananthan AH, Ratnam SS, Ng SC, et al. The sperm centriole: its inheritance, replication and perpetuation in early human embryos. Hum Reprod 1996; 11(2):345–356.

70. Takano H, Yanagimachi R, Urch UA. Evidence that acrosin activity is important for the development of fusibility of mammalian spermatozoa with the oolemma: inhibitor studies using the golden hamster. Zygote 1993; 1(1):79–91.

71. Bronson RA, Bronson SK, Oula L, et al. An investigation of the latency period between sperm oolemmal adhesion and oocyte penetration. Mol Reprod Dev 1999; 52(3):319–327.

72. Dozortsev D, Qian C, Ermilov A, et al. Sperm-associated oocyte-activating factor is released from the spermatozoon within 30 minutes after injection as a result of the sperm-oocyte interaction. Hum Reprod 1997; 12(12):2792–2796.

73. Parrington J, Lai FA, Swann K. A novel protein for Ca2+ signalling at fertilization. Cur Top Dev Biol 1998; 39:215–243.

74. Payne D, Flaherty SP, Barry MF, et al. Preliminary observations on polar body extrusion and pronuclear formation in human oocytes using time-lapse video cinematography. Hum Reprod 1997; 12(3): 532–541.

75. Bourgain C, Nagy ZP, De Zutter H, et al. Ultrastructure of gametes after intracytoplasmic sperm injection. Hum Reprod 1998; 13(suppl 1):107–116.

76. Sathananthan AH, Szell A, Ng SC, et al. Is the acrosome reaction a prerequisite for sperm incorporation after intra-cytoplasmic sperm injection (ICSI)? Reprod Fertil Dev 1997; 9(7):703–709.

77. Tarlatzis BC, Bili H. Survey on intracytoplasmic sperm injection: report from the ESHRE ICSI Task Force. Hum Reprod 1998; 13(suppl 1): 165–177.

78. Nygren KG, Andersen AN. Assisted reproductive technology in Europe, 1997. Results generated from European registers by ESHRE. Hum Reprod 2001; 16(2):384–391.

79. Silber SJ, Nagy Z, Devroey P, et al. The effect of female age and ovarian reserve on pregnancy rate in male infertility: treatment of azoospermia with sperm retrieval and intracytoplasmic sperm injection. Hum Reprod 1997; 12(12):2693–2700.

80. Moon SY, Kim SH, Jung BJ, et al. Influence of female age on pregnancy outcome in in vitro fertilizaton and embryo transfer patients undergoing intracytoplasmic sperm injection. J Obstet Gynaecol Res 2000; 26(1): 49–54.

81. Abdelmassih R, Sollia S, Moretto M, et al. Female age is important parameter to predict treatment outcome in intracytoplasmic sperm injection. Fertil Steril 1996; 65(3):573–577.

82. Bar-Hava I, Orvieto R, Ferber A, et al. Standard in vitro fertilization or intracytoplasmic sperm injection in advanced female age – what may be expected? Gynaecol Endocrinol 1999; 13(2):93–97.

83. Sherins RJ, Thorsell LP, Dorfmann A, et al. Intracytoplasmic sperm injection facilitates fertilization even in the most severe forms of male infertility: pregnancy outcome correlates with maternal age and number of eggs available. Fertil Steril 1995; 64(2):369–375.

84. Szamatowicz M, Grochowski D. Fertility and infertility in aging women. Gynaecol Endorinol 1998; 12(6): 407–413.

85. Osmanagaoglu K, Tournaye H, Camus M, et al. Cumulative delivery rates after intracytoplasmic sperm injection: 5 year follow-up of 498 patients. Hum Reprod 1999; 14(10):2651–2655.

86. Ron-El R, Raziel A, Strassburger D, et al. Outcome of assisted reproductive technology in women over the age of 41. Fertil Steril 2000; 74(3):471–475.

87. Loft A, Petersen K, Erb K, et al. A Danish national cohort of 730 infants born after intracytoplasmic sperm injection (ICSI) 1994–1997. Hum Reprod 1999; 14(8): 2143–2148.

88. Bonduelle M, Wilikens A, Buysse A, et al. A follow-up study of children born after intracytoplasmic sperm injection (ICSI) with epididymal and testicular spermatozoa and after replacement of cryopreserved embryos obtained after ICSI. Hum Reprod 1998; 13(suppl 1):196–207.

89. Wennerholm UB, Bergh C, Hamberger L, et al. Incidence of congenital malformations in children born after ICSI. Hum Reprod 2000; 15(4):944–948.

90. Aytoz A, Van den Abbeel E, Bonduelle M, et al. Obstetric outcome of pregnancies after the transfer of cryopreserved and fresh embryos obtained by conventional in-vitro fertilization and intracytoplasmic sperm injection. Hum Reprod 1999; 14(10):2619–2624.

91. Oehninger S, Kruger TF, Smith T, et al. A comparative analysis of embryo implantation potential in patients with severre teratozoospermia undergoing in-vitro fertilization with a high insemination concentration or intracytoplasmic sperm injection. Hum Reprod 1996; 11(5):1086–1089.

92. Hsu MI, Mayer J, Aronshon M, et al. Embryo implantation in in vitro fertilization and intracytoplasmic sperm injection: impact of cleavage status, morpholohy grade, and number of embryos transferred. Fertil Steril 1999; 72(4):679–685.

93. Lundin K, Soderlund B, Hamberger L. The relationship between sperm morphology and rates of fertilization, pregnancy and spontaneous abortion in an in vitro fertilization/intracytoplasmic sperm injection programme. Hum Reprod 1997; 12(12):2676–2681.

94. Miller JE, Smith TT. The effect of intracytoplasmic sperm injection and semen parameters on blastocyst development in vitro. Hum Reprod 2001; 16(5): 918–924.

95. Evenson DP, Darzynkiewicz Z, Melamed MR. Relation of mammalian sperm chromatin heterogeneity to fertility. Science 1980; 210(4474):1131–1133.

96. Foresta C, Zorzi M, Rossato M, et al. Sperm nuclear instability and staining with aniline blue; abnormal persistence of histones in spermatozoa in infertile men. Int J Androl 1992; 15(4):330–337.

97. Sailer BL, Jost LK, Evenson DP. Mammalian sperm DNA susceptibility to in situ denaturation associated with the presence of DNA strand breaks as measured by the terminal deoxynucleotidyl transferase assay. J Androl 1995; 16(1):80–87.

98. Obasaju M, Kadam A, Sultan K, et al. Sperm quality may adversely affect the chromosome constitution of embryos that result from intracytoplasmic sperm injection. Fertil Steril 1999; 72(6):1113–1115.

99. Oehninger S, Acosta AA, Morshedi M, et al. Corrective measures and pregnancy outcome in in vitro fertilization in patients with severe sperm morphology abnormalities. Fertil Steril 1988; 50(2):283–287.

100. Donnelly ET, Lewis SE, McNally JA, et al. In vitro fertilization and pregnancy rates: the influence of psperm motility and morphology on IVF outcome. Fertil Steril 1998; 70(2):305–314.

101. Fishel S, Aslam I, Lisi F, et al. Should ICSI be the treatment of choice for all cases of in-vitro conception? Hum Reprod 2000; 15(6):1278–1283.

102. Kent-First MG, Kol S, Muallem A, et al. The incidence and possible relevance of Y-linked microdeletions in babies born after intracytoplasmic sperm injection and their infertile fathers. Mol Hum Reprod 1996; 2(12): 943–950.

103. Jiang MC, Lien YR, Chen SU, et al. Transmission of de novo mutations of the deleted in azoospermia genes from a severely oligozoospermic male to a son via intracytoplasmic sperm injection. Fertil Steril 1999; 71(6):1029–1032.

104. Cram DS, Ma K, Bhasin S, et al. Y chromosome analysis of infertile men and their sons conceived through intracytoplasmic sperm injection: vertical transmission of deletions and rarity of de novo deletions. Fertil Steril 2000; 74(5):909–915.

105. Cooper TG. Maturation of spermatozoa in the eepididymis. In: Cooper TG, ed. The Epididymis, Sperm Maturation and Fertilization. New York: Springer-Verlag, 1986:1–8.

106. Amann RP, Hammerstedt RH, Veeramachaneni DNR. The epididymis and sperm maturation: a perspective. Reprod Fertil Dev 1993; 5(4):361–381.

107. Yanagimachi R. Fertilization mechanisms in man and other mammals. In: Tesarik J, ed. Frontiers in endocrinology. Male factor in human infertility. Ares-Serono Symposia, 1994:15–43.

108. Blash S, Melican D, Gavin W. Cryopreservation of epididymal sperm obtained at necropsy from goats. Theriogenology 2000; 54(6):899–905.

109. Fournier-Delpech S, Colas G, Courot M, et al. Epididymal sperm maturation in the ram: motility, fertilizing ability and embryonic survival after uterine insemination in the ewe. Ann Biol Anim Biochem Biophys 1979; 19:597–605.

110. Holtz W, Smidt D. The fertilizing capacity of epididymal spermatozoa in the pig. J Reprod Fert 1976; 46(1):227–229.

111. Morrell JM, Nowshari M, Rosenbusch J, et al. Birth of offspring following artificial insemination in the common marmoset, Callithrix jacchus. Am J Primatol 1997; 41(1):37–43.

112. Paufler SK, Foote RH. Morphology, motility and fertility of spermatozoa recovered from different areas of ligated rabbit epididymides. J Reprod Fert 1968; 17(1): 125–137.

113. Paz (Frenkel) G, Kaplan R, Yedwab G, et al. The effect of caffeine on rat epididymal spermatozoa: motility, metabolism and fertilizing capacity. Int J Androl 1978; 1:145–152.

114. Williamson BR, Shepherd BA, Martan J. Fertility of spermatozoa from the excurrent ducts of the guinea pig. J Reprod Fert 1980; 59(2):515–517.

115. Silber SJ, Ord T, Balmaceda J, et al. Congenital absence of the vas deferens. The fertilizing capacity of the epididymal sperm. N Engl J Med 1990; 323(26): 1788–1792.

116. Sankai T, Terao K, Yanagimachi R, et al. Cryopreservation of spermatozoa from cynomolgus monkeys (Macaca fascicularis). J Reprod Fertil 1994; 101(2):273–278.

117. Temple-Smith PD, Southwick GJ, Yates CA, et al. Human pregnancy by in vitro fertilization (IVF) using sperm aspirated from the epididymis. J In Vitro Fertil Embryo Transfer 1985; 2(3):119.

118. Hirsh AV, Mills C, Bekir J, et al. Factors influencing the outcome of in-vitro fertilization with epididymal spermatozoa in irreversible obstructive azoospermia. Hum Reprod 1994; 9(9):1710–1716.

119. Silber SJ. The use of epididymal sperm for the treatment of male infertility. Baillieres Clin Obstet Gynaecol 1997; 11(4):739–752.

120. de Kretser DM, Huidobro C, Southwick GJ, et al. The role of the epididymis in human infertility. J Reprod Fertil Suppl 1998; 53:271–275.

121. Patrizio P. Cryopreservation of epididymal sperm. Mol Cell Endocrin 2000; 169(1):11–14.

122. Pryor J, Parson J, Goswamy R. In vitro fertilisation for men with obstructive azoospermia. Lancet 1984; 2(8405):762.

123. Bladou F, Grillo JM, Rossi D, et al. Epididymal sperm aspiration in conjunction with in vitro fertilization and embryo transfer in cases with obstructive azoospermia. Hum Reprod 1991; 6(9):1284–1287.

124. Silber SJ, Nagy ZP, Liu J, et al. Conventional in vitro fertilization versus intracytoplasmic sperm injection for patients requiring microsurgical sperm aspiration. Hum Reprod 1994; 9(9):1705–1709.

125. Tournaye H, Devroey P, Liu J, et al. Microsurgical epididymal sperm aspiration and ICSI: a new effective approach to infertility as a result of congenital bilateral absence of the vas deferens. Fertil Steril 1994; 61(6):1045–1051.

126. Tsirigotis M, Pelekanos M, Beski S, et al. Cumulative experience of percutaneous epididymal sperm aspiration (PESA) with intracytoplasmic sperm injection. J Assist Reprod Genet 1996; 13(4):315–319.

127. Cha KY, Oum KB, Kim HJ. Approaches for obtaining sperm in patients with male factor infertility. Fertil Steril 1997; 67(6):985–995.

128. Nagy Z, Liu J, Cecile J, et al. Using ejaculated, fresh, and frozen-thawed epididymal and testicular spermatozoa gives rise to comparable results after intracytoplasmic sperm injection. Fertil Steril 1995; 63:808–815.

129. Oates RD, Lobel SM, Harris DH, et al. Efficacy of intracytoplasmic sperm injection using intentionally cryopreserved epididymal spermatozoa. Hum Reprod 1996; 11(1):133–138.

130. Holden CA, Fuscaldo GF, Jackson P, et al. Frozen-thawed epididymal spermatozoa for intracytoplasmic sperm injection. Fertil Steril 1997; 67(1):81–87.

131. Friedler S, Raziel A, Soffer Y, et al. The outcome of intracytoplasmic injection of fresh and cryopreserved epididymal spermatozoa from patients with obstructive azoospermia–a comparative study. Hum Reprod 1998; 13(7):1872–1877.

132. Hutchon S, Thornton S, Hall J, et al. Frozen-thawed epididymal sperm is effective for intracytoplasmic sperm injection: implications for the urologist. Br J Urol 1998; 81(4):607–611.

133. Van Steirteghem A, Nagy P, Joris H, et al. Results of intracytoplasmic sperm injection with ejaculated, fresh and frozen-thawed epididymal and testicular spermatozoa. Hum Reprod 1998; 13(suppl 1):134–142.

134. Tournaye H, Merdad T, Silber S, et al. No differences in outcome after intracytoplasmic sperm injection with fresh or with frozen-thawed epididymal spermatozoa. Hum Reprod 1999; 14(1):90–95.

135. Cayan S, Lee D, Conaghan J, et al. A comparison of ICSI outcomes with fresh and cryopreserved epididymal spermatozoa from the same couples. Hum Reprod 2001; 16(3):495–499.

136. Nudell DM, Conaghan J, Pedersen RA, et al. The mini-micro-epididymal sperm aspiration for sperm retrieval: a study of urological outcomes. Hum Reprod 1998; 13(5):1260–1265.

137. Hauser R, Temple-Smith PD, Southwick GJ, et al. Fertility in cases of hypergonadotropic azoospermia. Fertil Steril 1995; 63(3):631–636.

138. Tournaye H, Camus M, Goossens A, et al. Recent concepts in the management of infertility because of non-obstructive azoospermia. Hum Reprod 1995; 10(suppl 1):115–119.

139. Devroey P, Liu J, Nagy Z, et al. Pregnancies after testicular sperm extraction and intracytoplasmic sperm injection in non-obstructive azoospermia. Hum Reprod 1995; 10(6): 1457–1460.

140. Silber SJ, Van Steirteghem AC, Liu J, et al. High fertilization and pregnancy rate after intracytoplasmic sperm injection with spermatozoa obtained from testicle biopsy. Hum Reprod 1995; 10(1):148–152.

141. Oates RD, Mulhall J, Burgass C, et al. Fertilization and pregnancy using intentionally cryopreserved testicular tissue as the sperm source for intracytoplasmic sperm injection in 10 men with non-obstructive azoospermia. Hum Reprod 1997; 12(4):734–739.

142. Tash JA, Schlegel PN. Histologic effects of testicular sperm extraction on the testicle in men with nonobstructive azoospermia. Urology 2001; 57(2):334–337.

143. Gil-Salom M, Romero J, Minguez Y, et al. Testicular sperm extraction and intracytoplasmic sperm injection: a chance of fertility in nonobstructive azoospermia. J Urol 1998; 160(1):2063–2067.

144. Schlegel PN, Su LM. Physiological consequences of testicular sperm extraction. Hum Reprod 1997; 12(8):1688–1692.

145. Tournaye H, Verheyen G, Nagy P, et al. Are there any predictive factors for successful testicular sperm recovery in azoospermic patients? Hum Reprod 1997; 12(1):80–86.

146. Silber J, Johnson L. Are spermatid injections of any clinical value? Hum Reprod 1998; 13(3):509–515.

147. Edwards RG, Tarin JJ, Dean N, et al. Are spermatid injections into human oocytes now mandatory? Hum Reprod 1994; 9(12):2217–2219.

148. Aslam I, Fishel S, Green S, et al. Can we justify spermatid microinjection for severe male factor infertility? Hum Reprod Update 1998; 4(3):213–222.

149. Ogura A, Yanagimachi R. Round spermatid nuclei injected into hamster oocytes form pronuclei and participate in syngamy. Biol Reprod 1993; 48(2):219–225.

150. Ogura A, Yanagimachi R, Usui N. Behaviour of hamster and mouse round spermatid nuclei incorporated into mature oocytes by electrofusion. Zygote 1993; 1(1):1–8.

151. Ogura A, Matsuda J, Yanagimachi R. Birth of normal young after electrofusion of mouse oocytes with round spermatids. Proc Natl Acad Sci USA 1994; 91(16): 7460–7462.

152. Vanderzwalmen P, Lejeune B, Nijs M, et al. Fertilization of an oocyte microinseminated with a spermatid in an in-vitro fertilization programme. Hum Reprod 1995; 10(3):502–503.

153. Tesarik J, Mendoza C, Testart J. Viable embryos from injection of round spermatids into oocytes. N Engl J Med 1995; 333(8):525.

154. Fishel S, Green S, Bishop M, et al. Pregnancy after intracytoplasmic injection of spermatid. Lancet 1995; 345(8965):1641–1642.

155. Levran D, Nahum H, Farhi J, et al. Poor outcome with round spermatid injection in azoospermic patients with maturation arrest. Fertil Steril 2000; 74(3): 443–449.

156. Balaban B, Urman B, Isiklar A, et al. Progression to the blastocyst stage of embryos derived from testicular round spermatids. Hum Reprod 2000; 15(6): 1377–1382.

157. Tesarik J, Mendoza C, Greco E. In vitro culture facilitates the selection of healthy spermatids for assisted reproduction. Fertil Steril 1999; 72(5):809–813.

158. Ghazzawi IM, Alhasani S, Taher M, et al. Reproductive capacity of round spermatids compared with mature spermatozoa in a population of azoospermic men. Hum Reprod 1999; 14(3):736–740.

159. Vanderzwalmen P, Zech H, Birkenfeld A, et al. Intracytoplasmic injection of permatids retrieved from testicular tissue: influence of testicular pathology, type of selected spermatids and oocyte activation. Hum Reprod 1997; 12(6):1203–1213.

160. Araki Y, Motoyama M, Yoshida A, et al. Intracytoplasmic injection with late spermatids: a successful procedure in achieving childbirth for couples in which the male partner suffers from azoospermia due to deficient spermatogenesis. Fertil Steril 1997; 67(3): 559–561.

161. Antinori S, Versaci C, Dani G, et al. Fertilization with human testicular spermatids: four successful pregnancies. Hum Reprod 1997; 12(2):286–291.

162. Kahraman S, Polat G, Samli M, et al. Multiple pregnancies obtained by testicular spermatid injection in combination with intracytoplasmic sperm injection. Hum Reprod 1998; 13(1):104–110.

163. Bernabeu R, Cremades N, Takahashi K, et al. Successful pregnancy after spermatid injection. Hum Reprod 1998; 13(7):1898–1900.

164. Barak Y, Kogosowski A, Goldman S, et al. Pregnancy and birth after transfer of embryos that developed from single-nucleated zygotes obtained by injection of round spermatids into oocytes. Fertil Steril 1998; 70(1):67–70.

165. Sofikitis NV, Yamamoto Y, Miyagawa I, et al. Ooplasmic injection of elongating spermatids for the treatment of non-obstructive azoospermia. Hum Reprod 1998; 13(3):709–714.

166. Al-Hasani S, Ludwig M, Palermo I, et al. Intracytoplasmic injection of round and elongated spermatids from azoospermic patients: results and review. Hum Reprod 1999; 14(suppl 1):97–107.

167. Choavaratana R, Suppinyopong S, Chaimahaphruksa P. ROSI from TESE the first case in Thailand: a case report. J Med Assoc Thai 1999; 82(9):938–941.

168. Gianaroli L, Selman HA, Magli MC, et al. Birth of a healthy infant after conception with round spermatids isolated from cryopreserved testicular tissue. Fertil Steril 1999; 72(3):539–541.

169. Zech H, Vanderzwalmen P, Prapas Y, et al. Congenital malformations after intracytoplasmic injection of spermatids. Hum Reprod 2000; 15(4):969–971.

170. Testart J, Gautier E, Brami C, et al. Intracytoplasmic sperm injection in infertile patients with structural chromosome abnormalities. Hum Reprod 1996; 11(12): 2609–2612.

171. Van Assche E, Bonduelle M, Tournaye H, et al. Cytogenetics of infertile men. Hum Reprod 1996; 11(suppl 4):1–24.

172. Mau UA, Backert IT, Kaiser P, et al. Chromosomal findings in 150 couples referred for genetic counseling prior to intracytoplasmic sperm injection. Hum Reprod 1997; 12(5):930–937.

173. Chandley AC. Chromosome anomalies and Y chromosome microdeletions as causal factors in male infertility. Hum Reprod 1998; 13(suppl 1):45–50.

174. van der Ven K, Peschka B, Montag M, et al. Increased frequency of congenital chromosomal aberrations in female partners of couples undergoing intracytoplasmic sperm injection. Hum Reprod 1998; 13(1):48–54.

175. Meschede D, Lemcke B, Exeler JR, et al. Chromosome abnormalities in 447 couples undergoing intracytoplasmic sperm injection: prevalence, types, sex distribution and reproductive relevance. Hum Reprod 1998; 13(3):576–582.

176. Causio F, Fischetto R, LM Schonauer, et al. Intracytoplasmic sperm injection in infertile patients with structural cytogenetic abnormalities. J Reprod Med 1999; 44(10):859–864.

177. Meschede D, Lemcke B, Behre HM, et al. Clustering of male infertility in the families of couples treated with intracytoplasmic sperm injection. Hum Reprod 2000; 15(7):1604–1608.

178. Peschka B, Leygraaf J, Van der Ven K, et al. Type and frequency of chromosome aberrations in 781 couples undergoing intracytoplasmic sperm injection. Hum Reprod 1999; 14(9):2257–2263.

179. Zirkin BR, Santulli R, Awoniyi CA, et al. Maintenance of advanced spermatogenic cells in the adult rat

testis: quantitative relation to testosterone concentration within the testis. Endrocrinology 1989; 124(6): 3043–3049.

180. Lubahn DB, Joseph DR, Sullivan PM, et al. Cloning of human androgen receptor complementary DNA and localization to the X chromosome. Science 1988; 240(4850):327–330.

181. La Spada AR, Wilson EM, Lubahn DB, et al. Androgen receptor gene mutations in X-linked spinal and bulbar muscular atrophy. Nature 1991; 352(6330):77–79.

182. Edwards A, Hammond HA, Jin L, et al. Genetic variation at five trimeric and tetrameric tandem repeat loci in four human population groups. Genomics 1992; 12(2):241–253.

183. Tut TG, Ghadessy FJ, Trifiro MA, et al. Long polyglutamine tracts in the androgen receptor are associated with reduced trans-activation, impaired sperm production, and male infertility. J Clin Endocrinol Metab 1997; 82(11):3777–3782.

184. Mifsud A, Sim CKS, Boettger-Tong H, et al. Trinucleotide (CAG) repeat polymorphisms in the androgen receptor gene: molecular markers of risk for male infertility. Fertil Steril 2001; 75(2):275–281.

185. Foote S, Vollrath D, Hilton A, et al. The human Y chromosome: overlapping DNA clones spanning the euchromatic region. Science 1992; 258(5079):60–66.

186. Vollrath D, Foote S, Hilton A, et al. The human Y chromosome: a 43-interval map based on naturally occurring deletions. Science 1992; 258(5079):52–59.

187. Ma K, Inglis JD, Sharkey A, et al. A Y chromosome gene family with RNA-binding protein homology: candidates for the azoospermia factor AZF controlling human spermatogenesis. Cell 1993; 75(7):1287–1295.

188. Reijo R, Lee TY, Salo P, et al. Diverse spermatogenic defects in humans caused by Y chromosome deletions encompassing a novel RNA-binding protein gene. Nat Genet 1995; 10(4):383–393.

189. Vogt PH, Edelmann A, Kirsch S, et al. Human Y chromosome azoospermia factors (AZF) mapped to different subregions in Yq11. Hum Mol Genet 1996; 5(7):933–943.

190. Lahn BT, Page DC. Functional coherence of the human Y chromosome. Science 1997; 278(5338):675–680.

191. Elliot DJ, Millar MR, Oghene K, et al. Expression of RBM in the nuclei of human germ cells is dependent on a critical region of the Y chromosome long arm. Proc Natl Acad Sci USA 1997; 94(8):3848–3853.

192. Chai NN, Salido EC, Yen PH. Multiple functional copies of the RBM gene family, a spermatogenesis candidate on the Y chromosome. Genomics 1997; 45(2): 355–361.

193. Tiepolo L, Zuffardi O. Localization of factors controlling spermatogenesis in the non-fluorescent portion of the human Y chromosome long arm. Hum Genet 1976; 34(2):119–124.

194. Liow SL, Ghadessy FJ, Ng SC, Yong EL. Y chromosome microdeletions, in azoospermic or near-azoospermic subjects, are located in the AZFc (DAZ) subregion. Mol Hum Reprod 1998; 4(8):763–768.

195. Liow SL, Yong EL, Ng SC. Prognostic value of Y deletion analysis. How reliable is the outcome of Y deletion analysis in providing a sound prognosis? Hum Reprod 2001; 16(1): 9–12.

196. Kerem B, Rommens JM, Buchanan JA, et al. Identification of the cystic fibrosis gene: genetic analysis. Science 1989; 245(4922):1073–1080.

197. Riordan JR, Rommens JM, Kerem B, et al. Identification of the cystic fibrosis gene: cloning and characterization of complementary DNA. Science 1989; 245: 1066–1073.

198. Rommens JM, Iannuzzi MC, Kerem B, et al. Identification of the cystic fibrosis gene: chromosome walking and jumping. Science 1989; 245(4922):1059–1065.

199. Welsh MJ, Smith AE. Molecular mechanisms of CFTR chloride channel dysfunction in cystic fibrosis. Cell 1993; 73(7):1251–1254.

200. Welsh MJ, Tsui LC, Boat TF, et al. Cystic fibrosis. In: Scriver CR, Beaudet AL, Sly W, Valle D, eds. The Metabolic and Molecular Bases of Inherited Diseases. 7th ed. New York: McGraw-Hill Inc, 1995:3799–3876.

201. Hargreave TB. Genetic basis of male infertility. Br Med Bull 2000; 56(3):650–671.

202. Lewis-Jones DI, Gazvani MR, Mountford R. Cystic fibrosis in infertility: screening before assisted reproduction. Hum Reprod 2000; 15(11):2415–2417.

203. Patrizio P, Leonard DGB. Mutations of the cystic fibrosis gene and congenital absence of the vas deferens. In: McElreavey K, ed. The Genetic Basis of Male Infertility. Results and Problems in Cell Differentiation. Vol. 28. Berlin Heidelberg: Springer-Verlag, 2000:175–186.

204. Jequier AM, Ansell ID, Bullimore NJ. Congenital absence of the vasa deferentia presenting with infertility. J Androl 1985; 6(1):15–19.

205. Chillon M, Casals T, Mercier B, et al. Mutations in the cystic fibrosis gene in patients with congenital absence of the vas deferens. N Engl J Med 1995; 332(22): 1475–1480.

206. Zielenski J, Patrizio P, Corey M, et al. CFTR gene variant for patients with congenital absence of vas deferens. Am J Hum Genet 1995; 57(4):958–960.

207. Stuhrmann M, Dork T. CFTR gene mutations and male infertility. Andrologia 2000; 32(2):71–83.

208. Dumur V, Gervais R, Rigot JM, et al. Abnormal distribution of CF delta F508 allele in azoospermic men with congenital aplasia of epididymis and vas deferens. Lancet 1990; 336(8713):512.

209. Anguiano A, Oates RD, Amos JA, et al. Congenital bilateral absence of the vas deferens: a primarily genital form of cyctic fibrosis. JAMA 1992; 267(13): 1794–1797.

210. Jarvi K, Zielenski J, Wilschanski M, et al. Cystic fibrosis transmembrane conductance regulator and obstructive azoospermia. Lancet 1995; 345(8694):1578.

211. Meschede D, Dworniczak B, Behre HM, et al. CFTR gene mutations in men with bilateral ejaculatory-duct obstruction and anomalies of the seminal vesicles. Am J Hum Genet 1997; 61(5):1200–1202.

212. de Braekeleer M, Ferec C. Mutations in the cystic fibrosis gene in men with congenital bilateral absence of the vas deferens. Mol Hum Reprod 1996; 2(9):669–677.

213. Lissens W, Mercier B, Tournaye H, et al. Cystic fibrosis and infertility caused by congenital bilateral absence of the vas deferens and related clinical entities. Hum Reprod 1996; 11(suppl 4):55–78; discussion 79–80.

214. Boucher D, Creveaux I, Grizard G, et al. Screening for cystic fibrosis transmembrane conductance regulator gene mutations in men included in an intracytoplasmic sperm injection programme. Mol Hum Reprod 1999; 5(6):587–593.

215. Patrizio P, Salameh WA. Expression of the cystic fibrosis transmembrane conductance regulator (CFTR) mRNA in normal and pathological adult human epididymis. J Reprod Fertil Suppl 1998; 53:261–270.

216. Tuerlings JHAM, Mol B, Kremer JAM, et al. Mutation frequency of cystic fibrosis transmembrane regulator is not increased in oligozoospermic male candidates for intracytoplasmic sperm injection. Fertil Steril 1998; 69(5):899–903.

217. Mak V, Zielenski J, Tsui LC, et al. Cystic fibrosis gene mutations and infertile men with primary testicular failure. Hum Reprod 2000; 15(2):436–439.

218. Meng MV, Black LD, Cha I, et al. Impaired spermatogenesis in men with congenital absence of the vas deferens. Hum Reprod 2001; 16(3):529–533.

219. Denning CR, Sommers SC, Quigley HJ. Infertility in male patients with cystic fibrosis. Pediatrics 1968; 41(1):7–17.

220. Kaplan E, Shwachman H, Perlmutter AD, et al. Reproductive failure in males with cystic fibrosis. N Engl J Med 1968; 279(2):65–69.

221. Oppenheimer EH, Esterly JR. Observations on cystic fibrosis of the pancreas. V. Developmental changes in the male genital system. J Pediatr 1969; 75(5): 806–811.

222. Holsclaw DS, Permutter AD, Jockin H, et al. Genital abnormalities in male patients with cystic fibrosis. J Urol 1971; 106:568–574.

223. Gottlieb C, Ploen L, Kvist U, et al. The fertility potential of male cystic fibrosis patients. Int J Androl 1991; 14:437–440.

224. Goldstein M, Schlossberg S. Men with congenital absence of vas deferens often have seminal vesicles. J Urol 1988; 140(1):85–86.

225. Silber SJ, Patrizio P, Asch RH. Quantitative evaluation of spermatogenesis by testicular histology in men with congenital absence of the vas deferens undergoing epididymal sperm aspiration. Hum Reprod 1990; 5(1): 89–93.

226. Rule AH, Kopito L, Shwachman H. Chemical analysis of ejaculates from patients with cystic fibrosis. Fertil Steril 1970; 21(6):515–520.

227. Oates RD, Amos JA. The genetic basis of congenital bilateral absence of the vas deferens and cystic fibrosis. J Androl 1994; 15(1):1–8.

228. Olson JR, Weaver DK. Congenital mesonephric defects in male infants with mucoviscidosis. J Clin Pathol 1969; 22(6):725–730.

229. Gvakharia MO, Lipshultz LI, Lamb DJ. Human sperm microinjection into hamster oocytes: a new tool for training and evaluation of the technical proficiency of intracytoplasmic sperm injection. Fertil Steril 2000; 73(2):395–401.

230. Ahmadi A, Bongso A, Ng SC. Intracytoplasmic injection of human sperm into the hamster oocyte (hamster ICSI assay) as a test for fertilizing capacity of the severe male-factor sperm. J Assist Reprod Genet 1996; 13(8): 647–651.

231. Palermo GD, Colombero LT, Schattman GL, et al. Evolutions of pregnancies and initial follow-up of newborns delivered after intracytoplasmic sperm injection. JAMA 1996; 276(23):1893–1897.

232. Tournaye H, Van Steirteghem A. ICSI concerns do not outweigh its benefits. J NIH Res 1997; 9:35–40.

233. Bonduelle M, Wilikens A, Buysse A, et al. A follow-up study of children born after intracytoplasmic sperm injection (ICSI) with epididymal and testicular spermatozoa and after replacement of cryopreserved embryos obtained after ICSI. Hum Reprod 1998; 13(suppl 1): 196–207.

234. Zech H, Vanderzwalmen P, Prapas Y, et al. Congenital malformations after intracytoplasmic injection of spermatids. Hum Reprod 2000; 15(4): 969-971.

235. Macas E, Imthurn B, Keller PJ. Increased incidence of numerical chromosome abnormalities in spermatozoa injected into human oocytes by ICSI. Hum Reprod 2001; 16(1): 115–120.

236. Schatten H, Schatten G, Mazia D, et al. Behavior of centrosomes during fertilization and cell division in mouse oocytes and in sea urchin eggs. Proc Natl Acad Sci USA 1986; 83(1):105–109.

237. Szollosi D, Szollosi MS, Czolowska R, et al. Sperm penetration into immature mouse oocytes and nuclear changes during maturation: an EM study. Biol Cell 1990; 69(1):53–64.

238. Manandhar G, Sutovsky P, Joshi HC, et al. Centrosome reduction during mouse spermiogenesis. Dev Biol 1998; 203(2):424–434.

239. Wu GJ, Simerly C, Zoran SS, et al. Microtubule and chromatin dynamics during fertilization and early development in rhesus monkeys, and regulation by intracellular calcium ions. Biol Reprod 1996; 55(2):260–270.

240. Ng SC, Martelli P, Liow SL, et al. Intracytoplasmic injection of frozen-thawed epididymal spermatozoa in a nonhuman primate (*Macaca fascicularis*). Theriogenonology 2002; 58(9): 1385–1397.

38

Fertility Preservation in Males with Cancer

Paul J. Turek

Departments of Urology, Obstetrics, Gynecologic and Reproductive Sciences, Male Reproductive Laboratory, University of California, San Francisco, California, U.S.A.

□ INTRODUCTION

> When you go in search of honey, you must expect to be stung by bees.
>
> —*K. Kaunda (1983)*

Most children and young adults treated for cancer can expect to be cured. In fact, 70% of children with cancer survive their malignancies, in large part because of major advances in the field of oncology during the 1970s (1). Thus, clinical attention has begun to shift away from the problem of cure and toward refinements in the quality of life among cancer survivors. Fertility is certainly one quality-of-life issue very commonly affected by cancer treatment, and one that may have significant psychological consequences in adulthood.

This chapter reviews the factors that contribute to infertility in men with cancer and also discusses the treatment-specific risks to fertility that accompany cancer management. Contemporary methods of overcoming infertility in cancer patients are outlined. Finally, several exciting and promising experimental approaches to the preservation or restoration of fertility with cancer are discussed.

Evaluating the Male Cancer Patient for Infertility

The evaluation of male infertility in the setting of cancer is undertaken methodically to acquire four kinds of information. A thorough history reviews past medical and surgical problems, medications, and exposures and delineates the frequency and timing of intercourse, contraceptive use, and associated prior pregnancies. The physical examination investigates peritesticular pathology including cancer, cryptorchidism, varicocele, epididymitis, and palpable absence of the vas deferens. The evaluation proceeds with laboratory studies, which include serum follicle-stimulating hormone (FSH) and testosterone levels. A hormone assessment can detect deficiencies within or compensatory states of, the pituitary–gonadal axis. Lastly, at least two semen analyses are obtained to evaluate semen volume, sperm concentration, sperm motility, and the quality of motility and morphology.

In patients with cancer, analysis of the centrifuged pellet of semen is important if azoospermia is detected on gross examination, since sperm can be found in 23% of men with apparent azoospermia (2). When indicated, valuable adjunctive studies are available and include scrotal and transrectal ultrasound, assays of semen leukocytes or antisperm antibodies, sperm DNA fragmentation, and sperm-penetrating function by bioassay. Therapeutic choices rely on the information garnered from this basic evaluation.

□ WHAT IS THE IMPACT OF CANCER AND CANCER TREATMENT ON MALE INFERTILITY?

Fertility in men with cancer may be affected by both the disease and its treatment. For example, compromised semen quality is detected in 60% of men with Hodgkin's disease—an effect thought to be due to fever and other constitutional symptoms associated with the illness (3). Likewise, 50% of men with testis cancer present with abnormal semen quality, possibly because of tumor endocrine activity, autoimmune dysfunction, and contralateral organ involvement (4). Cancer treatment has profound effects on fertility, because spermatogenesis involves rapid cell division and is therefore exquisitely sensitive to the effects of chemotherapy and radiotherapy. A review of pre- and post-treatment semen quality associated with several common cancers is listed in Table 1.

Essential to any discussion of the literature on cancer and infertility is a review of the limitations inherent among studies. Many studies of fertility in cancer patients use semen analysis, and not necessarily paternity, as the measure of fertility. Further complicating the matter, semen parameters that define a "normal" semen analysis vary from report to report, making comparisons difficult. The assessment of fertility outcomes in cancer patients is often confounded by the fact that the treatment populations lack sufficient size and homogeneity for statistically meaningful analysis; in addition, there is often a lack of comparative control groups. Notably, fertility is a couple phenomenon, and many studies do not address, or control for,

Table 1 Pre- and Post-treatment Semen Quality in Men with Common Cancers

| | Semen quality | | | | |
| | Pretreatment | | Post-treatment (>2 yr) | | |
Type of cancer	Oligospermic patients (%)	Azoospermic patients (%)	Oligospermic patients (%)	Azoospermic patients (%)	Ref.
Testis cancer					
Stage I, surveillance	28	12	25	25	(5,6)
Stage I, chemotherapy	N/A	N/A	7	7	(7)
Stages II, III	69	69	48	48	(6)
Lymphoma (HD and NHL)[a]	27	0	22	33	(8)
Leukemia (ALL)	N/A	N/A	77	21	(9)
Sarcoma	N/A	N/A	29	59	(10)
Osteosarcoma	N/A	N/A	12	59	(11)

[a]Patients referred for sperm banking prior to therapy.
Abbreviations: ALL, acute myelogenous leukemia; HD, Hodgkin's disease; N/A, data not available; NHL, non-Hodgkins lymphoma.

the potential female-factor infertility. Finally, to some degree, cancer therapeutic regimens lack standardization, which can cloud meaningful observations on treatment-related effects on fertility. Yet, given these caveats, important clinical and scientific information has been garnered through these valuable investigations.

Specific Effects of Cancer Treatment on Fertility

All major forms of cancer therapy, including surgery, radiation therapy, and chemotherapy can have a major impact on male fertility. In fact, the impact of these therapies on infertility constitutes the major morbidity in young men with cancer and hence is worthy of discussion.

Surgery for Cancer
Radical Orchiectomy
Surgical removal of the testis is routinely performed in men with testis cancer. One study suggests that men with testis cancer and orchiectomy do not experience more gonadal dysfunction than men who undergo orchiectomy for other reasons (12). Among 54 men who received orchiectomy for various reasons, including cryptorchidism, torsion, cancer, and trauma, the fraction of men with normal sperm concentrations and those with azoospermia were no different (Fig. 1). Although paternity was not examined in this study, it appears that orchiectomy performed for any reason has a similar potential impact on male fertility.

Retroperitoneal Lymph Node Dissection or Pelvic Surgery
Two fertility-related complications can occur after retroperitoneal lymph node dissection (RPLND) or pelvic surgery: retrograde ejaculation and anejaculation. Both result from different degrees of injury to the postganglionic sympathetic fibers arising from the thoracolumbar region of the spinal cord. These autonomic nerves overlie the inferior aorta and coalesce to

form the hypogastric plexus within the pelvis and can be damaged in the retroperitoneum or pelvis during lymph node or tumor dissection. These nerves supply the ampullary vas deferens, seminal vesicle, periurethral glands, and the internal sphincter closure mechanism and thus control seminal emission. In addition, they supply the bulbourethral and periurethral musculature and affect ejaculation. Thus, damage to these nerves, especially in the area of the aortic bifurcation, can result in failure of seminal emission or ejaculation, or both. (For more detailed information on male reproductive anatomy, please refer to Chapter 2.)

Fortunately, surgical techniques have evolved in ways that have reduced these fertility complications. The earliest RPLND procedure for testis cancer involved a bilateral, extended suprahilar excision of retroperitoneal nodes and almost uniformly resulted in ejaculatory dysfunction and infertility. In the 1980s, the modified unilateral RPLND limited the dissection below the inferior mesenteric artery in patients without grossly node-positive disease (13). Subsequently,

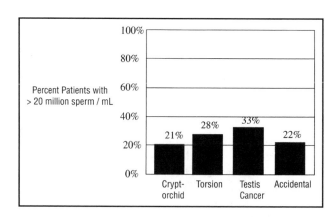

Figure 1 Semen quality after unilateral orchiectomy. The percent of patients with normal sperm concentrations (>20 million sperm/mL) after unilateral orchiectomy (n = 54 patients) for four different reasons is shown. No statistical differences are noted. *Source*: From Ref. 4.

nerve-sparing approaches further scaled down the dissection template as they prospectively targeted dissection of lymph nodes among sympathetic nerve fibers (14). With these advances, the incidence of postoperative antegrade ejaculation increased from 10% in men with the extended bilateral suprahilar dissection to well over 90% in men who underwent a nerve-sparing approach (Fig. 2) (14). Most recently, the introduction of the laparoscopic approach to retroperitoneal lymphadenectomy promises to reduce the morbidity from cancer surgery even further (15,16).

Radiation Therapy for Cancer
Effect on Spermatogenesis
The effects of ionizing radiation on testis sperm production are well described. These are derived mainly from a series of remarkable experiments performed 40 years ago but only recently published. Using data generated from a study of healthy prisoners in Oregon and Washington in the 1960s, Clifton et al. examined the effects of ionizing irradiation on semen quality and spermatogenesis (17). Prior to a vasectomy, each of 111 volunteers was exposed to a different level of radiation, from 7.5 to 600 rads (cGy). Sperm counts were analyzed weekly before, during, and after the exposure; each prisoner served as his own control. Testicular biopsies were performed when possible; most men had one biopsy prior to and one after irradiation. There was a distinct dose-dependent, inverse relationship between irradiation and sperm count. Significant reduction in sperm count manifested at doses of 15 cGy and was temporarily abolished at 50 cGy. Azoospermia was induced at 400 cGy in four of five patients; this persisted for at least 40 weeks. Despite these profound effects, sperm counts eventually rebounded to preirradiation levels in most patients.

Dose-Dependent Nature of Effect
Testis biopsy data from these experiments were also evaluated for the effects of radiation (17,18). From

examination of the testis biopsies, it was concluded that spermatogonia were the most sensitive germ cells to irradiation at all dose levels. Type A spermatogonia were obliterated to the degree that <1% remained at exposures >400 cGy. Even at higher doses of irradiation, however, spermatogenesis returned, indicating that a slowly dividing subpopulation of spermatogonia may exhibit a relative resistance to exposure. In addition, these studies revealed that the recovery time of spermatogenesis after radiation exposure increases with the dose received: with 20 cGy exposure, histologic and sperm count recovery occurred at a mean of six months postexposure, whereas doses of 400 cGy or more required more than five years for complete recovery.

Given the dramatic sensitivity of the testis to irradiation, what level of unintended radiation is encountered by the testes from "scatter" during infradiaphragmatic radiation for testis cancer? In a study of 26 seminoma patients subjected to 3200 cGy in 16 fractions over four weeks with gonadal shielding (please refer below for further information), Hahn et al. estimated the mean unintended gonadal exposure as 78 cGy (19). Semen quality after irradiation was also monitored (14 patients) and it was found that sperm counts fell between 1 to 4 months, that most men were azoospermic between 2.5 to 7.5 months after irradiation, and that the vast majority of men showed evidence of semen recovery within 7.5 to 20 months. In summary, although the testis is exquisitely sensitive to the effects of ionizing radiation, recovery of spermatogenesis is usually excellent in men receiving infradiaphragmatic templates. In addition, there does not appear to be an increase in congenital birth defects among offspring of irradiated men (20).

Chemotherapy for Cancer
Effect on Spermatogenesis
Chemotherapy regimens are designed to kill rapidly dividing cells; one undesired outcome of therapy is the cytotoxic effect on normally proliferating tissues such as those of the testis. Differentiating spermatogonia appear to be the most sensitive germ cells to the cytotoxic effects of chemotherapy (21), and alkylating agents are considered the most toxic agents to the testis. Obviously, toxic effects will vary, depending on dose and duration of chemotherapy, stage of disease, age and health of the patient, and baseline testis function prior to therapy. A list of various chemotherapeutic agents and relative toxicities to the testis is given in Table 2.

Agent-Specific Toxicity
Evidence suggests that both the exocrine and the endocrine compartments of the testis are affected by chemotherapy. Several chemotherapeutic agents are particularly toxic to the testis, including cisplatin and cyclophosphamide. Hansen et al. compared semen parameters from 22 patients with disseminated testis cancer in remission (median = five years) after

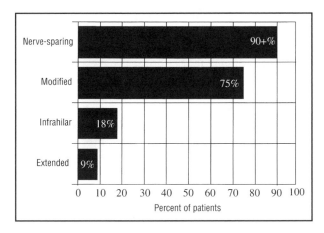

Figure 2 Incidence of normal ejaculation after RPLND. The percent of patients with antegrade ejaculation after four different RPLND techniques. *Abbreviation*: RPLND, retroperitoneal lymph node dissection. *Source*: From Ref. 4.

Table 2   Toxic Effects of Chemotherapeutic Agents on the Testis

Agent	Effect on testis	Recoverability	Recovery time
Mechlorethamine	Severe	Poor	>2–5 yr
Cyclophosphamide	Severe	Poor	1–5 yr
Chlorambucil	Severe	Poor	3–5 yr
Methotrexate	Minimal	Good	6–12 mo
Cytosine arabinoside	Moderate	Good	6–12 mo
6-Mercatopurine	Moderate	Good	6–12 mo
Thioguanine	Moderate	Good	9 mo
Vincristine	Moderate	Good	6–12 mo
Prednisone	Moderate	Good	6 mo
Androgens	Moderate	Good	6–12 mo
Estrogens	Moderate	Good	6–12 mo
Doxorubicin	Moderate	Good	1 yr
Procarbazine	Severe	Poor	>2–5 yr
Cisplatin	Moderate	Good	1–2 yr
Nitrogen mustard, vincristine, procarbazine, and prednisone	Severe	Very poor	>2–5 yr
Cyclophosphamide, vincristine, procarbazine, and prednisone	Moderate	Moderate	3 yr
Doxorubicin, bleomycin, vinblastine, and decarbazine	Moderate	Moderate	1–4 yr
Cisplatin, etoposide, and bleomycin	Moderate	Good	1–2 yr
Vinblastine, bleomycin, and cisplatin	Moderate	Good	1–2 yr

Note: Poor: <20% of patients will recover; moderate: 20% to 50% of patients will recover; good: >50% of patients will recover spermatogenesis.
Source: From Ref. 22.

cisplatin-based chemotherapy (total cisplatin = 600 mg/m^2), with nine patients diagnosed with stage I nonseminomatous germ cell tumors followed with surveillance (23). Mean sperm concentration was significantly lower in the chemotherapy group compared to surveillance patients: 0.35 million sperm/mL compared with 17 million sperm/mL. In addition, azoospermia was noted in 27% of chemotherapy patients but only 11% of surveillance patients. In another study, it was concluded that long-term effects of cisplatin on sperm production are unlikely to occur at doses below 400 mg/m^2 (24). Similarly, Meistrich et al. studied semen quality in males with sarcomas and concluded that the dose of cyclophosphamide was the single most significant determinant of recovery to normal sperm counts after cancer treatment (25). Most patients returned to normospermia if the cyclophosphamide dose was < 7.5 gm/m^2. In summary, the exocrine testis is particularly sensitive to chemotherapy for cancer.

Chemotherapy has also been shown to affect the endocrine compartment of the testis. In the same study mentioned above, Hansen et al. found elevated FSH levels in 86% of chemotherapy patients compared to 11% of men on surveillance (23). Elevations in luteinizing hormone (LH) occurred in 59% of men undergoing chemotherapy and 11% of men on surveillance. From these observations, it is apparent that chemotherapy may also induce Leydig cell dysfunction such that more pituitary LH and FSH are needed to maintain normal testosterone levels and spermatogenesis.

Studies of paternity in the setting of cancer reflect these observations of decreased testis function with chemotherapy. Hansen et al. found that the fertility in

men who received cisplatin-based chemotherapy for testis cancer was reduced compared to another cohort of men with testis cancer treated with orchiectomy alone (23). A subsequent study has suggested that the average paternity rates after therapy among patients who received one or more kinds of treatment (including chemotherapy) for testis cancer may indeed be half of that observed in the same population of couples before the diagnosis of cancer is made (26). Fortunately, there is evidence in the literature that the issue of fertility is gaining importance in the design of chemotherapy regimens for young men with cancer (7).

Does Cancer Treatment Cause Birth Defects in Offspring?

Given that chemotherapy can be toxic to the testis, are there measurable mutagenic effects in sperm? There is evidence to suggest that chromosomal damage occurs in the sperm of men who receive cancer chemotherapy. Robbins et al. examined the rate of chromosomal aneuploidy using fluorescence in situ hybridization in the ejaculated sperm of Hodgkin's disease patients receiving NOVP chemotherapy (Novantrone, Oncovin, vinblastine, prednisone) (27). When compared to prechemotherapy or baseline values, the incidence of abnormalities in sperm chromosomes 8, X, and Y increased fivefold during chemotherapy. Baseline levels of sperm aneuploidy were again achieved 100 days after therapy ended. In addition to chromosomal abnormalities, there is also evidence to suggest that sperm DNA fragmentation occurs with exposure to chemotherapy. In a single patient with chronic lymphocytic leukemia, undergoing fludarabine-based chemotherapy, Chatterjee et al. applied a single cell Comet assay to detect DNA strand breaks in sperm before, during, and after chemotherapy (28). High levels of sperm DNA fragmentation were observed during chemotherapy when compared to pretreatment. In addition, high levels of DNA damage persisted after treatment ended (up to 11 months), suggesting that such damage may not be fully reversible. Although the clinical significance of these findings is not established, this data suggests that sperm should not be banked while a patient is receiving chemotherapy; contraceptive intercourse is advised for the duration of chemotherapy and six months after completion.

Are these mutagenic events significant enough to increase the chance of congenital defects or genetically linked diseases among offspring of treated men? To better understand the potential heritable risk associated with chemotherapy, Marchetti et al. investigated the effects of etoposide on the induction of chromosomal abnormalities in spermatocytes and their transmission to zygotes in a mouse model (29). With the technique of chromosome painting, high frequencies of chromosomal aberrations in exposed male germ cells and significant increases in the percent of embryos with chromosomal structural aberrations were found. As the types of aberrations observed generally represented a loss of genetic material, these insults are expected to result in embryonic lethality. This study suggests that certain chemotherapeutic agents may produce unstable structural aberrations and aneuploidy and potentially transmit them to progeny. In a clinical study, Senturia et al. analyzed children born to 96 patients after chemotherapy treatment for testis cancer and found that the relative risk of birth defects was not increased compared with 44 age-matched men with testis cancer managed by surveillance and 52 healthy controls (20). Thus, it is currently unclear as to whether or not the genetic damage induced by chemotherapy significantly affects the survivor's offspring.

☐ CURRENT METHODS TO MAINTAIN FERTILITY WITH CANCER
Gonadal Shielding

The use of external beam radiotherapy to treat malignancy has led to the development of shielding devices to protect tissues outside the target area. Radiation affects organs distant from the intended target by (i) "leakage" through machine shielding, (ii) "scatter" from the collimator, or (iii) "scatter" of radiation from within the patient (30). Although several different gonadal shields have been fashioned, the ideal shield should allow <50 cGy to penetrate the testes (18,31). Foo et al. evaluated gonadal exposure during pelvic irradiation on unshielded phantoms and demonstrated that a 5000 cGy treatment would result in 632 cGy exposure to the testes—high enough to cause permanent azoospermia (30). The use of a pelvic shield, however,

can block as much as 99% of the 5000 cGy radiation dose. Therefore, it is critical that gonadal shielding be employed for all men receiving infradiaphragmatic radiation for cancer.

Sperm Cryopreservation

The most effective way to preserve fertility in patients who undergo cancer treatment is the cryopreservation of sperm, which can be performed on ejaculated semen after a routine semen analysis. The specimen is placed in plastic vials or "straws" and diluted 1:1 with cryoprotectants, usually glycerol and egg yolk–citrate buffer, after an initial wash. The straws are frozen in a very precise, stepwise, computer-controlled manner in liquid nitrogen (–96°C) or by exposure to liquid nitrogen vapor followed by submersion in liquid nitrogen. Specimens are thawed by room temperature exposure for 30 minutes after removal from liquid nitrogen, followed by warming in an incubator for 10 minutes. The thawed specimen is then washed free of cryoprotectants and then used for either intrauterine insemination or more sophisticated reproductive technologies. (For further information on assisted reproductive techniques, please refer to Chapters 33 and 37.) A "test thaw" is usually performed with a small amount of the first specimen from each patient to see how the cryopreservation process affects sperm quality. Several variables influence ability of sperm to survive the freeze–thaw process, including the rate of cooling and warming and the nature of the suspending medium. Damage to sperm with freezing is generally due to the formation of intracellular ice crystals that can grow to sizes sufficient to destroy the cell. Among men with normal semen quality prior to sperm cryopreservation, a 40% to 60% recovery of the motile sperm fraction is possible. In cancer patients with subnormal semen parameters, there is generally a poorer recovery of motile sperm (32,33). Sperm recoverability after thaw is generally independent of the length of time that sperm are cryopreserved.

In the past, it was commonly thought that the preservation of poor quality semen in men with cancer is not worthwhile. This was based on the limited technological resources available to assist in achieving a pregnancy. At present, even the poorest quality semen specimen (1–50 sperm) is capable of resulting in a pregnancy with highly refined techniques of in vitro fertilization (IVF) and intracytoplasmic sperm injection (ICSI). Therefore, all semen specimens that show motile or viable sperm should be considered for cryopreservation. In addition, techniques to retrieve viable sperm from the male reproductive tract before cancer treatment should also be considered, as the cryobiological behavior of this sperm is well defined and its clinical utility also well established (Table 3) (34).

Testis-Sparing Surgery for Cancer

There has been recent interest in organ-sparing, partial orchiectomy surgery as an alternative to radical

Table 3 Motility and Viability of Three Kinds of Surgically Retrieved Sperm

Aspirated sperm	Motility (%)		Vital stain (% viable)	
	Fresh	Thawed	Fresh	Thawed
Testicle	5	0.2	86	46
Epididymis	22	7	57	24
Vas deferens	71	38	91	51

Source: From Ref. 34.

orchiectomy in selected testis cancer cases in an attempt to preserve gonadal hormonal function, and possibly fertility (35–37). This development stems from fact that the surgical rationale associated with the well-established "radical" orchiectomy for testis cancer has a basis that is largely empirical. The partial orchiectomy seeks to provide similar cure rates but also has a secondary goal to preserve gonadal function. To date, impressive rates of cancer cure and hormone preservation have been described in men with solitary testes or bilateral testis cancer (36,37). Indeed, the author has performed organ-preserving testis surgery in six cases involving malignant intratesticular tumors that were approached inguinally using early vascular control. Good preservation of testis function (both exocrine and endocrine) was noted without evidence of disease recurrence at a mean of two years postoperatively. This approach to testis cancer treatment may be considered in patients with small (less than 2 cm) peripheral intratesticular tumors in a solitary testis, who also have normal preoperative LH and testosterone levels and are amendable to frequent and careful postoperative follow-up (37).

☐ CURRENT METHODS TO RESTORE FERTILITY AFTER CANCER
Electroejaculation

For men who are unable to perform antegrade ejaculation after pelvic or retroperitoneal surgery, several fertility treatment options should be considered. Retrograde ejaculation is diagnosed by the finding of sperm within the postejaculate bladder urine. Initially, a trial of sympathomimetic medication should be attempted as approximately 30% of men will respond with some degree of antegrade ejaculation. Imipramine-HCl 25 to 50 mg b.i.d. and Sudafed Plus (pseudoephedrine-HCl 60 mg) q.i.d. are begun several days before ejaculation and have been used with various degrees of success. The side effects associated with these medications usually limit efficacy. For those who fail medication, sperm-harvesting techniques can be used to retrieve sperm from the bladder with intrauterine insemination or IVF to achieve pregnancies (38). (For more details on electroejaculation, see Chapter 39.)

The absence of sperm in the voided bladder urine after ejaculation indicates more extensive damage to the autonomic nerves and is termed "anejaculation." In the vast majority of these men, rectal probe electroejaculation can induce ejaculation by electrically stimulating the contraction of the vas deferens, seminal vesicle, and prostate. With graded increases in voltage to the transrectal probe, the pelvic plexus of nerves can be bulk-stimulated to induce the ejaculatory reflex. Both antegrade and retrograde semen are collected. Washed sperm can then be used with assisted reproductive technologies to achieve biological pregnancies (39). Hultling et al. treated 10 anejaculatory men after testis cancer treatment with rectal probe electroejaculation (40). Successful recovery of sperm was possible in 9 of 10 patients. An examination of the ejaculates revealed that sperm motility was decreased in all patients, ranging from 0% to 25%. Six couples used electroejaculation in combination with IVF, and five were able to conceive. These findings have been confirmed by others, and pregnancy rates of 30% to 35% are common with assisted reproductive technology (39). Because of its success in anejaculatory adult men, rectal probe electroejaculation is now being considered for the purpose of procuring semen for banking in pubertal (pre-ejaculatory) boys before anticancer therapy (41).

Sperm Aspiration (IVF and ICSI)

In patients with anejaculation, sperm aspiration from the reproductive tract is a powerful tool to help achieve paternity. It is possible to aspirate sperm from the vas deferens, epididymis, and testis and retrieve sperm for use with assisted reproduction. It is important to realize, however, that IVF and ICSI are generally required to achieve a pregnancy with extracted sperm. Thus, success rates are intimately tied to a complex and complementary program of assisted reproduction for both partners.

Sperm can be retrieved from the reproductive tract by either percutaneous or incisional approaches. Common sources of sperm include the vas deferens, epididymis, and testis (Fig. 3). In cases of normal sperm production, vasal, epididymal, and testicular sperm retrieval are all possible. With abnormal spermatogenesis, however—similar to the state found

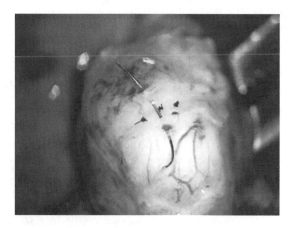

Figure 3 Microscopic view of two-layer vas deferens closure after vasal sperm aspiration in a patient with anejaculation.

in men after cancer treatment—the testes are the only viable site, and generally, a biopsy is needed. Sperm is aspirated into a nourishing fluid, and individual sperm are selected for IVF and ICSI in the laboratory. Patient recovery after sperm extraction is rapid and most procedures are performed under local anesthesia (42). Egg fertilization rates of 65% to 75% and pregnancy rates of approximately 30% to 50% have been reported with vasal and epididymal and testicular sperm (42,43), but the results vary widely among individuals because of differences in sperm and egg quality.

Testis Fine Needle Aspiration "Mapping"

As described above, IVF and ICSI have been used with great success in cancer patients with ejaculatory dysfunction. It is now possible, however, to use this technology in men with testis failure due to chemotherapy or radiation-induced injury, in whom very few sperm are obtainable from the testis (44). This urologic foray into the failing testis for sperm has allowed men with cancer, who have no sperm in the ejaculate, to father biological children. Problems encountered to date in the failing testis include the fact that sperm production is very low and that it may vary geographically within the testis, making the usual "blind" testis biopsy an inaccurate method to either diagnose or extract sperm. Consequently, there is a failure to obtain sufficient sperm for IVF and ICSI in 25% to 50% of men with testis failure (45,46). Several strategies have been developed to better detect and localize sperm within the failing testis, including a unique adaptation of the fine needle aspiration (FNA) technique (47). Taking advantage of the relatively atraumatic percutaneous technique of FNA, this method of detecting testicular sperm relies on multiple, systematic samplings of many areas of the testis (11 sites per testis) according to a "map," or template, under local anesthesia (Fig. 4). After sperm are located, testis tissue removal is then "directed" to the sites showing sperm, and sperm are obtained for IVF and ICSI (44,48). Such strategies improve the chances for paternity in many men who have undergone cancer treatment. Indeed, in a recent series, 11 men with various cancers, who had been treated with chemotherapy, were studied by FNA

mapping after no sperm was detected in the ejaculate (49). Residual spermatogenesis in the testis was detected in 8 of 11 (73%) men and subsequent pregnancies achieved by IVF and ICSI in six of the eight (75%) in this cohort. Thus, even men with no ejaculated sperm after chemotherapy for cancer are now candidates for biological paternity.

☐ PROMISING APPROACHES TO PRESERVING/RESTORING FERTILITY
Protecting the Testis Prior to Treatment

Since cancer therapy can deplete germ cells and cause infertility, studies have pursued ways to "protect" the delicate germ cells from such damage. In 1981, Glode et al. theorized that spermatogenesis might be slowed or suspended with hormones that suppress the hypothalamic–pituitary–gonadal axis (50). If this were done prior to chemotherapy for cancer, the testis might be protected from the devastating effects of chemotherapy on rapidly dividing germ cells. Since then, researchers have applied a variety of hormonal regimens, including estrogens, androgens, antiandrogens, gonadotropin-releasing hormone (GnRH) agonists, and GnRH antagonists in animal models to investigate this hypothesis. This research has met with varying levels of success in the preservation of the spermatogonial population in testes exposed to radiation or chemotherapeutic agents (51–56). Confounding variables have included (i) individual differences in the host response to cytotoxic agents, (ii) individual differences in the host response to "protective" hormonal manipulation, (iii) wide variability of hormonal regimens used for spermatogonial protection, (iv) lack of knowledge as to which germ cells types are affected by hormonal manipulation, and (v) variability in animal species studied. In the few studies with human subjects, the results have been largely disappointing (57,58). As these experiments are refined, however, it is conceivable that hormonal manipulation may emerge as a workable form of testis-protective therapy.

Restoring Spermatogenesis: Germ Cell Transplantation

An extremely exciting advance in the understanding of spermatogenesis may also have practical application for the restoration of spermatogenesis in men after cytotoxic cancer treatment: In an area of research termed "germ-cell transplantation," Brinster and Zimmerman successfully transplanted spermatogonial stem cells from fertile mice into genetically or chemically sterile mice (59). With the use of a genetics-based method to identify the donor germ cells, the authors were able to demonstrate colonization, active spermatogenesis, and sperm production of donor germ cells within recipient seminiferous tubules in a mouse–mouse model. Remarkably, offspring conceived by the recipient male mice were shown to be derived from donor germ cells (60). Further work has

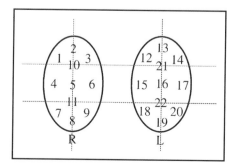

Figure 4 Testis fine needle aspiration "map" illustrating template of systematically placed sampling sites. Frequently, only a few sites might reveal sperm in men with testis failure. *Source*: From Ref. 48.

Table 4   Published Studies on Interspecies Germ Cell Transplantation

Study	Comment	Ref.
Hamster-to-mouse transplants	Hamster sperm found in all mice testes	(63)
	1–18% of the testis was colonized	
	Spermiogenic cells were visually abnormal	
Rabbit and dog-to-mouse transplants	Polyclonal antibody assay to detect donor cells	(64)
	Donor cells colonize and expand in mice (1 yr)	
	No postmeiotic donor cells seen	
Mouse-to-pig transplants	10/11 recipient testis had colonization (1 mo)	(65)
Boars-, bulls-, and stallion-to mouse transplants	Donor cells variably colonize and expand	(66)
	No postmeiotic donor cells seen	
Human-to-mouse transplants	73% of recipient testes were colonized (6 mo)	(67)
	No spermatogonial differentiation observed	

shown it is also possible to transplant rat spermatogonia into immunotolerant mouse testes (61), and that frozen–thawed germ cells can be transplanted from mice to mice (62). A current summary of studies that have used germ cell transplantation in other species, including humans, is given in Table 4 (63–67).

An innovative variation of germ cell transplantation involves grafting ectopic testis tissue from one species to another. Instead of using single dispersed cells, investigators have tried using intact testis to increase the "take" of donor cells in the recipient. Ectopic grafting of testis tissue has reportedly resulted in complete spermatogenesis when donor newborn mouse, rabbit, pig, and goat testes were transplanted subcutaneously into nude mice (68,69), and live progeny have resulted from tissue grafting with IVF–ICSI in animal models (69,70).

Despite the fact that interspecies transplantation of germ cells has encountered mixed success, the implications that arise from these studies are profound, as it may eventually be possible to biopsy and freeze normal testis tissue in men (or boys) before the initiation of cytotoxic cancer therapy and, subsequent to cure, perform an autologous transplant of thawed germ cells to repopulate the empty seminiferous tubules and reinitiate spermatogenesis and fertility.

Restoring Spermatogenesis: In Vitro Sperm Maturation

In another area of innovative research, several studies have attempted to develop in vitro culture systems that encourage spermatogenesis to proceed to completion (71,72). This technology may find future use in the preservation of testis tissue from prepubertal boys who are to receive potentially sterilizing cancer treatment. Fertility preservation may be possible if the explanted tissue can subsequently be "grown" in culture to the point of mature sperm development for use with IVF and ICSI.

□ CONCLUSION

Much progress is being made in the ability to preserve or restore fertility in males with cancer. Cancer treatment regimens are now taking quality-of-life issues such as future fertility into consideration during protocol redesign, including the reduction of chemotherapy doses or cycles and refinements in surgical techniques in order to preserve ejaculation. In addition, assisted reproduction has seen exciting advances with technology such as IVF and ICSI, so that men who were previously unable to have children because of the effects of cancer therapy are now enabled. Finally, exciting new technologies such as hormonal downregulation, germ cell transplantation, and in vitro sperm cell maturation are currently being studied with the promise of improving the odds of fertility in even more men who are currently unable to father children despite being cured of their cancers.

☐ REFERENCES

1. Robisin LL. Methodologic issues in the study of second malignant neoplasms and pregnancy outcomes. Med Pediatr Oncol Suppl 1996; 1:41–44.

2. Jaffe T, Kim ED, Hoekstra TH, et al. LI. Sperm pellet analysis: a technique to detect the presence of sperm in men considered to have azoospermia by routine semen analysis. J Urol 1998; 159(5):1548–1550.

3. Marmor D, Elefant E, Dauchez C, et al. Semen analysis in Hodgkin's disease before the onset of treatment. Cancer 1986; 57:1986–1987.

4. Turek PJ, Lowther DN, Carroll PR. Fertility issues and their management in men with testis cancer. Urol Clin N Am 1998; 25(3):517–531.

5. Nijman JM, Schraffordt Koops H, Kremer J, et al. Gonadal function after surgery and chemotherapy in men with stage II and III nonseminomatous testicular tumors. J Clin Oncol 1987; 5(4):651–656.

6. Jacobsen KD, Theodorsen L, Fossa SD. Spermatogenesis after unilateral orchiectomy for testicular cancer in patients following surveillance policy. J Urol 2001; 165(1):93–96.

7. Bohlen D, Burkhard FC, Mills R, et al. Fertility and sexual function following orchiectomy and 2 cycles of chemotherapy for stage I high risk non-seminomatous germ cell cancer. J Urol 2001; 165(2): 441–444.

8. Tal R, Botchan A, Hauser R, et al. Follow-up of sperm concentration and motility in patients with lymphoma. Hum Reprod 2000; 15(9):1985–1988.

9. Humpi T, Schramm P, Gutjahr P. Male fertility in long-term survivors of childhood ALL. Arch Androl 1999; 43(2):123–129.

10. Kenney LB, Laufer MR, Grant FD, et al. High risk of infertility and long term gondal damage in males treated with high dose cyclophosphamide for sarcoma in childhood. Cancer 2001; 91:613–621.

11. Siimes MA, Elomaa I, Koskimies A. Testicular function after chemotherapy for osteosarcoma. Eur J Cancer 1990; 26(9):973–975.

12. Ferreira U, Netto NR Jr, Esteves SC, et al. Comparative study of the fertility potential of men with only one testis. Scand J Urol Nephrol 1991; 25(4):255–259.

13. Richie JP. Clinical stage I testicular cancer: the role of modified retroperitoneal lymphadenectomy. J Urol 1990; 144(5):1160–1163.

14. Donohue JP, Foster RS, Rowland RG, et al. Nerve-sparing retroperitoneal lymphadenectomy with preservation of ejaculation. J Urol 1990; 144(2 Pt 1): 287–291.

15. Nelson JB, Chen RN, Bishoff JT, et al. Laparoscopic retroperitoneal lymph node dissection for clinical stage 1 nonseminomatous germ cell testicular tumors. Urology 1999; 54(6):1064–1067.

16. Janetschek G, Hobisch A, Peschel R, et al. Laparoscopic retroperitoneal lymph node dissection. Urology 2000; 55(1):136–140.

17. Clifton DK, Bremner WJ. The effect of testicular X-irradiation on spermatogenesis in man. J Androl 1983; 4(6):387–392.

18. Rowley MJ, Leach DR, Warner GA, et al. Effect of graded doses of ionizing radiation on the human testis. Radiat Res 1974; 59(3):665–678.

19. Hahn EW, Feingold SM, Simpson L, et al. Recovery from aspermia induced by low-dose radiation in seminoma patients. Cancer 1982; 50(2):337–340.

20. Senturia YD, Peckham CS, Peckham MJ. Children fathered by men treated for testicular cancer. Lancet 1985; 5(8458):766–769.

21. Meistrich ML. Relationship between spermatogonial stem cell survival and testis function after cytotoxic therapy. Br J Cancer Suppl 1986; 7:89–101.

22. Costabile A. The effects of cancer and cancer therapy on male reproductive function. J Urol 1993; 149(5 Pt 2): 1327–1330.

23. Hansen SW, Berthelsen JG, von der Maase H. Long-term fertility and Leydig cell function in patients treated for germ cell cancer with cisplatin, vinblastine, and bleomycin versus surveillance. J Clin Oncol 1990; 8(10):1695–1698.

24. DeSantis M, Albrecht W, Holtl W, et al. Impact of cytotoxic treatment on long-term fertility in patients with germ cell cancer. Int J Cancer 1999; 83(6):864–865.

25. Meistrich ML, Wilson G, Brown BW, et al. Impact of cyclophosphamide on long term reduction in sperm count in men treated with combination chemotherapy of Ewing and soft tissue sarcomas. Cancer 1992; 70(11): 2703–2712.

26. Hansen PV, Glavind K, Panduro J, et al. Paternity in patients with testicular germ cell cancer: pre-treatment and post-treatment findings. Eur J Cancer 1991; 27(11): 1385–1389.

27. Robbins WA, Meistrich ML, Moore D, et al. Chemotherapy induces transient sex chromosomal and autosomal aneuploidy in human sperm. Nature Gen 1997; 16:74–78.

28. Chatterjee R, Haines GA, Perera DMD, et al. Testicular and sperm DNA damage after treatment with fludarabine for chronic lymphocytic leukemia. Hum Reprod 2000; 15(4):762–766.

29. Marchetti F, Bishop JB, Lowe X, et al. Etoposide induces heritable chromosomal aberrations and aneuploidy during male meiosis in the mouse. Proc Natl Acad Sci USA 2001; 98(7):3952–3957.

30. Foo ML, McCullough EC, Foote RL, et al. Doses to radiation sensitive organs and structures located outside the radiotherapeutic target volume for four treatment situations. Int J Radiat Oncol Biol Phys 1993; 27(2):403–417.

31. Shapiro E, Kinsella TJ, Makuch RW, et al. Effects of fractionated irradiation on endocrine aspects of testicular function. J Clin Oncol 1985; 3(9):1232–1239.

32. Agarwal A, Tolentino MV, Sidhu RS, et al. Effect of cryopreservation on semen quality in patients with testicular cancer. Urology 1995; 46(3):382–389.

33. Padron OF, Sharma RK, Thomas AJ Jr, et al. Effects of cancer on spermatozoa quality after cryopreservation: a 12-year experience. Fertil Steril 1997; 67(2):326–331.

34. Bachtell N, Conaghan J, Turek PJ. The relative viability of human spermatozoa from the testis, epididymis and vas deferens before and after cryopreservation. Hum Reprod 1999; 14(12):101–104.

35. Houlgatte A, De la Taille A, Fournier R, et al. Paternity in a patient with seminoma and carcinoma in situ in a solitary testis treated by partial orchidectomy. Br J Urol Int 1999; 84(3):374–375.

36. Maneschg C, Rogatsch H, Neururer R, et al. Hobisch A. Follow-up of organ preserving tumor enucleation in testicular tumors. J Urol 2000; 163(suppl):642A.

37. van der Schyff S, Heidenreich A, Weibach L, et al. Organ preserving surgery in testicular cancer-long term results. J Urol 2000; 163(suppl):645A.

38. Silva PD, Larson KM, Van Every MJ, et al. Successful treatment of retrograde ejaculation with sperm recovered from bladder washings. A report of 2 cases. J Reprod Med 2000; 45(11):957–960.

39. Ohl DA. Electroejaculation. Urol Clin North Am 1993; 20(1):181–188.

40. Hultling C, Rosenlund B, Tornblom M, et al. Transrectal electroejaculation in combination with in-vitro fertilization: an effective treatment of anejaculatory infertility after testicular cancer. Hum Reprod 1995; 10(4): 847–850.

41. Schmiegelow ML, Sommer P, Carlson E, et al. Penile vibratory stimulation and electroejaculation before anticancer therapy in 2 pubertal boys. J Pediatr Hematol Oncol 1998; 20(5):429–430.

42. Nudell DM, Conaghan J, Pedersen RA, et al. Schriock ED, Turek PJ. The mini-MESA for sperm retrieval: a study of urological outcomes. Hum Reprod 1998; 13: 1260–1265.

43. Cha K-Y, Oum K-B, Kim H-J. Approaches for obtaining sperm in patients with male factor infertility. Fertil Steril 1997; 67(6):985–995.

44. Turek PJ, Givens CR, Schriock ED, et al. Testis sperm extraction and intracytoplasmic sperm injection guided by prior fine needle aspiration mapping in nonobstructive azoospermia. Fertil Steril 1999; 71(3): 552–558.

45. Kahraman S, Ozgur S, Alatas C, et al. Fertility with testicular sperm extraction and intracytoplasmic sperm injection in non-obstructive azoospermic men. Hum Reprod 1996; 11(4):756–760.

46. Tournaye H, Liu J, Nagy PZ, et al. Correlation between testicular histology and outcome after intracytoplasmic sperm injection using testicular spermatozoa. Hum Reprod 1996; 11(1):127–132.

47. Turek PJ, Cha I, Ljung B-M. Systematic fine-needle aspiration of the testis: correlation to biopsy and results of organ "mapping" for mature sperm in azoospermic men. Urology 1996; 49(5):743–747.

48. Turek PJ, Cha I, Ljung B-M, et al. Diagnostic findings from testis fine needle aspiration mapping in obstructed and non-obstructed azoospermic men. J Urol 2000; 163(6):1709–1716.

49. Master VA, Meng MV, Cha I, et al. Spermatogenesis after chemotherapy for cancer. J Urol 2000; 163(suppl):257.

50. Glode LM, Robinson J, Gould SF. Protection from cyclophosphamide induced testicular damage with an analog of gonadotropin-releasing hormone. Lancet 1981; 1(8230):1132–1134.

51. da Cunha MF, Meistrich ML, Nader S. Absence of testicular protection by a gonadotropin-releasing hormone analogue against cyclophosphamide-induced testicular cytotoxicity in the mouse. Cancer Res 1987; 47(4):1093–1097.

52. Velez de la Calle JF, Jegou B. Protection by steroid contraceptives against procarbazine-induced sterility and genotoxicity in male rats. Cancer Res 1990; 50(4): 1308–1315.

53. Kurdoglu B, Wilson G, Parchuri N, et al. Protection from radiation-induced damage to spermatogenesis by hormone treatment. Radiat Res 1994; 139(1): 97–102.

54. Meistrich ML, Parchuri N, Wilson G, et al. Hormonal protection from cyclophosphamide-induced inactivation of rat stem spermatogonia. J Androl 1995; 16(4): 334–341.

55. Meistrich ML, Wilson G, Ye W-S, et al. Hormonal protection from procarbazine-induced testicular damage is selective for survival and recovery of stem spermatogonia. Cancer Res 1994; 54(4):1027–1034.

56. Ward JA, Robinson J, Furr BJA, et al. Protection of spermatogenesis in rats from the cytotoxic procarbazine by the depot formulation of Zoladex, a gonadotropin-releasing hormone agonist. Cancer Res 1990; 50(3):568–574.

57. Johnson DH, Linde R, Hainsworth JD, et al. Effect of a luteinizing hormone releasing hormone agonist given during combination chemotherapy on post therapy fertility in male patients with lymphoma: preliminary observations. Blood 1985; 65:832–836.

58. Waxman JH, Ahmed R, Smith D, et al. Failure to preserve fertility in patients with Hodgkin's disease. Cancer Chemother Pharmacol 1987; 19(2):159–162.

59. Brinster RL, Zimmermann JW. Spermatogenesis following male germ-cell transplantation. Proc Natl Acad Sci USA 1994; 91(24):11298–11302.

60. Brinster RL, Avarbock MR. Germline transmission of donor haplotype following spermatogonial transplantation. Proc Natl Acad Sci USA 1994; 91(24): 11303–11307.

61. Clouthier DE, Avarbock MR, Maika SD, et al. Rat spermatogenesis in mouse testis. Nature 1996; 381(6581):418–421.

62. Avarbock MR, Brinster CJ, Brinster RL. Reconstitution of spermatogenesis from frozen spermatogonial stem cells. Nature Med 1996; 2(6):693–696.

63. Ogawa T, Dobrinski I, Avarbock MR, Brinster RL. Xenogenic spermatogenesis following transplantation of hamster germ cells to mouse testis. Biol Reprod 1999; 60:515–521.

64. Dobrinski I, Avarbock MR, Brinster RL. Transplantation of germ cells from rabbits and dogs into mouse testes. Biol Reprod 1999; 61(5):1331–1339.

65. Honaramooz A, Megee SO, Dobrinski I. Germ cell transplantation in pigs. Biol Reprod 2002; 66(1):21–28.

66. Dobrinski I, Avarbock MR, Brinster RL. Germ cell transplantation from large domestic animals into mouse testes. Mol Reprod Dev 2000; 57(3):270–279.

67. Nagano M, Patrizio P, Brinster RL. Long-term survival of human spermatogonial stem cells in mouse testes. Fertil Steril 2002; 78(6):1225–1233.

68. Honaramooz A, Snedaker A, Boiani M, et al. Sperm from neonatal mammalian testes grafted in mice. Nature 2002; 418(6899):778–781.

69. Shinohara T, Inoue K, Ogonuki N, et al. Birth of offspring following transplantation of cryopreserved immature testicular pieces and in-vitro microinsemination. Hum Reprod 2002; 17(12):3039–3045.

70. Schlatt S, Honaramooz A, Boiani M, et al. Progeny from Sperm Obtained after Ectopic Grafting of Neonatal Mouse Testes. Biol Reprod 2003; 68: 2331–2335.

71. Rassoulzadegan M, Paquis-Flucklinger V, Bertino B, et al. Transmeiotic differentiation of male germ cells in culture. Cell 1993; 75(5):997–1066.

72. Hue D, Staub C, Perrard-Sapori MH, et al. Meiotic differentiation of germinal cells in the 3 week culture of whole cell population from rat seminiferous tubules. Biol Reprod 1998; 59(2):379–387.

39

Treatment of Reproductive Dysfunction in Males with Spinal Cord Injury and Other Neurologically Disabling Diseases

Khashayar Hematpour
St. Luke's-Roosevelt Hospital Center, Columbia University College of Physicians and Surgeons, New York, New York, U.S.A.

Carol Bennett
Department of Urology, Greater Los Angeles VA Medical System and David Geffen School of Medicine, University of California, Los Angeles, California, U.S.A.

□ INTRODUCTION

Spinal cord injury (SCI) is a common, devastating condition that profoundly impacts the lifestyle of the affected individuals as well as their families. In the United States alone, 10,000 new cases are reported each year (1), of which 60% involve individuals aged 16 to 30 years. Further, the National Spinal Cord Injury Statistical Center has shown that approximately 82% of the 200,000 people in the United States who have SCI currently are men. Consequently, male sexual function and fertility are important areas that need to be addressed for these individuals. Only 5% of the men with SCI are likely to be able to achieve pregnancies with their partners without assistance (2). The two major reasons for this infertility following SCI are ejaculatory failure and poor semen quality (3–6).

□ EJACULATORY FAILURE

The ejaculatory process consists of three consecutive and possibly independently occurring phases: emission, which is the movement of the semen along the vas deferens to the posterior urethra; ejection, in which the sympathetic-mediated contraction of the posterior urethra and closure of the bladder neck occurs simultaneously with the rhythmic contraction of the bulbocavernosus, ischiocavernosus, and pelvic floor muscles, resulting in anterograde expulsion of the semen through the urethral meatus; and lastly, orgasm, which appears to be controlled centrally and is the least understood phase of ejaculation. (For further details on these physiologic processes, see the chapters within Part I.)

In general, any pharmacological agent or disease process that interrupts the aforementioned neurologic pathways can interfere with the peristaltic function of the vas deferens and closure of the bladder neck. After medications, however, the most common cause of ejaculatory failure is SCI (7). Other neurologic disorders, such as diabetes mellitus and multiple sclerosis, are also common causes. Retroperitoneal surgery may injure the sympathetic ganglia that control ejaculation, but current methods of nerve-sparing retroperitoneal lymph node dissection avoid this complication in the majority of patients (8,9). Typically, both ejaculation and orgasm are permanently lost in these patients. The result may be either failure of emission or retrograde ejaculation and, eventually, infertility. The majority of patients with complete SCI are unable to ejaculate. In fact, ejaculation is seen in less than 10 % of these cases, and spontaneous procreation without medical intervention is rare.

Absent ejaculation may be caused by either retrograde ejaculation or failure of emission. The complete absence of seminal fluid is called aspermia, and this disorder should be differentiated from azoospermia (absence of sperm in the seminal fluid). Other causes of aspermia include the psychologic disturbances associated with an inability to obtain orgasm.

□ POOR SPERM QUALITY

Ejaculate from patients with SCI is known to be poor in quality. Several studies have documented abnormal parameters in the semen analysis of these individuals, specifically with regard to poor sperm motility and viability. Brackett et al. (10) showed that sperm from spinal cord-injured men lose motility—particularly, linear motility—more rapidly than sperm from normal men. The same study demonstrated that despite the large proportion of dead sperm in the fresh ejaculates of the spinal cord-injured men, the rate of cell death is not faster than that of normal specimens. Interestingly, this is in contrast to a later study by Brackett et al. (11) that showed decreased sperm viability in this population.

Yet, despite these findings, sperm concentration is not reduced, and in fact, it has been reported as normal by several groups (5,12,13). One study even showed an increase in the sperm count of SCI patients (14). Other studies have suggested that seminal plasma is a major contributor to the semen abnormalities seen in these patients (15,16). Sperm motility of normal subjects was shown to decrease significantly when the sperm were exposed to seminal plasma obtained from spinal cord-injured patients. Conversely, when sperm from SCI patients were exposed to seminal plasma of normal individuals, they exhibited an increase in motility.

Currently, there is no generally accepted etiology for poor sperm quality in SCI patients that can completely explain all the abnormalities seen in the semen of these men.

Abnormal prostatic or secretory vesicle function, or both, may be the cause of these semen alterations. In this regard, Brackett et al. (15) have shown that sperm motility and viability are lower in ejaculated sperm versus aspirated sperm from the vas deferens. Similarly, Ohl et al. (14) found an abnormal pattern of sperm transport and storage in the seminal vesicles of men with SCI. Brackett et al. (15) demonstrated that men with SCI were shown to have elevated serum prostate-specific antigen and decreased seminal prostate-specific antigen compared with normal men. Additional animal studies have provided further evidence that alterations in the prostatic fluid constituents could be the result of changes in the autonomic innervation of this gland. It is possible that the inactivation of the seminal plasma motility inhibitor, a factor that originates from seminal vesicles and is supposed to be rapidly inactivated within a few minutes after ejaculation in normal men, is deficient in the seminal plasma of spinal cord-injured men (17).

This theory, however, is controversial. Although Randall et al. (18) showed that leukocyte concentrations were elevated in the semen of men with SCI when compared with controls, no signs of acute or chronic prostatitis were observed, casting doubt on the validity of the hypothesis that inflammation of the prostate is the source of seminal abnormalities.

Mallidis et al. (19) suggested that the basic defect in SCI patients could be the same as the defect in epididymal necrospermia (deficiency in epididymal sperm storage). Since both conditions have similar sperm qualities, in the first description of necrospermia, it was shown that frequent ejaculation (two ejaculations per day for five days) improves sperm motility and viability. This observation has led to the belief that frequent ejaculations will improve the quality of semen in SCI patients. Later studies, however, have shown that sperm quality of patients with SCI will continue to deteriorate over time, even with frequent ejaculations; thus, the previously observed improvement in sperm

quality with frequent ejaculations was considered to be temporary.

Subsequent studies in patients with SCI also showed that poor semen motility and viability could be the result of the collecting method used, for example, when a current is applied to the patient during electroejaculation (EEJ), which is a method for semen retrieval in these patients.

Semen abnormalities seen in SCI patients have also been attributed to many other factors, including testicular hyperthermia, possible changes in the hypothalamic–pituitary–testicular axis, and the excessive generation of reactive oxygen species (Table 1).

□ TREATMENT

The treatment of infertility in spinal cord-injured men may take one or more of several approaches: procedures to obtain sperm naturally through assisted ejaculation, the surgical retrieval of sperm, or procedures designed to assist in fertilizing the female egg (assisted reproductive techniques, or ART). This chapter will focus on the first group. (For further details on techniques for surgical retrieval of sperm and assisted reproductive techniques, see Chapters 33 and 37.)

Assisted Ejaculatory Procedures

Most individuals with a complete SCI cannot produce anterograde ejaculation either by masturbation or by sexual stimulation. This inability results from the traumatic interruption of the nerve pathways that control ejaculation. While spinal cord injuries at or below the level of T10 commonly lead to loss of erection and ejaculation, injuries above this level allow the spinal reflex arcs to remain intact, and thus the patients may be able to retain reflex erection, and, occasionally, ejaculation (20). Recently, the development and advancement of penile vibratory stimulation (PVS) and EEJ has significantly improved the outcome of treatment for ejaculatory dysfunction in spinal cord-injured men.

Table 1 List of the Postulated Mechanisms Contributing to Poor Sperm Quality in Spinal Cord-Injured Men

Sperm transport dysfunction in the seminal vesicles
Deficiency in epididymal sperm storage
Prostatic secretory dysfunction
Leukocytospermia
Retrograde ejaculation
Testicular hyperthermia
Reactive oxygen species generation
Changes in hypothalamic–pituitary–testicular axis
Elevation of TNF-α, IL-1β, and IL-6 in the seminal plasma
Recurrent urinary tract infection
Neurogenic bladder
Electrical stimulation
Sperm autoimmunity
General poor health

Abbreviations: IL, interleukin; TNF, tumor necrosis factor.

Penile Vibratory Stimulation

History

PVS was first introduced by Sobrero et al. (21) in 1965 as a method of inducing ejaculation in a group of normal men. The first therapeutic evaluation of PVS for ejaculatory failure in SCI patients was published by Brindley (20,22). In his initial studies, Brindley reported a success rate of 60% for inducing ejaculation in men with SCI. With current methods of vibratory stimulation, however, ejaculation can be produced in more than 80% of the cases, irrespective of patient age, level of injury, years since injury, and level of bladder management (23).

Procedure

PVS involves the stimulation of the penile dorsal nerve via the placement of a high-amplitude (1.5–2.5 mm) vibrating disc on the frenular region of the ventral penis for two minutes in order to induce ejaculation. If no ejaculation occurs, there will be a rest period of one to two minutes before the stimulation begins again. This stimulation leads to the activation of the ejaculatory reflex in the thoracolumbar area of the spinal cord. With this technique, ejaculation can be achieved in 83% of patients with cord lesions above T10. The required time to induce ejaculation by PVS in SCI patients ranges from 10 seconds to 45 minutes (24). It should be noted that the ejaculation may or may not be accompanied by an erection. During PVS, somatic reactions such as abdominal muscle contractions and leg spasms may also be seen. Although specially-designed equipment with specific vibration frequencies and amplitudes are available, many practitioners have found good results using the readily available vibrators intended for general use. In fact, it is possible that the wide range of reported ejaculation rates (19–91%) is attributable to the nonstandard design and output of these vibrators (25).

Indications

It is generally accepted that in order for PVS to be successful, the injury must have occurred above the thoracolumbar emission center, which lies between T10 and L2. Patients with lesions above the T10 spinal level generally have an intact ejaculatory reflex arc since the peripheral efferent nerves exiting from T10–L2 and S2–S4 are intact. The integrity of this reflex arc can be confirmed by the presence of an intact bulbocavernosus reflex and the ability to perform hip flexion, both of which predict successful ejaculation when sensory afferent input is increased to suprathreshold levels (26–30). Patients with spinal cord injuries involving the lower spinal cord or peripheral neural lesions resulting from, e.g., retroperitoneal surgery, are not likely to respond to vibratory stimulation (11).

Compared to EEJ (see below under "Problems"), PVS is generally safe, simple, inexpensive, and repeatable; it can be administered at home, and does not require anesthesia. PVS with vaginal insemination performed by the couple at home is a viable reproductive option for those SCI men with adequate semen parameters (29,31,32). Many investigators recommend that PVS should be the first-line treatment in patients with lesions above T10 (29). Brindley (22) reported 11 home pregnancies following PVS and vaginal self-insemination in 81 couples where the father had a complete or nearly complete spinal cord lesion. Recently, several additional pregnancies have been reported from PVS procedures combined with self-insemination at home. Most studies, however, have used multiple ovulation-induced cycles to achieve home pregnancies and that the overall pregnancy rate per couple ranged from 25% to 61% (29).

Problems

Occasionally, local skin abrasions may occur where the vibrator is applied to the skin. No further treatment is required other than the prevention of subsequent irritation. It should be noted, however, that in men with neurologic lesions above T6, the application of PVS may induce autonomic dysreflexia if they are prone to this condition (33). Lesions above T6 will disrupt the regulatory effects of higher sympathetic control centers in the brain; therefore, the spinal sympathetic neurons will function independently and elaborate an exaggerated and unopposed response (34). Men with a prior history of autonomic dysreflexia should be given pretreatment with 20 mg of sublingual nifedipine 15 minutes prior to the procedure. In the event of a sympathetic outflow (autonomic dysreflexia), termination of the procedure should be sufficient to break the response; however, it may be necessary to gain intravenous access in order to deliver sympatholytic agents.

Electroejaculation

History

EEJ is the word generally used to denote the acquisition of semen by electrical stimulation with the placement of electrodes inside the rectum. The name is somewhat misleading, however, as the semen is never actually ejaculated, but rather dribbles from the external urinary meatus without the force of ejection.

Electrical stimulation was first employed in an animal model in 1863 when Eckhardt applied an electrical current to the branches of the sacral nerves in dogs to induce penile erection (35). In 1936, Gunn was the first investigator who used electrical stimulation to produce actual ejaculation in sheep (36) with a rectal electrode and an alternation current of 50 cycles per second, electrically stimulating the seminal vesicles and vas deferens. EEJ in humans dates back to the work of Learmonth (37) and later Bucy et al. (38), who inserted a cystoscope into the male urethra while simultaneously stimulating the presacral nerves. On stimulation, the prostatic urethra became obscured by seminal-like fluid containing spermatozoa. In 1948, Horne et al. collected semen via electrical stimulation in 15 SCI patients with lesions lower than the level of C5.

The rates of successful seminal emission with EEJ range widely according to different studies, from 50%

to 70% (25) up to 80% to 100% (39–41). In general, EEJ produces an ejaculation in approximately 75% of the patients, regardless of whether the lesion is high or low, and complete or incomplete (20,24,25).

Procedure

EEJ is a reliable method of obtaining semen from men with anejaculation. The method has been modified over time in order to minimize the thermal and electrical damage to the rectal mucosa and adjacent reproductive structures. The procedure may be performed without anesthesia in spinal cord-injured patients who have complete cord lesions. In patients with incomplete cord lesions, who have some degree of pelvic sensation, however, general anesthesia is required (3).

First, the patient is put into a lithotomy position. A Foley catheter is inserted and the bladder is drained. A neutralizing solution is instilled into the bladder and the catheter is clamped off. Next, a rectoscopy is performed to ensure the health of the rectal wall. During the procedure, one must ensure that the Foley balloon remains tight against the bladder neck to prevent the semen from leaking into the bladder, as contact with the urine may adversely affect the sperm (41–44). The electrical probe is then placed inside the rectum and positioned toward the anterior rectal wall, adjacent to the area of the prostate gland and the seminal vesicles. The electrical stimulation is administered in a wave-like pattern, with the voltage increased in one-to-two-volt increments. The antegrade sample is milked out of the urethra. The probe is then removed and another rectoscopy is performed. The bladder is then drained, and a retrograde sample is collected. Both antegrade and retrograde samples are taken for analysis.

Until recently, a low level of electrical gradient was maintained between the voltage peaks and during ejaculation. More recently, it was suggested that interrupted current delivery appears to produce a more efficient ejaculate with more sperm available in the antegrade fraction (44). It was suggested that this change in current delivery may take advantage of the observed pressure differential of the internal and external sphincter, thus increasing the percent of antegrade semen obtained.

Indications

EEJ should be attempted as the second line of therapy in those patients who have failed to respond to PVS. It would, however, be appropriate to perform rectal probe EEJ as first-line therapy in patients with injury levels below T10 and/or lower extremity flaccidity (23). Since these patients have an impaired spinal reflex arc, PVS will not produce emission.

Patient age and the interval since injury have no effect on the outcome of EEJ. No historical feature is absolutely predictive of success or failure. Bladder management does have an effect on the success rate, with intermittently catheterized patients experiencing the best results. Patients with indwelling urethral catheters may perform poorly due to chronic urethritis,

prostatitis, and obstruction of the ejaculatory ducts. High-pressure reflex voiding also has a negative effect on outcomes that could be due to the reflux of urine into the ejaculatory ducts, seminal vesicles, and vas deferens, causing chronic inflammation (25).

As an additional benefit, Ohl et al. (25) reported a temporary reduction in lower extremity spasticity after EEJ. Although many patients appreciate this as a break from the bothersome spasm, this phenomenon potentially may cause a temporary urinary retention; thus, patients with spontaneous voiding need to be observed for urinary retention after EEJ.

Problems

It is rare not to be able to produce a semen sample from SCI men using the EEJ technique (25). The main reason for failure is usually related to abandonment of the procedure due to autonomic dysreflexia, the most worrying complication of the treatment.

As with PVS, EEJ may produce autonomic dysreflexia in men with SCI above T6 (33). This condition can present initially with headache, sweating, bradycardia, and elevated blood pressure, but may progress to life-threatening circulatory collapse and death. For this reason, heart rate and blood pressure need to be carefully controlled throughout the procedure in those prone to autonomic dysreflexia. Pretreatment of these patients with 10 to 20 mg of sublingual nifedipine 15 minutes before the procedure will usually allow EEJ to be performed safely (34).

If, however, autonomic dysreflexia should occur, the first step in its management is to sit the patient upright. This evokes an orthostatic drop in blood pressure (45). At the same time, any tight or restrictive clothing or devices should be removed. During treatment, blood pressure should be carefully monitored every two to five minutes. In many cases, draining the bladder alleviates the symptoms as well as the hypertension. If, after performing the steps outlined above, the systolic blood pressure is 150 mm Hg or greater, pharmacologic therapy should be undertaken.

There are few published studies evaluating antihypertensive therapy in patients with autonomic dysreflexia. In general, the best antihypertensive medications to use in this situation have a rapid onset and short duration of action. Oral nitrates and nifedipine (immediate-release form) are the most commonly used medications (46–48). In 1995, the Cardiorenal Advisory Committee of the Food and Drug Administration decided after a lengthy deliberation that sublingual nifedipine should not be approved for the treatment of hypertensive emergencies. A review of literature at that time revealed reports of serious adverse effects such as cerebrovascular ischemia, stroke, numerous instances of severe hypotension, acute myocardial infarction, conduction disturbances, fetal distress, and death (49). Despite this decision, the use of short-acting oral nifedipine for what is perceived as a hypertensive emergency remains widespread in the United States and indeed all over the globe (50).

Thus far, there have been no reported adverse events from the use of nifedipine in the treatment of autonomic dysreflexia (45); however, there have been such events in cases of hypertensive emergencies. Captopril is an alternative pharmacologic agent for the management of autonomic dysreflexia (51).

Pain described as a mild rectal discomfort during EEJ is experienced by some individuals with partially preserved rectal sensation. Brindley (20) reported that every patient who had pinprick sensation in the sacral or L4 or L5 dermatome was unable to tolerate EEJ. Those with intact sensation in the L1 to L3 dermatome were unpredictable in their tolerance.

Brindley (20) examined the rectal mucosa with a sigmoidoscope a few minutes after the procedure. The sites of stimulation were indistinguishable from the surrounding mucosa. He also reported blood staining of the next feces passed, in only 2 of 256 EEJs on 89 patients. Generally, no significant rectal mucosal injury has ever been noted in association with EEJ.

One of the major disadvantages of EEJ is that it must be performed in the physician's office due to the necessity of monitoring heart rate and blood pressure as well as performing anoscopy before and after the procedure.

Initial studies have suggested that the EEJ process itself might be harmful to the sperm (52–54). Other studies, however, have not supported this theory, and similar quality sperm is obtained after PVS (55,56).

Sperm Retrieval Techniques

All SCI patients who fail to produce semen after EEJ should be evaluated with a postprocedural urine specimen. The urine specimen is evaluated by centrifuging the urine for 10 minutes at 300 g or more. In patients with absent ejaculation, the finding of greater than 10 to 15 sperm per high-power field indicates retrograde ejaculation, and EEJ should be repeated. Prior to the EEJ procedure, the patient's bladder should be emptied of urine by a catheter to prevent urine from adversely affecting the retrograde ejaculate. A buffering medium can be instilled into the bladder before the procedure. After EEJ, the bladder should be catheterized again to empty the retrograde fraction (29). If no sperm are present, these patients should be evaluated for causes of azoospermia. Blood tests for hormonal profiles, including follicle-stimulating hormone (FSH), luteinizing hormone (LH), and testosterone are done to assess the testicular function. Similarly, ultrasonography of the testes, epididymes, and seminal vesicles may be used to evaluate for obstructive conditions, which could be treated with surgical retrieval of the sperm.

A few men will produce seminal fluid but are azoospermic. In these patients, especially if FSH is elevated and they have atrophic testes, testicular sperm extraction (TESE) is then performed (57,58). Conventional teaching has been that infertile men with azoospermia and a serum FSH greater than two to three times normal levels have severe testicular failure that is not amenable by any conventional therapy; however Kim et al. (59) noted that 30% of men who were previously advised against testicular biopsy if atrophy was present were able to initiate pregnancy by means of TESE with advanced micromanipulation techniques.

Vasal aspiration is performed in aspermic patients with normal testicular ultrasonography and endocrine profile or those with obstruction of the ejaculatory duct. Lewin et al. (60) successfully obtained sperm by this method in 100% of the cases. Another technique that has been employed for the retrieval of sperm in cases with obstruction is seminal vesicle aspiration (61,62).

Sperm may also be retrieved from the ductal system or from the testicular parenchyma. In contrast, only testicular sperm retrieval is applicable for azoospermic patients without an obstruction but with normal testicular function (63–67).

Microepididymal sperm aspiration (MESA) was first introduced to retrieve sperm in cases with obstructive azoospermia such as congenital bilateral absence of the vas deferens (68). Spermatozoa obtained by MESA with in vitro fertilization (IVF) have been used for more than 10 years (69). The fertilization and pregnancy rates with MESA and standard IVF, however, are low—not higher than 20% and 11%, respectively (68,69). The introduction of micromanipulation for assisted fertilization, however, has significantly improved the fertilization rate achieved using testicular spermatozoa with this method (70). (For further information on micromanipulation, see Chapter 37.) Ever since, new technologies of testicular sperm retrieval combined with intracytoplasmic sperm injection (ICSI) have been developed (71). Therefore, many patients with various pathologies of sperm production, including SCI leading to azoospermia, can be offered IVF. Although MESA and TESE are the most common retrieval procedures, percutaneous aspirating techniques are favored by some groups (72–74). Percutaneous epididymal sperm aspiration (PESA) is a less invasive technique (75). Pregnancy rates are likely comparable between open and percutaneous sperm retrieval techniques for patients with obstruction; however, many more sperm are retrieved by MESA than by PESA (76). Because excess sperm may be cryopreserved and used for subsequent IVF cycles, patients are likely to only need one MESA procedure, whereas multiple PESA procedures may be required for subsequent cycles.

Advantages and Disadvantages

A retrospective analysis by Pasqualotto et al. (77) showed no significant difference in the rate of fertilization or embryo transfer irrespective of the etiology of azoospermia (obstructive vs. nonobstructive) and the site of sperm retrieval (epididymal vs. testicular). Testicular sperm retrieval, however, resulted in both a lower pregnancy and a higher abortion rate than epididymal sperm retrieval. In an EEJ–ICSI cohort, Schatte et al. (78) reported a lower pregnancy rate than the 45% and 42% rates achieved with age-matched specimens obtained by MESA and TESE, respectively; however, the reason for the low pregnancy rates with sperm obtained by EEJ than with sperm resulting from normal ejaculation by patients with severe male factor infertility, epididymal aspiration, or testis biopsy remains unclear.

Further, it is unknown why there were no differences in fertilization rates between patients with obstructive (epididymal spermatozoa) and nonobstructive azoospermia (testicular spermatozoa), even though testicular spermatozoa were related to a higher abortion rate than epididymal spermatozoa. One explanation for the high abortion rate with testicular spermatozoa is that there may be severe impairment of spermatogenesis in these cases (79).

Donor Sperm Program

When the options for sperm retrieval techniques have been exhausted with no success, the patient and his partner may be counseled regarding the use of donor sperm. The donor is usually screened with a questionnaire and personal interview about any history of hereditary and sexually transmitted diseases. Blood tests are performed for blood type, Rh group, syphilis, hepatitis B surface antigen, and anti-human immunodeficiency virus antibodies. The semen samples are examined and cryopreserved. Six months after retrieval, blood tests are performed again for the latter three tests. If negative for infectious diseases, the semen is used for intrauterine insemination (IUI), IVF, or ICSI based on the sperm quality.

Assisting Oocyte Fertilization

Once sperm has been retrieved from the male patient, the next step in producing a successful pregnancy is the fertilization of the female oocyte. Several techniques now exist to achieve this goal.

Intrauterine Insemination
Indications
The first pregnancy achieved by combining EEJ and insemination was reported in 1975 by Thomas et al. (80), but the patient aborted spontaneously. The first live birth following treatment combining transrectal EEJ and IUI was reported by Bennett et al. in 1987. Standard insemination of the partners of spinal cord-injured men with the ejaculate obtained by either vibrator or EEJ has been shown to be unsuccessful because of the poor quality of the semen samples obtained (81). The more recently developed technique of IUI of washed and prepared semen is more successful. With this method, published pregnancy rates are between 5% and 9% per insemination cycle (81–83).

Outcomes
Traditionally, semen has been used for IUI with a relatively poor pregnancy rate of 2% to 36%, with most studies reporting figures of less than 10% (5,22,24,84–86). The low pregnancy rate achieved with sperm from these men is often attributed to poor semen quality. Although the semen of spinal cord-injured men typically contains a normal-to-high concentration of sperm, often low motility, poor viability, and perhaps other unidentified factors are present that are detrimental to sperm function (17,87,88).

In Vitro Fertilization

The combination of EEJ and IUI has given rise to several reports of successful pregnancies for couples in whom the male partner suffers from paraplegic anejaculation (3,89); however, it is common in such men for spermatozoal counts to be low and progressive motility to be poor, possibly because of either testicular hyperthermia or negative influences of the EEJ procedure on semen production. These factors reduce the success of timed IUI alone. IVF is a viable alternative for patients with anejaculation in whom IUI failed. Ayres et al. (6) reported the first successful application of IVF and embryo transfer in combination with EEJ in a couple with poor sperm quality.

Indications
Currently, most urologists perform vibratory stimulation or EEJ with four to six cycles of IUI before attempting IVF. Ohl suggested that it is cost-effective to bypass IUI and proceed directly to IVF with the spouse of men who require anesthesia for EEJ and who have a total inseminated motile sperm count less than 4 million. IVF has resulted in improved fertility rates in couples with anejaculation after multiple failed attempts at IUI (82). If the sperm sample produced by rectal probe EEJ is of poor quality but still has a sufficient number of motile and normal sperm cells, conventional IVF can be successful (90).

Many investigators have suggested that proceeding directly to IVF is more cost effective in the setting of severely reduced semen quality. Van Voorhis et al. (91) suggested that if the total motile sperm count was less than 10×10^6, IVF is more cost effective. Although there is no established threshold for a total motile sperm count below which IUI cannot be performed, the literature suggests that 5×10^6 to 10×10^6 is a safe estimate.

Outcomes
To improve pregnancy rates, IVF has been used with EEJ. Clinical pregnancy rates have been as high as 67% (32,43,78,85,90,92–95). To minimize the number of invasive procedures and the number of cycles of superovulation, a limited number of IUI procedures could be performed before proceeding to IVF. Alternatively, if the initial EEJ specimen was of very poor quality (e.g., a total motile sperm count less than 5×10^6), it would not be unreasonable to proceed directly to IVF.

Intracytoplasmic Sperm Injection

Subzonal sperm injection was the first gamete micromanipulation technique and was performed by either chemical or mechanical opening of the zona pellucida (Fig. 1) and the insertion of sperm under this layer (97,98). Subzonal insemination requires only a few spermatozoa but its success is highly dependent upon the ability of those spermatozoa to fuse with the oolemma. When this happens, penetration of more than one sperm cell often occurs, rendering the embryo genetically abnormal (99). Manipulation of the human fertilization process by deposition of a single sperm cell into the cytoplasm of the oocyte was preceded by experimental work in hamsters and mice using sperm nuclei and membrane relaxants (100,101).

Indications

The capability of injecting sperm directly into the cytoplasm of a human oocyte (bypassing the zona pellucida and oolemma), achieving decondensation and male pronucleus formation, has offered new possibilities for male gametes with poor motility and abnormal or absent acrosome (102,103). Studies by Palermo et al. (104) in which four human pregnancies were attained by ICSI also showed ICSI to have superior results to subzonal insemination. Schoysman et al. (105) were the first to report, in 1993, a successful fertilization and pregnancy after ICSI with spermatozoa obtained after TESE.

Since then, there has been a tendency to abandon the subzonal approach as the ICSI technique has become increasingly popular because of the higher

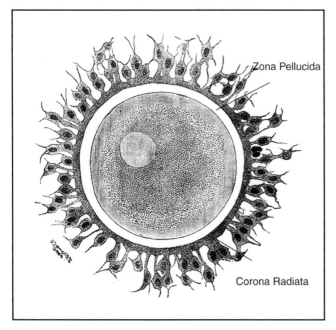

Figure 1 (*See color insert.*) Human ovum. The zona pellucida is seen as a thick clear girdle surrounded by the cells of the corona radiata. The egg itself shows a central granular deutoplasmic area and a peripheral clear layer, and encloses the germinal vesicle, in which is seen the germinal spot. *Source*: From Ref. 96.

fertilization rates (106). Since its introduction in 1992, ICSI has revolutionized the techniques of assisted reproduction and has become a popular fertilization procedure. The combined use of EEJ to overcome the barrier of sperm procurement and ICSI to overcome the functional deficiencies of electroejaculates has dramatically improved the prognosis of fertility in anejaculatory men (85). ICSI seems to be the only successful method of assisted reproduction in cases of severe male subfertility, in which low sperm count, extremely low motility, and poor morphology do not respond well to fertilization attempts by classic IVF. Even in cases of testicular failure, TESE can be used successfully to allow performing of ICSI (107). (For further details, see Chapters 25 and 33.)

In the presence of consistently poor semen samples, however, and in common with other (25,90,92), Brinsden et al. (94) opted for earlier recourse to IVF or ICSI in the presence of very poor samples. Another study performed by Schatte et al. (78) supports the use of ICSI after failed IUI in men with anejaculation who require EEJ. Brinsden et al. showed that early recourse to the use of the more sophisticated treatment methods, such as IVF and ICSI, is likely to achieve success for couples sooner than multiple attempts at simple insemination or even IUI. If semen quality after EEJ is consistently good, then up to three or four attempts at IUI may be recommended initially.

Outcomes

For spinal cord-injured patients with infertility secondary to nonobstructive azoospermia, no corrective treatment is available. ICSI, however, has enabled some of these couples to have genetic offspring using a small number of spermatozoa retrieved from the testicles. It seems that these patients have small foci of spermatogenesis in the testes, although they remain azoospermic overall. It is possible that a minimum quantitative threshold of spermatogenesis must be exceeded for any spermatozoa to reach the ejaculate, estimated at four to six mature spermatids per tubule (108).

Palermo et al. (109) demonstrated that ICSI results in higher fertilization and pregnancy in couples in whom sperm characteristics are severely impaired. The efficacy of this technique compares favorably with the rates of fertilization and pregnancies achieved with standard IVF in couples with no sperm abnormalities.

Despite the reported success with ICSI, no correlation has been found between sperm characteristics (density, motility, and morphology) and eventual fertilization after ICSI. Spermatozoa collected by epididymal aspiration (supposedly less mature) and those exposed to unfavorable conditions during collection by EEJ or after cryopreservation performed equally well with ICSI when compared with spermatozoa collected by masturbation. This fact raises the question of whether spermatozoon integrity is indeed necessary to achieve fertilization in humans.

Chung et al. (85) demonstrated that the use of ICSI for electroejaculates undoubtedly provides couples with anejaculation the highest chance of pregnancy as compared with standard IVF. Another advantage of this technique is that by use of ICSI, the number of necessary rectal probe EEJs is reduced—and, consequently (when indicated), the number of general anesthesia procedures.

With a poor sperm sample, cryopreservation is usually abandoned because motility is further impaired during freezing and thawing. Since ICSI does not depend on sperm motility, cryopreservation of poor semen is feasible (110). ICSI using previously frozen sperm achieves fertilization and pregnancy rates similar to those using fresh ejaculate.

Cryopreservation as a means of the storage of testicular spermatozoa is very important, because it allows the possible avoidance of a subsequent testicular biopsy if no pregnancy is achieved after a first ICSI cycle with fresh testicular spermatozoa. Particularly in patients with SCI who have nonobstructive azoospermia, cryopreservation can be of major benefit. De Croo et al. (111) showed that it is possible to achieve a high fertilization rate after ICSI with both fresh and frozen–thawed testicular spermatozoa, but implantation and live birth rates per transferred embryo are significantly lower after ICSI with frozen–thawed than with fresh testicular spermatozoa. In a study performed by Schwarzer et al. (112), there was no difference in the birth rates achieved with fresh and cryopreserved spermatozoa.

Many case reports on successful ICSI with frozen–thawed testicular spermatozoa have been published (113–115). Gil-Salom and coworkers (116) reported that the fertilization rate, embryo cleavage rate, and embryo quality after ICSI with fresh or frozen–thawed testicular spermatozoa were comparable in a group of 12 patients.

Although normal fertilization occurs in approximately 60% of surviving oocytes after ICSI, rare instances of abnormal fertilization may occur. Even though sperm dysfunction can be overcome by ICSI, the age of the female partner, as is seen in conventional IVF, continues to be a determinant in terms of pregnancy.

It is clear that for both MESA and TESE in combination with ICSI and the freezing of epididymal or testicular spermatozoa that remain after the injection with fresh collected spermatozoa is of benefit to the patient. Epididymal spermatozoa can be frozen more easily because of their higher concentration and motility compared with testicular spermatozoa. Imoedemhe et al. (117) indicated that the preservation of human sperm by air drying in the short term does not impair their ability to participate in pronuclear formation and development of cleavage state embryo. This cheap and simple sperm preservation technique requires further evaluation as it holds potential application in patients with transmissible viral conditions, such as HIV.

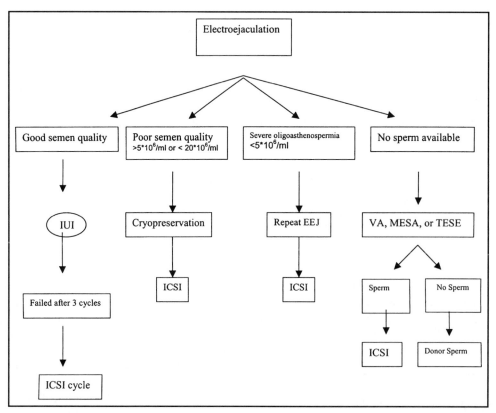

Figure 2 Algorithm for the selection of additional treatment after electroejaculation. *Abbreviations*: EEJ; electroejaculation; ICSI, intracytoplasmic sperm injection; IUI, intrauterine insemination; MESA, microepididymal sperm aspiration; TESE, testicular sperm extraction; VA, vasal aspiration.

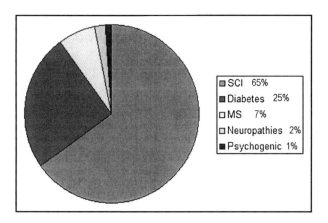

Figure 3 Different diseases that may benefit from ART due to anejaculation. *Abbreviations*: ART, assisted reproductive technology; MS, multiple sclerosis; SCI, spinal cord injury.

For the detection of viability of sperm of an immotile sample, pentoxifylline is added to the sperm suspension at a concentration of 3.5 mmol/L followed by incubation for 15 minutes at 37°C (117). The sample is then washed and centrifuged. Some sperm become motile, which facilitates recognition of viable sperm for ICSI.

It was proposed recently that by performing ICSI through a micro-hole, which is created by a laser beam on the zona pellucida, the damage to the oocyte or to its subcellular components may be reduced. As reported, laser-assisted ICSI can lead to more successful embryonic formation in selected patients with prior high oocyte degeneration rates. Nagy et al. (118) demonstrated that this technique may provide benefit to all patients requiring ICSI procedure (Figs. 2 and 3). (For further details on micromanipulation techniques, see Chapter 37.)

□ SUMMARY

Shieh et al. (119) designed a very comprehensive protocol for SCI patients who wanted to father a baby by using EEJ and assisted reproductive technology (ART). First, they performed EEJ twice with an interval of one month. Depending on the semen parameters, the

couples were counseled and treated with ART. A fair semen sample was considered to have a sperm concentration of 5×10^7/mL or more, progressive motility of 20% or higher, and normal morphology of 4% or higher by using Kruger's strict criteria (120). If at least one semen sample was considered fair, three cycles of IUI were suggested before entering into ICSI treatment (85,121). If both semen samples were poor, then ICSI was suggested. If no sperm were obtained from EEJ, the patient would be evaluated and surgical retrieval of the sperm was performed by using vasal aspiration, MESA, or TESE.

Candidates

Men with irreversible obstruction are candidates for MESA or TESE, both in conjunction with ICSI. In cases of nonobstructive azoospermia, TESE can also be used for sperm retrieval and subsequent ICSI.

Outcomes

In general, ICSI with spermatozoa from men with impaired semen quality achieves a delivery rate of up to 39% per cycle (122). Even in cases of azoospermia, ICSI can realize a couple's hopes of fertility. Men with normal spermatogenesis have good chances of achieving fertility. In contrast, patients with testicular lesions should be informed that their chances of achieving fertility are lower, and the probability of not detecting spermatozoa may be as high as 40%.

Schwarzer et al. (112) tried to evaluate the male factors relating to the outcome of ICSI. While it is well established that female partner's age is one of the most important prognostic factors (123), the age of the male partner did not seem to have an influence on birth rates.

□ CONCLUSION

In general, ICSI can be used successfully to treat couples who have failed IVF or who have too few spermatozoa for conventional methods of in vitro insemination. Sperm parameters do not clearly affect the outcome of this technique.

□ REFERENCES

1. Stover SL, DeLisa JA, Whiteneck GG. Spinal Cord Injury: Clinical Outcomes from the Model Systems. Gaithersburg, Maryland: Aspen Publishers Inc., 1995.

2. Mallidis C, Lim TC, Hill ST, et al. Collection of semen from men in acute phase of spinal cord injury. Lancet 1994; 343(8905):1072–1073.

3. Bennett CJ, Ayres JWT, Randolf JF Jr, et al. Electroejaculation of paraplegic males followed by pregnancies. Fertil Steril 1987; 48(6):1070–1072.

4. Bennett CJ, Seager SW, McGuire EJ. Electroejaculation for recovery of semen after retroperitoneal lymph node dissection: case report. J Urol 1987; 137(3): 513–515.

5. Bennett CJ, Seager SW, Vasher EA, et al. Sexual dysfunction and electroejaculation in men with spinal cord injury: review. J Urol 1988; 139(3):453–457.

6. Ayres JWT, Mionipanah R, Bennett CJ, et al. Successful combination therapy with electroejaculation and in vitro fertilization-embryo transfer in the treatment of paraplegic males with severe oligoasthenospermia. Fertil Steril 1988; 49(6):1089–1090.

7. Firisin WK, Rodriguez HF, Lynne C, et al. Severe male infertility associated with spinal cord injury (SCI) or extreme oligoasthenozoospermia (OAS) yields lower numbers of good quality embryos on day 3, but excellent pregnancy rates with blastocyst transfer. Fertil Steril 2002; 78(3) suppl 1:S191.

8. Foster RS, Bennett R, Bihrle R, et al. A preliminary report: postoperative fertility assessment in nerve-sparing RPLND patients. Eur Urol 1993; 23(1): 165–167.

9. Klein EA. Open technique for nerve-sparing retroperitoneal lyphadenectomy. Urology 2000; 55(1):132–135.

10. Brackett NL, Santa-Cruz C, Lynne CM. Sperm from spinal cord injured men lose motility faster than sperm from normal men: the effect is exacerbated at body compared to room temperature. J Urol 1997; 157(6): 2150–2153.

11. Brackett NL, Ferrell SM, Aballa TC, et al: an analysis of 653 trials of penile vibratory stimulation in men with spinal cord injury. J Urol 1998; 159(6):1931–1934.

12. Brackett NL, Nash MS, Lynne CM. Male fertility following spinal cord injury: fact and fiction. Phys Ther 1996; 76(11):1221–1231.

13. Linsenmeyer TA, Perkash I. Infertility in men with spinal cord injury. Arch Phys Med Rehabil 1991; 72(10): 747–754.

14. Ohl DA, Menge AC, Jarow JP. Seminal vesicle aspiration in spinal cord injured men: insight into poor semen quality. J Urol 1999; 162(11):2048–2051.

15. Brackett NL, Lynne CM, Aballa TC, et al. Sperm motility from the vas deferens of spinal cord injured men is higher than from the ejaculate. J Urol 2000; 163(3 Pt 1): 712–715.

16. Hirsch IH, Jeyendran RS, Sedor J, et al. Biochemical analysis of electroejaculates in spinal cord injured men: comparison to normal ejaculated. J Urol 1991; 145(1):73–76.

17. Brackett NL, Davi RC, Padron OF, et al. Seminal plasma of spinal cord injured men inhibits sperm motility of normal men. J Urol 1996; 155(5):1632–1635.

18. Randall JM, Evans DH, Bird VG, et al. Leukocytospermia in spinal cord injured patients is not related to histological inflammatory changes in the prostate. J Urol 2003; 170(3):897–900.

19. Mallidis C, Lim TC, Hill ST, et al. Necrospermia and chronic spinal cord injury. Fertil Steril 2000; 74(2): 221–227.

20. Brindley GS. Electroejaculation: its technique, neurological implications and uses. J Neurol Neurosurg Psychiatry 1981; 44(1):9–18.

21. Sobrero AJ, Stearns HE, Blair JH. Technique for the induction of ejaculation in humans. Fertil Steril 1965; 16(6):765–767.

22. Brindley GS. The fertility of men with spinal injuries. Paraplegia 1984; 22(6):337–348.

23. Nehra A, Werner MA, Bastuba M, et al. Vibratory stimulation and rectal probe electroejaculation as therapy for patients with spinal cord injury: semen parameters and pregnancy rates. J Urol 1996; 155(2): 554–559.

24. Shaban SF, Seager SW, Lipshultz LI. Clinical electroejaculation. Med Instrum 1988; 22(2):77–81.

25. Ohl DA, Bennett CJ, McCabe M, et al. Predictors of success in electroejaculation of spinal cord injured men. J Urol 1989; 142(6):1483–1486.

26. Piera JB. The establishment of a prognosis for genitosexual function in the paraplegic and tetraplegic male. Paraplegia 1973; 10(4):271–278.

27. National Spinal Cord Injury Statistical Center. Spinal cord injury: facts and figures at a glance. Birmingham, AL: National Spinal Cord Injury Statistical Center, July 1996. Information sheet.

28. Kamishke A, Nieschlag E. Update on medical treatment of ejaculatory disorders 1. Int J Androl 2002; 25(6):333–344.

29. Sonksen J, Ohl DA. Penile vibratory stimulation and electroejaculation in the treatment of ejaculatory dysfunction 1. Int J Androl 2002; 25(6):324–332.

30. Bird VG, Brackett NL, Lynne CM, et al. Reflexes and somatic responses as predictors of ejaculation by penile vibratory stimulation in men with spinal cord injury. Spinal Cord 2001; 39(10):514–519.

31. Rawicki HB, Hill S. Semen retrieval in spinal cord injured men. Paraplegia 1991; 29(7):443–446.

32. Ohl DA, Sonksen J, Menge AC, et al. Electroejaculation versus vibratory stimulation in spinal cord injured me: sperm quality and patient preference. J Urol 1997; 157(6):2147–2149.

33. Frankel HL, Mathias CJ. Cardiovascular aspects of autonomic dysreflexia since Guttmann and Whitteridge (1974). Paraplegia 1979; 17(1):46–51.

34. Steinberger RE, Ohl DA, Bennett CJ, et al. Nifedipine pretreatment for autonomic dysreflexia during electroejaculation. Urology 1990; 36(3): 228–231.

35. Eckhard C. Untersuchungen über die Erection des Penis beim Hunde. Beiträge zur Anat U Physiol 1863; 3:123–166.

36. Gunn RMC. Fertility in sheep, artificial production of seminal ejaculation and the characters of the spermatozoa contained therein. Bull Coun Sci Industr Res 1936:94.

37. Learmonth JR. Contribution to neurophysiology of urinary bladder in man. Brain 1931; 54:147–176.

38. Bucy PC, Huggins C, Buchanan DN. Sympathetic innervation of the external sphincter of the human bladder. Amer J Dis Child 1937; 54:1012–1015.

39. Lucas MG, Hargreave TB, Edmund P, et al. Sperm retrieval by electroejaculation. Preliminary experience in patients with secondary anejaculation. Br J Urology 1991; 67:191–194.

40. Matthews GJ, Gardner TA, Eid JF. In vitro fertilization improves pregnancy rates for sperm obtained by rectal probe ejaculation. J Urol 1996; 155(6):1934–1937.

41. Nehra A, Werner MA, Bastuba M, et al. Vibratory stimulation and rectal probe electroejaculation as therapy for patients with spinal cord injury: semen parameters and pregnancy rates. J Urol 1996; 155(2): 554–559.

42. Pagani RL, Lamb DJ, Lipshultz LI, et al. A multi-center study of the electroejaculation procedure. Fertil Steril 2001; 76(3) suppl 1:S40–S41.

43. Rutkowski SB, Geraghty TJ, Hagen DL, et al. A comprehensive approach to the management of male infertility following spinal cord injury. Spinal Cord 1999; 37(7):508–514.

44. Brackett NL, Ead DN, Aballa TC, et al. Semen retrieval in men with spinal cord injury is improved by interrupting current delivery during electroejaculation. J Urol 2002; 167(1):201–203.

45. Consortium for Spinal Cord Medicine. Acute Management of Autonomic Dysreflexia: Individuals with Spinal Cord Injury Presenting to Health Care Facilities (Clinical Practice Guideline). 2nd ed. Washington: The Consortium, Paralyzed Veterans of America, 2001.

46. Karlsson AK. Autonomic dysreflexia. Spinal Cord 1999; 37(6):383–391.

47. Naftchi NE, Richardson JS. Autonomic dysreflexia: pharmacological management of hypertensive crises in spinal cord injured patients. J Spinal Med 1997; 20(3):355–360.

48. Braddom RL, Rocco JF. Autonomic dysreflexia. A survey of current treatment. Am J Phys Rehabil 1991; 70(5):234–241.

49. Grossman E, Messerli FH, Grodzicki T, et al. Should the moratorium be placed on sublingual nifedipine capsules given for hypertensive emergencies and pseudoemergencies? JAMA 1996; 276(16):1328–1331.

50. Messerli FH, Grossman E. The use of sublingual nifedipine: a continuing concern. Arch Intern Med 1999; 159(19):2259–2260.

51. Blackmer J. Rehabilitation medicine: 1. Autonomic dysreflexia. CMAJ 2003; 169(9):931–935.

52. Linsenmeyer TA, Perkash I. Review article: infertility in men with spinal cord injury. Arch Phys Med Rehabil 1991; (10):747–754.

53. Rajasekaran M, Hellstrom WJ, Sparks RL, et al. Sperm-damaging effects of electric current: possible role of free radicals. Reprod Toxicol 1994; 8(5):427–432.

54. Sikka SC, Wang R, Kukuy E, et al. The detrimental effects of electric current on normal human sperm. J Androl 1994; 15(2):145–150.

55. Witt MA, Grantmyre JE, Lomas M, et al. The effect of semen quality of the electrical current and heat generated during rectal probe electroejaculation. J Urol 1992; 147(3):747–749.

56. Ohl DA, Denil J, Cummins C. Electroejaculation does not impair sperm motility in the beagle dog: a comparative study of electroejaculation and collection by artificial vagina. J Urol 1994; 152:1034–1037.

57. Negri L, Albani E, DiRocco M, et al. Testicular sperm extraction in azoospermic men submitted to bilateral orchidopexy. Hum Reprod 2003; 18(12): 2534–2539.

58. Jezek D, Knuth UA, Schulze W. Successful testicular sperm extraction (TESE) in spite of high serum follicle stimulating hormone and azoospermia: correlation between testicular morphology, TESE results, semen analysis and serum hormone values in 103 infertile men. Hum Reprod 1998; 13(5): 1230–1234.

59. Kim ED, Gilbaugh JH, Patel VR. et al. Testis biopsies frequently demonstrate sperm in men with azoospermia and significantly elevated follicle-stimulating hormone levels. J Urol 1997; 157(1):144.

60. Lewin A, Reubinoff B, Porat-Katz A, et al. Testicular fine needle aspiration: the alternative method for sperm retrieval in non-obstructive azoospermia. Hum Reprod 1999; 14(7):1785–1790.

61. Hovatta O, Reima I, Foudila T, et al. Vas deferens aspiration and intracytoplasmic injection of frozen-thawed spermatozoa in a case of anejaculation in a diabetic man. Hum Reprod 1996; 11(2):334–335.

62. Jarow JP. Seminal vesicle aspiration of fertile men. J Urol 1996; 156(3):1005–1007.

63. Belker AM, Sherins RJ, Dennison-Lagos L, et al. Percutaneous testicular sperm aspiration: a convenient and effective office procedure to retrieve sperm for in vitro fertilization with intracytoplasmic sperm injection. J Urol 1998; 160(6 Pt 1):2058–2062.

64. Schlegel PN. Testicular sperm extraction: microdissection improves sperm yield with minimal tissue excision. Hum Reprod 1999; 14(1):131–135.

65. Turek PJ, Cha I, Ljung BM. Systematic fine-needle aspiration of the testis: correlation to biopsy and results

of organ "mapping" for mature sperm in azoospermic men. Urology 1997; 49(5):743–748.

66. Silber SJ. Microsurgical TESE and the distribution of spermatogenesis in non-obstructive azoospermia. Hum Reprod 2000; 15(11):2178–2184.

67. Ezeh UI, Moore HD, Cooke ID. A prospective study of multiple needle biopsies versus a single open biopsy for testicular sperm extraction in men with non-obstructive azoospermia. Hum Reprod 1998; 13(11): 3075–3080.

68. Silber SJ, Balmaceda J, Borrero C, et al. Pregnancy with sperm aspiration from the proximal head of the epididymis: a new treatment for congenital absence of the vas deferens. Fertil Steril 1988; 50(3):525–528.

69. Temple-Smith PD, Southwick GJ, Yates CA, et al. Human pregnancy by in vitro fertilization (IVF) using sperm aspirated from the epididymis. J In Vitro Fertil Embryo Transfer 1985; 2(3):119–122.

70. Schoysman R, Bertin G, Vanderzwalmen P, et al. Utilisation du sperme epididymaire dans un programme de fecondation in vitro. Prog Androl 1990; 3: 137–134.

71. Silber SJ, Nagy ZP, Liu J, et al. Conventional in-vitro fertilization versus intracytoplasmic sperm injection for patients requiring microsurgical sperm aspiration. Hum Reprod 1994; 9(9):1705–1709.

72. Craft I, Tsirigotis M, Bennet V, et al. Percutaneous epididymal sperm aspiration and intracytoplasmic sperm injection in the management of infertility due to obstructive azoospermia. Fertil Steril 1995; 63(5): 1038–1042.

73. Levine LA, Lisek EW. Successful sperm retrieval by percutaneous epididymal and testicular sperm aspiration. J Urol 1998; 159(2):437–440.

74. Elliott SP, Orejuela F, Hirsch IH, et al. Testis biopsy findings in the spinal cord injured patient. J Urol 2000; 163(3):792–795.

75. Craft IL, Khalifa Y, Boulos A, et al. Factors influencing the outcome of in-vitro fertilization with percutaneous aspirated epididymal spermatozoa and intracytoplasmic sperm injection in azoospermic men. Hum Reprod 1995; 10(7):1791–1794.

76. Sheynkin YR, Ye Z, Menendez S, et al. Controlled comparison of percutaneous and microsurgical sperm retrieval in men with obstructive azoospermia. Hum Reprod 1998; 13(11):3086–3089.

77. Pasqualotto FF, Rossi-Ferragut LM, Rocha CC, et al. Outcome of in vitro fertilization and intracytoplasmic injection of epididymal and testicular wperm obtained from patients with obstructive and nonobstructive azoospermia. J Urol 2002; 167(4):1753–1756.

78. Schatte EC, Orejuela FJ, Lipshultz LI, et al. Treatment of infertility due to anejaculation in the male with electrejaculation and antracytoplasmic sperm injection. J Urol 2000; 163(6):1717–1720.

79. Martin RH, Greene C, Rademaker A, et al. Chromosome analysis of spermatozoa extracted from testes of men with non-obstructive azoospermia. Hum Reprod 2000; 15(5):1121–1124.

80. Thomas RJ, McLeish G, McDonald IA. Electroejaculation of paraplegic male followed by pregnancy. Med J Aust 1975; 2(21):789–789.

81. Rizk B, Doyle P, Tan SL, et al. Perinatal outcome and congenital malformations in in-vitro fertilization babies from the Bourn-Hallam group. Hum Reprod 1991; 6(9):1259–1264.

82. Toledo AA, Tucker MJ, Bennett JK, et al. Electroejaculation in combination with in vitro fertilization and gamete micromanipulation for treatment of anejaculatory male infertility. Am J Obstet Gynecol 1992; 167(2):322–325.

83. Ohl DA, Sonksen J. What are the chances of infertility and should sperm be banked? Semin Urol Oncol 1996; 14:36–44.

84. Chung PH, Verkauf BS, Mola R, et al. Correlation between semen parameters of electroejaculates and achieving pregnancy by intrauterine insemination. Fertil Steril 1997; 67(1):129–132.

85. Chung PH, Palermo G, Schlegel PN, et al. The use of intracytoplasmic sperm injection with electroejaculation from anejaculatory men. Hum Reprod 1998; 13(7):1854–1858.

86. Hurd WW, Randolph JF Jr, Ansbacher R, et al. Comparison of intracervical, intrauterine, and intratubal techniques for donor insemination. Fertil Steril 1993; 59(2):339–342.

87. Hirsch IH, McCue P, Allen J, et al. Quantitative testicular biopsy in spinal cord injured men: comparison to fertile controls. J Urol 1991; 146(2):337–341.

88. Denil J, Ohl DA, Menge AC, et al. Functional characteristics of sperm obtained by electroejaculation. J Urol 1992; 147(1):69–72.

89. Leeton J, Yates C, Rawicki B. Successful pregnancy using known donor oocytes fertilized in vitro by spermatozoa obtained by electroejaculation from a quadriplegic husband. Hum Reprod 1991; 6(3):384–385.

90. Hultling C, Rosenlund B, Tornblom M, et al. Transrectal electroejaculation in combination with in-vitro fertilization: an effective treatment of anejaculatory infertility after testicular cancer. Hum Reprod 1995; 10(4): 847–850.

91. Van Voorhis BJ, Barnett M, Sparks AE, et al. Effect of the total motile sperm count on the efficacy and cost-effectiveness of intrauterine insemination and in vitro fertilization. Fertil Steril 2001; 75(4): 661–668.

92. Denil J, Kupker W, Al-Hasani S, et al. Successful combination of transrectal electroejaculation and intracytoplasmic sperm injection in the treatment of anejaculation. Hum Reprod 1996; 11(6):1247–1249.

93. Kiekens C, Spiessens C, Duyck F, et al. Pregnancy after electroejaculationin combination with intracytoplasmic sperm injection in a patient with idiopathic anejaculation. Fertil Steril 1996; 66(5):834–836.

94. Brinsden PR, Avery SM, Marcus S, et al. Transrectal electroejaculation combined with in-vitro fertilization: effective treatment of anejaculatory infertility due to spinal cord injury. Hum Reprod 1997; 12(12): 2687–2692.

95. Rosenlund B, Westlander G, Wood M, et al. Sperm retrieval and fertilization in repeated percutaneous epididymal sperm aspiration. Hum Reprod 1998; 13(1):2805–2807.

96. Gray H (1821–1865). The ovum. Anatomy of the Human Body. 1918. Accessed online at <URL>www.bartleby.com</URL>, 2006.

97. Gordon JW, Grunfeld L, Garrisi GJ, et al. Fertilization of human oocytes by sperm from infertile males after zona pellucida drilling. Fertil Steril 1988; 50(1):68–73.

98. Malter HE, Cohen J. Partial zona dissection of the human oocyte: a nontraumatic method using micro-manipulation to assist zona pellucida penetration. Fertil Steril 1989; 51(1):139–148.

99. Cohen J, Alikani M, Malter HE, et al. Partial zona dissection or subzonal sperm insertion: microsurgical fertilization alternatives based on evaluation of sperm and embryo morphology. Fertil Steril 1991; 56(4): 696–706.

100. Uehara T, Yanagimachi R. Microsurgical injection of spermatozoa into hamster eggs with subsequent trans-formation of sperm nuclei into male pronuclei. Biol Reprod 1976; 15(4):467–470.

101. Market CL. Fertilization of mammalian eggs by sperm injection. J Exp Zool 1983; 228(2):195–201.

102. Lanzendorf SE, Maloney MK, Veeck LL, et al. A preclinical evaluation of pronuclear formation by microinjection of human spermatozoa into human oocytes. Fertil Steril 1988; 49(5):835–842.

103. Lanzendorf S, Maloney M, Ackerman S, et al. Fertili-zing potential of acrosome-defective sperm following microsurgical injection into eggs. Gamete Res 1988; 19(4):329–337.

104. Palermo G, Joris H, Devroey P, et al. Pregnancies after intracytoplasmic injection of a single spermatozoon into an oocyte. Lancet 1992; 340(8810):17–18.

105. Schoysman R, Vanderzwalmen P, Nijs M, et al. Pregnancy after fertilization with human testicular spermatozoa. Lancet 1993; 342(8881):1237.

106. Palermo GD, Schlegel PN, Sills ES, et al. Births after intracytoplasmic injection of sperm obtained by testic-ular extraction from men with nonmosaic Klinefelter's syndrome. N Engl J Med 1998; 338(9):588–590.

107. Devroy P, Nagy P, Tournaye H, et al. Outcome of intracytoplasmic sperm injection with testicular spermatozoa in obstructive and non-obstructive azoospermia. Hum Reprod 1996; 1(5):1015-1018.

108. Silber SJ, Nagy Z, Devroey P, et al. Distribution of spermatogenesis in the testicles of azoospermic men: the presence or absence of spermatids in the testes of men with germinal failure. Hum Reprod 1997; 12(11): 2422–2428.

109. Palermo GD, Cohen J, Alikani M, et al. Intracytoplasmic sperm injection: a novel treatment for all forms of male factor infertility. Fertil Steril 1995; 63(6): 1231–1240.

110. Chen SU, Shieh JY, Wang YH, et al. Pregnancy achieved by intracytoplasmic sperm injection using cryopreserved vassal-epididymal sperm from a man with spinal cord injury. Arch Phys Med Rehabil 1998; 79(2): 218–221.

111. De Croo I, Van der Elst J, Everaert K, et al. Fertilization, pregnancy and embryo implantation rates after ICSI with fresh or frozen-thawed testicular spermatozoa. Hum Reprod 1998; 13(7):1893–1897.

112. Schwarzer JU, Fiedler K, Hertwig IV, et al. Male factors determining the outcome of intracytoplasmic sperm injection with epididymal and testicular spermatozoa. Andrologia 2003; 35(4):220–226.

113. Graham F, Fisher R, Peck J. Intracytoplasmic sperm injection. NZ Med J 1996; 109(1029):345.

114. Hovatta O, Foudila T, Siegberg R, et al. Pregnancy resulting from intracytoplasmic injection of spermato-zoa from a frozen-thawed testicular biopsy specimen. Hum Reprod 1996; 11(11):2472–2473.

115. Khalifeh FA, Sarraf M, Dabit ST. Full-term delivery following intracytoplasmic sperm injection with sper-matozoa extracted from frozen-thawed testicular tissue. Hum Reprod 1997; 12(1):87–88.

116. Romero J, Remohi J, Minguez Y, et al. Fertilization after intracytoplasmic sperm injection with cryopre-served testicular spermatozoa. Fertil Steril 1996; 65(4):877–879.

117. Imoedemhe DA, Chan RC, Ramadan IA, et al. Changes in follicular fluid gas and pH during carbon dioxide pneumoperitoneum for laparoscopic aspiration and their effect on human oocyte fertilizability. Fertil Steril 1993; 59(1):177–182.

118. Nagy ZP, Oliveira SA, Abdelmassih V, et al. Novel use of laser to assist ICSI for patients with fragile oocytes: a case report. Reprod Biomed Online 2002; 4(1): 27–31.

119. Shieh JY, Chen SU, Wang YH, et al. A protocol of elec-troejaculation and systematic assisted reproductive technology achieved high efficiency and efficacy for pregnancy for anejaculatory men with spinal cord injury. Arch Phys Med Rehabil 2003; 84(4):535–540.

120. Check JH, Adelson HG, Schubert BR, et al. Evaluation of sperm morphology using Kruger's strict creiteria. Arch Androl 1992; 28(1):15–17.

121. Yang YS, Chen SU, Ho HN, et al. Correlation between sperm morphology using strict criteria in original semen and swim-up inseminate and human in vitro fertilization. Arch Androl 1995; 34(2):105–113.

122. Palermo GD, Neri QV, Hariprashad JJ, et al. ICSI and its outcome. Semin Reprod Med 2000; 18(2):161–169.

123. Nygren K, Andersen A. Assisted reproductive tech-nology in Europe. Results generated from European registers by ESHRE. Hum Reprod 2001; 16(2): 384–391.

Part V

Mass Lesions of the Male Reproductive System

The goal of this volume has been to review the entire spectrum of male reproductive dysfunction; however, the extremely complex subject of mass lesions of the male reproductive tract could be in itself an entire textbook. What further differentiates these lesions from the other pathologies discussed previously is that not only can malignancy impact the integrity of reproductive function, but its very presence often threatens life. Thus, the treatment of malignant lesions is focused primarily on saving the life of the individual, rather than preserving reproductive and sexual function. Therefore, the mass lesions of the male reproductive system have been allotted their own dedicated section so that the pathophysiology, diagnosis, and management of these diseases may be discussed in a unified manner for the sake of completeness, with the particular goal of addressing reproductive concerns that may arise during or in the aftermath of cancer treatment that may not be covered elsewhere.

Testicular and Penile Cancer

John W. Davis
Department of Urology, The University of Texas M.D. Anderson Cancer Center, Houston, Texas, U.S.A.

Donald F. Lynch
Department of Urology, East Virginia Medical School, Norfolk, Virginia, U.S.A.

Paul F. Schellhammer
Department of Urology, Eastern Virginia Medical School, Norfolk, Virginia and Prostate Cancer Center, Sentara Cancer Institute, Hampton, Virginia, U.S.A.

☐ TESTICULAR CANCER

Testis cancer is a rare disorder that mostly affects young males. In 2006, there will be an estimated 8250 new cases and an estimated 370 deaths in the United States (1). In Caucasian men aged 20 to 34 years, however, it has the distinction of being the most common solid tumor (2). Most testis cancers are germ-cell tumors (GCTs) and they have received significant attention from the medical community, despite their rarity, due to several features: the array of pathologic subtypes, the ability of multimodal therapy to cure metastatic disease, and the successful design and execution of multimodal clinical trials to refine treatment regimens. As a result, in the past few decades, testis cancer has gone from being a highly lethal disease to one in which multimodal therapies can provide over 99% cure rates for low-stage disease and over 70% cure rates for metastatic disease. These excellent survival statistics, plus the fact that surgical, radiation therapy, and chemotherapy treatments are being applied to a population of young men, makes GCTs a fascinating area of research. In addition to survival, quality of life, fertility, secondary cancers, and side effects of treatment are all important end points of the study.

Table 1 lists 10 "classic" papers in the history of testis cancer that demonstrate this revolution in cancer treatment.

Epidemiology and Risk Factors for GCT

The incidence of GCT is rising worldwide, but no definitive explanation has been provided (4). Reviews of the 1990s SEER data (5), a military cohort (6), and a cohort study from 1973 to 1995 (7) confirm that the incidence of GCT is rising and that the peak age at diagnosis has decreased.

Numerous explanations for the rising incidence of GCTs have been proposed (4). Although GCTs have been increasing, sperm counts have been purportedly decreasing. Testis atrophy may be a risk factor whereby increased serum follicle-stimulating hormone (FSH) production leads to clonal evolution from carcinoma-in-situ (CIS) to seminoma to nonseminoma. Wanderas et al. (8) found that elevated levels of FSH after orchiectomy predicted increased risk of contralateral GCT. Postpubertal endocrine effects may also contribute, as studies have correlated earlier sexual activity with earlier peak age incidence. Other epidemiological factors described include intrauterine estrogen excess, gonadal heat exposure, trauma, and mumps (4).

The most recognized risk factor for GCT is a history of cryptorchidism. Patients with a history of cryptorchidism have up to a tenfold increased risk of GCT, and 10% of patients with GCT have previously suffered from this condition (9). Abdominal cryptorchidism is associated with a higher risk of nonseminoma germ-cell tumor (NSGCT) compared to inguinal cryptorchism (4). Successful orchiopexy to the scrotum allows for easier physical examination and detection of GCT in an adult but is not known to alter the risk of GCT in men compared to those with no history of cryptorchidism unless corrected before puberty (10).

AIDS is a risk factor for GCT. Testicular tumors are the third most common AIDS-related malignancy after non-Hodgkins lymphoma and Kaposi's sarcoma (11). An increased proportion of seminomas have been reported (12), and increased incidence of bilateral disease with different histology has been reported (13). Immunosuppression may play a role, as organ transplant recipients have 20 to 50 times greater risk of GCT compared to the general male population (13).

Prevention and Screening for GCT

Currently, no dietary or pharmacologic preventive measures are available for GCT. The low prevalence combined with the successful results of treatment for early- and late-stage disease will likely make any mass screening for GCT impractical. Nevertheless, the testes are readily amenable to self-examination and self-referral for the evaluation of a suspicious mass. Both testis and penile cancers are commonly associated with delayed presentation to a physician—likely due to embarrassment and/or lack of awareness of the disease. Therefore, young men should be counseled to perform regular testicular self-examinations and to seek early evaluation for a mass or swelling.

Work-Up of a Solid Testicular Mass

Testis tumors are most often asymptomatic. Patients may infrequently report local symptoms such as a change in size, the presence of pain, or a history of trauma. Symptoms of metastatic disease may include shortness of breath, weight loss, fatigue, abdominal pain or distention, or tender breasts. GCT usually presents as an asymptomatic enlarged testis, and approximately 25% report a dull pain, usually due to hemorrhage and/or infarction (14). If testis pain is the chief complaint, however, the diagnoses of testicular torsion, infection, or infarction are all more likely than that of a tumor.

GCTs are right sided in 53% of cases, left sided in 44%, and bilateral in 0.4% (15). Testicular lymphoma is the most likely diagnosis if the patient is older (greater than 60 years of age) and has bilateral tumors (16). The testis should be examined by gentle palpation between the thumb and two forefingers and should be differentiated from the epididymis. Any solid mass distinctly localized to the testis is highly suspicious of cancer, unless it can be readily explained by infection or recent trauma. If a hydrocele is present, scrotal ultrasound can provide diagnostic information. Some metastatic testis cancers—especially choriocarcinoma—may have a "burned-out" testis lesion that is nonpalpable but evident on ultrasound and histopathology.

Standard blood counts, urinalysis, and serum electrolytes should be obtained to rule out other conditions. Three serum tumor markers, although not sensitive enough for screening use, are a part of the work-up:

- Beta-human chorionic gonadotropin (β-hCG) is secreted by syncytiotrophoblast cells and elevations occur in 40% to 60% of all GCTs: 100% with choriocarcinoma, 80% with embryonal tumors, and 10% to 25% with seminoma (17).
- Alpha fetoprotein (AFP) is associated with yolk sac and embryonal tumors, but not seminoma or choriocarcinoma (17). Its elevation occurs in 50% to 70% of GCTs and excludes the diagnosis of a pure seminoma (even if only seminoma is seen in the orchiectomy specimen), thereby directing therapy toward nonseminomatous GCT.
- Lactate dehydrogenase elevation may indicate bulky, advanced disease or relapse.

Ultrasound of the scrotum is a highly sensitive diagnostic tool for the work-up of most scrotal pathology. Imaging patterns can be diagnostic for solid versus cystic masses. Doppler imaging can differentiate low blood-flow patterns consistent with torsion from high blood-flow patterns consistent with epididymo-orchitis (18). With testis tumors, histologic subtype can be suggested. Seminomas tend to be homogenous, hypoechoic, intratesticular lesions, whereas nonseminomatous subtypes tend to have more cystic, calcified, and inhomogeneous areas, often due to hemorrhage. (For further information, please refer to Chapter 28.)

Radical Orchiectomy and Further Staging

At the conclusion of the work-up of a testicular mass, if other pathologies such as torsion, orchitis, and trauma are readily excluded, the patient with a solid mass is then assumed to have a tumor until proven otherwise. Due to the drainage of testicular lymphatics along their embryologic origins into the retroperitoneum, radical inguinal orchiectomy is the procedure of choice. Scrotal skin lymphatics drain to the inguinal areas; because a scrotal incision for testis cancer risks contaminating these lymphatics, this approach is contraindicated. If a patient is explored scrotally and a tumor is incidentally found, the patient may suffer no adverse effects if tumor spillage is avoided. Subsequent therapy for tumor spillage usually requires chemotherapy (19). By the same rationale, if a patient has a history of herniorrhaphy, orchiopexy, or other alteration in lymphatic drainage, subsequent radiation for stage I seminoma may include the ipsilateral inguinal region with testis shielding (20).

During inguinal exploration, it is sometimes reasonable to obtain frozen section biopsy of the tumor if trauma or a benign tumor is strongly suspected. For the majority, GCT is suspected, and the inguinal cord and vas deferens are separately ligated high and preferably above the internal inguinal ring. It is useful to leave a long nonabsorbable suture on the patient side of the cord, as this remaining stump of cord will need to be removed from the abdominal side if a retroperitoneal lymph node dissection (RPLND) is subsequently performed.

Even before a tissue diagnosis and staging are obtained, fertility and prosthesis questions may arise. Many patients with GCT are subfertile at diagnosis. If a patient is found to have severe oligospermia, Baniel et al. (21) have described sperm aspiration from the vas at the time of orchiectomy. Intracytoplasmic sperm injection (ICSI) was subsequently performed in two couples, and one delivered a healthy infant. (For further information on this topic, please refer to Chapter 33). Silicon testicular prostheses have been available in the past, but were removed from clinical application due to the problems associated with silicone breast implants. Saline-filled implants were recently approved by the FDA.

Staging work-up is completed by chest X ray (CXR) and computed tomography (CT) scanning of the abdomen. CT of the chest is indicated if disease is detected on the abdominal CT (22). Histologic subtype can direct staging as well. Seminoma, embryonal carcinoma, and teratoma tend to spread directly along lymphatic paths, whereas choriocarcinoma and yolk sac carcinoma spread preferentially by hematogenous routes to the lung, liver, and brain (23).

The overall analysis of histologic subtype, serum tumor markers, and location of metastatic disease (if present) has been incorporated into a consensus staging system that includes a designation of good risk, intermediate risk, or poor risk for response to treatment and overall cure rates. Tables 2, 3, and 4 demonstrate how a patient's tumor (T), lymph node (N), metastatic (M), and serum status (S) are classified, combined into a stage designation, and further stratified by risk.

Pathologic Classification

The pathologic distinction between pure seminoma and mixed GCT (NSGCT) is important and directs subsequent clinical decisions. Any GCT in which only seminoma histology is seen but is producing an elevated AFP marker must, by marker definition, have yolk sac elements and is therefore classified as NSGCT. Elevated β-hCG, however, is seen in approximately 10% to 25% of pure seminomas.

GCTs have the following subtypes and frequencies: seminoma, 40%; embryonal carcinoma, 25%; teratocarcinoma, 25%; teratoma, 5%; and choriocarcinoma (pure), 1%. GCTs are the most common tumor of the testis by far, and other tumors rarely occur.

Significance of Intratubular Germ-Cell Neoplasia

Intratubular germ-cell carcinoma, or CIS, is the premalignant condition to GCT, with a natural history of progression to seminoma or embryonal cancer. Giwercman (26) reported a 0.8% incidence among 399 men aged 18 to 50 years, who died of other cancers; a 2.8% incidence among 599 men with a history of cryptorchidism; and a 5% incidence in the contralateral testis of 1000 men with a history of treated GCT. Patients with infertility, intersex disorders, cryptorchidism, prior contralateral GCT, or atrophic testes more commonly have CIS. Once CIS is diagnosed, approximately 40% to 50% will develop GCT within five years (27), and with extended follow-up, this number may continue to increase (28,29).

Daugaard et al. (30) have argued that the contralateral testis should be biopsied at the time of orchiectomy. Patients diagnosed early can be treated effectively with radiation or surgery. Herr and Sheinfeld (31), however, argue that biopsy is unnecessary, as 95% of GCT patients do not have CIS, and the 5% with CIS can be effectively treated (cured) at a later time. In place of biopsy, they recommend patient education and close follow-up. This plan may be reasonable, but high-risk groups with a history of undescended, small, and/or

infertile testis should be considered for a contralateral testis biopsy.

Treatment of Stage I Seminoma

The vast majority of seminomas (approximately 90%) present as stage I and are cured by radical orchiectomy alone, but 25% harbor occult metastatic disease and will recur. Such recurrences are highly curable by platinum-based chemotherapy. Therefore, surveillance for stage I is a reasonable option for a patient who is motivated and reliable enough to go through a rigorous follow-up regimen that includes office visits and imaging studies. Unfortunately, tumor markers are not available to follow up for recurrence. The interval for the appearance of metastases is longer than for stage I NSGCT, and therefore, the time required for adequate follow-up is longer.

Warde et al. (32) reported on a pooled analysis of 638 patients with stage I seminoma placed on surveillance protocols. At seven years, 121 relapses were observed for an actuarial five-year relapse-free rate of 82.3%. Primary tumor size and rete testis invasion were important predictors of relapse. Although this option may be appropriate for well-selected patients, the majority will be referred for adjuvant radiation therapy (XRT) for stage I. This therapy involves 25 cGy delivered over three weeks. The fields comprise an area in the shape of a "hockey stick" that includes para-aortic, paracaval, bilateral common iliac, and external iliac nodal regions. Recent protocols are reducing the field to para-aortic only. Adjuvant XRT reduces relapse to 3%—usually outside the radiation field and still curable by chemotherapy. Short-term side effects include fatigue, nausea, vomiting, and GI upset. Long-term side effects are unusual with the dose of 25 cGy, ranging from 0% to 6% (33,34), and secondary malignancies are rare (34). Radiation is also utilized for stage IIA and IIB disease, and the technique is similar.

Treatment of Stage IIC (Bulky) and Stage III Seminoma

For patients with stage IIC or III disease, platinum-based chemotherapy is more effective than XRT. The optimum regimen is debatable but generally consists of four cycles of bleomycin, etoposide, and cisplatin (BEP). Ongoing clinical trials are evaluating the safety of eliminating the fourth cycle or bleomycin altogether to reduce toxicity further. For poor-risk and salvage cases, alternating regimens using ifosfamide and vinblastine, with dose escalation may be necessary. Table 5 reviews the prognosis for seminoma and nonseminoma based upon stage and risk factors.

Although most patients with bulky retroperitoneal disease have a complete response to chemotherapy, an occasional patient will have a residual mass. In contrast to NSGCT, the postchemotherapy seminoma retroperitoneum undergoes significant desmoplastic, fibrotic reaction that makes surgical excision of masses technically difficult and more prone to complications

Table 1   Historic Developments in Testicular Cancer: 10 "Classic" Papers

Year	Author	Institution	Findings	Significance
1974	Higby	Roswell Park Cancer Center	1st report of the efficacy of cisplatin	Cisplatin is now the cornerstone of metastatic germ-cell cancer therapy
1976	Samuels	MD Anderson Cancer Center	Combination chemotherapy works at different points in the cell cycle	Multiagent chemotherapy regimens designed for synergy are standard practice for most chemotherapy regimens
1977	Einhorn	Indiana University	Cisplatin, vinblastine, bleomycin (PVB) combination 74% CR, 26% PR, 85% disease-free after surgical removal of residual masses	PVB combination was a major advance and the concept of chemotherapy cytoreduction with subsequent surgical resection was established
1974	Ray	Memorial Sloan Kettering Cancer Center	321 RPLND cases reported	The groundwork for RPLND template surgery by mapping the landing sites for the spread of retroperitoneal lymph-node disease was laid
1980	Donohue	Indiana University	Study of 26 patients treated by postchemotherapy RPLND (full bilateral)	Surgery was curative in 50% of the patients overall and 85% of those with teratoma
1982	Peckham	Royal Marsden Hospital, London	53 patients with stage I NSGCT treated by orchiectomy and surveillance. 17% relapse on all were salvaged	Surveillance, rather than RPLND, with chemotherapy for relapse is an option for stage I NSGCT
1987	Freedman	Multicenter: Medical Research Council	Stage I NSGCT followed up with surveillance had a 68% relapse-free survival. Risk factors established	Most patients had one or more risk factors: vascular invasion, lymphatic invasion, absence of yolk sac elements, undifferentiated tumor. Postorchiectomy chemotherapy was proposed
1987	Williams	Multi-institutional	195 patients randomized between post RPLND chemotherapy vs. observation for stage II	2 courses of PVB after RPLND for stage II is curative, but observation with subsequent chemotherapy for relapse is also curative
1993	Giwercman	Rigshospitalet, Copenhagen, Denmark	CIS incidence—50% of men with CIS subsequently develop GCT	Intratubular CIS is the precursor for invasive GCT. Contralateral biopsy for men who presented with GCT
1997	Bosl		Review article	State of the art update

Abbreviations: CIS, carcinoma-in-situ; GCT, germ-cell tumor; CR, complete remission; NSGCT, nonseminoma germ-cell tumor; PR, partial response; PVB, cisplatin, vinblastine, bleomycin; RPLND, retroperitoneal lymph-node dissection.
Source: From Ref. 3.

Table 2 Tumor, Node, Metastases, and Serum Marker Staging for Germ-Cell Tumors

Primary tumor		Regional lymph nodes—clinical		Distant metastases		Serum tumor markers	
p0	Primary tumor cannot be assessed	N0	Nodes not assessed	M0	No mets	Sx	Not assessed
p0	No evidence of primary tumor	N1	Lymph node mass (s) ≤2 cm^a	M1a	Nonregional nodal or pulmonary mets	S0	LDH ≤ normal and hCG normal and AFP normal
pTis	Intratubular germ-cell neoplasia	N2	Lymph node (s) >2 cm ≤5 cm^a	M1b	Nonpulmonary visceral mets	S1	LDH >1.5 × normal and hCG <5000 and AFP <1000
pT1	Tumor limited to the testis and epididymis, no vascular/lymphatic invasion, may invade tunica albuginea, but not the tunica vaginalis	N3	Lymph node (s) >5 cm^a			S2	LDH 1.5–10 × normal or hCG 5000–50,000 or AFP 1000–10,000
		Regional lymph nodes—pathologic					
		PN0	No evidence of lymph nodes			S3	LDH >10 × normal or hCG >50,000 or AFP >10,000
pT2	Tumor limited to the testis and epididymis, vascular/lymphatic invasion or tumor extending through the tunica albuginea with vaginalis involvement	PN1	Lymph nodes ≤2 cm^a				
pT3	Tumor invades the spermatic cord with or without vascular/lymphatic invasion	PN2	Lymph node (s) >2 cm ≤5 cm^a, >5 positive nodes, or extranodal extension				
pT4	Tumor invades the scrotum with or without vascular/lymphatic invasion	PN3	Lymph node (s) >5 cm^a				

^{a}Greatest dimension.

Abbreviations: AFP, alpha fetoprotein; hCG, human chorionic gonadotropin; LDH, lactate dehydrogenase; M, metastatic; N, lymph node; S, serum status; T, tumor.

such as vascular or bowl injury. Motzer et al. (35) found that a residual mass greater than 3 cm had a 50% chance of harboring tumor, and they recommended the 3-cm size as the cutoff for exploration but cautioned that these cases are best performed at experienced referral centers due to the rarity of the situation and the potential morbidity. The Indiana group (36), however, recommends observation. In their series, most of these masses were necrosis, and with extended follow-up, observed patients had no further evidence of disease. Definitive recommendations are in the process of evaluation. Positron emission tomography (PET) scanning has emerged as a diagnostic tool to evaluate recurrent masses after chemotherapy, and with further experience may be utilized in addition to the 3-cm rule for deciding between salvage therapy and surveillance (37).

Treatment of Stage I NSGCT

One of the most fascinating and often debated topics in testis cancer is the optimum management of stage I NSGCT. The good news for patients is that they can expect a chance of cure of above 99% (38) as long as they undergo orchiectomy followed up with strict compliance with one of three treatment/management algorithms: RPLND, two cycles of immediate chemotherapy, or surveillance with four cycles of chemotherapy if and when disease recurrence becomes clinically detectable on follow-up imaging. There is no definitive data to prove which one is the best; rather, physicians must educate patients on the known outcomes, risks, and benefits of each treatment scheme and make decisions individualized to the patient.

Surveillance is the easiest protocol to describe first, as it introduces the important facts of the natural history of the disease and is the benchmark to compare the results of RPLND and initial chemotherapy. As Tables 2 and 3 show, stage I is defined as any pathologic T classification of the primary testis tumor (pT1-4) with no lymphadenopathy or metastatic disease on imaging studies. Serum markers may be elevated preorchiectomy, but the patient would only be treated as stage I if the markers normalize postorchiectomy consistent with their half-lives. Stage I patients have been enrolled in large clinical protocols of surveillance (39) since the initial 1982 study by Peckham et al. (40), and the overall recurrence rate is approximately 30% (38). Multiple imaging modalities have been evaluated for GCT including ultrasound, magnetic resonance imaging (MRI), and lymphangiogram. CT of the abdomen remains the most effective staging modality (41) but still misses 30% of the patients with occult metastatic disease. PET scanning is promising and may be an area of future improvement in GCT staging (42).

Subclinical metastases tend to become clinically evident within the first two years. During this time, patients must undergo evaluation every two to three months to include examination, serum markers, CXR, and CT of the abdomen. Follow-up intervals can be lengthened after two years, but should probably never cease altogether. Recurrences, usually in the retroperitoneum, are then effectively salvaged with four cycles of platinum-based chemotherapy. If compliance is achieved and salvage therapy promptly and appropriately delivered, cure rates are not compromised in the 30% that recur, and 70% are spared any subsequent surgical or systemic therapy. Compliance has

Table 3   Staging System for Testicular Germ-Cell Cancers

	T1-4	N0	M0	Sx
Stage I				
IA	T1	N0	M0	S0
IB	T2	N0	M0	S0
	T3	N0	M0	S0
	T4	N0	M0	S0
IS	Any T	N0	M0	S1-3
Stage II	Any T	Any N	M0	SX
IIA	Any T	N1	M0	S0
	Any T	N1	M0	S1
IIB	Any T	N2	M0	S0
	Any T	N2	M0	S1
IIC	Any T	N3	M0	S0
	Any T	N3	M0	S1
Stage III	Any T	Any N	M1a	SX
IIIA	Any T	Any N	M1a	S0
	Any T	Any N	M1a	S1
IIIB	Any T	Any N	M0	S2
	Any T	Any N	M1a	S2
IIIC	Any T	Any N	M0	S3
	Any T	Any N	M1a	S3
	Any T	Any N	M1b	Any S

Abbreviations: T, patient tumor; N, lymph node; M, metastatic; S, serum status.
Source: From Ref. 24.

Table 4   Risk Assessment for Testicular Germ-Cell Cancers

	Serum markers	Extent of disease
NSGCT		
Good risk	LDH < 1.5 × normal hCG < 5000 mIU/mL AFP < 1000 ng/mL	No evidence of nonpulmonary metastases
Intermediate risk	LDH 1.5–10 × normal hCG 5000–50,000 mIU/mL or AFP 1000–10,000 ng/mL	No evidence of nonpulmonary metastases
Poor risk	LDH > 10 × normal hCG > 50,000 mIU/mL AFP > 10,000 ng/mL	Evidence of nonpulmonary metastases
Seminomas		
Good risk		No evidence of nonpulmonary metastases
Intermediate		Evidence of nonpulmonary metastases

Abbreviations: AFP, alpha fetoprotein; hCG, human chorionic gonadotropin; LDH, lactate dehydrogenase; NSGCT, nonseminoma germ-cell tumor.
Source: From Ref. 25.

Table 5 Prognosis of Testicular Germ-Cell Tumors Treated by Orchiectomy and XRT or Platinum-Based Chemotherapy as Indicated

Seminoma	
Stage I	98–100%
Stage II (B1/B2 non-bulky)	98–100%
Stage II (B3 bulky) and III	90% complete response to chemotherapy and 86% durable response
Nonseminoma	
Stage I	>98%
Stage II	90–95%
Stage III	50–90% depending upon risk assessment

been shown to be inconsistent in many studies (43), resulting in potentially higher stage relapse, but a negative effect on survival has not been demonstrated.

RPLND is a common treatment pathway for stage I NSGCT. Cuneo first successfully performed the procedure in 1906, and subsequently, thoracoabdominal and transperitoneal midline abdominal approaches have been described (44). It has been shown to be both a staging and a therapeutic procedure (45) and has undergone numerous revisions in the past two decades. Based upon studies in which testicular lymphatics were injected with contrast, an early version of RPLND included complete bilateral dissections of all lymph-node tissue along the common iliacs, presacral, interaortocaval, para-aortic, paracaval, and suprahilar regions (46). Such dissections effectively upstaged 30% of stage I patients to stage II, while the remainder of the patients with negative nodes (pathological stage I) enjoyed more peace of mind that their chance of disease recurrence after a negative RPLND was very low.

Further studies demonstrated that the chance of suprahilar nodal disease was very low, and, therefore, this region was omitted from the dissection (47,48). Nevertheless, the bilateral dissection sacrificed the lumbar sympathetic chains and hypogastric plexus, and consequently about 90% of men had impaired sympathetic function manifested as retrograde or dry ejaculation (49). Erectile function and the ability to achieve a sexual climax were not affected. Since many men with GCT are still within the age that fertility is desired (50), further understanding of the anatomy of the retroperitoneal nerves and revision of the operation was desired. Extensive lymph-node mapping studies demonstrated that the potential "landing zones" for a right- versus left-sided GCT could be readily predicted (8,47). Therefore, dissection templates could be devised, whereby one side of the lumbar sympathetics and the hypogastric plexus could be left undisturbed. Ejaculation was preserved in 75% to 94% of the patients with these templates (49,51). Further description of the anatomy of the lumbar nerves led to the ability to "spare" these nerves on the side of the template dissection, while the other side continued to

remain undisturbed. Follow-up studies from centers of excellence have now shown that normal ejaculation can be preserved in nearly 100% of the cases (52), and while short-term morbidity and complications are present in 14% to 23% (38), long-term morbidity is negligible.

If patients have small-volume positive lymph nodes at RPLND, they can choose between two treatment options that offer the same >99% cure rate: two immediate cycles of chemotherapy, or observation and four cycles of chemotherapy are case of recurrence (45,53,54). If the patient opts for observation, approximately 50% will recur, and therefore the other 50% would be cured by their RPLND alone. If two immediate cycles of chemotherapy are selected, the cure rate is 99%, but 50% of the patients would have received unnecessary chemotherapy. If observation is selected, there is a 50% chance of not needing any further treatment but also a 50% chance of needing four cycles of chemotherapy, which is significantly more toxic both in the long and short term when compared to only two cycles. Under this observation scheme, recurrence in the retroperitoneum has been documented but is rare; therefore, the follow-up protocol can reasonably include only serum markers and a CXR.

Based on the data presented thus far, RPLND would seem to be the treatment of choice. RPLND is diagnostic, therapeutic for some, minimizes the need for chemotherapy (see toxicity discussion below), and has minimal long-term morbidity. Follow-up studies have shown, however, that approximately 10% of RPLND-negative patients will have a recurrence (55), including up to 2.7% in the retroperitoneum, according to a multicenter study (56). In these cases, four cycles of chemotherapy are required despite surgical efforts to avoid them. Of all treatment choices, four cycles of chemotherapy have the most significant long-term morbidity, including adverse effects on fertility, and cardiac, GI, peripheral nervous, renal, and secondary cancers. Therefore, minimizing the chance of needing four cycles of chemotherapy is a worthwhile goal. If 30% of surveillance patients need four cycles and 10% of RPLND patients need four cycles, then the net benefit of RPLND is reduced to 20%.

Immediate chemotherapy for stage I NSGCT was introduced with the idea of eliminating the need for RPLND and four cycles of chemotherapy. As mentioned, four cycles are associated with significant long-term morbidity and increased risk of secondary cancers. Two cycles are associated with fewer effects on spermatogenesis; however, the long-term morbidity and secondary cancers are far less studied. A few centers have designed trials whereby stage I NSGCT patients receive two cycles of immediate chemotherapy. At a median of 93 months of follow-up, Studer et al. (57) reported that 57 of 59 patients were recurrence-free and there were no disease-specific deaths in a cohort of patients with high-risk stage I (vascular invasion, embryonal cell predominant, primary tumor growth beyond the testis—see Risk Assessment below).

These results are equivalent to RPLND and observation; however, under this scheme, up to 70% of the patients received unnecessary chemotherapy.

An interesting, new combination of the above treatment paths is laparoscopic RPLND, which has been reported at a few high-volume centers of expertise (58,59). Both right and left template dissections have been performed. Since the therapeutic ability of the procedure has not been fully evaluated, patients with node-positive disease have undergone two cycles of chemotherapy. The learning curve for this procedure is very steep, and therefore more studies will be required to prove whether this minimally invasive procedure is an effective method of properly staging patients so that chemotherapy is only instituted when necessary (60). Currently, laparoscopic RPLND does provide an option whereby chemotherapy is given with histological documentation of node-positive disease. Future techniques will need to address the ability to spare nerves in addition to a template dissection.

What is the best treatment path for stage I NSGCT? As stated, there is no simple answer, but review articles elaborating these debates have recently been published (57,61). All three modalities have very high cure rates of greater than 99%. Therefore, side effects, long-term toxicity, and secondary cancers may be the determining issues. Currently, there is not enough data to know the long-term toxicity of immediate chemotherapy. Laparoscopic RPLND is a minimally invasive method of pathologic staging but has not been proven therapeutically. Therefore, these modalities should be restricted to clinical trials at this time. For motivated and compliant patients with low risk factors for node-positive disease, surveillance is a rational approach. For the remainder, RPLND offers staging and a chance for curing limited stage II disease. All patients need careful counseling, informed consent, and a careful follow-up for metastatic as well as contralateral testis recurrence.

Risk Assessment of Testicular Germ-Cell Cancer

The above discussion presents the overall data for each treatment plan and a simplified template to compare each one. A key statistic is the fact that 30% of patients with clinical stage I NSGCT who undergo surveillance will have a recurrence; however, additional data is now available that enables physicians to further stratify this risk based upon the specifics of the orchiectomy specimen. Four risk factors for metastatic disease have been identified: predominately embryonal cell histology, vascular invasion, lymphatic invasion, and absence of yolk sac elements (22,62). With multiple criteria present, patients may have above 50% chance of recurrence. No absolute prediction of occult metastatic disease is available. These risk factors may be utilized, however, to argue for one treatment path over another. Surveillance, for example, may not be the best treatment plan for higher risk patients. Such patients may be recommended for RPLND or immediate chemotherapy, depending upon one's evaluation of the risks/benefits of each treatment.

Treatment of Stage II–III NSGCT

Stage II is subclassified into IIA, IIB, and IIC, based upon the volume of positive lymph nodes and serum markers (Tables 2 and 3). RPLND is a treatment option for stages IIA and IIB for two reasons: (i) overstaging is possible (i.e., enlarged radiographic nodes were pathologically negative) in approximately 25% (45,63) of the cases and (ii) surgical removal of low-volume retroperitoneal disease is curative in 50% of the cases. At most centers, stage IIC is treated the same as stage III—cisplatin-based chemotherapy—and IIA and IIB may also be treated by primary chemotherapy.

Ideally, stage IIC and III disease treated with chemotherapy results in complete resolution of the mass on imaging and normalization of serum markers. If markers do not resolve, two more cycles and other high-risk protocols may be necessary. In select patients who undergo postchemotherapy RPLND with elevated markers, cure is possible, with a five-year overall survival of 53%. Predictors of poor survival included marker status, repeat RPLND, and viable germ-cell cancer in the specimen (64). Another scenario for nearly 50% of bulky abdominal masses is the normalization of serum markers but incomplete resolution of the mass. Resection of these postchemotherapy masses yields one of four entities: (i) necrosis, (ii) teratoma, (iii) germ-cell carcinoma, or (iv) non-germ-cell cancer (rare) (65). The typical distribution is 50% necrosis, 40% teratoma, and 10% GCT (66).

If GCT is found in the mass, surgery can be curative, but more often, two additional cycles of chemotherapy are given. RPLND is the only means of curing residual teratoma, as such masses are resistant to chemotherapy, may cause local tissue destruction, or worse, degenerate into non-germ-cell cancers, which are also chemotherapy resistant. If necrosis is found, the procedure may be considered diagnostic but nontherapeutic. Thus, it is desirable to be able to predict the pathology of a postchemotherapy residual mass. If teratoma was present in the orchiectomy specimen, the chance of teratoma in the postchemotherapy mass, despite normalized markers, is greater than 80% (67). Therefore, only patients with no teratoma in their orchiectomy specimens should be considered for observation of a postchemotherapy residual mass. This decision remains debatable, with different recommendations from major centers depending upon the amount of tumor shrinkage, prechemotherapy size, and postchemotherapy size (65,68). A less common scenario is the simultaneous presence of postchemotherapy abdominal and chest masses. Attempts have been made to show that if necrosis is found in the abdominal specimen, then necrosis is likely in the chest mass and may therefore be omitted. Unfortunately, the prediction of necrosis is not better than 90%, and therefore most centers will recommend surgical resection of all areas of radiographic disease (65).

Although staging systems are important in determining treatment strategies, experience has shown that patients can be categorized into good, intermediate, and poor-risk categories, with a dramatic effect on cure rates: 92%, 80%, and 48%, respectively (Table 4) (69). Thus, most patients can be started on standard cisplatin-based chemotherapy, but some intermediate- to poor-risk patients will need additional chemotherapy strategies available in the context of clinical trials (70).

Fertility Issues in GCT

The majority of men with GCT are subfertile at diagnosis, with postorchiectomy sperm counts of less than 20 million/mL (71). Possible explanations include underlying systemic disease, contralateral testis CIS, endocrine or autoimmune effects, and psychological issues (72). Petersen et al. (73) studied men with GCT, lymphoma (nontesticular), and normal controls and found that men with GCT had impaired spermatogenesis and higher serum FSH, but men with lymphoma and normal controls had neither. Thus, impaired spermatogenesis is often present in the contralateral testis, and a systemic tumor effect was not seen in the lymphoma controls. Sperm counts are also lower in men with only CIS (74). There is evidence that following orchiectomy, sperm counts can improve within the first year; however, an elevated FSH is associated with incomplete recovery of spermatogenesis (75).

Treatment for GCT also carries the risk of changes in fertility. RPLND is associated with significant ejaculatory dysfunction if a bilateral template is used. For stage I patients treated by modern nerve-sparing template dissection techniques, however, nearly 100% of ejaculatory function is preserved, and a 76% pregnancy rate was achieved in a large study (52). Ejaculatory function can also be spared after postchemotherapy RPLND in very select patients; however, the results are not as successful (76).

Three to four cycles of cisplatin-based chemotherapy have toxic effects on spermatogenesis, which vary by dose and duration of treatment, stage of disease, baseline testis function, and age and health of the patient (72). Cullen et al. (77), however, found no difference in pre- and posttreatment semen with only two cycles of BEP.

Spermatogenesis can recover after chemotherapy. Nijman et al. (78) found that in a group treated with chemotherapy with and without RPLND, 73% were oligospermic at baseline, with this figure increasing to 84% after one year but then decreasing to 48% at two years. The same trend was noted for azoospermia: 4% at baseline, 48% at one year, then 28% at two years. Hansen et al. (79) found that paternity was still negatively affected after chemotherapy compared to stage I NSGCT treated by orchiectomy alone. Analysis of

children born to patients treated by chemotherapy has not shown increased risk of birth defects compared to those with NSGCT managed by surveillance and controls (80). Genetic sperm abnormalities, however, were increased by five times during and 100 days after completing chemotherapy for Hodgkin's disease (81), and therefore, conception and sperm banking should be avoided during and three months after chemotherapy treatment (72).

Prior to chemotherapy or RPLND, patients should be counseled on the fertility effects of treatment and offered cryopreservation of sperm for future fertility. Hallak et al. (82) recently evaluated sperm cryopreservation in GCT patients and normal controls and found that GCT had lower prefreeze and post-thaw motile sperm counts compared to normal specimens, but the percentage change of pre- and post-thaw was not different. Histologic features and stage did not affect sperm quality. With or without cryopreservation, infertile males with a history of testis cancer have a number of infertility treatments available to them, such as rectal probe electroejaculation or sperm aspiration in conjunction with in vitro fertilization (IVF) or intracytoplasmic sperm injection (ICSI), as indicated.

Long-Term Side Effects of Treatment for Testis Cancer

An important issue that needs to be discussed with all patients undergoing chemotherapy is the long-term side effects. For patients with metastatic disease, chemotherapy offers remarkable cure rates compared to the pre-cisplatin era and greatly outweighs the risks of long-term side effects. Long-term side effects, however, may be of greater significance in cases of adjuvant therapy such as the proposed two cycles of chemotherapy for stage I, or low-volume resected stage II disease. Side effects may include nephrotoxicity, renovascular hypertension, peripheral vascular effects such as Raynaud's phenomena, cardiovascular events, peripheral neuropathy, hearing loss, and pulmonary toxicity. Radiation therapy patients typically have a low incidence of GI and cardiopulmonary side effects.

In addition to the fertility effects discussed, testis cancer may relapse (greater than two years after treatment) in 1.5% to 6% of patients (83). Having had an initial bulky teratoma may increase this risk (84). Contralateral germ-cell testicular tumor may develop in up to 4% of the patients (83). Patients are also at increased risk of secondary malignancies including leukemia (most common), lymphoma, sarcoma, melanoma and skin tumors, and solid tumors of the GI, lung, and urothelial tract (83). In a summary of 11 population-based registries, testis cancer survivors had 30% more tumors than expected for the general population (85).

Conclusion

Testicular carcinoma is a rare cancer in the overall scope of cancer incidence but is the most common type seen in men less than 35 years of age. The work-up consists of a careful history and physical examination, ultrasound of the scrotum, tumor markers, and imaging studies. Radical orchiectomy provides therapeutic and diagnostic benefit. Depending upon primary tumor pathologic stage, histology, markers, and imaging, patients may be carefully selected for close observation, radiation, chemotherapy, or RPLND. Overall cure rates are excellent, and much progress has been made to minimize treatment morbidity.

☐ CARCINOMA OF THE PENIS

In this section, the management of localized penile cancer will be reviewed. The treatment of the local lesion will be discussed and an approach formulated for managing the regional lymph nodes. It is critical to recognize that appropriate treatment of inguinal nodal metastatic deposits may achieve long-term cure, whereas delayed or inappropriate treatment may be lethal.

Epidemiology

The etiology of penile cancer is multifactorial, but the uncircumcised penis is predisposed to development of the disease. It is hypothesized that glandular secretions, termed smegma, which accumulate within the preputial sac, are irritating and carcinogenic. Although careful penile hygiene may reduce the risk of penile cancer, such hygiene is rarely achieved in many areas of the world. Consequently, in certain South American, Asian, and African countries, the incidence of penile cancer is quite high and may represent the most common male malignancy in those areas. Contrast this with the extraordinarily low incidence of carcinoma of the penis in the United States, where it comprises less than 1% of all male malignancies that occur annually. Because of the rarity of this disorder in the United States and Europe, much of the information about treatment of this cancer is based upon the experience of urologists in Puerto Rico, South America, Asia, and Africa.

With regard to circumcision, it is noted that a great deal of tension and conflict has long surrounded this neonatal surgical procedure. In 1971, the American Academy of Pediatrics stated that "there was no valid medical indication for neonatal circumcision." In 1988, this statement was modified, recognizing that neonatal circumcision lowered the incidence of urinary tract infection in the newborn male, reduced the incidence of sexually transmitted diseases (STDs) in the adult male, and had a role in preventing penile cancer. The American Academy of Pediatrics has therefore stated that parents need to be advised: "Newborn circumcision has potential medical advantages as well as disadvantages and risks" (86). Circumcision certainly represents the only surgical procedure that can prevent the development of cancer in an organ without sacrificing the organ itself.

Another important etiological factor is the human papilloma virus (HPV), specifically serotypes 16, 18, 31, 33, and 35 (87). Although the virus is not present in every penile cancer, about two-thirds of men with penile cancer do have evidence of HPV infection. In addition, there is a link between the incidence of HPV-related cervical cancer and HPV infection and penile cancer in the male consort.

Natural History

Carcinoma of the penis usually begins with a small ulcerative lesion on the glans, corona, or shaft that gradually extends to involve the entire glans, shaft, and corpora, with a necrotic, disfiguring process that if left untreated can lend to autoamputation. The initial lesion may be hidden by the foreskin and may range in appearance from a relatively nondescript area of abraded skin to a deeply excoriated ulcer.

CIS, sometimes referred to as *Erythroplasia of Queyrat* when it affects the glans or prepuce and as *Bowen's Disease* when it involves the shaft or scrotum, may also be the presenting lesion. This usually appears as a velvety, slightly raised pink or reddish area of skin. The epidemiology and natural history of penile CIS parallel those of early carcinoma of the penis.

The route of metastatic spread from penile cancer is quite predictable. Lesions of the prepuce or glans metastasize to the superficial inguinal nodes and those of the shaft or shaft structures to the deep inguinal and pelvic nodes. Among patients who have invasive carcinoma, 40% to 80% have palpable inguinal adenopathy at initial diagnosis. Because concurrent infection is often present, it may be difficult to delineate metastases from inflammatory lymphadenitis. Approximately 50% of adenopathy proves secondary to metastases; the balance is due to inflammatory reaction. Clinically detectable distant metastases to lung, liver, bone, and brain are uncommon and found in only 1% to 10% of the patients.

Carcinoma of the penis has a relentless, progressive course. Untreated, most patients die within two years of diagnosis. There have been no cases reported of spontaneous regression of this disease.

Making the Diagnosis

Critical to planning for treatment of carcinoma of the penis is first identifying the malignant histology, the grade of the tumor, and its depth of invasion. This requires microscopic analysis of a generous biopsy specimen that ideally includes adjacent normal skin for comparison. Biopsy and extirpative treatment can be separate procedures, but biopsy with confirmation of tumor by frozen section immediately followed by limited partial or total amputation is an accepted and efficient way to simultaneously diagnose and treat carcinoma of the penis. All patients undergoing such procedures should have full informed consent to permit proceeding with whatever appropriate surgery may be required.

Identification of the tumor stage and grade is essential to subsequent treatment and planning. Penile tumors that are low in stage and low in grade are associated with low metastatic potential and can be followed up with periodic examination of inguinal nodes for abnormality. High-grade tumors are frequently associated with regional nodal metastases (88). The strongest prognostic indicator for survival is the presence and extent of nodal metastasis and adequacy of their excision (89). Therefore, patients with high-grade or high-stage tumors are best treated with a prompt inguinal node dissection once control of the primary tumor and any associated infection has been achieved.

Recent developments in MRI imaging using a lymphotropic nanoparticle-enhanced technique shows promise in detecting inguinal metastases with an accuracy previously unavailable. Although not yet widely available, this technique may revolutionize the work-up and management of patients with invasive penile cancer (90).

Treating Local Penile Lesions by Stage of Presentation
CIS (Eryhtroplasia of Queyrat or Bowen's Disease)

Intraepithelial neoplasia or genital squamous CIS is, as mentioned previously, often labeled *Bowen's Disease* or *Erythroplasia of Queyrat*. The histopathology is identical (91). Enough (multiple) confirmatory punch biopsies should be taken to rule out invasive squamous carcinoma.

When CIS (Tis) lesions are small and noninvasive, local excision (sparing the anatomic structure and function of the penis) is usually curative. Circumcision suffices if the lesion is limited to the prepuce. Mohs' micrographic surgery (discussed in detail below) is another surgical option in selected cases. Radiation therapy can be successful in eradicating the lesion. Appropriately planned and delivered, it causes minimal morbidity. Topical 5-fluorouracil cream and laser therapies (CO_2 or Nd:YAG) have been used with good therapeutic and cosmetic success.

Treatment of Other Local Penile Lesions

Amputation by partial or total penectomy has been the gold standard for the management of localized penile cancers. The potential disfigurement and loss of function, however, has encouraged development of organ-sparing techniques such as partial excision or Mohs' surgery. Other noninvasive methods that employ X ray, laser, or cryosurgical destruction have also been explored. The primary goal of any treatment remains complete eradication of the primary tumor.

Conventional Surgery

For lesions that involve the glans and distal shaft, even when apparently superficial, partial amputation, with a 2-cm margin proximal to the tumor, has been advocated to minimize local recurrence. A recent series reported no local recurrences were seen after total amputation. After partial amputation, the rate of local recurrence remains acceptably low, at about 5%. Treatment by circumcision or local wedge excision has been associated with rates of recurrence that approach 50%.

Mohs' Micrographic Surgery

Mohs' micrographic surgery is a technique to remove skin cancer by excising tissue in thin layers (92). It includes color coding of the excised specimens with tissue dyes, accurate orientation of the excised tissue through construction of tissue maps, and microscopic examination of the horizontal frozen sections.

The Mohs' technique is an attractive therapy for selected cases of carcinoma of the penis. It can trace out silent tumorous extensions, its cure rate equals that of more radical surgical techniques, and it allows maximum preservation of normal, uninvolved tissue. This technique has been used frequently and successfully to excise squamous cell carcinoma from other areas—e.g., ear, nose, and lip—with excellent cosmetic results. Therefore, its application to the penis is logical and appropriate if performed by a surgeon skilled in the methodology and if thoughtful patient selection is observed.

Micrographic surgery has seemed ideally suited for treating small, distal carcinomas with a high cure rate in lesions less than 1 cm in diameter but decreasing in those greater than 3 cm in diameter (93). Healing after Mohs' micrographic surgery is by secondary intention. Meatal stenosis may complicate the postoperative course and may occasionally produce significant glans deformity.

If the proximal penile shaft is involved, total penectomy with perineal urethrostomy will be required. For more advanced tumors marked by local extension to the scrotum or pubis, combination chemotherapy followed by surgery may be successful in controlling the disease or in converting a potentially unresectable lesion into one amenable to surgery (94). In rare instances, hemipelvectomy may merit consideration (95).

Laser Surgery

This modality has been used to treat stages Tis, Ta (non-invasive carcinoma), T1, and some T2 penile cancers. A potential advantage of laser therapy is that it destroys the lesion while preserving normal structures and function. The depth of destruction by a laser beam may be difficult to determine, however, making accurate histologic documentation of the depth of malignant penetration impossible. The tumor must, therefore, be staged adequately by taking deep biopsies before applying the laser.

Tis tumors can be treated with any common surgical laser. The Nd-YAG laser, because of its greater penetration, has been used to treat T1 and T2 tumors (96).

Radiation Therapy

The sole advantage of initial radiation therapy over initial surgery is that it preserves penile anatomic structure and function. However, this may also be achieved with the aforementioned organ-sparing surgeries. The primary indications for radiation therapy are small lesions in those patients who refuse surgical treatment or for local palliation in patients with advanced disease.

In many patients, radiation therapy is not ideal for several reasons. Squamous cell carcinoma is characteristically radioresistant; consequently, the dose needed to sterilize deeply infiltrating penile tumors often causes complications—e.g., pain and meatal/urethral stricture—that may require secondary penectomy. Additionally, the lengthy treatment schedule of three to six weeks may be formidable for an elderly patient. In contrast, partial penectomy, which can be done under local anesthesia, is relatively simple and expeditious.

Furthermore, long-term follow-up to detect recurrence is challenging. It is often difficult to distinguish tissue changes from radiation from recurrent disease. Long-term close follow-up in conjunction with interval computerized tomography of the groins is mandatory. In a report of a small series of 11 patients treated with radiation, seven (63%) recurrences were detected after two years and two additional (18%) occurrences after five years (total rate of recurrence, 82%) (97).

Issues in Treating Inguinal Node Metastases

Nodal metastases affect the prognosis more than tumor grade, gross appearance, or morphologic and microscopic patterns of the tumor. The management has been a long-time surgical dilemma as controversy surrounds the timing and extent of inguinal surgery. Several important questions must be addressed:

What are the contemporary guidelines for proceeding with inguinal lymphadenectomy and for following up the patient with penile cancer expectantly?
Patients with well-differentiated tumors (Grade I or II) that are limited to the penile skin and do not involve the corpora or the spongiosal or urethral tissues and who have palpably negative inguinal lymph nodes are candidates for expectant follow-up. Patients must be absolutely reliable regarding close interval follow-up.

Patients with grade II (moderately differentiated) lesions that demonstrate any degree of invasion or any patient with grade III (poorly differentiated) tumor should undergo modified bilateral inguinal lymphadenectomy (98).

Should lymphadenectomy be performed in the presence of clinically palpable inguinal nodes after appropriate treatment of the primary lesion and resolution of inflammation?
Absolutely. Five-year disease-free survival occurs in 20% to 50% of patients who are treated by inguinal node lymphadenectomy in the presence of clinically palpable adenopathy and histologically proven inguinal node metastases. One U.S. study reported 82% five-year survival after lymphadenectomy in a series of patients who had one positive node (89); another study from Norway found 88% five-year survival after lymphadenectomy for patients who had minimal nodal metastases (97).

Should inguinal lymphadenectomy be routine in patients who have a clinically negative groin examination at presentation of the primary lesion?
This question invites the most controversy. Early complications of phlebitis, pulmonary embolism, wound infection, and flap necrosis as well as the long-term later complication of lymphedema can occur after inguinal lymphadenectomy and have traditionally made surgeons reticent about recommending groin dissection in every patient with penile cancer. In the last decade however, postoperative complications have been diminished by improved preoperative and postoperative care and modification of the extent of node dissection to include preservation of the dermis, Scarpa's fascia, and saphenous vein (98).

The incidence of occult metastases to inguinal nodes has been reported to be 2% to 25% in patients with penile carcinoma in whom inguinal examination is clinically negative. Which patients, then, should be subjected to groin dissection, and which can be followed up expectantly? Several recent studies comparing immediate adjunctive lymphadenectomy with delayed lymphadenectomy after expectant follow-up have helped to clarify this issue.

First, in a series of 23 patients who had invasive primary lesions and nonpalpable nodes, those patients who had immediate adjunctive lymphadenectomy and positive nodes had a survival rate of 88%. In the portion of the group followed up with surveillance, in which delayed lymph node dissection was performed only when nodes became palpable, only 38% survived five years. It is also important to note that patients in this study who presented with palpable inguinal nodes at diagnosis (and thus might be considered as having more advanced disease at presentation), who were treated with immediate lymphadenectomy had a five-year survival rate of 66% (99).

In a second study, immediate adjunctive lymphadenectomy resulted in a five-year, disease-free survival in six of nine (66%) node-positive patients, compared to 1 of 12 (8%) patients who had been followed up and treated by delayed therapeutic lymphadenectomy (100).

Finally, a study of patients at M.D. Anderson Cancer Center in Houston reported a five-year survival of 57% with early lymphadenectomy but only 13% when lymphadenectomy was delayed (101).

Should inguinal lymphadenectomy be bilateral, rather than unilateral, for patients who have unilateral adenopathy at first presentation of the primary tumor?
A bilateral inguinal lymphadenectomy should be performed. The anatomic crossover of lymphatics at the base of the penis is well established. Clinical

support for a bilateral procedure is based on the finding of subclinical contralateral metastases in more than 50% of the patients so treated (102).

Should pelvic lymphadenectomy be performed in patients who have positive inguinal metastases?
Yes. Iliac nodes have been found positive for tumor metastases in 15% to 30% of patients who have positive inguinal nodes (89). Survival among patients who have positive pelvic nodes, although limited, has been documented (86,95). The procedure is reasonable for a young man who is a good surgical risk.

How effective is chemotherapy?
Neoadjuvant and adjuvant protocols were employed in studies at the National Cancer Institute of Milan (103). A protocol of 12 weekly courses of vincristine, bleomycin, and methotrexate was instituted as adjuvant therapy for 12 patients after lymphadenectomy and for 5 patients before node dissection, as neoadjuvant therapy. Those treated with adjuvant chemotherapy were considered high risk—nine showed extranodal tumor growth, five had pelvic node involvement, and five had bilateral metastases. At follow-up (range 18–102 months), only one patient had had a recurrence. In the five patients who had large nodal tumor metastasis ranging from 6 to 11 cm in diameter, three achieved a partial response, were successfully resected, and were disease-free at follow-up between 20 and 72 months.

Reconstruction after Penectomy

Once the patient who has undergone partial or total penectomy is proved free of recurrent disease, he may be a candidate for penile reconstruction. At the Eastern Virginia Medical School, surgeons have been quite successful using free-flap reconstruction with an upper lateral arm flap. This flap is an excellent source of relatively nonhirsute thin epithelium that has a dependable cutaneous neural and vascular supply, which provides the reconstructed penis with erogenous sensibility (104). Furthermore, successful microvascular free-flap techniques for tissue transfer demonstrate that one-stage penile reconstruction is possible.

Inguinal Reconstruction Following Node Dissection

Changes in the technique of lymph-node dissection and the choice of incision have limited the complications that were once seen after lymph-node dissection. Skin loss is usually minimal; it can be covered with a split-thickness graft. When skin loss is deeper or when a large cuticular area must be excised, more substantial tissue transfer may be required. A number of local flaps can be transposed into these defects. The gracilis musculocutaneous unit is totally expendable and easily transposed into a groin defect.

When a large flap is required, the tensor fascia lata musculofascial cutaneous system is excellent. The vastus lateralis can be transferred as muscle flap separately from the tensor fascia lata flap. Other sources of tissue to cover a groin defect include the inferiorly based rectus abdominus musculocutaneous flap and the rectal femoris musculocutaneous flap for difficult groin problems. The pedical omental flap may also represent a viable alternative for coverage (105).

Conclusion

Squamous carcinoma of the penis is an uncommon but potentially devastating cancer that is often curable when involvement is limited to local disease and early nodal metastases. Success in treatment is achieved by careful initial pathologic evaluation, close follow-up, careful staging, and appropriate treatment of the inguinal and pelvic nodes when indicated. Management of advanced local disease and metastatic disease is difficult, although some survivals have been achieved with extensive surgery and with chemotherapy.

□ REFERENCES

1. Jemal A, Siegel R, Ward E, et al. Cancer statistics, 2006. CA Cancer J Clin 2006; 56(2):106–130.

2. Davies JM. Testicular cancer in England and Wales; some epidemiological aspects. Lancet 1981; 1(8226): 928–932.

3. Donohue JP. Testicular cancer. In: Gerharz EW et al., eds. Classic Papers In Urology. Oxford: Isis Medical Media Ltd., 1999:111–131.

4. Oliver RTD. Epidemiology of testis cancer: a clinical perspective. In: Vogelzang NJ et al., eds. Comprehensive Textbook of Genitourinary Oncology. Philldelphia: Lippincott, Williams and Wilkins, 2000: 880–890.

5. Pharris-Ciurej ND, Cook LS, Weiss NS. Incidence of testicular cancer in the United States: has the epidemic begun to abate? Am J Epidemiol 1999; 150(1):45–46.

6. Thompson IM, Optenberg S, Byers R, et al. Increased incidence of testicular cancer in active duty members of the Department of Defense. Urology 1999; 53(4):806–807.

7. McKiernan JM, Goluboff ET, Liberson GL, et al. Rising risk of testicular cancer by birth cohort in the United States from 1973 to 1995. J Urol 1999; 162(2): 361–363.

8. Wanderas EH, Fossa SD, Heilo A, et al. Serum follicle stimulating hormone—predictor of cancer in the remaining testis in patients with unilateral testicular cancer. Br J Urol 1990; 66(3):315–317.

9. Garner MJ, Turner MC, Ghadirian P, et al. Epidemiology of testicular cancer: an overview. Int J Cancer 2005; 116(3):331–339.

10. Forman D, Chilvers C, Oliver R, et al. The aetiology of testicular cancer: association with congenital abnormalities, age at puberty, infertility, and exercise. Br Med J 1994; 308(6941):1393–1399.

11. Monfardini S, Vaccher E, Pizzocaro G, et al. Unusual malignant tumors in 49 patients with HIV invection. AIDS 1989; 3:449–452.

12. Wilkinson M, Carroll PR. Testicular carcinoma in patients positive and at risk for human immunodeficiency virus. J Urol 1990; 144(5):1157–1159.

13. Leibovitch I, Baniel J, Rowland RG, et al. Malignant testicular neoplasms in immunosuppressed patients. J Urol 1996; 155(6):193–1942.

14. Hricak H, Hamm B, Kim B. Imaging of the Scrotum: Textbook and Atlas. New York, Raven Press, 1995: 49–95.

15. Kennedy BJ. Testis cancer. Clinical signs and symptoms. In: Vogelzang et al., eds. Comprehensive Textbook of Genitourinary Oncology. 2nd ed. Philadelphia, PA, Lippincott Williams and Wilkins, 2000:877–879.

16. Doll DC, Weiss RB. Malignant lymphoma of the testis. Am J Med 1986; 81(3):515–524.

17. Klein EA. Tumor markers in testis cancer. Urol Clin North Am 1993; 20(1):67–73.

18. Horstman WG. Scrotal imaging. Urol Clin North Am 1997; 24(3):653–671.

19. Leibovitch I, Baniel J, Foster RS, et al. The clinical implications of procedural deviations during orchiectomy for nonseminomatous testis cancer. J Urol 1995; 154(3):935–939.

20. Warde PR, Smalley SR. Radiation therapy for testicular seminoma. In: Volgelzang NJ et al., eds. Comprehensive Textbook of Genitourinary Oncology. 3rd ed. Philadelphia, PA, Lippincott Williams and Wilkins, 2006:629–637.

21. Baniel J, Sella A. Sperm extraction at orchiectomy for testis cancer. Fertil Steril 2001; 75(2):260–262.

22. Moul JW. Proper staging techniques in testicular cancer patients. Tech Urol 1995; 1(3):126–132.

23. Gatti JM, Stephenson RA. Staging of testis cancer. Combining serum markers, histologic parameters, and radiographic findings. Urol Clin North Am 1998; 25(3):397–403.

24. American Joint Committee on Cancer and the Union Internationale Contre Le Cancre. AJCC Cancer Staging Manual. Philadelphia, Lippincott-Raven, 1997.

25. Risk Assessment for Testicular Germ Cell Cancers (International Germ Cell Consensus classification: a prognostic factor-based staging system for metastatic germ cell cancers. J Clin Oncol 1997; 15:594–603.

26. Giwercman A, von der Maase H, Skakkebaek NE. Epidemiological and clinical aspects of carcinoma in situ of the testis. Eur Urol 1993; 23(1):104–114.

27. von der Maase H, Rorth M, Walbom-Jorgensen S, et al. Carcinoma in situ of contralateral testis in patients with testicular germ cell cancer: study of 27 cases in 500 patients. Br Med J Clin Res Ed 1986; 293(6559): 1398–1401.

28. Müller J, Skakkebaek NE, Nielsen OH, et al. Cryptorchidism and testis cancer: atypical infantile germ cells followed by carcinoma in situ and invasive carcinoma in adulthood. Cancer 1984; 54(4):629–634.

29. Engeler DS, Hosli PO, John H, et al. Early orchiopexy: prepubertal intratubular germ cell neoplasia and fertility outcome. Urology 2000; 56(1):144–148.

30. Daugaard G, Giwercman A, Skakkebaek NE. Should the other testis be biopsied? Semin Urol Oncol 1996; 14(1):8–12.

31. Herr HW, Sheinfeld J. Is biopsy of the contralateral testis necessary in patients with germ cell tumors? J Urol 1997; 158(4):1331–1334.

32. Warde P, Specht L, Horwich A, et al. Prognostic factors for relapse in stage I seminoma managed by surveillance: a pooled analysis. J Clin Oncol 2002; 20(22): 4448–4452.

33. Van Rooy EM, Sagerman RH. Long-term evaluation of postorchiectomy irradiation for stage I seminoma. Radiology 1994; 191(3):857–861.

34. Bauman GS, Venkatesan VM, Ago CT, et al. Postoperative radiotherapy for Stage I/II seminoma: results for 212 patients. Int J Radiat Oncol Biol Phys 1998; 42(2):313–317.

35. Motzer R, Bosl G, Heelan R. Residual mass: an indication for further therapy in patients with advanced seminoma following systemic chemotherapy. J Clin Oncol 1987; 5(7):1064–1070.

36. Schultz S, Einhorn L, Conces D, et al. Management of post chemotherapy residual mass in patients with advanced seminoma: Indiana University experience. J Clin Oncol 1989; 7:1497–1503.

37. De Santis M, Becherer A, Bokemeyer C. 2-18fluoro-deoxy-D-glucose Positron Emission Tomography is a reliable predictor for viable tumor in postchemotherapy seminoma: an update of the prospective multicentric SEMPET trial. J Clin Onc 2004; 22(6):1034–1039.

38. Lashley DB, Lowe BA. A rational approach to managing stage I nonseminomatous germ cell cancer. Urol Clin North Am 1998; 25(3):405–423.

39. Segal R, Lukka H, Klotz LH, et al. Surveillance programs for early stage non-seminomatous testicular cancer: a practice guideline. Can J Urol 2001; 8(1): 1184–1192.

40. Peckham MJ, Barrett A, Husband J, et al. Orchidectomy alone in testicular stage I non-seminomatous germ cell tumours. Lancet 1982; 2(8300):678–680.

41. Heiken JP, Forman HP, Brown JJ. Neoplasms of the bladder, prostate, and testis. Radiol Clin North Am 1994; 32(1):81–96.

42. Stephens A, Donohue J, Hutchins G, et al. Positron emission tomography (PET) evaluation of residual radiographic abnormalities in post-chemotherapy germ cell tumors (GCT). Proceedings of ASCD 1994; 13:239.

43. Hao D, Seidel J, Brant R, et al. Compliance of clinical stage I nonseminomatous germ cell tumor patients with surveillance. J Urol 1998; 160(3 Pt 1):768–771.

44. Staubitz W. Historical perspectives on node dissection. In: Donohue JP, ed. Testis Tumors. Baltimore: Williams & Wilkins, 1983:159.

45. Donohue JP, Thornhill JA, Foster RS, et al. The role of retroperitoneal lymphadenectomy in clinical stage B testis cancer: the Indiana University experience (1965–1989). J Urol 1995; 153(1):85–89.

46. Busch FM, Sayegh ES. Roentgenographic visualization of human testicular lymphatics: a preliminary report. J Urol 1963; 89:106–110.

47. Ray B, Hajdu SI, Whitmore WF Jr. Distribution of retroperitoneal lymph nodal metastases in testicular germ cell tumours. Cancer 1974; 33:340–348.

48. Donohue JP, Zachary JM, Maynard BR. Distribution of nodal metastases in nonseminomatous testis cancer. J Urol 1982; 128(2);:315–320.

49. Donohue JP, Foster RS. Retroperitoneal lymphadenectomy for clinical stage a testis cancer: modifications of technique and impact on ejaculation. Probl Urol 1994; 8:100.

50. Aass N, Fossa SS. Paternity in young patients with testicular cancer. Expectations and experience. In: EORTIC Genitorurinary Group Monograph 5: Progress and Controversies in Oncological Urology II. New York, Aln R. Liss, 1988:481-491.

51. Richie JP. Clinical stage I testicular cancer: the role of modified retroperitoneal lymphadenectomy. J Urol 1990; 144(5):1160–1163.

52. Foster RS, McNulty A, Rubin LR, et al. The fertility of patients with clinical stage I testis cancer managed by nerve sparing retroperitoneal lymph node dissection. J Urol 1994; 152(4):1139-1142.

53. Williams SD, Stablein DM, Einhorn LH, et al. Immediate adjuvant chemotherapy versus observation with treatment at relapse in pathologic stage II testicular cancer. NEJM 1987; 317(23):1433–1438.

54. Horwich A, Norman A, Fisher C, et al. Primary chemotherapy for stage II nonseminomatous germ cell tumours of the testis. J Urol 1994; 151:72–77.

55. Hermans BP, Sweeney CJ, Foster RS, et al. Risk of systemic metastases in clinical stage I nonseminoma germ cell testis tumor managed by retroperitoneal lymph node dissection. J Urol 2000; 163(6):1721–1724.

56. McLeod DG, Weiss RB, Stablein DM, et al. Staging relationships and outcome in early stage testicular cancer: a report from the Testicular Cancer Intergroup Study. J Urol 1991; 145(6):1178–1183.

57. Studer UE, Burkhard FC, Sonntag RW. Risk adapted management with adjuvant chemotherapy in patients with high risk clinical stage I nonseminomatous germ cell tumor. J Urol 2000; 163(6):1785–1787.

58. Janetschek G, Hobisch A, Peschel R, et al. Laparoscopic retroperitoneal lymph node dissection for clinical stage I nonseminomatous testicular carcinoma: long-term outcome. J Urol 2000; 163(6):1793–1796.

59. Bhayani SB, Ong A, Oh WK, et al. Laparoscopic retroperitoneal lymph node dissection for clinical stage I nonseminomatous germ cell testicular cancer: a long-term update. Urology 2003; 62(2):324–327.

60. Winfield HN. Laparoscopic retroperitoneal lymphadenectomy for cancer of the testis. Urol Clin North Am 1998; 25(3):469–473.

61. Foster RS, Donohue JP. Retroperitoneal lymph node dissection for the management of clinical stage I nonseminoma. J Urol 2000; 163:1788–1792.

62. Rodriguez PN, Hafez GR, Messing EM. Nonseminomatous germ cell tumor of the testicle: does extensive staging of the primary tumor predict the likelihood of metastatic disease? J Urol 1986; 136(3): 604–608.

63. Aass N, Kaasa S, Lund E, et al. Long–term somatic side-effects and morbidity in testicular cancer patients. Br J Cancer 1990; 61(1):151–155.

64. Beck SD, Foster RS, Bihrle R, et al. Outcome analysis for patients with elevated serum tumor markers at postchemotherapy retroperitoneal lymph node dissection. J Clin Oncol 2005; 23(25): 6149–6156.

65. Foster RS, Donohue JP. Can retroperitoneal lymphadenectomy be omitted in some patients after chemotherapy? Urol Clin North Am 1998; 25(3):479–484.

66. Sheinfeld J. Postchemotherapy retroperitoneal lymph node dissection and resection of residual masses for germ cell tumors of the tesis. In: Volgelzang NJ et al., eds. Comprehensive textbook of genitourinary oncology. 3rd ed. Philadelphia, PA, Lippincott Williams and Wilkins, 2006:616–623.

67. Debono D, Heilman D, Einhorn L, et al. Decision analysis for avoiding post chemotherapy surgery in patients with disseminated nonseminomatous germ cell tumors. J Clin Oncol 1997; 15(4):1455–1464.

68. Steyerberg EW, Keizer HJ, Sleijfer DT, et al. Retroperitoneal metastases in testicular cancer: role of CT measurements of residual mases in decision making for resection after chemotherapy. Radiology 2000; 215(2):437–444.

69. Frohlich MW, Small EJ. Stage II nonseminomatous testis cancer: the role of primary and adjuvant chemotherapy. Urol Clin North Am 1998; 25(3):451–459.

70. Dodd PM, Motzer RJ, Bajorin DF. Poor-risk germ cell tumors. Recent developments. Urol Clin North Am 1998; 25(3):485–493.

71. Lange PH, Change WY, Fraley EE. Fertility issues in the therapy of nonseminomatous testicular tumors. Urol Clin North Am 1987; 14(4):731.

72. Turek PJ, Lowther DN, Carroll PR. Fertility issues and their management in men with testis cancer. Urol Clin North Am 1998; 25(3):517–531.

73. Petersen PM, Skakkebaek NE, Vistisen K, et al. Semen quality and reproductive hormones before orchiectomy in men with testicular cancer. J Clin Oncol 1999; 17(3):941–947.

74. Petersen PM, Giwercman A, Hansen SW, et al. Impaired testicular function in patients with carcinoma-in-situ of the testis. J Clin Oncol 1999; 17(1):173–179.

75. Jacobsen KD, Theodorsen L, Fossa SD. Spermatogenesis after unilateral orchiectomy for testicular cancer in patients following surveillance policy. J Urol 2001; 165(1):93–96.

76. Coogan CL, Hejase MJ, Wahle GR, et al. Nerve sparing post-chemotherapy retroperitoneal lymph node dissection for advanced testicular cancer. J Urol 1996; 156(5):1656–1658.

77. Cullen MH, Stenning SP, Parkinson MC, et al. Short-course adjuvant chemotherapy in high-risk stage I nonseminomatous germ cell tumors of the testis: a Medial Research Council Report. J Clin Oncol 1996; 14(4):1106–1113.

78. Nijman JM, Koops HS, Kremer J, et al. Gonadal function after surgery and chemotherapy in men with stage II and III nonseminomatous testicular tumors. J Clin Oncol 1987; 5(4):651–656.

79. Hansen PV, Glavind K, Panduro J, et al. Paternity in patients with testicular germ cell cancer: pre-treatment and post-treatment findings. Eur J Cancer 1991; 27(11):1385–1389.

80. Senturia YD, Peckham GS, Peckham MJ. Children fathered by men treated for testicular cancer. Lancet 1985; 2(8458):766–769.

81. Robbins WA, Meistrich JL, Moore D, et al. Chemotherapy induces transient sex chromosomal and autosomal aneuoploidy in human sperm. Nature Gen 1997; 16(1):74–78.

82. Hallak J, Kolettis PH, Sekhon VS, et al. Sperm cryopreservation in patients with testicular cancer. Urology 1999; 54(5):894–895.

83. Grossfeld GD, Small EJ. Long-term side effects of treatment for testis cancer. Urol Clin North Am 1998; 25(3):503–515.

84. Roth BJ, Greist A, Kubilis PS, et al. Cisplatin-based combination chemotherapy for disseminated germ cell tmors: long-term follow-up. J Clin Oncol 1988; 6(8):1239–1247.

85. Kaldor JM, Day NE, Band P, et al. Second malignancies following testicular cancer, ovarian cancer, and Hodgkin's disease: an international collaborative study among cancer registries. Int J Cancer 1987; 39(5): 571–585.

86. Schoen EH, Anderson G, Bohon C, et al. Task force on circumcision report of the task force on circumcision. Pediatrics 1989; 84:388–391.

87. Cubilla AL, Reuter VE, Gregoire L, et al. Basaloid squamous cell carcinoma: a distinctive human papilloma virus-related penile neoplasm: a report of 20 cases. Am J Surg Pathol 1998; 22(6):755–761.

88. Theodorescu D, Russo P, Zhang Z, et al. Outcomes of initial surveillance of invasive squamous cell carcinoma of the penis and negative nodes. J Urol 1996; 155(5):1626–1629.

89. Srinivas V, Morse MJ, Herr HW, et al. Penile cancer: relation of extent of nodal metastases to survival. J Urol 1987; 137(5):880–882.

90. Tabatabaei S, Harisinghani M, McDougal WS. Regional lymph node staging using lymphotropic nanoparticle enhanced magnetic resonance imaging with Ferumoxtran-10 in patients with penile cancer. J Urol 2005; 174(3):923–927.

91. Graham JH, Helwig EB. Erythroplasia of Queyrat. A clinicopathologic and histochemical study. Cancer 1973; 32(6):1396–1414.

92. Mohs FE: Chemosurgery. A microscopically controlled method of cancer excision. Arch Surg 1941; 42:279–295.

93. Mohs FE, Snow SN, Messing EM, et al. Microscopically controlled surgery of the treatment of carcinoma of the penis. J Urol 1985; 133(6):961–968.

94. Block NL, Rosen P, Whitmore WF Jr. Hemipelvectomy for advanced penile cancer. J Urol 1973; 110(6): 703–707.

95. Malloy TR, Wein AJ, Carpiniello VL. Carcinoma of the penis treated with neodymium YAG laser. Urology 1988; 31(1):26–29.

96. Mazeron JJ, Langlois D, Lobo PA, et al. Interstitial radiation therapy for carcinoma of the penis using

iridium 192 wires: the Henri Mondor experience (1970–1979). Int J Radiat Oncol Biol Phys 1984; 10(10): 1891–1895.

97. Fossa SE, Hall KS, Johannessen MB, et al. Cancer of the penis: experience at the Norwegian Radium Hospital 1974–1985. Eur Urol 1987; 13(6):372–377.

98. Catalona WJ. Modified inguinal lymphadenectomy for carcinoma of the penis with preservation of saphenous veins: technique and preliminary result. J Urol 1988; 140(2):306–310.

99. McDougal WS, Kirchner FK Jr, Edwards RH, et al. Treatment of carcinoma of the penis: the case for primary lymphadenectomy. J Urol 1986; 136(1): 38–42.

100. Fraley EE, Zhang G, Manivel C, et al. The role of ilioinguinal lymphadenectomy and significance of histological differentiation in treatment of carcinoma of the penis. J Urol 1989; 142(6):1478–1482.

101. Johnson DE, Lo RK. Management of regional lymph nodes in penile carcioma. Five-year results following therapeutic groin dissections. Urology 1984; 24(4): 308–311.

102. Bouchot O, Auvigne J, Peuvrel P, et al. Management of regional lymph nodes in carcinoma of the penis. Eur Urol 1989; 16(6):410–415.

103. Pizzocaro G, Piva L. Adjuvant and neoadjuvant vincristine, bleomycin, and methotrexate for inguinal metastases from squamous cell carcinoma of the penis. Acta Oncol 1988; 27(6b):823–824.

104. Orticochea M. A new method of total reconstruction of the penis. Br J Plast Surg 1972; 25:347–366.

105. Nahai F. The tensor fascia lata flap. Clin Plast Surg 1980; 7(1):51–56.

Prostate Disease: Prostate Hyperplasia, Prostate Cancer, and Prostatitis

Stephen J. Assinder
Discipline of Physiology, School of Medical Sciences, University of Sydney, New South Wales, Australia

Helen D. Nicholson
Department of Anatomy and Structural Biology, Otago School of Medical Sciences, University of Otago, Dunedin, New Zealand

□ INTRODUCTION

Diseases of the prostate are remarkably common, especially in the older male. Benign enlargement of the prostate affects over 50% of the male population between the ages of 51 and 60 years, and more than 80% of men by age 80 (1,2). Prostate cancer is now the most commonly diagnosed malignancy and second most common cause of cancer death in men in the United States (3). As the male lifespan, at least in the Western world, continues to increase, diseases associated with the prostate are likely to become more significant. This chapter discusses the most common disorders of the prostate: hyperplasia, cancer, and prostatitis.

□ BENIGN PROSTATIC HYPERPLASIA

Benign prostatic hyperplasia (BPH) is the most common nonmalignant tumor in males. A disease associated with aging, this nonmalignant overgrowth of the gland obstructs bladder outflow due to narrowing of the urethra, disturbing micturition. The associated symptoms are a source of serious morbidity. Approximately one-fifth of all men who live into their eighth decade will require surgical intervention to alleviate the symptoms and complications that arise from this disease (4,5).

Incidence of BPH

More than 80% of men will develop hyperplastic changes of the prostate by the age of 80 (1). Of these men (6), 50% will have suffered urodynamic consequences, as defined by the "American Urology Association Symptom Score" (7), by middle age. Of all men who live to 80 years of age, 20% to 25% will require surgical intervention to alleviate these symptoms (4,5).

Racial and ethnic variations in symptom severity and need for surgery exist and are summarized in Table 1. No difference in risk of high-moderate to severe lower urinary tract symptoms (LUTS) was reported among black, Asian, and different white participants (Southern European, Scandinavian, and other white). Asian men are less likely to require surgical intervention. Southern European men had increased risk for surgery and high-moderate to severe symptoms compared to other white men (8,9).

Pathology of BPH

Hyperplastic changes begin to develop at approximately 30 years of age (2,10). Histologically, the normal prostate exhibits distinct differences in the appearance of the central zone, the transition zone, and the peripheral zone. In the central and transition zones, the stroma is interlaced with compact bundles of smooth muscle, while the peripheral zone exhibits a loose stroma (Fig. 1). Benign hyperplasia of the prostate is primarily the result of overgrowth of this stromal tissue in the transition and central zones of the prostate (Fig. 2). In the hyperplastic prostate, the stromal compartment can be fourfold heavier than that of normal tissue (11) and is nodular in distribution, causing a partially solid and partially micro- or macrocystic character. Stromal nodules of three distinct types have been described (12): (*i*) stromal, (*ii*) fibromuscular, and (*iii*) muscular. All three types can occur simultaneously (11). The majority of early periurethral nodules are purely stromal in character, resembling embryonic mesenchyme (13).

Glandular components of the normal prostate consist of secretory epithelium, separated from the stroma by a layer of flattened elongated basal cells (Fig. 1). Hyperplastic growth of the glandular components occurs secondary to development of the disease in the stroma. Hyperplasia of the secretory epithelium is characterized by two common patterns: (*i*) intraglandular papillae with projections supported by a very narrow stromal component (Fig. 3) and (*ii*) cribriform formations (Fig. 4). Secretory activity of the hyperplastic glandular component is reduced (14). Basal-cell hyperplasia may also occur in glandular nodules, with small foci of basal-cell proliferation within hyperplastic acini. The integrity of the basal-cell portion is always maintained, however, in contrast to incidences of prostate cancer, in which the basal-cell layer is often absent.

Table 1　Relative Risks for Surgery or Severe Symptoms Among Different Races/Ethnicities

	White	Afro-American	Asian	Southern European	Scandinavian	Other White
Relative risk of surgery	1.0	0.52	0.41	1.28	0.96	1.00
Relative risk of high moderate/severe symptoms	1.0	1.1	0.94	1.34	0.84	1.00

Note: Adjusted for age, smoking, alcohol consumption, body mass index, and level of physical activity.
Source: From Ref. 8.

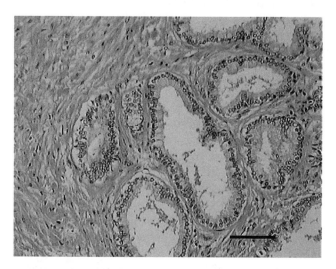

Figure 1　Histology of the normal prostate. Bar represents 100 μm.

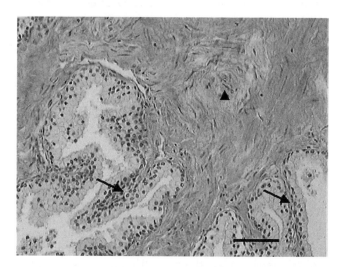

Figure 3　Histology of benign prostatic hyperplasia. *Arrows* indicate papillary epithelium and arrowhead indicates stromal nodule, bar represents 100 μm.

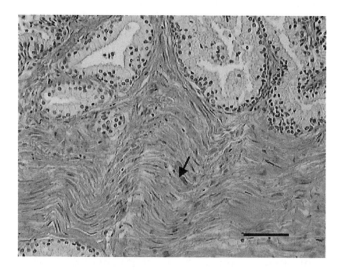

Figure 2　Histology of benign prostatic hyperplasia. *Arrow* indicates stromal hyperplasia. Bar represents 100 μm.

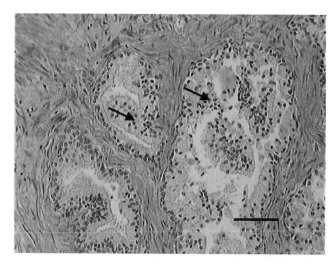

Figure 4　Histology of benign prostatic hyperplasia. *Arrows* indicate cribriform epithelium. Bar represents 100 μm.

Hyperplastic changes alone do not necessarily result in urinary symptoms. Additional factors are required, such as prostatitis, vascular infarcts, or an increase in the tensile strength of the glandular capsule (7). Most significantly, an increase in the stromal smooth-muscle tone is associated with benign prostatic disease. This contributes to bladder outflow obstruction (15) and may lead to bladder trabeculation and

associated chronic bladder infection. Approximately 50% of the total urethral pressure in BPH patients is due to α-adrenergic receptor–mediated increased muscle tone (16,17). The density of the α-adrenergic receptors that determines prostate tone (18) is increased in hyperplastic stroma (19,20).

Evidence indicates that BPH is not related to the development of prostate cancer, even though the two conditions share similar risk factors and hormonal environments. This may be a reflection of the fact that BPH is predominantly a disease of the transitional and central zones of the prostate, while prostate cancer develops in the peripheral zone (21).

Etiology of BPH

Several theories have been proposed to explain the etiology of BPH. The following were outlined by Isaacs and Coffey (2):

- Dihydrotestosterone (DHT) hypothesis: changes in androgen metabolism that occur with aging cause an increase in prostatic DHT.
- Stem-cell theory: increasing total stem-cell number.
- Embryonic reawakening theory: changes in the stromal–epithelial interactions occur with aging.

It is likely that the disease process involves all these factors, but it is presently unclear which of these is the most important.

Role of Steroids in BPH

It is well accepted that androgens have an important role in the pathogenesis of BPH. Regression of the fully developed disease is achieved by castration (11). Furthermore, castration prior to puberty prevents prostate growth as do androgen-related genetic disorders (22,23). The content of DHT in the prostate has been reported to be elevated three- or fourfold in cases of BPH (24,25). These studies, however, compared normal tissue obtained at autopsy with BPH tissue obtained by biopsy. Walsh et al. (26) showed that tissue taken at autopsy had artificially reduced DHT content. Subsequent studies have shown that total prostatic concentrations of DHT in BPH tissue are not elevated above those of normal tissue (26,27). In fact, DHT concentrations are reduced with age, and BPH may occur as a consequence of a decline in the ability of epithelial cells to convert testosterone to DHT (27,28). Epithelial DHT production decreases with age and BPH, while stromal DHT concentrations remain constant (27).

Androgens are thought to regulate the balance between cell proliferation and cell death in the normal prostate. A disturbance of this balance is apparent in BPH. Actions of DHT in maintaining this balance in all cells of the prostate are most likely mediated by growth factors produced by fibroblasts of the stroma (see below "Embryonic Reawakening"). Prostatic fibroblast proliferation is stimulated by both DHT and by basic fibroblast growth factor (bFGF). bFGF expression by fibroblasts is also stimulated by androgen (29); however, it is known that bFGF has opposing actions (growth arrest and proliferation) depending on dose (30) and cell-cycle stage (29). Further, transformation of fibroblasts to smooth-muscle cells by bFGF may also be regulated by estrogen (31). Androgens suppress the expression of transforming growth factor β (TGFβ) but stimulate the differentiation of fibroblasts

to smooth-muscle cells (29). This is paradoxical, as differentiation is thought to be a key step in formation of nodular BPH. DHT alone is not sufficient for inducing BPH. In the dog, only treatment with DHT plus estrogen or estrogen alone causes development of the disease (32–36), indicating that a change in the androgen-to-estrogen ratio is important in the development of the disease. Age-related changes in the ratio of serum steroids are known to occur. Free plasma testosterone (37) and DHT decrease with age (Fig. 5A and B), while estradiol concentrations increase (Fig. 5C) (38,39). More significantly, a decrease in prostatic DHT is seen with age (Fig. 5D), but concentrations of testosterone and estrogen do not change (28). Although changes in estrogen concentrations are debatable, there is clearly an age- and disease-associated increase in the ratio of prostatic estrogen to DHT (Fig. 5E). The change in this ratio is thought to be responsible for the induction of hyperplasia (40), with a correlation between the degree of steroid imbalance and the relative amounts of stromal tissue (28). This is supported by the stimulatory effects of estrogen on the stroma (41), consistent with BPH being primarily a disease of this tissue.

The conversion of testosterone and androstenedione to estrogen is mediated by aromatase. This enzyme is present primarily in the prostatic stroma (42), and its activity increases with age (43). Expression of estrogen receptors (ERs) is also altered in hyperplastic tissue. In the normal prostate, ERα is present only in stromal tissue; however, in hyperplastic tissue, 10% of the secretory epithelial cells also contain ERα. ERβ is expressed only in the epithelium of the healthy prostate, but expression of this receptor is more than doubled in the epithelium of hyperplastic tissue (44). The mechanisms by which estrogens contribute to the development of BPH remain unclear (45). Recent evidence indicates that estrogen may stimulate the growth of prostatic stromal cells through a pathway involving TGFβ (31). TGFβ is known to inhibit prostate epithelial growth, but it has both stimulatory and inhibitory effects on stromal growth depending on its concentration (30).

Although androgens are thought to mediate their actions on the prostate through the production of growth factors, there is no clear evidence that estrogens similarly modulate the production of growth factors in humans (46). Estrogen deprivation in humans has been shown to improve BPH-related symptoms and to reduce prostate volume significantly in BPH patients, indicating that estrogen has a role in established BPH (47).

Stem-Cell Theory and Apoptosis

Isaacs and Coffey (2) proposed that BPH results from an expansion of the native stem-cell population in the prostate. In the prostate, dormant stem cells divide to give rise to transiently proliferative daughter cells that are capable of differentiation. These rare events ensure that the normal cell complement of the prostate is

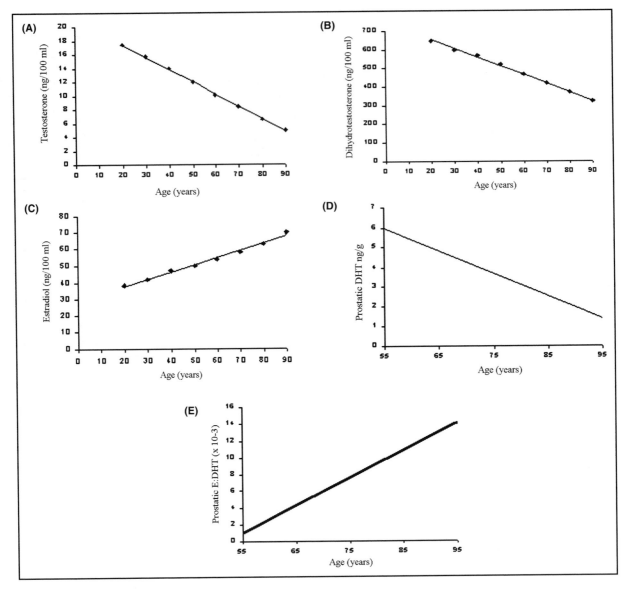

Figure 5 Hormone changes with age in men. In men, plasma concentrations of testosterone (**A**) and DHT (**B**) decrease with age, while levels of estradiol increase (**C**) (38,39). Within the prostate, concentrations of DHT also decrease with age (**D**), and as can be expected, the ratio of estrogen to DHT increases (**E**) (28). *Abbreviation*: DHT, dihydrotestosterone.

maintained. Once a proliferative cell is fully differentiated, it has a finite life span. The stem-cell theory suggests that in the aging prostate, the rate of progression toward the terminally differentiated state is slowed. This results in the overall rate of cell death being reduced. The rates of cell proliferation and cell death thus determine the overall volume of the prostate at any given time (48). In the normal prostate, there is equilibrium between cell proliferation and cell death, while in the hyperplastic prostate, the rate of cell death is reduced, resulting in a net increase in cell number (Fig. 6). This reduced rate of apoptosis is paralleled with increased cell proliferation in both the stromal and epithelial compartments (49,50). Whilst androgens and growth factors stimulate cell proliferation in vitro, they also actively inhibit cell death (48). Other studies have shown an increase in epithelial cell production but no change in apoptosis of epithelial cells (51).

Embryonic Reawakening

Androgen effects on prostate growth appear to be mediated by changes in growth factors. Deregulation of some growth factors combined with reactivation of the stroma is known to be involved in prostatic overgrowth (52). The majority of early small stromal nodules resemble embryonic mesenchyme (13). It has been demonstrated both during development and in the adult that differentiation of epithelial tissue is regulated by the mesenchyme (53). Thus, reactivation of embryonic-type stromal tissue growth in the adult stroma may stimulate growth of the glandular epithelium. This reemergence of the inductive potential of the stroma is described by the "embryonic reawakening theory." The complex interactions of growth factors of both stromal and epithelial origin integrate cell growth, apoptosis, and cell differentiation (11).

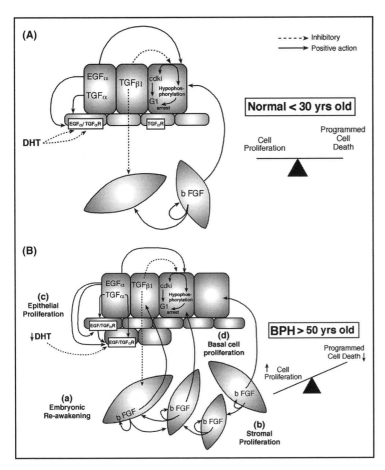

Figure 6 Stromal embryonic reawakening and growth factor imbalances that may result in BPH. (**A**) In the normal prostate (<30 years old), an equilibrium between cell proliferation and programmed cell death is maintained by paracrine actions of growth factors of both stromal (bFGF) and epithelial (TGF$_\beta$) origins. (**B**) In the aging prostate (>50 years), BPH exists due to an imbalance in favor of cell proliferation over cell death. In the embryonic reawakening hypothesis, this results from an earlier cascade of events. Stromal embryonic reawakening (a) results in increased bFGF secretion, causing an increased ratio of bFGF (positive):TGF$_\beta$ (negative) that results in further stromal proliferation. (b) Increased bFGF leads to epithelial cell activation increasing EGF$_\alpha$ expression. A net increase in epithelial-activating factors (bFGF and EGF$_\alpha$) to TGF$_\beta$ (which acts to arrest cell cycle at the G$_1$ phase) results in increased epithelial cell mitosis and thus epithelial proliferation (c). Similarly, basal-cell proliferation (d) is stimulated due to mitogenic effects of increased EGF$_\alpha$ and TGF$_\alpha$ on basal cells, enhanced by an increase in expression of their common receptor as inhibitory dihydrotestosterone levels are decreased in this 50-year-old subject. *Abbreviations*: bFGF, basic fibroblast growth factor; BPH, benign prostatic hyperplasia; DHT, dihydrotestosterone; EGF, epidermal growth factor; TGF, transforming growth factor.

Imbalance in these relationships caused by embryonic reawakening is probably involved in initiation, progression, and maintenance of BPH (Fig. 6).

Stromal growth is regulated by interactions between TGFβ and bFGF. In vitro bFGF stimulates mitosis of fibroblasts derived from human prostate tissue. In contrast, TGFβ inhibits fibroblast proliferation in vitro. bFGF is increased in BPH tissue, resulting in an imbalance between bFGF and TGFβ and thus potentially promoting stromal hyperplasia (54).

Epithelial growth is influenced by both TGFβ and epidermal growth factor α (EGFα). EGFα stimulates epithelial growth in vitro, while TGFβ inhibits it (55). Thus, it is possible to imagine that an increase in bFGF expression caused by reawakening of the mesenchyme could cause a cascade of changes resulting in an imbalance favoring cell proliferation of both stromal and epithelial tissues (Fig. 6).

Changes in the balance of growth factors and their effects are not limited to the stroma and the secretory epithelium of the acini. The growth factors EGFα and TGFα share a common receptor (56,57) that is expressed by basal cells. Interestingly, this receptor is downregulated by androgens.

Other Factors in the Etiology of BPH

Nonsteroid hormones including oxytocin and prolactin have also been implicated in BPH. Prostatic oxytocin concentrations are elevated in the hyperplastic prostate (58). Increased oxytocin expression may be of significance for several reasons. As in other regions of the male reproductive tract, oxytocin stimulates smooth-muscle contraction of the prostate, maintaining muscle tone (59). Thus, increased levels may contribute to the increased prostatic tone associated with BPH. Furthermore, oxytocin increases epithelial cell growth of the acini in rabbits (60) and in rats (61). The mechanism of this action is unclear; however, oxytocin has been shown to regulate androgen production in vitro by increasing the activity of 5-α-reductase (62), which converts testosterone to the biologically active DHT. In the rat, an animal in which BPH does not develop, a feedback mechanism involving regulation of local oxytocin concentration by androgens and estrogens is proposed (63). It is hypothesized that such a regulatory feedback mechanism is either absent in man or perturbed during the pathogenesis of BPH.

Prolactin is also synthesized in the secretory epithelium of the prostate (64). Transgenic mice that overexpress prolactin have been shown to develop dramatically enlarged prostates with significantly increased stromal growth (65). This peptide hormone acts as a direct growth and differentiation factor (66) and enhances the sensitivity of prostate tissue to androgen in vitro (67), possibly by increasing cell permeability to testosterone (68). Although circulatory prolactin levels are similar in BPH patients and disease-free men (69), it has been suggested that BPH tissue may be more sensitive to prolactin (45).

Diagnosis of BPH

Diagnosis of BPH is achieved from a detailed medical and physical examination, rectal examination, tests to exclude urinary tract infections, and urinary flow measurement. In men over 50, BPH is the most common cause of LUTS, but other conditions can cause similar symptoms. Men with either bladder or prostate cancer can also present with LUTS. LUTS are commonly classified into voiding and storage symptoms. Voiding symptoms include hesitancy, interruption of voiding, and decreased urinary flow rate resulting in prolonged micturition. Storage symptoms include increased voiding frequency, nocturia, urgency, and incontinence. Validated symptom scores such as the American Urological Association score index or the International Prostate Symptom Score (IPSS) are used to measure the severity of symptoms in patients presenting with LUTS (70).

A commonly applied case definition of BPH includes at least two of the following: moderate-to-severe LUTS (a score ≥8 on the IPSS), an enlarged prostate volume of greater than 30 mL, and a decreased peak urinary flow rate of less than 10 mL/sec (71).

Symptoms of BPH generally progress over a period of years. Sudden onset of symptoms usually suggests the presence of another condition, often a malignancy of prostate or bladder.

Digital rectal examination (DRE) is useful in assessing prostate volume, which is increased in BPH. An enlarged, firm (similar to the consistency of the tip of the nose) prostate is a common finding in BPH (72). The size of the gland in BPH is relevant to the type of surgery offered (see section "Clinical Management of BPH"). Discrete nodules or asymmetry is suggestive of prostate cancer (72). A DRE can often detect locally advanced but not early prostate cancer.

A raised level of prostate-specific antigen (PSA) is used as a marker for prostate cancer, but many patients presenting with LUTS and BPH will also have a raised PSA level. Conversely, men with early prostate cancer will often have normal levels of PSA. PSA testing is controversial. Thorpe and Neal (71) have suggested that it should not be used as a routine screening procedure.

Measurement of urodynamics and postflow residual urine can be used to confirm a diagnosis of BPH and to assess the level of symptom severity. These are optional tests for men with LUTS, but when the history and physical examination tests are inconclusive or conflict, they may be useful. A low flow rate of less than 10 mL/sec is a reasonable predictor of outlet obstruction (71). Urine analysis and renal function tests can be performed to exclude renal damage and urinary tract infections as causes of LUTS. Table 2 summarizes symptoms and diagnostic options and the results that allow BPH and prostate cancer to be distinguished from each other.

Clinical Management of BPH

Several strategies using either a surgical or a pharmacological approach have been utilized to reduce the symptoms of BPH (73). Treatment options range from "watchful waiting" (the regular monitoring of patients who wish to delay active therapy) and transurethral resection of the prostate (TURP) to minimally invasive surgical techniques such as laser therapy, transurethral needle ablation, and transurethral microwave therapy. Medical therapies involving androgen blockade are also used. Table 3 summarizes available treatment options for BPH as well as their indications and potential risks.

Transurethral Resection of the Prostate

In men with severe symptoms or complications arising from BPH, TURP is considered the gold standard to which other therapies are compared. This procedure first involves the stepwise removal of fibers at the bladder neck followed by resection of the midprostatic fossa, with the prostatic capsule forming the limit to the depth of the resection (81). Finally, tissue

Table 2 Symptoms and Diagnostic Test Results Indicative of BPH Vs. Prostate Cancer

	BPH	**Prostate cancer**
History of lower urinary tract symptoms	Slowly progressive symptoms, often over a number of years	Rapid onset of symptoms
International Prostate Symptom Score	≥8	≥20
Digital rectal examination	Enlarged prostate (>30 mL), but firm and symmetrical	Nodules and/or hard areas; asymmetrical shape is indicative of locally advanced cancer
Measurement of PSA levels	Can be elevated in BPH	Can be elevated in advanced disease, but also found within normal range in early stages of prostate cancer
Peak urinary flow rate	Decreased, <10 mL/sec (Ref. 71)	Not appropriate, as prostate cancer may often be asymptomatic

Abbreviations: BPH, benign prostatic hyperplasia; PSA, prostate-specific antigen.

Table 3 Treatment Approaches for Benign Prostatic Hyperplasia: Indications and Potential Risks

Approach	Indications	Possible complications
Watchful waiting	Mild symptoms	None
TURP	Prostate >30 g	Mortality (0.2–0.4% for elective operations), incontinence (3%), erectile dysfunction (5–10%), retrograde ejaculation (60–80%), bladder neck contracture (3–5%) (Ref. 71)
TUIP	Prostate ≤25 g (Ref. 74), moderate bladder outflow obstruction (Ref. 75)	Incontinence (1%), erectile dysfunction (0–4%), retrograde ejaculation (15–20%), bladder neck contracture (1%)
TUNA	Moderate to severe symptoms, with minimal bladder obstruction	Significantly fewer complications reported for TUNA (Ref. 76) compared to TURP (Ref. 77). Incidence of incontinence, erectile dysfunction, and bladder stricture are 1.5% less than TURP
TUMT	Prostate >30 g, high-grade bladder obstruction. Patients with high operative risk for invasive procedures (Ref. 78)	Limited durability of outcomes, urinary tract infections, urinary retention, reintervention, erectile dysfunction, retrograde ejaculation
Finasteride (5-α-reductase inhibitor)	Prostate >40 g (Ref. 79)	Erectile dysfunction (3–16%), decreased libido (2–10%), abnormal ejaculation (0–8%) (Ref. 80)

Abbreviations: TUIP, transurethral incision of the prostate; TUMT, transurethral microwave treatment; TURP, transurethral resection of the prostate; TUNA, transurethral needle ablation.

immediately proximal to the external sphincter mechanism is removed. As up to 20% of the prostate projects distal to the verumontanum, it is often necessary to leave part of the adenoma in order to avoid sphincter injury and subsequent urinary incontinence (81). Resection of the bladder neck can result in retrograde ejaculation. There is conflicting evidence regarding the level of morbidity associated with TURP, which is often dependent on the outcome measures selected. A recent review estimates that TURP morbidity can be as high as 20% (82).

Alternative Surgical Interventions

Simpler and less intrusive surgical methods of control are also available. Transurethral incision of the prostate is simpler than TURP in that only one or two incisions, starting at the urethral orifice and continuing to the verumontanum, are made. Laser prostatectomy and prostatic stents are other less common interventions that may be considered. Laser therapy has been shown to be effective in decreasing LUTS and has the benefit of shorter hospital stay and lower

risk of complications; however, TURP has been shown to be superior to laser therapy in terms of effectiveness (83,84).

Hormone Therapy

Pharmacological methods of androgen deprivation (Table 4) have been shown to be effective in decreasing prostate size; however, these methods may take up to six months for a significant decrease in prostate size to be achieved, probably due to the fact that incomplete androgen blockade is achieved. 5-α-reductase inhibition by finasteride has few significant side effects, although decreased libido in 5% to 10% of patients (85) and reduced semen volume have been reported (86). The decrease in prostate size following finasteride treatment appears to be related to apoptosis as do all androgen ablation therapies (87).

Since estrogens may be involved in the etiology of BPH, antiestrogens or aromatase inhibitors may be useful in the treatment of the disease; however, studies thus far have not indicated any positive improvements with such treatment. This may be due to the

Table 4 Pharmacological Methods of Androgen Ablation Therapy and Associated Side Effects

Method of androgen blockade	Example of agents	Side effects
Antiandrogens		
Progestational antiandrogens	Cyproterone acetate	Severe loss of libido
Non-steroid antiandrogen	Flutamide	Gynecomastia, gastrointestinal disturbance
GnRH/LHRH agonists	Leuprolide acetate Triptoreline pamoate Histrelin implant	Decreased libido, hot flushes, erectile dysfunction
5-α-reductase inhibitors	Finasteride	Decreased libido, reduced semen volume

Abbreviation: GnRH/LHRH, gonadotropin-releasing hormone/luteinizing hormone-releasing hormone.

concomitant increase in the concentration of androgens caused by this treatment counterbalancing any effect of the treatment (46).

α_1-Adrenoreceptor Blockers

The tone of prostatic smooth muscle is controlled by adrenergic nerve activity. To relieve symptoms, a reduction in the increased tone associated with BPH may be achieved through the use of α_1-adrenoreceptor blockers (e.g., alphazosin and doxazosin). These treatments have the added advantage of a rapid onset of action, with optimum symptom relief being achieved within the first month of treatment (88). These drugs have some common side effects including postural hypotension, dizziness, and light-headedness. In addition to relaxation of muscle tone, α_1-blockers may also increase rates of apoptosis of prostate cells without affecting cell proliferation (89).

Herbal Remedies

Phytotherapeutic agents extracted from herbs and plants are increasing in popularity for the treatment of BPH symptoms. These agents account for half of the medications dispensed in Italy (90) and 90% of all drugs prescribed in Germany and Austria (91). Two of the most widely used phytotherapeutic agents are those that contain β-sitosterols (91) and the extract of *Serenoa repens*. Their exact mechanisms of action are unknown. It is proposed that β-sitosterols may affect cholesterol metabolism and thus subsequent steroid production or have anti-inflammatory effects (92). Systematic reviews of the available literature have shown that β-sitosterols improve urological conditions, but there is a lack of comparison with other agents (93). *S. repen* produces symptomatic improvements similar to finasteride (94). A recent meta-analysis of all published trials of *S. repens* for treating BPH showed a significant improvement in flow rate and a reduction in nocturia compared with placebo, and also a reduction of five points in the IPSS (95). No data exists, however, on the long-term effectiveness and side effects of these phytotherapeutic agents.

□ PROSTATE CANCER

Carcinoma of the prostate is now the most frequently diagnosed cancer and the second most common cause of cancer-related death in men. It is typically a disease of older men, with an interesting natural history. Postmortem studies have demonstrated that approximately 40% of 50-year-old men have evidence of microscopic prostate cancer. Less than 20% of men, however, will develop clinical disease, and only 2% to 4% will subsequently die from the malignancy (96). As a result, there is considerable controversy concerning the appropriate clinical management of prostate cancer, with debate existing over the necessity of screening, and when and how to treat the disease.

Incidence of Prostate Cancer

There are worldwide variations in the incidence of prostate cancer that appear to be related to race and geography. Within the United States, the incidence is highest in the African-American population and lowest in those of Asian descent (97). Geographically, the incidence of prostate cancer in Europe is higher than that seen in Asia or Egypt (98). Even within Europe, there are marked differences, with the incidence of prostate cancer in northern Europe being almost twice that in the southern part of the continent (98).

Perhaps more worrying is the fact that the incidence of prostate cancer has drastically increased over the last 30 years (99). It has been argued that the rise in incidence may be due to the introduction of screening programs in the mid-1980s (100). Certainly, evidence from the United States suggests that screening may have had some impact as there was a slow increase in the incidence of prostate cancer from 1974 and a more rapid increase between 1988 and 1992 (101). Since 1992, there has been a decline in the incidence of prostate cancer in the United States. The evidence from England and Wales presents a slightly different picture, showing a steady increase in incidence since 1971 with only a small increase in incidence following the availability of PSA testing (99).

Recent changes in the incidence of prostate cancer have been accompanied by alterations in the mortality rate of the disease. Death rates have risen during the last 30 years, but there is evidence that peak rates may have been reached in the mid-1990s. Nevertheless, carcinoma of the prostate is still responsible for approximately 3% of all deaths in men over the age of 55 in the United States. (102). Table 5 summarizes worldwide death rates from prostate cancer.

Etiology of Prostate Cancer

The etiology of prostate cancer is poorly understood. Prostate cancer is a disease of the aging male, with 96% of all cases occurring in men over the age of 60 (99). Prostate cancer is an androgen-dependent disease (103), and androgen withdrawal has been used as a

Table 5   Worldwide Death Rates from Prostate Cancer in 2000

Country	Age-adjusted death rates for prostate cancer per 100,000 population
United States	17.9
Australia	18.0
China	1.0
Denmark	23.0
France	19.2
Greece	10.7
Japan	5.5
New Zealand	21.2
Sweden	27.3
Trinidad and Tobago	32.3
United Kingdom	18.5

Source: Adapted from Ref. 101.

major treatment of the malignancy. The role of testosterone in the development of the disease, however, is unclear. Prostate cancer rarely occurs in men who have been castrated, but there is conflicting evidence as to whether circulating levels of the androgen are increased or decreased in patients with carcinoma of the prostate. Thus, androgens may be actively involved in the initiation of the disease or may play a permissive role, being necessary for the maintenance of the malignant changes.

Family history also plays a role in the development of the disease. Patients who have a first- or second-degree relative with the disease have an increased risk of developing prostate cancer (104,105), and the risk is higher if the relatives were diagnosed with the disease at an early age. There is also an association between breast cancer and prostate cancer. Men who have female relatives with carcinoma of the breast have a higher incidence of prostate cancer (106). A hereditary form of prostate cancer has also been identified. This form of the disease tends to have an earlier age of onset and accounts for approximately 9% of all cases of prostate cancer (107). The hereditary form of the disease has an autosomal dominant mode of inheritance and has a frequency of 0.36% in the Caucasian population (107). Several predisposing loci have been mapped. Hereditary prostate cancer 1 was the first predisposing gene locus to be identified (107), and recent evidence suggests that within Europe, predisposing for cancer of the prostate (PCaP) is the major predisposing locus for hereditary prostate cancer (108).

Prostate cancer is also associated with significant racial and environmental factors. Within the United States, the incidence of prostate cancer is greatest among the African-American population, who also have the poorest survival rates (96). Some of the variation between races may be due to genetic differences. It has been suggested that the increase in incidence may, in part, be related to the length of the androgen-receptor gene, since in African-Americans, the mean number of androgen-receptor gene CAG repeats is lower than other races (109).

Even within a single race, variations in the incidence of the disease occur. Carcinoma of the prostate is less common in Japanese men living in Japan than in Hawaii; however, amongst Japanese men who migrate to Hawaii, the incidence of the disease significantly increases within one generation (110). The relatively rapid increase in incidence of the disease in these men suggests that environmental, rather than genetic, influences are involved. A variety of dietary factors have been implicated over the years. Of these, a diet high in dairy products and red meat has been reported to increase the incidence of prostate cancer, while dietary phytoestrogens (i.e., soy), vitamin E, and selenium may be protective (111).

In the early 1990s, concern was raised that vasectomy may increase the risk of developing prostate cancer (112). Recent studies confirm that vasectomy does not increase the risk of prostate cancer even 25 years or longer after vasectomy (113,114), although vasectomized men may present with earlier-stage prostate tumors (115).

Natural History of Prostate Cancer

The development of prostate cancer appears to occur in several stages (Fig. 7). First, there is an initiation process that leads to the development of focal lesions of high-grade prostatic intraepithelial neoplasia (PIN). These focal lesions are characterized by proliferation of the epithelial cells within existing ducts and acini. Unlike poorly differentiated prostate carcinoma, however, in which the basal-cell layer of the acini is absent, basal cells are present in PIN, although the layer may be fragmented. The development of PIN and localized cancer is due to a continuum of changes. During this process, there is a gradual loss of the basal-cell layer, increased numbers of abnormalities in the expression of cell adhesion molecules, and increasing cell proliferation and genetic instability (116). The progression to metastatic disease is accompanied by further changes in the expression of extracellular matrix molecules (e.g., E-cadherin). In the final stages of the disease, the prostate may become insensitive to androgens.

There is a high rate of focal lesions worldwide, and the incidence of such lesions does not appear to be related to race or ethnicity; however, the presence of focal lesions is age dependent (117). The incidence of focal lesions approximately doubles every five years and affects approximately 30% of 45-year-old men.

Two theories exist with respect to the progression of focal lesions to clinical disease. One hypothesis, proposed by Stamey (118), suggests that when histological carcinoma of the prostate is detected, all the cells in the lesion have already completed the necessary steps to produce a fully malignant and invasive tumor. Thus, progression of the disease is determined by the time it takes for the tumor to grow. This might suggest that there is a relatively fixed period of time between the appearance of focal lesions and the development of clinical disease. This, however, does not seem to be the case. Although the factors leading to

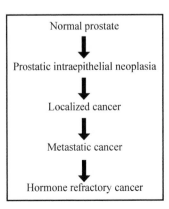

Figure 7 The progression of prostate cancer.

initiation of prostate cancer appear to be independent of race, the progression of these focal lesions to invasive disease is affected by environmental conditions.

A second theory by Carter et al. (119) proposes that not all cells in focal lesions have undergone the changes necessary to transform them into malignant cells. It suggests that a series of further steps are required and these can occur at any time and may be modified by other factors. This "multistep" theory could explain how the initiation of prostate cancer and the development of focal lesions are independent of race or geography, while the promotion of the disease to localized cancer can be influenced by genetic makeup and the environment. It also raises the possibility that modification of diet and lifestyle may influence the progression of prostate cancer.

Pathology of Prostate Cancer

More than 95% of all prostate cancers are adenocarcinomas. The remaining tumors represent a wide variety of epithelial and nonepithelial malignancies. Carcinoma of the prostate occurs more commonly in the peripheral zone of the prostate, with approximately 70% of tumors occurring in this region. An additional 20% of tumors occur in the transition zone and 10% in the central zone. (For further information on normal function of the prostate, see Chapter 7.)

Carcinoma of the prostate is associated with altered prostatic function. The secretory pattern of the epithelial cells may be changed, resulting in fewer corpora amylacea and often an increase in mucin secretion (120). Altered prostatic levels of zinc, choline, and citrate have also been observed (121–124). As mentioned earlier, expression of many cell adhesion proteins and constituents of the extracellular matrix are also altered in the malignant tissue (116).

Androgens appear to be necessary for the maintenance of normal prostate function and the continuing growth of prostate cancer; however, evidence suggests that these steroids may act indirectly via various growth factors. Changes in the expression of growth factors and their receptors occur in carcinoma of the prostate. TGFα, which promotes growth in the normal prostate, is increased both in prostate cancer cell lines (125) and tissue from patients with prostate cancer (126). Similarly, the EGF receptor, which TGFα utilizes, is upregulated (127). The inhibitory response to growth by TGFβ is also reported to be diminished in some cancer cells (128). In addition to changes in expression of growth factors, alterations in receptors for other hormones, such as estrogen and growth hormone, also occur in the malignant tissue. Thus, while only ERβ is expressed in normal epithelial cells, both ERα and ERβ are seen in malignant cell lines (129).

It remains unclear whether these changes are important in the development of the tumor or whether they result as a consequence of the malignant change. The identification of these factors, however, provides new avenues for the development of effective treatment for prostate cancer.

Clinical Manifestation of Prostate Cancer

Localized prostate cancer may be asymptomatic, although patients commonly present with obstructive urinary symptoms. DRE at this time may reveal an area of induration or a palpable prostatic nodule. Initially, there is usually local growth of the tumor, followed by lymphatic and hematogenous spread. Within the gland, there may be a single area or multiple foci of the disease. Local extension of the tumor through the capsule may result in involvement of the seminal vesicles, bladder neck, and ureters. Lymphatic spread commonly involves the obturator nodes but may also spread to a variety of other nodes including the hypogastric, external iliac, common iliac, sacral, and inguinal nodes. Hematogenous spread typically results in bony metastases. The pelvis and lumbosacral vertebrae are commonly affected. This is thought to be due to the communication between the prostatic and vertebral venous plexi and the lack of valves in the latter, which allows retrograde spread.

Detection of Prostate Cancer

The natural history of prostate cancer, with an early latent phase followed by clinical disease some years later, makes it a candidate for a screening program. Whether to screen or not, however, is still a matter for debate. The controversy exists in several areas including the accuracy and sensitivity of available markers to detect the tumor and how tumors should subsequently be treated.

DRE can be used to detect and stage prostate cancer; however, DRE is subjective, and suffers from both under and overstaging of tumors. PSA is commonly used to screen for prostate cancer. PSA is a serine protease (kallikrein 3) that is secreted by the epithelial cells of the prostate. In the normal prostate, most PSA is secreted into the seminal fluid, but with breakdown of the basal-cell layer that occurs with prostate cancer, PSA "leaks" into the circulation. Elevated levels of PSA are associated with both prostate-confined and extraprostatic disease, with a value of above 4 ng/mL being suggestive of malignancy. Although PSA levels may be useful in studying large groups of patients, there is significant variation in normal PSA secretion between individuals. Furthermore, in poorly differentiated tumors, PSA secretion may be less elevated. Thus, a few patients with a PSA below 4 ng/mL may have carcinoma of the prostate, and a sizeable number of those patients with a PSA above 4 ng/mL will not have clinical prostate cancer. The combination of PSA measurement and DRE increases the positive predictive value of screening from 31.5% to 48.5%, and the addition of transrectal ultrasound has a further additive effect (130). The diagnosis of prostate cancer should be confirmed by systematic needle biopsy of the prostate.

Staging and Grading

Assessment of the nature of the tumor and its degree of spread are critical to the management of patients with prostate cancer and depend on the accurate staging of the disease.

The tumor, nodes, metastases (TNM) method of staging classifies the disease according to the characteristics of the primary tumor and the degree to which it has spread locally (T stage), or if there is lymph node involvement (N stage), or distant metastases (M stage) (Table 6). Another method of staging is the modified Jewett system (131), which uses the information obtained from DRE as well as the degree of metastasis (Table 7). The biological behavior of the tumor is also important. Well-differentiated malignancies with a slower rate of cell division and growth usually have a better prognosis than poorly differentiated tumors.

The Gleason system is commonly used to grade the tumor (132). This system assesses the low-power light microscopic appearance of the glandular architecture of the prostate. The pathologist assigns a grade (from 1 to 5) to the pattern of cancer that is most commonly seen within the specimen and another grade to the second most common pattern of disease observed. The two grades are then added together to give the "Gleason score." An area of well-differentiated tumor is assigned a "1," and a poorly differentiated, a "5." Thus, scores range from 2 (1 + 1) to 10 (5 + 5). A score of "2" indicates a well-differentiated tumor, while "5–6" signifies a moderately differentiated cancer, and "8–10" indicates poorly differentiated cancer. The Gleason score is a measure of how aggressive the cancer may be.

Taken with clinical stage and PSA level, it is used to assess the likelihood of progression of the cancer and is useful in helping patients and their clinicians choose between treatment options. In general, survival following diagnosis of prostate cancer is linked to the Gleason score. Men between the ages of 65 and 75 years with conservatively treated, low-grade prostate cancer (Gleason score of 2–4) have no loss of life expectancy, but those with scores between 5 and 10 have a progressively decreased life expectancy (133).

Clinical Management of Prostate Cancer

The management of carcinoma of the prostate is influenced by a variety of factors including the age of the patient, the stage of the disease, and the histological grade of the tumor. It is also affected by whether the treatment is intended to be curative or palliative. In a younger man (aged 55–74 years) with organ-confined tumor, curative treatment might include radical prostatectomy or radiotherapy. Radical prostatectomy, as its name infers, involves removal of the whole prostate. It has a 10-year survival rate of approximately 60%, but the operation itself carries a 0% to 2% mortality rate as well as the risks of impotence and incontinence (134). Radiotherapy can be administered either by external beam radiation or by brachytherapy, which is the local delivery of high doses of radiation by the implantation of radioactive seeds.

Table 6 Tumor, Nodes, Metastases (TNM) Staging System for Prostate Cancer

T (primary tumor)		N (regional lymph nodes)[a]		M (distant metastasis)	
Tx	Cannot be assessed	Nx	Cannot be assessed	Mx	Cannot be assessed
T0	No evidence of primary tumor	N0	No regional lymph node metastasis	M0	No distant metastasis
Tis	Prostatic intraepithelial neoplasia			M1	Cancer has metastasized to distant organs, bones, or other organs
T1	Clinically unapparent tumor, not detected by DRE nor visible by imaging	N1	Metastasis in regional lymph node(s)		
T1a	≤5% of tissue in resection for BPH has cancer, normal DRE			M1a	Distant metastasis in nonregional lymph nodes
T1b	>5% of tissue in resection for BPH has cancer, normal DRE			M1b	Distant metastasis to bone
T1c	Cancer detected from needle biopsy due to elevated PSA alone, normal DRE and TRUS			M1c	Distant metastasis to other sites
T2	Tumor confined to prostate (detectable by DRE, not visible on TRUS)				
T2a	Tumor limited to one lobe				
T2b	Tumor involves both lobes				
T3	Tumor extends through the prostate capsule but without metastasis				
T3a	Extracapsular extension of tumor				
T3b	Involvement of seminal vesicles				
T4	Tumor extends into the bladder neck, sphincter, rectum, pelvic floor or wall				

[a]Regional lymph nodes = obturator, external and internal iliac, presacral.
Abbreviations: DRE, digital rectal examination; PRA, prostate-specific antigen; TRUS, transrectal ultrasound.

Table 7   Modified Jewett Staging System for Prostate Cancer

A1	≤5% of tissue in resection for BPH has cancer
A2	>5% of tissue in resection for BPH has cancer
B1	Palpable nodule ≤1.5 cm, confined to prostate
B2	Palpable nodule >1.5 cm, confined to prostate
C1	Palpable extracapsular extension
C2	Palpable involvement of seminal vesicle
D0	Clinically localized disease, elevated prostate-specific antigen
D1	Pelvic lymph node metastasis
D2	Metastasis to bone
D3	Hormone refractory disease

Abbreviation: BPH, benign prostatic hyperplasia.

Cancer confined to the prostate in an elderly man (>75 years) is often "treated" by "watchful waiting," since death is more likely to be due to causes other than prostate cancer. It has been recently recommended that the term "watchful waiting" be replaced by a more accurate description, "active monitoring" (135).

In patients in whom the tumor has spread outside of the prostate, hormonal treatment is aimed at either depleting androgens or reducing their effects. Orchidectomy provides a safe method of reducing testicular androgens but is accompanied by loss of libido and potency. Gonadotrophin-releasing hormone analogues provide an alternative means of reducing androgen production. The addition of an antiandrogen (e.g., flutamide) maximizes the androgen blockade. Alternatively, treatment may be directed to specific problems related to the disease (e.g., local radiotherapy for bony metastases).

As prostate cancer progresses, the disease may become refractory or insensitive to androgens, and the tumor may escape the effects of androgen suppression or androgen blockade therapy. This refractoriness was initially thought to be due to a loss of androgen receptor expression by the cancer. Although androgen receptor expression is reduced in some prostate cancer cell lines, this does not always appear to be the case in vivo. In fact, recent data suggests that in hormone refractory disease, antiandrogens may activate rather than inhibit the androgen receptor (136).

☐ PROSTATITIS

Prostatitis is the most common urological complaint seen by the general practitioner in men aged less than 50 years and the third most common urological diagnosis in men older than 50 years (137). A survey in the United States showed that there were more consultations for prostatitis than either BPH or prostate cancer, and that it was diagnosed in 25% of all genitourinary related complaints (138). The disease is associated with chronic pelvic pain, sexual disturbance, and psychological disturbance (139,140). Although it is a debilitating disease that causes significant morbidity, prostatitis has been somewhat neglected in the literature.

Prostatitis can also be difficult and frustrating to treat. According to Nickel, "in terms of time, resources, and finances being expended on management and research in prostatitis, it really seems to be the 'poor cousin' when compared to prostate cancer and benign prostatic hyperplasia" (138).

Prostatitis as a Risk Factor for BPH and Prostate Cancer

There is little available data that suggests a causative link between prostatitis and BPH or prostate cancer; however, there does appear to be an increase in risk of developing BPH in men with a history of prostatitis (141). There is also evidence to suggest that prostatitis is associated with an increased risk of prostate cancer. This risk appears to be lower than that associated with BPH (142). To date, there is no clear mechanism of causality in either case.

Symptoms of Prostatitis

Symptoms of prostatitis vary. The most common presenting complaints are those relating to pain and discomfort. Pain is often perceived in the penis and urethra but can also be felt in the perineum, groin, testes, lower back, and suprapubic areas. Irritative and obstructive voiding dysfunctions also occur. These commonly include increased urinary urgency and frequency, dysuria, nocturia, and abnormal urinary flow (e.g., hesitancy, interrupted flow, and reduced force and volume).

Classification and Etiology of Prostatitis

Prostatitis has traditionally been divided into four clinical classifications according to Drach et al. (143):

- Acute bacterial prostatitis (ABP) resulting in prostatic abscess formation
- Chronic bacterial prostatitis (CBP)
- Non/abacterial prostatitis (NBP)
- Prostatodynia

While the clinical symptoms of ABP, CBP, and NBP are all accepted as being the result of inflammation, prostatodynia describes a painful condition in which no signs of inflammation or bacterial infection exist, despite clinical symptoms. A slight modification of this classification system (Table 8) was later adapted by the National Institute of Health and summarized by Nickel (138).

The most common causes of bacterial prostatitis are the gram-negative pathogens. *Escherichia coli* is by far the most common isolate, being identified in 65% to 80% of all cases. Other gram-negative bacteria including *Pseudomonas aeruginosa*, Serratia, Klebsiella, and *Enterobacter aerogenes* are isolated less frequently and account for 10% to 15% of all bacterial cases (144). The significance of gram-positive bacteria is unclear. *Staphylococcus saprophyticus, Staphylococcus*

Table 8 National Institute of Health Classification of Prostatitis and Suggested Management

Classification	Definition	Management
Category I: Acute bacterial prostatitis	Acute infection of the prostate	Broad-spectrum antibiotic cover (initially, parenteral antibiotics)
Category II: Chronic bacterial prostatitis	Recurrent infection of the prostate	Trimethroprin or quinolone suppressive antibiotic therapy in relapsing phase. Recurrent phase control with long-term, low-dose prophylactic antibiotic treatment
Category III: CPPS		
IIIA: Inflammatory CPPS	White blood cells in semen/expressed prostatic secretions/post-prostatic massage urine but no demonstrable infection	Trial broad range antibiotic (4–6 wk). Anti-inflammatory agents, α-blocker for obstructive voiding, phytotherapy, repetitive prostate massage (2–3 times weekly). Consider transurethral microwave therapy
IIIB: Noninflammatory CPPS	No white blood cells in semen/expressed prostatic secretions/post-prostatic massage urine and no demonstrable infection	α-blocker therapy, muscle relaxant therapy, analgesics, relaxation exercises
Category IV: Asymptomatic inflammatory prostatitis	No subjective symptoms detected either by prostate biopsy or presence of white blood cells in semen/expressed prostatic secretions during evaluation for other disorders	No therapy

Abbreviation: CPPS, Chronic pelvic pain syndrome.
Source: Adapted from Ref. 138.

aureus, coagulase-negative staphylococci, hemolytic streptococci, *Neisseria gonorrheae*, *Mycobacterium tuberculosis*, Salmonella, and *Chlamydia trachomatis* have all been implicated (145). It has been suggested that an immunocompromised state leads to an increased risk of prostatitis due to these uncommon pathogens (146).

The significance of enterococci, coagulase-negative staphylococci, chlamydia, and anaerobic pathogens in the etiology of prostatitis remains unresolved. Although the diagnosis of acute prostatitis and CBP is not usually problematic, the classification of Drach et al. (143) does not readily grade those patients who present with uncommon pathogens. Furthermore, patients with recurrent prostatitis often fail to produce a positive bacterial culture. Such cases, diagnosed as chronic NBP, are most likely to be false negatives (147) and reflect the changes in bacterial growth caused by inefficient antibacterial challenge used in the treatment of ABP. High concentrations of antibiotic are difficult to achieve in the prostate (148) such that low concentrations drive the formation of bacterial biofilms in the prostatic ducts and acini (149,150). These biofilms present mechanisms of protection against further challenge from antimicrobial agents (151), resulting in persistent infection.

In true chronic NBP, the etiology is more difficult to classify, with many cases being misclassified. In many patients in whom no bacterial culture can be achieved, antibodies to common uropathogens are present (152). Indeed, molecular biology techniques have shown the presence of bacteria in men experiencing chronic pelvic pain, in whom bacteria were undetectable by traditional methodology (153). While the involvement of *C. trachomatis* in nonbacterial prostatitis remains the subject of debate, its detection using nonconventional screening methods has shown it to be commonly present (154,155).

By definition, patients with prostatodynia have symptoms of prostatitis but no previous history of urinary tract infection, no identifiable infection, and normal prostatic secretions. Most patients, however, will show evidence of an immune response and the same urodynamic abnormalities associated with nonbacterial prostatitis (156). These similarities are not considered in the classification of Drach et al. (143). Likewise, the asymptomatic inflammation noted in prostate biopsies and resections of BPH tissue is not considered (138).

To address these problems, acquire a better understanding of prostatitis etiology, and provide clearer definitions of the disease, the National Institute of Diabetes and Digestive and Kidney Disorders has proposed a new system of classification (Table 8). In categories I and II, traditional ABP and CBP are defined by the presence of culturable uropathogenic bacteria in specific specimens of prostatic fluid from patients with definite prostatic inflammation. Chronic pelvic pain syndrome (CPPS) is defined by the presence of prostatitis-like symptoms with no uropathogenic bacteria demonstrable in specific specimens of prostatic fluid. This classification is subdivided into inflammatory and noninflammatory CPPS. Inflammatory CPPS is defined as leukocytosis in expressed prostatic secretions or urine after prostate massage. Noninflammatory CPPS is indicated when there is no evidence of an inflammatory response.

Asymptomatic prostatitis describes those situations where there is pathological evidence of inflammation without symptoms being evident.

Diagnosis of Prostatitis

It is generally accepted that the presence of leukocytes at a concentration of 10^6/mL indicates an active infection of the prostate (157); however, this only gives an indication of prostatic inflammation. The gold standard method for diagnosing prostatitis is the "Meares-Stamey four glass test" (Fig. 8) (158). This test differentiates bacterial from nonbacterial prostatitis by sequential and quantitative bacteriological culturing of the urethra/bladder urine and prostatic secretions. When bacterial counts in the urethral specimen [first and midstream urine samples, or voided bladder (VB)

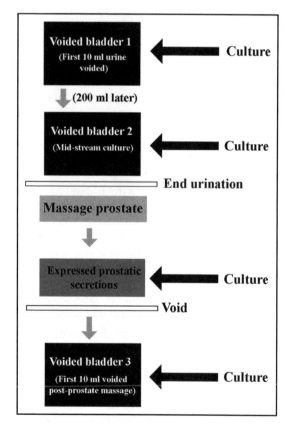

Figure 8 The Meares–Stamey four-glass test. The test requires the patient to have a full bladder. If uncircumcised, the foreskin must be retracted throughout. The glans is washed with an antiseptic (followed by water to avoid false negatives) prior to collection. The patient is instructed to stop urinating after VB1 and VB2 are collected. Expressed prostate fluid for microscopic examination is collected on a glass slide during digital massage. Additional expressed fluid is collected for culture. Immediately after prostatic massage, the patient voids again and the VB3 fraction is collected. Specimens are routinely cultured on blood agar (gram-negative and gram-positive bacteria) and MacConkey agar (gram-negative). *Abbreviation*: VB, voided bladder. *Source*: Adapted from Ref. 158.

(VB1 and VB2)] are greater than that in the expressed prostatic fluid or the postprostatic massage urine sample (VB3), then bacterial urethritis is present. If the prostatic fluid and VB3 bacterial loads exceed that in the VB1 specimen by at least a factor of 10, then bacterial prostatitis can be accurately diagnosed. When prostatic secretions are unobtainable, quantitative cultures of the ejaculate have been used; however, this is not recommended, as semen contains a mix of secretions from varying sites and sex accessory glands. The procedure is cumbersome, time-consuming, has a low yield, can give false positives and negatives, and has poor therapeutic predictive value; therefore, it is not routinely used (159,160).

Nickel (161) has proposed a simpler technique for prostate screening that provides almost as accurate a classification of prostatitis patients as that of Meares and Stamey. In this pre- and postmassage test, urine specimens are produced before and after prostate massage. These specimens are compared by microbiological culture and microscopic examination. The presence or absence of bacteria and/or leukocytes in the postprostatic massage urine as compared with the preprostatic massage urine allows for accurate diagnosis, with a sensitivity and specificity of 91% (161).

Clinical Management of Prostatitis

Currently, there is very little in the way of evidence-based treatment guidelines for the care and management of prostatitis, and this is reflected in the poor outcome of many patients. Although most patients are treated with antibiotics, the cause of their disease will probably not be fully determined, and many of these patients will have continual recurrence throughout their lives (162). Management of chronic prostatitis is usually focused on relieving symptoms through the use of antibiotics, anti-inflammatory drugs, normalization of urine flow, and changes in general and sexual behaviors (163). Nickel (138) has proposed a recommended scheme for treating the various categories of prostatitis (Table 8); however, until there is a validated symptom-scoring system accepted for common use, evaluation of such treatment strategies will be difficult.

☐ CONCLUSIONS

Diseases of the prostate are complex, multifactorial processes that continue to pose intriguing and fundamental questions that serve to illustrate the relative lack of understanding of the biology and physiology of this accessory sex gland. For example:

- Why is BPH restricted to the transitional zone of the prostate and prostate cancer to the peripheral zone?
- How do the interactions between stromal and epithelial components differ between the normal prostate, BPH, and prostate cancer?

- Why does overproliferation of epithelial cells not result in malignant phenotypes in BPH?
- How is a history of prostatic inflammation (prostatitis) related to increased risks of BPH and prostate cancer?

The development of prostate disease is clearly a matter of balance between hormones and growth-factor effects. Changing the homeostasis that exists in the normal gland leads to disease. A full understanding of the events that lead to this imbalance is the key to better diagnosis and prognosis and development of novel therapies. In both benign and malignant prostate disease, these advances may come from comprehensive studies of altered gene expressions in diseased states and the discovery of novel prostate-specific genes. The completion of the human genome project has been a major advance in providing a resource ripe for mining. Indeed, a database of expressed genes (expressed sequence tags) derived from normal and diseased human tissues is publicly available at the National Center for Biotechnology Information (164) as is the Prostate Expression DataBase (PEDB). The PEDB was developed as a resource of genes expressed in the normal and neoplastic human prostate (available online) (165). As well as these bioinformatic resources, the advent of cDNA microarray technology has provided a powerful tool to investigate gene-expression profiles from individual samples, whilst proteomics allows the study of gene expression at the protein level. These molecular biology approaches, along with advances in noninvasive functional imaging (e.g., magnetic resonance imaging/magnetic resonance spectroscopy) of the diseased prostate, will have a major impact on biomarker development, early diagnosis, and end-point assessment in prostate cancer. Chemoprevention of prostate cancer is a continually active field. Many chemoprevention trials are underway or nearing completion and involve an array of agents including steroid antagonists, selenium, and phytoestrogens (166). Natural remedies such as phytoestrogens are also now receiving greater interest in their use for symptomatic relief of LUTS associated with BPH (167). More conventional treatments involving inhibitors of 5-α-reductase have led to the introduction of dutatsteride, an inhibitor of both type I and II isoforms (168). A recent study of the effect of finasteride, a 5-α-reductase type II inhibitor, demonstrated that finasteride can delay or prevent the development of prostate cancer; however, men in the trial had an increased risk of high-grade prostate cancer (169).

Developments of minimally invasive surgical techniques are continually evolving for the treatment of BPH (e.g., surgical endoscopic laser treatment) (170), as are microwave thermotherapies for LUTS (78).

As the average age of populations in the developed world increases, age-related diseases will become an even greater burden to health care services. Prostate disease will be no exception. The challenge facing biomedical research is to answer those questions relating to prostate disease that continue to be perplexing. In doing so, clinicians will be provided with more substantial armories to enable effective management tailored to the individual needs of the increased number of men presenting with prostate disease.

□ REFERENCES

1. Berry SJ, Coffey DS, Walsh PC, et al. The development of human benign prostatic hyperplasia with age. J Urol 1984; 132(3):474–479.

2. Isaacs JT, Coffey DS. Etiology and disease process of benign prostatic hyperplasia. Prostate 1989; 2:33–50.

3. Greenlee RT, Hill-Harmon MB, Murray T, et al. Cancer statistics 2001. CA Cancer J Clin 2001; 51(2):15–36.

4. Lepor H. Nonoperative management of benign prostatic hyperplasia. J Urol 1989; 141(6):1283–1289.

5. Cunningham GR. Overview of androgens on the normal and abnormal prostate. In: Bhasin S, Gebelnick HL, Spieler JM, et al., eds. Pharmacology, Biology and Clinical Applications of Androgens: Current Status And Future Prospects. New York: Wiley-Liss Inc., 1996:79–93.

6. Garraway WM, Collins GN, Lee RJ. High prevalence of benign prostatic hypertrophy in the community. Lancet 1991; 338(8765):469–471.

7. Isaacs JT. Etiology of benign prostatic hyperplasia. Eur Urol 1994; 25(suppl 1):6–9.

8. Platz EA, Kawachi I, Rimm EB, et al. Race, ethnicity and benign prostatic hyperplasia in the health professionals follow-up study. J Urol 2000; 163(2):490–495.

9. Watanabe H. Natural history of benign prostatic hypertrophy. Ultrasound Medl Biol 1986; 12(7):567–571.

10. Arenas MI, Romo E, Royuela M, et al. Morphometric evaluation of the human prostate. Int J Andr 2001; 24(1):37–47.

11. Helpap B. Benign prostatic hyperplasia. In: Foster CS, Bostwick DG, eds. Pathology of the Prostate. Philadelphia: WB Saunders Co., 1998:66–94.

12. Franks LM. Benign nodular hyperplasia of the prostate: A review. Ann R Coll Surg Engl 1954; 14:92–106.

13. McNeal JE. Origin and evolution of benign prostatic enlargement. Invest Urol 1978; 15(4):340–345.

14. Foster CS. Pathology of benign prostatic hyperplasia. Prostate Suppl 2000; 9:4–14.

15. Caine M, Raz S, Zeigler M. Adrenergic and cholinergic receptors in the human prostate, prostatic capsule and bladder neck. Br J Urol 1975; 47(2):193–202.

16. Appell RA, England HR, Hussell AR, et al. The effects of epidural anesthesia on the urethral closure pressure profile in patients with prostate enlargement. J Urol 1980; 124(3):410–411.

17. Furuya S, Kumamoto Y, Yokoyama E, et al. Alpha-adrenergic activity and urethral pressure in prostatic zone in benign prostatic hypertrophy. J Urol 1982; 128(4):836–839.

18. Lepor H, Gup DI, Baumann M, et al. Laboratory assessment of terazosin and alpha-1 blockade in prostatic hyperplasia. Urology 1988; 32(suppl 6):21–26.

19. Kobayashi S, Tang R, Shapiro E, et al. Characterization and localization of prostatic alpha 1 adrenoreceptors using radioligand receptor binding on slide-mounted tissue section. J Urol 1993; 150(6):2002–2006.

20. Nasu K, Moriyama N, Kawabe K, et al. Quantification and distribution of alpha1-adrenoreceptor subtype mRNAs in human prostate: comparison of benign hypertrophied tissue and non-hypertrophied tissue. Br J Pharmacol 1996; 119(5):797–803.

21. Young JM, Muscatello DJ, Ward JE. Are men with lower urinary tract symptoms at increased risk of prostate cancer? A systematic review and critique of the available evidence. BJU Int 2000; 85(9):1037–1048.

22. Imperato-McGinley J, Peterson RE, Gautier T, et al. Androgens and the evolution of male-gender identity among male pseudohermaphodites with 5alpha-reductase deficiency. N Engl J Med 1979; 300(22):1233–1237.

23. McPhaul MJ, Marcelli M, Zoppi S, et al. Genetic basis of endocrine disease. 4. The spectrum of mutations in the androgen receptor gene that causes androgen resistance. J Clin Endocrinol Metab 1993; 76(1):17–23.

24. Siiteri P, Wilson JD. Dihydrotestosterone in prostatic hypertrophy. I. The formation and content of dihydrotestosterone in the hypertrophic prostate of man. J Clin Invest 1970; 49(9):1737–1745.

25. Geller J, Albert J, Lopez D, et al. Comparison of androgen metabolites in benign prostatic hypertrophy (BPH) and normal prostate. J Clin Endocrinol Metab 1976; 43(3):686–688.

26. Walsh PC, Hutchins GM, Ewing LL. Tissue content of dihydrotestosterone in human prostatic hyperplasia is not supranormal. J Clin Invest 1983; 72(5):1772–1777.

27. Krieg M, Nass R, Tunn S. Effect of aging on endogenous level of 5 alpha-dihydrotestosterone, testosterone, estradiol and estrone in epithelium and stroma of normal and hyperplastic prostate. J Clin Endocrinol Metab 1993; 77(2):375–381.

28. Shibata Y, Ito K, Suzuki K, et al. Changes in the endocrine environment of the human prostate transition zone with aging: simultaneous quantitative analysis of prostatic sex steroids and comparison with human prostatic histological composition. Prostate 2000; 42(1):45–55.

29. Niu Y, Xu Y, Zhang J, et al. Proliferation and differentiation of prostatic stromal cells. BJU Int 2001; 87(4):386–393.

30. Zhou W, Park I, Pins M, et al. Dual regulation of proliferation and growth arrest in prostatic stromal cells by transforming growth factor-β1. Endocrinology 2003; 144(10):4280–4284.

31. Hong JH, Song C, Shin Y, et al. Estrogen induction of smooth muscle differentiation of human prostatic stromal cells is mediated by transforming growth factor-beta. U Urol 2004; 171:1965–1969.

32. Walsh PC, Wilson JD. The induction of prostatic hypertrophy in the dog with androstanediol. J Clin Invest 1976; 57(4):1093–1097.

33. Trachtenberg J, Hicks LL, Walsh PC. Androgen- and estrogen-receptor content in spontaneous and experimentally induced canine prostatic hyperplasia. J Clin Invest 1980; 65(5):1051–1059.

34. Habenicht UF, Schwartz K, Schweikert HU, et al. Development of a model for the induction of estrogen-related prostatic hyperplasia in the dog and its response to aromatase inhibitor 4-hydroxy-4-androstene-3,17-dione: preliminary results. Prostate 1986; 8(2):181–194.

35. Winter ML, Bosland MC, Wade DR, et al. Induction of benign prostatic hyperplasia in intact dogs by near physiological levels of 5 α-dihydrotestosterone and 17 β-estradiol. Prostate 1995; 26(6):325–333.

36. Rhodes L, Ding VDH, Kemp R, et al. Estradiol causes a dose-dependent stimulation of prostate growth in castrated beagle dogs. Prostate 2000; 44(1):8–18.

37. Gray A, Feldman HA, McKinlay JB, et al. Age, disease, and changing sex hormone levels in middle-aged men: results of the Massachusetts Male Aging Study. J Clin Endocrinol Metab 1991; 73(5):1016–1025.

38. Pirke KM, Doerr P. Age related changes and interrelationships between plasma testosterone, oestradiol and testosterone-binding globulin in normal adult males. Acta Endocrinol (Copenh) 1973; 74(4):792–800.

39. Pirke KM, Doerr P. Age related changes in free plasma testosterone, dihydrotestosterone and oestradiol. Acta Endocrinologica 1975; 80(1):171–181.

40. Levine AC, Kirschenbaum A, Gabrilove JL. The role of sex steroids in the pathogenesis and maintenance of prostatic hyperplasia. Mount Sinai J Med 1997; 64(1):20–25.

41. El-Alfy M, Pelletier G, Hermo LS, et al. Unique features of the basal cells of human prostate epithelium. Microsc Res Tech 2000; 51(5):436–446.

42. Matzkin H, Soloway MS. Immunohistochemical evidence of the existence and localization of aromatase in human prostatic tissues. Prostate 1992; 21(4):309–314.

43. Hemsell DL, Grodin JM, Brenner PF, et al. Plasma precursors of estrogen. II. Correlation of the extent of conversion of plasma androstenedione to estrone with age. J Clin Endocrinol Metab 1974; 38(3):476–479.

44. Royuela M, de Miguel MP, Bethencourt FR, et al. Estrogen receptors alpha and beta in the normal,

hyperplastic and carcinomatous human prostate. J Endocrinol 2001; 168(3):447–454.

45. Farnsworth WE. Estrogen in the etiopathogenesis of BPH. Prostate 1999; 41(4):263–274.

46. Sciarra F, Toscano V. Role of estrogens in human benign prostatic hyperplasia. Arch Androl 2000; 44(3):213–220.

47. Schweikert HU, Tunn UW, Habenicht UF, et al. Effects of estrogen deprivation on human benign prostatic hyperplasia. J Steroid Biochem Mol Biol 1993; 44(4–6): 573–576.

48. Isaacs JT. Antagonistic effect of androgen on prostatic cell death. Prostate 1984; 5(5):545–557.

49. Claus S, Berges R, Senge T, et al. Cell kinetic in epithelium and stroma of benign prostatic hyperplasia. J Urol 1997; 158(1):217–221.

50. Kyprianou N, Tu H, Jacobs SC. Apoptotic versus proliferative activities in human benign prostatic hyperplasia. Hum Pathol 1996; 27(7):668–675.

51. Colombel M, Vacherot F, Diez SG, et al. Zonal variation of apoptosis and proliferation in the normal prostate and in benign prostatic hyperplasia. Br J Urol 1998; 82(3):380–385.

52. Steiner MS. Role of peptide growth factors in the prostate: a review. Urology 1993; 42(1):99–110.

53. Cunha GR, Alarid ET, Turner T, et al. Normal and abnormal development of the male urogenital tract. Role of androgens, mesenchymal-epithelial interactions, and growth factors. J Androl 1992; 13(6): 465–475.

54. Story MT, Hopp KA, Meier DA, et al. Influence of transforming growth factor beta 1 and other growth factors on basic fibroblast growth factor level and proliferation of cultured human prostate-derived fibroblasts. Prostate 1993; 22(3):183–197.

55. Jones EG, Harper ME. Studies on the proliferation, secretory activities, and epidermal growth factor receptor expression in benign prostatic hyperplasia explant cultures. Prostate 1992; 20(2):133–149.

56. Harper ME, Goddard L, Glynne-Jones E, et al. An immunocytochemical analysis of TGF alpha expression in benign and malignant prostatic tumors. Prostate 1993; 23(1):9–23.

57. Yang Y, Chisholm GD, Habib FK. Epidermal growth factor and transforming growth factor alpha concentrations in BPH and cancer of the prostate: their relationships with tissue androgen levels. Br J Cancer 1993; 67(1):152–155.

58. Nicholson HD. Oxytocin: a paracrine regulator of prostatic function. Rev Reprod 1996; 1(2):69–72.

59. Bodanszky M, Sharaf H, Roy JB, et al. Contractile activity of vasotocin, oxytocin, and vasopressin on mammalian prostate. Eur J Pharmacol 1992; 216(2):311–313.

60. Armstrong DT, Hansel W. Effects of hormone treatment on testis development and pituitary function. Int J Fertil 1958; 3:296–306.

61. Plecas B, Popovic A, Jovovic D, et al. Mitotic activity and cell deletion in ventral prostate epithelium of intact and castrated oxytocin-treated rats. J Endocrinol Invest 1992; 15(4):249–253.

62. Nicholson HD, Jenkin L. Oxytocin and prostatic function. Adv Exp Med Biol 1995; 395:529–538.

63. Nicholson HD, Jenkin L. Evidence for the regulation of prostatic oxytocin by gonadal steroids in the rat. J Androl 1999; 20(1):80–87.

64. Nevalainen MT, Valve EM, Ingleton PM, et al. Prolactin and prolactin receptors are expressed and functioning in human prostate. J Clin Invest 1997; 99(4):618–627.

65. Wennbo H, Kindblom J, Isaksson OG, et al. Transgenic mice overexpressing the prolactin gene develop dramatic enlargement of the prostate gland. Endocrinology 1997; 138(10):4410–4415.

66. Bole-Feysot C, Goffin V, Edery M, et al. Prolactin (PRL) and its receptor: actions, signal transduction pathways and phenotypes observed in PRL receptor knockout mice. Endocr Rev 1998; 19(3):225–268.

67. Ben-Jonathan N, Mershon JL, Allen DL, et al. Extrapituitary prolactin: distribution, regulation, functions, and clinical aspects. Endocrin Rev 1996; 17 (6): 639–669.

68. Farnsworth WE, Slaunwhite WR Jr, Sharma M, et al. Interaction of prolactin and testosterone in the human prostate. Urol Res 1981; 9(2):79–88.

69. Farnsworth WE. Prolactin. J Urol 1985; 133(3):488.

70. Barry MJ, Fowler FJ Jr, O'Leary MP, et al. The American Urological Association symptom index for benign prostatic hyperplasia. The Measurement Committee of the American Urological Association. J Urol 1992; 148(5):1549–1557.

71. Thorpe A, Neal D. Benign prostatic hyperplasia. Lancet 2003; 361(9366):1359–1367.

72. Barry M, Roehrborn C. Management of benign prostatic hyperplasia. Annu Rev Med 1997; 48:177–189.

73. Oesterling JE. Benign prostatic hyperplasia. Medical and minimally invasive treatment options. N Engl J Med 1995; 332(2):99–109.

74. Yang Q, Peters TJ, Donovan JL, et al. Transurethral incision compared with transurethral resection of the prostate for bladder outlet obstruction: a systematic review and meta-analysis of randomized controlled trials. J Urol 2001; 165(5):1526–1532.

75. Tkocz M, Prajsner A. Comparison of long-term results of transurethral incision of the prostate with transurethral resection of the prostate, in patients with benign prostatic hypertrophy. Neurolurol Urodyn 2002; 21(2):112–116.

76. Campo B, Bergamaschi F, Corrada P, et al. Transurethral needle ablation (TUNA) of the prostate: a clinical and urodynamic evaluation. Urology 1997; 49(6):847–850.

77. Hill B, Belville W, Bruskewitz R, et al. Transurethral needle ablation versus transurethral resection of the prostate for the treatment of symptomatic benign prostatic hyperplasia: 5-year results of a prospective, randomized, multicenter clinical trial. J Urol 2004; 171(6 Pt 1): 2336–2340.

78. Gravas S, Laguna P, de la Rosette J. Thermotherapy and thermoablation for benign prostatic hyperplasia. Curr Opin Urol 2003; 13(1):45–49.

79. Boyle P, Gould AL, Roehrborn CG. Prostate volume predicts outcome of treatment of benign prostatic hyperplasia with finasteride: meta-analysis of randomized clinical trials. Urology 1996; 48(3):398–405.

80. Schulman CC. Lower urinary tract symptoms/benign prostatic hyperplasia: minimizing morbidity caused by treatment. Urology 2003; 62(3 suppl 1):24–33.

81. Mebust WK. Transurethral resection of the prostate and transurethral incision of the prostate. In: Lepor H, Lawson R, eds. Prostate Diseases. Philadelphia: WB Saunders, 1993:150–163.

82. Hoffman RM, MacDonald R, Wilt TJ. Laser prostatectomy for benign prostatic obstruction. Cochrane Database Syst Rev 2005; 1:CD001987.

83. Donovan JL, Peters TJ, Neal DE, et al. A randomized trial comparing transurethral resection of the prostate, laser therapy and conservative treatment of men with symptoms associated with benign prostatic enlargement: the CLasP study. J Urol 2000; 164(1):65–70.

84. Gujral S, Abrams P, Donovan JL, et al. A prospective randomized trial comparing transurethral resection of the prostate and laser therapy in men with chronic urinary retention: the CLasP study. J Urol 2000; 164(1):59–64.

85. Gormley GJ, Stoner E, Bruskewitz RC, et al. The effect of finasteride in men with benign prostatic hyperplasia. The Finasteride Study Group. N Engl J Med 1992; 327(17):1185–1191.

86. Bluestein DL, Oesterling JE. Hormonal therapy in the management of benign prostatic hyperplasia. In: Lepor H, Lawson R, eds. Prostate Diseases. Philadelphia: WB Saunders, 1993:182–198.

87. Isaacs JT, Lundmo PI, Berges R, et al. Androgen regulation of programmed death of normal and malignant prostatic cells. J Androl 1992; 13(6):457–464.

88. Roehrborn C, Oesterling JE, Auerbach S, et al. The Hytrin Community Assessment Trial study: a one year study of terazosin versus placebo in the treatment of men with symptomatic benign prostatic hyperplasia. HYCAT Investigator Group. Urology 1996; 47(2):159–168.

89. Chon JK, Borkowski A, Partin AW, et al. Alpha 1-adrenoreceptor antagonists terazosin and doxazosin induce prostate apoptosis without affecting cell proliferation in patients with benign prostatic hyperplasia. J Urol 1999; 161:2002–2008.

90. Di Silverio F, Flammia GP, Sciarra A, et al. Plant extracts in BPH. Minerva Urolog Nefrol 1993; 45(4):143–149.

91. Buck AC. Phytotherapy for the prostate. Br J Urol 1996; 78(3):325–326.

92. Lowe FC, Ku JC. Phytotherapy in treatment of benign prostatic hyperplasia: a critical review. Urology 1996; 48(1):12–20.

93. Wilt T, Ishana A, MacDonald R, et al. Beta-sitosterols for benign prostatic hyperplasia. Cochrane Database Syst Rev 2000; (2):CD001043.

94. Wilt T, Ishana A, Stark G, et al. *Seronoa repens* for benign prostatic hyperplasia. Cochrane Database System Rev 2000; (2):CD001423.

95. Boyle P, Robertson C, Lowe F, et al. Updated meta-analysis of clinical trials of *Serenoa repens* extract in the treatment of symptomatic benign prostatic hyperplasia. BJU Int 2004; 93(6):751–756.

96. Neal DE, Leung HY, Powell PH, et al. Unanswered questions in screening for prostate cancer. Eur J Cancer 2000; 36(10):1316–1321.

97. Mebane C, Gibbs T, Horm J. Current status of prostate cancer in North American black males. J Natl Med Assoc 1990; 82(11):782–788.

98. Zaridze DG, Boyle P. Cancer of the prostate: epidemiology and aetiology. Br J Urol 1987; 59(6):493–502.

99. Majeed A, Babb P, Jones J, et al. Trends in prostate cancer incidence, mortality and survival in England and Wales 1971–1998. BJU Int 2000; 85(9):1058–1062.

100. Mettlin C. Impact of screening on prostate cancer rates and trends. Microsc Res Tech 2000; 51(5):415–418.

101. American Cancer Society. Cancer Facts and Figures 2004. (www.cancer.org), 16–17.

102. Seidman H, Mushinski MH, Gelb SK, et al. Probabilities of eventually dying of cancer—United States, 1985. CA Cancer J Clin 1985; 35(1):36–56.

103. Huggins C, Hodges CV. Studies on prostate cancer. I. The effect of castration, of estrogen and of androgen injection on serum phosphatases in metastatic carcinoma of the prostate. 1941. J Urol 2002; 168(1):9–12.

104. Steinberg GD, Epstein JI, Piantadosi S, et al. Management of stage D1 adenocarcinoma of the prostate: the Johns Hopkins experience 1974 to 1987. J Urol 1990; 144(6):1425–1432.

105. Spitz MR, Currier RD, Fueger JJ, et al. Familial patterns of prostate cancer: a case-control analysis. J Urol 1991; 146(5):1305–1307.

106. Thiessen EU. Concerning a familial association between breast cancer and both prostatic and uterine malignancies. Cancer 1974; 34(4):1102–1107.

107. Carter BS, Bova GS, Beaty TH, et al. Hereditary prostate cancer: epidemiologic and clinical features. J Urol 1993; 150(3):797–802.

108. Cancel-Tassin G, Latil A, Valeri A, et al. PCAP is the major known prostate cancer predisposing locus in families from south and west Europe. Eur J Human Genet 2001; 9(2):135–142.

109. Platz EA, Rimm EB, Willett WC, et al. Racial variation in prostate cancer incidence and in hormonal system markers among male health professionals. J Natl Cancer Inst 2000; 92(24):2009–2017.

110. Yatani R, Chigusa I, Akazaki K, et al. Geographic pathology of latent prostatic carcinoma. Int J Cancer 1982; 29(6):611–616.

111. Schulman CC, Zlotta AR, Denis L, et al. Prevention of prostate cancer. Scand J Urol Nephrol Suppl 2000; 205:50–61.

112. Giovannucci E, Ascherio A, Rimm EB, et al. A prospective cohort study of vasectomy and prostate cancer in US men. JAMA 1993; 269(7):873–877.

113. Bernal-Degredo E, Latour-Perez J, Pradas-Arnal F, et al. The association between vasectomy and prostate cancer: a systematic review of the literature. Fert Steril 1998; 70(2):191–200.

114. Cox B, Sneyd MJ, Paul C, et al. Vasectomy and the risk of prostate cancer. JAMA 2002; 287(23):3111–3115.

115. Stanford JL, Wicklund KG, McKnight B, et al. Vasectomy and risk of prostate cancer. Cancer Epidemiol Biomarkers Prev 1999; 8(10):881–886.

116. Bostwick DG, Pacelli A, Lopez-Beltran A. Molecular biology of prostatic intraepithelial neoplasia. Prostate 1996; 29(2):117–134.

117. Breslow N, Chan CW, Dhom G, et al. Latent carcinoma of prostate at autopsy in seven areas. The International Agency for Research on Cancer, Lyons, France. Int J Cancer 1977; 20(5):680–688.

118. Stamey TA. Cancer of the prostate: an analysis of some important contributions and dilemmas. Monogr Urol 1982; 3:67–94.

119. Carter HB, Piantadosi S, Isaacs JT. Clinical evidence for and implications of the multistep development of prostate cancer. J Urol 1990; 143(4):742–746.

120. Cohen RJ, McNeal JE, Redmond SL, et al. Luminal contents of benign and malignant prostatic glands: correspondence to altered secretory mechanisms. Hum Pathol 2000; 31(1):94–100.

121. Saini MS, Van Etten RL. A clinical assay for prostatic acid phosphatase using choline phosphate as a substrate: comparison with thymolphthalein phosphate. Prostate1981; 2(4):359–368.

122. Gyorkey F, Min KW, Huff JA, et al. Zinc and magnesium in human prostate gland: normal, hyperplastic, and neoplastic. Cancer Res 1967; 27(8): 1348–1353.

123. Costello LC, Franklin RB. The intermediary metabolism of the prostate: a key to understanding the pathogenesis and progression of prostate malignancy. Oncology 2000; 59(4):269–282.

124. Costello LC, Franklin RB, Narayan P. Citrate in the diagnosis of prostate cancer. Prostate 1999; 38(3): 237–245.

125. Derynck R, Goeddel DV, Ullrich A, et al. Synthesis of messenger RNAs for transforming growth factors alpha and beta and the epidermal growth factor receptor by human tumors. Cancer Res 1987; 47(3): 707–712.

126. Leav I, McNeal JE, Ziar J, et al. The localization of transforming growth factor alpha and epidermal growth factor receptor in stromal and epithelial compartments of developing human prostate and hyper-plastic, dysplastic, and carcinomatous lesions. Hum Pathol 1998; 29(7):668–675.

127. De Miguel P, Royuela M, Bethencourt R, et al. Immunohistochemical comparative analysis of transforming growth factor alpha, epidermal growth factor, and epidermal growth factor receptor in normal, hyperplastic and neoplastic human prostates. Cytokine 1999; 11(9):722–727.

128. Moses HL, Yang EY, Pietenpol JA. TGF-beta stimulation and inhibition of cell proliferation: new mechanistic insights. Cell 1990; 63(2):245–247.

129. Lau KM, LaSpina M, Long J, et al. Expression of estrogen receptor(ER)-alpha and ER-beta in normal and malignant prostatic epithelial cells: regulation by methylation and involvement in growth regulation. Cancer Res 2000; 60:3175–3182.

130. Catalona WJ, Richie JP, Ahmann FR, et al. Comparison of digital rectal examination and serum prostate specific antigen in the early detection of prostate cancer: results of a multicenter clinical trial of 6630 men. J Urol 1994; 151(5):1283–1290.

131. Jewett HJ. The present status of radical prostatectomy for stages A and B prostatic cancer. Urol Clin North Am 1975; 2(1):105–124.

132. Gleason DF, Mellinger GT. Prediction of prognosis for prostatic adenocarcinoma by combined histological grading and clinical staging. J Urol 1974; 111(1):58–64.

133. Albertsen PC, Fryback DG, Storer BE, et al. Long-term survival among men with conservatively treated localised prostate cancer. JAMA 1995; 274(8):626–631.

134. Steineck G, Helgesen F, Adolfsson J, et al. Quality of life after radical prostatectomy or watchful waiting. N Engl J Med 2002; 347(11):790–796.

135. Donovan J, Mills N, Smith M, et al. Quality improvement report: improving design and conduct of randomised trials by embedding them in qualitative research: ProtecT (prostate testing for cancer and treatment) study. BMJ 2002; 325(7367):766–770.

136. Packman K, Zhan P, Walker J, et al. Antiandrogen-induced invasion in prostate cancer cells. In: Robaire B, Chemes H, Morales CR, eds. Andrology in the 21st Century. Englewood, NJ: Medimond, 2001:185–195.

137. Collins MM, Stafford RS, O'Leary P, et al. How common is prostatitis? A national survey of physician visits. J Urol 1998; 159(4):1224–1228.

138. Nickel JC. Prostatitis: myths and realities. Urology 1998; 51(3):362–366.

139. Krieger JN, Egan KJ, Ross SO, et al. Chronic pelvic pains represent the most prominent urogenital symptoms of "chronic prostatitis". Urology 1996; 48(5):715–721.

140. de la Rosette JJ, Ruijgrok MC, Jeuken JM, et al. Personality variables involved in chronic prostatitis. Urology 1993; 42(6):654–662.

141. Collins MM, Meigs JB, Barry MJ, et al. Prevalence and correlates of prostatitis in the health professionals follow-up study cohort. J Urol 2002; 167(3):1363–1366.

142. Krieger JN, Riley DE, Cheah PY, et al. Epidemiology of prostatitis: new evidence for a world-wide problem. World J Urol 2003; 21(2):70–74.

143. Drach GW, Fair WR, Meares EM, et al. Classification of benign disease associated with prostatic pain: prostatitis or prostatodynia? J Urol 1978; 120(2):266.

144. Weidner W, Schiefer HG, Krauss H, et al. Chronic prostatitis: a thorough search for etiologically involved microorganisms in 1,461 patients. Infection 1991; 19(suppl 3):S119–S125.

145. Weidener W, Krause W, Ludwig M. Relevance of male accessory gland infection for subsequent fertility with special focus on prostatitis. Human Reprod Update 1999; 5(5):421–432.

146. Ludwig M, Schroeder-Printzen I, Schiefer HG, et al. Diagnosis and therapeutic management of 18 patients with prostatic abscess. Urology 1999; 53(2):340–345.

147. Berger RE, Krieger JN, Rothman I, et al. Bacteria in the prostate tissue of men with idiopathic prostatic inflammation. J Urol 1997; 157(3):863–865.

148. Nickel JC, Downey J, Clark J, et al. Antibiotic pharmacokinetics in the inflamed prostate. J Urol 1995; 153(2):527–529.

149. Nickel JC, Costerton JW. Bacterial localization in antibiotic-refractory chronic bacterial prostatitis. Prostate 1993; 23(2):107–114.

150. Nickel JC, Costerton JW, McLean RJ, et al. Bacterial biofilms: influence on the pathogenesis, diagnosis and treatment of urinary tract infections. J Antimicro bChemother 1994; 33(suppl A):31–41.

151. Dibdin GH, Assinder SJ, Nichols WW, et al. Mathematical model of beta-lactam penetration into a biofilm of *Pseudomonas aeruginosa* while undergoing simultaneous inactivation by released beta-lactamases. J Antimicrob Chemother 1996; 38(5):757–769.

152. Shortliffe L, Elliot K, Sellers RG. Measurement of urinary antibodies to crude bacterial antigen in patients with chronic bacterial prostatitis. J Urol 1989; 141(3):632–636.

153. Krieger JN, Riley DE, Roberts MC, et al. Prokaryotic DNA sequences in patients with chronic idiopathic prostatitis. J Clin Microbiol 1996; 34(12):3120–3128.

154. Bruce AW, Reid G. Prostatitis associated with *Chlamydia trachomatis* in 6 patients. J Urol 1989; 142(4):1006–1007.

155. Corradi G, Bucsek M, Pánovics J, et al. Detection of *Chlamydia trachomatis* in the prostate by in-situ hybrid-ization and by transmission electron microscopy. Int J Androl 1996; 19(2):109–112.

156. Meares EM. Nonbacterial prostatitis and prostatodynia. In: Lepor H, Lawson RK, eds. Prostate Diseases. Philadelphia: WB Saunders & Company, 1993: 419–424.

157. World Health Organization. WHO Laboratory Manual for the Examination of Human Semen and Semen-Cervical Mucus Interaction. Cambridge: Cambridge University Press, 1992.

158. Meares EM, Stamey TA. Bacteriologic localization patterns in prostatitis and urethritis. Invest Urol 1968; 5(5):492–518.

159. Moon TD. Questionnaire survey of urologists and primary care physicians' diagnostic and treatment practices for prostatitis. Urology 1997; 50(4):543–547.

160. Nickel JC, Nigro M, Valiquette L, et al. Diagnosis and treatment of prostatitis in Canada. Urology 1998; 52(5):797–802.

161. Nickel JC. The pre and post massage test (PPMT): a simple screen for prostatitis. Tech Urol 1997; 3(1): 38–43.

162. Bennett BD, Richardson PH, Gardner WA. Histopathology and cytology of prostatitis. In: Lepor H, Lawson RK, eds. Prostate Diseases. Philadelphia: WB Saunders & Company, 1993:399–413.

163. Weidner W, Ludwig M, Miller J. Therapy in male accessory gland infection—what is fact, what is fiction? Andrologia 1998; 30(suppl 1):87–90.

164. http://www.NCBI.NIH.GOV/dbEST.

165. http://www.pedb.org.

166. Greenwald P, Lieberman R. Chemoprevention trials for prostate cancer. In: Chung LWK, Isaacs WB, Simons JW, eds. Prostate Cancer: Biology, Genetics and the New Therapeutics. Totowa, NJ: Humana Press, 2001.

167. Klingler HC. New innovative therapies for benign prostatic hyperplasia: any advance? Curr Opin Urol 2003; 13(1):11–15.

168. Foley CL, Kirby RS. 5 alpha-reductase inhibitors: what's new? Curr Opin Urol 2001; 13(1):31–37.

169. Thompson IM, Goodman PJ, Tangen CM, et al. The influence of finasteride on the development of prostate cancer. N Engl J Med 2003; 349(3):215–224.

170. Aho TF, Gilling PJ. Laser therapy for benign prostatic hyperplasia: a review of recent developments. Curr Opin Urol 2003; 13(1):39–44.

Gynecomastia

Ronald S. Swerdloff
Division of Endocrinology and Metabolism, Harbor-UCLA Medical Center, Torrance, California and Department of Medicine, David Geffen School of Medicine, University of California, Los Angeles, California, U.S.A.

Jason Ng
Division of Endocrinology, Department of Medicine, Queen Elizabeth Hospital, Hong Kong Special Administration Region, P.R. China

Fouad R. Kandeel
Department of Diabetes, Endocrinology and Metabolism, City of Hope National Medical Center, Duarte, California and David Geffen School of Medicine, University of California, Los Angeles, California, U.S.A.

□ INTRODUCTION

In pubertal females, a complex hormonal interplay occurs that results in the appearance of the secondary sex characteristics, including the growth and maturation of the adult female breast. Male breast development occurs in an analogous fashion to female breast development, but at a much reduced level due to the markedly lower levels of estrogens in men compared to women. This chapter will review the general ontogeny and physiology of breast development, the factors that influence breast enlargement in the male, the differential diagnosis of gynecomastia, the process of diagnostic investigation, and the treatment of gynecomastia.

□ BREAST DEVELOPMENT

In both male and female fetuses, epithelial cells proliferate into ducts that will eventually form the areola of the nipple at the surface of the skin. The blind ends of these ducts bud to form alveolar structures in later gestation. With the decline in fetal prolactin, placental estrogen, and progesterone at birth, the infantile breast regresses until early puberty (1).

During thelarche, the period of prepubertal breast enlargement, the initial clinical appearance of the breast bud, growth, and division of the ducts occur, eventually giving rise to club-shaped terminal end buds, which then form alveolar buds. Approximately, a dozen alveolar buds will cluster around a terminal duct, forming the type-1 lobule. Eventually, the type-1 lobule will mature into type-2 and 3 lobules, called ductules, by increasing its number of alveolar buds to as many as 50 in type-2 and 80 in type-3 lobules. The entire differentiation process takes years after the onset of puberty and, in the female, if pregnancy is not achieved, may never be completed (2).

□ HORMONAL REGULATION OF BREAST DEVELOPMENT

At puberty, the initiation and progression of breast development involve a coordinated effort of pituitary and gonadal hormones, as well as local mediators (Fig. 1).

□ ESTROGEN, GH, INSULIN-LIKE GROWTH FACTOR, PROGESTERONE, AND PROLACTIN

Estrogen and progesterone act integratively to stimulate normal adult female breast development. Estrogen promotes duct growth via its receptor, estrogen receptor (ER), while progesterone, also acting through its receptor, progesterone receptor (PR), supports alveolar development (1). This is demonstrated by experiments in ER-knockout mice that display grossly impaired ductal development, while PR-knockout mice possess significant ductal development but lack alveolar differentiation (3,4).

Although estrogens and progestogens are vital to mammary growth in the female, they are ineffective in the absence of anterior pituitary hormones (5). Thus, neither estrogen alone nor estrogen plus progesterone can sustain breast development without other mediators. This has been confirmed by studies involving the administration of estrogen and growth hormone (GH) to hypophysectomized and oophorectomized female rats, which resulted in breast ductal development. The GH effects on ductal growth are mediated through stimulation of insulin-like growth factor-1 (IGF-1): estrogen and GH administration to IGF-1–knockout rats showed significantly decreased mammary development when compared to age-matched IGF-1-intact controls. Combined estrogen and IGF-1 treatment in these IGF-1–knockout rats restored mammary growth

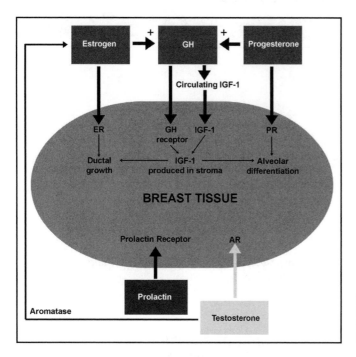

Figure 1 Hormones affecting growth and differentiation of breast tissue. *Abbreviations*: AR, androgen receptor; ER, estrogen receptor; GH, growth hormone; PR, progesterone receptor; +, stimulatory (*dark arrows*); –, inhibitory (*light arrow*).

(6,7). In addition, Walden et al. demonstrated that GH stimulated production of IGF-1 mRNA in the mammary gland itself, suggesting that IGF-1 production in the stromal compartment of the mammary gland acts locally to promote breast development (8). Furthermore, other data indicate that estrogen promotes GH secretion and increased GH levels, stimulating the production of IGF-1, which synergizes with estrogen to induce ductal development.

Like estrogen, progesterone has minimal effects on breast development without concomitant anterior pituitary hormones. For example, prolonged treatment of dogs with progestogens such as depot medroxyprogesterone acetate or proligestone caused increased GH and IGF-1 levels, suggesting that progesterone may also have an effect on GH secretion (9). Maximal cell proliferation has also been correlated to specific phases in the female menstrual cycle. For example, maximal proliferation occurs during the luteal phase, when progesterone reaches levels of 10 to 20 ng/ml (31–62 nnmol) and estrogen levels are two to three times lower than that in the follicular phase (2). Furthermore, immunohistochemical studies of ER and PR showed that the highest percentage of proliferating cells, found almost exclusively in the type-1 lobules, contained the highest percentage of ER and PR positive cells (2). Similarly, there is immunocytological presence of ER, PR, and androgen receptors (AR) in gynecomastia and male breast carcinoma. ER, PR, and AR expression was observed in 100% (30/30) of gynecomastia cases (10). Given these data and the fact that PR-knockout mice lack alveolar development in breast tissue, it appears as if progesterone, in an analogous mechanism to that of estrogen, may increase GH secretion via action at its receptor in mammary tissue in order to enhance breast development—specifically, alveolar differentiation (4,11).

Prolactin is another anterior pituitary hormone integral to breast development. Prolactin may also be produced in the epithelial cells of normal mammary tissue as well as in breast tumors (12,13). Prolactin stimulates epithelial cell proliferation only in the presence of estrogen and enhances lobulo-alveolar differentiation only with concomitant progesterone. Recently, receptors for luteinizing hormone and human chorionic gonadotropin have been found in both male and female breast tissues, although its function remains to be determined (14). The male breast is similar in embryonic development to the female but undergoes much less stimulation in the peripubertal period (thelarche and puberty).

☐ ANDROGEN AND AROMATASE

Estrogen effects on the breast may be the result of either circulating estradiol levels or locally produced estrogens. Since aromatase P450 catalyzes the conversion of the C19 steroids (androstenedione, testosterone, and 16-α -hydroxyandrostenedione) to estrone, estradiol-17β, and estriol, an overabundance of substrate or an increase in enzyme activity can increase estrogen concentrations, thus initiating the cascade that produces abnormal breast development in males. For example, in the more complete forms of androgen insensitivity syndromes in genetically male (XY) patients, excess androgen aromatizes into estrogen that causes not only gynecomastia but also a phenotypic female appearance. Furthermore, the biologic effects of overexpression of the aromatase enzyme in female and male mice transgenic for the aromatase gene result in increased breast proliferation. In female transgenetics, overexpression of aromatase promotes the induction of hyperplastic and dysplastic changes in breast tissue. Overexpression of aromatase in male transgenics caused increased mammary growth and histological changes similar to gynecomastia, with an increase in ER and PR and an increase in downstream growth factors such as TGF-β and bFGF (15). Interestingly, treatment with an aromatase inhibitor leads to involution of the mammalian gland phenotype (16). Thus, although androgens do not stimulate human breast development directly, they may do so if they aromatize to estrogen. This occurs in cases of androgen excess or in patients with increased aromatase activity.

□ PHYSIOLOGIC GYNECOMASTIA

Enlargement of the male breast is termed "gynecomastia," and this process can occur normally during three different phases of life. The first occurrence of gynecomastia may be in both male and female newborns. This is typically caused by the high maternal levels of hCG, estradiol, and progesterone during pregnancy, which stimulates breast tissue. This type of gynecomastia can persist for several weeks after birth and can cause mild breast discharge that is colloquially called "witch's milk" (2).

Puberty marks the second stage at which gynecomastia can occur physiologically. In fact, up to 60% of boys have detectable gynecomastia by the age of 14. This is mostly bilateral, although it can occur unilaterally, and usually resolves within three years of onset (2). Interestingly, in early puberty, the pituitary gland releases gonadotropins in order to stimulate testicular production of testosterone, mostly at nighttime. Estrogens, however, rise throughout the entire day. Some studies have shown that a decreased androgen to estrogen ratio exists in boys with pubertal gynecomastia when compared with boys who do not develop gynecomastia (17). Furthermore, another study showed increased aromatase activity in the skin fibroblasts of boys with gynecomastia. Thus, the mechanism by which pubertal gynecomastia occurs may be due either to decreased production of androgens or to increased aromatization of circulating androgens, thus increasing the estrogen to androgen ratio (18).

The third age range in which gynecomastia is frequently seen is during older age (greater than 60 years). Although the exact mechanisms have not been fully elucidated, evidence suggests that this may result from increased peripheral aromatase activity secondary to the increase in total body fat, coupled with mild age-associated hypogonadism. For instance, increased urinary estrogen levels have been observed in obese individuals, as well as aromatase expression in adipose tissue (19). Thus, like the gynecomastia of obesity, the gynecomastia of aging may partly result from increased aromatase activity, causing increased circulating estrogen levels (20). As aromatase activity tends to increase with age in the adipose tissue already present, the typical increase in total body fat with age will serve to increase circulating estrogens even further. Lastly, sex hormone–binding globulin (SHBG) increases with age in men. Since SHBG binds estrogen with less affinity than testosterone, the bioavailable estradiol to bioavailable testosterone ratio may increase in the obese older male.

□ PATHOLOGIC GYNECOMASTIA
Increased Estrogen

Since the development of breast tissue in males occurs in an analogous manner to that in females, the same hormones that affect female breast tissue can cause gynecomastia (please see above). Serum levels of estradiol and estrone in the adult male are principally the product of peripheral aromatization of testosterone and androstenedione (21). Direct secretions of estrogens by the testes comprise only a small fraction of estrogens in circulation (i.e., 15% of estradiol and 5% of estrone). Thus, any cause of estrogen excess can lead to increased breast development.

Tumors

Testicular tumors can lead to increased blood estrogen levels by estrogen overproduction, androgen overproduction with peripheral aromatization to estrogens, and ectopic secretion of gonadotropins that stimulate otherwise normal Leydig cells. Tumors that cause an overproduction of estrogen represent an unusual but important cause of estrogen excess. Examples of estrogen-secreting tumors include Leydig cell tumors, Sertoli cell tumors, granulosa cell tumors, and adrenal rest tumors (Table 1).

Interstitial cell tumors, or Leydig cell tumors, constitute 1% to 3% of all testis tumors. These usually occur in men between the ages of 20 and 60, although up to 25% may occur prepubertally. When the tumor occurs prior to puberty, isosexual precocity, rapid

Table 1 Examples of Estrogen-Secreting Tumors

Tumor type	Hormone produced	Aromatase over-activity
Leydig cell tumor	Testosterone, estrogen	
Sertoli cell tumor	Estrogen	+ (in Peutz–Jegher syndrome), + (in Carney complex)
Germ cell tumor	β-hCG, estrogen	
Granulosa cell tumor	Estrogen	
Adrenal tumors	Dehydroepiandrosterone, dehydroepiandrosterone sulfate, and androstenedione, which are converted in the periphery to estrogens	

somatic growth, and increased bone age with elevated serum testosterone and urinary 17-ketosteroid levels are the presenting features. In adults, elevated estrogen levels may develop, coupled with a palpable testicular mass and gynecomastia. Although mostly benign, Leydig cell tumors may be malignant, and metastatic sites include the lung, liver, and retroperitoneal lymph nodes (22,23).

Sertoli cell tumors comprise less than 1% of all testicular tumors and may present at all ages, but about one-third occur in patients less than 13 years—often in boys under six months of age. Although they may arise in young boys, they usually do not produce endocrinologic effects in children. Gynecomastia occurs in one-third of cases, presumably due to increased estrogen production. Up to 10% of Sertoli cell tumors are malignant (23).

Granulosa cell tumors are rare testicular neoplasms that can also overproduce estrogen. Only 11 cases have been reported in the literature, with gynecomastia, a presenting feature in half of them (24).

Germ cell tumors are the most common cancer in males between the ages of 15 and 35. These tumors are divided into seminomatous and nonseminomatous subtypes and include embryonal carcinoma, yolk sac carcinoma, choriocarcinoma, and teratomas. Elevated alpha-fetoprotein and β-hCG function as reliable markers in some tumors. Increased levels of β-hCG stimulate the Leydig cell luteinizing hormone (LH) receptor, producing increased testicular androgen and estrogen. The estrogens from direct secretion and by aromatization of testosterone and androstenedione can cause gynecomastia. Although germ cell tumors generally arise in the testes, they can also originate extra-gonadally—for example, in the mediastinum. These extragonadal tumors also possess the capability of producing β-hCG, but they must be differentiated from a multitude of other tumors, such as large cell carcinomas of the lung, which can synthesize ectopic β-hCG (25).

Some neoplasms that overproduce estrogens also possess aromatase overactivity. Sertoli cell tumors in boys with Peutz–Jegher syndrome, an autosomal dominant disease characterized by pigmented macules on the lips, gastrointestinal polyposis, and hormonally active tumors in males and females, for instance, have repeatedly demonstrated aromatase over activity. Presenting features will include gynecomastia, rapid growth, and advanced bone age (26–28). Feminizing Sertoli cell tumors with increased aromatase activity can also be seen in the Carney complex, an autosomal dominant disease characterized by cardiac myxomas, cutaneous pigmentation, adrenal nodules, and hypercortisolism. Other than sex-cord tumors, fibrolamellar hepatocellular carcinoma has also been shown to possess ectopic aromatase activity, causing severe gynecomastia in a 17-year-old boy (29). Furthermore, adrenal tumors can secrete excess dehydroepiandrosterone, dehydroepiandrosterone sulfate, and androstenedione that can then be aromatized peripherally to estradiol.

Nontumor Causes of Estrogen Excess
Increased Aromatase Activity

Besides tumors, other conditions associated with excessive aromatization of testosterone and androgens to estrogen also result in gynecomastia. For instance, a familial form of gynecomastia has been discovered in which affected family members have an elevation of extragonadal aromatase activity (30). More recently, novel gain-of-function mutations in chromosome 15 have been reported to cause gynecomastia, possibly by forming cryptic promoters that lead to over-expression of aromatase (31). As stated above, obesity may cause estrogen excess through increased aromatase activity in adipose tissue. Furthermore, hyperthyroidism induces gynecomastia through several mechanisms, including increased aromatase activity (2).

Displacement of Estrogens from SHBG

Another cause of gynecomastia is estrogen displacement from its carrier protein SHBG, Since SHBG binds androgens more avidly than estrogen, any condition or drug that can displace steroids from SHBG will more easily displace estrogen, allowing for higher circulating levels of free estrogens relative to free androgens.

Decreased Testosterone and Androgen Resistance

Breast development requires the presence of estrogen. Androgens, on the other hand, oppose the estrogenic effects. Thus, equilibrium exists between the higher serum levels of androgens relative to estrogens in the adult male to prevent growth of breast tissue, whereby either an increase in estrogen or a decrease in androgen can tip the balance toward gynecomastia.

Any pathologic state that results in increased estrogen levels will also increase glandular proliferation by several mechanisms, including the direct stimulation of glandular tissue and the suppression of LH, therefore decreasing testicular testosterone secretion and exaggerating the already high estrogen to androgen ratio.

Primary hypogonadism reduces serum testosterone levels and increases serum LH levels; increased LH stimulates aromatase activity in the testes resulting in increased testicular estradiol production and an increased estrogen to androgen ratio (21). Klinefelter's syndrome (KS) (occurring in 1 in 500 males who possess an XXY karyotype and primary testicular failure) is an example of a form of primary hypogonadism gynecomastia secondary to decreased testosterone production, compensatory increased LH secretion, over stimulation of the Leydig cells, and relative estrogen excess. Lastly, enzyme deficiencies in the testosterone synthesis pathway from cholesterol also result in depressed testosterone levels, and, hence, a relative increase in estrogen. For example, a deficiency of 17-oxosteroid reductase, the enzyme that catalyzes the conversion of androstenedione to testosterone and estrone to estradiol, will cause both a decrease in circulating testosterone levels and an elevation in estrone and androstenedione that are then further aromatized to estradiol (20).

Secondary hypogonadism, if severe enough, results in low serum testosterone and an unopposed estrogen effect from the normal conversion of adrenal precursors to estrogens (21). Thus, patients with Kallmann's syndrome (a form of congenital secondary hypogonadism with anosmia) also develop gynecomastia.

The androgen-resistance syndromes, including complete and partial testicular feminization (e.g., Reifenstein's syndrome), are characterized by gynecomastia and varying degrees of pseudohermaphroditism. Kennedy syndrome, a neurodegenerative disease, is also associated with decreased effective testosterone due to a defective androgen receptor (2). In this group of androgen-resistance syndromes, androgens are not recognized by the peripheral tissues, including the breast and pituitary. Androgen resistance at the pituitary results in elevated serum LH levels and increased circulating testosterone. The increased serum testosterone is then aromatized peripherally, promoting gynecomastia. Thus, gynecomastia is the result of increased estradiol levels that arise due to androgen unresponsiveness.

Other Diseases

Other disease states have also resulted in gynecomastia. Men with end-stage renal disease may have reduced testosterone and elevated gonadotropins. This apparent primary testicular failure may then lead to increased breast development (11).

The gynecomastia of liver disease, however—particularly cirrhosis—does not have a clear etiology. Some have speculated that this type of gynecomastia is the result of estrogen overproduction, possibly secondary to increased extraglandular aromatization of androstenedione, which may have decreased hepatic clearance in cirrhotics. Testosterone administration to cirrhotic patients, however, causes a rise in estradiol, but decreases the prevalence of gynecomastia (5,32,33). Therefore, although the association of gynecomastia with liver disease is apparent, current data are conflicting, and the mechanism by which this occurs remains unclear.

Thyrotoxicosis is also associated with gynecomastia. Patients often have elevated estrogen that may result from a stimulatory effect of thyroid hormone (TH) on peripheral aromatase. Testosterone may also be increased due to a TH-stimulated increase in SHBG, as free testosterone is usually normal. Since SHBG binds testosterone more avidly than estradiol, there is a higher ratio of free estradiol to free testosterone. Thus, with normal testosterone and increased estrogen, there is an elevated estrogen to testosterone ratio. In addition, LH is also increased, which may also stimulate testicular aromatase activity and estrogen synthesis (11,34).

Gynecomastia can also follow the occurrence of spinal cord disorders. Most patients with spinal cord disorders display depressed testosterone levels, and, in fact, can develop testicular atrophy with resultant hypogonadism and infertility. It has been speculated that this may result from recurrent urinary tract infections, increased scrotal temperature, and a neuropathic bladder, which ultimately cause acquired primary testicular failure. The exact mechanism, however, remains elusive (35). (For further information on infertility and spinal cord injury, refer to Chapter 39.)

"Refeeding gynecomastia" refers to the breast development that may occur in men recovering from a malnourished state (1). Although most cases regress within seven months, the etiology of this phenomenon has not been fully elucidated.

HIV patients can also develop gynecomastia. This is likely due to the high incidence of androgen deficiency in these patients due to multiple factors, including primary and secondary hypogonadism (21).

Drugs

A significant percentage of gynecomastia is caused by medications or exogenous chemicals that result in increased estrogen effect. This may occur by several mechanisms: (i) synergistic action with estrogen due to intrinsic estrogen-like properties of the drug, (ii) the production of increased endogenous estrogen, or (iii) the excess supply of an estrogen precursor (e.g., testosterone or androstenedione) that can be aromatized to estrogen. Examples of drugs that cause gynecomastia are listed in Tables 2 and 3. Contact with estrogen vaginal creams, for instance, can elevate circulating estrogen levels in both men and women. These may or may not be detected by standard estrogenic quantitative assays. An estrogen-containing embalming cream has been reported to cause gynecomastia in morticians (36,37). Recreational use of marijuana, a phytoestrogen, has also been associated with gynecomastia. It has been suggested that digitalis causes gynecomastia due to its ability to bind to ERs (11,38). The appearance of gynecomastia has been described in body builders and athletes after the administration of aromatizable androgens. This latter type of gynecomastia is presumably caused by an excess of circulating estrogens due to the conversion of androgens to estrogen by peripheral aromatase enzymes (39).

In general, drugs and chemicals that cause decreased testosterone levels by causing direct testicular damage, blocking testosterone synthesis, or blocking androgen action can produce gynecomastia. For instance, phenothrin, a chemical component in delousing agents that possesses antiandrogenic activity, has been attributed as the cause of an epidemic of gynecomastia among Haitian refugees in U.S. detention centers in 1981 and 1982 (40). Chemotherapeutic drugs such as alkylating agents may cause Leydig cell

Table 2 Drugs that Induce Gynecomastia by Known Mechanisms

Estrogen-like, or binds to estrogen receptor	Stimulate estrogen synthesis	Supply aromatizable estrogen precursors	Direct testicular damage	Block testosterone synthesis	Block androgen action	Displace estrogen from sex hormone–binding globulin
Estrogen (i.e., vaginal cream, estrogen-containing embalming cream) Delousing powder Digitalis Clomiphene Marijuana	Gonadotropins Growth hormone	Exogenous androgen Androgen precursors (i.e., androstenedione and dehydroepiandrosterone)	Busulfan Nitrosurea Vincristine Ethanol	Ketoconazole Spironolactone Metronidazole Etomidate	Flutamide Bicalutamide Finasteride Cyproterone Zanoterone Cimetidine Ranitidine Spironolactone	Spironolactone Ethanol

and germ cell damage, resulting in primary hypogonadism. Flutamide, an antiandrogen used as treatment for prostate cancer, blocks androgen action in peripheral tissues, while cimetidine blocks androgen receptors. Ketoconazole, on the other hand, can inhibit steroidogenic enzymes required for testosterone synthesis. Spironolactone causes gynecomastia by several mechanisms; like ketoconazole, it can block androgen production by inhibiting enzymes in the testosterone synthetic pathway (i.e., 17α-hydroxylase

and 17-20-desmolase), but it can also block receptor binding of testosterone and dihydrotestosterone (41). Spironolactone also can displace estradiol from SHBG, increasing free estrogen levels. Ethanol increases the estrogen to androgen ratio, and as it is associated with increased SHBG, it decreases free testosterone levels. Ethanol also increases hepatic clearance of testosterone and has a direct toxic effect on the testes (21).

Besides the agents discussed above, a multitude of other pharmaceutical and recreational drugs may cause gynecomastia, albeit by unknown mechanisms (Table 3).

Table 3 Drugs that Cause Gynecomastia by Uncertain Mechanisms

Cardiac and antihypertensive medications
　Calcium channel blockers (verapamil, nifedipine, diltiazem)
　Angiotensin-converting enzyme inhibitors (captopril, enalapril)
　β blockers
　Amiodarone
　Methyldopa
　Reserpine
　Nitrates
Psychoactive drugs
　Neuroleptics
　Diazepam
　Phenytoin
　Tricyclic antidepressants
　Haloperidol
Drugs for infectious diseases
　Indinavir
　Isoniazid
　Ethionamide
　Griseofulvin
Drugs of abuse
　Amphetamines
Others
　Theophylline
　Omeprazole
　Auranofin
　Diethylpropion
　Domperidone
　Penicillamine
　Sulindac
　Heparin

□ MALE BREAST CANCER

Male breast cancer is rare, comprising only 0.2% of all male cancers and a very small percentage of men with gynecomastia. Factors that may increase the risk for male breast cancer include KS, exogenous estrogen exposure, a previous family history, and the presence of testicular disorders. It is unclear if these factors are specific risks for breast cancer or if they are linked to the stimulatory process responsible for gynecomastia. Since breast cancers occur much more frequently in KS than in other forms of hypogonadal gynecomastia states, it is presumed that the risk of breast cancer in KS is an integral part of the XXY chromosome state. New evidence suggests that obesity and the consumption of red meat may also raise the risk for the development of male breast cancer (42).

Patient Evaluation
History and Physical Examination

At presentation, all patients require a thorough history and physical exam. Particular attention should be given to medications, drug and alcohol abuse, as well as other chemical exposures. Symptoms of underlying systemic illness, such as hyperthyroidism, liver disease, or renal failure should be sought. Notably, the clinician must recall neoplasm as a possible etiology and should establish the duration and timing of breast development. Rapid, recent breast growth should be more concerning than a history of chronic gynecomastia. Additionally, the clinician should inquire about fertility, erectile dysfunction, and libido in order to rule out hypogonadism, either primary or secondary, as a potential cause.

In the authors' experience, the breast examination is best performed with the patient supine and with the examiner palpating from the periphery to the areola. The glandular mass should be measured in diameter. Gynecomastia is diagnosed by finding subareolar breast tissue of 2 cm in diameter or greater. Malignancy is suspected if an immobile firm mass is found on physical examination. Skin dimpling, nipple retraction or discharge, and axillary lymphadenopathy further support malignancy as a possible diagnosis.

A thorough testicular exam is essential. Bilaterally small testes imply testicular failure, while asymmetric testes or a testicular mass suggest the possibility of a testicular neoplasm. Visual field impairment may suggest pituitary disease. Physical findings of underlying systemic conditions such as thyrotoxicosis, HIV disease, liver, or kidney failure should also be assessed.

Laboratory Evaluation

All patients who present with gynecomastia should have serum testosterone, estradiol, LH, and β-hCG measured. Further testing should be tailored according to the history, physical examination and the results of these initial tests. An elevated β-hCG or a markedly elevated serum estradiol suggests neoplasm, and a testicular ultrasound is warranted to identify a testicular tumor, all the while keeping in mind, however, that other nontesticular tumors can also secrete β-hCG. A low testosterone level with elevated LH and normal-to-high estrogen level indicates primary hypogonadism. If the history suggests KS, then a karyotype should be performed for definitive diagnosis. Low testosterone, low LH, and normal estradiol levels imply secondary hypogonadism, and hypothalamic or pituitary causes should be sought. If testosterone, LH, and estradiol levels are all elevated, then the diagnosis of androgen resistance should be entertained. Liver, kidney, and thyroid function should be assessed if the physical examination suggests any of these conditions. Furthermore, if examination of the breast tissue raises a suspicion for malignancy, a biopsy should be performed. This is of particular importance in patients with KS, who harbor an increased risk of breast cancer.

Treatment

Treatment of the underlying endocrinologic or systemic cause of gynecomastia is mandatory. Testicular tumors such as Leydig cell, Sertoli cell, or granulosa cell tumors should be surgically removed. In addition to surgery, germ cell tumors are further managed with chemotherapy involving cisplatin, bleomycin, and either vinblastine or etoposide (22,23). Should underlying thyrotoxicosis, chronic renal failure, or hepatic failure be discovered, appropriate therapy should be initiated. Medications that cause gynecomastia should also be discontinued whenever possible, based on their roles in management of the underlying condition. If a breast biopsy indicates malignancy, then mastectomy should be performed (please see below).

If no pathogenic mechanism is uncovered and the degree of gynecomastia is modest, then close observation is the appropriate treatment. A careful breast exam should be done every three months until the gynecomastia regresses or stabilizes, after which a breast exam may be performed yearly. It is important to remember that some cases of gynecomastia, especially that which occurs in pubertal boys, can resolve spontaneously.

Medical Treatment

If the gynecomastia is severe, does not resolve, and does not have a treatable underlying cause, some medical therapies may be attempted. There are three classes of medical treatment for gynecomastia: androgens (testosterone, dihydrotestosterone, and danazol), antiestrogens (clomiphene citrate and tamoxifen), and aromatase inhibitors (testolactone).

Unfortunately, testosterone treatment of hypogonadal men with gynecomastia often fails to produce breast regression once gynecomastia is established, and it may actually produce the adverse side effect of further gynecomastia. Thus, although testosterone is used to treat hypogonadism, its use to counteract gynecomastia specifically is limited (43).

Dihydrotestosterone, a nonaromatizable androgen (i.e., does not get converted to estrogens), has been used in patients with prolonged pubertal gynecomastia with good response rates (44). Since dihydrotestosterone is given either intramuscularly or percutaneously, however, this may restrict its usefulness.

Danazol, a weak androgen that inhibits gonadotropin secretion and results in decreased serum testosterone levels, has been used as a treatment of gynecomastia. In one trial, it resolved gynecomastia in 23% of patients as opposed to placebo (12%) (45). Unfortunately, the undesirable side effects of edema, acne, and cramps have limited the use of danazol (21).

Clomiphene citrate is both a weak estrogen and an antiestrogen. Investigators have reported a 64% response rate with 100 mg/day of clomiphene citrate. Lower doses of clomiphene have shown varied results, indicating that higher doses may need to be administered (46).

Tamoxifen is a more potent antiestrogen than clomiphene and has been studied in two randomized, double-blind studies in which a statistically significant regression in breast size was achieved, although complete regression was not documented (47). One study compared tamoxifen with danazol in the treatment of gynecomastia. Although patients taking tamoxifen had a greater response, with complete resolution occurring in 78% as against 40% in the danazol-treated group, the relapse rate was higher (48). Although complete breast regression may not be achieved due to the risk of recurrence with tamoxifen, due to the relatively lower side effect profile, this drug may be a more reasonable choice when compared to the other therapies. Tamoxifen should be given at a dose of 10 mg twice a day for at least three months (21).

An aromatase inhibitor, testolactone, has also been studied in an uncontrolled trial with promising effects (49). Further studies must be performed on this drug before any recommendations can be established on its usefulness in the treatment of gynecomastia.

Newer aromatase inhibitors such as anastrozole and letrozole may have therapeutic potential (50,51), but recent randomized, double-blind, placebo-controlled trials involving patients receiving bicalutamide therapy for prostate cancer showed that tamoxifen, but not anastrozole, significantly reduced the incidence of gynecomastia/breast pain when used prophylactically and therapeutically (52,53).

Surgical Treatment

Surgical therapy is appropriate when medical therapy is ineffective (particularly in cases of long-standing gynecomastia), when the patient's activities of daily living are compromised, or when there is suspicion of malignancy of breast. This includes removal of glandular tissue, and, if needed, liposuction. In the authors' experience, the use of delicate cosmetic surgical techniques is warranted to prevent unsightly scarring.

□ PREVENTION OF GYNECOMASTIA IN MEN WITH PROSTATE CANCER

Because androgen deprivation is one of the commonly used treatment modalities for advanced prostate cancer, its possible role in the development of gynecomastia is of particular concern to clinicians. Low-dose prophylactic irradiation has been variably reported to reduce the rate of gynecomastia in men receiving estrogens or antiandrogens for advanced prostate cancer (54,55).

□ CONCLUSION

In summary, gynecomastia is a relatively common disorder that may be caused by a vast range of mechanisms, from benign physiologic processes to rare neoplastic disorders. Thus, in order to properly diagnose the etiology of the gynecomastia, the clinician must understand the hormonal factors involved in breast development. Parallel to female breast development, estrogen, along with GH and IGF-1, is required for breast growth in males. Since a balance exists between estrogen and androgens in males, any disease state or medication that can increase circulating estrogen or decrease circulating androgen, thus causing an elevation in the estrogen to androgen ratio, can also induce gynecomastia. Due to the diversity of possibly etiologies, particularly malignant neoplasm, the performance of a careful history and physical examination is imperative. Once gynecomastia has been diagnosed, treatment of the underlying cause is warranted. If no underlying cause is discovered, then close observation is appropriate. If the gynecomastia is severe, however, medical therapy can be attempted, and if this is ineffective, glandular tissue can be removed surgically.

□ REFERENCES

1. Franz A, Wilson J. Williams Textbook of Endocrinology, ninth edition. 1998; 877–885.
2. Santen R. Endocrinology, fourth edition. 2001; 3: 2335–2341.
3. Bocchinfuso WP, Korach KS. Mammary gland development and tumorigenesis in estrogen receptor knockout mice. J Mammary Gland Biol Neoplasia 1997; 90: 323–334.
4. Lubahn DB, Moyer JS, Golding TS. Alteration of reproductive function but not prenatal sexual development after insertional disruption of the mouse estrogen receptor gene. Proc Soc Natl Acad Sci USA 1993; 90: 11162–11166.
5. Edman DC, Hemsell DL, Brenner PF. Extraglandular estrogen formation in subjects with cirrhosis. Gastroenterology 1975; 69:819.
6. Kleinberg DL, Feldman M, Ruan W. IGF-1: an essential factor in terminal end bud formation and ductal morphogenesis. J Mammary Gland Biol Neoplasia 2000; 5(1):7–17.
7. Ruan W, Kleinberg DL. Insulin-like growth factor i is essential for terminal end bud formation and ductal morphogenesis during mammary development. Endocrinology 1999; 140(11):5075–5081.
8. Walden PD, Ruan W, Feldman M, et al. Evidence that the mammary fat pad mediated the action of growth hormone in mammary gland development. Endocrinology 1998; 139(2):659–6628.
9. Mol JA, Van Garderen E, Rutteman GR, et al. New insights in the molecular mechanism of progestin-induced proliferation of mammary epithelium: induction of the local biosynthesis of growth hormone in the mammary gland of dogs, cats, and humans. J Steroid Biochem Mol Biol 1996; 57(1–2):67–71.

10. Sasano H, Kimura M, Shizawa S, et al. Aromatase and steroid receptors in gynecomastia and male breast carcinoma: an immunohistochemical study. J Clin Endocrinol Metab 1996; 81(8):3063–3067.

11. Glass AR. Gynecomastia. Endocrinol Metab Clin North Am 1994; 23(4):825–837.

12. LeProvost F, Leroux C, Martin P, et al. Prolactin gene expression in ovine and caprine mammary gland. Neuroendocrinology 1994; 60:305–313.

13. Steinmetz R, Grant A, Malven P. Transcription of prolactin gene in milk secretory cells of the rat mammary gland. J Endocrinol 1993; 36:305–313.

14. Carlson HE, Kane P, Lei ZM, et al. Presence of luteinizing hormone/human chorionic gonadotropin receptors in male breast tissues. J Clin Endocrinol Metab 2004; 89(8):4119–4123.

15. Gill K, Kirma N, Tekmal RR. Overexpression of aromatase in transgenic male mice results in the induction of gynecomastia and other biochemical changes in mammary gland. J Steroid Biochem Mol Biol 2001; 77(1):13–18.

16. Li X, Warri A, Makela S, et al. Mammary gland development in transgenic male mice expressing human P450 aromatase. Endocrinology 2002; 143(10): 4074–4083.

17. Moore DC, Schlaepfer LP, Sizonenko PC. Hormonal changes during puberty: transient pubertal gynecomastia; abnormal androgen-estrogen ratios. J Clin Endocrinol Metab 1984; 58:492–499.

18. Mahoney CP. Adolescent gynecomastia. Differential diagnosis and management. Pediatr Clin North Am 1990; 37(6):1389–1404.

19. Niewoehner CB, Nuttall FQ. Gynecomastia in hospitalized male population. Am J Med 1984; 77:633–638.

20. Braunstein. Aromatase and Gynecomastia. Endocr Relat Cancer 1999; 6:315–324.

21. Mathur R, Braunstein. Gynecomastia: pathomechanisms and treatment strategies. Hor Res 1997; 48: 95–102.

22. Gana BM. Leydig cell tumor. Br J Urology 1995; 75(5): 676–678.

23. Richie J. Campbell's Urology, seventh edition. 1998:2439–2443.

24. Matoska J, Ondrus D, Talerman A. Malignant granulosa cell tumor of the testes associated with gynecomastia and long survival. Cancer 1992; 69(7):1769–1772.

25. Moran CA, Suster S. Primary mediastinal choriocarcinoma: a clinicopathologic and immunohistochemical study of eight cases. Am J Surg Pathol 1997; 21(9): 1007–1012.

26. Coen P, Kulin H, Ballantine T, et al. An aromatase-producing sex-cord tumor resulting in prepubertal gynecomastia. N Engl J Med 1991; 324 (5):317–322.

27. Hertl MC, Wiebel J, Schafer H, et al. Feminizing sertoli cell tumors associated with peutz-jeghers syndrome: an increasingly recognized cause of prepubertal gynecomastia. Plasc Reconstr Surg 1998; 102(4): 1151–1157.

28. Young S, Gooneratne S, Straus FH II, et al. Feminizing sertoli cell tumors in boys with peutz-jehgers syndrome. Am J Surg Pathol 1995; 19(1):50–58.

29. Agarwal VR, Takayama K, Van Wyk JJ, et al. Molecular basis of severe gynecomastia associated with aromatase expression in a fibrolamellar hepatocellular carcinoma. J Clin Endocrinol Metab 1988; 83(5): 1797–1800.

30. Berkovitz GD, Guerami, Brown TR, et al. Familial gynecomastia with increased extraglandular aromatization of plasma carbon 19-steroids. J Clin Invest 1985; 75: 1763–1769.

31. Shozu M, Sebastian S, Takayama K, et al. Estrogen excess associated with novel gain-of-function mutations affecting the aromatase gene. N Engl J Med 2003; 348(19):1855–1865.

32. Bahnsen M, Gluud C, Johnsen SG. Pituitary-testicular function in patients with alcoholic cirrhosis of the liver. Eur J Clin Invest 1981; 11:473–479.

33. Olivo J, Gordon GG, Raifi F. Estrogen metabolism in hyperthyroidism and in cirrhosis of the liver. Steroids 1975; 26:47–56.

34. Chan WB, Yeung VT, Chow CC, et al. Gynecomastia as a presenting feature of thyrotoxicosis. Postgrad Med J 1999; 75(882):229–231.

35. Herito RJ, Dankner R, Berezin M, et al. Gynecomastia following spinal cord disorder. Arch Phys Med Rehab 1997; 78(5):534–537.

36. Bhat N, Rosato E, Gupta P. Gynecomastia in a mortician: a case report. Acta Cytol 1990; 34:31.

37. Finkelstein J, McCully W, MacLaughlin D, et al. The mortician's mystery: gynecomastia and reversible hypogonadotropic hypogonadism in an embalmer. N Eng J Med 1988; 319:961.

38. Rifka SM, Pita JC, Vigersky RA, et al. Interaction of digitalis and spironolactone with human sex steroid receptors. J Clin Endocrinol Metab 1977; 46:228–244.

39. Calzada L, Torres-Calleja JM, Martinez N. Measurement of androgen and estrogen receptors in breast tissue from subjects with anabolic steroid-dependent gynecomastia. Life Sci 2001; 69(2110):1465–1479.

40. Brody SA, Loriaux DL. Epidemic of gynecomastia among haitian refugees: exposure to an environmental antiandrogen. Endocr Pract 2003; 9(5):370–375.

41. Thompson DF, Carter J. Drug-induced gynecomastia. Pharmacotherapy 1993; 13(1):37–45.

42. Hsing A, McLaughlin J, Cocco P, et al. Risk factors for male breast cancer. Cancer Causes Control 1998; 9:269–275.

43. Treves N. Gynecomastia: the origins of mammary swelling in the male: and analysis of 406 patients with breast hypertrophy, 525 with testicular tumors, and 13 with adrenal neoplasms. Cancer 1958; 11: 1083–1102.

44. Kuhn JM, Roca R, Laudat MH, et al. Studies on the treatment of idiopathic gynecomastia with percutaneous dihydrotestosterone. Clin Endo 1983; 19: 513–520.

45. Jones DJ, Holt SD, Surtees P, et al. A comparison of danazol and placebo in the treatment of adult idiopathic gynecomastia: results of a prospective study in 55 patients. Ann R Coll Surg Engl 1990; 72: 296–298.

46. Leroith D, Sobel R, Glick SM. The effect of clomiphene citrate on pubertal gynecomastia. Acta Endocrinol (Copenh) 1980; 95:177–180.

47. Alagaratnam TT. Idiopathic gynecomastia treated with tamoxifen; a preliminary report. Clin Ther 1987; 9:483–487.

48. Ting AC, Chow LW, Leung YF. Comparison of tamoxifen with danazol in the management of idiopathic gynecomastia. Am Surg 2000; 66(1): 38–40.

49. Zachmann M, Eiholzer U, Muritano M, et al. Treatment of pubertal gynecomastia with testolactone. Acta Endocrinol Suppl (Copenh) 1986; 279:218–226.

50. Miller WR, Jackson J. The therapeutic potential of aromatase inhibitors. Expert Opin Investig Drugs 2003; 12(3):337–351.

51. Riepe FG, Baus I, Wiest S, et al. Treatment of pubertal gynecomastia with the specific aromatase inhibitor anastrozole. Horm Res 2004; 62(3):113–118.

52. Boccardo F, Rubagotti A, Battaglia M, et al. Evaluation of tamoxifen and anastrozole in the prevention of gynecomastia and breast pain induced by bicalutamide monotherapy of prostate cancer. J Clin Oncol 2005; 23(4):808–815.

53. Saltzstein D, Sieber P, Morris T, et al. Prevention and management of bicalutamide–induced gynecomastia and breast pain: randomized endocrinologic and clinical studies with tamoxifen and anastrozole. Prostate Cancer Prostatic Dis 2005; 8(1):75–83.

54. Chou JL, Easley JD, Feldmeier JJ, et al. Effective radiotherapy in palliating mammalgia associated with gynecomastia after DES therapy. Int J Radiat Oncol Biol Phys 1988; 15(3):749–751.

55. Trump DL. Does prophylactic breast irradiationprevent antiandrogen-induced gynecomastia? Evaluation of 253 patients in the randomized Scandinavian trial SPCG-7/SFUO-3. Urology 2003; 61:145–151.

Male Breast Cancer

Sandeep K. Reddy
Los Alamitos Hematology/Oncology Medical Group, Inc., Los Alamitos, California, U.S.A.

Lucille Leong
Division of Medical Oncology, City of Hope National Medical Center, Duarte, California, U.S.A.

□ INTRODUCTION

Cancer of the male breast is an uncommon diagnosis, accounting for less than 0.1% of all malignancies in men and only 1% of total breast cancers (1). It is estimated that approximately 2000 new cases of male breast cancer are diagnosed and 400 deaths do occur from that disease each year in the United States. The first description of male breast cancer dates back to 3000 B.C. and can be found on the Edwin Smith Papyrus, the world's earliest known medical document (2). In the 14th century, the English surgeon, John of Aderne, reported on a priest of Colstone with a slowly growing wound of the right nipple—an entity that is now recognized as Paget's disease (3). It was not until 1927, however, that Wainwright reported an actual diagnosis of male breast cancer (4).

□ EPIDEMIOLOGY

The incidence of male breast cancer has remained relatively steady over the past 50 years (5); this is in sharp contrast to the rising rate of female breast cancer. The incidence of breast cancer in men is one-hundredth of that in women and accounts for less than 1% of the annual cancer deaths in men. The prevalence of male breast cancer increases with age: it is rare before the fourth decade of life and most common in the sixth decade of life (6). The geographic variance in incidence is striking, ranging from 0.1 cases per 100,000 in Hungary and Japan to 3.4 cases per 100,000 in Brazil (7). Sparse registry data from Africa suggest an even higher male/female ratio of breast cancer in a narrow band through the center of the continent from Angola to Tanzania (8). Interestingly, this is consistent with the male/female ratio of breast cancer in African-Americans, which is 1.4 to 100 versus 1 to 100 in American whites (9).

Several risk factors have been identified for male breast cancer through a meta-analysis of case–control studies, including: men who have a family history of breast cancer as well as those who have never been married, are of Jewish descent, or have liver disease, testicular pathology, prior benign breast disease, including gynecomastia, or prior chest wall irradiation.

Hormonal Factors

The best explanation for the origin of male breast cancer is that of hormonal imbalance caused by androgen deficiency and a relative increase in endogenous estrogen levels or by the presence of excess estrogen. Such hormonal imbalances may occur in individuals with a history of testicular pathology such as undescended testes, mumps at an age greater than 20 years (thus increasing the risk of mumps orchitis), and testicular trauma (10). The presence of excess estrogen may be due to the use of medications or the intake of exogenous chemicals that result in an increased estrogen effect. (For further information, see Chapter 42.)

Perhaps the strongest hormonal risk factor for the development of male breast cancer is a history of Klinefelter's syndrome, a rare condition with a frequency of 1 or 2 per 1000 men that results from the inheritance of an additional X chromosome. The characteristic clinical findings include atrophic testes, low plasma testosterone, high plasma follicle-stimulating hormone and luteinizing hormone (LH), and gynecomastia. The relative risk for male breast cancer in these men is 50:1 when compared to men with a normal genotype. Approximately 4% of men with breast cancer have Klinefelter's syndrome. Most of these are associated with gynecomastia and have a mean age at diagnosis of 58 years (11,12). The late age of onset may suggest that prolonged exposure to an abnormal hormonal milieu is required for the development of male breast cancer. Given the increased risk of male breast cancer in these patients, any palpable breast mass should receive a thorough evaluation.

Chronic liver disease—notably bilharziasis and alcoholism—represents another hormonal risk factor for male breast cancer (13), probably via altered estrogen metabolism. Bilharziasis is the term applied to the infestation with schistosomiasis that can lead to liver damage and is responsible for a doubling of male breast cancer risk in Egypt, Sudan, and Zambia (14). Chronic alcoholism is associated with a twofold relative risk (15,16) independent of cirrhosis, which conveys only a slight increase in risk (9). It is important to note that these studies addressed patients with liver disease who also had coexisting gynecomastia, which has been linked to male breast cancer in its own right. Although the association between gynecomastia and male breast cancer remains unclear, it is thought that an increased estrogen/testosterone ratio may play a role in causing malignancy. The underlying process that leads to the development of gynecomastia in an individual, however, may actually be of more significance than the mere presence of gynecomastia itself. Some agents known to cause gynecomastia, such as marijuana use and thyroid disease, have not been linked to an increased risk of male breast cancer, whereas male breast cancer has been reported in three patients who used finasteride, a competitive and specific inhibitor of Type II 5-α-reductase for the treatment of benign prostatic hyperplasia (17). It is possible that the association between gynecomastia and male breast cancer may be overreported in the literature as it is subject to recall bias on the part of the patient and diagnostic-awareness bias on the part of the physician. It is certain, however, that both the incidences of gynecomastia and male breast cancer increase with age.

Family History/Genetics

A positive family history is a significant risk factor for female breast cancer. Male breast cancer appears to be no exception although there is a paucity of information on accurate pedigrees. Familial male breast cancer was first reported in 1889 (18) and fewer than 20 cases of related men with breast cancer are found in the literature (19). Retrospective series, however, have reported a positive family history in 5% to 27% of cases, predominantly in first-degree female relatives (20). Also, sisters and daughters of male breast cancer patients have a relative risk of two to three of developing breast cancer (21). When two or more family members are affected (either male or female), the possibility of hereditary breast cancer should be evaluated and genetic screening initiated.

A variety of specific genetic mutations have been identified in association with male breast cancer and the most significant appears to be linkage to the BRCA2 gene on chromosome 13q12-13 (22). BRCA2 accounts for up to 35% of inherited breast cancer in men and women. BRCA2 mutations were found in 40% of male breast cancers in Iceland over the past 40 years (23). In a study of 34 male breast cancers in Sweden, 20% had BRCA2 mutations (24).

Conversely, mutations of the BRCA1 gene do not appear to be linked to male breast cancer (25), and mutations of the p53 gene account for only a small fraction of patients with male breast cancer (26). Other non-BRCA1/2 gene mutations such as loss of heterozygosity at chromosome 11q13 and the short arm of chromosome 8 suggest that tumor-suppressor gene mutations may be involved (27). A mutation in exon 3 (G to A substitution) of the androgen receptor gene

was observed in two brothers with male breast cancer, hypospadias, and undescended testes (28).

□ DIAGNOSIS

Clinical awareness of male breast cancer is essential to its diagnosis and early treatment. Most patients will present with a palpable mass that is more commonly fixed to the underlying tissue or skin than in women. Nipple discharge is frequent, occurring in 80% of patients. Bloody discharge is highly sensitive for malignancy, with an incidence of 13.7% in malignant lesions versus 2.1% in benign lesions in one series (29). The left breast is more commonly involved than the right breast in most series (20).

Although mammography is technically more difficult secondary to small breast size, it can help to differentiate between gynecomastia and breast cancer (30). It is also useful in follow-up screening of the contralateral breast, which, like in females, has an increased risk of developing new primary cancers. Ultrasound with high-frequency linear transducers has been shown to be as effective as mammography at evaluating breast masses (31). Fine needle aspiration (FNA), however, has proved to be the diagnostic test of choice when in the hands of an experienced clinician and cytopathologist. No false negatives were seen in two large series (32,33), and the combination of FNA and physical examination was shown to be as accurate as and more cost-effective than open biopsy (34).

Although the National Comprehensive Cancer Network has developed detailed algorithmic guidelines for the evaluation and treatment of breast masses and breast cancer in women, no consensus exists for male breast lesions.

The evaluation of the unilateral breast mass in the male poses an unusual challenge for the clinician. Traditionally, patients were routinely subjected to open biopsy; however, the high false-negative rate of over 90% has led to the proposal of several algorithms for the improved evaluation of a male breast mass. A proposed algorithm for the evaluation of a male breast mass is presented in Figure 1. Highly suspicious characteristics include firmness, fixation to pectoralis fascia or skin, subareolar location, skin changes (peau d'orange, edema, and erythema), and the presence of predisposing risk factors.

□ PATHOLOGY

The most common histologic type of male breast cancer is invasive or infiltrating ductal carcinoma, which accounts for 85% of cases (35). Generally, the same types of breast carcinoma described in the female have also been reported in the male, but there are some notable differences. Although lobular carcinoma accounts for 15% of cases in women, it is quite rare in males (36). This rarity has been explained by the lack of

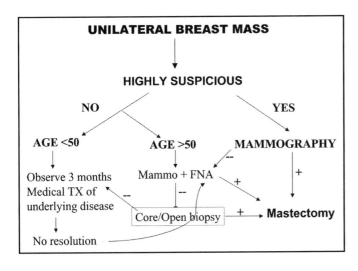

Figure 1   Proposed algorithm for the evaluation of a male breast mass. *Abbreviations*: FNA, fine needle aspiration; TX, treatment.

true acini and lobules in the normal male breast. Yet, male breast tissue can be induced to form lobules and acini under estrogenic stimulation, as seen in Klinefelter's syndrome and exogenous estrogen administration. Similarly, ductal carcinoma in situ [(DCIS); also referred to as noninvasive or intraductal] accounts for 20% of all female cases of breast cancer; in men, it represents only 10% to 15% of cases (37,38). As in women, the prognosis of male DCIS is excellent following mastectomy. In one series of 31 patients, there was a predominance of the papillary subtype, and comedocarcinoma was observed in only three patients. All lymph nodes sampled in 19 patients were negative (39). Lobular carcinoma in situ, once thought not to occur in males, has indeed been reported, albeit only a handful of times (36,37). Inflammatory, medullary, papillary, and tubular carcinomas account for less than 10% of the cases. Breast sarcomas, including cystosarcoma phylloides, liposarcomas, and leiomyosarcomas, have also been described infrequently. Paget's disease accounts for up to 5% of female breast tumors but is far less common in the male, with fewer than 50 cases reported (40).

Interestingly, invasive male breast cancers express estrogen receptors (ERs) far more commonly than in women; between 80% and 90% of men have ER-positive tumors (41–43). Progesterone receptors (PRs) are positive 25% to 75% of the time. Greater variability has been reported for c-erb B-2 (her-2-neu) in male breast cancer, with cytoplasmic immunopositivity 2+ or higher ranging between 9% and 81% in several small series (44–46), compared to 30% in female breast cancer. Similarly, nuclear staining for p53 has also varied widely—between 0% and 58% in several series (47–49). Other cellular differentiation markers that have been associated with male breast cancer include epidermal growth factor receptor, present in 14% to 76% of the cases (50,51), Cathepsin D, in 46% to 86% of the cases (52,53), and pepsinogen C, in 76% of the cases (54). Pepsinogen C scores were higher in well-differentiated tumors than poorly differentiated tumors and higher in ER-positive than ER-negative tumors. A trend

toward improved survival was seen in a single study amongst patients with pepsinogen C–positive tumors, but this was not statistically significant.

The special circumstance of breast metastasis in the case of prostate carcinoma must also be considered. The incidence of this occurrence is high—up to 5% of patients with advanced prostate carcinoma (55). Hence, distinguishing metastasis from a primary breast cancer can be difficult. Only seven primary breast cancers concurrent with prostate cancers have been reported in the English literature (56). Bilateral cases with multiple foci can be clues to a metastatic disease. Immunohistochemical staining for acid phosphatase and prostate-specific antigen can also help to resolve uncertainty (57).

□ PROGNOSTIC FEATURES

Although it has been argued that male breast cancers have a poorer prognosis than female breast cancers, when matched for stage, there does not appear to be a difference between the two (58,59). Historically, higher stage at presentation has characterized male breast cancer, suggesting a biologically aggressive, hormone receptor–negative, and high-grade tumor; however, the opposite case is true. The relatively aggressive behavior of male breast cancer occurs despite a lower histologic grade, a higher frequency of hormone receptor positivity, and an overall smaller size. A possible explanation for this phenomenon may be the result of the anatomic difference between male and female breasts. Due to the relatively reduced amount of breast tissue in males, the resultant proximity of even a small tumor to the skin of the male breast allows for a greater incidence of dermal lymphatic involvement in male breast cancer (60,61). In women, dermal lymphatic invasion is associated with a significantly worse prognosis and is in fact pathognomonic for inflammatory breast cancer.

As in women, the most important prognostic factors for male breast cancer are stage, tumor size, and the presence of lymph node metastasis. A series of 335 male breast cancers over a 20-year period reported a 10-year survival rate of 84% for patients with negative nodes, 44% for patients with one to three positive nodes, and 14% for those with four or more positive nodes (62). Histologically, the presence of higher ploidy and S-phase cellular fractions do not affect prognosis, with aneuploidy commonly found in 57% of the cases and an S-phase fraction in 9% of the cases (63,64).

□ TREATMENT

The treatment of male breast cancer does not differ significantly from that of female breast cancer. Historically, male breast cancer patients have tended to present at a later stage of the disease, presumably secondary to a delay in diagnosis (65). Nevertheless, the rates of node positivity and outcomes have remained similar to those of female breast cancer (66).

Surgery

As with female breast cancer, radical mastectomy (removal of the entire breast, all axillary lymph nodes, and the chest wall muscles under the breast) was the treatment of choice in earlier years, but this has given way to modified radical mastectomy (which removes the entire breast and levels I and II (of three levels) of the axillary lymph nodes) and simple (total) mastectomy (which removes the entire breast but not any axillary lymph nodes or chest wall muscles). No survival advantage was seen with more radical surgical procedures in limited studies (67). Unlike surgical therapy in female breast cancer, segmental resection of the involved quadrant of the breast has not been a high priority in males due to the lack of concern regarding cosmesis. Clinical examination of the axilla is inferior to definitive surgical exploration, but sentinel lymph node sampling with radionucleotide injection has been as effective in men as in women (68). Radiation therapy to the chest wall and regional draining lymph nodes has reduced locoregional recurrence but has had no impact on survival (69). Some authors have suggested routine irradiation of the internal mammary nodes since most male breast cancers arise in the central, subareolar area (70). Given the higher rate of cardiovascular disease in men, particular attention regarding radiation planning should be given to men with left breast cancer to minimize the subsequent risk of cardiomyopathy, coronary artery disease, and carotid vascular disease.

Sites of metastatic disease are similar in men and women, and median survival from presentation with metastatic disease is 27 months (71).

Hormonal Therapy

Hormonal approaches to male breast cancer have been particularly successful. Steroid hormone-receptor estrogen receptor/progesterone receptor (ER/PR) positivity is high (70–90%) in male breast cancer, which is higher than the rate seen in women. The response rate to hormonal manipulation is 51% in unselected men and 71% in ER-positive patients (56), with the respective response rates in women being 30% and 70%.

Response to hormonal therapy is more common and longer lasting in men than in women. As with prostate cancer, hormone ablative strategies are the first approach. Orchiectomy has a response rate of 45% to 80% (72–75), adrenalectomy has a response rate of 80% (75–77), and hypophysectomy has a response rate of 56% (78,79). Despite the proven benefit of castration, many men have been reluctant to pursue this option secondary to the psychological effect of surgical orchiectomy. Following the examples of prostate cancer and female breast cancer, chemical castration with an leutinizing hormone-releasing hormone (LHRH) analog has also been employed successfully as an adjuvant therapy (80) and for the treatment of metastatic (81) disease.

Tamoxifen has also been used effectively in both adjuvant and metastatic settings. Thirty-nine patients with stage II or stage III breast cancer were given adjuvant tamoxifen without any chemotherapy; the five-year survival rate was 61% in the treatment group versus 44% in the historical control group (82).

Chemotherapy

Chemotherapy has generally been reserved for patients with advanced disease, who are ER negative or whose cancers have continued to progress despite hormonal therapy. The response rates to combination chemotherapy appear to be similar in male and female breast cancer.

Adjuvant chemotherapy has been studied in a limited series of patients with stage II and stage III breast cancer. Twenty-four patients with stage II breast cancer were treated with cyclophosphamide, methotrexate, and 5-fluorouracil, with a projected 80% survival rate at five years (83). A smaller series of 11 men were treated with cyclophosphamide, adriamycin, and 5-fluorouracil, with a reported 91% overall survival rate at 52 months (84). The results of high-dose chemotherapy followed by autologous bone-marrow or stem-cell transplant in the adjuvant or responsive-metastatic setting appear to be similar in both men and women (85).

Recently, the short- and long-term sequelae of female breast cancer therapy and its effects on quality of life have come under increased scrutiny from both patient advocates and physicians. These sentiments, however, have not been expressed as vocally regarding male patients. The lack of concern over cosmetic effects of surgical treatment has led to a preponderantly aggressive surgical approach to male breast cancer management. The effects of hormonal therapy, decreased libido, hot flushes, and impotence have been generally accepted by elderly men as preferable to orchiectomy. Data regarding hormone replacement therapy in this population are not available.

□ CONCLUSION

Male breast cancer is an uncommon disease in which the management is generally similar to female breast cancer. Risk factors include all forms of hypotestosteronism and hyperestrogenism, particularly Klinefelter's syndrome, testicular and liver pathology, and bilharziasis. Genetic susceptibility has been identified in association with BRCA2 but not BRCA1. The prognosis for male breast cancer patients is equivalent to that for females when controlled for stage. Treatment has followed guidelines for female breast cancer with the exception of the expectation of a significantly higher response to hormonal manipulation in male breast cancer. Few randomized studies exist and most information has been obtained from small retrospective case series. Male patients with breast cancer should be encouraged to participate in clinical trials to advance the knowledge of this disease.

□ REFERENCES

1. Parker SL, Tong T, Bolden S, et al. Cancer statistics, 1997. CA Cancer J Clin 1997; 47(1):5–27.

2. Lewison EF. The Surgical treatment of breast cancer. An historical and collective review. Surgery 1953; 34(5):904–953.

3. Holleb AL, Freeman HP, Farrow JH. Cancer of the male breast. NY State Med J 1968; 68(5):544–553.

4. Wainwright JM. Carcinoma of the male breast. Arch Surg 1927; 14:836–859.

5. LaVecchia C, Levi F, Lucchini F. Descriptive epidemiology of male breast cancer in Europe. Intl J Cancer 1992; 51(1):62–66.

6. Ewertz M, Holmberg L, Kajalainen S, et al. Incidence of male breast cancer in Scandinavia, 1943–1982. Intl J Cancer 1989; 43(1):27–31.

7. Muir C, Waterhous J, Mack T, et al. Cancer Incidence in Five Continents. Vol. 5. Lyon: IARC Scientific Publications, 1987:882.

8. Parkin D. Cancer Occurrence in Developing Countries. Lyon: IARC Scientific Publications, 1986.

9. Sasco AJ, Lowenfels AB, Pasker-de Jong P. Review article: epidemiology of male breast cancer. A meta-analysis of published case-control studies and discussion of selected aetiological factors. Int J Cancer 1993; 53(4):538–549.

10. Mabuchi K, Bross DS, Kessler II. Risk factors for male breast cancer. J Natl Cancer Inst 1985; 74(2):371–375.

11. Hultborn R, Hanson C, Kopf I, et al. Prevalence of Klinefelter's syndrome in male breast cancer patients. Anticancer Res 1997; 17(6D):4293–4397.

12. Scheike O, Visfeldt J, Petersen B. Male breast cancer. 3. Breast carcinoma in association with Klinefelter's syndrome. Acta Path Microbiol Scand 1973; 81:352–358.

13. Lenfant-Pejovic MH, Mlika-Cabanne N, Bouchardy C, et al. Risk factors for male breast cancer: a Franco-Swiss case-control study. Intl J Cancer 1990; 45(4):661–665.

14. Abdel Aziz MT, Abdel-Kader MM, Khattab M, et al. Urinary oestrogens in normal Egyptian subjects and in patients with bilharzial hepatosplenomegaly. Acta Med Acad Sci Hung 1973; 30(1):79–90.

15. Keller A. Demographic, clinical and survivorship characteristics of males with primary cancer of the breast. Am J Epidemiol 1967; 85(2):183–199.

16. Olsson H, Ranstam J. Head trauma and exposure to prolactin-elevating drugs as risk factors for male breast cancer. J Natl Cancer Inst 1988; 80(9):679–683.

17. Green L, Wysowski DK, Fourcroy JL. Gynecomastia and breast cancer during finasteride therapy. N Engl J Med 1996; 335(11):823.

18. Kozak F, Hall J, Baird P. Familial breast cancer in males. A case report and review of the literature. Cancer 1986; 58(12):2736–2739.

19. Demeter J, Waterman N, Verdi S. Familial male breast carcinoma. Cancer 1990; 65(10):2342–2343.

20. Whooley B, Borgen P. Male Breast Cancer. In: Roses DF, ed. Breast Cancer. Elsevier 1999; p.613–622.

21. Anderson D, Badzioch M. Breast cancer risk in relatives of male breast cancer patients. JNCI 1992; 84(4):1114–1117.

22. Thorlacius S, Tryggvadottir L, Olafsolottir GH, et al. Linkage to BRCA2 region in hereditary male breast cancer. Lancet 1995; 346(8974):544–545.

23. Thoralacius S, Olafsdottir GH, Tryggvadottir L, et al. A single BRCA2 mutation in male and female breast cancer families from Iceland with varied cancer phenotypes. Nat Genet 1996; 13(1):117–119.

24. Haraldsson K, Loman N, Zhang QX, et al. BRCA2 germ-line mutations are frequent in male breast cancer patients without a family history of the disease. Cancer Res 1998; 58(7):1367–1371.

25. Stratton M, Ford D, Neuhasen S, et al. Familial male breast cancer is not linked to the BRCA1 locus on chromosome 17q. Nat Genet 1994; 7(1):103–107.

26. Borreseen A, Andersen T, Garber J, et al. Screening for germline TP53 mutations in breast cancer patients. Cancer Res 1992; 52(11):3234–3236.

27. Chuaqui R, Sanz-Ortega J, Vocke C, et al. Loss of heterozygosity on the short arm of chromosome 8 in male breast carcinomas. Cancer Res 1995; 55(21):4995–4998.

28. Wooster R, Mangion J, Eeles R, et al. A germline mutation in the androgen receptor gene in two brothers

with breast cancer and Reifenstein syndrome. Nat Genet 1992; 2(2):132–134.

29. Crichlow R. Carcinoma of the male breast. Surg Gyn/ Obstet 1972; 134(6):1011–1019.

30. Applebaum A, Evans G, Levy K, et al. Mammographic appearances of male breast disease. Radiographics 1999; 19(3):559–568.

31. Stewart R Howlett D, Hearn F. Pictorial review: the imaging features of male breast disease. Clin Radiol 1997; 52(10):739–744. Review.

32. Joshi A, Kapila K, Verma K. Fine needle aspiration cytology in the management of male breast masses. Nineteen years of experience. Acta Cytol 1999; 43(3): 334–338.

33. Lilleng R, Paksoy N, Vual G. et al. Assessment of fine needle aspiration cytology and histopathology for diagnosing male breast masses. Acta Cytol 1995; 39(5): 877–881.

34. Vetto J, Schmidt W, Pommler R, et al. Accurate and cost-effective evaluation of breast masses in males. Am J Surg 1998; 175(5):383–387.

35. Norris HJ, Taylor HB. Carcinoma of the male breast. Cancer 1969; 23(6):1428–1435.

36. Sanchez AG, Villanueva AG, Redondo C. Lobular carcinoma of the breast in a patient with Klinefelter's syndrome. A case with bilateral, synchronous, histologically different breast tumors. Cancer 1986; 57(6): 1181–1183.

37. Nance KV, Reddick RL. In situ and infiltrating lobular carcinoma of the male breast. Hum Pathol 1989; 20(12): 1220.

38. Camus MG, Joshi MG, Mackarem G, et al. Ductal carcinoma in situ of the male breast. Cancer 1994; 74(4):1289–1293.

39. Cutuli B, Dilhuydy J, De Lafontan B, et al. Ductal carcinoma in situ of the male breast. Analysis of 31 cases. Eur J Cancer 1997; 33(1):35–38.

40. Gupta S, Khanna NN, Khanna S. Paget's disease of the male breast: a clinicopathologic study and a collective review. J Surg Oncol 1983; 22(3):151–156.

41. Leclercq G, Verhest A, Deboel MC, et al. Oestrogen receptors in male breast cancer. Biomedicine 1976; 25(9):327–330.

42. Heller KS, Rosen PP, Schottenfeld D, et al. Male breast cancer: a clinicopathologic study of 97 cases. Ann Surg 1978; 188(1):60–65.

43. Everson RB, Lippman ME, Thompson EB, et al. Clinical correlations of steroid receptors and male breast cancer. Cancer Res 1980; 40(4):991–997.

44. Willshir P, Leach H, Ellis I, et al. Male breast cancer: pathological and immunohistochemical features. Anticancer Res 1997; 173:2335–2338.

45. Moore J, Frieman M, Gansler T, et al. Prognostic indicators in male breast cancer. The Breast J 1998; 4:261–269.

46. Leach IH, Ellis IO, Elston CW. c-erb-B-2 expression in male breast carcinoma. J Clin Pathol 1992; 45(10):942.

47. Dawson PJ, Schroer KR, Wolman SR. ras and p53 genes in male breast cancer. Mod Pathol 1996; 9(4):367–370.

48. Hecht JR, Winchester DJ. Male breast cancer. Am J Clin Pathol 1994; 102(4 suppl 1):S25–S30.

49. Pich A, Margaria E, Chiusa L. Oncogenes and male breast carcinoma: c-erbB-2 and p53 coexpression predicts a poor survival. J Clin Oncol 2000; 18(16): 2948–2956.

50. Fox SB, Harris AL. The epidermal growth factor receptor in breast cancer. J Mammary Gland Biol Neoplasia 1997; 2(2):131–141.

51. Salvadori B, Saccozzi R, Manzari A, et al. Prognosis of breast cancer in males: an analysis of 170 cases. Eur J Cancer 1994; 30A(7):930–935.

52. Rogers S, Day CA, Fox SB. Expression of cathepsin D and estrogen receptor in male breast carcinoma. Hum Pathol 1993; 24(2):148–151.

53. Bruce D, Heys S, Payne S, et al. Male breast cancer: clinicopathologic features, immunocytochemical characteristics and prognosis. Eur J Surg Onc 1996; 22:42–46.

54. Serra Diaz C, Vizoso F, Rodriguez JC, et al. Expression of pepsinogen C in gynecomastias and male breast carcinomas. World J Surg 1999; 23(5):439–445.

55. Salyer W, Salyer D. Metastases of prostatic carcinoma to the breast. J Urol 1973; 109(4):671–675.

56. Tavassoli FA. Pathology of the Breast. 2nd ed. Appleton & Lange: Stamford, CN, 1999:843.

57. Green L, Klima M. The use of immunohistochemistry in metastatic prostatic adenocarcinoma to the breast. Hum Pathol 1991; 22(3):242–246.

58. Borgen PI, Senie R, McKinnon W, et al. Carcinoma of the male breast: analysis of prognosis compared with matched female patients. Ann Surg Onc 1997; 4(5):385.

59. Willsher P, Leach I, Ellis I, et al. A comparison outcome of male breast cancer with female breast cancer. Am J Surg 1997; 173:185.

60. Treves N. Inflammatory carcinoma of the breast in the male patient. Surgery 1953; 34(5):810–820.

61. Joshi M, Lee A, Loda M, et al. Male breast carcinoma: an evaluation of prognostic factors contributing to a poorer outcome. Cancer 1996; 77(3):490–498.

62. Guinee VF, Olsson H, Moller T, et al. The prognosis of breast cancer in males. A report of 335 cases. Cancer 1993; 71(1):154.

63. Hultborn R, Friberg S, Hultborn KA, et al. Male breast carcinoma. II. A study of the total material reported to the Swedish Cancer Registry 1958–1967 with respect to treatment, prognostic factors and survival. Acta Oncol 1987; 26(5):327–341.

64. Hatschek T, Wingren S, Carstensen J, et al. DNA content and S-phase fraction in male breast carcinomas. Acta Oncol 1994; 33(6):609–613.

65. Scheike O. Male Breast Cancer. 6. Factors influencing prognosis. Br J Cancer 1974; 30(3):261–271.

66. Ouriel K, Lotze MT, Hinshaw JR. Prognostic factors of carcinoma of the male breast. Surg Gyn Obst 1984; 159(4):373–376.

67. Robison R, Montague ED. Treatment results in males with breast cancer. Cancer 1982; 49(2):403–406.

68. Erlichman C, Murphy K, Elhakim T. Male breast cancer: a 13 year review of 89 patients. JCO 1984; 2(8):903–909.

69. Cutulli B, Lacroze M, Dilhuydy JM, et al. Male breast cancer: results of the treatments and prognostic factors in 397 cases. Eur J Cancer 1995; 31A(12):1960–1964.

70. Kinne D. Male breast cancer. In: Harris J, Hellman S, Henderson I, et al., eds. Breast Disease. Philadelphia: Lippincott, 1987:577–583.

71. Sandler B, Carman C, Perry R. Cancer of the male breast. Am Surg 1994; 60(11):816–820.

72. Crichlow RW, Galt SW. Male breast cancer. Surg Clin North Am 1990; 70(5):1165–1177.

73. Farrow J, Adair F. Effect of orchiectomy on skeletal metastases from cancer of the male breast. Science 1942; 95:964.

74. Gupta N, Cohen JL, Rosenbaum C, et al. Estrogen receptors in male breast cancer. Cancer 1980; 46(8):1781–1784.

75. Meyskens FL Jr, Tormey DC, Neifeld JP. Male breast cancer: a review. Cancer Treat Rev 1976; 3(2):83–93.

76. Patel JK, Nemoto T, Dao TL. Metastatic breast cancer in males. Assessment of endocrine therapy. Cancer 1984; 53(6):1344–1346.

77. Stephens RL, Muggia FM. Breast cancer in men. Report illustrating the value of endocrine ablation. Am J Med 1974; 57(4):679–682.

78. Kennedy B, Kiang D. Hypophysectomy in the treatment of advanced cancer of the male breast. Cancer 1972; 29(6):1606–1612.

79. Tindall GT, Ambrose SS, Christy JH, et al. Hypophysectomy in the treatment of disseminated carcinoma of the breast and prostate gland. South Med J 1976; 69(5):579–583.

80. Doberauer C, Niederle N, Schmidt C. Advanced male breast cancer treatment with the LH-RH analogue buserelin alone or in combination with the antiandrogen flutamide. Cancer 1988; 62(3):474–478.

81. Lopez M, Natali M, Di Lauro L, et al. Combined treatment with buserelin and cyproterone acetate in metastatic male breast cancer. Cancer 1993; 72(2):502–505.

82. Ribiero G, Swindell R. Adjuvant tamoxifen in male breast cancer. Br J Cancer 1992; 65(2):252–254.

83. Bagley CS, Wesley MN, Young RC, et al. Adjuvant chemotherapy in males with cancer of the breast. JCO 1987; 10(1):55–60.

84. Patel H, Buzdar A, Hortabagyi G. Role of adjuvant chemotherapy in male breast cancer. Cancer 1989; 64(8):1583–1585.

85. McCarthy Pl, Hurd D, Rowlings P, et al. Autotransplants in men with breast cancer. ABMTR Breast Cancer Working Committee. Autologous Blood and Marrow Transplant Registry. BMT 1999; 24(4):365–368.

Index